T0309341

# BLACKWELL'S
# FIVE-MINUTE
# VETERINARY
# CONSULT

# BLACKWELL'S FIVE-MINUTE VETERINARY CONSULT

# AVIAN

**Second Edition**

Edited by

*Hugues Beaufrère, DVM, PhD, DACZM, DECZM (Avian), DABVP (Avian)*
*Associate Professor of Companion Zoological Medicine and Surgery, Department of Veterinary Medicine and Epidemiology, School of Veterinary Medicine, University of California, Davis, Davis, CA, USA*

*Jennifer E. Graham, DVM, DACZM, DABVP*
*Graham Veterinary Consulting, LLC, Madison, AL, USA*

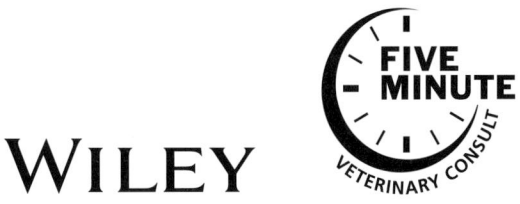

Published by John Wiley & Sons, Inc., Hoboken, New Jersey.
Published simultaneously in Canada.

For general information on our other products and services or for technical support, please contact our Customer Care Department within the United States at (800) 762-2974, outside the United States at (317) 572-3993 or fax (317) 572-4002.

Wiley also publishes its books in a variety of electronic formats. Some content that appears in print may not be available in electronic formats. For more information about Wiley products, visit our web site at www.wiley.com.

*Library of Congress Cataloging-in-Publication Data Applied for:*

Hardback ISBN: 9781119870579

Cover Design and Image: Wiley

Set in 9/10pt GaramondPro by Straive, Pondicherry, India

Printed in Singapore
M120757_011024

This book is dedicated to my flock. First, my wife, Mélanie, for her unwavering support as I "revolutionize the field of avian medicine as we know it," as I often put it when having a significant finding with a $p = 0.0499$. She knows it really means to "overcomplicate things to have fun using birds in the process." I also wanted to mention my sons, Armand "Larmi" and Arthur "Larti," who probably will never open this book, but who are always on my mind, especially since they literally have a 5-minute attention span.

Hugues Beaufrère

This second edition is dedicated to the students and house officers I have mentored through the years. I am so proud of your accomplishments and grateful to be a part of the journey. If only I had a dime for every time I asked, "did you look in the *5-Minute Consult?*"

Jennifer E. Graham

# CONTENTS

Contributors                                                                              xvi

Preface                                                                                   xix

Acknowledgements                                                                          xx

About the Companion Website                                                               xxi

## TOPICS

Adenoviruses                                                                              1

Adrenal Gland Diseases                                                                    4

Aggression *see* Problem Behaviors: Aggression, Biting and Screaming                      (374)

Air Sac Mites                                                                             8

Air Sac Rupture                                                                           10

Airborne toxicosis *see* Toxicosis (Airborne)                                             (434)

Algal Biotoxins                                                                           13

Amyloidosis                                                                               15

Anemia                                                                                    17

Angel Wing                                                                                20

Angular Limb Deformity (Splay Leg)                                                        22

Anorexia                                                                                  24

Anticoagulant rodenticide toxicosis *see* Toxicosis (Anticoagulant Rodenticides)         (436)

Arboviruses *see* Eastern and Western Equine Encephalitis Viruses; Usutu Virus;          (145)

West Nile Virus                                                                           (478)

Arthritis *see* Joint Diseases                                                            (241)

Ascites                                                                                   27

Aspergillosis                                                                             30

Aspiration Pneumonia                                                                      33

Atherosclerosis                                                                           36

Atoxoplasmosis *see* Coccidiosis (Systemic)                                               (104)

Avian Influenza                                                                           40

Avian Vacuolar Myelinopathy                                                               43

Avocado poisoning *see* Toxins (Ingested, Gastrointestinal)                               (448)

Avulaviruses *see* Othoavulaviruses                                                       (323)

Baylisascaris *see* Neural Larva Migrans                                                  (300)

Beak Injuries                                                                             45

Beak Malocclusion (Lateral Beak Deformity)                                                48

Beak Malocclusion (Mandibular Prognathism)                                                51

Behavior *see* Problem Behaviors: Aggression, Biting and Screaming                        (374)

Bite wounds *see* Wounds (Including Bite Wounds, Predator Attacks)                         (481)

 *Client education handouts are available at www.wiley.com/go/Beaufrère/2e for you to download and use in practice*

| | |
|---|---|
| Bordetellosis | 53 |
| Bornaviral Disease (Aquatic Birds) | 56 |
| Bornaviral Disease (Psittaciformes) | 58 |
| Botulism | 62 |
| Brachial Plexus Injury | 64 |
| Brain tumors *see* Neoplasia (Neurological) | (305) |
| Bumblefoot *see* Pododermatitis | (358) |
| Bursa of Fabricius Diseases | 66 |
| Campylobacteriosis | 70 |
| Candidiasis | 72 |
| Capture Myopathy (Exertional Rhabdomyolysis) | 74 |
| Cardiac disease *see* Congestive Heart Failure, Myocardial Diseases | (114) |
| Carbamate toxicity *see* Toxicosis (Environmental, Pesticides) | (439) |
| Central nervous system tumors *see* Neoplasia (Neurological) | (290) |
| Cere and Skin Color Changes | 77 |
| Cervicocephalic diverticulum rupture *see* Air Sac Rupture | (10) |
| Chlamydiosis | 79 |
| Cholera *see* Pasteurellosis | (345) |
| Chronic Egg Laying | 82 |
| Circovirus (Psittacines) | 85 |
| Circoviruses (Non-Psittacine Birds) | 87 |
| Cloacal bursa diseases *see* Bursa of Fabricius Diseases | (66) |
| Cloacal Diseases | 89 |
| Cloacal Prolapse | 92 |
| Clostridiosis | 95 |
| Coagulopathies and Coagulation | 98 |
| Coccidiosis (Intestinal) | 101 |
| Coccidiosis (Systemic) | 104 |
| Coelomic Distension | 107 |
| Colibacillosis | 111 |
| Congestive Heart Failure | 114 |
| Conjunctivitis *see* Ocular Lesions | (313) |
| Constricted toe *see* Toe and Nails (Diseases of) | (426) |
| Coxiellosis | 116 |
| Crop Burn | 118 |
| Crop stasis *see* Ileus (Functional Gastrointestinal, Crop Stasis) | (233) |
| Cryptococcosis | 120 |
| Cryptosporidiosis | 122 |
| Degenerative joint disease *see* Joint Diseases | (241) |
| Dehydration [*see also* Hypotension] | 125 |
| Dermatitis | 127 |
| Diabetes Insipidus | 130 |

 *Client education handouts are available at www.wiley.com/go/Beaufrère/2e for you to download and use in practice*

Diabetes Mellitus and Hyperglycemia                                              132

Diarrhea                                                                         134

Discospondylitis                                                                136

Dyslipidemia/Hyperlipidemia                                                     139

Dyspnea *see* Respiratory Distress                                             (386)

Dystocia and Egg Binding                                                        142

Eastern and Western Equine Encephalitis Viruses (EEV/WEEV)                     145

Ectoparasites (Mites)                                                          148

Ectoparasites (Ticks, Lice, Dipterans)                                        151

Egg Abnormalities                                                             154

Egg binding *see* Dystocia and Egg Binding                                    (142)

Egg Yolk and Reproductive Coelomitis                                          158

Electrocution                                                                 160

Emaciation                                                                    162

Embryonic death/hatching failure *see* Egg Abnormalities                      (154)

Endoparasites *see* Helminthiasis; Coccidiosis; Neural Larva Migrans          (300)

Enteritis and Gastritis                                                       165

Enterococcal spondylitis *see* Discospondylitis                              (136)

Exertional rhabdomyolysis *see* Capture Myopathy                              (74)

Feather Cyst                                                                  168

Feather-Damaging and Self-Injurious Behavior                                  170

Feather Disorders                                                             174

Flagellate Enteritis [*see also* Trichomoniasis]                             177

Foreign Bodies (Gastrointestinal)                                            180

Foreign Bodies (respiratory) *see* Tracheal Diseases                         (457)

Fractures                                                                     183

Frostbite *see* Hypothermia                                                  (231)

Gastrointestinal foreign bodies *see* Foreign Bodies (Gastrointestinal)      (180)

Gastritis *see* Enteritis and Gastritis                                      (165)

Giardiasis *see* Flagellate Enteritis                                        (177)

Goiter *see* Thyroid Diseases                                                (424)

Gout *see* Renal Disease and Hyperuricemia                                   (380)

Head trauma *see* Neurologic Trauma                                          (305)

Heart failure *see* Congestive Heart Failure                                 (114)

Heat Stroke                                                                   186

Heavy metal toxicity *see* Toxicosis (Heavy Metals)                          (443)

Helminthiasis (Body Cavity and Cardiovascular)                               188

Helminthiasis (Gastrointestinal)                                             190

Helminthiasis (Neurological) *see* Neural Larva Migrans                      (300)

Helminthiasis (Respiratory)                                                   193

Hemochromatosis *see* Iron Storage Disease                                   (239)

Hemoparasites                                                                 196

 *Client education handouts are available at www.wiley.com/go/Beaufrère/2e for you to download and use in practice*

| | |
|---|---|
| Hemorrhage | 199 |
| Hepatic Lipidosis | 203 |
| Hepatitis *see* Liver Disease | (250) |
| Hernia/Pseudohernia | 206 |
| Herpesvirus (chicken) *see* Marek's Disease; | (261) |
| Respiratory Infections of Backyard Chickens | (389) |
| Herpesvirus (Columbid Herpesvirus 1 in Pigeons and Raptors) | 208 |
| Herpesvirus (Duck Viral Enteritis) | 210 |
| Herpesvirus (Passerine Birds) | 213 |
| Herpesvirus (Psittacid Herpesviruses) | 215 |
| Histomoniasis | 218 |
| Horner Syndrome | 220 |
| Hypercholesterolemia *see* Dyslipidemia | (139) |
| Hyperglycemia *see* Diabetes Mellitus and Hyperglycemia | (132) |
| Hyperlipidemia *see* Dyslipidemia/Hyperlipidemia | (139) |
| Hyperparathyroidism *see* Metabolic Bone Disease | (263) |
| Hyperthermia *see* Heat Stroke | (186) |
| Hyperuricemia | 222 |
| Hypocalcemia (and Hypomagnesemia) | 225 |
| Hypotension and Hypovolemia | 228 |
| Hypothermia | 231 |
| Hypothyroidism *see* Thyroid Diseases | (424) |
| Hypovitaminosis A *see* Nutritional Imbalances | (308) |
| Ileus (Functional Gastrointestinal, Crop Stasis) | 233 |
| Infectious bronchitis *see* Respiratory Infections of Backyard Chickens | (389) |
| Infectious laryngotracheitis *see* Respiratory Infections of Backyard Chickens | (389) |
| Infertility | 236 |
| Ingested toxicosis *see* Toxicosis (Ingested) | (448) |
| Ingluvial hypomotility *see* Ileus (Functional Gastrointestinal, Crop Stasis) | (233) |
| Iron Storage Disease | 239 |
| Joint Diseases | 241 |
| Knemidocoptic mites *see* Ectoparasites (Mites) | (148) |
| Lameness | 243 |
| Lead *see* Toxicosis (Heavy Metals) | (443) |
| Leukemia *see* Neoplasia | (284) |
| Leukocytosis | 247 |
| Leukosis virus (avian) *see* Retroviruses in Galliformes | (393) |
| Lice *see* Ectoparasites (Ticks, Lice, Dipterans) | (151) |
| Lipoma *see* Neoplasia (Integument) | (284) |
| Liver Disease | 250 |
| Lung Diseases [*see also* Pneumonia; Toxicosis (Airborne and Respiratory Distress)] | 253 |
| Luxations | 256 |
| Lymphosarcoma *see* Neoplasia (Lymphoproliferative) | (286) |

 *Client education handouts are available at www.wiley.com/go/Beaufrère/2e for you to download and use in practice*

| | |
|---|---|
| *Macrorhabdus Ornithogaster* | 259 |
| Malaria *see* Hemoparasites | (196) |
| Malnutrition *see* Emaciation | (162) |
| Mandibular prognathism *see* Beak Malocclusion (Mandibular Prognathism) | (51) |
| Marek's Disease | 261 |
| Metabolic Bone Disease | 263 |
| Microsporidiosis/Encephalitozoon | 266 |
| Mites *see* Ectoparasites (Mites) | (148) |
| Mycobacteriosis | 268 |
| Mycoplasmosis | 271 |
| Mycotoxicosis | 274 |
| Myiasis | 277 |
| Myocardial Diseases | 279 |
| Nails (diseases of) *see* Toes and Nails (Diseases of) | (426) |
| Neoplasia (Gastrointestinal and Hepatic) | 282 |
| Neoplasia (Integument) | 284 |
| Neoplasia (Lymphoproliferative) | 286 |
| Neoplasia (Neurologic) | 290 |
| Neoplasia (Renal) | 293 |
| Neoplasia (Reproductive) | 295 |
| Neoplasia (Respiratory) | 298 |
| Neural Larva Migrans | 300 |
| Neurologic (Non-Traumatic Diseases) | 302 |
| Neurologic (Trauma) | 305 |
| Newcastle disease *see* Orthoavulaviruses | (323) |
| Nutritional Imbalances [*see also* Hypovitaminosis A] | 308 |
| Obesity | 311 |
| Ocular Lesions | 313 |
| Oil Exposure | 316 |
| Oral Plaques | 320 |
| Organophosphate toxicity *see* Toxicosis (Environmental, Pesticides) | (439) |
| Orthoavulaviruses | 323 |
| Osteomyelosclerosis *see* Polyostotic Hyperostosis | (367) |
| Otitis | 327 |
| Ovarian Diseases | 330 |
| Overgrown beak *see* Beak Malocclusion | (48) |
| Oviductal Diseases | 334 |
| Pacheco's disease *see* Herpesviruses (Psittacids) | (215) |
| Pain | 337 |
| Pancreatic Diseases | 340 |
| Papillomatosis (Cutaneous) | 343 |
| Papillomatosis, internal *see* Herpesvirus | (208) |
| Paramyxoviruses *see* Orthoavulaviruses | (323) |

 *Client education handouts are available at www.wiley.com/go/Beaufrère/2e for you to download and use in practice*

Parasites (external) *see* Ectoparasites (148)

Parasites (internal) *see* Helminthiasis; Coccidiosis; Neural Larva Migrans (300)

Pasteurellosis 345

Patagium Diseases 347

Perosis/Slipped Tendon 349

Phallus Prolapse 351

Pituitary tumors *see* Neoplasia (Neurological) (290)

Plant toxins *see* Toxicosis (Ingested, Gastrointestinal) (448)

Pneumonia 354

Pododermatitis 358

Polydipsia 362

Polyfolliculitis *see* Dermatitis (127)

Polyomavirus 365

Polyostotic Hyperostosis 367

Polyuria 369

Poxvirus 371

Predator attack *see* Wounds (Including Bite Wounds, Predator Attacks) (481)

Problem Behaviors: Aggression, Biting and Screaming 374

Prolapses (*see* Cloacal Prolapse) (92)

Proventricular Dilatation Disease (*see* Bornaviral Diseases) (56)

Proventricular diseases (*see* Enteritis and Gastritis) (165)

Psittacine beak and feather disease (*see* Circoviruses) (85)

PTFE toxicosis *see* Toxicosis (Environmental/Pesticides) (439)

Regurgitation and Vomiting 378

Renal Diseases 380

Reovirus 384

Respiratory Distress 386

Respiratory foreign bodies *see* Tracheal Diseases (457)

Respiratory Infections of Backyard Chickens [*see also* Mycoplasmosis] 389

Retroviruses in Galliformes 393

Rhinitis and Sinusitis 395

Rotavirus 398

Salmonellosis 400

Salpingitis *see* Oviductal Diseases (334)

Sarcocystosis 402

Scissors beak *see* Beak Malocclusion (Lateral Beak Deformity) (48)

Seizures 405

Self-injurious behavior *see* Feather-Damaging and Self-Injurious Behavior (170)

Sepsis 408

Sick-Bird Syndrome 411

Smoke inhalation injury *see* Toxicosis (Airborne) (434)

Spinal trauma *see* Neurologic Trauma (305)

Spirochete Infection 413

 *Client education handouts are available at www.wiley.com/go/Beaufrère/2e for you to download and use in practice*

Spironucleus *see* Flagellate (Intestinal)                                      (177)

Splay Leg *see* Angular Limb Deformities                                        (22)

Spleen (Diseases of)                                                            415

Squamous Cell Carcinoma *see* Neoplasia (Integument)                           (284)

Squamous metaplasia *see* Hypovitaminosis A                                    (308)

Stroke *see* Atherosclerosis                                                    (36)

Syringeal disease *see* Tracheal and Syringeal Diseases                        (457)

Tendinitis and Tenosynovitis                                                    418

Thymus (Diseases of)                                                            422

Thyroid Diseases                                                                424

Toe and Nail Diseases                                                           426

Togaviruses *see* Eastern and Western Equine Encephalitis Viruses             (145)

Tongue Diseases                                                                 431

Toxicosis (Airborne)                                                            434

Toxicosis (Anticoagulant Rodenticide)                                          436

Toxicosis (Environmental, Pesticides)                                          439

Toxicicosis (Heavy Metals)                                                      443

Toxicosis (Iatrogenic)                                                          445

Toxicosis (Ingested, Gastrointestinal)                                         448

Toxicosis (Vitamin D)                                                           452

Toxoplasmosis                                                                   454

Tracheal and Syringeal Diseases                                                457

Trauma [*see also* Neurologic Trauma]                                          461

Trichomoniasis                                                                  465

Tumors *see* Neoplasia                                                         (284)

Undigested Food in Droppings                                                    468

Urate and Fecal Discoloration                                                   471

Uropygial Gland Disease                                                         474

Usutu Virus                                                                     476

Viral diseases *see* individual named viral diseases                           (56)

Vitamin D toxicosis *see* Toxicosis (Vitamin D)                               (452)

West Nile Virus                                                                 478

Wing droop *see* Brachial Plexus Avulsion; Fractures; Luxations               (64)

Wounds (Including Bite Wounds, Predator Attacks)                               481

Xanthoma/Xanthogranulomamatosis                                                484

Yersiniosis                                                                     486

Yolk Sac Retention and Infection                                               488

Young pigeon syndrome *see* Circovirus                                         (85)

Zinc *see* Toxicosis (Heavy Metals)                                           (443)

Appendix I: Common Dosages for Birds                                           490

Appendix II: Avian Hematology Reference Values                                 497

Appendix III: Laboratory Testing (USA)                                         499

Appendix IV: Viral Diseases of Concern                                         504

 *Client education handouts are available at www.wiley.com/go/Beaufrère/2e for you to download and use in practice*

Appendix V: Selected Zoonotic Diseases of Concern and Personal Protection     511

Appendix VI: Common Avian Toxins and Their Clinical Signs     513

Appendix VII: Avian Taxonomy     516

Appendix VIII: Clinical Algorithms     523

    Algorithm 1: Sick-Bird Syndrome     523

    Algorithm 2: Diarrhea     524

    Algorithm 3: Regurgitation/Vomiting     525

    Algorithm 4: Respiratory Distress     526

    Algorithm 5: Coelemic Distension     527

    Algorithm 6: Egg Binding     528

    Algorithm 7: Anemia     529

    Algorithm 8: Oropharyngeal Lesions     530

    Algorithm 9: Neurologic Signs     531

    Algorithm 10: Polydipsia     532

    Algorithm 11: Polyuria     533

    Algorithm 12: Feather Loss     534

    Algorithm 13: Lameness     535

    Algorithm 14: Hyperuricemia     536

    Algorithm 15: Hepatopathy     537

    Algorithm 16: Wing Droop     538

    Algorithm 17: Respiratory Distress in Chickens     539

    Algorithm 18: Cloacal Prolapse     540

Index     541

## ONLINE MATERIALS

**Procedures**

Air Sac Cannula

Beak and Nail Trimming

Blood Transfusion

Bone Marrow Aspiration

Choanal Swab

Cloacal Swab

Coelomocentesis

Conjunctival Swab

Deslorelin Implant

Elizabethan Collar

Fecal Wet Mount and Gram Stain

Figure of Eight Bandage

Handling and Restraint

Indirect Blood Pressure Monitoring

Ingluvial gavage

 *Client education handouts are available at www.wiley.com/go/Beaufrère/2e for you to download and use in practice*

Intramuscular Injection

Intraosseous Catheter

Intravenous Catheter

Microchip Placement

Nasal Flush

Oral medications

Sinus Aspiration

Subcutaneous injection

Tracheal Swab or Wash

Venipuncture

Ventplasty

Wing Trimming

**Client Education Handouts**

Airborne Toxins

Angel Wing

Arthritis

Aspergillosis

Avocado/Plant Toxins

Bornaviral Disease (Psittaciformes)

Chlamydiosis

Chronic Egg Laying

Cloacal Disease

Cystic Ovarian Disease

Feather-Damaging Behavior

Heavy-Metal Toxicity

Hypocalcemia and Hypomagnesemia

Liver Disease

Macrorhabdosis

Nutritional Deficiencies

Ovarian Neoplasia

Overgrown Beak and Nails

Obesity

Oophoritis

Pododermatis (Bumblefoot)

Polyomavirus in Psittacines

Regurgitation and Vomiting

Renal Disease

Rhinitis and Sinusitis

Sick-Bird Syndrome

Ten Things Your Parrot Wants You to Know about Behavior

Trauma

 *Client education handouts are available at www.wiley.com/go/Beaufrère/2e for you to download and use in practice*

# CONTRIBUTORS

MELANIE AMMERSBACH, DVM, DACVP
(Clin Path)
Associate Professor in Clinical Pathology
Department of Pathology, Microbiology, and
Immunology
UC Davis School of Veterinary Medicine
Davis, CA, USA

NATALIE ANTINOFF, DVM, DABVP (Avian)
Texas Avian and Exotic Hospital
Grapevine, TX, USA

HANNAH ATTARIAN, DVM
Department of Avian and Exotics Pets
ACCESS Specialty Animal Hospitals – Los
Angeles
Culver City, CA, USA

PANAGIOTIS AZMANIS, DVM, PhD, DECZM
(Avian), Dip ZooMed
Dubai Falcon Hospital/Wadi al Safa
Wildlife Center
Dubai, UAE

TRINITA BARBOZA, DVM, DVSc, DACZM
Assistant Professor, Zoological Companion
Animal Medicine Service
Department of Clinical Sciences
Cummings School of Veterinary Medicine at
Tufts University
North Grafton, MA, USA

HEATHER W. BARRON, DVM, DABVP
(Avian), CertAqV
Loggerhead Marinelife Center
Juno Beach, FL, USA

HUGUES BEAUFRÈRE, DVM, PhD,
DACZM, DABVP (Avian), DECZM (Avian)
Associate Professor, Companion Zoological
Medicine and Surgery
Department of Veterinary Medicine and
Epidemiology
UC Davis School of Veterinary Medicine
Davis, CA, USA

JOÃO BRANDÃO, LMV, MS, DECZM
(Avian), DACZM
Associate Professor, Zoological Medicine
Department of Veterinary Clinical Sciences
College of Veterinary Medicine, Oklahoma
State University
Stillwater, OK, USA

JAMES W. CARPENTER, MS, DVM, DACZM
Professor Emeritus, Zoological Medicine
Department of Clinical Sciences
College of Veterinary Medicine, Kansas
State University
Manhattan, Kansas, USA

ERIKA CERVASIO, DVM, DABVP
(Avian, Feline, Canine)
Norton Animal Hospital
Mansfield, MA, USA

SUNOH CHE, DVM, MSc, PhD, DACVPM
Assistant Professor of Poultry Management
Department of Animal and Avian Sciences
University of Maryland
College Park, MD, USA

SUE CHEN, DVM, DABVP (Avian)
Gulf Coast Veterinary Specialists
Houston, TX, USA

LEIGH ANN CLAYTON, DVM, DABVP
(Reptile/Amphibian), eMBA
Wildlife Conservation Society's New York
Aquarium
Brooklyn, NY 11224, USA

LORENZO CROSTA, DVM, PhD, DECZM
(Zoo Health Management), ACEPM, GP Cert
(ExAp), FNOVI (Zoo-Avian)
Università di Milano
Dipartimento di Medicina Veterinaria e
Scienze Ambientali
Milano, Italy

RYAN S. DE VOE, DVM, DABVP
(Avian, Reptile/Amphibian), DACZM
Disney's Animal Kingdom
Bay Lake, FL, USA

MARION DESMARCHELIER, DMV,
IPSAV, DES (Zoological Medicine), MSc,
DACZM, DECZM (Zoo Health Management),
DACVB
Department of Clinical Sciences
Faculté de médecine vétérinaire,
Université de Montréal
Saint-Hyacinthe QC, Canada

STEPHEN DYER, DVM, DABVP (Avian)
North Paws Veterinary Center
Greenville, RI, USA

BRENNA COLLEEN FITZGERALD, DVM,
DABVP (Avian Practice)
Colorado Exotic Animal Hospital
Denver, CO, USA

HILLARY G. FRANK, DVM, DABVP (Avian)
North Central Animal Hospital
Phoenix, AZ, USA

SUSAN G. FRIEDMAN, PhD
Psychology Department
Utah State University, Logan, UT, USA

SARA GARDHOUSE, DVM, DABVP
(Exotic Companion Mammal), DACZM
Evolution Veterinary Specialists
Lakewood, CO, USA

JENNIFER E. GRAHAM, DVM, DABVP
(Avian/Exotic Companion Mammal),
DACZM
Graham Veterinary Consulting, LLC
Madison, AL, USA.

KATHARINA B. HAGEN, DVM
Exoticus Veterinary Clinic
Adliswil, Switzerland

DAVID E. HANNON, DVM, DABVP (Avian)
Animal Emergency Center
Memphis, TN, USA

TARA M. HARRISON, DVM, MPVM,
DACZM, DACVPM, DECZM (Zoo Health
Management), CVA
College of Veterinary Medicine, North
Carolina State UniversityRaleigh, NC, USA

J. JILL HEATLEY, DVM, MS, DABVP
(Avian, Reptilian, Amphibian), DACZM
Department of Small Animal Clinical
Sciences
College of Veterinary Medicine and
Biomedical Sciences, Texas A&M University
College Station, TX, USA

HEIDI L. HOEFER, DVM, DABVP (Avian)
Island Exotic Veterinary Care
Huntington Station, NY, USA

MINH HUYNH, DVM, MRCVS, DECZM
(Avian), DACZM
William R. Pritchard Veterinary Medical
Teaching Hospital
UC Davis School of Veterinary Medicine
Davis, California, USA

ALISON JEFFREY, DVM
Zoological Medicine Resident
College of Veterinary Medicine,
University of Georgia
Athens, GA, USA

MICHAEL P. JONES, DVM, DABVP (Avian)
University of Tennessee College of
Veterinary Medicine
Pigeon Forge, TN, USA

ERIC KLAPHAKE, DVM, DACZM
Cheyenne Mountain Zoo
Colorado Springs, CO, USA

ISABELLE LANGLOIS, DMV, DABVP
(Avian)
Centre hospitalier universitaire vétérinaire
Faculté de médecine vétérinaire - Université
de Montréal
Saint Hyacinthe, QC, Canada

DELPHINE LANIESSE, DVM, DVSc,
DECZM (Avian)
Eläinsairaala Evidensia Tammisto
Vantaa, Finland

ANGELA M. LENNOX, DVM, DABVP
(Avian and Exotic Companion Mammal),
DECZM (Small Mammal)
Avian and Exotic Animal Clinic of
Indianapolis
Indianapolis IN, USA

MICHAEL LIERZ, Prof Dr Med Vet,
DZooMed, DECZM (Wildlife Population
Health) DECPVS
Clinic für Birds, Reptiles Amphibians and Fish
Faculty of Veterinary Medicine
Justus-Liebig.University Giessen
Germany

SHACHAR MALKA, DVM, DABVP (Avian),
DACEPM
Long Island Bird & Exotics Veterinary Clinic
Great Neck, NY, USA

RUTH M. MARRION, DVM, DACVO, PhD
[no current affiliation]

KEMBA L. MARSHALL, MPH, DVM,
DABVP (Avian)
PetSmart SSG
Phoenix, AZ, USA

CRYSTAL MATT, DVM
Avian and Exotic Animal Clinic of
Indianapolis
Indianapolis IN, USA

BRYNN MCCLEERY, DVM, DABVP
(Avian Practice)
Redbank Veterinary Hospital
Tinton Falls, NJ, USA

ALICIA MCLAUGHLIN, DVM, CertAqVet
Center for Bird and Exotic Animal Medicine
St Bothell, WA, USA
Seattle Aquarium
Seattle, WA, USA

BIANCA MURPHY, DVM, DABVP (Avian)
Moichor Reference Laboratory
San Francisco, CA, USA

MAUREEN MURRAY, DVM, DABVP (Avian)
Director, Tufts Wildlife Clinic
Clinical Associate Professor
Cummings School of Veterinary Medicine at
Tufts University
North Grafton MA, USA

GLENN H. OLSEN, DVM, MS, PhD
USGS Patuxent Wildlife Research Center
Laurel, MD, USA

ANTHONY A. PILNY, DVM, DABVP (Avian)
Arizona Exotic Animal Hospital
Phoenix, AZ, USA

CHRISTAL POLLOCK, DVM, DABVP
(Avian Practice)
Lafeber Company Veterinary Consultant

LAUREN V. POWERS, DVM, DABVP
(Avian Practice / Exotic Companion
Mammal Practice)
Carolina Veterinary Specialists
Huntersville, North Carolina, USA

GREGORY RICH, DVM, BS Medical
Technology
Avian and Exotic Animal Hospital of
Louisiana
Metairie, LA, USA

SHANNON M. RIGGS, DVM, DABVP
(Avian)
Pacific wildlife care
Morro Bay, CA, USA

VANESSA ROLFE, DVM, ABVP (Avian)
The Bird and Exotic Hospital
Greenacres, FL, USA

DAVID SANCHEZ-MIGALLON GUZMAN, LV,
MS, DECZM (Avian, Small Mammal), DACZM
Professor of Clinical Zoological Companion
Animal Medicine and Surgery
Department of Veterinary Medicine and
Epidemiology
UC Davis School of Veterinary Medicine
Davis, CA, USA

VOLKER SCHMIDT, PD Dr Med Vet,
DECZM (Avian and Herpetological)
Universität Leipzig
Veterinärmedizinische Fakultät
Klinik für Vögel und Reptilien
Leipzig, Germany

RODNEY W. SCHNELLBACHER, DVM,
DACZM
Zoo Miami
Miami, FL, USA

PETRA SCHNITZER, Med Vet, MANZCVS
(Medicine of Australasian Wildlife), ACEPM,
Gp-Cert ExAP
Free University of Bolzano
Bolzano, Italy

NICO J. SCHOEMAKER, DVM, PhD,
DECZM (Small Mammal, Avian),
DABVP (Avian)
Department of Clinical Sciences of
Companion Animals Division of Zoological
Medicine
Faculty of Veterinary Medicine,
Utrecht University
Utrecht, Netherlands

JULIA SHAKERI, DVM, DABVP (Avian),
ACEPM
Avian and Exotic Animal Department
Central Hospital for Veterinary Medicine
North Haven, CT, USA

KRISTIN M. SINCLAIR, DVM, DABVP
(Avian Practice, Exotic Companion
Mammal Practice)
Kensington Bird and Animal Hospital
Kensington, CT, USA

KURT K. SLADKY, MS, DVM, DACZM,
DECZM (Zoo Health Management and
Herpetology)
Department of Surgical Sciences
School of Veterinary Medicine,
University of Wisconsin
Madison, WI, USA

MARIANA SOSA HIGAREDA, DVM
Department of Veterinary Clinical Medicine
College of Veterinary Medicine,
University of Illinois
Urbana, IL, USA

MARCY J. SOUZA, DVM, MPH, MPPA,
DABVP (Emeritus, Avian), DACVPM
College of Veterinary Medicine,
University of Tennessee
Knoxville, TN, USA

BRIAN SPEER, DVM, DABVP
(Avian Practice), DECZM (Avian)
Medical Center for Birds
Oakley, CA, USA

JONATHAN STOCKMAN, DVM, DACVIM
(Nutrition)
Department of Clinical Veterinary Sciences,
College of Veterinary Medicine
Long Island University, Brookville, NY, USA

ANNELIESE STRUNK, DVM, Dipl. ABVP
(Avian Practice)
Center for Bird and Exotic Animal Medicine
Bothell, WA, USA

NOÉMIE SUMMA, DMV, IPSAV
(Zoological Medicine), DACZM
Centre hospitalier universitaire vétérinaire
Faculté de médecine vétérinaire - Université
de Montréal
Saint Hyacinthe, QC, Canada

LEONARDO SUSTA, DVM, PhD, DACVP
Department of Pathobiology
Ontario Veterinary College,
University of Guelph
Guelph, ON, Canada

LAUREN THIELEN, DVM, ABVP
(Avian Practice)
Cornell University College of Veterinary
Medicine
Ithaca, NY, USA

FLORINA S. TSENG, DVM
Department of Infectious Disease and
Global Health
Cummings School of Veterinary Medicine at
Tufts University
North Grafton, MA, USA

YVONNE R. A. VAN ZEELAND, DVM,
MVR, PhD, DECZM (Avian, Small Mammal),
CPBC
Department of Clinical Sciences of
Companion Animals, Division of Zoological
Medicine
Faculty of Veterinary Medicine,
Utrecht University
Utrecht, Netherlands

KENNETH R. WELLE, DVM, DABVP
(Avian)
College of Veterinary Medicine,
University of Illinois
Urbana-Champaign, IL, USA

NICOLE R. WYRE, DVM, DABVP
(Avian and Exotic Companion Mammal),
CVA, CTPEP
Zodiac Pet and Exotic Hospital
Fortress Hill, Hong Kong

MIKE ZICCARDI, DVM, MPVM, PhD,
DACZM
UC Davis School of Veterinary Medicine
Davis, CA, USA

GRAHAM ZOLLER, DVM, IPSAV,
DECZM (Avian)
Exotic Pet Department, Centre Hospitalier
Veterinaire OnlyVet
Saint-Priest, France

PETRA ZSIVANOVIS, Dr Med Vet,
DECZM (Avian)
Tierärztliche Praxis für Vogelmedizin
Wahlstedt, Germany

# PREFACE

In the wake of the success of the first edition of this *5-Minute Veterinary Consult: Avian*, we are pleased to unveil the second edition, a result of much work, dedication, and love for birds by the 71 authors and experts in the field who took on the challenge to update, rewrite, expand, or produce new chapters. Avian medicine is a dynamic field, with constant advancements in research and knowledge, and this new edition fills a particular niche for easily digestible information that can be accessed on the fly (pun intended) in a busy veterinary practice environment. Simply put, this book is about finding specific information without wading through paragraphs and paragraphs of reference textbooks. Do not get us wrong, having reference textbooks available is also recommended to better understand the pathophysiology of diseases and more complex aspects of disease management. However, access to a practical book using standardized organization of short chapters with key information on most common avian medicine topics goes a long way to learning and maintaining one's knowledge and skills. A patient-side microlearning approach provides information in a direct care context, ensuring better retention of key concepts applicable to future cases.

The second edition builds on the first, with many of the same chapters updated, expanded, or consolidated into different chapters. For instance, the previous chapters on viruses have been split into individual viruses of importance and the previous chapter on tumors has been expanded into organ system-associated neoplasia. The same approach has been adopted for other topics, to provide targeted information on parasites, beak disorders, cardiology, toxicology, and many others. We have also expanded the range of species covered beyond psittacine birds whenever applicable. The result is an overall increase of approximately 50% in content with now close to 200 separate chapters.

Additionally, new appendices, clinical algorithms, and client education materials are available in the second edition. An avian taxonomy appendix is a valuable inclusion. This resource on rapidly changing avian classification can aid when extrapolating information across species.

We hope this new edition will be as successful as the first one, offering you valuable insights to care for the planet's most extraordinary creatures—birds.

Hugues Beaufrère
Jennifer E. Graham

# Acknowledgements

Thank you to all of the authors who updated or created new material for the second edition. We couldn't have done it without your contributions!

# ABOUT THE COMPANION WEBSITE

Don't forget to visit the companion web site for this book:

www.wiley.com/go/Beaufrère/2e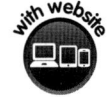

There you will find valuable materials, including:

• Client Handouts
• Online resources

# BASICS

## DEFINITION
Adenoviruses are double-stranded nonenveloped DNA viruses that are known to infect and cause disease in passerine birds, Psittacines, Columbiformes, Falconiformes, Strigiformes, and gallinaceous birds.

## PATHOPHYSIOLOGY
Wide range of virulence; even within the same serotype. Subclinical infections are the most common, where birds remain latent and become persistent shedders for life. Outbreaks can result in considerable morbidity and mortality. Overall, younger and immunocompromised birds tend to have more severe infections. Concurrent diseases are common. Poor hygiene and high stocking densities may play a role in mortality. Cellular damage is caused by virus replication and viral structural proteins that are thought to be cellularly toxic.

## SYSTEMS AFFECTED
**Gastrointestinal**: Falcons, finches, hawks, owls, pigeons, psittacine birds, turkeys.
**Hemic/lymphatic/immune**: Falcons, finches, pheasants, pigeon, psittacine birds, owls, pigeon, turkeys.
**Hepatobiliary (necrosis)**: Pigeons, psittacine birds, falcons, hawks, owls.
**Renal/urologic**: Finches, pigeons, psittacine birds.
**Reproductive**: Chickens (egg drop syndrome).
**Respiratory**: Pheasants.
**Respiratory**: Quail.

## GENETICS
Many outbreaks of adenoviruses in mixed collections of birds are likely caused by cross-species infection. At least one falcon adenovirus is believed to subclinically infect peregrine falcons and is more likely to cause disease in other species. The adenoviruses causing marble spleen disease in pheasants and hemorrhagic enteritis in turkeys are asymptomatically carried by waterfowl.

## INCIDENCE/PREVALENCE
**Falcons**: Rare outbreaks have been described. Prevalence of infection in peregrine falcons may be high.
**Hawks and owls**: Two outbreaks have been described. Prevalence is unknown.
**Pigeons**: Outbreaks occur sporadically, prevalence is unknown, but subclinical infections are likely to be common.
**Psittacine birds**: Prevalence is variable. There have been extensive outbreaks in budgerigars and lovebirds. Individual infections and outbreaks in other psittacine birds are sporadic.

**Chickens**: Prevalence is variable, but can be high.
**Turkeys**: Prevalence is variable, but can be high.
**Pheasants**: Prevalence is variable.
**Quail**: High prevalence of infection.

## GEOGRAPHIC DISTRIBUTION
**Finches**: Described in North America.
**Falcons**: Described in North America.
**Hawks and owls**: Described in the United Kingdom.
**Pigeons**: Worldwide.
**Psittacine birds**: Outbreaks have occurred on multiple continents, not all adenoviruses have been adequately characterised. The distribution of each adenovirus therefore is not fully known.
**Chickens**: Worldwide, but not in North America.
**Turkeys**: Worldwide.
**Pheasants**: Worldwide.
**Quail**: Worldwide.

## SIGNALMENT
**Finches**: Adult finches, multiple species, both sexes.
**Falcons**: Nestling northern aplomado falcon, peregrine falcon, Taita falcon, orange-breasted falcon, adult American kestrel, both sexes.
**Hawks and owls**: Harris hawk, Bengal eagle owl, Verreaux's eagle owl, both sexes various ages.
**Pigeons**: Less than 1 year old, both sexes.
**Psittacine birds**: Most common in budgerigars, lovebirds, Senegal parrots and related species; occurs sporadically in other parrot species.
**Chickens**: Laying hens.
**Turkeys**: Growing birds of both sexes 6–12 weeks old.
**Pheasants**: 3–8 months old, both sexes.
**Quail**: 1–6 weeks old, both sexes.

## SIGNS
### Historical Findings
**Finches**: Unexpected deaths in a flock.
**Falcons**: Death after a short duration of non-specific signs.
**Hawks and owls**: Death without premonitory signs or a short duration of non-specific signs.
**Pigeons**: Type 1: Vomiting, watery diarrhea and depression, rapid spread through the loft, increased mortality; type 2: Multiple unexpected deaths.
**Psittacine birds**: Unexpected mortality in nestling parrots.
**Chickens**: Sudden drop in egg production, abnormally colored eggs, shell-less eggs.
**Turkeys**: Sudden onset of hemorrhagic enteritis and depression.
**Pheasants**: Dyspnea and death.
**Quail**: Sudden and dramatic increase in mortality, nonspecific signs of illness,

increased respiratory effort and increased respiratory sounds.

### Physical Examination Findings
**Hawks and owls**: Birds die before they can be presented for examination.
**Pigeons**: Type 1: Vomiting, watery diarrhea, depression, weight loss; type 2: N/A.
**Chickens**: Abnormally colored eggs, shell-less eggs. Chickens appear normal.
**Turkeys**: Bloody diarrhea and depression.
**Pheasants**: Dyspnea, cyanosis.
**Quail**: Nasal discharge, open-mouthed breathing, respiratory sounds.
**All other species**: N/A

## CAUSES
Three genera of adenoviruses (*Aviadenovirus*, *Siadenovirus*, and *Atadenovirus*) have been shown to cause disease in birds. The signs associated with infection depend on the organ targeted by the virus and the host's immune response.

## RISK FACTORS
Failure to quarantine new birds. Housing multiple species together in the same collection. High stocking densities. Concurrent infections (circovirus, aspergillosis, coccidiosis, Marek's disease virus, etc.). Pheasants, turkeys, chickens: exposure to waterfowl.

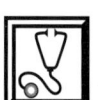

# DIAGNOSIS

## DIFFERENTIAL DIAGNOSIS
All species: Other systemic viral infections, septicemia, gross management errors.

## CBC/BIOCHEMISTRY/URINALYSIS
In birds experiencing hepatitis, elevations in the AST, SDH, GLDH are expected.

## OTHER LABORATORY TESTS
Dependent on strain of virus. Virus neutralization assay. Antibodies can be detected by hemagglutination inhibition and enzyme-linked immunoassays. PCR (DNA probes).
Virus isolation and electron microscopy.

## IMAGING
Possible hepatomegaly and splenomegaly enlargement.

## DIAGNOSTIC PROCEDURES
N/A

## PATHOLOGIC FINDINGS
Intranuclear inclusion will be observed in infected tissues.
**Finches**: Grossly, liver and spleen enlargement. Microscopically, multiple round-to-irregular pale tan (necrotic) foci. Hepatic, splenic, and intestinal mucosal necrosis with varying numbers of large intranuclear basophilic to amphophilic inclusion bodies.

**Falcons**: Grossly, liver and spleen enlargement. Microscopically, hepatic and splenic necrosis with a mild-to-moderate lymphoplasmacytic inflammatory response. Varying numbers of large intranuclear basophilic to amphophilic inclusion bodies are present.

**Hawks and owls**: Grossly, liver and spleen enlargement. Microscopically, hepatic necrosis and mild-to-moderate inflammatory response, splenic necrosis, and proventricular and ventricular necrosis resulting in ulceration. Varying numbers of large intranuclear basophilic to amphophilic inclusion bodies are present in all affected tissues.

**Pigeons**: Type 1: Grossly, fibrinous and hemorrhagic enteritis, variable liver enlargement with necrotic foci. Microscopically, villus atrophy of the duodenum, characteristic inclusion bodies are found in intestinal epithelial cells. Hepatic necrosis may occur, but it is infrequent. Inclusion bodies are infrequently found in the liver. Type 2: Grossly, hepatic and possibly splenic enlargement are seen. There may be multifocal discoloration of the liver. Microscopically, there is a moderate to massive necrosis of the liver with intranuclear eosinophilic inclusion bodies.

**Psittacine birds**: Lesions depend on the virus and species of bird. Grossly, there may be evidence of one or more of: conjunctivitis, hepatitis, pancreatitis, enteritis, and splenic enlargement. The virus causes necrosis of the affected tissues, which will be accompanied by inflammation depending on how long the bird lives after the lesions develop. Intranuclear inclusions are generally common, but may be difficult to find. Inclusions in the tubular epithelial cells of the kidneys may be incidental findings in birds dying of other causes.

**Chickens**: Grossly, inactive ovaries and atrophied oviducts. Microscopically, severe chronic active inflammation of the shell gland with intranuclear inclusion bodies in the epithelial cells. Microscopically, there is expansion of the histiocytic population surrounding the sheathed arteries of the spleen with lymphoid necrosis with pannuclear inclusion bodies. Digestive tract lesions include epithelial sloughing, hemorrhage within the villi and the submucosa, a variable degree of inflammation which can include heterophils and mononuclear cells and the presence of intranuclear inclusion bodies. Lesions are most severe in the duodenum.

**Turkeys**: Grossly, well muscled but pale, may have still been eating, hemorrhage into the intestine, hepatomegaly and splenomegaly. Lesions resemble those seen in the chicken, but do not involve the digestive tract.

**Pheasants**: Pulmonary edema and enlarged mottled spleens. Lesions resemble those seen in the chicken, but do not involve the digestive tract.

**Quail**: Exudate in the nasal passages and in the trachea with tracheal mucosal thickening. Exudate may extend into the mainstem bronchi. Microscopically, there is necrosis and sloughing of the tracheal epithelium and the presence of intranuclear inclusion bodies and nuclear enlargement. There will be varying degrees of inflammation, which may be complicated by secondary bacterial infections. Multifocal hepatic necrosis may also occur.

 **TREATMENT**

**NURSING CARE**
Supportive care with fluids, supplemental heat, and assist feeding. Broad-spectrum antibiotics to prevent secondary bacterial infections. Hepatoprotectants.

**DIET**
N/A

**CLIENT EDUCATION**
N/A

**SURGICAL CONSIDERATIONS**
N/A

 **MEDICATIONS**

**DRUG(S) OF CHOICE**
N/A

**CONTRAINDICATIONS**
N/A

**PRECAUTIONS**
N/A

**POSSIBLE INTERACTIONS**
N/A

**ALTERNATIVE DRUGS**
N/A

 **FOLLOW-UP**

**PATIENT MONITORING**
N/A

**PREVENTION/AVOIDANCE**
**Falcons**: Do not raise other species of falcons with peregrine falcons.
**Chickens, turkeys, pheasants**: Avoid contact with waterfowl.
**Chickens**: Disease has been eradicated from laying stock. Infection is prevented by strict quarantine and hygiene methods. Inactivated vaccines have been developed and used effectively.

**Turkeys**: Vaccination by water administration.
**Quail**: Strict biosecurity measures.

**POSSIBLE COMPLICATIONS**
Secondary infections.

**EXPECTED COURSE AND PROGNOSIS**
**Finches**: Overall low level or sporadic mortality; symptomatic birds high mortality.
**Falcons**: Clinically diseased birds high mortality.
**Hawks and owls**: The only known infected birds died.
**Pigeons**: Type 1: High levels of morbidity (up to 100%), low mortality unless secondary *Escherichia coli* infections occur. Type 2: Sporadic mortality, most birds that develop the disease die.
**Psittacine birds**: Birds with clinical systemic disease have a high mortality. Likely that there are many subclinically infected birds. Nestling deaths may occur in subsequent clutches.
**Chickens**: A 10–40% reduction in egg production.
**Turkeys**: Average mortality of 10–15%, but may be higher. Secondary *E.coli* infections may increase the morbidity and mortality.
**Pheasants**: Flock mortality ranges from 2% to 15%.
**Quail**: Mortality rates may exceed 50% of susceptible birds.

 **MISCELLANEOUS**

**ASSOCIATED CONDITIONS**
N/A

**AGE-RELATED FACTORS**
N/A

**ZOONOTIC POTENTIAL**
N/A

**FERTILITY/BREEDING**
N/A

**SYNONYMS**
N/A

**SEE ALSO**
Colibacillosis
Herpesvirus (Columbid Herpesvirus 1 in Pigeons and Raptors)
Herpesvirus (Duck Viral Enteritis)
Herpesvirus (Passerine Birds)
Herpesvirus (Psittacid Herpesviruses)
Liver Disease
Also individual named viral diseases
Appendix 3: Laboratory Testing

**ABBREVIATIONS**
AST—aspartate aminotransferase
GLDH—glutamate dehydrogenase
PCR—polymerase chain reaction
SDH—sorbitol dehydrogenase

## INTERNET RESOURCES
N/A

*Suggested Reading*
Gerlach, H. (1994) Viruses. In: *Avian Medicine: Principles and Applications* (ed. B.W. Ritchie, G.J. Harrison, L.R. Harrison), 862–948. Lake Worth, FL: Wingers Publishing.

Marlier, D., Vindevogel, H. (2006). Viral infections in pigeons. *Veterinary Journal*, 172:40–51.

Oaks, J.L., Schrenzel, M., Rideout, B., Sandfort, C. (2005). Isolation and epidemiology of Falcon Adenovirus. *Journal of Clinical Microbiology*, 43:3414–3420.

Saif, Y.M. (ed.) (2008). *Diseases of Poultry*, 12th edn. Oxford, UK: Blackwell Publishing.

Schmidt, R., Reavell, D., Phalen, D.N. (2003). *Pathology of Exotic Birds*. Ames, IA: Iowa State University Press.

Zsivanovits, P., Monks, D.J., Forbes, N.A., et al. (2006). Presumptive identification of a novel adenovirus in a Harris hawk (*Parabuteo unicinctus*), a Bengal eagle owl (*Bubo bengalensis*), and a Verreaux's eagle owl (*Bubo lacteus*). *Journal of Avian Medicine and Surgery*, 20:105–112.

**Author**: Rodney W. Schnellbacher DVM, DACZM

**Acknowledgement**: Updated from first edition chapter authored by David N. Phalen, DVM, PhD, DABVP (Avian)

# ADRENAL GLAND DISEASES

 **BASICS**

## DEFINITION

Adrenal gland diseases are characterized by a dysfunction or pathology of the adrenal glands and may include inflammatory (adrenalitis), hyperplastic, and neoplastic changes (adenoma, carcinoma, pheochromocytoma), hypofunction (hypoadrenocorticism, Addison's disease) and hyperfunction (hyperadrenocortisism, Cushing syndrome, hyperaldosteronism).

## PATHOPHYSIOLOGY

The avian adrenal glands are paired organs situated at the anterior medial poles of the left and right kidneys, just caudal to the lungs. Unlike mammals, there is no distinct histologic division between the inner medulla and outer cortex, as the cortical (interrenal) and medullary (chromaffin) cells are intermingled. Nevertheless, the cortical cells are arranged in linear cords radiating outward from the center, thereby resulting in a structural and functional layout in which two zones can be recognized (i.e. the subcapsular zone, reminiscent of mammalian zona glomerulosa cells, and an inner zone, reminiscent of mammalian zona fasciculata/reticularis). The chromaffin cells are mostly concentrated centrally in the adrenal gland and gather in clusters (medullary islets), which are each innervated by a single nerve bundle, similar to mammals. Production of hormones by the cortical cells is stimulated by pituitary ACTH, whereby the subcapsular zone cells mostly produce aldosterone (involved with electrolyte and hemodynamic balance), and the inner zone cells mostly produce corticosterone (the predominant glucocorticoid hormone in birds, which has widespread effects on many tissues). In addition, aldosterone secretion is affected by activation of the renin–angiotensin system, where aldosterone is released in response to angiotensin II. The chromaffin cells are under direct neural control and synthesize and release norepinephrine and epinephrine, which are involved in regulation of blood pressure and heart rate. Adrenal gland tumors can be functional or non-functional. In case of functional tumors or hyperplasia, depending on the cell type involved, corticosterone, aldosterone, or adrenaline may be produced in excess, leading to Cushing syndrome, hyperaldosteronism, or pheochromocytoma crisis (adrenaline surge). Additionally, hyperfunction may result from overstimulation of the adrenal glands by excess ACTH in case of pituitary neoplasia (Cushing's disease). Hypofunction with inadequate production of glucocorticoids

(corticosterone) and mineralocorticoids (aldosterone) can also occur (e.g. due to immune-mediated disease, infections or intoxications), which leads to development of Addison's disease. Carcinomas can become very large and may metastasize.

## SYSTEMS AFFECTED

**Endocrine/metabolic:** Increased or decreased production of corticosterone, aldosterone, or epinephrine, disruption of electrolyte balance and fluid homeostasis (Addison's disease), altered fat, protein, glucose metabolism, polyphagia and obesity or weight gain (Cushing syndrome), secondary diabetes mellitus (Cushing syndrome), increased blood pressure (hyperaldosteronism), periodic epinephrine release (pheochromocytoma).
**Hemopoeietic/immune:** Altered immune function with increased risk for secondary infections (Cushing syndrome); increased risk of hemorrhage (hyperaldosteronism).
**Renal/urologic:** Polyuria/polydipsia (Cushing syndrome); possible secondary renal failure (hyperaldosteronism).
**Cardiovascular:** Increased blood pressure with possible secondary cardiomyopathy (hyperaldosteronism); tachycardia and hypertension (pheochromocytoma); hypovolemia, dehydration and shock (Addison's disease).
**Respiratory:** Dyspnea due to space-occupying effects (adrenal neoplasia).
**Hepatic:** Liver lipidosis (Cushing syndrome).
**Skin/exocrine:** Alopecia, subcutaneous fat deposits (Cushing syndrome).
**Sensory:** Blindness (pituitary tumor), retinal hemorrhage (hyperaldosteronism).
**Nervous:** Central nervous signs such as ataxia (pituitary tumor).
**Musculoskeletal:** Lameness, paresis, paralysis due to sciatic compression (adrenal tumor); possible osteoporosis or altered calcium metabolism (Cushing syndrome).

## GENETICS

There are no indications for an underlying genetic basis for adrenal disease in birds.

## INCIDENCE/PREVALENCE

Adrenal lesions had a relatively high prevalence (41/150; 27%) in a retrospective study on adrenal pathology found during postmortem examinations in psittacine birds. Another study focusing on endocrine lesions found adrenal degeneration in about 30% of cases with adrenal disease and adenitis in another 27% of cases. However, clinical diagnoses of adrenal disease are only rarely reported, possibly due to the difficulties in recognizing the signs or achieving an antemortem diagnosis, as well as the quick progression of disease, leading to death (as may be the case for hypoadrenocorticism). Of the neuroendocrine tumors that are

reported in birds, pituitary adenomas are the most common.

## GEOGRAPHIC DISTRIBUTION
N/A

## SIGNALMENT

**Species predilections:** Pituitary adenomas are most prevalent in budgerigars (*Melopsittacus undulatus*) and cockatiels (*Nymphicus hollandicus*), but have also been reported in other species of birds including a Moluccan cockatoo (*Cacatua moluccensis*), Amazon parrot (*Amazona* sp.), lovebird (*Agapornis* sp.), canary (*Serinus canaria*), and chicken (*Gallus gallus domesticus*). For primary adrenal lesions, there are no known species predilections, although adrenal degeneration was frequently observed in grey parrots (*Psittacus erithacus*) and Amazon parrots. Primary adrenal gland neoplasia has been reported in various bird species including budgerigars, macaws, chicken, pheasants, peafowl, pigeons, and ducks. Signs of hyperadrenocorticism have been reported in a few psittacine birds (Senegal parrot, *Poicephalus senegalus*; scarlet macaw, *Ara macao*; Moluccan cockatoo, *Cacatua moluccensis*). Postmortem diagnosis of pheochromocytoma has been reported in a nicobar pigeon (*Caloenas nicobarica*) and budgerigar.
**Mean age and range:** Adrenal neoplasia is more likely to occur in middle-aged to older birds.
**Predominant sex:** No sex predilection is known.

## SIGNS

### Historical Findings
**Hypoadrenocorticism/Addison's disease:** Clinical signs are probably similar to those reported in other species and may include episodic weakness, chronic debilitation, collapse, gastrointestinal signs such as periodic diarrhea, anorexia and generalized abdominal tenderness, feather loss. Birds may also be found dead without premonitory signs.
**Hyperadrenocorticism/Cushing syndrome:** Polyuria/polydipsia, polyphagia, coelomic distension with respiratory distress, weight gain, obesity, feather changes or loss. In case of pituitary tumors, clinical signs may result from the space-occupying effect of the tumor and include cere and feather color changes, ataxia/circling/loss of balance, head tremors, decreased vocalization, depression, lethargy, visual impairment/blindness, and exophthalmos.
**Hyperaldosteronism:** Restlessness, weakness, neurologic signs (e.g. epilepsy/seizures, ataxia, altered mentation, coma), visual impairment, signs associated with cardiac or renal dysfunction.
**Adrenal neoplasia:** Wide-base stance, signs related to the mass effect and compression of

surrounding structures (e.g. paresis/paralysis or lameness, respiratory distress, abdominal distension, reduced fecal output).

### Physical Examination Findings
**Pituitary tumor**: Unilateral or bilateral exophthalmia, visual impairment (lack of response to light and poor response in obstacle test), lethargy, depression, ataxia, head tremors, and other neurologic deficits.
**Adrenal tumor**: Wide-legged stance, abdominal distension with mass effect, unilateral or bilateral paresis/paralysis with weakened grip, and abnormal reflexes.
**Hyperadrenocorticism**: Polyuria/polydipsia, obesity, subcutaneous fat deposits, coelomic distension, hepatomegaly, possible muscle wasting, feather loss, or other feather changes.
**Hyperaldosteronism**: Subjectively strong pulse, retinal hemorrhage, neurologic deficits, signs associated with cardiac or renal disease.
**Pheochromocytoma**: May not show any signs other than episodic tachycardia, hypertension, possible coelomic distension due to space-occupying effects of the growing mass.
**Hypoadrenocorticism**: Weak pulse, increased CRT, slow skin turgor, dehydration, generalized or episodic weakness, bradycardia (due to hyperkalemia), coelomic tenderness, diarrhea.

## CAUSES
Primary hypoadrenocorticism results from inadequate production of glucocorticoids and/or mineralocorticoids by adrenocortical cells, which is seen if > 90% of the adrenal cortex is damaged. Cell atrophy or necrosis can be induced by autoimmune diseases, neoplasia, inflammation, infectious diseases (sepsis, chlamydiosis, mycobacteriosis, viral diseases such as polyomavirus, paramyxovirus, avian ganglioneuritis), amyloidosis, trauma, pesticides, pollutants, or drugs (mitotane, trilostane). Secondary hypoadrenocorticism results from deficient production and secretion of ACTH, leading to atrophy and reduced glucocorticoid secretion. This can occur in cases of large pituitary tumors or in cases of prolonged therapy with glucocorticoids or progestogens. Primary hyperadrenocorticism results from functional neoplasia or hyperplasia of the adrenal cortex (e.g. adenoma, carcinoma). Secondary hyperadrenocorticism occurs due to ACTH-secreting pituitary neoplasia or exogenous glucocorticoid administration.

## RISK FACTORS
Exogenous corticosteroids can lead to hyperadrenocorticism and associated signs. Chronic exposure of herring gulls (*Larus argentatus*) to crude oil was reported to result in adrenal hypertrophy and short-term increases in circulating corticosterone, possibly as a response to acute stress.

Exposure to sublethal levels of lead in young white storks (*Ciconia ciconia*) lead to a higher stress response and circulating corticosterone after handling compared to non-exposed birds. Exposure of nestling bald eagles (*Haliaeetus leucocephalus*) to organochlorides depresses corticosterone levels and response to ACTH stimulation.

## DIAGNOSIS
### DIFFERENTIAL DIAGNOSIS
**Hypoadrenocorticism**: Renal disease, acute renal insufficiency, gastrointestinal and hepatic disease, sepsis, other causes of collapse or weakness.
**Hyperadrenocorticism**: Exogenous corticosteroid administration; obesity due to excessive feeding or low activity; hypothyroidism; other causes of polyuria and/or polydipsia.
**Hyperaldosteronism**: Chronic stress; other diseases leading to increased blood pressure and its associated complications, most notably atherosclerosis.
**Adrenal neoplasia**: Other types of neoplasia and conditions leading to abdominal distension and paresis and paralysis, including renal neoplasia, gonadal neoplasia.

### CBC/BIOCHEMISTRY/URINALYSIS
Hypoadrenocorticism—hyperkalemia, hyponatremia, hyperuricemia, azotemia, low fasting blood glucose, anemia.
Hyperadrenocorticism—hyperglycemia, elevated liver enzymes (ALP, ALT, AST), increased bile acids, elevated cholesterol and triglyceride concentrations, hypophosphatemia, changes in the hemogram (white blood cell count)—stress leukogram (heterophilia, lymphopenia, monocytosis).
Hyperaldosteronism—hypernatremia.
Pheochromocytoma, usually non-specific hematologic and biochemical changes.

### OTHER LABORATORY TESTS
In humans and other animals, renin and aldosterone are measured in patients suspected of hyperaldosteronism. These tests have not been validated for clinical use in birds. Corticosterone values could be measured for birds suspected of hyperadrenocorticism, but levels may fluctuate significantly (corticosterone levels are reported to rise < 2 minutes following restraint). Epinephrine levels could be determined in patients suspected of pheochromocytoma, but due to fluctuating blood levels values are difficult to interpret. In dogs, measurement of free metanephrines in urine and saliva have been used to screen for pheochromocytoma but these tests have

not been validated in birds. Decreased urine specific gravity (hypoadrenocorticism, hyperadrenocorticism), glucosuria (secondary diabetes mellitus). (In)direct blood pressure measurement may be helpful to diagnose hypertension in case of hyperaldosteronism or pheochromocytoma; however, indirect/non-invasive blood pressure measurement in birds has not been found to be reliable.

### IMAGING
In case of a large tumor, a space-occupying mass may be detected in the region of the kidneys and gonads on radiography or ultrasound. Advanced imaging techniques (e.g. contrast enhanced CT) may potentially be useful to detect smaller masses and/or pituitary neoplasia. Endoscopy may be considered to collect adrenal biopsies and obtain a histopathological diagnosis.

### DIAGNOSTIC PROCEDURES
ACTH stimulation test is predominantly useful to diagnose hypofunction of the adrenal gland. Various protocols have been developed for psittacines, raptors, pigeons, chickens, cranes, and ducks. In general, a baseline blood sample is collected, followed by ACTH 15–50 IU administered IM and a second blood sample is collected between 1 and 2 hours after ACTH administration. Depending on the protocol, route of administration, and species involved, increases in baseline corticosterone concentrations in healthy birds can be 10- to 100-fold (pigeons), 16-fold (chicken), 4- to 14-fold (cockatoos, macaws, Amazon parrots, and lorikeets), 5-fold (cranes), or 2- to 6-fold (ducks). Dexamethasone suppression test is useful to diagnose hyperfunction of the adrenal gland. In birds, this test has been used to successfully diagnose Cushing syndrome in a Senegal parrot. For this purpose, dexamethasone was administered IV at a dosage of 0.5 µg/kg, with blood collected for corticosterone concentrations at t = 0 and t = 90 minutes following administration of the dexamethasone. In healthy birds, this resulted in at least 2-fold reduction of corticosterone concentrations, whereas no decrease in corticosterone was observed in the bird with Cushing syndrome.

### PATHOLOGIC FINDINGS
Adrenal degeneration is characterized by swelling and vacuolation of adrenocortical cells. Cell necrosis can also be seen. Pituitary or adrenal neoplasia may be detected upon gross postmortem examination. In pituitary tumors, the gland will be enlarged and possibly the surrounding brain tissue may be discolored and distorted. Bilateral enlargement of the adrenal glands can be observed, although in case of a primary adrenal tumor, changes will usually be

unilateral. Histology of the pituitary or adrenal may reveal an adenoma or carcinoma. In malignant tumors, metastases may be found in other organs (e.g. liver, lung). Pheochromocytoma can be benign or malignant. Tumors are often composed of cords and packets of neoplastic round cells separated by delicate fibrous stroma. Neoplastic cells can show pale eosinophilic to vacuolated cytoplasm with anisokaryosis, dark cytoplasmic granules and mitotic figures. Special stains (Churukian–Schenk stain) can be used to detect neuroendocrine granules, confirming neuroendocrine origin of the cells.

 **TREATMENT**

### APPROPRIATE HEALTH CARE
**Hypoadrenocorticism/adrenal insufficiency**: Intravenous saline therapy (see Nursing Care section) and glucocorticoid administration for collapsed animals in Addison's crisis, followed by lifelong replacement therapy with mineralocorticoids alone or in combination with glucocorticoids. Replacement therapy may be achieved using deoxycorticosterone acetate 4 mg/kg q24h PO, cortisone acetate 10 mg/kg q24h PO, or dexamethasone 0.1–0.2 ml of a 2 mg/ml solution, and fludrocortisone ¼ to 1 tablet of 0.1 mg dissolved in 4 oz drinking water. Careful monitoring of the patient would be warranted, as insufficient replacement can be lethal but overreplacement could potentially also result in serious problems.
**Hyperadrenocorticism**: medical management is aimed at alleviating signs of hyperadrenocorticism through administering mitotane (Lysodren®, Corden Pharma Latina, Sermoneta, Italy; o,p′-DDD), trilostane (Vetoryl®, Dechra, Overland Park, KS), selegine hydrochloride (Anipryl®, Zoetis,) or ketoconazole in dogs, with the latter two options being considered less effective. Of these, only trilostane has been used to treat Cushing syndrome in a Senegal parrot (1 mg/kg q12–24h PO). Additional treatment may be aimed at eliminating secondary infections and other secondary complications from hyperadrenocorticism (diabetes mellitus, hepatic lipodosis).
**Hyperaldosteronism**: Treatment is likely similar to that described in humans, and consists of limiting salt intake and use of drugs that block the action of aldosterone and help to manage fluid buildup in the body. Additionally, secondary complications that arise from hypertension may be managed through supportive care and symptomatic treatment.

**Other adrenal disease**: Mostly supportive, directed at alleviating clinical signs.

### NURSING CARE
Patients with Addison's disease may present acutely with an adrenal crisis, which is a life-threatening situation requiring aggressive fluid therapy with intravenous physiologic saline. Patients with complications from hemorrhage/organ damage due to high blood pressure might require additional supportive care and husbandry adaptations (e.g. subdued lighting and adjusted housing with soft bedding to prevent trauma for patients with cerebrovascular incidents or retinal hemorrhage).

### ACTIVITY
N/A

### DIET
Limiting dietary salt intake is recommended for patients with high blood pressure and hyperaldosteronism. For patients with Cushing's disease, dietary recommendations are similar for those with high blood pressure and diabetes mellitus, with additional recommendations to ensure adequate calcium and vitamin D intake. Similar recommendations may apply to birds.

### CLIENT EDUCATION
Clients should be made aware that adrenal disease is rare in birds and little data exists on their diagnosis and management. As a result, information on treatment is mostly derived from other animals, and warrants gradual titration of the dose while carefully monitoring for adverse effects.

### SURGICAL CONSIDERATIONS
Surgical intervention (partial or total adrenalectomy) is applied in humans and other animals with adrenal neoplasia. Similarly, pituitary neoplasms have been surgically removed in companion animals with Cushing's disease, although following surgery, lifelong hormone therapy is indicated due to the lack of endogenous production. In birds, none of these procedures have been reported.

 **MEDICATIONS**

### DRUG(S) OF CHOICE
Trilostane successfully resolved clinical signs in a Senegal parrot in a dose of 1 mg/kg q12–24h PO. Dose should be gradually titrated to effect. Alternative medications used in humans and other animals to treat Cushing syndrome include osilodrostat, mitotane, levoketoconazole, and metyrapone, but no (clinical) data exist on their use on birds. Medications that could be useful to treat hyperaldosteronism include

spironolactone, eplerenone, and amiloride. These drugs help to manage fluid buildup in the body and block the action of aldosterone. Treatment of Addison's disease involves lifelong supplementation with glucocorticoid hormones—hydrocortisone, prednisone, or methylprednisolone. As no antemortem diagnoses of Addison's disease exist in birds there are no data available on the efficacy or complications of these medications in birds.

### CONTRAINDICATIONS
Trilostane is metabolized by the liver, and therefore generally not used in patients with impaired liver function. Additionally, trilostane should be used with caution in patients with kidney problems or those that are anemic.

### PRECAUTIONS
Trilostane may affect the levels of some of the other hormones produced in the adrenal gland. As this could increase the risk for metabolic problems (e.g. dehydration, weakness, and abnormal serum electrolyte levels), owners should carefully monitor their bird when initiating therapy.

### POSSIBLE INTERACTIONS
Combined use of trilostane with potassium-sparing diuretics is best avoided because of potential high serum potassium levels.

### ALTERNATIVE DRUGS
N/A

 **FOLLOW-UP**

### PATIENT MONITORING
Hyperadrenocorticism—regular rechecks of CBC, glucose, liver enzymes, bile acids, and electrolytes are advised. Patients with Addison's disease may benefit from regular monitoring of electrolyte levels and for features indicating over- or underreplacement. In patients with hyperaldosteronism, blood pressure measurement is warranted, but this is often difficult to achieve in the awake bird as non-invasive techniques are not very reliable (low accuracy and reproducibility). Additional monitoring may involve evaluation of retinal hemorrhage, cardiac and renal function.

### PREVENTION/AVOIDANCE
N/A

### POSSIBLE COMPLICATIONS
Cushing's disease may increase the risk for diabetes mellitus, liver lipidosis and secondary infections. Chronic elevation of blood pressure, as could be observed with hyperaldosteronism may increase the risk of damage to the retina, brain, heart, and

kidneys. Large adrenal tumors may lead to dyspnea due to compression of the air sacs and/or to lameness, paresis, or paralysis due to compression of the sciatic nerve.

## EXPECTED COURSE AND PROGNOSIS

Most adrenal diseases have mostly, if not exclusively, been diagnosed postmortem, hence making it difficult to provide details regarding its prognosis. Due to the scarcity of reported cases on hyperadrenocorticism in birds, prognosis is hard to predict. A Senegal parrot was successfully treated with trilostane for approximately 1 year and then died due to bleeding out from a liver rupture after clinical signs recurred. Hypoadrenocorticism/adrenal insufficiency likely leads to rapidly progressing, life-threatening disease without appropriate replacement therapy.

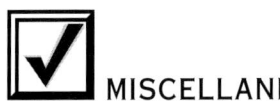 **MISCELLANEOUS**

## ASSOCIATED CONDITIONS

Glucocorticoids have a widespread effect on metabolism, immune function, behavior, and electrolyte balance; hence, excess amounts of corticosterone produced in birds with Cushing syndrome will produce a range of signs. Cushing syndrome is known to increase the risk for diabetes mellitus in humans and may have similar effects in birds. In addition, glucocorticoids have immunosuppressive effects and may increase the risk for secondary (bacterial or fungal) infections or metabolic and immunogenic effects. Due to altered fat metabolism, hepatic lipidosis and obesity are common sequela to excess amounts of glucocorticoids. In humans and other animals, hyperaldosteronism has been associated with increased risk for retinal

damage, cerebrovascular incidents and dysfunction of the heart and kidneys. Similar consequences may apply to birds.

## AGE-RELATED FACTORS

Neoplastic changes are more likely to occur in middle-aged to older birds.

## ZOONOTIC POTENTIAL

N/A

## FERTILITY/BREEDING

Cushing syndrome may induce a variety of metabolic disturbances that are known to negatively affect fertility in humans. A similar effect can therefore be anticipated in birds.

## SYNONYMS

Hyperadrenocorticism—Cushing syndrome; hypoadrenocorticism—Addison's disease, adrenal insufficiency.

## SEE ALSO

Coelomic Distension
Congestive Heart Failure
Diabetes Mellitus and Hyperglycemia
Hyperuricemia
Liver Disease
Myocardial Diseases
Polydipsia
Polyuria
Renal Diseases
Thyroid Diseases

## ABBREVIATIONS

ACTH—adrenocorticotropic hormone
ALP— alkaline phosphatase
ALT—alanine aminotransferase
AST—aspartate aminotransferase
CRT—capillary refill time

## INTERNET RESOURCES

N/A

*Suggested Reading*
Campbell-Ward, M.L. (2013). Hyperadrenocorticism and primary functioning adrenal tumors in other species (excluding horses and ferrets). In: *Clinical Endocrinology of Companion Animals* (ed. J. Rand), 95–99. Ames, IA: Wiley.

Cornelissen, H., Verhofstad, A. (1998). Hyperadrenocorticism caused by an adrenal carcinoma in a parrot. *Veterinary Quarterly*, 20(Suppl 1): S111.

De Matos, R. (2008). Adrenal steroid metabolism in birds: anatomy, physiology, and clinical considerations. *Veterinary Clinics of North America: Exotic Animal Practice*, 11:35–57.

Hahn, K.A., Jones, M.P., Petersen, M.G., et al. (1997). Metastatic pheochromocytoma in a parakeet. *Avian Diseases*, 41:751–754.

Lothrop, C.D. Jr. (1984). Diagnosis of adrenal diseases in caged birds. In: *Proceedings of the 1984 International Conference on Avian Medicine (AAV)*, 95–100.

Rae, M. (1995). Endocrine disease in pet birds. *Seminars in Avian and Exotic Pet Medicine*, 4:32–38.

Sonnenfield, J.M., Carpenter, J.W., Garner, M.M., et al. (2002). Pheochromocytoma in a nicobar pigeon (*Caloenas nicobarica*). *Journal of Avian Medicine and Surgery*, 16:306–308.

Starkey, S.R., Morrisey, J.K., Stewart, J.E., Buckles, E.L. (2008). Pituitary-dependent hyperadrenocorticism in a cockatoo. *Journal of the American Veterinary Medical Association*, 232:394–398.

Van Zeeland, Y.R.A., Bastiaansen, P., Schoemaker, N.J. (2013). Diagnosis and treatment of Cushing's syndrome in a Senegal parrot. In: *Proceedings of the 1st International Conference on Avian, Herpetologic and Exotic Mammal Medicine (ICARE)*, Wiesbaden, Germany, 303–304.

**Author**: Yvonne van Zeeland, DVM, MVR, PhD, Dip. ECZM (Avian, Small Mammal)

# BASICS

## DEFINITION
Infection with mites (mainly *Sternostoma tracheacolum*; other species, such as within the family Rhinonyssidae, e.g. *Ptilonyssus*, and less commonly *Cytodites nudus*, can be involved) in the upper and lower respiratory systems (including nasal passages, trachea, smaller air passages, and air sacs). Some mite species (especially *Cytodites*) have also invaded other visceral areas including the coelom.

## PATHOPHYSIOLOGY
Mites transmitted from infected birds travel throughout the respiratory system, restricting air flow by being present within narrowed spaces as well as causing inflammation and increased mucous production.

## SYSTEMS AFFECTED
**Respiratory**: Because of a foreign body response, inflammation, and increased fluid/mucous production.
**Behavioral**: Bird's reaction to the respiratory system being affected.

## GENETICS
None known other than species predilections.

## INCIDENCE/PREVALENCE
Common.

## GEOGRAPHIC DISTRIBUTION
Worldwide both in captive and wild individuals.

## SIGNALMENT
**Species**: Finches (especially Australian species), canaries, pigeons, small psittacine birds (budgerigars and cockatiels), poultry, and waterfowl. Many wild species.
**Breed predilections**: Gouldian finches, other finch spp., and canaries most likely; society finches may be resistant to infection.
**Mean age and range**: None.
**Predominant sex**: None.

## SIGNS
### Historical Findings
No signs may have been noted by the owner. Vocalization changes (cessation or tonal change of singing, clicking sounds). Non-specific signs of illness (lethargy, fluffed feathers, reduced appetite). Head shaking. Frequent swallowing, coughing or sneezing. Open-mouth breathing and tail bobbing.

### Physical Examination Findings
Normal in mild cases. Dyspnea (open-mouth breathing, tailbobbing, increased respiratory rate and effort). Clicking while breathing (may be variously loud; may require bird being close to ear to hear this sound). Frequent swallowing motions and increased oral mucous. Beak rubbing (upper and lower together or both on perch), head shaking.

Nasal or oral discharge. Moist breathing sounds ausculted. Weight loss. Various degrees of general lethargy/reduced activity/"fluffing" of feathers. Death.

## CAUSES
Mites or mite eggs eliminated in sneezes, coughs, and feces of infected birds. Mites will also crawl onto feathers around face for direct transmission. Water, food, and environment may become contaminated. Also delivered while infected parents feed chicks. There is no intermediate host required. Very fast (6 days in vitro) development from egg to adult shows how quickly cases can develop and can influence medication timing protocols.

## RISK FACTORS
Poor quarantine and flock management.

# DIAGNOSIS

## DIFFERENTIAL DIAGNOSIS
Any other cause of respiratory distress: Bacterial respiratory infection (*Enterococcus fecalis*), fungal infection (aspergillosis), other parasitic infection (*Syngamus* or *Trichomonas* infection), viral infection (poxvirus), space-occupying lesions in or around the respiratory system (including obesity, masses, dystocia), airborne irritants and toxicants (PTFE). Susceptible species have higher infection rate and mites are more likely with any respiratory signs.

## CBC/BIOCHEMISTRY/URINALYSIS
There are usually no changes in biochemical or urinalysis tests; reported hematological changes include eosinophilia and/or a basophilia with infection.

## OTHER LABORATORY TESTS
The eggs of the mites, or the mites themselves, may be seen in oral swab samples or in fecal samples (via direct wet mount microscopy), or may be flushed during nasal flushes. Test results may be falsely negative. Sometimes, success of treatment will confirm a presumed diagnosis.

## IMAGING
A respiratory mite infection may have generalized, nonspecific radio-opacity changes to the pulmonary and air sac fields with radiology.

## DIAGNOSTIC PROCEDURES
Transilluminate the neck/trachea with bright light source after moistening skin with alcohol. Dark specks can be seen in the tracheal lumen, with the dimensions 0.7 × 0.4 mm. The mites may be in the lower respiratory areas instead and may not be seen here. Tracheal endoscopy (using as small as 1–1.2 mm endoscope) can be useful.

## PATHOLOGIC FINDINGS
At necropsy, dark specks may be seen in the mucus at any location of the respiratory system. Pneumonia, thickened and opaque air sac membranes, and tracheitis can be seen. Mites embed their legs into the connective tissue and live in the mucus layer. Histopathology may show mucous epithelial necrosis, mucosal epithelial hyperplasia, and multiple inflammatory cellular responses.

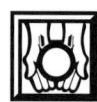

# TREATMENT

## APPROPRIATE HEALTH CARE
Mild to moderate signs: supportive care given at home is usually sufficient. Very dyspneic, lethargic, inappetent, or thin/weak birds may require hospital care. Infection with concurrent primary or secondary infectious agents may need additional therapy. Frequent disinfection of the caging and water supply during treatment will help to decrease reinfestation after treatment.

## NURSING CARE
If severe dyspnea is present, oxygen and humidity supplementation might be useful. If weight loss and/or reduced self-feeding is present, the bird may require supplemental/assisted feeding and crystalloid fluid administration (usually delivered subcutaneously).

## ACTIVITY
If respiratory distress is present, the bird's exercise range should be limited and agitation/stress should be carefully limited/monitored.

## DIET
Although nutritional needs must be met in all species, caloric intake must be aggressively maintained in species with a high metabolic rate that may have decreased intake with illness, as well as addressing any longer-term nutritional deficiencies that might be concurrent.

## CLIENT EDUCATION
The owner should be advised to expect possible exaggerated symptoms after therapy, as this has been reported with heavy infections; the massive die-off of the mites may cause symptoms to worsen shortly after treatment, before improving.

## SURGICAL CONSIDERATIONS
It is best to fully treat these mites before surgery; in the case of emergency surgical needs, there is a higher risk of airway maintenance difficulties because of the increased mucous production and mite blockage of the respiratory passageways. The species affected tend to be small, which may affect endotracheal tube use.

# MEDICATIONS

## DRUG(S) OF CHOICE
Drugs of the avermectin class, especially ivermectin at 0.2 mg/kg treated topically, orally, or parenterally, repeated as often as weekly, for as long as several months. Other avermectins used include moxidectin and doramectin of unknown regimen.

## CONTRAINDICATIONS
None known.

## PRECAUTIONS
Drugs that depress respiration should be used with caution such as sedatives and opioids.

## POSSIBLE INTERACTIONS
None likely.

## ALTERNATIVE DRUGS
Some texts describe the use of a dichlorvos or a "no pest" strip near the affected birds, or an aerosol of rotenone, malathion, or pyrethrin sprays. These pesticides have risks of toxicity since precise dosing is impossible and this is not a currently recommended option.

# FOLLOW-UP

## PATIENT MONITORING
Recheck examination performed within weeks for mild symptoms, sooner or later as symptom degree necessitates. Hemogram changes can be followed.

## PREVENTION/AVOIDANCE
Quarantine, examine and treat new arrivals into the flock to prevent spread to birds already treated.

## POSSIBLE COMPLICATIONS
Acaricide may worsen symptoms due to mite die-off. Insufficient therapy or resistance may allow recurrence of symptoms if all mites are not killed. Secondary infections may progress even with resolution of primary issue. Anesthesia and tracheoscopy higher risk in very symptomatic birds.

## EXPECTED COURSE AND PROGNOSIS
Resolution of symptoms with therapy; prognosis is good unless symptoms are severe.

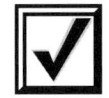

# MISCELLANEOUS

## ASSOCIATED CONDITIONS
N/A

## AGE-RELATED FACTORS
N/A

## ZOONOTIC POTENTIAL
N/A

## FERTILITY/BREEDING
Heavy air sac mite infections can decrease breeding success. Some finch breeders will use surrogate parents of less-susceptible species (such as society finches) to foster the chicks of more-susceptible species(such as Gouldian finches) to limit the spread of this organism to new chicks.

## SYNONYMS
Nasal mite
Respiratory acariasis
Respiratory mite
Tracheal mite
Visceral mite

## SEE ALSO
Respiratory Distress
Sick-Bird Syndrome
Tracheal/Syringeal Disease

## ABBREVIATIONS
PTFE— polytetrafluoroethylene

## INTERNET RESOURCES
PetMD. Air sac mite infection in birds (2008). www.petmd.com/bird/conditions/respiratory/ c_bd_respiratory_parasites-air_sac_mites

*Suggested Reading*
Altman, R., Clubb, S., Dorrestein, G., Quesenberry, K. (1997). *Avian Medicine and Surgery*. Philadelphia, PA: WB Saunders.
Ritchie, B., Harrison, G., Harrison, L. (1994). *Avian Medicine: Principles and Application*. Lake Worth, FL: Wingers Publishing.
Rosskopf, W., Woerpel, R. (1996). *Diseases of Cage and Aviary Birds*, 3rd edn. Baltimore, MD: Williams and Wilkins.
Samour, J. (ed.) (2016). *Avian Medicine*, 3rd edn. London, UK: Mosby.
**Author**: Vanessa Rolfe, DVM, ABVP (Avian Practice)

# AIR SAC RUPTURE

## BASICS

### DEFINITION
The cervicocephalic diverticulum of the infraorbital sinus, the abdominal air sacs, or caudal thoracic air sacs can contribute to subcutaneous air accumulation when ruptured. Affected birds show emphysematous enlargement of various body parts depending on which air sac is leaking. The infraorbital sinus has a very large cervicocephalic diverticulum in psittacine birds that can lead to air leakage around the neck. The cervicocephalic diverticulum is not strictly an air sac, but its rupture is commonly referred to as air sac rupture and will be included under that general term in this chapter for the sake of simplicity, as management is similar.

### PATHOPHYSIOLOGY
This condition occurs when the air sac lining is disrupted secondary to a traumatic event, allowing air to accumulate under the skin. While the location of the rupture can be identified in rare cases, it is generally not identifiable. Less commonly, air sac rupture may be associated to a respiratory infectious process. The cervicocephalic diverticula appear most commonly involved, with subcutaneous emphysema affecting the head, neck and extending over the dorsum/ventrum in severe cases. The cervicocephalic diverticula do not communicate directly with the pulmonary/air sac system. They communicate with the infraorbital sinuses. No oxygen exchange occurs within the cervicocephalic diverticula.

### SYSTEMS AFFECTED
**Respiratory**: Rupture of the cervicocephalic diverticula and sometimes the abdominal/caudal thoracic air sacs.
**Skin/exocrine**: Subcutaneous emphysema leading to skin expansion over the affected area; the degree of skin tension varies with the quantity of air present in the subcutaneous space.
**Musculoskeletal**: Air accumulation under the skin may restrict body movement.

### GENETICS
None.

### INCIDENCE/PREVALENCE
Unknown, but relatively common.

### GEOGRAPHIC DISTRIBUTION
N/A

### SIGNALMENT
No specific species, age or sex predilection. Commonly reported in Amazon parrots, macaws, and cockatiels.

## SIGNS

### General Comments
Rupture of an air sac is not life-threatening in most cases. However, fatalities may occur. Subcutaneous emphysema causes discomfort to the avian patient and likely affects the bird's quality of life.

### Historical Findings
Traumatic event reported by the owner. "Ballooning" under the skin of various body parts, most often affecting the head, neck, ventrum, and dorsum.

### Physical Examination Findings
Subcutaneous emphysema is seen in large species; the accumulation of air is most often confined to the dorsal aspect of the neck, whereas generalized subcutaneous emphysema may be seen more commonly in small species.

## CAUSES
**Traumatic**: Air sacs generally rupture secondary to a traumatic event. Fractures of pneumatized bones may cause or contribute to the emphysema.
**Infectious**: Chronic upper respiratory infection may also be involved. A pathologic process in the vicinity of the narrow connecting passage between the infraorbital sinus and the cervicocephalic diverticulum can act as a one-way valve, trapping air in the lumen of the diverticulum.
**Nutritional**: Nutritional deficiencies such as hypovitaminosis A may predispose birds to respiratory infection.

## RISK FACTORS
**Environmental**: Birds free-flying outside their cage present a higher risk of traumatic events, especially if the environment presents some dangers (ceiling fan, large mirror, wide unprotected windows, etc.).
**Medical conditions**: Malnutrition may predispose to upper respiratory disease.

## DIAGNOSIS

### DIFFERENTIAL DIAGNOSIS
• Fracture of a pneumatized bone.
• Luxation or subluxation of the humeroscapular joint causing disruption of the clavicular air sac.
• Distension of the cervicocephalic diverticula without rupture. With upper respiratory disease involving the infraorbital sinuses, air may become entrapped within the cervicocephalic diverticula leading to their distension.
• Infection with gas-producing bacteria.

### CBC/BIOCHEMISTRY/URINALYSIS
No specific abnormalities are seen with air sac rupture. CBC/biochemistry—indicated to rule out concurrent disease.

## OTHER LABORATORY TESTS
**Bacterial/fungal culture**: To evaluate the presence of respiratory disease. The rostral aspect of the choana may be sampled. Nasal or sinus flush may be considered to obtain a more representative sample of the upper respiratory tract microbial flora. Skin culture if subcutaneous infection is suspected.
**Chlamydia testing**: May be considered if respiratory signs are present.
**Aspergillus testing**: May be considered if respiratory signs are present.

## IMAGING
Whole body radiographs to identify respiratory or musculoskeletal abnormalities. CT examination to assess the respiratory system for disease processes or musculoskeletal abnormalities. Location of rupture may be identified on CT. Endoscopic examination of the air distention may also help localize the rupture.

## DIAGNOSTIC PROCEDURES
No additional diagnostic procedures are indicated.

## PATHOLOGIC FINDINGS
Air sac distention with concurrent signs of inflammation.

## TREATMENT

### APPROPRIATE HEALTH CARE
**Outpatient medical management**: Patient otherwise normal; diagnostic approach may require brief hospitalization.
**Inpatient medical management**: Patient presenting with severe subcutaneous emphysema with depression/lethargy or concurrent disease that requires close monitoring.
**Surgical management**: If relapse occurs following air aspiration.

### NURSING CARE
**Air aspiration**: Air can easily be removed using a syringe and hypodermic needle to decrease skin tension. However, the space often quickly refills as the patient breathes since the breach within the respiratory system is still patent. The procedure may be repeated multiple times. This technique may be used initially, especially if severe emphysema is present to decrease skin tension and improve patient's comfort. Elizabethan collar may be considered if a Teflon® (McAllister Technical Services, Coeur d'Alene, ID) dermal stent is used in an area that the bird can reach with its beak.

## ACTIVITY
Exercise may exacerbate the subcutaneous emphysema. Activity level recommendations should be adjusted to each individual avian patient.

## DIET
Suboptimal diets should be improved.

## CLIENT EDUCATION
Spontaneous resolution is possible but the problem may be chronic and recurrent.

## SURGICAL CONSIDERATIONS
**Fistula**: Using a 2–6 mm skin biopsy punch or a scapel blade, a piece of skin is removed over the inflated area and the wound is left to heal by second intention. This opening will allow the skin to lie against the traumatized tissue and allow the rupture site to heal properly. In many cases, there is no reinflation of the subcutaneous space by the time the skin wound has healed.
**Teflon dermal stent**: Non-absorbable sutures are preplaced in the four pairs of holes found around the stent. Then, a skin incision is performed over the distended skin ideally in an area that the bird is unable to reach with its beak. The bird's skin will deflate once the skin is incised and skin tension will decrease. The incision size should be just large enough to insert the stent into the subcutaneous space. A hypodermic needle is used to retrieve the sutures through the skin and tie the stent in place. The four sutures should be placed two on each side of the incision and two at both ends of the incision. A purse-string suture may be placed around the rim of the stent that remains above the skin. The stent is generally left in place permanently.
**Cervicocephalic–clavicular air sac shunt**: Possible when one of these two air sacs is ruptured. A skin incision is performed in the left lateral thoracic inlet area to avoid the esophagus. A small endotracheal tube is inserted in the hyperinflated air sac. The tube is then directed caudally along the esophagus to the cranial aspect of the clavicular air sac. The tube is sutured to the longus coli muscle to prevent migration before skin closure. The shunt is generally left in place permanently.
**Closure of the rupture**: In the rare cases where the location of the rupture can be identified, it can be closed with cruciate or interrupted sutures. The rupture is typically large and the diverticulum/air sac lining very thin.

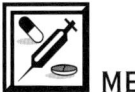 MEDICATIONS

## DRUG(S) OF CHOICE
Consider broad-spectrum antibiotic perioperatively and until cleaning of the stent is minimal postoperatively.

NSAIDs (meloxicam 0.5–1.0 mg/kg PO/SQ q12–24h in most species) may be considered to alleviate inflammation at the surgical site. Opioids (butorphanol 1–4 mg/kg q2–4h) is recommended perioperatively.

## CONTRAINDICATIONS
None.

## PRECAUTIONS
None.

## POSSIBLE INTERACTIONS
N/A

## ALTERNATIVE DRUGS
Consider doxycycline hyclate to attempt pleurodesis. Air sac lining of birds is similar to the pleural lining of mammals. Medication instilled in the air sac will cause irritation between the air sac surfaces, closing off the space between them and preventing further air from accumulating. This procedure may be considered for cervicocephalic diverticulum rupture only to avoid dissemination of the instilled product to the lower respiratory system. Pleurodesis has been described in one Amazon parrot. A study in chickens showed that doxycycline hyclate was superior to 1% polidocanol and absolute ethanol to induce cutaneous and subcutaneous fibrosis.

 FOLLOW-UP

## PATIENT MONITORING
**Aspiration**: Recurrence of emphysema indicates the rupture site is not healed. The procedure may be repeated or surgical approach may be considered.
**Fistula**: Recurrence of emphysema indicates the rupture site is not healed. Depending on the location, placement of a dermal stent or cervicocephalic–clavicular air sac shunt may be considered.
**Teflon dermal stent**: Postoperative care requires cleaning of the stent opening to prevent obstruction by debris and tissue fluids. Sterile swabs or needles are recommended to decrease bacterial contamination. Initially, cleaning twice daily is recommended. The cleaning frequency should be adjusted to each patient and decrease progressively. Recurrence of emphysema indicates that the stent is no longer patent.
**Cervicocephalic–clavicular air sac shunt**: Recurrence of emphysema may indicate that the shunt is no longer patent and surgical exploration is indicated.

## PREVENTION/AVOIDANCE
**Environment**: Ensure that the bird's environment is safe to decrease the likelihood of trauma.

## POSSIBLE COMPLICATIONS
**Teflon dermal stent**: Occlusion of the stent opening by debris and tissue fluids is common initially. On rare occasions, bird may pick at the stent.
**Cervicocephalic–clavicular air sac shunt**: Occlusion of the shunt. Unable to achieve complete resolution of the emphysema despite all therapeutic measures.

## EXPECTED COURSE AND PROGNOSIS
**Aspiration**: If performed rapidly following the traumatic event, chances that the air will continue to accumulate in the subcutaneous space may be decreased. This technique is expected to provide only a temporary relief in chronic cases of air sac rupture.
**Fistula**: If performed rapidly following the traumatic event, chances that the air will continue to accumulate in the subcutaneous space are decreased. This technique is expected to provide only a temporary relief in chronic cases of air sac rupture.
**Teflon dermal stent**: Complete resolution of the subcutaneous emphysema in most birds, partial resolution of the subcutaneous emphysema in some birds; minimally invasive procedure associated with a good prognosis.
**Cervicocephalic–clavicular air sac shunt**: Complete resolution of the subcutaneous emphysema in most birds based on scant literature; moderately invasive procedure associated with a good prognosis.

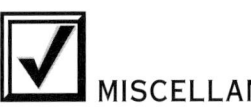 MISCELLANEOUS

## ASSOCIATED CONDITIONS
None.

## AGE-RELATED FACTORS
None.

## ZOONOTIC POTENTIAL
None.

## FERTILITY/BREEDING
Avoid teratogenic antibiotics in laying hens.

## SYNONYMS
N/A

## SEE ALSO
Fractures
Luxations
Respiratory Distress
Rhinitis and Sinusitis
Tracheal Disease and Syringeal Disease
Trauma
Wounds (Including Bite Wounds, Predator Attacks)

## ABBREVIATIONS
CT—computed tomography
NSAIDs—non-steroidal anti-inflammatory drugs

## INTERNET RESOURCES
N/A

*Suggested Reading*

Antinoff, N. (2008). Attempted pleurodesis for an air sac rupture in an Amazon parrot. Proceedings of the Association of Avian Veterinarians Annual Conference, August 11–14, Savannah, GA, p. 437.

Browing G.R., Eshar D., Tucker-Mohl K. (2019). Diagnosis and surgical repair of a chronic ruptured cervical air sac in a double yellow-headed Amazon parrot (*Amazona Ochrocephala Oratrix*). *Journal of Exotic Pet Medicine*, 29:45–50.

Harris, J.M. (1991). Teflon dermal stent for the correction of subcutaneous emphysema. Proceedings of the Association of Avian Veterinarians Annual Conference, September 23–28, Chicago, IL, pp. 20–21.

Levine, B.S. (2005). Cervicocephalic–clavicular air sac shunts to correct cervicocephalic–clavicular air sac emphysema. Proceedings of the Association of Avian Veterinarians Annual Conference, August 9–11, Monterey, CA, pp. 59–60.

Petevinos, H. (2006). A method for resolving subcutaneous emphysema in a griffon vulture chick (*Gyps fulvus*). *Journal of Exotic Pet Medicine*, 15:132–137. https://doi.org/10.1053/j.jepm.2006.02.009

Scagnelli, A.M. (2021). Effects of doxycycline hyclate, one percent polidocanol, and absolute ethanol on the cutaneous and subcutaneous tissues of chicken (*Gallus gallus domesticus*) and the potential implications in treating cervicocephalic diverticula rupture. *Journal of Zoo and Wildlife Medicine*, 52:117–125. https://doi.org/10.1638/2020-0098

**Author:** Isabelle Langlois, DVM, DABVP (Avian Practice)

BASICS

## DEFINITION
Harmful algal blooms (HABs) produce phycotoxins linked to mass mortalities in fish, birds, and other wildlife. These biotoxins are poisons that are produced by certain kinds of microscopic algae (a type of phytoplankton) that are naturally present in both marine and fresh waters, normally in amounts too small to be harmful. However, a combination of warm temperatures, sunlight, and nutrient-rich waters can cause rapid plankton reproduction, or "blooms." These blooms are commonly referred to as harmful algal blooms or "HABs" because of their potential to cause illness. These blooms may or may not discolor the water.

## PATHOPHYSIOLOGY
Common algal toxins affecting birds include domoic acid (DA), cyanotoxins (especially saxitoxin and microcystin), and brevetoxins. Birds exhibit a range of sensitivities to algal toxins, with pathophysiology and symptoms varying depending upon species of bird, age, the algal toxin, and route of exposure (ingestion, dermal, or inhalation).

## SYSTEMS AFFECTED
Brevetoxins, saxitoxins, and DA are all neurotoxins. Affected systems may potentially include:
• **Respiratory**: Direct inhalant exposure to aerosolized toxin, as well as blocking the passage of nerve impulses and leading to death via respiratory paralysis.
• **Nervous**: Neurotoxin that activates voltage-sensitive sodium channels in nerve cells.
• **Cardiovascular**: Secondary to neurotoxic effect.
• **Ocular**: Inflammation, irritation, as well as effect on innervation.
• **Gastrointestinal**: Ileus secondary to neurotoxic effects on GI innervation.

## GENETICS
N/A

## INCIDENCE/PREVALENCE
Regional and species specific for the different toxins described. Toxic thresholds for all HAB toxins that may affect seabirds are not currently known. DA was found in 70% and saxitoxin was found in 23% of all tested samples in one study in birds. Overall, in the past few decades, the numbers of microalgal species in marine and freshwater environments that are known to produce phycotoxins, and thus HABs, have increased.

## GEOGRAPHIC DISTRIBUTION
Several decades ago, relatively few countries appeared to be affected by HABs, but now most countries are threatened (especially coastal ones), in many cases over large geographic areas and by more than one harmful algal species. Approximately 80 toxic marine and 55 toxic freshwater species belonging to 10 classes of microalgae have been recognized worldwide. Toxic blooms of *Karenia brevis* found worldwide, but occur most frequently in Gulf of Mexico, and occasionally on the Southeast coast of the United States, where it is known as Florida red tide. Saxitoxins are found worldwide in both marine and freshwater blooms.

## SIGNALMENT
No sex predilections have been described. Affected animals are often juveniles (first year birds). It is possible that older birds have learned avoidance of intoxicated prey items and will change their foraging behavior in response to a bloom. Most HAB events affect piscivorous species.

## SIGNS
### Historical Findings
Harmful algal blooms documented in area. Fish kills or other marine wildlife morbidity and mortality. Occurrence of cases is not always correlative with documented HAB alerts in the area. Algal blooms may occur in another area that is not being monitored, birds may pick the toxins up along their migratory route, or blooms may occur offshore where there is no monitoring. Additionally, a bloom may have occurred several weeks earlier, and shellfish may harbor these toxins for weeks to months before the birds ingest them and are finally exposed.

### Physical Examination Findings
• Clinical signs vary depending on the species, the toxin, and route of exposure and may include ataxia, depression, muscle tremors, rear limb weakness or paresis, cloacal atony, nystagmus, opisthotonos, torticollis, dyspnea, tachypnea, coughing, vomiting, diarrhea, melena, hematochezia, bradycardia, loss of the palpebral reflex, and subsequent conjunctivitis and/or corneal ulcers.
• Clinical signs are not correlative with the level of toxin, but generally occur rapidly after ingestion. In one documented occurrence, a red tide caused by a bloom of non-toxic dinoflagellate *Akashiwo sanguinea* still caused debilitation and even death in a variety of seabirds by producing a surfactant that impaired waterproofing of plumage.
• In birds, DA primarily attacks the brain, causing lethargy, disorientation, fine motor tremors, opisthotonos, seizures, scratching (pelicans will scratch their pouch), vomiting, and death. Behavior may remain altered in affected birds for up to 2 weeks, according to one report.

## CAUSES
HABs are most commonly caused by diatoms and dinoflagellates, which are two kinds of phytoplankton (single-celled organisms). Birds are exposed to HAB toxins through biomagnification of toxins up the food chain, swimming in or drinking affected waters, or breathing in aerosolized droplets. Brevetoxins are produced primarily by marine dinoflagellates belonging to the genus *Karenia*. Brevetoxins are a group of more than 10 lipid-soluble neurotoxins that activate sodium ion channels, causing nerve membrane depolarization. DA is an excitatory amino acid analogue of glutamate, a neurotransmitter in the brain that activates glutamate receptors. It is thought to damage neurons by causing a rapid influx of calcium, which causes brain cells to degenerate. Saxitoxin is produced by marine dinoflagellates as well as freshwater cyanobacteria. The toxin causes blockage of neuronal sodium channels which produces a flaccid paralysis. Death often occurs from respiratory failure.

## RISK FACTORS
Seabirds affected by DA commonly include pelicans, murres, loons, grebes, cormorants, and shearwaters. Species commonly affected with brevetoxicosis include double-crested cormorants, brown pelicans, herons, common loons, and a variety of gulls, terns, and shorebirds.

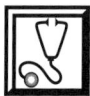 DIAGNOSIS

## DIFFERENTIAL DIAGNOSIS
• Respiratory compromise caused by trauma, bacterial (botulism), fungal or viral infections (especially West Nile virus, highly pathogenic avian influenza, Newcastle disease virus), neoplasia, or ascites.
• Primary heart disease, artherosclerosis causing left heart failure, congenital heart disease.
• Ataxia and weakness secondary to other neurologic disease (see neurologic conditions), metabolic derangements, or systemic disease.

## CBC/BIOCHEMISTRY/URINALYSIS
May be anemic or hypoproteinemic. Biochemistry profile varied based on toxin and systems affected. Serum blood urea nitrogen, uric acid, and creatinine. Point of care blood gas analysis (e.g. iSTAT®, Abbot Point of Care Inc., Princeton, NJ) to determine acid–base status, oxygen saturation, and electrolytes may be indicated.

## OTHER LABORATORY TESTS
N/A

## IMAGING
N/A

## DIAGNOSTIC PROCEDURES
Current laboratory diagnostic methods for HAB intoxication are challenging as the toxin is often eliminated from affected animal's system within 48 hours, depending on the toxin (especially DA, which is highly water soluble), amount ingested, and species of bird. Brevetoxin can be assayed by using a mouse bioassay, ELISA, or antibody radioimmunoassay on tissue, fecal or GI contents, plasma or serum samples.

## PATHOLOGIC FINDINGS
Many birds have no significant pathologic findings at necropsy. Variable but may include: gastrointestinal ulcers, melena, and pulmonary edema,

 ## TREATMENT

### APPROPRIATE HEALTH CARE
Toxins are processed by the liver and excreted by the kidneys and in bile. Treatment often includes parenteral fluids, nutritional support, antimicrobials, anti-ulcer medications, antiparasitic medications, blood or plasma transfusions, B-vitamin and iron supplementation, ocular medications (in patients unable to blink or with corneal ulcers), manual evacuation of cloacal contents as required. For fat-soluble toxins, such as brevetoxins, ILE therapy. Clearance of the toxin in birds typically takes 1–7 days.

### NURSING CARE
Oxygen therapy—40% $O_2$ at a flow rate of 3 L/minute. Fluid therapy to maintain hydration or correct dehydration. Thermal support as indicated.

### ACTIVITY
No restrictions.

### DIET
Ingluvial gavage or assisted alimentation for anorectic patients.

### CLIENT EDUCATION
N/A

### SURGICAL CONSIDERATIONS
N/A

 ## MEDICATIONS

### DRUG(S) OF CHOICE
Anticonvulsants: Midazolam 0.5–1.0 mg/kg IM. Anxiolytics: Diazepam (0.5–2.0 mg/kg PO q12h). Iron dextran 10 mg/kg IM once, repeat if

necessary. Antimicrobial eye ointment if loss of palpebral reflex or corneal ulcers + dexamethasone if no ulcers but conjunctivitis. Antibiotics often include metronidazole (25 mg/kg PO q12h) and enrofloxacin (10–20 mg/kg PO q12–24h). NSAIDs are generally contraindicated. Antiulcer medications—omeprazole (20 mg/kg PO q24h) with sucralfate (25 mg/kg PO q8h) if ulcers already present.

### CONTRAINDICATIONS
N/A

### PRECAUTIONS
Consider concurrent use of antifungals as many seabirds susceptible to aspergillosis.

### POSSIBLE INTERACTIONS
N/A

### ALTERNATIVE DRUGS
ILE therapy for brevetoxicosis: initial bolus – 2 ml/kg over 15 minutes; if no problems, start CRI – 15 ml/kg over 1 hour. Obtain PCV/TS 3–4 hours post ILE look for lipemia. If lipemia noted, wait 2 hours and recheck. If no lipemia, can repeat up to 3×, q4–6h. Rapid efficacy for lipid soluble toxins (brevetoxins) but no efficacy for water-soluble toxins (DA, saxitoxin).

 ## FOLLOW-UP

### PATIENT MONITORING
CBC as indicated to monitor for anemia and hypoproteinemia (useful as a prognostic indicator).

### PREVENTION/AVOIDANCE
Hazing birds away from smaller bodies of water affected by blue-green algae may be a viable strategy.

### POSSIBLE COMPLICATIONS
Gastrointestinal ulcers, anemia, septicemia, hypoproteinemia and hypoalbuminemia, liver failure, renal failure, death.

### EXPECTED COURSE AND PROGNOSIS
In the case of exposure to HAB toxins, many wild birds will drown or be predated. Cormorants treated with ILE for brevetoxicosis had a survival rate of over 85% in one study.

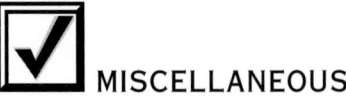 ## MISCELLANEOUS

### ASSOCIATED CONDITIONS
N/A

### AGE-RELATED FACTORS
Juvenile birds appear to be more frequently affected.

### ZOONOTIC POTENTIAL
None.

### FERTILITY/BREEDING
N/A

### SYNONYMS
N/A

### SEE ALSO
Toxicosis (Environmental/Pesticides)

### ABBREVIATIONS
CBC—complete blood count
DA—domoic acid
ELISA—enzyme-linked immunosorbent assay
GI—gastrointestinal
HABs—harmful algal blooms
ILE—intravenous lipid emulsion
PCV—packed cell volume
TS—total solids

### INTERNET RESOURCES
N/A

*Suggested Reading*
Atwood, K.E. (2008). Brevetoxin body burdens in seabirds of Southwest Florida. Graduate school theses and dissertations. Master thesis. University of South Florida. http://scholarcommons.usf.edu/etd/124.
Barron, H.W., Bartleson, R.D., McKinnis, K.B., et al. (2013). Hematologic and biochemical parameters in seabirds with brevetoxicosis. 7th Symposium on Harmful Algae in the US, Sarasota, FL (27–31 October). p. 33.
Bast, R.L., Barron, H.W., Ingraham, H., et al. (2013). Brevetoxicosis in seabirds and sea turtles of southern Florida. Proceedings of the Association of of Avian Vets Annual Conference; p. 361.
Brand, L.E., Compton, A. Long-term increase in *Karenia brevis* abundance along the Southwest Florida Coast. *Harmful Algae*, 2007;6:232–252.
Kreuder, C., Mazet, J.A.K., Bossart, G.D., et al. (2002). Clinicopathologic features of suspected brevetoxicosis in double-crested cormorants (*Phalacrocorax auritus*) along the Florida Gulf coast. *Journal of Zoo and Wildlife Medicine*, 33:8–15.
**Author:** Heather W. Barron, DVM, DABVP (Avian), CertAqV

# BASICS

## DEFINITION
Amyloidosis is defined as spontaneous extracellular deposition of reactive fibrillar amyloid proteins or precursor proteins in various organs, leading to tissue dysfunction. Amyloid proteins possess low solubility and are resistant to proteolytic digestion. The fibrils are rigid, non-branching, 7–10 nm in diameter, and found in varying lengths.

## PATHOPHYSIOLOGY
Pathophysiology is poorly understood. Increased concentration of hepatic acute phase serum amyloid A (SAA) combined with other factors causes increased concentrations of amyloid protein A (AA) deposits and fibrillogenesis. Deposition of amyloid proteins occurs systemically and results in functional disruption of the associated tissues. Amyloidosis has not been defined as either a primary or secondary disease; it is usually associated with concurrent medical disorders, but it is difficult to determine the timeline of disease in many cases.
Affected animals almost always have exposure to predisposing environmental factors such as stress or overcrowding.

## SYSTEMS AFFECTED
Amyloid deposits are most commonly found in the liver, spleen, kidneys, and small intestine. Joints and blood vessels are a common deposition site for affected Galliformes. The proventriculus, large intestine, heart, gonads, and endocrine organs may also be affected. Amyloid deposition in the brain (especially in flamingos), lungs, and skin is rare.

## GENETICS
A genetic cause has not been identified, although it is likely that one exists, as there are genera and species that are predisposed.

## INCIDENCE/PREVALENCE
While this is considered primarily a disorder of captivity, amyloidosis has also been reported in free-ranging wild birds.

## GEOGRAPHIC DISTRIBUTION
Worldwide.

## SIGNALMENT
Species that are prone to high stress associated with captivity are more predisposed to amyloidosis. Waterfowl have the highest reported incidences (up to 77% in one population). Amyloidosis may occur spontaneously in Pekin ducks. The disease is also particularly common in flamingos and gyrfalcons. Columbiformes and psittacines are less susceptible to amyloidosis than other species. Amyloidosis is usually diagnosed in middle-aged to older birds. There is no sex predilection.

## SIGNS

### Historical Findings
Clinical history may include an overcrowded enclosure, birds that seem particularly stressed, and one or more birds with evidence of systemic disease. Seasonal variation has been noted in Anseriformes, with peaks in winter and spring reported. Vaccination with oil-emulsified bacterins has been associated with amyloid outbreaks in some poultry flocks.

### Physical Examination Findings
Clinical signs may include chronic weight loss, pododermatitis, swelling of peripheral limbs, coelomic distention, ascites, dyspnea, polyuria, polydipsia, claudication syndrome, or sudden death. There is no specific clinical sign associated with amyloidosis, and this disease cannot be diagnosed on a physical exam. Affected birds may have other clinical diseases noted in their history or identified during diagnostic workup.

## CAUSES
- Environmental factors (stress, overcrowding, etc.) and species susceptibility appear to be the most important causes of amyloidosis.
- Chronic bacterial infections (such as cases of pododermatitis) may trigger amyloid deposition as their associated inflammation can cause persistent acute phase protein responses, thereby producing high serum concentrations of SAA.
- Viral infections do not have the same impact on acute phase proteins and are less likely to be associated with amyloidosis. However, there is a report of fowlpox associated with an amyloidosis outbreak.
- Mycobacteriosis has been associated with amyloidosis in humans and is also commonly (but not always) diagnosed in birds with amyloidosis.
- *Mycoplasma synoviae* has been identified concurrently in poultry flocks affected by amyloidosis.
- Aspergillosis and atherosclerosis are commonly found as concurrent disorders in affected birds.
- Chronic hepatitis and nephropathy of non-amyloid origin are often identified concurrently (may be age related).
- Vaccination with oil-emulsified bacterins may predispose some poultry to amyloid deposition.
- Amyloidosis can be artificially induced in laboratory settings by injecting poultry with a variety of infectious organisms and adjuvants and by administering amyloid fibrils to poultry via injection and orally.
- Amyloidosis is generally considered to be non-communicable, although there have been multiple reported "outbreaks" of amyloidosis in flocks with concurrent infectious, inflammatory, or stressful conditions.

## RISK FACTORS
Chronic stress, overcrowding, pododermatitis, other systemic diseases (mycobacteriosis, aspergillosis, atherosclerosis, chronic bacterial infections, etc.), and vaccination with oil-emulsified bacterins.

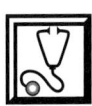

# DIAGNOSIS

## DIFFERENTIAL DIAGNOSIS
Because symptoms of amyloidosis are completely non-specific, a wide variety of differential diagnoses exist. These should include systemic infections (bacterial, viral, fungal, parasitic), organ dysfunction (hepatic, renal, cardiac), neoplasia, and nutritional deficiencies.

## CBC/BIOCHEMISTRY/URINALYSIS
Biopsy and histopathology of affected tissues is the only way to diagnose amyloidosis. This may occur premortem through endoscopic exam or exploratory coeliotomy, or postmortem at necropsy.

## OTHER LABORATORY TESTS
Other laboratory tests, bloodwork (CBC, chemistry, infectious disease testing), and microbiology testing should be performed to rule out other systemic disorders. Amyloidosis may be mistaken for atherosclerosis as AA can be deposited within blood vessels.

## IMAGING
Diagnostic imaging (radiographs, ultrasound, CT) can rule out other systemic disorders.

## DIAGNOSTIC PROCEDURES
Amyloid deposits can be detected using polarized light and display an apple-green birefringence and stains positively with Congo red.

## PATHOLOGIC FINDINGS
Affected organs may be enlarged, firm, and waxy; amyloid deposits are found in extracellular spaces. Common locations for amyloid deposits include the perisinusoidal spaces in the liver, blood vessels, basement membranes, and joint spaces.

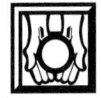

# TREATMENT

## APPROPRIATE HEALTH CARE
Effective treatment of amyloidosis in birds has not been described. Treatment of concurrent illnesses and symptomatic

management of diseases associated with amyloidosis should be implemented.

## NURSING CARE
Fluid support and nutritional support.

## ACTIVITY
N/A

## DIET
N/A

## CLIENT EDUCATION
As amyloidosis is almost always diagnosed postmortem, education should focus on prevention of the disease in other animals within the collection.

## SURGICAL CONSIDERATIONS
N/A

## MEDICATIONS

### DRUG(S) OF CHOICE
Treatment of concurrent inflammatory disease may help to slow the deposition of amyloid in tissues. In chickens with vaccine-induced amyloidosis, it has been shown that existing amyloid deposits may slowly regress in some animals if there is not a source of ongoing inflammation, which mirrors findings in human research. Colchicine and DMSO have been used to treat other species with amyloidosis, but appropriate dosage, treatment interval, and treatment duration are unknown for birds with this condition. Reported avian dosages of colchicine range from 0.01 mg/kg PO q12h to 0.2 mg/kg PO q12h, but none of these dosages are described as treatment of amyloidosis. Reported avian dosage of DMSO is 1 ml/kg applied topically to the affected area q4–7 days.

### CONTRAINDICATIONS
Colchicine is contraindicated in patients with serious renal, gastrointestinal, and/or cardiac dysfunction. Safety and efficacy is unknown in avian species. DMSO should not be administered to patients with known mast cell tumors. It should be used cautiously in animals that are dehydrated, in shock, or in renal or hepatic failure.

### PRECAUTIONS
Colchicine may potentiate gout formation. Adverse effects may include vomiting, anorexia, melena/hematochezia, paralytic ileus, renal failure, hepatoxicity, pancytopenia, paralysis, shock, and vascular collapse. DMSO can be easily absorbed through the skin and should not be handled without gloves. DMSO can degranulate mast cells and has diuretic and vasodilatory effects. It can cause hepatoxicity, renal toxicity, hemolysis, and hemoglobinuria in some species. Local effects of DMSO include discomfort at the site of administration, dry skin, and bad breath (garlic/oyster). High doses of DMSO can cause changes to ocular lens that are potentially reversible with discontinuation of the drug.

### POSSIBLE INTERACTIONS
Unknown.

### ALTERNATIVE DRUGS
Unknown.

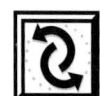

## FOLLOW-UP

### PATIENT MONITORING
Other species of animals that have previously developed amyloidosis are predisposed to aggressive amyloid deposition if another trigger occurs in the future; survivors of amyloidosis should be considered prone to recurrence of symptoms.

### PREVENTION/AVOIDANCE
Provide adequate spacing for housing, decrease stress, treat other concurrent diseases.

### POSSIBLE COMPLICATIONS
N/A

### EXPECTED COURSE AND PROGNOSIS
Death is a likely outcome for severe cases of amyloidosis.

## MISCELLANEOUS

### ASSOCIATED CONDITIONS
Chronic stress, overcrowding, pododermatitis, other systemic diseases (mycobacteriosis, aspergillosis, atherosclerosis, chronic bacterial infections, etc.), and vaccination with oil-emulsified bacterins.

### AGE-RELATED FACTORS
N/A

### ZOONOTIC POTENTIAL
N/A

### FERTILITY/BREEDING
Unknown.

### SYNONYMS
N/A

## SEE ALSO
N/A

## ABBREVIATIONS
AA—amyloid A
DMSO—dimethyl sulfoxide
SAA—serum amyloid A

## INTERNET RESOURCES
N/A

*Suggested Reading*
Hawkins, P.N., Pepys, M.B. (1990). A primed state exists in vivo following histological regression of amyloidosis. *Clinical and Experimental Immunology*, 81:325–328.
Hawkins, P.N., Richardson, S., Vigushin, D.M., et al. (1993). Serum amyloid P component scintigraphy turnover studies for diagnosis and quantitative monitoring of AA-amyloidosis in juvenile rheumatoid arthritis. *Arthritis and Rheumatism*, 36:842–851.
Ibi, K., Murakami, T., Goda, W.M., et al. (2015). Prevalence of amyloid deposition in mature healthy chickens in the flock that previously had outbreaks of vaccine-associated amyloidosis. *Journal of Veterinary Medical Science*, 77:1241–1245.
Jansson, D.S., Bröjer, C., Neimanis, A., et al. (2018). Post mortem findings and their relation to AA amyloidosis in free-ranging Herring gulls (*Larus argentatus*). *PLOS One*, 13: e.0193265.
Landman, W.J., Gruys, E., Gielkens, A.L. (1998). Avian amyloidosis. *Avian Pathology*, 27:437–449.
Landman, W.J.M., Feberwee, A. (2001). Field studies on the association between amyloid arthropathy and Mycoplasma synoviae infection, and experimental reproduction of the condition in brown layers, *Avian Pathology*, 30:629–639.
Murakami, T., Muhammad, Y.I., Yanai, T., et al. (2013). Experimental induction and oral transmission of avian AA amyloidosis in vaccinated white hens. *Amyloid*, 20:80–85.
Nakamura, K., Waseda, K., Yamamoto, Y., et al. (2006). Pathology of cutaneous fowlpox with amyloidosis in layer hens inoculated with fowlpox vaccine. *Avian Diseases*, 50:152–156.
Ono, A., Nakayama, Y., Inoue, M., Yanai, T., et al. (2020). AA Amyloid deposition in the central and peripheral nervous systems in flamingos. *Veterinary Pathology*, 57(5):700–705.
Sato, A., Koga, T., Inoue, M., Goto, N. (1981). Pathological observations of amyloidosis in swans and other Anatidae. *Japanese Journal of Veterinary Science*. 43:509–519.

**Author**: Alicia McLaughlin, DVM, CertAqVet

# BASICS

## DEFINITION
Anemia is defined as an abnormally low number of red blood cells (low PCV, hematocrit and/or red blood cell count) or low hemoglobin concentration, resulting in dimished oxygen-carrying capacity of the blood.

## PATHOPHYSIOLOGY
Anemia can be divided into four broad categories based on the mechanism, although multiple mechanisms may be occurring concurrently. Listed here are the top causes of anemia in birds.

**Decreased production of erythrocytes**: This occurs when erythropoiesis is absent or impaired. This can be due to disease of hematopoietic organs (e.g. bone marrow) or there is interference with normal hematopoiesis: Anemia of chronic disease; iron deficiency; metal toxicity (eg: lead, zinc); hemic neoplasia (e.g. acute leukemia, bone marrow invasion by lymphoma); viral diseases (e.g. circoviruses including PBFD and infectious chicken anemia, cobalamin deficiency, kidney disease).

**Any mechanism that shortens the lifespan of the erythrocytes**: This includes any mechanism which shortens the lifespan of the erythrocytes and includes predominantly hemolytic anemias, whether intravascular or extravascular: Hemoparasites (e.g. *Plasmodium*); heavy metal toxicity (lead, zinc, copper); ingestion or exposure to petroleum products (e.g. oiled birds) causing oxidative damage; anemia of chronic disease (shortened lifespan); immune-mediate hemolytic anemia (rare).

**Blood loss, which may be chronic or acute**: Trauma; blood feather; coagulopathy (e.g. rodenticide poisoning); neoplasia (e.g. ulcerated and/or bleeding tumor); heavy load of GI parasites or ectoparasites; GI ulceration and bleeding; spurious results; excessive preheparinizing of syringe for volume of blood collected; improper mixing of tube (e.g. settling of erythrocytes to bottom or tube); hemolysis (e.g. freezing, excessive heat, shaking).

Evaluating the body's response to anemia can help to identify the cause. This is done by counting the number of immature erythrocytes either on a regular bloodsmear (polychromatophils) or through staining with NMB (reticulocytes). Anemia is either regenerative (increased number of reticulocytes) or non-regenerative (no or low (normal) numbers of reticulocytes) anemia. Anemia caused by decreased production of erythrocytes is typically non-regenerative or poorly regenerative, whereas anemia caused by increased destruction or loss is typically regenerative, except in the first 1–2 days, during which regeneration may be occurring in the hematopoietic organs but not yet visible in blood. Regardless of the mechanism for the anemia, not enough functioning erythrocytes are produced. Without enough competent, hemoglobin-rich cells, the tissues of the avian body lack sufficient oxygen to properly carry out necessary functions leading to an overall weakness and lethargy of the patient. Depending on the chronicity and severity of the anemia, the lack of oxygen to tissues can lead to eventual organ failure and death of the patient.

## SYSTEMS AFFECTED
**Behavioral**: Anemia may not change the behavior, per se, of the patient, but if the patient is weakened from anemia, the typical behaviors of the pet may be dampened or non-existent due to lack of energy.

**Cardiovascular**: Chronic anemia can lead to increased cardiac output, increased blood flow, and cardiac murmurs. Acute blood loss may lead to hypotension and shock.

**Hepatobiliary**: The liver and/or spleen may enlarge in cases of hemic neoplasia and hemolytic anemia.

**Musculoskeletal**: Skeletal tissue may appear pale due to decreased erythrocyte population. Weakness may also be present.

**Ophthalmic**: Conjunctiva will appear pale with anemia. Intraocular hemorrhage can occur with coagulopathies.

**Renal/urologic**: The color of urine/urates can change if there is blood present (red), increased hemoglobin (red), or increased increased biliverdin (green) from hemolysis.

**Reproductive**: Breeding hens may have a disruption in breeding cycle if anemia is present.

**Respiratory**: Respiratory rate and depth may be increased significantly.

**Skin**: The skin and mucous membranes can take on a very pale appearance with severe anemia. Hematomas or petecchiation may be visible with coagulopathies.

## GENETICS
N/A

## INCIDENCE/PREVALENCE
Anemia is common in birds, with anemia of chronic disease (inflammation) being most common, and other causes such as trauma, metal poisoning, and parasites being variably common depending on the species.

## GEOGRAPHIC DISTRIBUTION
Anemia can occur anywhere geographically.

## SIGNALMENT
Birds of all species, ages, and sex can become anemic.

## SIGNS

### Historical Findings
If anemia is due to blood loss, owners may report trauma and blood loss due to trauma. If there is hemolytic anemia, owners may report darkened urine and urates in the droppings. Although unusual, frank blood or melena can be seen in the fecal portion of the droppings, or there may be frank blood not associated with the droppings but seen emanating from the cloaca, as could be the case with ulcerated lesions associated with cloacal papilloma disease.

### Physical Examination Findings
Lethargy. Pale mucous membranes. Increased respiratory rate and effort. Color change or blood in plasma, feces, urine/urates. Evidence of trauma and subsequent blood loss. Petechia and ecchymosis. Evidence of GI parasites or ectoparasites. Cardiac murmur, low ulnar refilling time.

## CAUSES
Most of the causes of anemias are listed above are self-explanatory, but additional details on some specific causes of anemia are presented here.

**Heavy metal toxicosis**: Lead poisoning often occurs secondary to direct ingestion, including ingestion of spent ammunition in food, lead paint, or costume jewelry, or secondary to being shot with lead ammunition. Zinc can be found in the metal of cages and aviaries, and metal parts of many objects, including bird toys.

**Iron deficiency**: Most often due to chronic blood loss.

**Hemoparasites**: The most common hemoparasites include *Leukocytozoon*, *Hemoproteus* and *Plasmodium* and they are vector borne. *Plasmodium* is most likely to cause clinical disease but this is species specific, with penguins being exquisitely sensitive. *Leukocytozoon* and *Hemoproteus* are often subclinical diseases, but can be problematic in some species or with a heavy parasite load.

**Chronic disease**: Common chronic diseases causing significant inflammation include chlamydiosis, aspergillosis, mycobacteriosis, egg yolk coelomitis, and neoplasia.

## RISK FACTORS
Risk factors are highly variable and depend on species, sex, age, housing, diet etc.

# DIAGNOSIS

## DIFFERENTIAL DIAGNOSIS
Trauma, heavy metal ingestion, reproductive disease, neoplasia, masses or organomegaly from neoplasia, or infectious diseases.

## CBC/BIOCHEMISTRY/URINALYSIS

At the minimum, a PCV or hemoglobin concentration must be found to be low for a diagnosis of anemia. A CBC is recommended, as it may provide erythrocyte indices that could provide additional information about the erythrocytes (e.g. hypochromasia, microcytosis), but also about other cell lines that could indicate inflammation (leukocytosis, left shift, toxic changes), hemic neoplasia (atypical cells in circulation), or evidence of bone marrow disease (multiple cytopenias). The number of polychromatophils may help in assessing the presence of regeneration. A review of blood smear morphology is also recommended as it may identify abnormal erythrocyte morphology (metal toxicity), evidence of oxidative damage (oiling etc.), hemoparasites, agglutination and so on. A biochemistry profile can provide information about other organs (renal failure, liver disease, evidence of reproductive activity). While full urinalysis is often not done in birds (due to contamination, post renal modifications etc.), gross evaluation may identify a color change. Urinary dipstick testing may also identify blood. Fecal evaluation, including gross evaluation for frank blood, melena and parasites, is recommended. In addition, a wet mount in clinic to identify flagellates and evaluation for parasites is recommended.

## OTHER LABORATORY TESTS

Staining the blood with NMB allows for counting of reticulocytes, which are equivalent to the polychromatophils seen with the regular stains use for bloodsmears (Diff-Quik™, Wright–Giemsa), as for other species, but generally considered easier to identify and count, with lesser subjectivity. Unlike in mammals, many bird erythrocytes will have visible dark structures in their cytoplasm. The cells in which they form a ring around 50% or more of the periphery of the nucleus are counted as reticulocytes. Unfortunately, reference intervals for reticulocytes are generally not available for most bird species and submitting a healthy bird of the same species for comparison may be considered. Heavy metals can be measured in blood, with > 0.5 ppm considered diagnostic for lead toxicosis (> 0.2 ppm also consistent if accompanied by clinical signs), and > 2 ppm considered diagnostic for zinc toxicosis. Occult blood testing on feces may be indicated if a gastrointestinal cause for the bleeding is suspected. Bone marrow evaluation may be indicated in cases of chronic non-regenerative anemia (± other cytopenias) and in patients with large atypical cells in circulation. Bone marrow may be collected from the tibiotarsus and directly smeared on a slide.

## IMAGING

Whole-body radiographs or CT may be necessary, depending on the differential diagnoses.

## DIAGNOSTIC PROCEDURES

Additional diagnostics may be necessary, depending on the list of differentials after initial physical examination and baseline tests.

## PATHOLOGIC FINDINGS

Depends on the cause of the anemia.

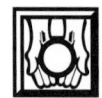

# TREATMENT

## APPROPRIATE HEALTH CARE

Management will depend on the cause of the anemia and includes treating parasites, infectious diseases, nutritional deficiencies, or neoplasia. The patient may also need supportive care including fluid therapy with crystalloids or a transfusion with whole blood from a member of the same species. Heterologous transfusion (from different species of birds) is generally poorly effective, as the lifespan of transfused red blood cells may be very short (hours). However, heterologous transfusions from birds of the same genus may be tried. Hypovolemic shock caused by acute trauma and hemorrhage can be treated with regular fluid resuscitation unless the PCV is extremely low, in which case, a transfusion is required during resuscitation treatment. Assisted feedings may be necessary. In severe cases, activity should be limited until oxygen carrying capacity is restored to normal.

## NURSING CARE

See Appropriate Health Care section.

## ACTIVITY

N/A

## DIET

N/A

## CLIENT EDUCATION

N/A

## SURGICAL CONSIDERATIONS

If anemia is due to heavy metal ingestion, in some cases surgical or endoscopic retrieval of the metal objects can be performed. Some cases of trauma, especially those causing internal bleeding, may require surgical intervention.

# MEDICATIONS

## DRUG(S) OF CHOICE

**Heavy metal toxicity**: Calcium edetate disodium 30–35 mg/kg, SC or IM, q12h for 3–5 days (or until asymptomatic), followed by oral treatment with dimercaptosuccinic acid 25–35 mg/kg, orally, q12h.
**Iron deficiency**: Iron dextran 10 mg/kg IM once, repeat if necessary. For treatment of parasites and other infectious diseases, see appropriate chapters.

## CONTRAINDICATIONS

Iron supplementation in species prone to iron storage disease (e.g. mynahs, toucans).

## PRECAUTIONS

N/A

## POSSIBLE INTERACTIONS

N/A

## ALTERNATIVE DRUGS

N/A

# FOLLOW-UP

## PATIENT MONITORING

PCV should be closely monitored and can be checked on a daily basis during the acute phase of treatment. The entire CBC should be evaluated on a regular basis until the patient is stable.

## PREVENTION/AVOIDANCE

Depends on the cause of anemia.

## POSSIBLE COMPLICATIONS

Severe anemia can lead to death.

## EXPECTED COURSE AND PROGNOSIS

Depends on the cause of the anemia.

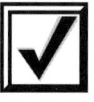

# MISCELLANEOUS

## ASSOCIATED CONDITIONS

N/A

## AGE-RELATED FACTORS

Young chicks and geriatric birds will be more susceptible to the severe complications of anemia than healthy adult birds.

## ZOONOTIC POTENTIAL

Depends on the cause of anemia.

## FERTILITY/BREEDING

Anemia can disrupt egg production.

## SYNONYMS

N/A

## SEE ALSO

Circovirus (Psittacines)
Coagulopathies and Coagulation
Hemoparasites
Hemorrhage
Hypotension and Hypovolemia
Liver Disease
Nutritional Imbalances
Oil Exposure
Polyomavirus

**(CONTINUED)**

Renal Diseases
Sick-Bird Syndrome
Toxicosis (Anticoagulant Rodenticide)
Toxicosis (Heavy Metals)
Trauma
Urate and Fecal Discoloration
Appendix 8, Algorithm 7: Anemia

## ABBREVIATIONS
CBC—complete blood count
GI—gastrointestinal

NMB—new methylene blue
PBFD—psittacine beak and feather disease
PCV—packed cell volume

## INTERNET RESOURCES
Cornell University College of Veterinary
Medicine. eClinPath: https://eclinpath.com

*Suggested Reading*
Brooks, M.B., Harr, K.E., Seelig, D.M.,
  Wardrop, K.J., Weiss D.J. (2022).
*Schalm's Veterinary Hematology*, 7th edn.
  Hoboken, NJ: Wiley.
Campbell, T., Grant, K. (2022). *Exotic
  Animal Hematology and Cytology*, 5th edn.
  Hoboken, NJ: Wiley.
Pendl H., Samour, J. (2016). *Avian Medicine,
  Hematology Analyses*. St. Louis, MO:
  Elsevier.
**Author**: Melanie Ammersbach, DVM,
DACVP (Clin Path)

**A** | ANGEL WING

 BASICS

## DEFINITION
Angel wing is a commonly used term to describe the condition of carpal valgus in avian patients resulting from malnutrition and captive mismanagement.

## PATHOPHYSIOLOGY
Angel wing is the result of the plumage developing at a faster rate than the musculoskeletal structures of the wing. The immature musculoskeletal structures of the wing are not strong enough to support the weight of the blood-filled quills of the rapidly developing plumage. The weight of the developing feathers increasingly pulls the wing into a deformed position.

## SYSTEMS AFFECTED
Musculoskeletal
Integument

## GENETICS
There is information to suggest a genetic predisposition to angel wing in certain lines of birds. In a study of white Roman geese, angel wing severity was worse in certain lines of birds regardless of diet.

## INCIDENCE/PREVALENCE
Angel wing is typically a disorder of birds under managed care being fed artificial diets (including wild water fowl in parks that receive significant amounts of bread from well-meaning bird lovers). Incidence is rare in well-managed captive animals. Occasionally, outbreaks of angel wing are noted in the nestlings of certain wild populations.

## GEOGRAPHIC DISTRIBUTION
N/A

## SIGNALMENT
**Species**: All species. Birds belonging to the orders Anseriformes and Otidiformes are most frequently affected. Slower growing species from temperate regions of the world are especially susceptible.
**Mean age and range**: Varies according to species. Occurs when initial set of primary wing feathers develop.
**Predominant sex**: No sex predilection.

## SIGNS
Angel wing presents as unilateral or bilateral drooping of the wing at the carpi and elbows with outward (valgus) rotation of the wing distal to the carpi. The primary remiges are often deviated dorsally and laterally with the wing in a relaxed, flexed position. In young birds with immature musculoskeletal structures, the wing(s) can usually be manually manipulated into normal conformation. In older birds, bone mineralization and maturation of soft tissue structures result in permanent deformities that cannot be corrected manually.

## CAUSES
Carpal valgus occurs when the weight of the developing primary feathers exceeds the musculoskeletal structure's ability to hold the wing in a normal position. Diets containing excessive protein and carbohydrates result in inappropriately rapid feather development leading to angel wing. This often occurs in populations of birds in parks that are fed large amounts of high-energy foods such as bread. Lack of exercise and musculoskeletal fitness can also result in angel wing even when the diet is appropriate.

## RISK FACTORS
There are a number of other factors thought to be involved in the development of angel wing. Excessive dietary protein and energy are most commonly associated with angel wing. However, lack of adequate exercise, genetic predisposition, interruption of egg incubation, excessive heat during early development, vitamin D, E, and manganese deficiency are also implicated in some cases.

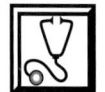 DIAGNOSIS

## DIFFERENTIAL DIAGNOSIS
Occasionally fractures (traumatic or pathologic) of the distal wing(s) will mimic angel wing.

## CBC/BIOCHEMISTRY/URINALYSIS
N/A

## OTHER LABORATORY TESTS
N/A

## IMAGING
Radiography of the affected wing(s) may help rule out traumatic injury, osteopenia, etc.

## DIAGNOSTIC PROCEDURES
The diagnosis of angel wing in birds is usually quite straightforward and is made via signalment, history, physical examination and sometimes radiography. Rarely will other diagnostic modalities be necessary.

## PATHOLOGIC FINDINGS
Abnormalities are limited to the gross anatomic deformities. Histologic lesions are not typically appreciated.

 TREATMENT

## APPROPRIATE HEALTH CARE
Early intervention is key to correction of angel wing in young, growing birds. In cases where clinical signs are limited to a mild wing droop and valgus has not begun to develop, trimming of the primary feathers to relieve weight on the distal wing can be corrective. In more severe cases where valgus of the distal wing has begun to develop, intervention usually requires fixing the wing in a normal resting position with or without weight relief by primary feather trimming. The wing is placed into a normal, resting position and immobilized temporarily. In some cases, taping the humerus, radius/ulna, and phalanges in line is sufficient; other cases require a more substantial bandage such as a figure-of-eight. A body wrap is not usually required. Holding the wing in a normal position for 3–5 days is typically sufficient to correct the deformity. If not caught early and musculoskeletal maturation has progressed to the point where the wing cannot be manually manipulated easily back into normal position, treatment via wing taping is usually ineffective.

## NURSING CARE
N/A

## ACTIVITY
Activity and exercise are encouraged in young birds to stimulate development of strong wings capable of supporting mature plumage. Typically, exercise can be encouraged simply by providing spacious quarters for the young birds to move about in.

## DIET
A balanced diet with appropriate protein and energy levels for the species is paramount to preventing angel wing and other development deformities in young, growing birds. Relatively slow-growing avian species should not be fed high-energy and high-protein diets as this practice can create mismatches between musculoskeletal and plumage development, leading to angel wing. In waterfowl, northern/arctic species are adapted to essentially feed around the clock on high-quality foods to maximize growth in the small window of time available. Conversely, temperate/tropical species typically have a much longer window of time in which to achieve the necessary growth, so they do not have the need for a constant intake of high-energy food. Dietary protein levels between 8% and 15% are recommended during the first 3 weeks of life in slow-growing waterfowl.

## CLIENT EDUCATION
Clients who are interested in breeding bird species predisposed to developing angel wing should be well versed in their dietary and husbandry requirements. Exact diet and husbandry requirements will depend on the species in question, but in general protein and energy levels should be kept at the minimum acceptable level and opportunity for exercise maximized.

## SURGICAL CONSIDERATIONS

Mature birds with angel wing typically require surgical correction. Phalangeal amputation ("pinioning") or osteotomy with rotation and fixation are typically required to create a comfortable and cosmetic wing. Pinioning of older birds can result in significant complications as the resultant stumps are often prone to injury.

## MEDICATIONS

### DRUG(S) OF CHOICE

Although typically not indicated, analgesic and/or anti-inflammatory medications may be prescribed for relief of discomfort at the discretion of the clinician.

### CONTRAINDICATIONS

Birds affected by angel wing are usually young, but otherwise there are usually no unique contraindications for analgesic/anti-inflammatory medications.

### PRECAUTIONS

N/A

### POSSIBLE INTERACTIONS

N/A

### ALTERNATIVE DRUGS

N/A

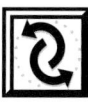

## FOLLOW-UP

### PATIENT MONITORING

Wing bandages/tape should not be left in place beyond 72 hours if possible. If bandaging is going to be successful, it will typically only need to be in place for 48–72 hours prior to removal. In adult birds with mature deformities, primary wing feathers can be periodically trimmed to make the abnormal conformation less obvious.

### PREVENTION/AVOIDANCE

Most cases of angel wing can be easily prevented with appropriate diet and husbandry. Proper nutrition during early development is key to prevention of angel wing. Neonatal birds should be provided with adequate opportunity to exercise and strengthen the developing musculoskeletal system. Removal from the breeding population of affected birds or birds with significant occurrence of the deformity in offspring may be warranted.

### POSSIBLE COMPLICATIONS

If intervention is not initiated early enough, usually within 3–5 days of first noticing clinical signs, bandaging will fail to correct carpal valgus. In cases of permanent deformity, the wing can sometimes become traumatized if the bird cannot manipulate it appropriately.

### EXPECTED COURSE AND PROGNOSIS

Birds that develop angel wing are often incapable of normal flight as adults despite intervention. Angel wing deformities are not life-threatening and many birds will survive and thrive if the deformities are not corrected. The birds will obviously continue to display the abnormal conformation and will be unable to fly. Complications can occur if the bird is not able to manipulate the wing to keep it from being traumatized.

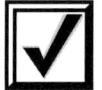

## MISCELLANEOUS

### ASSOCIATED CONDITIONS

Angular limb deformities of the pelvic limbs are sometime encountered in conjunction with angel wing deformities.

### AGE-RELATED FACTORS

Angel wing only occurs in young birds with developing plumage.

### ZOONOTIC POTENTIAL

N/A

### FERTILITY/BREEDING

As the role that genetics plays in the occurrence of angel wing is not understood, in some cases it may be prudent to avoid breeding affected birds.

### SYNONYMS

Carpal valgus, airplane wing, dropped wing, crooked wing

### SEE ALSO

Angular Limb Deformity (Splay Leg)
Feather Disorders
Fractures
Joint Diseases
Lameness
Metabolic Bone Disease
Nutritional Imbalances
Trauma

### ABBREVIATIONS

N/A

### INTERNET RESOURCES

N/A

*Suggested Reading*
Olsen, J.H. (1994). Anseriformes. In: *Avian Medicine: Principles and Application* (ed. B.W. Ritchie, G.J. Harrison, L.R. Harrison, eds.), 1237–1275. Lake Worth, FL: Wingers Publishing.
**Author**: Ryan S. De Voe, DVM, DABVP (Avian, Reptile/Amphibian), DACZM

**Client Education Handout available online**

# ANGULAR LIMB DEFORMITY (SPLAY LEG)

## BASICS

### DEFINITION
Angular limb deformities are rotational malformations of long bones (femur, tibiotarsometatarsal) or ligament abnormalities affecting various avian species. Possible etiologies includes trauma, nutrition, genetics, and lack of or excessive exercise.

### PATHOPHYSIOLOGY
The underlying mechanisms of angular limb deformity conditions of avian chicks are not fully understood and are extrapolated to early research in poultry. Several dietary factors may play a role, but manganese deficiency either through inadequate diet or excess calcium supplementation, is a possible primary predisposing factor. Limb deformities result in deviation along the limb, leading to a negative cascade affecting the other bones and joints of the limb. Other factors, such as deficiencies in calcium and vitamin $D_3$, may lead to weaker bones and growth plates that are affected by outside forces, such as slipping on smooth surfaces, trauma from handling, and so on. Leaving significant angular limb deformities untreated may result in irreparable limb misalignment that can result in joint abnormalities, muscle contracture, and ulcerative pododermatitis,

### SYSTEMS AFFECTED
Musculoskeletal, affecting the coxofemoral joint, femur, stifle joint, tibiotarsus, tarsal joint, and/or tarsometatarsus.

### GENETICS
None definitively known. Suspected in poultry to have some genetic relationships but not definitively proven.

### INCIDENCE/PREVALENCE
Rare in adults, uncommon in chicks with proper diet, common in chicks with improper diet or growth/weight monitoring.

### GEOGRAPHIC DISTRIBUTION
None.

### SIGNALMENT
**Species**: All avian species. Seen in Anseriformes, ratites, Galliformes, Passerines, and Psittaciformes species.
**Mean age and range**: Young chicks at or around fledging. Appears to be more common in growing hand-raised long-legged birds.
**Predominant sex**: None.

### SIGNS

#### Historical Findings
Signs reported by the owner.

#### Physical Examination Findings
Acute lameness and inability to stand and/or walk. Most commonly diagnosed in young chicks and those species with relatively long legs and those with a combination of larger body and shorter legs. Upon palpation, deviated of the limb laterally or medially. Edema is present in the acute phase leading to progressive joint inflammation, tendonitis, and bone bruising. Legs will be malpositioned when the patient is placed on a flat surface.

### CAUSES
Trauma. Vitamin E deficiency. Selenium deficiency. Valgus/varus malposition.

### RISK FACTORS
Typically seen in chicks prior to and around fledging due to rapid physical development and growth. Species with longer lengths of legs in relation to body size may also be at increased risk. Heavy-bodied species with relatively shorter legs (i.e. waterfowl) are also at an increased risk. Poor husbandry and substrate conditions. High gastrointestinal parasitic loads. Lack of exercise.

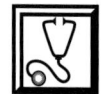

## DIAGNOSIS

### DIFFERENTIAL DIAGNOSIS
Joint infection, trauma/fractures, degenerative joint disease.

### CBC/BIOCHEMISTRY/URINALYSIS
Often will be within normal limits unless secondary inflammation or infection has developed to a point where the white blood cell count begins to increase.

### OTHER LABORATORY TESTS
None.

### IMAGING
Radiographs and CT should be performed to rule out any underlying pathology to the joint or bones.

### DIAGNOSTIC PROCEDURES
None.

### PATHOLOGIC FINDINGS
Inflammation of the tissues around the affected joint.

## TREATMENT

### APPROPRIATE HEALTH CARE
Initially, the patient needs to be assessed and the affected limb(s) stabilized. Once diagnostics are performed, the patient may be managed as an outpatient in mild cases. More severe cases should be managed in hospital initially until the limb(s) appear to be properly aligned.

### NURSING CARE
Bandaging. Hydrotherapy. Hobbles may be used to correct deformities if caught early enough, a few days. In some cases, housing the chick in a deep nesting cup may facilitate proper positioning of the limbs for corrective growth.

### ACTIVITY
Slick surfaces in the brooder/nest box should be avoided with the proper use of substrates, such as shaving, carpet, and so on. Should encouraged to exercise and hydrotherapy through.

### DIET
A well-balanced diet should be provided, avoiding excessive protein/calorie intake. Since excessive caloric intake is a risk factor, monitoring daily weight gain is vital in prevention and therapeutics. The daily weight gain should be appropriate for the species but on average is around 10% daily. Leg and tendon issues may be exacerbated with excessive calcium supplementation leading to decreased manganese absorption.

### CLIENT EDUCATION
Due to the varying levels of prognosis, client education about expectations of outcome is very important.

### SURGICAL CONSIDERATIONS
Corrective surgical techniques have been described in multiple avian species consisting of physeal retardation techniques, transphyseal bridging, and hinged transarticular external fixators.

## MEDICATIONS

### DRUG(S) OF CHOICE
NSAIDs and opioids may be used in management of the pain and inflammation associated with the stresses on the joints/bones.

### CONTRAINDICATIONS
None.

### PRECAUTIONS
None.

### POSSIBLE INTERACTIONS
None.

### ALTERNATIVE DRUGS
None.

 FOLLOW-UP

PATIENT MONITORING
Patients should be monitored daily for progress of therapy. Weekly radiographs may allow visual monitoring of return to normal positioning of bones or the development of additional lesions.

PREVENTION/AVOIDANCE
Most of the nutritional deficiencies can be prevented by placing chicks on a balanced and appropriate diet for the species. Daily monitoring of weight (same time of day before feeding) is extremely important to adjust the caloric input to regulate a slow, steady weight gain.

POSSIBLE COMPLICATIONS
Use of bandages and splints may lead to abnormal angles or pressures on the joints or constrictive blood flow, which may lead to edema and/or discomfort. Surgical corrections may break down due to the high forces and mobility of the joint.

EXPECTED COURSE AND PROGNOSIS
Depends on the severity presented during the initial examination. Mild cases may be managed medically with a fair prognosis but more advanced cases that require surgical correction have a guarded to poor prognosis.

 MISCELLANEOUS

ASSOCIATED CONDITIONS
Valgus/varus deformity. Angel wing. Curled toes.

AGE-RELATED FACTORS
Most commonly diagnosed in young chicks. Seen most commonly in species with relatively long legs and those with a combination of larger body and shorter legs.

ZOONOTIC POTENTIAL
N/A

FERTILITY/BREEDING
N/A

SYNONYMS
Splay leg, spraddle leg, bow leg, valgus/varus deformity.

SEE ALSO
Angel Wing
Toe and Nail Diseases

ABBREVIATIONS
CT—computed tomography
NSAIDs—non-steroidal anti-inflammatory drugs

INTERNET RESOURCES
N/A

*Suggested Reading*
Meij, B.P., Hazewinkel, H.A.W., Westerhof, I. (1996). Treatment of fractures and angular limb deformities of the tibiotarsus in birds by type II external skeletal fixation. *Journal of Avian Medicine and Surgery*, 10:153–162.
Mushi, E.Z., Binta, M.G., Chabo, R.G., et al. (1999). Limb deformities of farmed ostrich (*Struthio camelus*) chicks in Botswana. *Tropical Animal Health and Production*, 31:397–404.
Naldo, J.L., Bailey, T.A. (2001). Tarsometatarsal deformities in 3 captive-bred houbara bustards (*Chlamydotis undulata macqueenii*). *Journal of Avian Medicine and Surgery*, 15:197–203.
Samour, J. (2008). Management-related diseases. In: *Avian Medicine*, 2nd edn. (ed. J. Samour), 260–261. St. Louis, MO: Elsevier Inc.
Tully, T.N., Dorrenstein, G.M., Jones, A. (eds) (2009). *Handbook of Avian Medicine*, 2nd edn. St. Louis, MO: Elsevier.
Zollinger, T.J., Backues, K.A., Burgos-Rodriguez, A.G. (2005). Correction of angular limb deformity in two sub-species of flamingo (*Phoenicopterus ruber*) utilizing a transphyseal bridging technique. *Journal of Zoo and Wildlife Medicine*, 36:689–697.

**Author:** Rodney W. Schnellbacher, DVM, DACZM

**Acknowledgements:** updated from first edition chapter authored by Rob L. Coke, DVM, DACZM, DABVP (Reptile and Amphibian), CVA

## BASICS

### DEFINITION
Anorexia is defined as a complete lack of appetite. Hyporexia and dysorexia refer to a partial lack and a lack of consistent appetite, respectively. Anorexia can be the only complaint in a critically ill bird, especially in prey species, which tend to hide their clinical signs.

### PATHOPHYSIOLOGY
Food intake is initiated by numerous metabolic, sensory, and environmental signals that are integrated by different areas of the central nervous system. Anorexia results from interference with initiation of food intake, possibly associated with inflammatory cytokines (from infectious or neoplastic disorders), stress hormones (from the hypothalamic–pituitary–adrenal axis), or accumulation of toxins from endogenous (e.g. organ failure) or exogenous (e.g. toxic material) origin. Pain and nausea are other negative stimuli leading to anorexia. In case of anorexia, glycogen stores in the liver and muscles are depleted within the first few hours. Fat is then preferentially metabolized in birds. Ultimately, protein catabolism occurs. Typically, birds that are anorexic also have decreased fluid intake and can become dehydrated.

### SYSTEMS AFFECTED
All body systems. Anorexia is associated with denutrition, dehydration, and potentially malnutrition affecting all body systems.

### GENETICS
N/A

### INCIDENCE/PREVALENCE
Anorexia is a common complaint in birds and may be more prevalent during the warmer months.

### GEOGRAPHIC DISTRIBUTION
N/A

### SIGNALMENT
Seen in all species of birds. Anorexia is a normal physiologic response in some wild birds, especially birds that migrate.

### SIGNS

#### General Comments
Anorexia should be suspected in any sick bird.

#### Historical Findings
Owners will report decreased food intake with a loss of interest toward the food. Prey species (e.g. parrots) can pretend to eat; they will hull seeds but not consume the kernel. Duration and magnitude of patient's reduction in food intake should be evaluated. A weight loss and a decrease in size or frequency of the droppings are other signs associated with anorexia. Anorexic birds may produce green droppings secondary to bile staining. Reproductive and environmental history (toxin exposure, recent changes in the environment) may provide helpful diagnostic clues.

#### Physical Examination Findings
Physical examination may reveal weight loss and decreased body condition, characterized by loss of pectoral muscle mass. In severe cases, the keel is easily palpated and can be termed a "butterknife" keel. Dehydration and weakness are usually associated with anorexia. A thorough physical examination may reveal variable findings depending on the underlying cause.

### CAUSES
Anorexia is a nonspecific sign of illness. Primary anorexia can be associated with food aversion or stress induced by environmental changes (e.g. hospitalization, high temperature, dietary change, or modification of feeding management). Anorexia can be secondary to systemic diseases and diseases associated with pain or nausea, including neoplasia, inflammation (parasitic, bacterial, viral, fungal), toxicosis (lead, zinc), nutritional diseases (hypovitaminosis), metabolic disorders (e.g. kidney, liver or heart failure), trauma (e.g. crop burn), gastrointestinal foreign body, intracoelomic mass effect (e.g. egg binding, severe effusion), iatrogenic disorders (drug-induced anorexia associated with doxycycline, D-penicillamine, itraconazole, voriconazole, haloperidol).

### RISK FACTORS
N/A

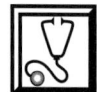

## DIAGNOSIS

### DIFFERENTIAL DIAGNOSIS
Pseudoanorexia refers to the situation where patients with a normal appetite are unable to eat due to lesions causing painful or dysfunctional prehension, mastication, or swallowing. These include disorders of the beak (fracture of the rhamphotheca or mandible), oropharynx (stomatitis, glossitis, dysphagia), and esophagus (foreign body). Pseudoanorexic birds will appear interested in food but attempts to eat will be interrupted. Careful examination of the oral cavity and cranial nerve function may reveal halitosis and nervous deficit, respectively. Disabled animals suffering from motor impairment (e.g. nervous, musculoskeletal, or feather disorders) or ophthalmic diseases may experience difficulties to reach food.

### CBC/BIOCHEMISTRY/URINALYSIS
**CBC:** Leukocytosis may be observed in case of stress or inflammatory reaction. Hypochromic regenerative anaemia may be observed in case of lead toxicity.
**Biochemistry:** Independent from the specific cause, chronic anorexia can be associated with hypoglycemia or hypoproteinemia. Increased bile acids, AST, CK and LDH may be observed in case of hepatic lipidosis.

### OTHER LABORATORY TESTS
Additional tests may be performed depending on the history and physical examinations, including blood lead and zinc levels, serology and/or PCR testing (e.g. *Chlamydia psittaci*, avian polyomavirus, avian bornavirus, psittacine beak and feather disease, herpesvirus). Fecal parasitologic examination. Culture and sensitivity of crop and cloaca.

### IMAGING
Diagnostic imaging may be necessary to diagnose the primary disease process.

#### Radiographic Findings
Survey whole body radiographs are indicated as a screening test and may reveal foreign body, organomegaly and space-occupying lesions. Additional diagnostic imaging exams may be performed depending on the history and physical examination. Contrast radiography can be used to improve visualization of the gastrointestinal tract and diagnose obstruction, compression or displacement of the digestive structures.

#### Ultrasonography
Coelomic ultrasonography is often informative in cases of coelomic distension.

#### Advanced Imaging
Whole-body CT is indicated in case of mass effect of unknown origin. Fluoroscopy allows for a better evaluation of the gastrointestinal motility.

### DIAGNOSTIC PROCEDURES
Additional diagnostic procedures may be performed depending on the history and physical examination. Endoscopy of the upper gastrointestinal tract is indicated to evaluate pharyngeal, oesophageal and crop appearance. Air sac endoscopy may be indicated to evaluate and sample coelomic organs. Biopsy or fine-needle aspiration with histology and cytological evaluation may be indicated (e.g. in case of hepatic lipidosis).

### PATHOLOGIC FINDINGS
Pathologic findings depend on the underlying cause. Independent of the primary disease, anorexia can induce the following lesions:
- Decreased muscle mass
- Decreased fat storage
- Enlarged gallbladder

• Hepatic lipidosis
• Liver atrophy
• Serous atrophy of fat.
On histopathology, atrophy of the bursa of Fabricius (in young birds) and hepatic hemosiderosis are common findings in anorexic birds.

# TREATMENT

## APPROPRIATE HEALTH CARE
The therapeutic goals are to improve nutritional status and manage any complications secondary to anorexia while efforts are directed at identifying and treating any underlying conditions. Anorexic birds should be initially treated as inpatient because complications of persistent anorexia can occur rapidly and underlying cause may require intensive care or surgical management.

## NURSING CARE
Hydration, acid-base abnormalities and electrolyte imbalance (especially hypokalemia) should be corrected before refeeding the patient because dehydrated and hypokalemic patients usually develop gastrointestinal ileus and the latter are at a higher risk of developing refeeding syndrome. Warmed crystalloid fluids are preferentially used (*see* Dehydration). Hypothermic patients and patients with a fluffed and ruffled appearance will be hospitalized in a humidified and heated incubator (29–32°C) as hypothermia is associated with poor perfusion of the gastrointestinal tract. A stress-free environment should be provided to stimulate voluntary food consumption. Minimize stressful conditions (e.g. administration of treatments) around meal times to avoid development of food aversion.

## ACTIVITY
Anorexic birds should have a limited activity to reduce energy deficits.

## DIET
**Enteral nutrition**: Preferred route of nutrition in birds once hypothermia, hydration, and electrolyte imbalances have been corrected. It is recommended that the patient be initially given access to its usual diet and food with high palatability, even if the nutrition is not balanced to stimulate spontaneous food intake. The food should be easily accessible and the bird should be stimulated to eat. If fresh food is distributed, it should be regularly replaced as dried food is less palatable.
**Assisted feeding**: Indicated if the patient is not eating enough to meet its energetic requirements with the BMR (kcal) = $(k \times W)^{0.75}$ where W is body weight

in kg and $k$ is a constant ($k$ = 78 for psittacine birds, $k$ = 129 for passerine birds).
**Type and quantity of food**: Depends on the species and age of the patient. Elemental diets that are calorically dense owing to fat content are appropriate to meet patient intake with a minimal quantity of food. The quantity of required food is divided into 2–4 meals and fed a temperature of 38–40°C.
**Syringe-feeding**: Can be used initially. Esophagostomy/duodenostomy tube can be considered when anorexia is expected to be protracted and/or situations where specific part of the gastrointestinal tract should be bypassed. Esophagostomy tubes are indicated in cases of severe beak trauma and disease of the oral cavity. They can also be used to bypass the crop in cases of severe crop disease. Duodenostomy tubes are indicated in cases of delayed crop emptying or gastric distension.

## CLIENT EDUCATION
Owners are advised to monitor food intake, body weight in grams, volume of droppings, and appearance daily as long as the bird is ill. A veterinarian should be contacted in case of decreased appetite, body weight, or fecal output.

## SURGICAL CONSIDERATIONS
Surgical treatment may be necessary to treat the underlying cause of anorexia, such as foreign body, neoplasia, crop burn, trauma, or egg retention. Anorexic patients should be stabilized before surgical intervention because cachectic or hypoglycemic patients are at a higher risk of anesthetic mortality.

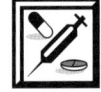

# MEDICATIONS

## DRUG(S) OF CHOICE
• Appetite-stimulants can be considered but should not replace diagnostic efforts to identify the underlying cause of anorexia. These include diazepam (0.2 mg/kg PO q24h in raptors), midazolam (1 mg/kg IM in budgerigars) or lorazepam (1 mg/kg IM in budgerigars).
• Symptomatic therapy may include management of inflammatory processes with NSAIDs (e.g. meloxicam 1 mg/kg PO, IM, IV q12h), ileus with prokinetic drugs (e.g. metoclopramide 0.1–2 mg/kg PO, IM, IV), nausea with antiemetic drugs (e.g. maropitant 1 or 2 mg/kg SQ q12–24 h) and pain (e.g. opiates such as tramadol 30 mg/kg PO q8–12h).
• In cases of hepatic lipidosis, S-adenyl methionine (10 mg/kg PO q12h), silymarin (100–150 mg/kg PO divided q8–12h) and B complex vitamins can be considered.

• Specific treatments will be provided depending on the underlying cause and special attention should be given to active ingredients that can contribute to anorexia.

## CONTRAINDICATIONS
Avoid antiemetics and prokinetics if gastrointestinal obstruction is present or suspected.

## PRECAUTIONS
Complications associated with assisted feeding include:
• Crop burn: Feeding formula should be slightly lower than body temperature and should not be heated with a microwave.
• Delayed emptying: Before each episode of assisted feeding, the crop should be palpated to ensure that no material remains from the previous feeding.
• Laceration of the oropharynx.
• Perforation of the cervical esophagus.
• Aspiration and regurgitation: Assisted feeding should be performed in birds that are able to maintain their head up. Dyspneic patients should be fed with caution, because feeding them can lead to choking.

## POSSIBLE INTERACTIONS
None.

## ALTERNATIVE DRUGS
N/A

# FOLLOW-UP

## PATIENT MONITORING
Food intake, body weight, body condition score, hydration and fecal output should be monitored twice daily. Depending on the primary disease, radiographs, CBC, plasma biochemistry and heavy metal levels in the blood may be monitored.

## PREVENTION/AVOIDANCE
All aspects of preventive medicine will decrease the risk of disease and anorexia in birds. Special attention should be directed to providing adequate nutrition, appropriate husbandry, safe and stress-free environment as well as vaccination (e.g. polyomavirus).

## POSSIBLE COMPLICATIONS
Liver disorders including hepatic lipidosis or hepatic atrophy: Caloric deficit leads to fat mobilization in order to maintain homeostasis and fat becomes stored in the liver.
• Gastrointestinal disorders including hemorrhagic diathesis, hypomotility, villous atrophy, bacterial translocation and endotoxemia.
• Fluid and electrolyte imbalance including dehydration and hypokalemia.
• Metabolic disorders including hypoglycemia and hypothermia.

• Decreased immunocompetence.
• Neuromuscular complications including sarcopenia, weakness, ataxia, confusion, seizure and death.
• Cardiac dysfunction can occur in cases of severe sarcopenia.

### EXPECTED COURSE AND PROGNOSIS

Depends on the cause and the duration of anorexia. Resolution can be simple for acute anorexia if the etiology is readily treatable. When anorexia is secondary to a cause difficult or impossible to treat, the management is challenging. The prognosis worsens when consequences of denutrition occur (e.g. hepatic lipidosis, cachexia, hemorrhagic diathesis). Anorexia can quickly become life-threatening in smaller birds due to their higher metabolic rate and potential hypermetabolic state associated with critical illness.

 MISCELLANEOUS

### ASSOCIATED CONDITIONS

Anorexia is often associated with weight loss or asthenia in the syndrome of impaired general condition.

### AGE-RELATED FACTORS

None.

### ZOONOTIC POTENTIAL

Diseases with a zoonotic potential can be responsible of anorexia (e.g. mycobacteriosis and chlamydiosis).

### FERTILITY/BREEDING

Reproductively active hens that are anorexic may be poor breeders or may not be able to normally oviposit. Developing eggs in the oviduct may be affected if anorexia occurs during that episode.

### SYNONYMS

Inappetence

### SEE ALSO

Beak Injuries/Trauma
Bornaviral Diseases
Chlamydiosis
Coelomic Distension
Dehydration
Emaciation
Enteritis and Gastritis
Foreign Bodies (Gastrointestinal)
Hepatic Lipidosis
Ileus (Functional Gastrointestinal, Crop Stasis)
Liver Disease
Mycotoxicosis
Regurgitation And Vomiting
Renal Diseases
Sick-Bird Syndrome
Toxicosis (Heavy Metals)

### ABBREVIATIONS

AST—aspartate aminotransferase
BMR—basal metabolic rate
CK—creatine kinase
CT—computed tomography
LDH—lactate dehydrogenase
PCR—polymerase chain reaction
NSAID—non-steroidal anti-inflammatory drug

### INTERNET RESOURCES

None.

*Suggested Reading*
Hollwarth, A.J., Pestell, S.T., Byron-Chance, D.H., et al. (2022). Mortality outcomes based on ASA grade in avian patients undergoing general anesthesia. *Journal of Exotic Pet Medicine*, 41:14–19.
Lumeij, J.T. (1994). Gastroenterology. In: *Avian Medicine: Principles and applications* (ed. B.W. Ritchie, G.J. Harrison, L.R. Harrison), 482–521. Brentwood, TN: HBD International.
Martel, A., Berg, C., Doss, G. et al. (2022). Effects of midazolam on food intake in budgerigars (*Melopsittacus undulatus*). *Journal of Avian Medicine and Surgery*, 36:53–57.
Scagnelli, A., Titel, C., Doss, G., et al. (2022). Effects of midazolam and lorazepam on food intake in budgerigars (*Melopsittacus undulatus*). *Journal of Exotic Pet Medicine*, 41:42–45.

**Author**: Graham Zoller, DVM, DECZM (Avian)

**BASICS**

## DEFINITION
Accumulation of fluid within the peritoneal cavities. Birds have five distinct peritoneal cavities: the intestinal peritoneal cavity, right and left ventral hepatic peritoneal cavities, and the right and left dorsal hepatic peritoneal cavities; fluid can accumulate within any one or more of these five cavities.

## PATHOPHYSIOLOGY
The accumulation of fluid in the peritoneal cavities usually results from a combination of reduced lymphatic drainage and increased vascular permeability and is often a sequela of congestive heart failure, liver failure, or inflammatory processes in the coelomic cavities. Increased capillary and lymphatic hydrostatic pressure may be due to portal hypertension from a chronic hepatopathy or pulmonary hypertension from congestive heart failure. Decreased albumin levels lead to the inability to maintain oncotic pressure to keep fluid in the circulatory system. Hypoproteinemia can be due to a loss of proteins (e.g. protein-losing enteropathy or protein-losing nephropathy) or from decreased production (e.g. hepatopathy). Compromise of vasculature from inflammation or infection can lead to leakage of fluid into the coelom. Neoplasms and carcinomatosis can lead to the accumulation of malignant ascites.

## SYSTEMS AFFECTED
**Respiratory**: Compression of the air sacs by the accumulated fluid can lead to increased respiratory effort.
**Integument**: Increased visualization of skin around the caudal coelom, either from distension of the coelom or localized plucking of feathers in response to discomfort from the distension.
**Reproductive**: Egg yolk peritonitis and cystic hyperplasia of the oviduct or ovary can lead to significant fluid accumulation.

## GENETICS
Direct and maternal genetic effects play a role in the development of broiler ascites syndrome. Heritable cardiac conditions have been described in neonatal and juvenile parrots.

## INCIDENCE/PREVALENCE
Common clinical sequela for congestive heart failure, hepatopathies, pancreatitis, and neoplasms within the coelomic cavity.

## GEOGRAPHIC DISTRIBUTION
N/A

## SIGNALMENT
**Species predilections**:
• Cockatiels—egg yolk peritonitis, ovarian neoplasms, cystic ovarian disease

• Toucans and mynah birds—hemochromatosis (iron storage disease)
• Broiler chickens—pulmonary arterial hypertension (ascites syndrome)
• Turkeys—spontaneous cardiomyopathy (round heart disease)
**Mean age and range and predominant sex**:
• Cardiomyopathies—atherosclerosis and congestive heart failure are more commonly diagnosed in middle-aged to geriatric birds; however, congenital heart conditions have been reported in juvenile birds.
• Egg-yolk peritonitis, cystic ovarian disease, and ovarian neoplasms—occur in sexually mature hens.
• Hepatopathies—hepatic neoplasms and cirrhosis usually seen in older birds; toxins and infectious causes of hepatitis can affect any age.

## SIGNS
### Historical Findings
• Tail bob and/or open mouth breathing.
• Distended abdomen.
• Generalized lethargy and depression; owner may note that patient is staying on the bottom of the cage.
• Decreased appetite.
• Exercise intolerance.
• Decreased ability to fly.

### Physical Examination Findings
• Swollen coelom that is compressible.
• Increased respiratory effort.
• Wheezing or crackles auscultated over lungs and caudal air sacs.
• Lethargic and depressed.
• Anorexic.
• Fecal and/or urate accumulation over vent and tail feathers.
• Exercise intolerance.
• Wide-based stance or drooped wings.
• Holosystolic heart murmur (cardiomyopathy).
• Yellow or green urates (hepatopathy).

## CAUSES
**Cardiovascular**: Congestive heart failure.
**Reproductive**: Ovarian neoplasia, salpingitis, metritis, oophoritis, egg yolk coelomitis, oviduct rupture, cystic hyperplasia of the oviduct or ovary, ectopic ovulation, testicular neoplasia.
**Neoplasia**: Neoplastic effusion, carcinomatosis.
**Gastrointestinal**: Protein-losing enteropathy, pancreatitis.
**Hepatic**: Cirrhosis (aflatoxins, chlamydiosis,); iron storage disease/hemochromatosis.
**Infectious**: Aspergillosis (granulomatous pneumonia leading to pulmonary hypertension); mycobacteriosis (liver failure and protein-losing enteropathy); polyomavirus.

## RISK FACTORS
The lungs of birds are more rigid and noncompliant than that of mammals, thus possibly making them more predisposed to pulmonary hypertension. Ingestion of moldy peanuts and grain may lead to aflatoxicosis, which can result in hepatic cirrhosis and ascites. Birds in the Ramphastidae (toucan) and Sturnidae (mynah) families are at greater risk for iron storage disease. Obesity and hypercholesterolemia due to high-calorie diets compounded with a sedentary lifestyle can lead to congestive heart failure/atherosclerosis.

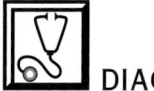 **DIAGNOSIS**

## DIFFERENTIAL DIAGNOSIS
### Coelomic Distension
• Egg binding or dystocia (common).
• Obesity and lipomas (common).
• Body-wall hernias.
• Coelomic masses (i.e. neoplasms, abscesses, or granulomas of any of the coelomic organs).
• Generalized ileus or severely enlarged proventriculus.
• Organomegaly (hepatomegaly, splenomegaly).

### Dyspnea/Increased Respiratory Effort
• Primary respiratory conditions such as pneumonia, sinusitis, or tracheal obstruction (common).
• Pain (common).
• Organomegaly or space-occupying masses in the coelomic cavity (common).
• Heat exhaustion.
• Cardiac disease.

## CBC/BIOCHEMISTRY/URINALYSIS
Leukocytosis, with or without a monocytosis and toxic heterophils, may be noted in patients with associated systemic infection; severe leukocytosis if an infectious disease process such as mycobacteria or chlamydia is involved. Moderate to severe hypoalbuminemia and decreased A:G ratio. Elevated bile acids if a hepatopathy is present. Damage to skeletal or smooth musculature may lead to elevated aspartate aminotransferase and creatine phosphokinase levels.

## OTHER LABORATORY TESTS
**Fluid analysis and cytology of aspirated fluid** allow for the characterization of the fluid and aid in the diagnosis of the underlying cause:
• Transudate—clear and odorless with low cellularity ($< 1 \times 10^9$/L), low specific gravity $< 1.020$, low protein $< 30$ g/L; may contain macrophages and mesothelial cells; due to hepatic cirrhosis, cardiac insufficiency, or hypoproteinemia.

• Modified transudate—serosanguineous, may be clear to slightly cloudy with moderate cellularity ($1–5 \times 10^9$/L), specific gravity usually < 1.020, low protein usually < 30 g/L; mesothelial cells and rare heterophils present, mesothelial cells may be reactive, neoplastic cells may be noted; may be associated with vascular leakage from increase capillary hydrostatic pressure or neoplasms.

• Exudates—frequently viscous and tend to clot, have increased cellularity (> $5 \times 10^9$/L), high specific gravity > 1.020, and high protein > 30 g/L; mixed cellularity that is predominately heterophils and macrophages if acute, lymphocytes and plasma cells are present if more chronic; can be characterized as septic or nonseptic; yolk or fat globules may be present in cases of egg yolk peritonitis; may be associated with inflammatory, necrotizing, infectious, or neoplastic disorders.

**Hemorrhagic effusion**: Bloody effusion with measurable hematocrit representing 10–25% of systemic blood PCV, erythrophagocytosis present, and no platelets noted; should be differentiated from peripheral blood contamination.

• Neoplastic cells may be noted in cases of malignant effusions or carcinomatosis.

• Bacterial culture and sensitivity of aspirated fluid should be performed if infection suspected.

### IMAGING

*Radiographic Findings*
Poor serosal detail of the distended coelomic cavity is usually present on survey films. Upper gastrointestinal contrast study may help to evaluate whether a mass effect is also present in the coelomic cavity. Cardiomegaly and enlarged hepatic silhouette may be present in cases of CHF.

*Ultrasonography*
Coelomic ultrasound is the preferred method of diagnostic imaging for the evaluation of ascites. Fluid distension enhances visualization of a bird's coelomic cavity. Multiple cystic structures of varying size or a single large cystic structure may be noted in the left craniodorsal region of the coelom with cystic ovarian disease. A large heart and valvular regurgitation are often noted in cases of CHF. The liver may also be large and hypoechoic with dilated portal veins. Hepatic changes associated with hepatic cirrhosis include small hyperechoic liver with nodular margins.

### DIAGNOSTIC PROCEDURES
Centesis of the coelomic cavity is both diagnostic and therapeutic. Removal of coelomic fluid before performing other diagnostic procedures can significantly improve the bird's ability to breathe. Ultrasound and/or transillumination may be beneficial in determining best area to tap.

**Note**: During centesis of the coelom, the needle must be directed midline to avoid puncturing through an air sac.

### PATHOLOGIC FINDINGS
Pathologic lesions will vary depending on the cause of the ascites:

• Fluid may fill the entire coelomic cavity or may surround a specific liver lobe; fluid may be transudative, exudative, or serosanguineous. The membranes of the hepatic and peritoneal cavities may be thickened, especially in cases of chronic ascites.

• CHF—cardiomegaly with right-sided, left-sided, or biventricular enlargement; enlarged and congested liver with rounded edges; moist pulmonary parenchyma.

• Hepatic cirrhosis—small fibrotic hepatic parenchyma; may be pale tan, firm, and nodular.

• Ovarian/testicular neoplasia—cystic and/or soft tissue mass may be noted at the cranial pole of the kidney.

• Egg yolk peritonitis—inspissated egg yolk and adhesions noted in the peritoneal cavity.

• Carcinomatosis—neoplastic nodules and tissue may be disseminated throughout the coelomic cavity.

• Polyomavirus—cardiomegaly, myocardial/epicardial hemorrhage, hepatomegaly with yellow-white foci, GI hemorrhage, splenomegaly, and pale swollen kidneys; large, clear, basophilic or amphophilic intranuclear inclusion bodies on histology.

• Mycobacteriosis—enlarged and mottled pale liver and spleen, thickening of the small intestinal wall with numerous pale miliary nodules on the mucosal surface; on histology, macrophages and giant cells containing acid-fast bacteria noted through multiple organs.

## TREATMENT

### APPROPRIATE HEALTH CARE
• Measures should be undertaken to improve the patient's ability to breathe. Treatments include diuretics, centesis of the coelom, and oxygen supplementation.

• Centesis of excessive fluid can be repeated as necessary on an outpatient basis.

• Control of infection and inflammation needs to be addressed when medically managing cases of egg yolk peritonitis; surgical intervention may be required once the patient is stabilized.

• Cystic ovarian disease, ovarian neoplasia, and testicular neoplasia are rarely treated surgically due to the vascular supply to the gonads; periodic coelomocentesis and medical management with hormone therapy may provide symptomatic treatment.

• Surgical excision of some neoplasms may alleviate symptoms if the neoplasm has not already metastasized.

• Phlebotomy (1% of body weight q7d) can be performed in birds with iron storage disease to reduce stored liver iron levels.

### NURSING CARE
Measures to improve respiratory function including oxygen supplementation and therapeutic coelomic centesis should be performed prior to undertaking procedures that may compromise the bird. Midazolam may be beneficial to help calm the bird down to avoid hyperventilation. Nutritional support is necessary if the patient is not eating or has lost muscle mass.

### ACTIVITY
Minimize stress and activity since the patient has limited ability to breathe.

### DIET
Gavage feed if the patient is not eating. Species susceptible to ISD should be on a specially formulated low-iron diet.

### CLIENT EDUCATION
Coelomocentesis may need to be repeated as needed to provide relief for dyspnea.

### SURGICAL CONSIDERATIONS
Compromised ability to breathe due to compression of air sacs. If performing surgery, intubation with positive pressure ventilation is strongly recommended. Extra care must be taken to prevent damaging the air sacs during the surgical approach to minimize the risk of fluid aspiration through the air sacs.

## MEDICATIONS

### DRUG(S) OF CHOICE
• Meloxicam (0.5–2 mg/kg PO, IM q12–24h): Administration of anti-inflammatory medication is indicated if an inflammatory or painful condition is present.

• Furosemide (1–5 mg/kg IM q2–12h for acute treatment, then 1–10 mg/kg PO q 8–12h for maintenance): Diuretic to remove excess fluid in cases of CHF or liver insufficiency.

• Broad-spectrum antibiotics should be administered if a septic exudate is noted and/or an infectious process is suspected until culture and sensitivity results of the aspirated fluid are available.

*For reproductive-related disorders*
• Leuprolide acetate (1500–3500 µg/kg IM q2–4w): Synthetic GnRH agonist.

• Deslorelin (4.7 mg implant SQ q2–5m): Synthetic GnRH agonist; long-term implant. **Note**: use of this implant in birds is considered off-label use and as an FDA-indexed drug is prohibited in the United States for the use in poultry.

### For congestive heart failure
- Furosemide (see above).
- Benazepril HCl (0.5 mg/kg PO q24h) or enalapril (1.25 – 5 mg/kg PO q12h): ACE inhibitors used in the management of CHF and hypertension.
- Pimobendan (6–10 mg/kg PO q12h): Inodilator (has inotropic and vasodilator effects) used in the management of CHF.

### For iron storage disease
Deferoxamine (100 mg/kg SQ/IM q24h); iron chelator for birds with ISD.

### For hepatic cirrhosis/fibrosis
Colchicine (0.02–0.2 mg/kg PO q12–24h); antifibrotic used in the treatment of cirrhosis of the liver.

## CONTRAINDICATIONS
- Furosemide is contraindicated in patients with anuria.
- Colchicine is contraindicated in patients with serious renal, GI, or cardiac dysfunction.
- Deferoxamine should not be used in patients with severe renal failure.

## PRECAUTIONS
Furosemide should be used with caution in patients with hepatic dysfunction or pre-existing electrolyte or water imbalances.

## POSSIBLE INTERACTIONS
Colchicine may cause additive myelosuppression when used in conjunction with medications with bone marrow depressant effects (i.e. antineoplastics, immunosuppressants, chloramphenicol, amphotericin B).

## ALTERNATIVE DRUGS
Hepatoprotective medication such as silymarin may be beneficial if a hepatopathy is suspected.

 FOLLOW-UP

## PATIENT MONITORING
Frequency of monitoring will vary depending on how quickly fluid reaccumulates in the coelomic cavity. Daily to weekly weight checks (either at home or at the clinic) evaluate for increases in body weight, which may indicate that fluid has refilled the coelomic cavity. Repeating coelomic ultrasound can be helpful in confirming and evaluating the amount of fluid in the coelomic cavity.

## PREVENTION/AVOIDANCE
Birds that are prone to developing ISD should be placed on a low-iron diet.

## POSSIBLE COMPLICATIONS
Lateral puncture of the coelomic cavity when performing coelomic centesis may result in leakage of fluid directly into the air sac and can result in the drowning of the patient.

## EXPECTED COURSE AND PROGNOSIS
Depends on the cause of the ascites; in general prognosis is guarded, especially if the respiratory system is severely compromised. Ascites from congestive heart failure can be managed with medical treatment; however, this condition is usually progressive over time. Yolk coelomitis, cystic ovarian disease, ovarian neoplasia, and testicular neoplasia have a guarded prognosis but some have been managed long-term with periodic coelomocentesis and hormone therapy. Hepatic insufficiency from hepatic cirrhosis generally carries a guarded long-term prognosis. Cases of mycobacteriosis require prolonged treatment; treatment of this disease in avian species is controversial.

 MISCELLANEOUS

## ASSOCIATED CONDITIONS
Peripheral edema may also be noted if ascites is due to hypoalbuminemia. Unilateral or bilateral hind limb lameness may be noted if the ascites is due to a neoplasm that is compressing the ischiatic nerve.

## AGE-RELATED FACTORS
N/A

## ZOONOTIC POTENTIAL
Although no cases of bird-to-human mycobacteriosis have been reported, owners must be advised of the potential zoonotic risk, especially to immunocompromised individuals.

## FERTILITY/BREEDING
Birds with ascites associated with reproductive disease may be infertile or produce abnormal eggs.

## SYNONYMS
Coelomic effusion
Hydroperitoneum

## SEE ALSO
Atherosclerosis
Congestive Heart Failure

Coelomic Distention
Egg Yolk and Reproductive Coelomitis
Liver Disease
Mycobacteriosis
Neoplasia (Reproductive)
Ovarian Diseases
Oviductal Disorders
Polyomavirus

## ABBREVIATIONS
ACE—angiotensin-converting enzyme
CHF—congestive heart failure
GI—gastrointestinal
GnRH—gonadotropin-releasing hormone
ISD—iron storage disease
PCV—packed cell volume

## INTERNET RESOURCES
Pollock, C., Powers, L. (2015). Abdominocentesis in birds. *LafeberVet.* https://lafeber.com/vet/abdominocentesis-in-birds

*Suggested Reading*
Antinoff, N. (2021). Birds with big bellies: What do I need to know? *ExoticsCon Virtual* 2021 Proceedings, 676–679.
Juan-Sallés, C., Soto, S., Garner, M.M., et al. (2011). Congestive heart failure in 6 African grey parrots (*Psittacus e erithacus*). *Veterinary Pathology,* 48:691–697.
Keller, K.A., Beaufrère, H., Brandão, J., et al. (2013). Long-term management of ovarian neoplasia in two cockatiels (*Nymphicus hollandicus*). *Journal of Avian Medicine and Surgery,* 27:44–52.
Scagnelli, A.M., Tully, T.N. Jr. (2017). Reproductive disorders in parrots. *Veterinary Clinics of North America. Exotic Animal Practice,* 20:485–507.
Sedacca, C.D., Campbell, T.W., Bright, J.M., et al. (2009). Chronic cor pulmonale secondary to pulmonary atherosclerosis in an African grey parrot. *Journal of the American Veterinary Medical Association,* 234:1055–1059.
Taylor, W.M. (2016). Pleura, pericardium, and peritoneum: The coelomic cavities of birds and their relationship to the lung-air sac system. In: *Current Therapy in Avian Medicine and Surgery* (ed. B.L. Speer), 345–362. St. Louis, MO: Elsevier.
Wheeler, C.L., Webber, R.A. (2002). Localized ascites in a cockatiel (*Nymphicus hollandicus*) with hepatic cirrhosis. *Journal of Avian Medicine and Surgery,* 16:300–305.
**Author:** Sue Chen, DVM, DABVP (Avian)

# ASPERGILLOSIS

 **BASICS**

## DEFINITION
Opportunistic mycotic disease, caused by the fungus *Aspergillus*, that can produce illness varying in severity, chronicity, and affected body systems.

## PATHOPHYSIOLOGY
The *Aspergillus* spp. spores are saprophytic, ubiquitous, and widespread within a given environment or inside the avian body. Birds manifest disease when they become immunocompromised. The spores will settle in respiratory epithelium with poor vascularization and reduced mucociliary function. The thermophilic environment of the avian air sac system is ideal growth environment. Spore infiltration will cause neovascularization, focal microcystic lesions that will develop to plaques, granulomas, hyphae, and sporulating conidia. In chronic forms, encapsulated granulomas will be formed and dissemination to the lungs, trachea, heart, and abdominal organs may occur. Production of mycotoxins such as gliotoxin and ergoline alkaloid fumigaclavine A play a role in pathogenesis.

## SYSTEMS AFFECTED
**Respiratory**: Increased respiratory rate and effort, respiratory distress; mycotic tracheitis, air sacculitis, rhinitis, and sinusitis.
**Behavioral**: Usually the first signs that owners note are listlessness, depression, and lethargy.
**Gastrointestinal**: Regurgitation, diarrhea, and abnormal droppings.
**Hemic/lymphatic/immune**.
**Hepatobiliary**: Biliverdinuria and hepatomegaly.
**Central nervous system**: Encephalitic and meningoencephalic lesions may occur with disseminated disease.
**Ophthalmic**: Rare, but ocular fungal granulomas and blepharitis have been reported.
**Renal/urologic**: Polyuria, polydipsia, and renomegaly.
**Skin/exocrine**.

## GENETICS
Specific turkey and chicken lineages are more susceptible. Hybridization or inbreeding (in captive falcons or other species) could produce individuals with outbreeding depression which are thus more susceptible.

## INCIDENCE/PREVALENCE
Most frequent cause of respiratory disease and most diagnosed fungal disease in pet birds, zoo birds, and falconry raptors. Most common, non-traumatically induced medical problem in free-ranging/rehabilitated birds. High prevalence in rehabilitated (20–42%) and captive penguins (40–61%). Seabirds and waterfowl prevalence can vary from 3–30%. In juvenile falcons in the Middle East prevalence is 28%, but in raptors in Belgium has reached up to 38%. Prevalence in captive psittacines in North America is 9%.

## GEOGRAPHIC DISTRIBUTION
Global distribution, except Antarctica. Latitude-related decrease of antibody seroprevalence in Subantarctic to Antarctic penguins. Seasonality, especially in autumn and spring, and high humidity.

## SIGNALMENT
Lack of evidence-based studies to highlight species predisposition, mostly empirical/population-based data. Juveniles in all species are more susceptible than adults. Male swans have twice the probability to be affected than females. Quails and turkeys were found to be more susceptible than chickens after an experimental trial. Upland, Arctic and Antarctic species are speculated to be more sensitive (i.e. gyrfalcon, snowy owl, goshawk, golden/bald/white-tailed sea eagles, osprey, rough-legged buzzard, penguins, loons, northern geese/duck species). Ground-dwelling species (e.g. kiwis) might be more easily exposed. Empirically, specific species such as grey parrots (*Psittacus erithacus*), Pionus parrots (*Pionus* spp.), Amazon parrots (*Amazona* spp.), swans (*Cygnus* spp.), and sea birds (gulls, guillemots, razorbills, albatross).

## SIGNS
### General Comments
Non-specific signs involving all possible differential conditions for respiratory distress, biliverdinuria, chronic weight loss, reduction of stamina/activity.

### Historical Findings
• Use of particulate bedding (corn cob or walnut-shell bedding, hay, wood shavings, etc.) within enclosure/mew.
• Inappropriate sanitation, ventilation, air circulation.
• Change in voice/call, with or without breathing abnormalities.
• Depression/weakness—reluctance to fly or perch, drooped wings.
• Inappetence.

### Physical Examination Findings
• Lethargy.
• Increased respiratory rate and/or effort—tail bobbing, dyspnea, tachypnea, cyanosis, vocalization when breathing, harsh breathing sounds on auscultation.
• Reduction of flight stamina.
• Weight loss.
• Polyuria/polydipsia/biliverdinuria.

## CAUSES
In avian cases, 90% caused by *A. fumigatus*; in other species, *A. flavus, A. terreus, A. niger, A. lentulus, A. nidulans* also frequently isolated. Avian isolates are phylogenetically diverse, with no clear distinction from human clinical isolates, and no sign of host or geographic specificity. High humidity and warm environment—abrupt weather changes. Sudden exposure to inhaled fungal spores.

## RISK FACTORS
Environmental factors: Poor husbandry/ventilation, use of particular bedding. Overcrowding. Nutritional disorders/deficiencies (e.g., hypovitaminosis A). Stress, in both captive birds of prey and *Psittacine* spp. Intense exercise or lack of exercise. Impaired immune function due to migration exhaustion. Prolonged antibiotic use and steroids. Prophylactic use of antifungals and azole resistance. Underlying disease condition (traumatic, toxic, microbiological, anatomic).

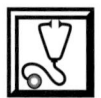 **DIAGNOSIS**

## DIFFERENTIAL DIAGNOSIS
Avian chlamydiosis. Environmental toxicosis or chronic exposure to respiratory irritant. Allergic pneumonitis or noninfectious pneumonitis. Fowl cholera. Mycobacteriosis. Mycoplasmosis. Airsacculitis. Foreign body obstruction within respiratory tract. Neoplasia. Avian influenza. Herpes virus. Hepatopathy.

## CBC/BIOCHEMISTRY/URINALYSIS
Profound heterophilic leucocytosis (25,000–100,000 cells/µl). A left shift may be present, and quite often white blood cells are very reactive. Chronic inflammation may also produce a non-regenerative anemia. Serum biochemistry analysis may reveal elevations in AST, LDH, and serum bile acids if liver involvement is present. Hypoalbuminemia and hypergammaglobulinemia can also be characteristic of the disease. Biliverdinuria.

## OTHER LABORATORY TESTS
Protein electrophoresis needs standardization per species and per disease. May support diagnosis, screening of large flocks and treatment monitoring. In psittacines and falcons, an increase in β-globulins, hypoalbuminemia, a decreased albumin: globulin ratio and lower prealbumin values may be indicative of aspergillosis. Higher sensitivity if combined with acute phase proteins in penguins. Acute phase proteins (serum amyloid, haptoglobin, 3-hydroxybutyrate). As with electrophoresis, may indicate inflammatory response and need standardization per species, disease, age, sex and stage. 3-hydroxybutyrate produced promising results in penguins and in falcon metabolomics. *Aspergillus* biomarkers (galactomannan, β-glucan, gliotoxin, fumiglavamine A, TAFC) show low sensitivity per avian order and lack of standardization. β-glucan was more sensitive in seabirds than raptors. Serology is often of limited value due to ubiquitous nature of *Aspergillus* spp. and there is low sensitivity with false positive and negatives to relate to disease status. Molecular

detection (PCR) is mostly used for research identification of *Aspergillus* genome, species, resistant genes, while the ubiquitous nature of *Aspergillus* limits its use as reliable antemortem diagnostic tool.

## IMAGING

### Radiographic Findings

May reveal the distribution and severity of fungal lesions in the lungs and air sacs, but of limited value for early disease detection and confirmation. There is species variation on the alterations. Common radiologic findings are a bronchopneumonia with marked parabronchial patterns, asymmetry, hyperinflation, or consolidation of the air sacs, as well as soft-tissue densities. Even after a successful resolution of clinical infection, the respiratory tract may remain thickened and irregular.

### Advanced Imaging

CT is more readily available and cheaper than in the past. It is non-invasive, helps to identify dissemination/invasiveness of aspergillosis (intra-abdominal, pericardial, intrapulmonary), and more accurately predicts the prognosis and treatment success. Still produces false positives and does not enable sample collection. High rate of false negatives in early cases. Excellent when combined with endoscopy, cytology, and culture.

## DIAGNOSTIC PROCEDURES

### Endoscopy (Rigid or Flexible)

Best antemortem diagnostic tool to confirm diagnosis of aspergillosis. An effective way for visualization of the trachea, syrinx, and lower respiratory tract (air sacs and lungs). Allows sample collection for cytology/culture/histopathology, antifungal application, and lesion debridement.

### Cytology/Culture/Histopathology

Quick, cheap diagnostic tool used for diagnosis and treatment monitoring. False negatives, depending on the sample site and size. Experience is crucial. Growth in Sabouraud agar takes 2–15 days (98.6°F/37°C) confirms diagnosis, species, and antifungal sensitivity. Calcium oxalate crystals can be seen in histopathology, apart from the other lesions.

## PATHOLOGIC FINDINGS

Air sacculitis is the most common form of the disease, sometimes extending into the lungs or blocking the ostia or bronchi. Thickened, milky air sac membranes infiltrated with large numbers of inflammatory cells and germinating conidia are usually observed. Germinating conidia may also be observed within macrophages. Fluid, plaques, adhesions, encapsulated granulomas tearing and invading different air sacs and body cavities in chronic form. Localised granulomas in trachea or around organs (heart, kidney, gonads).

# TREATMENT

## APPROPRIATE HEALTH CARE

The patient's overall stability will determine in-hospital management or outpatient care. The main goals of treatment are to stabilize, reduce stress, and improve patient's physical condition until complete resolution of infection.

## NURSING CARE

Maintain environmental temperature at 85–90°F (29–32°C) while providing a humidified environment. In some cases, Arctic species may benefit from low temperature. Supplemental oxygen support may be indicated in some advanced stages of disease. Fluid therapy: Warmed crystalloid fluids SQ, IV, IO (50–150 ml/kg/day maintenance plus dehydration deficit if needed) at a rate of 10–25 ml/kg over a 5-minute period or at a continuous rate of 100 ml/kg/q24h. Nutritional support if patient remains anorexic throughout treatment. Hepatoprotective products (milk thistle, lactulose, curcumin). Bronchodilator drugs (salbutamol) if needed.

## ACTIVITY

Stress reduction. Restricted activity should be maintained during this time to allow for complete resolution.

## DIET

Appropriate caloric intake should be closely monitored in the patient to maintain the overall health during treatment.

## CLIENT EDUCATION

Aspergillosis is generally a preventable disease when appropriate husbandry and dietary needs are met. Definitive diagnosis and successful treatment requires patience and persistence. Prolonged antifungal therapy (1–3 months) is often necessary and, despite various treatment approaches, failure to respond is not uncommon. Relapse common. Trained falconry raptors might lose their stamina.

## SURGICAL CONSIDERATIONS

Air sac cannulation, in cases of tracheal/syringeal blockage, may be performed within the caudal thoracic air sacs. Vacuum suction could help in the removal of tracheal/syringeal granulomas. Large granulomatous lesions that occlude air flow within the respiratory tract or are resistant to medical therapy (due to poor drug penetration) may require surgical/endosurgical debulking or, when possible, complete resection. Infections involving the sinus cavities may require trephination of the frontal sinuses permitting direct access for topical treatments and debridement as needed.

# MEDICATIONS

## DRUG(S) OF CHOICE

There is emerging azole resistance. Four avian *A. fumigatus* isolates were found resistant to both itraconazole and voriconazole; 22 isolates from penguins in the UK were resistant to itraconazole but sensitive to voriconazole and terbinafine. Based on various pharmacokinetic studies, the following drugs are recommended: **Gamebirds:** Itraconazole 10 mg/kg PO q12–24h terbinafine 15 mg/kg PO q12h. **Psittacines:** Amphotericin B (can be administered intratracheally, intravenously, in sinus flushes, and through nebulization). Systemic therapy: 1.5 mg/kg IV q8h for 3–5 days. Topical therapy: intratracheal use at 1 mg/kg q8–12h. Nebulization therapy: 1 mg/ml sterile water for 15 minutes q12h. Itraconazole—effective when administered with nebulized clotrimazole and/or amphotericin B (intravenous or nebulized): 5–10 mg/kg, PO q12–24h (not for grey parrots). Fluconazole—useful for treating ocular and CNS mycoses; less effective against aspergillosis than itraconazole systemically: 5–15 mg/kg PO q12h. Clotrimazole—used as topical/nebulization therapy in conjunction with other antifungals: Used as a 1% aqueous solution for 30 minutes q24h. Voriconazole 12–18 mg/kg, PO q12h (drug of choice for grey parrots). **Seabirds:** Itraconazole 10–20 mg/kg PO q24h. **Waterfowl:** Itraconazole 5–10 mg/kg PO q24h. Amphotericin B 3.25 mg/kg IV (in fluids) over 24h; 7.5 mg/kg intratracheally q8h; nebulization therapy: 12.5 mg diluted with 2.5 ml sterile water q24h for 7 days. **Raptors:** Terbinafine hydrochloride—excellent ability to penetrate mycotic granulomas; usually used in combination with itraconazole; lengthy treatment. Systemic therapy:10–15 mg/kg PO q12h. Nebulization therapy: 1 mg/ml (500 mg terbinafine plus 1 ml acetylcysteine plus 500 ml distilled water). Itraconazole 5–10 mg/kg PO q24h. Voriconazole 12.5 mg/kg, PO q12h for 3 days then q24h until resolution in falcons. Voriconazole 10–18 mg/kg PO q12h in hawks. Voriconazole 12.5 mg/kg IM q24h in falcons (empirical use based on PK study) faster resolution, easy application, no adverse effects.

## CONTRAINDICATIONS

N/A

## PRECAUTIONS

Amphotericin B is potentially nephrotoxic and should be used for a short duration. When nebulizing amphotericin B, a well-ventilated area should be used for the safety of staff members. Amphotericin B can be irritating when applied topically and should be diluted in water (saline inactivates amphotericin B) to reduce iatrogenic inflammation. African grey parrots are known to potentially be sensitive to itraconazole, sometimes exhibiting anorexia and depression. If used with this species, lower dosing and close monitoring of the patient is required. Itraconazole should be used with extreme caution in patients with liver impairment. Itraconazole can cause anorexia and liver impairment in falcons. Administration of fluconazole at 10 mg/kg q12h has been known to cause death in budgerigars. Administration of voriconazole can rarely cause blindness in falcons.

## POSSIBLE INTERACTIONS
Itraconazole: Coadministration with other drugs primarily metabolized by cytochrome enzyme system may lead to increased plasma concentrations of itraconazole and could increase or prolong both therapeutic and adverse effects. Voriconazole absorption is delayed by food, while posaconazole absorption is enhanced with a fatty meal and oil dilution.

## ALTERNATIVE DRUGS
Oral posaconazole pharmacokinetic model in falcons recommended at 20 mg/kg, diluted in plant oil 2:1. Itraconazole nanosuspension nebulization in quails and falcons has good tissue penetration. Antifungal subcutaneous implants may improve in future. Empirical use of oral/intramuscular isavuconazole in falcons did not produce superior results compared with voriconazole and exhibited liver impairment. Essential oil carvacrol produced prophylaxis and treatment in challenged chicken.

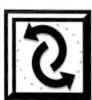

## FOLLOW-UP

## PATIENT MONITORING
Repeated survey radiographs, endoscopy, and CT may be used to assess treatment response. Serial biochemistry profiles (including protein electrophoresis) to monitor patient's condition during administration of antifungal medications are important.

## PREVENTION/AVOIDANCE
Minimizing exposure risk by proper diet, husbandry practices. Preventative health checks. Avoid OTC use or prescribed overuse of antifungals/antibiotics. Removal of old debris material from ground/aviary. Reducing stressors. Using HEPA filters regular cleaning and disinfection of aviaries/incubators/crates/transport boxes/nest boxes with essential oils and enilconazole prophylactic treatment of

susceptible species with essential oils, terbinafine or itraconazole before shipment, ownership/husbandry changes and extreme heat conditions, juvenile growth stage. Vaccination strategies so far are unsuccessful.

## POSSIBLE COMPLICATIONS
Long-term respiratory impairment or sensitivity may be observed after treatment, dependent upon severity of initial clinical disease. These changes may be noted on radiographs for the life of the bird. Birds might relapse after treatment. Ruptured air sacs might impair stamina and athletic performance in falconry raptors/free-flying birds.

## EXPECTED COURSE AND PROGNOSIS
Uncomplicated cases with early detection have a good prognosis; however, the prognosis is generally dependent upon the immune status, species, and chronicity of the illness. Infections affecting the nasal passageways may cause anatomical deformities to nares.

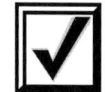

## MISCELLANEOUS

## ASSOCIATED CONDITIONS
N/A

## AGE-RELATED FACTORS
N/A

## ZOONOTIC POTENTIAL
Aspergillosis has been reported in humans but only acquired from the environment, not from contact with infected birds. It is considered non-contagious but recent studies imply contagiousness with airborne transmission among hospitalized human and avian patients.

## FERTILITY/BREEDING
N/A

## SYNONYMS
None.

## SEE ALSO
Aspiration Pneumonia
Mycobacteriosis
Oil Exposure
Oral Plaques
Pneumonia
Poxvirus
Respiratory Distress
Rhinitis and Sinusitis
Sick-Bird Syndrome
Tracheal and Syringeal Diseases
Trichomoniasis

## ABBREVIATIONS
AST—aspartate aminotransferase
CNS—central nervous system

HEPA—high-efficiency particulate air
LDH—lactate dehydrogenase
OTC—over the counter
PCR—polymerase chain reaction
PK—pyruvate kinase
PTFE—polytetrafluoroethylene
TAFC—triacetylfusarinine C

## INTERNET RESOURCES
N/A

*Suggested Reading*
Arné, P., Risco-Castillo, V., Jouvion, G., et al. (2021). Aspergillosis in wild birds. *Journal of Fungi*, 7:241.
Azmanis P., Anzoategui A., Di Somma A., et al. (2022). A retrospective study on prevalence of aspergillosis in juvenile falcons in United Arab Emirates and the effect of hybridization. Proceedings of 5th International Conference for Avian, Reptilian, Exotic Mammal Medicine, Budapest.
Azmanis, P., Pappalardo, L., Sara, Z.A., et al. (2021). Disposition of posaconazole after single oral administration in large falcons (*Falco* spp): Effect of meal and dosage and a non-compartmental model to predict effective dosage. *Medical Mycology*, 59:901–908.
Azmanis, P., Pappalardo, L., Sara, Z.A., et al. (2020). Pharmacokinetics of voriconazole after a single intramuscular injection in large falcons (*Falco* spp.). *Medical Mycology*, 58:661–666.
Hauck, R., Cray, C., França, M. (2020). Spotlight on avian pathology: aspergillosis. *Avian Pathology*, 49:115–118.
Lofgren, L.A., Lorch, J.M., Cramer, R.A., et al. (2022). Avian-associated *Aspergillus fumigatus* displays broad phylogenetic distribution, no evidence for host specificity, and multiple genotypes within epizootic events. *G3 (Bethesda)*, 12(5):jkac075.
Melo, A.M., Stevens, D.A., Tell, L.A., et al. (2020). Aspergillosis, avian species and the One Health perspective: the possible importance of birds in azole resistance. *Microorganisms*, 8:2037.
Savelieff, M.G., Pappalardo, L., Azmanis, P. (2018). The current status of avian aspergillosis diagnoses: Veterinary practice to novel research avenues. *Veterinary Clinical Pathology*, 47:342–362.
**Authors**: Panagiotis Azmanis, DVM, PhD, ECZM (Avian)
**Acknowledgement**: Gregory J. Costanzo, DVM, author of this chapter in the first edition.

 **Client Education Handout available online**

 BASICS

## DEFINITION
Injury to the lungs and air sacs caused by inhalation of fluid, food material, barium or vomitus.

## PATHOPHYSIOLOGY
Aspirated materials may follow air flow pattern in the avian respiratory system: First inspiration: Air moves into caudal thoracic and abdominal air sacs. First exhalation: Air moves into lungs. Second inspiration: Air moves in cranial thoracic and intraclavicular air sacs. Second exhalation: Air moves out. Aspiration: Due to unidirectional airflow, aspiration most often occurs in the caudal thoracic and abdominal air sacs. Triggers inflammatory response in the lower respiratory tract. Causes physical obstruction of the airway system. If bird survives acute episode, they can develop chronic weight loss, abscessation, secondary infections and persistent leukocytosis. Damages the respiratory epithelium.

## SYSTEMS AFFECTED
Respiratory. Cardiac—secondary to respiratory changes. Upper GI tract—as a primary cause of aspiration.

## GENETICS
N/A

## INCIDENCE/PREVALENCE
Not reported.

## GEOGRAPHIC DISTRIBUTION
N/A

## SIGNALMENT
Leading cause of respiratory disease in hand-fed psittacines that are near weaning. Common occurrence in ducks and geese in the foie gras industry. Aspiration occurs in budgerigars on a seed diet or those fed a diet low in iodine. Some birds including New World vultures vomit upon capture and restraint.

## SIGNS
### General Comments
The more chronic form of aspiration pneumonia is more likely to result in weight loss.

### Historical Findings
Cough-like sound shortly after syringe feeding. Death shortly after feeding. Recent history of eating. Poor weight gain in chicks. Recent history of anesthesia. Regurgitation/vomiting. Chronic weight loss. Recent barium administration, oral medication administration or gavage feeding.

### Physical Examination Findings
Acute death, anorexia, clicking/crackles in air sac auscultation, cough after feeding, crop distention, cyanosis, depression, dyspnea, fluffed appearance, frictional rubs on auscultation, intermittent dyspnea, lethargy, loud inspiratory sound, mass effect in the neck, open-mouthed breathing, prolonged exercise tolerance test. Respiratory rate should return to normal within 2 minutes in normal patient. Regurgitation/vomiting, sitting at bottom of cage, tachypnea, tail bobbing, thin body condition, vomitus crusted around nares or face, weakness.

## CAUSES
**Iatrogenic**: Hand feeding—resisted attempts at feeding; performed by inexperienced individuals. Overflow/overfilling of barium, supplemental feeding or oral medications. Improper restraint and capture of vultures.
**GI disease**: Any GI disease that causes vomiting or regurgitation or an esophageal motility disorder—heavy metal toxicosis, foreign body ingestion, infectious gastrointestinal disease (PDD, parasites crop mycoses), ingestion of oral irritants, rancid diet, pancreatitis, renal failure, hepatopathy, septicemia, polyoma virus–GI hypomotility.
**Courtship behavior**.
**Neoplasia**: Intraluminal or extraluminal neoplasia of the mouth, esophagus, neck, gastrointestinal disease.
**Goiter**: In budgerigars, secondary to a diet low in iodine.
**Neurologic or cardiac disease**: Any disease that causes generalized weakness and loss of aspiration-protective mechanisms.
**Near drowning**.

## RISK FACTORS
Gastrointestinal disease, weakness and debilitation, anesthesia, weaning.

 DIAGNOSIS

## DIFFERENTIAL DIAGNOSIS
Infectious respiratory disease: fungal (aspergillosis), bacterial, viral, parasitic; ascites; reproductive disease; neoplasia; anemia; respiratory toxins/irritants (PTFE, smoke, aerosols, candles, $CO_2$); vitamin A deficiency (thinning and weakening of respiratory epithelium); pulmonary hypersensitivity; tachypnea from pain or metabolic disease; normal behavior (growl of grey parrots; hiss of cockatoo species; normal moist respiratory sounds in the Pionus spp.; mimicry of human cough or sneeze); pneumoconiosis; ruptured air sac.

## CBC/BIOCHEMISTRY/URINALYSIS
**Biochemistry**: Globulin elevations and decreased A:G ratio; other non-specific changes.
**Hemogram**: Leukocytosis with heterophilia and monocytosis; polycythemia of 60–80% (chronic hypoxia); lead toxicosis; anemia; basophilic stippling; cytoplasmic vacuolization of red blood cells; hemolytic anemia and icterus in zinc toxicosis.

## OTHER LABORATORY TESTS
**Microbiology**: Culture of bacteria and fungi; blood culture may be positive with concurrent sepsis.
**Electrophoresis**: Inflammatory pattern; differentiates between acute and chronic.
**Lead levels**: 0.3–0.6 µg/ml highly suggestive; > 0.6 µg/ml diagnostic.
**Transtracheal wash**: Mild sedation can be used; instill and aspirate 1–2 ml/kg sterile saline (expect 25–50% recovery rate).
**Air sac lavage**: Place IVC or red rubber catheter (in larger birds) in last intercostal space; alternatively, use endoscope. Enter the caudal thoracic or abdominal air sacs; instill and aspirate 3–5 ml/kg sterile saline.

## IMAGING
### Radiographic Findings
Ventrodorsal and lateral radiographic projections recommended. May be normal in acute presentations. General anesthesia is often required for proper positioning. Balance risk/benefit to patient based on patient stability. Results: Neoplasia—space occupying lesions, soft-tissue densities. GI disease—crop distention, dilated proventriculus, generalized ileus. Aspiration pneumonia and airsacculitis—increased radiodensity or accentuation of the honeycomb pattern of the lungs; focal to diffuse abnormal densities of the abdominal air sacs; loss of definition of the air sacs or change in size; air sac hyperinflation. Toxicosis—metal densities.

### Ultrasonography
Soft-tissue masses, ascites, reproductive tract abnormalities.

### Advanced Imaging
**MRI/CT**: Provide more detailed information especially lesions that are too small to identify radiographically. Prevents superimposition of structures. MRI has disadvantage of long scanning time.

## DIAGNOSTIC PROCEDURES
Endoscopy: Provides direct visualization of lesions. Minimally invasive. Obtain air sac wash, culture or tissue biopsies. Removal of metallic foreign bodies.

## PATHOLOGIC FINDINGS
**Air sacs**: Vomitus or barium; airsacculitits; variable necrosis, yellow-white or grey exudate. Chronic: Caseous masses.

**Lungs**: Generally edematous, firm, fibrin accumulation and congested ± haemorrhage. Loss of the sharp honeycomb pattern. Irregular areas appear opaque red to brown. On cut surface, it may be possible to see the aspirated material within larger airways.

**Bone marrow changes**: Chronic hypoxia leads to increased erythrocyte precursors and polycythemia.

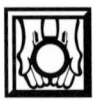

## TREATMENT

### APPROPRIATE HEALTH CARE
Inpatient or outpatient care depends on patient status. Acute aspiration or those with multisystemic signs (anorexia, lethargy, weight loss) are more likely to require hospitalization. Stabilize all compromised patients prior to diagnostic procedures. Airsac tube may partially improve respiration.

### NURSING CARE
Immediately place all dyspneic birds in 78–85% $O_2$ concentration at a flow rate of 5 L/minute. Supplemental heat at 85–90°F (29–32°C). Minimize tissue bruising from injections in neonates.

### ACTIVITY
Activity should be restricted until symptoms resolve.

### DIET
If the patient is vomiting, regurgitating or has an esophageal motility disorder, feed multiple small meals of easily digestible diet. Nutritional support via gavage feeding for anorexic patients: Gavage 5% of body weight initially and slowly increase up to 8–10% to avoid aspiration; crop emptying can take 2–4 hours. Use IV/IO routes in very debilitated birds. Complete the weaning process in psittacine chicks.

### CLIENT EDUCATION
Discourage hand feeding in novice aviculturalists. Discourage mating behavior. Iodine deficiency: change to an appropriate diet with the proper amount of iodine. Airborne toxin exposure: immediately remove to fresh oxygen. Prevent access to toxins and toxic metals. Warn owners that birds in severe respiratory distress or barium aspiration have a poor prognosis.

### SURGICAL CONSIDERATIONS
Fasting: Ensure an empty crop prior to surgery, typically 2–3 hours (up to 4 hours) in parrots; raptors can require up to 12 hours. Fasting may not be recommended in birds under 200 g. Aspirate crop contents if fasting

is not possible. Be cautious with anesthesia due to respiratory compromise and the inability to measure oxygen saturation in avian species. Surgical removal of space occupying masses and metallic foreign bodies.

## MEDICATIONS

### DRUG(S) OF CHOICE
Start **broad-spectrum antibiotics** (fluoroquinolone, trimethroprim-sulfamethoxazole, amoxicillin/clavulanic acid). Choose antibiotics based on culture when possible. Add antifungal medications for secondary yeast and fungal infections—nystatin, itraconazole, voriconazole, fluconazole.

**Bronchodilators**: Beta-agonists—both relax smooth muscle and decrease airway inflammation; less toxic in aerosolized form; terbutaline 0.01 mg/kg IM q6h followed by nebulization at 0.01 mg/kg in 9 cc saline. Methylxanthines—theophylline has been used at a dose of 2 mg/kg PO q12h. Aminophylline 10 mg/kg IV q6–8h, 4 mg/kg IM q6–12h, and 5 mg/kg PO q12h. Adverse effects include CNS excitation, vomiting and tachycardia. May be less effective at bronchodilation in birds, but clinical improvement has been noted with their use. Use limited to birds that fail to respond to beta-agonist treatment.

**Anti-anxiety analgesic**: Butorphanol 1–2 mg/kg IM q2–3h.

**Chelation and bulking agents for lead toxicosis**: Succimer 25–35 mg/kg PO q12h × 5 of 7 days, for 3–5 weeks. CaEDTA 35 mg/kg IM q12h × 5 days, discontinue for 3–4 days then repeat as necessary. Give concurrent fluid therapy to prevent renal injury. Broad-spectrum antibiotics due to immunosuppression of lead.

**Fluid therapy**: Warm fluids to 100-104°F (37.8–40°C). Hypotonic fluids contraindicated in birds with salt glands. Subcutaneous or oral fluids indicated for mild levels of blood loss and maintenance. Crystalloids should be sufficient. Correct for 4–5% of fluid loss (0.04–0.05 × body weight kg × 1000) in addition to maintenance. Divide into multiple doses as dictated by volume. SQ fluids—Place up to 10 cc/kg in each SQ injection site. Use the inguinal web, intrascapular and axillary areas. LRS absorbs well.

**IO/IV fluids**: Indicated for moderate levels of blood loss, surgery or hypothermia. Allows for rapid administration and dissemination of fluids.

**IV catheter** (22–26 g catheter in jugular, basophilic, ulnar or medial metatarsal vein); may be difficult in birds < 100 g.

**IO catheter**: Distal ulna or proximal tibiotarsus. Confirm placement with radiographs. Correct for 4–8% of fluid loss (0.04–0.08 × body weight kg × 1000) in addition to maintenance. 80% of fluid deficit should be replaced over 6–8 hours in acute loss and over 12–24 hours in chronic loss. Consider adding a colloid (3–5 ml/kg), especially if hypotensive, hypovolemia or hypoproteinemia. Plasmalyte A closest to avain plasma.

**Nebulization**: Non-invasive, non-stressful technique. Equipment must produce particles < 3µg in diameter to reach air capillaries. Equipment that produces larger particles can be used to reach the air sacs caudal to the lungs. Remove particles from feathers of birds to minimize oral ingestion. In one study with pigeons, nebulization of 30 minutes to 1 hour resulted in minimal particles in lower airway. Nebulization for 2–4 hours resulted in better penetration; 0.9% saline; 0.1% terbutaline within saline; antibiotics.

### CONTRAINDICATIONS
Fluid therapy contraindicated in hypovolemia, hypothermia, and shock due to peripheral vasoconstriction. Hypertonic fluids and colloids and fluids containing > 2.5% dextrose contraindicated in brown pelicans and turkey vultures. Colloids contraindicated in coagulopathy, CHF, renal disease, pneumonia. LRS contraindicated for rapid effusion. IO catheter contraindicated in the ulna of Cathartiformes. Steroids. Careful use of oral medications if the patient has been vomiting, regurgitation or motility disorder. Propranolol, other beta-blockers.

### PRECAUTIONS
N/A

### POSSIBLE INTERACTIONS
N/A

### ALTERNATIVE DRUGS
N/A

## FOLLOW-UP

### PATIENT MONITORING
CBC for resolution of leukocytosis. Radiologic resolution of signs (less reliable).

### PREVENTION/AVOIDANCE
Avoid hand feeding chicks by an inexperienced individual. Discourage mating behavior. Feed chicks 10% of body

weight per feeding. Frequency of feeding varies with species.

## POSSIBLE COMPLICATIONS
Granuloma formation in lungs or air sacs. Poor weight gain of chicks. Acute death.

## EXPECTED COURSE AND PROGNOSIS
Depends on the severity of the disease. Prognosis is more guarded in young or immune compromised individual.

 MISCELLANEOUS

## ASSOCIATED CONDITIONS
Polycythemia, crop burn, pharyngeal or esophageal punctures.

## AGE-RELATED FACTORS
Condition more common in young (weaning) birds.

## ZOONOTIC POTENTIAL
N/A

## FERTILITY/BREEDING
N/A

## SYNONYMS
None.

## SEE ALSO
Enteritis and Gastritis
Foreign Bodies (Gastrointestinal)
Ileus (Functional Gastrointestinal, Crop Stasis)
Pneumonia

Regurgitation and Vomiting
Respiratory Distress
Sick-Bird Syndrome
Thyroid Disease
Toxicosis (Heavy Metals)
Toxicosis (Ingested, Gastrointestinal)

## ABBREVIATIONS
CaEDTA—calcium disodium ethylenediamine tetraacetate
CNS—central nervous system
CT—computed tomography
GI—gastrointestinal
IVC—intravenous catheter
LRS—lactated Ringer's solution
MRI—magnetic resonance imaging
PDD—proventricular dilatation disease
PTFE—polytetrafluoroethylene

## INTERNET RESOURCES
N/A

*Suggested Reading*
Chitty, J. (2009). The use of nebulization in avian respiratory disease. *AAVAC Annual Conference, Adelaide, Proceedings*. Association of Avian Veterinarians, Australasian Committee. https://www.aavac.com.au/files/2009-01.pdf (accessed 31 December 2023).
Crosta, L. (2021). Respiratory diseases of parrots: Anatomy, physiology, diagnosis and treatment. *Veterinary Clinics of North America: Exotic Animal Practice*, 24:397–418.
Carpenter, J.W., Harms, C.A. (2022). *Exotic Animal Formulary*, 6th edn. St. Louis, MO: Elsevier.
Doneley, B. (2016). *Avian Medicine and Surgery in Practice*. Boca Raton, FL: CRC Press.
Fordham, M., Roberts, B.K. (eds.) (2016). Exotic pet and wildlife emergency medicine for the small animal practitioner. *Veterinary Clinics of North America: Exotic Animal Practice*, 19(2): xiii–xiv. https://doi.org/10.1016/j.cvex.2016.02.001
Gage, L.J., Duerr, R.S. (2007). *Hand-Rearing Birds*. Ames IO: Blackwell Publishing.
Harrison, G.J., Lightfoot, T.L. (2011). *Clinical Avian Medicine*. Palm Beach, FL: Spix Publishing.
Orosz, S.E., Lichtenberger, M. (2011). Avian respiratory distress: Etiology, diagnosis and treatment. *Veterinary Clinics of North America: Exotic Animal Practice*, 14:241–255.
Petritz, O.A. (2014). Approach to the Dyspneic Bird. *Exotic Animal Medicine for the Clinical Practitioner Conference*, AAZV 2014. https://www.vin.com/apputil/content/defaultadv1.aspx?id=6852135&pid=12132& (accessed 31 December 2023).
Schmidt, R.E. (2013). The avian respiratory system. Western Veterinary Conference.
Schmidt, R.E., Reavill, D.R., Phalen, D.N. (eds.) (2015). *Pathology of Pet and Aviary Birds* 2nd edn. Hoboken, NJ: Wiley.
**Author**: Erika Cervasio, DVM, DABVP (Avian, Feline, Canine)
**Acknowledgement/s**: Kristin Vyhnal, DVM, MS, DACVP; Barbara Oglesbee, DVM

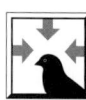
# BASICS

## DEFINITION
Atherosclerosis is an inflammatory and degenerative disease of the arterial wall characterized by the disorganization of the arterial wall due to the accumulation of fat, cholesterol, calcium, cellular debris, and inflammatory cells, and potentially leading to complications such as stenosis, ischemia, thrombosis, hemorrhage, and aneurysm. Atherosclerotic diseases include a spectrum of disease processes caused by atherosclerotic lesions such as coronary arterial disease, ischemic conditions, strokes, and peripheral arterial disease.

## PATHOPHYSIOLOGY
Response-to-injury hypothesis: Oxidative damage of the vascular endothelium and endothelial dysfunction promoted by risk factors set the stage for atherogenesis. Subendothelial retention of oxidized lipoproteins and other compounds, proliferation and accumulation of macrophages and other inflammatory cells, proliferation of vascular smooth muscle cells and formation of fibrous tissue. Histologic lesions progressed from subendothelial and medial accumulation of lipid vacuoles and foam cells to atheromatous plaque formation further expanding in a large lipidonecrotic core that may be covered by a fibrous cap (fibroatheromatous lesion). Progressive flow-limiting stenosis of the arterial lumen (advanced lesion types) is the main mechanism of atherosclerotic diseases in birds. It leads to chronic hypoperfusion and chronic ischemia of the supplied anatomical areas such as the heart, neurological system, and locomotory muscles. The increased vascular resistance at the great vessels may lead to increased afterload and cardiac failure. The chronic cardiac ischemia may lead to cardiac arrhythmias. Atherothrombosis (rupture of the fibrous cap and exposure of the thrombotic material to the circulation) and emboli may also occur but are rare in birds in comparison to mammals, particularly humans. This seems to be associated with the decreased ability of avian thrombocytes to form shear-resistant three-dimensional aggregates compared with mammalian platelets. Ruptured vascular aneurysm may be due to atherosclerotic lesions. In most birds the brachiocephalic arteries, ascending aorta, and carotid arteries are most frequently affected but lesions in the abdominal aorta, pulmonary arteries (cor pulmonale), coronary arteries, and peripheral arteries are not uncommon. Distribution of lesions may be different between avian species.

## SYSTEMS AFFECTED
**Cardiovascular**: Atheromatous, fibroatheromatous, and atherothrombotic lesions of the arteries. Chronic or acute ischemia of the myocardium potentially leading to cardiac arrhythmias, ischemic cardiomyopathy, coronary arterial disease, increased afterload. Peripheral arterial disease.
**Endocrine/Metabolic**: Associated with multiple endocrine factors (metabolic syndrome) and dyslipidemia.
**Hepatobiliary**: Frequently associated with liver lipid disorders.
**Musculoskeletal**: May be associated with ischemic muscle lesions and resulting muscular signs.
**Nervous**: May cause central neurological signs due to carotid atherosclerosis, central ischemia, hypoperfusion, or strokes.
**Respiratory**: Respiratory signs are common.

## GENETICS
A genetic basis has been demonstrated in several research breeds of birds: White Carneau pigeon—autosomal recessive trait. This pigeon breed has constitutive differences in the arterial wall compared with racing pigeons. Susceptible to experimental atherosclerosis: Japanese quail. Restricted ovulatory chicken: mutation in the VLDL receptor gene.

## INCIDENCE/PREVALENCE
Only the postmortem prevalence has been determined. Antemortem prevalence of atherosclerotic diseases or subclinical atherosclerosis is not well known. Reported in most avian groups and common in a variety of species of falconiformes, accipitriformes, bucerotiformes, coraciiformes, piciformes, galliformes, columbiformes, and sphenisciformes. Turkeys have high prevalence of atherosclerosis in the wild.
**Psittaciformes**: Common, raw prevalence around 7% but depends on many risk factors (see below), prevalence of atherothrombotic disease is low, approximately 0.1% (2% of advanced atherosclerotic lesions). In susceptible psittacine species, a 50% prevalence of advanced lesions is observed at 30–40 years.

## GEOGRAPHIC DISTRIBUTION
N/A

## SIGNALMENT
**Species**: Most species are susceptible but the following have been found to be particularly predisposed: Cockatiels, quaker parrots, Amazon parrots, grey parrots, kite species, turkeys, pigeons, and falcons (gyrfalcons and insectivorous falcons).
**Mean age and range**: Atherosclerosis has been reported in all ages but is more common in older birds, particularly in susceptible psittacine birds older than 20 years.

**Predominant sex**: Female psittaciformes have a higher risk than males (except Quaker parrots, for which males are at higher risks), the prevalence of which lags behind that of females by an average of 4 years. In poultry, males seem more commonly affected than females. A study in Californian raptors found a higher prevalence in female raptors.

## SIGNS
### General Comments
Atherosclerotic lesions are generally silent until either flow-limiting stenosis ensues (common and depends on the degree of narrowing) or lesion complications (rare) such as plaque rupture and thrombosis occur. The impact of subclinical atherosclerosis is unknown in birds and is likely a comorbid lesion to a variety of metabolic and endocrine disorders. Clinical signs partly depend on the affected arteries and the types of atherosclerotic lesions such as large fibroatheromatous, thrombotic plaques or aneurysms.

### Historical Findings
Sudden death. Nonspecific signs: lethargy, anorexia, weight loss, decreased activity.
• Muscular signs: permanent or intermittent leg weakness (intermittent claudication), falling off perches, ataxia, gangrene of the legs.
• Neurologic signs: obtundation, altered consciousness, seizures, ataxia, central neurological signs.
• Cardiac signs: abdominal distention, exercise intolerance, dyspnea, syncopes.
• Respiratory signs: dyspnea.

### Physical Examination Findings
No specific signs are detected on the physical examination in most instances but this depends on the type of atherosclerotic disease and the location of the lesions. The bird may be overconditioned or thin. Signs consistent with impaired cardiovascular function may be noticed such as abdominal distention, cardiac murmur and arrhythmias upon cardiac auscultation, cyanosis and dyspnea upon restraint. Abnormalities during a neurological examination may be noted and are usually related to central lesions such as cranial nerves deficits, altered consciousness, and postural abnormalities. Intermittent claudication-like signs have been seen in Amazon parrots and other birds.

## CAUSES
Risk factors associated with captive lifestyle may promote the occurrence and severity of atherosclerotic lesions (see Pathophysiology and Risk Factors sections for further details).

## RISK FACTORS
Few studies have adequately investigated the epidemiology and risk factors of avian atherosclerosis and most information is found

in psittaciformes. Findings in psittacine birds may not translate well to other avian groups, especially those with markedly different biology such as carnivorous birds. Likewise, the large body of human scientific information may not always be relevant to avian atherosclerosis, but some risk factors are anticipated to be similar when considering similarities in lesion progression, structure, and pathogenesis. In addition, risk factors are usually related to clinical atherosclerotic disease and not necessarily to subclinical atherosclerosis. Since atherosclerotic lesions are challenging to diagnose, atherosclerotic disease is usually a rule out diagnosis suggested by supportive epidemiology and risk factors.

**Epidemiologic risk factors**: Age. Psittaciformes: Female gender (males in Quaker parrots). This may be associated with vitellogenesis, high plasma lipid levels, and cholesterol transportation to the egg in reproductively active females. Species: Quaker parrots, cockatiels, grey parrots, Amazon parrots, gyrfalcons, lesser kestrel, black kites, Brahminy kites, pigeons, turkeys. Species predisposition may only reflect inadequate captive diet. In psittaciformes, susceptible species were found to have higher cholesterol than less susceptible species. Atherosclerosis has been reported in virtually all avian groups.

**Lifestyle risk factors**: A captive lifestyle characterized with ad libitum provision of food, unnatural diet, restricted exercise, increased stress may promote atherosclerosis. In some species, wild birds show a lower prevalence than their captive counterparts. Second-hand smoking in a household may be a risk factor in companion birds. Diet. Psittaciformes: A high fat and nutrient-deficient diet such as all-seed diet may promote atherogenesis. Saturated fat, in particular from animal-based diet, may also be deleterious as most psittacine birds have evolved to eat seeds, fruits, and flower products. A lack of polyunsaturated fatty acids (omega 3 and 6) has also been implicated. Birds of prey: The feeding of day-old chicks may promote atherosclerosis in susceptible species. Feeding unnatural prey items such as day-old chicks or mice to insectivorous species or limited fish to fish-eating species may also be atherogenic.

**Physiopathological risk factors**: Elevated blood pressure: Indirect blood pressure measurement is not reliable in most small to medium sized parrots. Turkeys have extremely high blood pressure. Obesity. Reproductive activity and diseases in female birds. Chlamydia psittaci infection: Controversial and likely not a major risk factor. Marek's disease (gallid herpesvirus 2 and 3) in chickens.

**Dyslipidemic risk factors**: In humans, dyslipidemic risk factors are the most important by far and include raised total, LDL, and non-LDL cholesterol, and low-HDL cholesterol. Other dyslipidemic risk factors of lesser importance include raised triglycerides, lipoprotein(a), apolipoprotein B, "small, dense" LDL, increased LDL particle number, and postprandial lipemia. In birds, dyslipidemic risk factors and their importance have not been well characterized. Total cholesterol level has been found to be a risk factor in multiple species and predisposed species tend to have higher blood cholesterol levels. Lipoprotein risk factors are unknown and are suspected to differ from humans owing to different lipoprotein metabolism in birds. Quaker parrots seem to be extremely susceptible to dyslipidemia in captivity and have higher cholesterol levels than most other psittacine species. Female birds may exhibit physiological increase in total cholesterol, tryglycerides, VLDL, total calcium, total proteins during reproductive activity and vittelogenesis. While physiological, maladaptive and unregulated reproductive activity is common in captive female psittacine birds, which may be atherogenic.

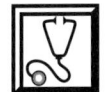 **DIAGNOSIS**

### DIFFERENTIAL DIAGNOSIS
Any cardiovascular or neurological disease may be a differential diagnosis. Since the diagnosis of atherosclerotic diseases is rarely achieved antemortem, all differential diagnosis must be ruled out first.
**Cardiac disease**: Dilated cardiomyopathy, valvular insufficiency, myocarditis, arrhythmias, other causes of congestive heart failure.
**Hind limb paresis**: Trauma, spinal disease, muscular disease, egg binding, viral neuritis.

### CBC/BIOCHEMISTRY/URINALYSIS
Hematologic and biochemistry tests are only intended to diagnose and assess the associated risk factors or consequences of atherosclerotic lesions but have limited value for atherosclerosis diagnosis itself. Only demonstration of the lesions is diagnostic.
**Dyslipidemia**: Elevated total cholesterol, elevated triglycerides, variable lipoprotein abnormalities (LDL, non-HDL increase). Needs to be differentiated from physiological increase in blood lipids in female birds.
**Liver enzymes and bile acids**: May be elevated in case of concurrent hepatic lipidosis, bile acids may be mildly elevated in hepatic congestion consecutive to congestive heart failure.
**Creatinine kinase**: May be elevated in repeated falling, ischemic myositis, or seizures.

### OTHER LABORATORY TESTS
Lipoprotein profiles may be useful for diagnosis or management of the associated dyslipidemia, if any. The recommended panel includes total cholesterol, HDL-cholesterol, triglycerides with calculated values of non-HDL-cholesterol, and total cholesterol/HDL-cholesterol ratio. LDL-cholesterol cannot be reliably measured using standard analyzers in birds and the indirect estimation (e.g. Friedewald formula) are inaccurate (see Dyslipidemia/Hyperlipidemia chapter). Inflammatory (acute phase proteins) and cardiac (troponins) markers have not been investigated in relation to avian atherosclerosis but may be useful.

### IMAGING
Diagnostic imaging is presently the only mean to diagnose atherosclerotic lesions, all laboratory tests focusing on dyslipidemic and inflammatory risk factors. Antemortem confirmed diagnosis is rarely achieved. There are two strategies to image atherosclerotic lesions: detecting arterial luminal stenosis and detecting arterial calcification.

#### Radiographic Findings
Radiographic findings: Calcification of the large arteries at the base of the heart or along the abdominal aorta is very specific for advanced atherosclerotic lesions, susceptible to cause clinical signs. However, it is seldom detected on radiographs. Enlargement and increased radiodensity of the large vessels at the base of the heart may be noticed but is highly subjective. The pulmonary veins, which are not susceptible to atherosclerosis, should not be confused with other vessels on the lateral view. Abnormalities associated with congestive heart failure: pulmonary edema (uncommon), ascites, hepatomegaly, reduced air sac volume.

#### Advanced Imaging
**Angiographic findings**: Can be performed using radiography, fluoroscopy (a fluoroscopic protocol has been published in Amazon parrots), and CT (a CT angiography protocol has been published in Amazon parrots and grey parrots). Arterial luminal narrowing. Aneurysmal dilation. Cardiomegaly.
**CT findings**: Calcification of the large arteries, more sensitive than radiographs at detecting calcification. A calcium score may be performed using free imaging softwares. Cardiomegaly and other signs of congestive heart failure.
**MRI findings**: Indicated in case of brain lesion, especially in the diagnosis of ischemic and hemorrhagic strokes.
**Echocardiographic findings**: Hyperechogenicity at the base of the ascending aorta may indicate mineralization.

Note that there are normal cartilages that can be mineralized at the base of the aorta and pulmonary arteries in birds. Evidence of cardiac dysfunction and congestive heart failure—valvular insufficiency, decreased ventricular fractional shortening, chamber enlargement, pericardial effusion. Evidence of stenosis and increased arterial velocities on pulse-wave/continuous wave spectral Doppler.
**Positron emission tomography**: Has been used to detect microcalcification in research parrots using 18F sodium fluoride as a specific radiotracer.

### DIAGNOSTIC PROCEDURES
**Rigid endoscopy**: Atherosclerotic lesions may be visualized on various arteries during a coelioscopic examination. The interclavicular approach allows the assessment of the brachiocephalic arteries and ascending aorta, but fat accumulation may be present in overweight birds at this location.
**Electrocardiography**: Arrhythmias consecutive to chronic ischemia and secondary cardiac effects of atherosclerotic lesions may be detected but have not been well characterized.

### PATHOLOGIC FINDINGS
This may not be obvious in small birds. Lesions occur most commonly on the brachiocephalic arteries, ascending aorta, carotid arteries but are also frequently found on the pulmonary arteries and intramyocardial coronary arteries. The thoracic and abdominal aorta, and other peripheral arteries may also be affected. Vascular aneurysm may occur and rupture leaving blood in the coelomic cavity.
**Histopathology**: A classification system has been proposed for psittacine atherosclerotic lesions with seven lesion types: Type I and II: Minimal changes characterized by isolated foam cells or multiple foam cell layers. Type III: Preatheromatous lesion with isolated pools of extracellular lipid forming confluent areas with minimal disruption of the arterial architecture. Type IV: Atheromatous lesion with the presence of a large lipid core with significant disruption of the arterial architecture, narrowing of the lumen, and calcification. Type V: Fibroatheroma characterized by the formation of a fibrous cap over the lipid core. Type VI: Complicated lesion by hematoma, fissure, or thrombosis. Type VII: Calcific lesion, osseous metaplasia, large calcium plaques but with minimal lipid deposition. Nonvascular lesions have also been found in association with atherosclerosis: Myocardial fibrosis, myocardial hypertrophy, myocardial infarction. Hepatic diseases. Pulmonary lesions.

 **TREATMENT**

### APPROPRIATE HEALTH CARE
When clinical signs of atherosclerotic diseases are evident, the prognosis is usually guarded and treatment of limited efficacy. Overall treatment is divided into the reduction of risk factors and the treatment of cardiovascular and ischemic consequences. Drastic reduction of risk factors is advised and has shown to reduce vascular atherosclerotic burden in mammalian species.

### NURSING CARE
Nursing care depends on the clinical presentation and the reader is referred to corresponding sections on cardiac and neurological diseases. Supportive care should be provided such as fluid replacement therapy, nutritional support, heat support, and oxygen therapy if dyspnea is present. Ascitic fluid should be drained to improve breathing.

### ACTIVITY
Increased physical activity may be beneficial in prevention and treatment of dyslipidemia and atherosclerosis.

### DIET
The provision of a balanced diet supplemented with fruits and vegetables is probably the most important aspect of the treatment in captive parrots. Decreasing the overall amount of food may be beneficial, especially in overconditioned birds. Discontinue the feeding of animal products to psittacine birds. Non-animal items do not contain any cholesterol. Switch to a pelletized diet if the bird is on an all-seed diet. Low-fat pelletized diet such as Roudybush® (Roudybush, Inc., Woodland, CA) Low Fat may be beneficial in some cases. Omega-3 fatty acids may help. They can be provided, among other items, with flaxseeds, walnuts, flaxseed oil, and fish oil. Fish oil has been found to be more effective than flaxseed oil at lowering blood lipids in cockatiels. In birds of prey, day-old chicks should probably be limited or avoided in highly susceptible species such as gyrfalcons, insectivorous species, and kites.

### CLIENT EDUCATION
Atherosclerosis is a chronic disease with a long latency period that develops over decades. Offering a healthy captive lifestyle to pet birds and other captive birds may significantly reduce the likelihood of developing atherosclerotic diseases later on in life. Owners should promote physical

exercises by limiting time spent in a cage environment and providing increased physical space and complexity (e.g., free flying in the house, foraging tree, playground areas). As most birds are flying animals and their heart rate increase by more than four times during flight, flight activities may be beneficial. The diet should be balanced and adapted to the species. Captive psittacine birds should preferentially be fed a pelletized diet supplemented with fruits and vegetables and omega-3 polyunsaturated fatty acids. Some species are adapted to consume higher fat diet than others (e.g., macaws, palm cockatoos). Decreasing reproductive stimuli in pet birds. Owners should be made aware of major epidemiologic factors such species and gender susceptibility and increase frequency with age. It is wise to remind owners that older parrots may have severe subclinical lesions that may significantly impact medical management and anesthesia.

### SURGICAL CONSIDERATIONS
N/A

 **MEDICATIONS**

### DRUG(S) OF CHOICE
Only limited information is available for most drugs listed below. Most is empirical and pharmacological information has rarely been obtained in birds. For treatment of heart failure, please see corresponding section.
**Statins**: Lipid lowering agents, which are competitive inhibitors of the HMG-CoA reductase enzyme in hepatic cholesterol synthesis. Pharmacokinetic studies on rosuvastatin in Amazon parrots failed to reach therapeutic concentrations at 10–25 mg/kg. Atorvastatin 20 mg/kg PO q12–24h can be recommended in Amazon parrots and cockatiels based on pharmacokinetic studies. Atorvastatin 20 mg/kg PO q12h for 2 weeks in Quaker parrots and atorvastatin 10 mg/kg PO q12h in Amazon parrots did not lead to significant decrease in blood lipids. Additional pharmacological studies on statins are ongoing. Other statins of interest include simvastatin, lovastatin, pravastatin, and fluvastatin. Should not be taken while feeding grapefruits and concurrently with azole antifungals. Statins also have non-lipid effects such as beneficial properties on endothelial function, vascular inflammation, immune modulation, oxidative stress, thrombosis, and plaque stabilization.
**Fibrates**: Hypolipidemic drugs, which are agonists of PPARα that stimulates β-oxidation

of fatty acids. Fibrates mainly cause a decrease in blood triglycerides. Gemfibrozil and fenofibrate. No pharmacokinetic information are available in companion birds.

**Other lipid lowering agents**: Include cholesterol absorption inhibitors (ezetimibe) and nicotinic acid.

**Blood pressure medications**: In case systemic hypertension can be documented, ACE-inhibitors (enalapril 1.25–5 mg/kg q12h PO or benazepril) or beta-blockers may be used. Beta-blockers have also been shown to reduce the progression of atherosclerosis in poultry.

**Antithrombotic medications**: Due to the low prevalence of atherothrombosis and emboli, preventive antithrombotic treatment is probably not warranted in birds. Aspirin, cilostazol, and clopidogrel may be employed.

**Peripheral vasodilators**: For the treatment of signs attributable to peripheral arterial disease (e.g., intermittent claudication). Cilostazol is the drug of choice in humans and also inhibits platelet aggregation. Pentoxifylline 15 mg/kg q12h PO and isoxsuprine may also be used.

**GnRH agonists**: (Leuprolide acetate, subcutaneous deslorelin implant) may be given to decrease reproductive hyperlipidemia and as part of the treatment of reproductive conditions.

## CONTRAINDICATIONS
N/A

## PRECAUTIONS
Statins and fibrates may cause rhabdomyolysis and myalgia.

## POSSIBLE INTERACTIONS
The combination of statins with fibrates may increase the risk of rhabdomyolysis. Some statins (e.g. atorvastatin) interact with drugs metabolized through the cytochrome P450 pathway such as azole antifungals. Grapefruit should not be fed to birds receiving statins, which may increase plasma levels.

## ALTERNATIVE DRUGS
N/A

 FOLLOW-UP

## PATIENT MONITORING
The lipid panel should be monitored at regular intervals in case of dyslipidemia. Peak effects of statins may not be evident for several weeks. The bird's weight should be monitored.

## PREVENTION/AVOIDANCE
Reduction of risk factors: Balanced and healthy diet, physical activity, reduction of stress in captivity, reduction of reproductive stimuli (see sections on Risk Factors and Client Education).

## POSSIBLE COMPLICATIONS
N/A

## EXPECTED COURSE AND PROGNOSIS
The long-term prognosis is guarded for birds displaying signs of atherosclerotic or cardiac diseases and most of them die in the next few weeks/months. The prognosis for subclinical atherosclerosis is variable and depends on the modifications of risk factors. Birds may live decades with clinically silent atherosclerotic lesions.

 MISCELLANEOUS

## ASSOCIATED CONDITIONS
Reproductive disease, hepatic disease, cardiac disease.

## AGE-RELATED FACTORS
Increased incidence with increasing age.

## ZOONOTIC POTENTIAL
N/A

## FERTILITY/BREEDING
N/A

## SYNONYMS
Arteriosclerosis, coronary arterial disease, peripheral arterial disease.

## SEE ALSO
Arrhythmias
Congestive Heart Failure

Dyslipidemia/Hyperlipidemia
Lameness
Myocardial Diseases
Neoplasia (Lymphoproliferative)
Neurologic (Non-Traumatic Diseases)
Seizures

## ABBREVIATIONS
ACE—angiotensin-converting enzyme
CT—computed tomography
GnRH—gonadotropin-releasing hormone
HDL—high density lipoprotein
HMG-CoA—3-hydroxy-3-methylglutaryl coenzyme A
LDL—low density lipoprotein
MRI—magnetic resonance imaging
PPAR—peroxisome proliferator-activated receptor
VLDL—very low density lipoprotein

## INTERNET RESOURCES
None.

*Suggested Reading*
Beaufrère, H. (2013). Atherosclerosis: Comparative pathogenesis, lipoprotein metabolism and avian and exotic companion mammal models. *Journal of Exotic Pet Medicine*, 22:320–335.
Beaufrère, H., Ammersbach, M., Reavill, D.R., et al. (2013). Prevalence of and risk factors associated with atherosclerosis in psittacine birds. *Journal of the American Veterinary Medical Association*, 242:1696–1704.
Beaufrère, H. (2013). Avian atherosclerosis: parrots and beyond. *Journal of Exotic Pet Medicine*, 22:336–347.
St Leger, J. (2007). Avian atherosclerosis. In: *Zoo and Wild Animal Medicine Current Therapy*, 6th edn. (ed. M.E. Fowler, R.E. Miller), 200–205. St Louis, MO: Saunders.
Lujan-Vega, C., Keel, M.K., Barker, C.M. et al. (2021). Evaluation of atherosclerotic lesions and risk factors of atherosclerosis in raptors in Northern California. *Journal of Avian Medicine and Surgery*, 35:295–304.
**Author**: Hugues Beaufrère, DVM, PhD, ACZM, ECZM (Avian), ABVP (Avian)

**Client Education Handout available online**

**A** | **AVIAN INFLUENZA**

# BASICS

## DEFINITION
Avian influenza viruses (AIVs) are enveloped, segmented, single-stranded, negative sense RNA viruses in the family Orthomyxoviridae, genus *Influenzavirus A*. They are grouped into subtypes based on the surface glycoproteins HA and NA. There are 18 known HA subtypes (H1–H18) and 11 NA subtypes (N1–N11); birds have been shown to be susceptible to H1–H16. AIV virions express one HA and one NA, in any combination. Subtyping is denoted by listing HA and NA antigens together (e.g. H5N1). AIVs are classified as low (LPAI) or highly pathogenic (HPAI), based on genetic structure and ability to cause disease in chickens (*Gallus gallus*). HPAI viruses have historically been restricted to the H5 or H7 subtypes (therefore all H5 and H7 subtypes regardless of virulence are notifiable avian influenza) LPAI may be caused by any subtype (including non-HPAI H5 and H7).

## PATHOPHYSIOLOGY
Host-cell entry gained by viral HA attachment to receptors on host cell membrane, followed by receptor-mediated endocytosis, acidification of the endosome, fusion of the envelope with the endosome membrane, release of viral ribonucleoprotein, and transport thereof to the nucleus where replication occurs. Virions are released by budding. LPAI virions bud from the host cell in a noninfectious state and are activated afterwards by extracellular host proteases (e.g. trypsin-like enzymes). This limits proliferation to areas where these proteases are present (e.g. GI and respiratory tracts). HPAI infectivity is activated by intracellular proteases prior to budding, allowing release of fully infectious virions in most tissues and systemic virus infection. Novel AIV result from two processes: 1) Antigenic drift—random mutations in the HA or NA genes, which can accrue over time resulting in antigenic and functional changes; 2) Antigenic shift—reassortment of genetic material with other influenza A viruses; this occurs when the same animal is infected with different AIV types (i.e. mixing vessel). Virus is shed in feces, saliva, and respiratory secretions. Transmission is by fecal–oral and aerosol routes. Fomites may enhance transmission. Incubation is approximately 1–14 days but may vary by host species.

## SYSTEMS AFFECTED
Varies with host species.
LPAI—gastrointestinal, respiratory, ophthalmic, renal/urologic, reproductive.
HPAI—cardiovascular, endocrine/metabolic, gastrointestinal, hemic/lymphatic/immune, hepatobiliary, musculoskeletal, neuromuscular, nervous, ophthalmic, reproductive, respiratory, skin/exocrine.

## GENETICS
N/A

## INCIDENCE/PREVALENCE
Varies greatly by geographic region, species, age, time of year, and environment. Common in Anseriformes (ducks, geese, swans) and Charadriiformes (gulls, terns, and shorebirds). Many of these species are reservoirs of LPAI. Rare in Columbiformes (pigeons and doves), psittacines, raptors, and ratites. There were 11 HPAI epizootics in North America from 1966 to 2022. Since 1996, HPAI has been reported from over 110 countries, affecting poultry, wild birds, wild and captive mammals, and/or humans.

## GEOGRAPHIC DISTRIBUTION
**LPAI**: Worldwide.
**HPAI**: Epidemic ongoing in parts of Asia, Africa, the Middle East, and Pacific. In fall 2020, HPAI H5Nx clade 2.3.4.4.b spread from Central Asia to Europe, Eastern Asia, the Middle East, and Africa; it moved to North America in fall 2021 and to Central and South America in fall 2022. Spread of Eurasia H5Nx into North America across the Atlantic or Pacific is becoming more common.

## SIGNALMENT
**Species:** Any avian species may be infected. Anseriformes and Charadriiformes are reservoirs of AI.
**Mean age and range:** All ages susceptible, juveniles may show more severe disease.
**Predominant sex:** Both are susceptible.

## SIGNS
### General Comments
History, physical examination findings may vary markedly by host species.

### Historical Findings
**LPAI**: Combination of GI and respiratory signs generally noted. Columbiformes, Anseriformes, and Charadriiformes are generally asymptomatic. Domestic ducks or geese may show respiratory signs. Poultry show high morbidity (> 50%) and low mortality (< 20%). General malaise, decreased egg production, malformed eggs, diarrhea, and/or respiratory signs may be reported. Psittacine birds may show general malaise and GI signs. Ratites primarily show respiratory signs with green diarrhea.
**HPAI**: GI, respiratory, and/or neurologic signs in combination with high mortality. Columbiformes, Passerines: Often asymptomatic, may show sporadic mortality. Domestic ducks and geese: Respiratory and neurologic signs. Poultry: Severe increase in mortality. Chickens and turkeys may be more severely affected than other Galliformes. Respiratory signs less prominent than in LPAI. May manifest in two phases: Peracute: Marked drop in egg production, malaise, diarrhea, birds die before clinical signs noted. Acute: As in peracute phase, but clinical signs noted prior to death. Neurologic signs common. 3- to 7-day average survival.

### Physical Examination Findings
**LPAI**: Columbiformes and wild waterfowl usually asymptomatic. Domestic ducks and geese: Often asymptomatic, malaise, oculonasal discharge, coughing, sneezing, rales. Poultry: Malaise, underweight, oculonasal discharge, sinusitis (esp. infraorbital sinuses), conjunctivitis, coughing, sneezing, rales, dyspnea, subcutaneous emphysema following air sac rupture. Psittacines: Rarely seen. A case in a juvenile red-lored Amazon (*Amazona autumnalis autumnalis*) reported malaise, dehydration, melena, crop stasis, subcutaneous edema, and inability to stand. Ratites: Oculonasal discharge, conjunctivitis, coughing, sneezing, rales, dyspnea.
**HPAI**: Columbiformes often asymptomatic. Domestic ducks and geese: Possibly asymptomatic, ataxia, excitation, nystagmus, head tilt, circling, opisthotonus, tremors, convulsions, paresis, paralysis, coughing, sneezing, rales, dyspnea, pulmonary crackles, death. Passerines: Malaise, conjunctivitis, neurologic signs, death. Poultry: Death, ataxia, excitation, cyanotic to necrotic wattles/combs/snoods, nystagmus, head tilt, circling, opisthotonus, tremors, convulsions, paresis, paralysis, petechiae/ecchymoses, multifocal subcutaneous edema, rales, coughing, sneezing. Psittacines: Rarely seen. A case in budgerigars (*Melopsittacus ungulatus*) reported anorexia, malaise, neurologic signs, death. Raptors: A report of AI in American kestrels (*Falco sparverius*) described anorexia, acute weight loss, fluffed feathers, head tilt, ataxia, tremors. Ratites: Malaise, subcutaneous edema of head and neck, ataxia, head tilt, tremors of head and neck, paralysis of wings, sneezing, open-mouth breathing. Wild waterfowl: May be asymptomatic, emaciation, diarrhea, sinusitis, death; wood ducks (*Aix sponsa*): Cloudy eyes, rhythmic myosis and mydriasis, unkempt feathers, ataxia, tremors, seizures, death; swans (mute [*Cygnus olor*] and whooper [*C. cygnus*]): Neurologic signs, death.

## CAUSES
Influenza virus A.

## RISK FACTORS
Exposure to the outdoors, wild birds, live bird markets, illegally acquired birds, drinking water used by wild birds. Turkeys—exposure to swine. Residence along

wild waterfowl migration routes. Seasons with high waterfowl migratory activity.

## DIAGNOSIS

### DIFFERENTIAL DIAGNOSIS
Newcastle disease (clinically indistinguishable from HPAI). Avian metapneumovirus. Infectious laryngotracheitis. Infectious bronchitis. *Chlamydia. Mycoplasma.* Acute respiratory infections.

### CBC/BIOCHEMISTRY/URINALYSIS
Results dependent on systems affected and severity of infection.

### OTHER LABORATORY TESTS
**Serology**: Indications: evaluate for flock-level exposure to AIV (often for trade purposes to certify as AI-free). Contraindications: Determine individual bird immune status. Positive results using one modality should be confirmed using another. AGID: Pros—gold standard for exposure detection; early post-exposure antibody detection, high specificity; cons—moderate sensitivity, inconsistent results in some non-poultry species; testing period 24–48 hours. ELISA: Pros—rapid results, quantitative; cons—moderate sensitivity and specificity. HI and NI (for subtype identification of AIV antibody-positive sample): Pros—high specificity, rapid results, gold standard for subtyping; cons—moderate sensitivity, specificity dependent on quality of reference sera.
**Virus detection**: Virus isolation. Indications: Rule-out AI in actively infected birds. Pros—gold standard for diagnosis of AI, very high sensitivity; cons—moderate specificity, requires confirmation with other tests, requires BSL-3 laboratory, expensive, lengthy test period (1–2 weeks). Antigen detection immunoassays (aka antigen capture). Indications: Rule-in AI in sick or recently dead birds (low viral load of asymptomatic birds may hinder detection). Pros—high specificity, rapid results, small and self-contained ("pen-side"); cons—moderate sensitivity, false positives caused by bacterial/blood contamination. AGID: Indications: Rule-in AI in suspect birds. Pros—high specificity, reasonable cost; cons—moderate sensitivity, testing period 24–48 hours. Molecular diagnostics (e.g. rt-PCR). Indications: Rule-out AI in suspect birds. Pros—high sensitivity and specificity, reasonable cost, rapid results; cons—does not differentiate between live and inactivated virus (contamination may reduce specificity for active disease), false negatives possible due to viral genetic mutation. HI and NI: Indications: Subtype identification of influenza A-positive sample. Pros—high specificity, rapid results; cons—specificity dependent on quality of reference antisera.
**Further virus characterization**: Sequence analysis: Characterization of HA gene cleavage site. In vivo pathotyping: Inoculation of chicks to characterize an isolate as LPAI or HPAI. Usually only performed for H5 and H7 isolates due to expense, facility requirements BSL-3.

### IMAGING
Findings dependent on systems affected and severity of infection.

### DIAGNOSTIC PROCEDURES
N/A

### PATHOLOGIC FINDINGS
Vary markedly by species and systems affected.

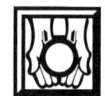

## TREATMENT

### APPROPRIATE HEALTH CARE
**Flock level**: Cull exposed poultry, quarantine other exposed birds.
**Individual level**: Strict isolation, therapy directed by affected systems. Reduce stocking density, improve ventilation, and remove manure frequently. Environment: AIV survives best in moist environments at low temperatures. May survive indefinitely when frozen. Remove litter, manure, and carcasses—burial, incineration, or composting for at least 10 days are acceptable methods. Disinfection of equipment and affected premises: Oxidizing agents (e.g. bleach), povidone iodine, quaternary ammonium compounds, 70% ethanol, phenols, and lipid solvents. Buildings may be heated to 90–100°F (32–38°C) for 1 week to inactivate virus. Ionizing radiation or heating to 133°F (56°C) for ≥ 60 minutes will inactivate AIV.

### NURSING CARE
Symptomatic care indicated by patient, situation. Fluid therapy, oxygen therapy, hand feeding, supplemental heat may all be indicated.

### ACTIVITY
N/A

### DIET
N/A

### CLIENT EDUCATION
Biosecurity measures appropriate to geographic location should be instituted. Educate owners on risk factors for AI exposure and zoonotic potential.

### SURGICAL CONSIDERATIONS
N/A

## MEDICATIONS

### DRUG(S) OF CHOICE
Secondary infections are common, especially in the respiratory tract. Select antimicrobials based on pathogen, sensitivity, location of infection, and patient species.

### CONTRAINDICATIONS
Use of anti-influenza drugs (e.g. amantidine, oseltamivir) in non-humans is highly discouraged to prevent emergence of resistance.

### PRECAUTIONS
Make drug selection for food animals in compliance with regulatory statutes.

### POSSIBLE INTERACTIONS
N/A

### ALTERNATIVE DRUGS
N/A

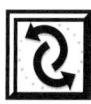

## FOLLOW-UP

### PATIENT MONITORING
Consult regulatory statutes for quarantine and follow-up testing requirements. HPAI and LPAI of H5 or H7 subtypes are considered notifiable diseases by the World Organization for Animal Health.

### PREVENTION/AVOIDANCE
Vaccination against HPAI has been employed in poultry and domestic waterfowl in countries where HPAI is enzootic (i.e. China, Vietnam, Egypt, Indonesia, Bangladesh, Mexico). Countries vaccinating poultry against HPAI for prevention are Mongolia, Kazakhstan, France, and the Netherlands. Countries vaccinating poultry against HPAI for emergency are Cote d'Ivoire, Sudan, North Korea, Israel, Russia, and Pakistan. Vaccination of wild birds with poultry AI vaccines has been performed—effectiveness unknown. Avoid exposure to most common potential virus sources: Manure, respiratory secretions, carcasses, unwashed eggs and associated packing material, and people/equipment contaminated by the above. Proper biosecurity is essential.

### POSSIBLE COMPLICATIONS
Secondary infections (especially respiratory).

### EXPECTED COURSE AND PROGNOSIS
Varies by species and pathogenicity of virus.

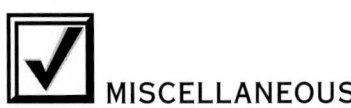

# MISCELLANEOUS

## ASSOCIATED CONDITIONS
Influenza in non-avian species. Acute respiratory infections.

## AGE-RELATED FACTORS
Juveniles may be more susceptible to disease.

## ZOONOTIC POTENTIAL
HPAI infection in humans has been extensively documented since the outbreak of Asian lineage H5N1 HPAI. Severe respiratory disease results. Mortality rate is high, approximately 60% at the time of this writing. Infection is commonly a result of direct/close contact with sick/dead infected poultry. Person-to-person transmission is rare, usually from prolonged contact with infected people. Transmission from wild birds to humans has not been documented. Poultry products—pasteurization or cooking to an internal temperature of 165°F (74°C) will inactivate AIV.

## FERTILITY/BREEDING
May cause substantial drops in egg production.

## SYNONYMS
Fowl plague, bird flu, avian flu, fowl pest.

## SEE ALSO
Infertility
Neurologic (Non-Traumatic Diseases)
Orthoavulaviruses
Pneumonia
Respiratory Distress

## ABBREVIATIONS
AGID—agar gel immunodiffusion
AI—avian influenza
AIV—avian influenza virus
BSL—biosecurity level
GI—gastrointestinal
HA—hemagglutinin
HI—hemagglutinin inhibition
HPAI—high pathogenicity avian influenza
LPAI—low pathogenicity avian influenza
NA—neuraminidase
NI—neuraminidase inhibition
rt-PCR—reverse transcriptase polymerase chain reaction

## INTERNET RESOURCES
US Department of Agriculture—Defend the Flock Program: http://www.aphis.usda.gov/animal_health/birdbiosecurity
Centers for Disease Control and Prevention—Influenza Type A Viruses: https://www.cdc.gov/flu/avianflu/influenza-a-virus-subtypes.htm
World Organisation for Animal Health—Technical meeting on HPAI vaccination, March 3, 2023: https://rr-americas.woah.org/en/events/technical-meeting-on-hpai-vaccination

*Suggested Reading*
Capua, I., Alexander, D.J. (eds.) (2009). *Avian Influenza and Newcastle Disease: A field and laboratory manual.* Milan, Italy: Springer-Verlag Italia.
Swayne, D.E. (2008). *Avian Influenza.* Ames, IA: Blackwell.
Swayne, D.E, Suarez, D.L., Sims, L.D. (2020). Influenza. In: *Diseases of Poultry*, 14th edn. (ed. D.E. Swayne), 210–256. Ames, IA: Wiley.

**Authors:** Sunoh Che, DVM, PhD, DACVPM; Leonardo Susta, DVM, PhD, DACVP
**Acknowledgements:** Previous author (first edition): Andrew D. Bean, DVM, MPH, CPH

# BASICS

## DEFINITION
Avian vacuolar myelinopathy (AVM) is a fatal neurologic disease that affects water birds and the raptors that prey upon them.

## PATHOPHYSIOLOGY
Disease caused by neurotoxin called aetokthonotoxin, produced by the cyanobacteria *Aetokthonos hydrillicola*. Toxin causes widespread, bilaterally symmetrical vacuolation of white matter of brain and spinal cord.

## SYSTEMS AFFECTED
Central nervous system.

## GENETICS
No genetic predispositions identified to date.

## INCIDENCE/PREVALENCE
Most common in the bald eagle and American coot. Some reports show 50–95% prevalence of disease in coots on affected lakes. Sporadically seen in killdeer, bufflehead, northern shoveler, American wigeon, Canada goose, great horned owl, mallard, and ring-necked duck.

## GEOGRAPHIC DISTRIBUTION
Index cases described in bald eagles (*Haliaeetus leucocephalus*) and American coots (*Fulica americana*) at DeGray Lake, Arkansas, in the winters of 1994–96. Now implicated in deaths of hundreds of eagles, thousands of American coots, and many other species of water birds and raptors in five southeastern states.

## SIGNALMENT
Most common in adult bald eagle and American coots of either sex. Sporadically seen in both sexes of other adult waterbirds or the raptor predators that consume them.

## SIGNS
Ataxia, difficulty swimming or flying, weakness or dragging of limbs, head tremors, weakness of beak and tongue, weight loss, decreased responsiveness to sounds, death.

## CAUSES
Novel pentabrominated biindole alkaloid toxin, known as aetokthonotoxin, produced by epiphytic cyanobacterium, *A. hydrillicola*. Aetoktonos grows on aquatic plants, particularly invasive *Hydrilla* sp. found in freshwater lakes. Coots and other water birds consume vegetation contaminated with this neurotoxin. Eagles and other raptors prey on impaired water birds, ingesting the toxin.

## RISK FACTORS
Late fall and winter. Not contagious. AVM disease acquired directly in coots and waterfowl by ingestion of aquatic vegetation with

*A. hydrillicola* growing on it. Neurologically impaired coots and waterfowl make easy targets for birds of prey. Toxin bioaccumulates in animal tissues and predators/scavengers may also be exposed to AVM toxin through ingestion of gut contents of prey.

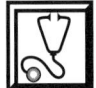

# DIAGNOSIS

## DIFFERENTIAL DIAGNOSIS
Trauma; infectious diseases: Viral (e.g. West Nile virus, avian influenza, Newcastle disease virus), fungal (e.g. aspergillosis), bacterial (e.g. pasteurellosis), parasitic (e.g. toxoplasma); metabolic derangements (e.g. hypokalemia, hypoglycemia, etc), other neurotoxins: botulism, heavy metals (lead, zinc, mercury), harmful algal bloom toxins (brevetoxins, etc), organochlorines (e.g. DDT, chlordane), organophosphates, and carbamates.

## CBC/BIOCHEMISTRY/URINALYSIS
CBCs and profiles are typically within stated reference ranges for the species.

## OTHER LABORATORY TESTS
N/A

## IMAGING
N/A

## DIAGNOSTIC PROCEDURES
No specific test for AVM in live animals. PCR assay for *A. hydricolla* on aquatic vegetation.

## PATHOLOGIC FINDINGS
Only way to confirm AVM is by histological examination of brain tissue in dead birds. Characteristic neurospinal vacuolar lesions. Vary in severity and location, but most frequently observed in white matter of optic lobe and cerebellum. Lesions develop due to fluid buildup between the layers of the myelin sheath surrounding nerve cells (intramyelinic edema).

# TREATMENT

## APPROPRIATE HEALTH CARE
There is no known treatment at this time.

## NURSING CARE
N/A

## ACTIVITY
N/A

## DIET
N/A

## CLIENT EDUCATION
N/A

## SURGICAL CONSIDERATIONS
N/A

# MEDICATIONS

## DRUG(S) OF CHOICE
N/A

## CONTRAINDICATIONS
N/A

## PRECAUTIONS
N/A

## POSSIBLE INTERACTIONS
N/A

## ALTERNATIVE DRUGS
N/A

# FOLLOW-UP

## PATIENT MONITORING
N/A

## PREVENTION/AVOIDANCE
Take the time to thoroughly wash fomites (equipment, boats, nets, etc) after time in fresh water to reduce the likelihood of transferring cyanobacteria. Report ill or deceased wildlife to local or state agencies. There are several management strategies currently being tested to control invasive aquatic plants associated with AVM. Herbicides containing bromide may potentially make the problem worse, creating more aetokthonotoxin.

## POSSIBLE COMPLICATIONS
Hydrilla continues to spread and new AVM sites continue to be identified annually. With every new AVM positive location, more avian deaths are documented and potential for other species to be affected increases.

## EXPECTED COURSE AND PROGNOSIS
All symptomatic eagles have died within days after capture. Removing animals from the source and giving supportive care may stop progression of neurologic impairment, but brain lesions persist.

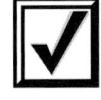

# MISCELLANEOUS

## ASSOCIATED CONDITIONS
N/A

## AGE-RELATED FACTORS
N/A

## ZOONOTIC POTENTIAL
Fish, turtles, amphibians, and invertebrates may be affected, but the threat to mammals, including humans, is unknown.

# AVIAN VACUOLAR MYELINOPATHY (CONTINUED)

**FERTILITY/BREEDING**
N/A

**SYNONYMS**
N/A

**SEE ALSO**
N/A

**ABBREVIATIONS**
AVM—avian vacuolar myelinopathy
DDT—dichlorodiphenyltrichloroethane
PCR—polymerase chain reaction

**INTERNET RESOURCES**
None.

*Suggested Reading*
Breinlinger, S., Phillips, T.J., Haram, B.N., et al. (2021). Hunting the eagle killer: A cyanobacterial neurotoxin causes vacuolar myelinopathy. *Science*, 371: eaax9050.
Dodd, S., Haynie, R., Williams S., Wilde, S. (2016). Alternate food-chain transfer of the toxin linked to avian vacuolar myelinopathy and implications for the endangered Florida snail kite (*Rostrhamus sociabilis*). *Journal of Wildlife Diseases*, 52:335–344.
Fischer, J.R., Lewis-Weis, L., Tate, C.M., et al. (2006). Avian vacuolar myelinopathy outbreaks at a southeastern reservoir. *Journal of Wildlife Diseases*, 42:501–510.
Wilde, S.B., Johansen, J.R., Wilde, H.D., et al. (2014). *Aetokthonos hydrillicola gen. et sp. nov*: Epiphytic cyanobacteria on invasive aquatic plants implicated in avian vacuolar myelinopathy. *Phytotaxa* 181(5):243–260.

**Author**: Heather W. Barron, DVM, DABVP (Avian), CertAqV

# BASICS

## DEFINITION
Traumatic injuries to the beak are common clinical presentations. These injuries often are most often seen following bite wounds from other birds or predators, or household/aviary traumatic accidents.

## PATHOPHYSIOLOGY
Injuries to the beak, including damage to the keratin, its underlying dermis, and bone. Primary and secondary involvement of the prokinetic and mandibular muscles and their innervation, and the multiple kinetic joints of the skull can also occur, resulting in abnormal form and function of the beak. With altered structure and force vector delivery, continuing keratin growth can lead to further deformities and functional deficits.

## SYSTEMS AFFECTED
**Skin/exocrine**: The beak is covered by integument, including keratin and dermis.
**Musculoskeletal**: The integumentary structures are supported by bone, and dynamic function of the upper and lower beak requires that all of these structures function in concert to maintain balanced force vector delivery.
**Respiratory**: Portions of the maxillary and mandibular beaks are pneumatized by the infraorbital sinus.
**Behavioral and welfare**: Beak injuries may lead to the need for recurrent trimming procedures, which may result in undesired learned fear and impairment to quality of life due to their perceived intrusiveness and adverse effects on the bird.

## GENETICS
N/A

## INCIDENCE/PREVALENCE
The incidence of traumatic beak injuries is not known; however, varying injuries to beaks are relatively commonly encountered in private practice and in zoological settings.

## GEOGRAPHIC DISTRIBUTION
No specific distribution is recognized.

## SIGNALMENT
All avian species. Likely more prevalent in companion bird species because of their more immediate availability for recognition; however, beak injuries are also encountered in wildlife because of collisions with glass/buildings.

## SIGNS
Visible injuries to the structures or function of the beak. Altered behaviors: Hyporexia, altered food selection (softer foods), avoidance of hard food items. Acute injuries to the distal rhinothecal tomium may present with blood in the oral cavity. Chronic injuries may be visibly apparent with healed injuries to the structures or function of the beak or may manifest with abnormal keratin growth due to altered force vector delivery and uneven wear.

## CAUSES
**Traumatic (primary)**: Crushing injuries: bite wounds (predator attacks, injuries from cage or house mates), blunt trauma (household, aviary or anthropogenic accidents) or handling/restraint associated injuries to the upper or lower bill.
**Secondary potential contributing causes**: Degenerative/metabolic—metabolic bone disease, abnormal keratin overgrowth secondary to hepatic functional deficits. Nutritional—chronic malnutrition, with secondary metabolic bone disease or keratin malformation. Neoplastic—squamous cell carcinoma, keratoacanthoma, melanoma, xanthoma, osteoma, fibrosarcoma. Infectious: Keratitis or osteomyelitis—bacterial (multiple organisms) or mycotic (*Aspergillus* sp., *Cryptococcus* sp.), or parasitic keratitis (*Knemidocoptes*); sinusitis with or without direct extension to the structures of the beak. Viral infections of beak and associated tissues—Psittacine beak and feather disease, polyomavirus, pox.

## RISK FACTORS
**Environmental**: Husbandry—free-ranging activities in the home, cage, or aviary hazards for entrapment and/or trauma.
**Behavioral**: Aggressive behaviors resulting in inadvertent injury because of the bird's behavior.
**Medical conditions**: Metabolic bone disease, chronic malnutrition, pre-existing pathology of the structures of the beak.

# DIAGNOSIS

## DIFFERENTIAL DIAGNOSIS
There are comparatively few differential diagnoses for an acutely evident beak injury. The presence of soft or abnormally flexible bone of the beak(s), abnormal keratin, or apparent pre-existing deformities should open the possibility of a beak injury that is secondary to a primary disease process.

## CBC/BIOCHEMISTRY/URINALYSIS
There are no hematologic or serum biochemistry abnormalities that are helpful in diagnosis of an acute traumatic injury to the beak. Anemia (regenerative) may occur secondary to blood loss. Serum bile acids: May be elevated in some species with beak keratin overgrowth associated with hepatic dysfunction

## OTHER LABORATORY TESTS
Where there is reason to suspect underlying Psittacine beak and feather disease as a contributing factor, whole blood PCR is indicated and serology (HI) in parts of the world where this test is available. Where polyomavirus may be suspected (finch species), whole blood and cloacal swab PCR may be indicated.

## IMAGING
Radiographic findings (plain radiography or CT): Traumatic amputation of maxillary and/or nasal bones or mandibular rami; penetration to the rostral diverticulum of the frontal sinus or into the nasofrontal hinge in psittacine species; fractures and luxations of the jugal, palatine and/or pterygoids, quadrate and regionally decreased bone density of the bony skull. Multiple orthopedic injuries are common in many cases and may not be detectable on standard projection radiographs. A skull CT is recommended to have a more thorough assessment of all bones.

## DIAGNOSTIC PROCEDURES
Where pre-existing pathology may be suspected as a primary contributing factor in a specific case, biopsy and histopathology may be indicated. Samples may be obtained by deep scalpel blade or punch biopsy methods. Samples can also be submitted for aerobic culture, cytology or other testing modalities as indicated.

## PATHOLOGIC FINDINGS
Gross: Visible traumatic amputation or other injuries to the upper and lower bills, avascular necrosis of remaining distal beak, secondary opportunistic infections. Some avascular injuries may take 1–3 weeks or even longer to declare themselves.

# TREATMENT

## APPROPRIATE HEALTH CARE
Where it is uncertain whether the bird can feed normally due to the injury, inpatient management is important until it demonstrates ability for homeostasis. Comparatively minor and stable injuries may be treated on an outpatient basis.

## NURSING CARE
**Outpatient**: Should not require nursing or supportive care.
**Inpatient**: Fluid therapy—LRS or physiological saline (0.9%), 25–50 ml/kg maintenance SQ q12–24h. LRS, physiological saline or colloid fluids IV or IO if patient has sustained considerable blood loss or is in shock. Force/gavage feeding as needed to assist in daily caloric intake.

# BEAK INJURIES

Appropriate pain management: (NSAIDs, opioids, gabapentin) are indicated with most acute and painful injuries. Antibiosis may be indicated (antibacterials, antifungals), depending on the severity of the injury. Exposed tissues should be kept moist to prevent dessication with topical treatments.

### ACTIVITY
Where the beak is deemed to be painful, feeding activities should be modified to minimize reinjury. Psittacine species may benefit from restriction from climbing activities that require the use of the upper bill.

### DIET
Where the beak is deemed to be painful, the diet may need to be altered to softer items to minimize the amount of force required for prehension and chewing behaviors.

### CLIENT EDUCATION
Keys to treatment success are in large part dependent on the severity of the injuries sustained, and the ultimate probability of the bird regaining ability to feed on its own. Most birds, but not all, with injuries to the upper and lower beaks are ultimately capable of learning to feed on their own. Assurance that the bird can eat and drink on its own and maintain body condition are important prior to outpatient management. Secondary opportunistic infections are comparatively less common with many beak injuries, but possible. Comparatively minor injuries to the maxillary beak typically heal well with conservative treatments. Surgical attempts at repairs of large fractures, reattachments of avulsed beaks and application of prostheses can offer some individual birds an opportunity to return to normal function, however initial patient stabilization, monitoring and assessment is often required prior to most of these techniques. Historically, these more significant injuries have carried an overall poor prognosis in most cases, although newer methods may offer more potential options in some select cases.

### SURGICAL CONSIDERATIONS
Most unilateral or bilateral compression fractures and penetrating injuries to the maxillary beak can be treated as open wounds, although some may benefit from the application of an acrylic cap. Damage to the vascular integrity of the beak(s) may not be initially apparent at the time of presentation, and there is some risk of avascular necrosis should a surgical repair be performed too soon. Where bone has been traumatically amputated, regrowth is unlikely. Normal force vector delivery is still possible in maxillary beak amputations, as long as the keratin occlusal ledge remains intact, enabling normal occlusion with the rostral gnathothecal tomium. In acute injuries with partial fractures through the maxillary beak, surgical stabilization may have success. Lower beak symphyseal fractures have historically had a poor prognosis for successful repair, although some newer techniques may offer more options than have been used in the past. Stabilization often requires the use of extraskeletal fixators, acrylic caps with care to make sure that the acrylic is not in direct contact with the injured tissues to best stabilize the entire upper beak while maintaining normal function. Fractures of the mandibular rami and symphyseal/diaphyseal splits may be successfully repaired in some cases, typically the more acute injuries. KE fixation of unilateral or bilateral mandibular fractures, with cross pins through both mandibular rami provides best stability in most. Symphyseal/diaphyseal mandibular splits can be stabilized with wire and the careful use of acrylic with an avoidance of direct acrylic contact with the injury site. Pharyngostomy tubes may be indicated in severe craniofacial trauma for maintaining nutritional support for the injured bird. In select cases where normal prehension, beak function and quality of life cannot be restored, the use of prosthetics can have value once the initial injuries have been healed.

## MEDICATIONS

### DRUG(S) OF CHOICE
**Bimodal Pain management**: Psittaciformes: Meloxicam 1 mg/kg IM q12–24h, 1.6 mg/kg PO q12–24h; butorphanol 1–4 mg/kg IM q6h; tramadol 30 mg/kg PO q8–12h. Galliformes: Carprofen 1 mg/kg IM q8–12h; ketoprofen 12 mg/kg IM q8–12h; tramadol 7.5 mg/kg PO q12–24h. Accipitriformes: Tramadol 5 mg/kg PO q12h (bald eagles), 11 mg/kg PO q4h (red-tailed hawks).
**Amtimicrobial management**: Antibacterial choices are based on culture and sensitivity data, antifungals may include itraconazole 5–10 mg/kg q12–24h, voriconazole 12–18 mg/kg q12h.

### CONTRAINDICATIONS
N/A

### PRECAUTIONS
N/A

### POSSIBLE INTERACTIONS
N/A

### ALTERNATIVE DRUGS
N/A

## FOLLOW-UP

### PATIENT MONITORING
Critical assessment of effectiveness of analgesia daily for in-patients. Physical assessment of outpatient form and function, the presence of normal maintenance behaviors (feeding, preening, social interaction) and degree of healing on loosely a weekly basis.

### PREVENTION/AVOIDANCE
Reduce or eliminate household traumatic risks and hazards. Prevent exposure to predators, aggressive birds. Controlled, supervised observation in the home while out of cage.

### POSSIBLE COMPLICATIONS
In the acute injury, anorexia without proper support, leading to starvation and death. In more chronic injuries, secondary infection, exposure of sinuses; exposure of tongue (Galliformes, Anseriformes) and desiccation following amputation of upper bill; avascular necrosis and loss of distal anatomy to the site of injury; abnormal beak alignment leading to keratin overgrowth problems in the future.

### EXPECTED COURSE AND PROGNOSIS
**Compressive or penetrating injuries to the maxillary beak**: Typically healed within weeks in psittacine species; prognosis is good for normal return of appearance and function.
**Amputation of maxillary beak distal to its occlusal ledge (Psittacines)**: Good for ability to feed on own and a lack of necessary follow-up trimming of the rostral gnathothecal tomium overgrowth.
**Amputation of maxillary beak proximal to its occlusal ledge (Psittacines)**: fair for ability to feed on own, but will require regular trimming of the rostral gnathothecal tomium overgrowth.
**Amputation of the lower beak**: guarded for ability to feed on own; probable necessity for trimming of rhinothecal overgrowth required. The potential use of a prosthesis may be considered.
**Lower bill mandibular ramus symphyseal split**: Heals quickly, but typically fails to reunite without effective surgical stabilization. Prognosis for ability to prehend and eat is good, but there will be probable be necessary trimming of rhinothecal and gnathothecal overgrowth.

(CONTINUED)

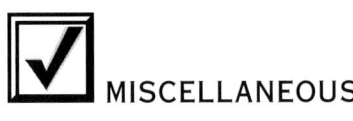

## MISCELLANEOUS

**ASSOCIATED CONDITIONS**
None.

**AGE-RELATED FACTORS**
N/A

**ZOONOTIC POTENTIAL**
N/A

**FERTILITY/BREEDING**
N/A

**SYNONYMS**
N/A

**SEE ALSO**
Beak Malocclusion

Cere and Skin, Color Changes
Hemorrhage
Liver Disease
Problem Behavior: Aggression,
Biting and Screaming
Trauma
Wounds (Including Bite Wounds, Predator
Attacks)

## ABBREVIATIONS
CT—computed tomography
HI—hemagglutinin inhibition
LRS— lactated Ringer's solution
NSAIDs—non-steroidal anti-inflammatory
drugs
PCR—polymerase chain reaction

## INTERNET RESOURCES
None.

*Suggested Reading*
Speer, B.L., Feccio, R., Holliday, C. (2024).
  The beak: form, function and problems.
  In: *Current Veterinary Therapy in Avian
  Medicine and Surgery*, Volume 2.
  St. Louis, MO: Elsevier. In press.
Speer, B.L. (2014). Beak deformities:
  form, function, and treatment methods.
  *Proceedings of the Association of Avian
  Veterinarians Annual Conference*, New
  Orleans, LA, August 2–6, pp. 213–219.
Speer, B.L., Echols, M.S. (2013). Surgical
  procedures of the Psittacine skull.
  *Proceedings of the Association of Avian
  Veterinarians Annual Conference*,
  Jacksonville, FL, August 4–7, pp. 99–109.
**Author**: Brian Speer, DVM, DABVP (Avian
practice), DECZM (Avian)

B

# BEAK MALOCCLUSION (LATERAL BEAK DEFORMITY)

# BASICS

## DEFINITION
Lateral (scissors) beak deformities are characterized by a bending of the upper beak and/or the maxilla to one side to varying degrees, with bending of the lower beak to the opposing side. These deformities often are self-augmenting, due to abnormal force delivery and unchecked and imbalanced keratin growth of the rhinothecal and gnathothecal tomia.

## PATHOPHYSIOLOGY
Not clearly understood. It is hypothesized by many that bruising of the rictal phalanges of the upper beak on one side or the other leads to a transient uneven growth in young hand-fed parrots, resulting in the ultimate development of a scissoring deformity. Possible causal factors that can lead to the onset of lateral asymmetrical growth of the upper beak include hand feeding technique flaws resulting in bruising of the rictal phalanges; incubation or hatching problems; genetic predisposition; subclinical malnutrition; infectious sinusitis; trauma; nutritional deficits.

## SYSTEMS AFFECTED
**Skin**: The beak is covered by integument, including keratin and dermis.
**Musculoskeletal**: The integumentary structures are supported by bone, and dynamic function of the upper and lower beak requires that all work in concert to maintain balanced force vector delivery.
**Behavioral**: Scissors beak deformities will lead to the need for recurrent trimming procedures, which may be accompanied by undesired learned fear and impairment to quality of life as a result.

## GENETICS
There is no evidence of any genetic predisposition for this condition in young parrot species.

## INCIDENCE/PREVALENCE
The true incidence or prevalence of scissors beak deformities is not known; however, this specific acquired beak developmental deformity is probably most encountered in young hand reared psittacine species.

## GEOGRAPHIC DISTRIBUTION
No specific distribution is recognized. The problem is most encountered in settings where young parrots are being hand reared, as opposed to parent reared.

## SIGNALMENT
**Species**: All Psittacine species, but more commonly seen in the large macaws (*Ara* sp.) and hyacinth macaws (*Anodorhynchus*), and

less commonly in other species. This deformity is also seen on occasion in other taxonomic orders, including but not limited to Piciformes, Galliformes, Columbiformes, Strigiformes, and Accipitiriformes.
**Mean age and range**: Onset of the problem is in subadults, typically prior to fledging; however, it can be an acquired problem as an adult, and adults with chronic deformities that have been present for years are not uncommonly encountered.

## SIGNS
Deviation of the rostrum maxillare away from the midline (right or left), and away from a perpendicular angle with the nasofrontal hinge joint. Secondary overgrowth of rhinothecal and gnathothecal tomia on opposing sides of the beaks, due to lack of opposing wear from normal occlusion. Secondary overgrowth or abnormal wear of occlusal ledge keratin of the rhinotheca in psittacine species, where the gnathothecal rostral tomium is normally intended to contact. Tertiary abnormal boney angles and growth of the upper and lower bills.

## CAUSES
Any event that causes anatomically uneven growth of the rhinothecal structures, resulting in abnormal force vector delivery and keratin overgrowth of the rhinotheca and gnathothecal tomia. Handfeeding-associated bruising of the rictal phalanges. Unilateral traumatic injuries to the maxillary beak. Incubation flaws, typically with dehydration and secondary injury to the developing beak tissues.

### Secondary potential contributing causes
**Nutritional**: Chronic malnutrition with secondary metabolic bone disease or keratin malformation. Infectious—unilateral bacterial (multiple organisms), mycotic (*Aspergillus* sp, *Cryptococcus* sp), parasitic (*Knemidocoptes*) or viral (Psittacine beak and feather disease virus), all which can result in abnormal and uneven keratin growth, originating from the keratin, dermis, bone, or sinuses.
**Degenerative/Metabolic**: Metabolic bone disease, asymmetric and abnormal keratin overgrowth secondary to hepatic functional deficits
**Neoplastic**: Squamous cell carcinoma, keratoacanthoma, melanoma, xanthoma, osteoma, fibrosarcoma, all of which can result in abnormal and uneven keratin growth.

## RISK FACTORS
**Behavioral**: Aggressive feeding behaviors, inattentive handfeeding technique resulting in inadvertent injury to the rictal phalanges.
**Medical conditions**: Inadequate nutritional support, resulting in hungry or varying

degrees of stunting in chicks with stronger than normal feeding reflexes and a greater predisposition to traumatic injury of the rictus.

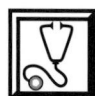

# DIAGNOSIS

## DIFFERENTIAL DIAGNOSIS
Primary deformities of the lower beak that may result in abnormal force vector delivery and secondary deformity of the upper beak.

## CBC/BIOCHEMISTRY/URINALYSIS
There are no hematologic or serum biochemistry abnormalities that are helpful in diagnosis of a lateral beak deformity.

## OTHER LABORATORY TESTS
N/A

## IMAGING
Radiographic findings (plain radiography or computed tomography): Asymmetrical rhinothecal overgrowth, lateral deviation of the maxillary bone, pathologic changes to the bone, dermis or keratin.

## DIAGNOSTIC PROCEDURES
Physical assessment and rule out of contributing underlying pathology.

## PATHOLOGIC FINDINGS
Gross: Visible deviation of the maxillary beak away from its normal perpendicular articulation at the nasofrontal hinge joint. Lateral exposure of the rostral gnathothecal tomium outside of its normal point of contact at the occlusal ledge of the maxillary beak in psittacine species. Absence of paired and opposing occlusion of upper and lower beak tips in other species.

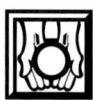

# TREATMENT

## APPROPRIATE HEALTH CARE
Where the deformity is noted in young handfeeding chicks, lateral pressure that is applied during hand feeding to direct the maxillary beak towards the midline may be effective for correction or slowing progress of minor scissors deformities. Corrective procedures in young birds are designed to alter the forces that direct the direction of rostral growth of the rhinotheca. The goal with supportive health care is to enable normal growth until a more definitive corrective procedure can be done shortly before or after weaning or lead to correction outright.

## NURSING CARE
Outpatient: Most birds should not require nursing or supportive care, although those birds with marked keratin overgrowth may

benefit from strategic, serial corrective rhampothecal grinding procedures.
Inpatient: N/A

## ACTIVITY
There are no indicated alterations in activity, pending planned surgical corrective maneuvers for correction of a lateral beak deformity should intervention of that manner be indicated.

## DIET
There are no indicated dietary alterations.

## CLIENT EDUCATION
It is important to try to correct scissors beak deformities younger in life where at all possible, to try to reduce if not eliminate the need for corrective trimming or grinding procedures for the remainder of the bird's life.

## SURGICAL CONSIDERATIONS
In young psittacine birds that are at or close to weaning age, there are two procedures that can be considered for correction of this deformity: Transfrontal pin and tension band, or the use of a mandibular ramp orthosis. The transfrontal pin and tension band procedure is generally the preferred method for correction, offering less time for the surgical procedure and a shorter duration of time until correction can be achieved.

### Transfrontal Pin and Tension Band
The patient is premedicated and then induced under general anesthesia with isoflurane, desflurane or sevoflurane, maintained via endotracheal tube in dorsal recumbency. The feathers are plucked, and skin is aseptically prepared rostral to the eye and up to the junction of skin and rhinotheca. Use a positive or negative profile threaded pin, 0.035–0.045 mm (in large macaw species), to drill through the frontal bone (lacrimal bone which is functionally fused with the frontal) just caudal and parallel to the nasofrontal hinge and parallel to it, caudal and ventral to the nares. Insert the pin from the side of the head that the maxillary beak is deviated away from, towards the side that it is deviated to. The pin is placed with careful attention to the angle of entry, as an incorrect angle of entry can result in inadvertent penetration of the nasofrontal kinetic joint or the eye. A handheld pin driver may facilitate passage of the pin. Pass the pin evenly through the frontal bone, and out the opposite side of the skull and skin at an identical exit site as the entrance location. On the side of the beak which the upper beak is deviated towards, cut the point from the threaded pin, and back it up to where it is seated in the frontal bone, but beneath the skin. On the opposite side, grasp the pin where it exits the skin with a firm clamp to prevent applying force to the bone itself, and bend the pin to a 90-degree angle, parallel

with the rostral-caudal axis of the upper beak. Do not bend the pin with direct pressure directly against the bone, as there is a greater risk of causing injury to the bone and loosening of the pin. At approximately the same length as the maxillary beak, cut the pin off with wire cutters. This produces an "L" shaped pin, with the short portion placed through the frontal sinuses, and the longer portion angling down the lateral length of the upper beak. Curl the end of this pin, at least 360 degrees, producing a circle, which will enable fixation of your tension band. Variable sized rubber bands can be used to apply tension from the K-wire to the tip of the beak. An important key to keep in mind is that gentle tension is usually all that is needed with young birds. More aggressively applied tension may have a higher failure rate with these young birds. In some birds, a dremmel may be used to score a groove in the rhinotheca where the tension band is to rest. Adjust the tension by bending the angle of the pin or tightening the rubber band as needed to lightly pull the deviated upper beak towards midline. No placement of Elizabethan or other restraint collars are needed, and the bird should be enabled to feed normally, using normal prokinetic function during the period when there is a tension band in place. Most young birds will be able to be straightened in a matter of a few days to approximately 2 weeks. When straightened alignment appears to have been achieved, cut the rubber tension band, and observe for another 24 hours to assure that your functional goal has been attained, prior to removal of the transfrontal pin itself.

### Mandibular Ramp Orthosis
A mandibular ramp orthosis is also used for the surgical correction of lateral beak deformities in some large parrots, specifically where it is deemed that the trans sinus pin technique above is not a feasible option, and the mandible should be capable of supporting the apparatus. The principle on which this method rests is by forming a mechanism that opposing force can be applied against the maxillary lateral deformity, from an apparatus affixed to the lower mandible. This procedure is also typically used in young birds. A method using dental composites has been described, which does not use anesthesia, and this method may offer advantages in some select cases. If this is not feasible, general anesthesia is used. The patient is premedicated and induced under general anesthesia with isoflurane, desflurane or sevoflurane, maintained via endotracheal tube in dorsal recumbency. The first component of this procedure is one of corrective grinding of the pressure bearing keratin surfaces and tomia of the upper and lower rhamphotheca. The rostral

gnathothecal tomium is ground and trimmed in an angle that is opposite the direction of overgrowth seen in a more chronic lateral maxillary beak deformity, leaving the highest point on the same side of the lateral deformity. Concurrently, any overgrowth of the occlusal ledge of rhinotheca is ground, to enable a more normal force vector delivery when the two beaks are closed together. A wire mesh foundation may then be cut and shaped, specifically designed to fit over the entire outer aspect of the mandibular beak and extending upward in a ramp on the same side that the upper beak is deviated towards. This wire base is attached to the lower beak using fine cerclage wires, which are applied by lacing through 22-gauge needles that are inserted through the wire and entire mandible and into the oral cavity, and then back out a second hole. These wires are lightly twisted tight enough to hold the wire mesh in place. Layers of light sensitive acrylic are then placed and hardened to produce a functional cap that encompasses the entire outer and inner aspects of the lower beak and extends up the vertical ramp. As the ramp is cured, it is positioned against the maxillary beak carefully, to apply enough force to the upper so that the two beaks show normal occlusion when opened and closed. The height of the ramp is designed to be great enough to prevent the upper beak from extending up and over it. Potential complications from the use of this ramp prosthesis include the development of abnormal lower beak angulation, fractures of the delicate mandibular ramus in young birds, or mechanical damage to the prosthesis caused by the bird's own behaviors. Functional correction of lateral beak deformities with this method may require 1–3 weeks on average in large macaw species. When the prosthesis is removed, a dremmel is used to cut the acrylics, and suture removal scissors can be used to cut the wire mesh.

### Ramp Orthotics
In other taxonomic orders, the use of ramp orthotics has been described (Strigiformes), tension band methods affixed to the maxillary beak (Piciformes, Rhamphastidae), as well as distraction osteogenesis and mandibular wedge resections (Galliformes).

## MEDICATIONS
### DRUG(S) OF CHOICE
Bimodal pain management (pre and post procedure): Psittaciformes: Meloxicam 1 mg/kg IM Q 12–24h, 1.6 mg/g PO Q 12–24h, butorphanol 1–4 mg/kg IM q1–4h, tramadol 30 mg/kg PO q8–12h.

**B**

## CONTRAINDICATIONS
N/A

## PRECAUTIONS
N/A

## POSSIBLE INTERACTIONS
N/A

## ALTERNATIVE DRUGS
N/A

## FOLLOW-UP

### PATIENT MONITORING
Critical assessment of effectiveness of analgesia daily for in-patients. Regular physical assessment of outpatient form and function on a weekly basis or more frequently as needed. There may be need to bend the transfrontal pin or tighten/loosen the rubber band tension band as needed to facilitate correction in the transfrontal pin technique. There may be the need to add more acrylic to the medial side of the ramp to maintain contact with the upper beak as it begins to move towards the midline, should the orthotic ramp technique be used.

### PREVENTION/AVOIDANCE
Avoid or minimize the risk of traumatic bruising of the rictal phalanges during hand feeding. When upper beak lateral deviations are first detected, apply digital pressure to counter continued growth during hand feeding and hopefully avoid development of more significant deviations in time. Use a surgical procedure to correct alignment once the gnathothecal rostral tomium continually rests laterally, outside of its normal contact point with the rhinothecal occlusal ledge.

### POSSIBLE COMPLICATIONS
Loosening of the transfrontal pin in the frontal bone and inability to apply adequate lateral tension as a result. Abnormal angulation of the lower beak towards the side bearing the ramp in the orthotic correction method, and potential for worsened malocclusion as a result.

### EXPECTED COURSE AND PROGNOSIS
Transfrontal pin tension band placement should be expected to have successful correction in a few days to 2 weeks in most large macaws, with an excellent return to normal for and function. Ramp orthosis should require 1–3 weeks for correction, with a good prognosis for a permanent return of normal form and function.

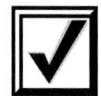

## MISCELLANEOUS

### ASSOCIATED CONDITIONS
None.

### AGE-RELATED FACTORS
None.

### ZOONOTIC POTENTIAL
N/A

### FERTILITY/BREEDING
N/A

### SYNONYMS
Scissors beak.

### SEE ALSO
Beak Malocclusion (Mandibular Prognathism)
Beak Injuries

### ABBREVIATIONS
N/A

### INTERNET RESOURCES
None.

*Suggested Reading*
Speer, B.L., Feccio, R., Holliday, C. (2024). The beak: form, function and problems. In: *Current Veterinary Therapy in Avian Medicine and Surgery*, Volume 2. St. Louis, MO: Elsevier. In press.
Speer, B.L. (2014). Beak deformities: form, function, and treatment methods. *Proceedings of the Association of Avian Veterinarians Annual Conference*, New Orleans, LA, August 2–6, pp. 213–219.
Speer, B.L., Echols, M.S. (2013). Surgical procedures of the Psittacine skull. *Proceedings of the Association of Avian Veterinarians Annual Conference*, Jacksonville, FL, August 4–7, pp. 99–109.
**Author**: Brian Speer, DVM, DABVP (Avian Practice), DECZM (Avian)

 **Client Education Handout available online**

# BEAK MALOCCLUSION (MANDIBULAR PROGNATHISM)

 BASICS

## DEFINITION
Mandibular prognathism is characterized by the mandible being functionally longer than the maxilla (undershot), resulting in the distal maxillary beak resting caudal to the rostral margin of the mandibular beak, within the oral cavity ("underbite").

## PATHOPHYSIOLOGY
Inward growth and curvature of the rostral rhinothecal keratin, paired with retraction of the maxillary beak. Contracture of the prokinetic musculature responsible for maxillary beak retraction and mandibular beak elevation and protraction (pterygoideus, ethmomandibularis, pseudomasseter, pseudotemporalis superficialis). Secondarily elongated or deformed mandibular beak structures.

## SYSTEMS AFFECTED
**Skin/exocrine**: The beak is covered by integument, including keratin and dermis.
**Musculoskeletal**: The integumentary structures are supported by bone, and dynamic function of the upper and lower beak requires that all work in concert to maintain balanced force vector delivery.
**Behavioral**: Prognathic deformities may lead to the need for recurrent trimming procedures, which in turn may result in undesired learned fear and impairment to quality of life as a result.

## GENETICS
N/A

## INCIDENCE/PREVALENCE
The incidence and prevalence are not known, however mandibular prognathism problems are most encountered in handfeeding psittacine species.

## GEOGRAPHIC DISTRIBUTION
No specific distribution is recognized.

## SIGNALMENT
Psittacine species; most commonly cockatoos and cockatiels. Most often start at a young age, prior to weaning.

## SIGNS
The maxillary beak is placed and rests inside the mandibular beak, although some birds may be able to retract the maxillary beak and place it normally, with the distal upper beak outside of the mandibular beak. Progressive, curled inward growth of the rostral rhinothecal tomial edges. Rostral deviations of growth of the rostral—most gnathothecal structures and in some cases, the entire mandibular beak.

## CAUSES
Unknown. It is hypothesized that this deformity may be seen more often in handfeeding chicks that are stunting or stressed, and more constantly vocalizing with beaks held open.

## RISK FACTORS
**Signalment factors**: Handfeeding, subadults, cockatoos, cockatiels.
**Medical conditions**: Inflammatory conditions within the infraorbital sinuses resulting in prokinetic muscle contracture. Acquired injuries to the maxillary beak and its normal prokinetic function. Nutritional deficiencies, especially metabolic bone disease may lead to bone deformities including the skull.

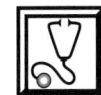 DIAGNOSIS

## DIFFERENTIAL DIAGNOSIS
There are comparatively few differential diagnoses for an apparent mandibular prognathism.

## CBC/BIOCHEMISTRY/URINALYSIS
There are no hematologic or serum biochemistry abnormalities that are helpful in diagnosis of a typical mandibular prognathism deformity. Hematologic changes (leukocytosis, heterophilia) may be seen in those cases secondary to infraorbital sinusitis.

## OTHER LABORATORY TESTS
Where there is reason to suspect the presence of infraorbital sinusitis, aerobic culture, and PCR for specific pathogens (*Bordetella avium*) may be indicated.

## IMAGING
Radiographic findings (plain radiography or CT): Bony deformities of the maxillary and mandiubular beaks, rhinosinusitis.

## DIAGNOSTIC PROCEDURES
Infraorbital sinus sampling, aerobic culture, *Bordetella* PCR if indicated.

## PATHOLOGIC FINDINGS
Gross: Visible traumatic amputation or other injuries to the upper and lower bills, avascular necrosis of remaining distal beak, secondary opportunistic infections.

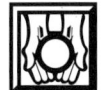 TREATMENT

## APPROPRIATE HEALTH CARE
Where the deformity is first noted in young handfeeding chicks, regular elevation (protraction) of the maxillary beak may aid in reduction of the severity of the problem if not elimination of it.

## NURSING CARE
Outpatient: Most birds should not require nursing or supportive care, although those birds with marked keratin overgrowth may benefit from strategic, serial corrective rhamphothecal grinding procedures.

## ACTIVITY
There are no indicated alterations in activity, pending planned surgical corrective maneuvers for correction of a mandibular prognathism problem, if indicated.

## DIET
There are no indicated dietary alterations.

## CLIENT EDUCATION
It is important to try to correct mandibular prognathism deformities younger in life where at all possible, to try to reduce if not eliminate the need for corrective trimming or grinding procedures for the remainder of the bird's life.

## SURGICAL CONSIDERATIONS
Where the deformity is first noted in young handfeeding chicks, regular elevation (protraction) of the maxillary beak may aid in reduction of the severity of the problem if not elimination of it.

### Orthotic Maxillary Beak Extension Procedure
The patient is premedicated and then induced under general anesthesia with isoflurane, desflurane or sevoflurane, maintained via endotracheal tube in dorsal recumbency. A variety of acrylic or dental composite products can be used. A functional cap, extending from the cere distally, and encompassing the pressure bearing keratin at the occlusal ledge of the upper beak, is progressively constructed. The orthosis is structured to duplicate and exaggerate the relative dimensions of a normal upper beak, so that the bird can function normally when it is applied. The lower bill must not be able to extend out and beyond this prosthesis, and the rostral tomium of the gnathotheca should be capable of applying normal force at the area of the occlusal ledge of the rhinotheca. A small sterile pin may be placed in the maxillary beak or the lateral aspects of the rhinothecal occlusal ledge to facilitate stabilization of the orthotic. This process functionally extends the upper beak, preventing placement of the maxillary beak into the lower beak, enabling normal occlusion and a normalization of the range of motion of the hyperflexed and hyperextended prokinetic joints. A method using dental composites has been described, which does not utilize anesthesia and may

## BEAK MALOCCLUSION (MANDIBULAR PROGNATHISM)    (CONTINUED)

**B**

offer advantages in some cases. Potential complications with this procedure are few. Should the orthosis loosen prior to resolution of the problem, it can be cleaned and readhered to the maxillary beak with tissue glue or other similar adhesives.

### Tension Band Technique
The patient is premedicated and then induced under general anesthesia with isoflurane, desflurane or sevoflurane, maintained via endotracheal tube in dorsal recumbency. Transverse placement of a pin through the frontal bone is like that described for correction of lateral beak deviation. A second small pin or small threaded screw is placed in the bone of the maxillary beak along the mid culmen at the point where inward rotation of the maxillary beak is most severe. Structural adhesive resins can be applied to support the second pin. An elastic band is placed from either exposed end of the transfrontal bone pin to the premaxilla pin. The band can be removed after normal alignment is restored, and the pins removed once this correction is assured. Potential complications with this procedure are related to the risks of trauma to bony and vascular tissues.

## MEDICATIONS
### DRUG(S) OF CHOICE
Bimodal pain management may be indicated should a transfrontal pin or tension band with screws used. Psittaciformes: Meloxicam 1 mg/kg IM q12–24h, 1.6 mg/g PO q12–24h, butorphanol 1–4 mg/kg IM q1–4h, tramadol 30 mg/kg PO q8–12h.

### CONTRAINDICATIONS
N/A

### PRECAUTIONS
N/A

### POSSIBLE INTERACTIONS
N/A

### ALTERNATIVE DRUGS
N/A

## FOLLOW-UP
### PATIENT MONITORING
Regular physical assessment of outpatient form and function on a weekly basis or more frequently as needed. There may be need to reapply the orthosis should it loosen or come off prior to correction of the deformity. Tension bands may require adjustment to facilitate optimal outcome.

### PREVENTION/AVOIDANCE
Handfeed optimally, so that chicks are resting with their beaks closed in normal occlusion. If prognathism is detected early, regular protraction (elevation) of the maxillary beak may help reduce, if not eliminate, the problem prior to a need for surgical intervention. Use a surgical procedure to correct alignment if the deformity persists following manipulation.

### POSSIBLE COMPLICATIONS
Potential of trauma to bony and vascular tissues caused by transfrontal pin placement or screws.

### EXPECTED COURSE AND PROGNOSIS
Orthotic extension technique as well as transfrontal tension band techniques should be expected to achieve successful correction in 1–3 weeks in most cases, with an excellent return to normal for and function.

## MISCELLANEOUS
### ASSOCIATED CONDITIONS
None.

### AGE-RELATED FACTORS
Typically, this is a problem of sub-adults.

### ZOONOTIC POTENTIAL
None.

### FERTILITY/BREEDING
N/A

### SYNONYMS
None.

### SEE ALSO
Anorexia
Beak Injuries
Beak Malocclusion (Lateral Beak Deformity)

### ABBREVIATIONS
CT—computed tomography
PCR—polymerase chain reaction

### INTERNET RESOURCES
None.

*Suggested Reading*
Speer BL, Feccio R, Holliday C. (2024). The beak: form, function and problems. In: *Current Veterinary Therapy in Avian Medicine and Surgery*, Volume 2. St. Louis, MO: Elsevier. In press.
Speer, B.L. (2014). Beak deformities: form, function, and treatment methods. *Proceedings of the Association of Avian Veterinarians Annual Conference*, New Orleans, LA, August 2–6, pp. 213–219.
Speer, B.L., Echols, M.S. (2013). Surgical procedures of the Psittacine skull. *Proceedings of the Association of Avian Veterinarians Annual Conference*, Jacksonville, FL, August 4–7, pp. 99–109.
**Author**: Brian Speer, DVM, DABVP (Avian Practice), DECZM (Avian)

 **Client Education Handout available online**

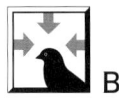 **BASICS**

## DEFINITION
Bordetellosis is a contagious disease affecting birds which typically causes low mortality but high morbidity, mainly in turkeys. Historically, the most common cause of bordetellosis was *Bordetella avium*, however, *Bordetella hinzii* has also been increasingly recognized. These organisms are similar to other *Bordetella* species, as they tend to infect the tissues of the upper respiratory tract.

## PATHOPHYSIOLOGY
In cockatiels, and occasionally other psittacines, bordetellosis presents as a syndrome known as "lockjaw", wherein the young birds are unable to open their mouths due to extension of sinusitis into the various surrounding tissues, often resulting in death unless aggressively treated. A dermonecrotic toxin produced by *B. avium* may play an important role in producing rhinitis, sinusitis, and "temporomandibular osteomyelitis" in these birds. It must be noted, however, that any serious sinus infection can result in this syndrome and that it is not always caused by *B. avium*. In young turkeys, *B. avium* is a well-known cause of coryza, a disease of high morbidity and low mortality, manifested mostly by tracheitis and sinusitis with excess mucous production. Some strains of *B. hinzii* cause disease in poults similar to *B. avium*. Bordetellosis has also been reported in ostrich chicks and quail and can be an opportunistic infection in chickens infected with bronchitis virus or exposed to poor conditions.

## SYSTEMS AFFECTED
**Upper respiratory tract**: Rhinitis, frontal sinusitis (can be severe and necrotizing), tracheitis.
**Lower respiratory tract**: Pneumonia and airsacculitis in turkeys can be seen with secondary colibacillosis or other coinfections.
**Ophthalmic**: Conjunctivitis.
**Musculoskeletal**: In lockjaw syndrome, inflammation of all tissues in contact with the frontal sinus, muscles, nerves and bones and possibly joints.

## GENETICS
N/A

## INCIDENCE/PREVALENCE
Bordetellosis is reported sporadically in cockatiels, usually associated with a "lockjaw" type of presentation; it can manifest as an outbreak in some aviaries; more rarely it is reported in other psittacines. It is a significant problem in young turkeys and can be associated with outbreaks in turkey flocks.

## GEOGRAPHIC DISTRIBUTION
Worldwide; in turkeys it appears in focal outbreaks. The disease is most common where turkeys are extensively reared.

## SIGNALMENT
**Species**: Most commonly seen in cockatiels as lockjaw syndrome; occasionally in other psittacines; turkeys (coryza) and quail are susceptible; opportunistic in chickens; has been reported in ostriches.
**Mean age and range**: Turkeys, generally less than 6 weeks of age. Cockatiels and other psttacines, usually 2–4 weeks.
**Predominant sex**: Both sexes are susceptible.

## SIGNS
### Historical Findings
In young turkeys, sudden onset after 7- to 10-day incubation period, up to 40% affected; low mortality. Cockatiels with lockjaw may initially have nasal or sinus signs, rhinitis, sinusitis, and temporomandibular joint rigidity, followed by gradual starvation due to inability to open the mouth. May be seen in one or more birds; untreated birds die.

### Physical Examination Findings
**Turkeys**: Swelling of sinuses. Sneezing and nasal discharge. Foamy eyes/ocular discharge. Dyspnea, cough or "snick," loss or change of voice, excessive/abnormal respiratory sounds. Decreased appetite and poor weight gain, thin, unthrifty.
**Psittacine birds**: In young cockatiels and other psittacine birds with lockjaw, temporomandibular rigidity, inability to open the mouth (trismus) with resultant accumulation of material in the mouth; food and exudate, weight loss, anorexia, vocalizing due to hunger, sneezing, coughing, serous nasal discharge, emaciation, dehydration, and swollen infraorbital sinuses.

## CAUSES
Infection with *Bordetella* sp. in susceptible (young) birds.

## RISK FACTORS
Unknown, but the age and general health status of each patient plays a role in whether it will become infected and, if infected, how sick the patient will become. Co-infections could play a role, as could environmental and genetic factors.

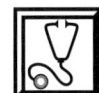 **DIAGNOSIS**

## DIFFERENTIAL DIAGNOSIS
**Turkeys with respiratory disease**: Mycoplasmosis, fowl cholera (pasteurellosis), aspergillosis (brooder pneumonia), avian influenza, Newcastle disease, chlamydiosis.

**Psittacines with lockjaw**: There are unlikely to be too many differential diagnoses to be considered when a young psittacine, especially a cockatiel, is presented with the typical clinical signs and findings. However, many different bacteria have been isolated in these cases. *Enterococcus* sp. infections may be overrepresented. In theory, fungal infection, foreign bodies and introduction of irritants (food, etc.) into the nasal cavity could cause similar pathology.

## CBC/BIOCHEMISTRY/URINALYSIS
Most avian patients would not be subjected to blood or urine testing, but if they were, there would likely be non-specific findings. An inflammatory leukogram would be expected in patients with significant inflammation. In cases of lockjaw, there could be elevations in muscle enzymes.

## OTHER LABORATORY TESTS
**Turkeys**: Culture and sensitivity of affected tissues may reveal *B. avium* or *B. hinzii*, but it can be difficult to isolate if there are other faster-growing bacteria present. Serologic tests are available for turkeys.
**Lockjaw cases**: Cytology of choana and or nasal/sinus flush material. C/S of choana or sinus flush. PCR testing for *B. avium* and *B. hinzii* is also available in some specialized laboratories.

## IMAGING
**Lockjaw cases**: Radiogaphs and skull CT might be helpful and may allow ruling out orthopaedic lesions.

## DIAGNOSTIC PROCEDURES
**Turkeys**: Sampling of infected tissues; swab of or flush from nasal/sinus/trachea to procure samples for C/S, cytology, PCR, plus necropsy and histopathology of tissues of dead birds.
**Lockjaw**: Sampling of infected tissues; swab of or flush from nasal/sinus/trachea to procure samples for C/S, cytology, PCR.

## PATHOLOGIC FINDINGS
**Turkeys**: Watery eyes, extensive mucous in sinuses and trachea, softening and flattening of the trachea; lesions rarely extend past the tracheal bifurcation. Pneumonia and airsacculitis in secondary infections (esp. colibacillosis).
**Lockjaw cases**: Moderate subacute necrotizing to mucopurulent to fibrinosuppurative rhinitis, sinusitis, and osteomyelitis. Mild to moderate subacute necrotizing and fibrosing myositis, tendonitis, and perineuritis. Some birds have inflammation of the quadrate pterygoid apparatus and jugal arch, characterized by periosteal fibrosis and irregular lysis, and mixed inflammatory infiltrates. Rarely, peracute hepatic necrosis, chronic hepatic fibrosis, lymphocytic depletion, and subacute pneumonia with air sacculitis are present.

## TREATMENT

### APPROPRIATE HEALTH CARE
Turkeys with coryza will generally get better unless co-infected with other viruses or bacteria. Psittacines with sinusitis and secondary lockjaw syndrome need aggressive therapy; antibiotics orally or parenterally, nasal/sinus flushing, supportive care such as fluid therapy and gavage feeding, pain management and anti-inflammatory medications, as well as physical therapy of the complex masticatory apparatus.

### NURSING CARE
Turkeys with coryza need little nursing care. Individual cases may need supportive care, depending on whether they have secondary or co-infections. Psittacines with lockjaw need extensive nursing care as mentioned above; they are generally young and need frequent feeding and medicating, as well as vigilant monitoring of clinical signs and body weight. Physical therapy can be done several times a day by massaging the muscles of mastication and by opening the beak. This can be done digitally or with the use of hemostats or, in the case of larger birds, a thumbscrew small-mammal oral speculum, so that the fibrotic muscles can be gradually stretched. This is difficult to do in an awake patient; it can be done carefully in an anesthetized patient, but care must be taken to avoid aspiration.

### ACTIVITY
N/A

### DIET
**Turkeys**: N/A.
**Lockjaw**: Generally gavaged with hand rearing formula; can be difficult due to difficulty passing the tube. Alternatively, an esophagostomy tube can be placed.

### CLIENT EDUCATION
**Turkeys**: General conversation about the illness and course to be expected; do not overtreat with antibiotics. Bring in recently deceased patients for necropsy to further evaluate the health of the flock.
**Lockjaw cases**: Depends on the situation. If the owner is going to be treating the patient, they need a lot of guidance and should be given a poor prognosis in general. In aviary situations, the breeder needs to be educated about general aviary health management, cleanliness, disinfection, biosecurity, traffic flow, etc.

### SURGICAL CONSIDERATIONS
N/A

## MEDICATIONS

### DRUG(S) OF CHOICE
**In turkeys**: Antibiotics have generally not been very effective and the disease will run its course.
**In lockjaw cases**: Selection of antibiotic should be based upon results of antimicrobial C/S. However, this organism can be difficult to grow in the laboratory and, despite the selection of a proper antibiotic based on C/S, there may be minimal response to treatment due to various factors such as difficulty in achieving proper antibiotic concentration in the areas that are infected, presence of excess mucous. Various medications can be added to saline to flush the infraorbital sinus at least twice a day. Anti-inflammatory medications such as meloxicam are essential: 1–1.6 mg/kg q12–24h. PO or by gavage. Additional analgesics such as opioids as needed for pain.

### CONTRAINDICATIONS
N/A

### PRECAUTIONS
N/A

### POSSIBLE INTERACTIONS
N/A

### ALTERNATIVE DRUGS
N/A

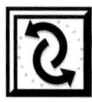

## FOLLOW-UP

### PATIENT MONITORING
**Turkeys with coryza**: N/A
**Lockjaw cases**: Quite a bit of follow up is needed, depending on whether the patient is treated in-house or by the client. Several months of treatment are likely to be needed. If the patient improves, and the bird is able to eat, the prognosis is much better and there is less need for continual follow-up.

### PREVENTION/AVOIDANCE
N/A

### POSSIBLE COMPLICATIONS
N/A

### EXPECTED COURSE AND PROGNOSIS
In turkeys, the disease is usually self-limiting and will resolve with time, unless there are secondary infections such as *Escherischia coli*, in which case there could be airsacculitis and pneumonia, and higher mortality.
In psittacines with lockjaw, the disease is usually fatal unless aggressively treated. Since treatment is labor intensive, the risks and benefits of attempted treatment must be considered. With aggressive treatment, some birds can be saved, especially larger psittacines, but in general the prognosis is poor since most patients are cockatiels; thus, the amount of pathology is great when compared with patient size and there are more difficulties in trying to perform physical therapy in these patients.

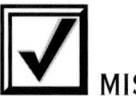

## MISCELLANEOUS

### ASSOCIATED CONDITIONS
N/A

### AGE-RELATED FACTORS
In turkeys and cockatiels, bordetellosis is generally seen in younger birds, but it is possible that older and/or recovered birds may be carriers.

### ZOONOTIC POTENTIAL
*B. avium* is characterized as an opportunistic pathogen that presents a risk to public health by its zoonotic potential. *B. hinzii*, potentially secondary to exposure to positive birds, has been reported in two cases of pulmonary disease in immunodeficient human patients.

### FERTILITY/BREEDING
N/A

### SYNONYMS
In cockatiels, lockjaw, or lockjaw syndrome. In turkeys, infectious coryza or rhinotracheitis.

### SEE ALSO
Anorexia
Aspergillosis
Aspiration Pneumonia
Beak Injuries
Beak Malocclusion (Lateral Beak Deformity)
Beak Malocclusion (Mandibular Prognathism)
Chlamydiosis
Mycoplasmosis
Pasteurellosis
Rhinitis and Sinusitis

### ABBREVIATIONS
C/S—culture and sensitivity
PCR—polymerase chain reaction

### INTERNET RESOURCES
There are multiple good poultry disease websites, including the online *Merck Veterinary Manual*:
https://www.msdvetmanual.com.

*Suggested Reading*

Clubb, S.L., Homer, B.L., Pisani, J., Head, C. (1994). Outbreaks of bordetellosis in psittacines and ostriches. *Proceedings of the Association of Avian Veterinarians Annual Conference, Reno NV, September 28–30*, 63–68. Association of Avian Veterinarians.

Fabre, A., Dupin, C., Bénézit, F., et al. (2015). Opportunistic pulmonary *Bordetella hinzii* infection after avian exposure. *Emerging Infectious Diseases*, 21:2122.

Fitzgerald, S.D., Hanika, C., Reed, W.M. (2001). Lockjaw syndrome in cockatiels associated with sinusitis. *Avian Pathology*, 30:49–53.

Grespan, A., Camera, O., Knöbl, T., et al. (2012). Virulence and molecular aspects of *Bordetella avium* isolated from cockatiel chicks (*Nymphicus hollandicus*) in Brazil. *Veterinary Microbiology*, 160:530–534.

Moreno, L.Z., Knöbl, T., Grespan, A.A., et al. (2015). Draft genome sequence of *Bordetella avium* Nh1210, an outbreak strain of lockjaw syndrome. *Genome Announcements* 3(2):e00120-15.

Raffel, T.R., Register, K.B., Marks, S.A., Temple, L. (2002). Prevalence of *Bordetella avium* infection in selected wild and domesticated birds in the eastern USA. *Journal of Wildlife Diseases* 38(1):40–46.

Register, K.B. (2013) Development of a PCR for Identification of *Bordetella hinzii*. *Avian Diseases* 57:307–310.

Skeeles, J.H., Arp, L.H. (1977). Bordetellosis (turkey coryza). In: *Diseases of Poultry*, 10th edn. (ed. B.W. Calnek), 275–288. Ames, IA: Iowa State Press.

Schmidt, R.E., Reavill, D.R., Phalen, D.N. (2003). Respiratory system. *Pathology of Pet and Aviary Birds*. Ames, IA: Iowa State Press, pp. 17–40.

Schmidt R.E., Reavill D.R., Phalen D.N. (2015). Respiratory system. In: *Pathology of Pet and Aviary Birds*, 2nd edn. (ed. R.E. Schmidt, D.R. Reavill, D.N. Phalen), 21–53. Ames, IA: Wiley.

**Author**: João Brandão, LMV, MS, DECZM (Avian), DACZM

**Acknowledgement/s**: updated from first edition chapter authored by George Messenger.

## BORNAVIRAL DISEASE (AQUATIC BIRDS)

# BASICS

## DEFINITION
Orthobornaviruses are enveloped, non-segmented, single-stranded, negative-sense RNA viruses in the order *Mononegavirales*, family *Bornaviridae*, and genus *Orthobornavirus*. Orthobornaviruses circulating in avian species are divided into five species (*Orthobornavirus alphapsittaciformes*, *betapsittaciformes*, *serini*, *estrlididae*, *avisaquaticae*), which encompass 15 unique viruses, namely parrot bornavirus (PaBV) 1–8, canary bornavirus (CnBV) 1–3, munaica bornavirus (MuBV) 1, estrid finch bornavirus (EsBV) 1, and aquatic bird bornavirus (ABBV) 1 and 2. While orthobornaviruses of birds have been indicated as ABVs, this is a descriptive and not a taxonomical term. In psittacine species, PaBVs are the cause of PDD, which is a chronic, frequently lethal disease that presents with wasting, GI motility impairment, and variable neurological symptoms. PDD-like disease has been described in birds naturally infected with ABBV-1 in wild waterfowl. Avian ganglioneuritis has been proposed as a more appropriate name for PDD, as multiple organs in the body can be affected, and proventricular dilation may not always be present.

## PATHOPHYSIOLOGY
Orthobornaviruses are neurotropic viruses that cause chronic (persistent) infection without inducing cell lysis (non-cytolytic). Most of the basic virology for this group of viruses derived for studies of borna disease virus 1 (a mammalian orthobornavirus that is the type species of the *Bornaviriade* family). Orthobornaviruses enter the cell via attachment of the surface G protein receptor-mediated endocytosis, acidification of the endosome, fusion of the envelope with the endosome membrane, release of viral RNP, which is then transported into the nucleus, where virus replication occurs. In the nucleus, the virus uses the splicing machinery of the host cell. The RNP becomes associated with nuclear histone proteins, allowing virus persistence in the nucleus. Viral spread is believed to occur by direct cell-to-cell contact, and, to a lesser extent, by the release from the plasma membrane. Transmission is thought to occur via the fecal–oral and respiratory routes, although virus shedding is often intermittent and mucosal infection (i.e. oral) has not been reproduced experimentally. Rare congenital infection of embryos with PaBVs has been documented, although vertical transmission has not been formally proven.

## SYSTEMS AFFECTED
Orthobornavirus are neurotropic, and infect both the CNS and PNS; as part of the PNS, the ganglia throughout the GI tract are often affected.

## GENETICS
N/A

## INCIDENCE/PREVALENCE
ABBV-1 appears to be endemic in wild waterfowl in North America, as tested by molecular methods in tissues or swabs, as well as seroprevalence studies. Infection rates in studies from North America has been shown to be < 25%, although seroprevalence in certain populations of Canada geese in Ontario, Canada, has been described to be up to 70% in mute swans (*Cygnus olor*). Experimental infection through intracranial or intramuscular inoculation showed that domestic chickens (*Gallus gallus*), Muscovy (*Cairina moschata*) and Pekin (*Anas plathyrinchus*) ducks are permissive to ABBV-1 infection, although waterfowl species showed a broader tissue distribution and higher magnitude of virus replication compared with chickens. Despite this evidence, natural cases of ABBV-1 infection in have not been documented.

## GEOGRAPHIC DISTRIBUTION
ABBV-1 has predominantly been observed in wild bird populations. ABBV-1 has been detected in several species in the order Anseriformes, including Canada geese (*Branta canadensis*) and mute swans (*Cygnus olor*) in the USA, Canada, Denmark, Germany, and Poland. Infection by ABBV-1 has been documented also in birds of the order Charadriiformes. Transcontinental transmission between America and Europe has not been confirmed.

## SIGNALMENT
**Species**: Orthobornaviruses have been discovered in pet and wild birds, including both psittacine (order Psittaciformes) and non-psittacine species like birds in the orders Passeriformes, Anseriformes, and Charadriiformes. Disease development has been exclusively associated with PaBVs and ABBV-1 infection. Canada geese, trumpeter swans, and mute swans are overrepresented for ABBV-1 infection.
**Mean age and range**: No age predilection has been identified.
**Predominant sex**: Both are susceptible.

## SIGNS
Clinical signs have not been reproduced experimentally with ABBV-1 infection. Retrospective studies have shown that ABBV-1 infection in waterfowl was associated with wasting, proventricular dilation, and paresis/paralysis. In these cases, postmortem revealed mononuclear infiltrations in the CNS and PNS (encephalitis, myelitis, ganglioneuritis). Upper GI impaction has been seen in association with bornavirus infection in Canada geese.

## CAUSES
ABBV-1

## RISK FACTORS
N/A

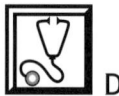

# DIAGNOSIS

## DIFFERENTIAL DIAGNOSIS
**GI signs**: Mycobacteriosis, GI parasites, gastroenteritis, food or foreign body impaction.
**CNS signs**: Heavy metal poisoning, viral, bacterial, and fungal infections of the CNS. Viral (West Nile virus), bacterial, and fungal infections of the CNS. Hydrocephalus.

## CBC/BIOCHEMISTRY/URINALYSIS
CBC and serum chemistry findings are typically non-specific.

## OTHER LABORATORY TESTS
Diagnosis of ABBV-1 infection is carried out by rt-qPCR in tissues, virus isolation, or immunohistochemistry for N protein (nuclear or nuclear and cytoplasmic reactivity).
**Serology**: Indirect fluorescent antibody and Western blot tests are employed, but cannot differentiate between diseased birds and healthy carriers because not all birds shedding the virus have detectable antibodies.
**Molecular diagnostics**: (e.g. rt-PCR) Laboratories offering rt-PCR lack a standardized testing method. Urine, feces, and cloacal swabs are the most likely sources of the virus. A combination of whole blood and choanal/cloacal swabs improves sensitivity although fecal swabs are less desirable and cloacal sampling may underestimate ABV infection. Primers have been developed to target the nucleocapsid (N) gene, matrix (M) gene, phosphoprotein (P) gene, and polymerase (L) gene. Assays designed for the detection of M and immunodominant N gene sequences possess a similar, high level of sensitivity. However, those for the L and P genes demonstrate lower accuracy.
**Immunohistochemistry**: Used to detect virus proteins in infected tissues. Brain, spinal cord, adrenal, pancreas, and kidney, as well as anterior GI tract, heart, testes, ovary, and thyroid have been shown to be positive for ABBV-1.

## IMAGING
Whole-body radiography: evidence of upper GI impaction.

## DIAGNOSTIC PROCEDURES
N/A

## PATHOLOGIC FINDINGS
Vary markedly by species and systems affected.

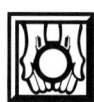

# TREATMENT

## APPROPRIATE HEALTH CARE
No cure is available, and few treatments are available.

## NURSING CARE
Symptomatic care indicated by patient, situation. Fluid therapy, oxygen therapy, hand feeding, supplemental heat may all be indicated.

## ACTIVITY
N/A

## DIET
N/A

## CLIENT EDUCATION
N/A

## SURGICAL CONSIDERATIONS
N/A

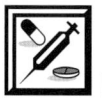

# MEDICATIONS

## DRUG(S) OF CHOICE
N/A

## CONTRAINDICATIONS
N/A

## PRECAUTIONS
N/A

## POSSIBLE INTERACTIONS
N/A

## ALTERNATIVE DRUGS
N/A

# FOLLOW-UP

## PATIENT MONITORING
PCR tests and serologic antibody tests can be used to detect the presence of ABV in the sample.

## PREVENTION/AVOIDANCE
There is no available vaccine.

## POSSIBLE COMPLICATIONS
N/A

## EXPECTED COURSE AND PROGNOSIS
Once GI impaction occurs, the prognosis for wild geese is typically poor.

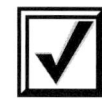

# MISCELLANEOUS

## ASSOCIATED CONDITIONS
Vomiting, weight loss, passing undigested seeds in the stool or show neurologic signs.

## AGE-RELATED FACTORS
N/A

## ZOONOTIC POTENTIAL
Borna disease virus 1 has been detected in human patients, with severe to fatal encephalitis in Germany. However, the incidence of avian bornavirus infection in humans has not been reported.

## FERTILITY/BREEDING
The presence of PaBVa RNA has been detected in eggs derived from wild-sourced eggs from Canada geese. However, relationship between orthobornavirus infection and fertility in birds is currently unknown.

## SYNONYMS
N/A

## SEE ALSO
Algal Biotoxins
Bornaviral Disease (Psittaciformes)
Eastern and Western Equine Encephalitis Viruses
Neural Larva Migrans
Neoplasia (Neurologic)
Neurologic (Non-Traumatic Diseases)
Neurologic (Trauma)
Toxicosis (Heavy Metals)
West Nile Virus

## ABBREVIATIONS
ABBV—aquatic bird bornavirus
ABV—avian bornavirus
CnBV—canary bornavirus
CNS—central nervous system
GI—gastrointestinal
MuBV—munaica bornavirus
NSAIDs—nonsteroidal anti-inflammatory drugs
PaBV—parrot bornavirus
PCR—polymerase chain reaction
PDD—proventricular dilatation disease
PNS—peripheral nervous system
RNP—ribonucleoprotein
rt-PCR—reverse transcriptase polymerase chain reaction

## INTERNET RESOURCES
N/A

*Suggested Reading*
Ampuero, F., Leacy, A., Pham, P.H., et al. (2023). Experimental pathogenesis of aquatic bird bornavirus 1 in Pekin ducks. *Scientific Reports*, 13:18094.
Delnatte, P., Ojkic, D., Delay, J. et al. (2013). Pathology and diagnosis of avian bornavirus infection in wild Canada geese (*Branta canadensis*), trumpeter swans (*Cygnus buccinator*) and mute swans (*Cygnus olor*) in Canada: a retrospective study. *Avian Pathology*, 42:114–128.
Iverson, M., Leacy, A., Pham, P.H., et al L. (2022). Experimental infection of aquatic bird bornavirus 1 in domestic chickens. *Veterinary Microbiology*, 275:109602.
Iverson, M., Leacy, A., Pham, P.H., Che S, et al. (2022). Experimental infection of aquatic bird bornavirus in Muscovy ducks. *Scientific Reports*, 12:16398.
Rubbenstroth, D. (2022). Avian bornavirus research: A comprehensive review. *Viruses*, 14:1513.

**Authors:** Sunoh Che, DVM, PhD, DACVPM; Leonardo Susta, DVM, PhD, DACVP

# BORNAVIRAL DISEASE (PSITTACIFORMES)

## BASICS

### DEFINITION
Bornaviral disease of Psittaciformes is an inflammation of the neurologic system characterized by lymphoplasmacytic infiltrations, mainly in the ganglia. It affects the central nervous system as well as the peripheral nerves. One main target organ system is the GI tract. Formerly known as proventricular dilatation disease (PDD), it is now known that it can affect also other organ systems leading to various clinical signs. Avian ganglioneuritis is caused by the avian orthobornavirus and it is assumed that it triggers an autoimmune response rather than a direct cell damage by the virus. It has been speculated that other infectious agents may cause a similar pathological picture, but evidence is lacking so far, although the Henle–Koch postulates have been fulfilled for avian orthobornavirus.

### PATHOPHYSIOLOGY
The pathophysiology of a bornaviral infection leading to clinical disease is poorly understood. In mammals (rats), a T-cell mediated disease has been shown. The neural invasion of CD8 T-lymphocytes seems to cause the cellular damage rather than the virus itself. It is assumed that the pathogenesis in birds is similar and a delayed-type hypersensitivity effect has been suggested, which supports the hypothesis of clinical disease resulting from a T cell mediated response. This is further underlined by a reduction and even prevention of clinical signs after cyclosporine A treatment (which reduces T cell activity) and the observation that birds infected when very young (immature immune system) do not develop clinical signs compared with birds infected as adults. It is presently unknown whether viral factors play a role in the pathogenesis of a bornaviral infection in psittacines. It is known that different parrot bornavirus strains act differently within the same host, demonstrating various replication patterns and clinical signs. The inflammation of the neural ganglia leads to a functional impairment of the innervated organs. Smooth musculature of the gastrointestinal tract is especially affected, in particular the proventriculus, leading to a loss of function and ultimately to proventricular dilatation. Central nervous signs, peripheral tremors, blindness, and other neural associated signs can also occur.

### SYSTEMS AFFECTED
Nervous
GI
Cardiovascular

Ophthalmic
Integument (suspected feather damaging behavior)

### GENETICS
N/A

### INCIDENCE/PREVALENCE
In Psittaciformes, mainly PaBV-4 and PaBV-2 are found. In captive populations, prevalence varies between 4% and 33% of clinically healthy birds. It thus seems likely that many larger parrot facilities do have infected birds, except those which have aimed for virus clearance in recent years. In free-ranging populations, prevalence seems to be much lower, with only a very few birds found to be positive. The prevalence of clinical disease after infection is presently unknown.

### GEOGRAPHIC DISTRIBUTION
Worldwide in captive birds and also likely in free-ranging populations.

### SIGNALMENT
Parrot bornavirus has been documented in many different psittacine species and it seems likely that it may occur in all Psittaciformes. Infection with PaBV or clinical disease does not seem to be associated with the sex of the birds. However, it seems that there is an age-related occurrence of the clinical disease. Birds infected during first week after hatch remain carrier birds with no clinical apparent disease compared with birds infected as adults at the same time, which display severe clinical symptoms. So far, there are no reports about affected budgerigars (*Melopsittacus undulatus*), so resistance to the disease is speculated.

### SIGNS
Clinical signs can be restricted to one organ system or can affect multiple systems. CNS—tremor, head shaking, opisthotonos, ataxia, seizures, blindness. GI—weight loss, muscle wasting, emaciation, dilation of the proventriculus and/or ventriculus. Vomiting, diarrhea, undigested food in feces. Cardiac arrest. It is speculated that some case of feather damaging behavior are associated with PaBV infection.

### CAUSES
Psittaciform orthobornavirus 1 and 2. Psittaciform bornavirus 1 includes PaBV-1,2,3,4,7, whereas Psittaciform bornavirus 2 includes only PaBV-5. To date, PaBV-6 and PaBV-8 have not been classified. It seems that the different strains might cause different clinical disease with varying severity and course of disease. However, only PaBV-2 and -4 have been closely studied. Birds can be infected concurrently with different genotypes and there are reports that in carrier birds of one genotype, clinical disease occurred after being infected with a second genotype.

### RISK FACTORS
Transmission of the virus between birds seems not that easy. Despite shedding of the virus through feces and urine, oral and nasal infections were not successful in an experimental setup. Horizontal transmission occurs through wounds, followed by neural migration of the virus to the CNS and back to other organ systems. Experimental intracerebral and intravenous inoculation has also led to a successful infection. Recently, vertical transmission has been proven. The factors influencing vertical transmission are not well understood, but carrier birds infected at young age seems to support vertical transmission compared with birds infected as adults. It therefore seems reasonable to assume that indirect vectors do not support transmission between flocks and that carrier birds mainly contribute to virus distribution. Exchange of untested birds between collections or release of untested birds back into free-ranging populations seems to be a major risk. The immune status at time of infection seems to represent a risk factor to develop clinical disease. Birds with an immature immune system seem not to develop clinical disease as easily as birds infected as adults with a fully developed immune system.

## DIAGNOSIS

### DIFFERENTIAL DIAGNOSIS
**CNS signs**: Any infectious disease affecting the CNS. Examples include West Nile virus, paramyxovirus, avian influenza virus, *Sarcocystis* spp., also heavy metal toxicosis such as lead and zinc.
**GI signs**: Foreign bodies, heavy metal toxicosis, *Macrorhabdus ornithogaster*, *Candida* spp., neoplasia.
**General emaciation**: Any chronic disease with infectious or non-infectious background, severe parasitic infection, avian mycobacteriosis. Nutritional deficiencies.
**Feather-damaging behavior**: Psychogenic causes, bacterial feather folliculitis, management related causes, dermatitis.

### CBC/BIOCHEMISTRY/URINALYSIS
Alterations in CBC/biochemistry values are not specific and depend on the cause of clinical disease. Regularly PaBV diseased birds do not demonstrate any alterations. The pathogen itself does not cause alterations. In gastrointestinal chronic cases, elevation of creatine phosphokinase, anemia, hypoproteinemia. Hyperuricemia if neurologic signs result in difficulty drinking.

## OTHER LABORATORY TESTS
### General Considerations
The goals of diagnostic testing should first be clarified; are protocols adequate for viral infection only or also for the confirmation of clinical disease? As carrier birds occur regularly, birds with clinical signs caused by one of the differential diagnoses can still be detected as being PaBV positive, even though the virus may not be responsible for the clinical signs. Detection of viral infection does not therefore always lead to the cause of the clinical signs. Demonstration of the infection of the bird is important for a pre-purchase exam, transfer or release of birds, pairing of birds, establishment of flocks that are free from PaBV or to include PaBV as a potential cause of the clinical disease. However, in clinical disease, other causes need to be excluded to support the diagnosis of bornaviral disease.

### Molecular Testing
Birds that are PaBV positive might shed the virus intermittently and sometimes do not seroconvert, as the virus might hide from the immune system. Detection of the virus and serological testing is important for a complete diagnostic investigation. Direct demonstration of the virus is by PCR using a pooled swab from the crop and the cloaca. In deceased birds, brain and retina as well as adrenal tissue are the best tissues for PCR. Feces, feather, and blood are poor sample material and are not preferred. For psittacine birds, commercial laboratories commonly use real-time PCR protocols to detect PaBV-2 and/or PaBV-4 as the most common strains. In suspected bornaviral clinical cases with a negative PCR in those protocols, additional protocols involving other bornavirus genotypes might be used. Serological screening for anti-PaBV antibodies is important for a complete investigation. Gold standard is the immunofluorescence assay based on an infected cell culture. Alternatively, ELISA or Western blot tests are described. If the latter two tests use a single protein as antigen, it is required that this protein demonstrates cross-reaction between different ABV genotypes, to ensure a positive reaction when antibodies against any ABV–subtypes are detected. Comparison of such serological tests with tests based on infected cell cultures (providing several antigens) point toward a higher sensitivity for Western blot, especially when low antibody titers are present, even though all methods are congruent in birds with high antibody titers. As high antibody titers can regularly be found in clinically sick birds, the ELISA or Western blot might be adequate for diagnosing clinically ill birds. For the detection of carrier birds,

immunofluorescence might be advantageous. Birds with positive test results in both PaBV PCR and serology should be considered as positive. Those found to be positive by PCR alone should be retested 4–6 weeks later to confirm the result and exclude contamination of the sample, and also perhaps to detect seroconversion. In case of seroconversion or repeatedly positive PCR results, birds should be considered positive. Birds only positive by serology are likely to be infected, even though lifelong infection has not been proven and single cases have been suspected to have cleared infection.

## IMAGING
Imaging techniques are helpful in cases of bornaviral clinical disease in the GI tract. An enlarged, dilated proventriculus and/or ventriculus can be seen in radiography, best by using GI contrast media. A very thin proventricular wall, typical in a PaBV-related disease, can be seen during endocopy. If the contents of the proventriculus are visible, it is usually the terminal stage of the disease. Fluoroscopy has been described to detect an impaired motility of the proventricular wall. However, diagnostic alterations cannot be linked to PaBV infection as other causes demonstrate similar alterations. Other clinical courses linked to PaBV infection cannot be made visible in any imaging technique.

## DIAGNOSTIC PROCEDURES
While molecular testing only detects the virus, histopathology confirms the presence of lesions compatible with bornaviral diseases. In live birds, biopsy of affected organs, most commonly a crop biopsy if PDD is suspected, can be done. However, as this is very invasive, the detection of a PaBV infection is preferred. The sensitivity of crop biopsies for the detection of avian ganglioneuritis is variable and likely low when GI signs are absent. A piece of crop tissue may also be submitted for tissue PCR to increase the sensitivity of the test. High antibody titers are often seen in association with disease and might be useful for diagnosis. However, the exclusion of other potential causes in PaBV-positive birds is recommended. One theory describes the occurrence of antiganglioside antibodies in association with clinical disease (avian ganglioneuritis) independently from PaBV. Even though this theory has some merit, proof of the occurrence of antiganglioside antibodies in affected birds is lacking, as well as a validation of the tests.

## PATHOLOGIC FINDINGS
Gross pathological alterations are only linked to GI signs of a PaBV infection. The enlarged proventriculus is visible, commonly with a very thin wall allowing sight of food particles in the proventrulus. Further findings can be

emaciation and atrophy of ventricular muscles and dilation of the GI tract. In cases of CNS lesions, adrenal gland dysfunction, or myocardial lesions or arrhythmias, gross pathology is usually without visible alterations. Histopathologic lesions are characterized by lymphoplasmacytic ganglioneuritis. Lesions may be seen in the CNS as well as in peripheral nerves.

## TREATMENT
### APPROPRIATE HEALTH CARE
There is no direct treatment for PaBV infection. In vitro studies have demonstrated the effectiveness of ribavirin and favipiravir (T-705) against PaBV but in vivo studies have raised doubts about clinical efficiency. Treatment is currently focused on supportive care and reduction of clinical signs.
1) Immunosuppressive drugs might reduce the ABV-immune mediated lesions.
2) Reducing inflammatory lesions associated with the disease might reduce clinical signs. For immunosuppression, cyclosporine A as a selective T-cell suppressor has been used, either alone or with a COX-2 inhibitor. The anti-inflammatory drug meloxicam is widely used with variable success. At present, the use of the selective COX-2 inhibitor celecoxib remains the treatment of choice for birds. A novel yet interesting approach includes the use of gabapentin, a gamma-amino butyric acid agonist. Especially in cases with GI disease, a highly digestible diet and nutritional antioxidants should be used. Metoclopramide can assist to increase intestinal motility. Antiseizure medications can also be used.

### NURSING CARE
Nursing care will be necessary for months or years, consisting of therapy and nutritional management. Probiotics or antibiotics may be helpful to prevent/treat secondary enteric infections. In cases with severe GI disease, the feeding of supportive mush (critical care diet) might be required.

### ACTIVITY
Activity should not be limited if the patient is physically capable. In birds with CNS signs, especially with seizure, cages should not contain high perches and high density of branches where birds can be injured during seizuring.

### DIET
In cases with GI signs, the diet needs to be adapted. It should be highly digestible and preferably contain higher than normal fibre foods to aid in intestinal motility. Birds on a seed diet may have more difficulty

digesting foods. Conversion to a formulated diet may be very difficult in an ill bird, but if successful can advantageous. Supplemental feeding of highly digestible foods will be beneficial. Supplementation with foods high in antioxidants may be beneficial.

## CLIENT EDUCATION
The potential for exposure and disease in contact birds in the home or aviary is of concern. Infected or clinical birds should ideally be isolated from other birds. Breeders should be encouraged to sanitize their breeding flock, not to create and distribute carrier birds after vertical transmission. Bird-care centers should require negative testing before birds are accepted. Mixing untested birds from private owners at birds days, bird exhibition or free-flying events should be avoided.

## SURGICAL CONSIDERATIONS
A crop biopsy.

## MEDICATIONS
### DRUG(S) OF CHOICE
Celecoxib: 13–30 mg/kg PO q12h for several weeks; in case with severe CNS signs 30–40 mg/kg PO q12h. Meloxicam 0.5–1 mg/kg q12–24h IM or PO. Gabapentin: for CNS signs 10–25 mg/kg q12h. PO might be tried, up to 50 mg/kg PO. Cyclosporine 10 mg/kg q12h. PO in combination with a COX-2 inhibitor. Levetiracetam 100 mg/kg q8–12h. PO for seizures.

### CONTRAINDICATIONS
NSAIDs: GI ulcerations. Hypersensitivity to NSAIDs. Renal disease. Immunosuppressive drugs: Any other infection, especially aspergillosis.

### PRECAUTIONS
Renal disease, hepatic disease, cardiac disease, hemorrhagic disorders.

### POSSIBLE INTERACTIONS
Possibly interactions with NSAIDs include furosemide and fluconazole. Combination with antidepressants such as fluoxetine may cause bleeding or bruising.

### ALTERNATIVE DRUGS
N/A

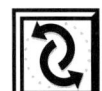

## FOLLOW-UP
### PATIENT MONITORING
After start of treatment, the bird's body weight needs to be closely monitored.

Any further weight reduction needs to be avoided. The severity of CNS signs should be monitored and birds no longer able to perch or with an increase in frequency of seizures should be taken as signs of terminal stage. The vision of the bird should be regularly assessed. The bird should be able to take food and water, which needs to be monitored. Weight gains can be misleading if the GI tract becomes dilated and filled with ingesta. Owners should be aware of signs that may indicate secondary infections, especially with spore-forming bacterial infections or yeast due to prolonged intestinal transit times. These risks may be higher with immunosuppressive treatments. If treating with NSAIDs, feces should be monitored for melena or fresh blood, which may indicate proventricular ulceration. Cases of proventricular dilatation can be monitored by radiography for increase in proventricular size. Monitoring of anti-PaBV antibody titers might be helpful for clinical prognosis as birds with a sudden increase in antibodies may be developing clinical disease.

### PREVENTION/AVOIDANCE
Any birds taken into a collection should test negative for PaBV. Positive birds, or a pair with one positive partner, should be isolated. Creating positive flocks separated from negative flocks should be considered. It seems to be possible to get negative offspring from positive parents. Vaccines against ABV have been experimentally tested. The success varied between the studies. However, in a few experimental setups, clinical signs were reduced after challenge of vaccinated birds, but infection with the challenge virus remained. No sterile immunization could be reached. Thus, clearance of the virus from the flock is currently the main strategy to combat the pathogen.

### POSSIBLE COMPLICATIONS
Foreign body ingestion. Secondary aspiration pneumonia. Injuries due to ataxia and seizures.

### EXPECTED COURSE AND PROGNOSIS
Birds infected with PaBV might stay healthy for years or even a lifetime. A prognosis for infected birds is thus impossible. In case anti-PaBV antibody titers increase, clinical disease becomes more likely. Once clinical signs have developed after infection, clinical prognosis is poor and leads sooner or later to death of the bird. With supportive treatment and care, affected birds can survive clinically, even for a few years. If symptoms become more severe, prognosis is very poor.

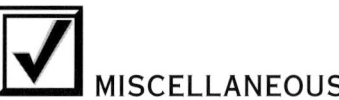

## MISCELLANEOUS
### ASSOCIATED CONDITIONS
N/A

### AGE-RELATED FACTORS
Age of the bird at time of infections, and presumably the stage of development of the immune system, seems to play a role in the development of clinical disease. Birds infected when very young do not develop clinical symptoms compared with birds infected as adults.

### ZOONOTIC POTENTIAL
Mammalian bornavirus, in particular squirrel bornavirus, does have a zoonotic potential. However, avian orthobornaviruses are divergent from those of mammals and, to date, a zoonotic potential has not been demonstrated or suspected.

### FERTILITY/BREEDING
PaBV is vertically transmitted. From PaBV-positive parents, not every egg contains the virus. It is therefore fair to assume that separate incubation and hand rearing might lead to some negative offspring, However, this requires the testing of all chicks raised.

### SYNONYMS
Avian ganglioneuritis, proventricular dilatation disease, macaw wasting disease, bornaviral ganglioneuritis.

### SEE ALSO
Anorexia
Candidiasis
Coelomic Distension
Emaciation
Enteritis and Gastritis
Feather-Damaging and Self-Injurious Behavior
Foreign Bodies (Gastrointestinal)
Ileus (Functional Gastrointestinal, Crop Stasis)
*Macrorhabdosis ornithogaster*
Neoplasia (Gastrointestinal and Hepatic)
Neoplasia (Neurologic)
Neurologic (Non-Traumatic Diseases)
Neurologic (Trauma)
Polyuria
Regurgitation and Vomiting
Seizures
Sick-Bird Syndrome
Toxicosis (Heavy Metals)
Undigested Food in Droppings

### ABBREVIATIONS
ABV—avian bornavirus
CBC—complete blood count
CNS—central nervous system
COX—cyclooxygenase
ELISA—enzyme-linked immunosorbent assay

**B**

GI—gastrointestinal
NSAIDs—non-steroidal anti-inflammatory drugs
PaBV—parrot bornavirus
PDD—proventricular dilatation disease

## INTERNET RESOURCES
None.

*Suggested Reading*
Lierz, M. (2016). Infectious diseases: Avian bornavirus and proventricular dilatation disease. In: *Current Therapy in Avian Medicine and Surgery*, 28–46. St. Louis, MO: Elsevier.

**Author**: Michael Lierz, DZooMed, DECZM (Wildlife Population Health) DECPVS, Prof Dr. Med Vet

 **Client Education Handout available online**

# BOTULISM

## BASICS

### DEFINITION
*Clostridium botulinum* is the main causative agent of botulism, a neurological disease caused by the neurotoxin produced by *C. botulinum*. It is an anaerobic, Gram-positive spore-forming, motile rod that commonly prospers in decaying organic matter and decomposing tissue. The disease is in essence a food poisoning caused by the ingestion of neurotoxin-laden food. In some cases, the disease can be caused by enterotoxicosis caused by bacteria that colonized the GI tract of an individual bird and produced the neurotoxin. This form of the disease usually occurs in birds that can normally carry the bacteria in their GI tract, such as chickens and ostriches. It is usually the result of preceding compromise to the normal gut flora. Nine serotypes of botulinum neurotoxins have been described but the majority of avian botulism outbreaks are caused by type C and fewer by D toxins, with sporadic die-off caused by types E and A toxins. *C. botulinum* spores are found in soil and wetland worldwide, while type C spores are primarily found in freshwater and marine environment. The carcass–maggot cycle of botulism is also recognized; the disease occurs secondary to the ingestion of fly larvae from decomposing carrion that is loaded with the neurotoxin. This route of poisoning is identified in some outbreaks in waterfowl but it is the prominent route in raptors that are otherwise considered less susceptible to the disease. Vultures are considered resistant. Botulism is the most significant population disease in migratory birds, especially waterfowl and shorebirds and has important ecological effect. Yearly massive die-off occurs in localized outbreaks in wetlands all around the world. Deaths of tens of thousands of birds or more are common in a single outbreak. However, underestimation is likely where the detection of dead birds can be challenging. Its epizoolotiological patterns are very complex and diverse, depending on numerous factors such as high environmental temperature and alkaline water pH, fly density, carcass density, and foraging patterns. Botulism causes flaccid paralysis followed by death within hours or days.

### PATHOPHYSIOLOGY
The *C. botulinum* exotoxin is a neurotoxin called BoNT and causes flaccid paralysis of the neck and limbs, pharyngeal, and respiratory muscles, and subsequent death. Botulism toxins are the most toxic known in nature. A protein complex against proteolysis in the GI tract protects the neurotoxin.

Once in the systemic circulation, all BoNT types have the same mode of action and enter into demyelinated terminal nerve endings, targeting the peripheral cholinergic nervous system. The extreme toxicity level is a result of its high affinity to the presynaptic membrane and specific and prolonged inhibition of neurotransmitter release from the nerve ending. The neurotoxin irreversibly binds to the neuronal membrane. It is then internalized into the cell by endocytosis, with the final step in the intoxication being the prevention of acetylcholine release, resulting in flaccid neuromuscular paralysis. GI tract toxicosis is less common but occurs in chickens and may also occur occasionally in wild birds such as raptors, waterfowl, and songbirds. Correlation with lead poisoning, vitamin A deficiency, or other factors debilitating the host GI tract function and flora has been made. This route of exposure is important in individual birds in captive situations but is insignificant in the massive wild bird die-offs. Another pathogenic mechanism of *C. botulinum* type C is caused by C2 toxin. This is not a neurotoxin but rather a lethal hemorrhagic toxin. Its role in avian botulism is unclear although the toxin is prevalent in wetlands. BoNTs do not cross the blood–brain barrier.

### SYSTEMS AFFECTED
Neuromuscular. Respiratory—paralysis of the respiratory muscles is usually the cause of death. Cardiovascular. Endocrine—the neurotoxin affects the adrenal glands. Gastrointestinal—severe ileus, megacolon, megacloaca. Renal/urologic—dehydration, dysuria and acute renal failure are common. Hemic—recumbent birds are rapidly infected with leeches and other parasites and suffer severe anemia.

### GENETICS
N/A

### INCIDENCE/PREVALENCE
Outbreaks in wild birds involve thousands to millions of birds in a single event. Most outbreaks are seasonal and occur in the summer or fall when the temperatures are higher than 79°F (26°C).

### GEOGRAPHIC DISTRIBUTION
Worldwide except the Antarctic. Most of the largest die-offs have occurred in North America and the frequency of outbreaks is higher in the USA and Canada compared with other countries. Avian botulism type C is frequently associated with wetland sediments in the USA and Canada.

### SIGNALMENT
All migratory waterfowl and shorebirds are highly sensitive. Botulism occurs less frequently in raptors and passerines and

vultures are considered resistant. Outbreaks have been described in farmed chickens and ostriches and in zoos.

### SIGNS

#### General Comments
Neuromuscular paralysis is the main mechanism; secondarily, all other organ systems are affected.

#### Historical Findings
Massive acute die-offs with no earlier warnings. Within the flocks individual birds can show flaccid paralysis, inability to walk or fly, diarrhea, and shallow and slow breathing, all of which would be evident to field agents detecting and monitoring the outbreaks.

#### Physical Examination Findings
Progressive paresis: flaccid neck and limbs. Ataxia, dysphagia, dyspnea, dehydration, green diarrhea, acute death.

### CAUSES
*C. botulinum* neurotoxin type C (A, D, and E in some cases) that binds irreversibly to the peripheral cholinergic nervous system.

### RISK FACTORS
Complex association among environmental factors and conditions is presumed to correlate with avian botulism outbreaks. However contradicting evidence makes this association rather unclear. High environmental temperatures, hence the summer and fall, are correlated with the massive die-offs but some outbreaks have been reported in the winter and spring. Stagnant or brackish water in wetlands are optimal for proliferation of the bacteria in decaying matter; again, few outbreaks occur in areas of cold, well-oxygenated running water. Bird crowdedness during migration and insect abundance are also important risk factors.

## DIAGNOSIS

### DIFFERENTIAL DIAGNOSIS
In the individual bird, any systemic neurological disease can be considered as a differential diagnosis. Other toxicities such as those caused by carbamates, organophosphorous, heavy metals, or algae should be considered.

### CBC/BIOCHEMISTRY/URINALYSIS
Hematological and biochemical changes are often absent, owing to the acute nature of the disease. Heterophilia, elevated liver enzymes, and hyperuricemia may be present.

### OTHER LABORATORY TESTS
Presumptive diagnosis can be made based on the typical history and clinical signs alone. Definitive diagnosis is made by tissue toxin analysis, usually from blood, kidney, or liver tissue. Mouse inoculation neutralization assay is

Avian

63

(CONTINUED)

BOTULISM

B

still considered the most sensitive assay in BoNT detection. Next-generation DNA sequencing is becoming more readily available; PCR and rt-PCR can identify the bacteria if present. Culture may be difficult due to the anaerobic and fastidious nature of *C. botulinum*. ELISA may be used to detect the neurotoxin.

## IMAGING
N/A

## DIAGNOSTIC PROCEDURES
N/A

## PATHOLOGIC FINDINGS
Gross pathology of dead birds is often consistent with no obvious lesions. Marked pulmonary congestion and edema have been described. Maggots and leeches can be found in the GI tract.

## TREATMENT

### APPROPRIATE HEALTH CARE
Treatment can be rewarding and most birds, if caught early, recover well with supportive care. Emphasis should be placed on protecting the patient from the elements, rehydration, and nutritional support.

### NURSING CARE
Aggressive fluid therapy is imperative. Recumbent birds should be provided with appropriate cushiony support.

### ACTIVITY
Birds are usually recumbent or weak and have limited ability to walk or fly.

### DIET
Providing easy access to food or gavage feeding in paralyzed birds is necessary.

### CLIENT EDUCATION
N/A

### SURGICAL CONSIDERATIONS
N/A

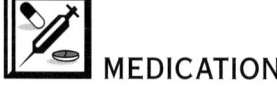

## MEDICATIONS

### DRUG(S) OF CHOICE
Type A and type C antitoxin injections are available and are very effective in facilitating

recovery and preventing the progression of clinical signs in affected birds. Antibiotics against anaerobes such as metronidazole, penicillin, and amoxicillin are useful in eliminating the bacteria from the GI tract.

### CONTRAINDICATIONS
N/A

### PRECAUTIONS
N/A

### POSSIBLE INTERACTIONS
N/A

### ALTERNATIVE DRUGS
A vaccine against type C botulism during an outbreak has been shown to aid in the healing process.

## FOLLOW-UP
Botulism is a disease of wild birds and, much more infrequently, of smaller captive populations such as chickens and zoological collections. Once recovered, follow-up is usually not necessary.

### PATIENT MONITORING
N/A

### PREVENTION/AVOIDANCE
Vaccine derived from neurotoxin C has been developed and can be useful in captive birds kept in zoological collections. Other measures that can aid in prevention include carcass removal and drainage of prone wetlands prior to the warm seasons.

### POSSIBLE COMPLICATIONS
Treatment of large numbers of birds is cost prohibitive.

### EXPECTED COURSE AND PROGNOSIS
In the individual birds that receive intensive supportive care, the survival rate ranges between 75% and 90%. Full recovery can take several weeks.

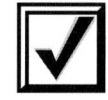

## MISCELLANEOUS

### ASSOCIATED CONDITIONS
N/A

### AGE-RELATED FACTORS
N/A

### ZOONOTIC POTENTIAL
N/A

### FERTILITY/BREEDING
N/A

### SYNONYMS
Limberneck, Western duck disease, alkali poisoning.

### SEE ALSO
Clostridiosis
Dehydration
Diarrhea
Emaciation
Ileus (Functional Gastrointestinal, Crop Stasis)
Neurologic (Non-Traumatic Diseases)
Neurologic (Trauma)
Toxicosis (Environmental/Pesticides)
Toxicosis (Heavy Metals)
Urate and Fecal Discoloration

### ABBREVIATIONS
BoNT—botulinum neurotoxins
ELISA—enzyme-linked immunosorbent assay
GI—gastrointestinal
PCR—polymerase chain reaction
rt-PCR—reverse transcriptase polymerase chain reaction

### INTERNET RESOURCES
Centers for Disease Control and Prevention. Botulism: https://www.cdc.gov/botulism
Merck & Co. MSD Manuals: www.merckmanuals.com
National Library of Medicine: www.ncbi.nlm.nih.gov

*Suggested Reading*
Meurens, F., Carlin, F., Federighi, M., et al. (2023). Clostridium botulinum type C, D, C/D, and D/C: An update. *Frontiers in Microbiology*, 13:1099184.
Rocke, T.E., Bollinger, T.K. (2007). Avian botulism. In: Infectious Diseases of Wild Birds (ed. N.J. Thomas, B. Hunter, B., C.T. Atkinson), 377–416. Oxford: Blackwell.
**Author:** Shachar Malka, DVM, DABVP (Avian), DACEPM

## BRACHIAL PLEXUS INJURY

B

# BASICS

## DEFINITION
Brachial plexus injury can be classified in four categories: (1) Avulsion is the separation of nerve root from its origin in the spinal cord. (2) Rupture is when the nerve is torn but not from its spinal root. (3) Neuroma is when scar tissue has grown around the injury site, putting pressure on the injured nerve and preventing the nerve from sending signals to the muscles. (4) Neurapraxia is when there is stretching and damage without the nerve being torn. In human, lesions can be classified as pre-ganglionic, post-ganglionic or mixed.

## PATHOPHYSIOLOGY
Trauma caused either by forceful impaction or penetrating wound at the area of thoracic girdle, which is the result of severe abduction of the scapula and thoracic limb, or displacement of the shoulder and scapula caudally with subsequent nerve damage (entrapment, total or partial tearing/detachment). Shoulder joint arthritis could also affect the nerves of the plexus. Soft-tissue infection and osteomyelitis could expand to neuritis. In neoplasia of the air sac, the bone structures could apply pressure/entrapment of the plexus nerves. Intraneural neoplasia (perineurioma of viral etiology).

## SYSTEMS AFFECTED
Neuromuscular system: Species variation on the origin of the plexus. In common buzzard. two plexuses the accessory brachial plexus (C10–C11) and the original brachial plexus (C11–T2); in merlin, swan, swift, it has five ventral neural origins; in the chicken and roadside hawk (*Rupornis magnirostris*) originated from C9–T3; in Amazon parrots (C9–C11); in turkey vulture, barn owl, burrowing owl, blue fronted Amazon, cardinal, white-throat sparrow, song sparrow, four nervous origin but within different vertebral spaces; in pigeon, duck, geese, turkey, blue and gold macaw, common sparrow, and northern ground hornbill had three nervous origins; in ostrich, originates from the last cervical and the first thoracic vertebrae.

## GENETICS
N/A

## INCIDENCE/PREVALENCE
Unknown global incidence. Rare; 32% of raptors with Horner syndrome also had wing paralysis.

## GEOGRAPHIC DISTRIBUTION
N/A

## SIGNALMENT
All avian species. Described in crow, gull, owls, pelican, cockatoo, red-tailed hawk. Mostly in free-living birds after collision trauma. Species variation of the plexus origin.

## SIGNS
Inability to fly. Wing dropping. Muscle atrophy. Joint ankylosis. Possibly accompanied by Horner syndrome (ptosis of eyelid, asymmetrically raised feathers, miosis). Good body condition.

## CAUSES
Penetration injury in the axillary area. Blunt (collision) trauma of thoracic girdle. Neoplasia of the axillary area or the nervous system. Shoulder arthritis. Possibly radiation therapy (human).

## RISK FACTORS
Rapidly flowing water (for waterbirds).

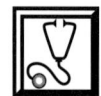

# DIAGNOSIS

## DIFFERENTIAL DIAGNOSIS
Shoulder luxation/fracture; chronic shoulder degenerative joint disease; proximal humeral fracture; damage of tendon of supracoracoideus muscle; radial nerve paralysis; central Horner syndrome; secondary to neoplasia.

## CBC/BIOCHEMISTRY/URINALYSIS
Often within normal limits unless secondary inflammation or infection has developed to a point where the WBC count begins to increase.

## OTHER LABORATORY TESTS
N/A

## IMAGING
Radiographs should be performed to rule out fracture or luxation of the thoracic girdle or the wing. CT (or CT myelography) and MRI are more useful to detect other conditions (e.g. spinal dislocation/fracture, osteomyelitis, degenerative disease, neoplasia, spinal cord injury).

## DIAGNOSTIC PROCEDURES
Orthopedic/neurologic examination. Electromyography. Nerve conduction study.

## PATHOLOGIC FINDINGS
Extensive fragmentation and loss of axons. Complete demyelination. Multifocal perivascular lymphocytic inflammation within the nerves. Connective tissue proliferation around nerve fiber bundles. Demyelination and axon loss in the left dorsal white matter at the origin of the brachial plexus of the spinal cord. Loss of cell bodies of the ventral grey column myofiber atrophy.

# TREATMENT

## APPROPRIATE HEALTH CARE
Initial stabilisation of the overall condition (trauma). Stabilization of the paretic wing until further diagnostics. Figure-of-eight bandage and around the body. Outpatient care.

## NURSING CARE
Care should include proper drug administration, movement restriction, bandage change and control.

## ACTIVITY
Restricted; cage rest.

## DIET
Assisted feeding if patient is anorectic.

## CLIENT EDUCATION
If a pet bird, owner should be informed of the poor prognosis and salvage wing amputation. Changes in the bird's environment/aviary should be made to facilitate the bird's welfare after wing amputation.

## SURGICAL CONSIDERATIONS
Salvage wing amputation (scapular dislocation or proximal humerus) could provide a chance to life. Novel technique described by Latney et al. (1) An elliptical approach that isolates shoulder joint specifically. (2) Minimal major muscle belly resection prior to intraoperative axillary nerve block. (3) A neurectomy technique employed to reduce nerve injury and neuroma formation (11–14). (4) Use of a minute capsular disarticulation with the use of bipolar cautery that serves to limit clavicular air sac damage.

# MEDICATIONS

## DRUG(S) OF CHOICE
NSAIDs, vitamin B complex.

## CONTRAINDICATIONS
N/A

## PRECAUTIONS
N/A

## POSSIBLE INTERACTIONS
N/A

## ALTERNATIVE DRUGS
Electrostimulation, gabapentin, neuromodulation/neuroablative techniques (human).

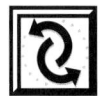

## FOLLOW-UP

### PATIENT MONITORING
Monitor the overall condition, CNS and PNS reflexes.

### PREVENTION/AVOIDANCE
N/A

### POSSIBLE COMPLICATIONS
Muscle atrophy, joint ankylosis.

### EXPECTED COURSE AND PROGNOSIS
In most cases, prognosis to return to full wing use is poor. Prognosis for survival is guarded depending on the severity of original cause of the wing paralysis. In a cockatoo, complete wing paralysis was reversed after 11 weeks but with 50% abduction loss. Salvage wing amputation could be applicable.

## MISCELLANEOUS

### ASSOCIATED CONDITIONS
Horner's syndrome, muscle atrophy, shoulder/spinal trauma, radial nerve damage, trauma of tendon of supracoracoideus muscle.

### AGE-RELATED FACTORS
N/A

### ZOONOTIC POTENTIAL
N/A

### FERTILITY/BREEDING
N/A

### SYNONYMS
N/A

### SEE ALSO
N/A

### ABBREVIATIONS
CNS—central nervous system
CT—computed tomography
MRI—magnetic resonance imaging
NSAIDs—non-steroidal anti-inflammatory drugs
PNS—peripheral nervous system
WBC—white blood cell

### INTERNET RESOURCES
N/A

*Suggested Reading*
Latney, L., Runge, J., Wyre, N., et al. (2018). Novel technique for scapulohumeral amputations in avian species: a case series. *Israel Journal of Veterinary Medicine*, 73:35–45.
Machado, D.L., Lezardo, T., Guimarães, J.P., et al. (2021). Origin and insertion of the nerves constituting the braquial plexus of the roadside hawk. *Anais da Academia Brasileira de Ciências*, 93(Suppl 3):e20191209.
McLelland, J.M., McLelland, D.J., Massy-Westropp, N., et al. (2020). Horner syndrome with ipsilateral wing paresis in a wild, juvenile yellow-tailed black cockatoo (*Calyptorhynchus funereus*). *Journal of Avian Medicine and Surgery*, 34(2):186–191.
Orosz, S., Antinoff, N. (2016). Clinical avian neurology and neuroanatomy. In: *Current Therapy in Avian Medicine and Surgery* (ed. B. Speer), 363–377. St. Louis, MO: Elsevier.

**Author**: Panagiotis Azmanis, DVM, PhD, DECZM (Avian)

# BURSA OF FABRICIUS DISEASES

## BASICS

### DEFINITION

The bursa of Fabricius (cloacal bursa or bursa), is a round sac located in the roof of the cloacal proctodeum, found only in birds. It is a primary lymphoid organ that is a critical part of the developing immune system in juvenile birds. The bursa is the site of beta-lymphocyte priming and production, so lymphocytes originating in the bursa are called B cells. In the rock pigeon, the structure grows slowly over the first 20 days after hatch and reaches it largest size (approx. 1–1.5 cm) by 60 days after hatching. In the chick, the bursa reaches its greatest size in about 1–2 weeks after hatching. Internally, the structure has a pentagonal appearance, with lymphoid cells grouped in follicular arrays separated by epithelial septa. Antigens drawn into the proctodeum enter the bursa and are presented to the fundic openings of the follicles, where they can make direct contact with beta-lymphocytes. Once matured and primed, the B cells disperse via the bloodstream throughout the body, leading to the involution and disappearance of all lymphoid tissue in the bursa. The time of involution varies with species, but typically occurs between 2 and 6 months of age, prior to sexual maturation. Involution leaves behind the empty epithelial "sac" of the structure, which is difficult to identify in mature birds. The ostium of the bursa and its chambers frequently persist as reasonably sized chambers that can sometimes be located endoscopically. The bursa may be destroyed either surgically or by infecting newborn chicks with IBDV. Bursal atrophy can also be incited by administration of testosterone. Bursectomized birds have very low levels of antibodies in their blood, but still possess circulating lymphocytes and have minimal cell-mediated immune responses. Bursectomized birds are more susceptible to bacterial infections, such as leptospirosis and salmonellosis, but not to intracellular bacterial infection such as *Mycobacterium avium*.

### PATHOPHYSIOLOGY

**IBDV:** A birnavirus that affects poultry (chickens, turkeys, ducks, guinea fowl), ostriches, and cranes. IBDV is highly infectious; transmission is primarily through the fecal–oral route. It is very stable in the environment outside a host for several months. In poultry, it kills immature B cells, leading to extensive necrosis, bursal swelling, and B cell destruction. As a result of B cell depletion, affected birds are often severely immunocompromised. Secondary splenic hypoplasia may ensue. As a result of decreased antibody levels and reduced inflammatory response, there is increased susceptibility to bacterial and fungal infections.

**ARV:** In infected birds, the virus is found in large mononuclear cells within the bursa. Affected birds show significant lymphoid depletion, and they can suffer from secondary mycotic infections, such as *Aspergillus* spp. and Zygomycetes.

**DEV:** A herpesvirus (anatid herpesvirus-1) that causes massive depletion of bursal and thymic lymphocytes, resulting in profound bursal and thymic atrophy, and multiple secondary bacterial infections. In white Pekin ducks, thymic atrophy is temporary, but bursal atrophy is irreversible. In addition, lymphoid depletion is seen in the spleen and harderian gland.

**Avian circovirus:** Causes virus-induced immunosuppression accompanied by wasting. The virus attacks both T and B cells and depletion of both cell types is common, therefore resulting in ill thrift and predisposition to secondary infections.

**PBFDV:** A circovirus. One of the portals of entry is the bursa of Fabricius. Depending on the time of infection, atrophy and necrosis of lymphoid tissues, including the bursa, in addition to beak abnormalities, feather dystrophies, liver atrophy, and liver necrosis can be seen in varying severity histologically. Immunosuppression with subsequent fatal secondary infections is seen in juvenile birds before bursal regression. Because the virus attacks and kills B cells, it can cause extensive necrosis of bursal follicles and lymphocytolysis. These areas of necrosis can develop into cysts containing proteinaceous fluid and cell debris. Bursal haemorrhage may be seen due to blood vessel disruption. Circoviral inclusion bodies are restricted to bursal follicles only.

**PiCV:** Distinct from PBFDV; the presence of circovirus inclusion in the bursa of pigeons is associated with lymphoid depletion in the bursa, spleen, and bone marrow. The lesions in the bursa range from mild lymphocellular necrosis to severe cystic bursal atrophy, and are accompanied by concurrent bacterial, viral, fungal, and parasitic infections.

**Premature bursal atrophy:** Can occur with severe non-specific stress mediated through increased blood levels of corticosteroids. This stress can induce bursal cell necrosis. Stressors include poor nutrition, chronic infections, poor management, and environmental stressors (i.e. inappropriate temperature and humidity, etc). Premature bursal atrophy, if it prevents maximum expansion of the B cell repertoire, will not only result in decreased antibody levels, but the diversity of those immunoglobulins will also be reduced, resulting in birds with increased susceptibility to secondary infections.

### SYSTEMS AFFECTED

Lymphoid system: Bursa of Fabricius—viral infection can lead to bursal atrophy, bursal cell necrosis, cyst formation, and bursal haemorrhage. Chronic, severe stress or provocation with exogenous testosterone can cause premature bursal atrophy that can induce bursal cell necrosis. Secondary to the resulting B cell depletion and destruction leading to decreased antibody levels, decreased immunoglobulin differentiation, and decreased inflammatory response, affected birds have increased susceptibility to secondary bacterial, mycotic, viral, and parasitic infections, resulting in general ill-thrift, wasting, and weakened immune-system.

### GENETICS

N/A

### INCIDENCE/PREVALENCE

**IBDV:** Affects poultry (chickens, turkeys, ducks, guinea fowl), ostriches, and cranes.
**ARV:** Can affect Psittaciformes, Galliformes, and numerous wild bird species.
**Avian circovirus:** Has been reported in Psittaciformes, Anseriformes, Columbiformes, Passeriformes, Charadriiformes, and Struthioniformes.
**PBFDV:** Psittaciformes—all species and ages are considered susceptible (cockatiels are less susceptible).
**PiCV:** Pigeons.

### GEOGRAPHIC DISTRIBUTION

No specific geographic distribution is noted with these conditions.

### SIGNALMENT

Young birds may be more predisposed to infectious causes. IBDV, which exists as serotypes 1 and 2, is frequently seen in chicks 3–6 weeks of age, when immature B cells populate the bursa and maternal immunity has waned, causing high mortality. The subclinical form of infection is established in older birds, with increased morbidity (up to 100%). Both serotypes naturally infect poultry and ostriches, with pathogenicity only being reported in chickens by serotype 1. Serotype 2 viruses are isolated from turkeys and are avirulent to chickens. ARVs, such as viral arthritis and/or tenosynovitis, can infect both domestic and wild birds. Infection is most common in young or immune-incompetent individuals. Infection is particularly important in heavier bodied or rapidly growing poultry meat breeds, where inflammation within the joints and tendons can manifest as poor mobility, lameness, and decreased growth rates. DEV (anatid herpesvirus-1) is an acute, highly contagious disease of ducks, geese, and swans of all ages.

It has an incubation period of 3–7 days, and is characterized by hemorrhage and necrosis in internal organs, sudden death, and high mortality (5–100%), particularly in older ducks. Adult ducks may die in good flesh. Ducklings that are infected frequently show dehydration, weight loss, blue beaks, and blood-stained vents. PBFDV is most commonly seen in parrots of African and Australasian origins and in birds less than 3 years of age.

## SIGNS

### Historical Findings
Flocks, especially those of younger birds, may develop acute onset of ataxia, lethargy, diarrhea, soiled vent, vent picking, inflammation of vent, high morbidity and mortality (clinical IBDV, ARV—higher morbidity than mortality). Poor feed efficiency, ill-thrift, decreased growth rates, cachexia (subclinical IBDV, avian circovirus, anatid herpesvirus-1, premature bursal atrophy). Acute high and persistent mortality in waterfowl flocks, especially adult ducks in good flesh (anatid herpesvirus-1).

### Physical Examination Findings
In clinical IBD, may include cloacal bursa that is swollen, edematous, yellowish in color, and occasionally hemorrhagic. Sometimes hemorrhages seen on serosal and mucosal surfaces. Clinical symptoms include prostration, watery diarrhea, cloacal inflammation. In subclinical IBD, may include atrophy of the bursa, cachexia, weakness. Viremia with ARV may see lameness, poor mobility, tenosynovitis, arthritis, edema of hock joints, digital flexor tendon, and/or gastrocnemius tendon, gastrocnemius tendon damage or rupture, tendon fibrosis, hydropericardium if spread to heart. In duck viral enteritis, may include inability to stand, weakness, depression, light sensitivity, inappetence, extreme thirst, ataxia, nasal discharge, soiled vent, watery or hemorrhagic diarrhea, blue beaks, bloodstained vent, acute drop in egg production of hens. In PBFDV, may include lack of powder down on the beak, abnormal beak growth (overgrowth, breakage, delaminations), abnormal feather growth (pinched or clubbed at feather base, may have hemorrhage within the shaft), feathers falling out easily, feathers slow to grow back or do not grow back at all, pigment loss in colored feathers, stunted growth, wasting. In pigeon circovirus, may include ill thrift, diarrhea, upper GI signs. Concurrent secondary infections are common.

## CAUSES
Fecal–oral transmission, shed in feces and transferred from house to house by fomites (IBDV), stable and difficult to eradicate in environment. IBDV serotype 1 causes disease in chickens. IBDV serotype 2 infects chickens and turkeys but does not cause clinical disease or immunosuppression. Direct contact from infected to susceptible birds (DEV). Indirect contact with a contaminated environment; water seems to be a natural route of viral transmission, outbreaks frequent in duck flocks with access to bodies of water cohabitated with free-living waterfowl (DEV). A carrier condition is suspected in wild ducks with DEV, recovered birds may become latently infected carriers and shed the virus periodically. Infection via oral exposure or ingestion (ARV, PBFDV). Ingestion or inhalation of contaminated viral particles in feces and/or feather dust, ingestion of regurgitated food (PBFDV). Ingestion of crop milk (PiCV). Vertical transmission (ARV, PBFDV). Chronic severe stressors, including poor nutrition, chronic infections, poor management, and environmental stressors (premature bursal atrophy). See also Pathophysiology section.

## RISK FACTORS
See Signalment and Causes sections.

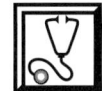 **DIAGNOSIS**

## DIFFERENTIAL DIAGNOSIS
### Differentiating Similar Signs
Diagnosis of IBDV can be achieved by observation of the cloacal bursa for macroscopic lesions (swelling, yellowish coloration, hemorrhage, atrophy) followed by microscopic analysis for lymphocyte depletion in the follicles and detection of the viral VP2 gene using rt-PCR. ARV infection causing viral tenosynovitis/arthritis cannot be differentiated without virus isolation in affected tissue, tendon, or synovial fluid and rt-PCR. Formalin-fixed tendon samples for histopathologic examination can confirm inflammatory changes consistent with reoviral infection, but with chronicity microscopic changes become indistinguishable from other joint pathologies that results in tendon fibrosis. Duck viral enteritis can be presumptively diagnosed based on clinical history and lesions. Lesions include multifocal ulcerations/necrosis of the mucosa and submucosa of the GI tract and lymphoid tissues, free blood in body cavities, petechial and ecchymotic "paint brush" hemorrhages on the heart, liver, pancreas, mesentery, and other organs. The cloacal bursa may be severely congested or hemorrhagic. Eosinophilic intranuclear inclusions may be seen in epithelial cells of the GI tract, thymus, bursa, spleen, esophagus, cloaca, liver, conjunctiva, and harderian gland. Occasional intracytoplasmic inclusions are also seen in the epithelial cells of the conjunctiva, esophagus, bursa, and cloaca. Definitive diagnosis is via viral isolation, viral detection molecular techniques, and PCR. Serologic tests are not useful for diagnosis in acute infections. Feather changes with PBFDV infection can be present for months to years, but as disease progresses, the immune system becomes affected and most birds die of secondary infections. With young birds with peracute infection, enteritis, pneumonia, weight loss, and death can occur. Grey parrots may develop pancytopenia. Viral inclusions are found in the thymus, bursa, and bone marrow.

### Differentiating Causes
There can be several overlapping clinical symptoms/exam findings with diseases of the bursa. Differential diagnoses can be excluded by diagnostic testing with viral PCR, biopsy sampling, serology, bacterial culture and sensitivity, mycobacterial culture, and fungal culture, Gram stain, and necropsy findings.

### Differential Diagnoses to Consider
**IBDV**: gastrointestinal parasites (i.e. coccidiosis), dysbiosis, Gram negative bacterial infection, or clostridial infection, given common finding of bloody droppings and diarrhea, other bacterial, viral, or mycotic infection/septicemia.
**ARV**: Bacterial or mycotic joint infection/septicemia, trauma, Marek's disease.
**DEV**: Duck viral hepatitis, pasteurellosis, other bacterial infection (mycoplasmosis, staphyloccosis, colibacillosis), necrotic and hemorrhagic enteritis, trauma, toxicosis, other viral infection (Newcastle disease, avian influenza, fowlpox), nutritional deficiencies (calcium:phosphorus imbalance, rickets).
**Avian circovirus**: Endocrinopathy, feather folliculitis, metabolic imbalance, nutritional deficiency, polyomavirus, behavioral/stress-induced feather plucking, ectoparasites.

## CBC/BIOCHEMISTRY/URINALYSIS
In non-systemic cases, the hemogram and biochemical profile may be normal. Leukocytosis may occur with secondary or concurrent systemic infection. Leukopenia may occur with circovirus infection. Anemia seen with severe gastrointestinal ulceration and bleeding and psittacine circovirus. Hypoglycemia seen with prolonged anorexia or secondary sepsis.

## CYTOLOGY
Lymphocyte depletion in the follicles of the bursa of Fabricius with IBDV, ARV, and circovirus infections. Eosinophilic intranuclear inclusions may be seen in the epithelial cells of the gastrointestinal tract, thymus, bursa, spleen,

esophagus, cloaca, liver, conjunctiva, and harderian gland, and occasional intracytoplasmic inclusions scattered in epithelial cells of the conjunctiva, esophagus, bursa, and cloaca with DEV. Basophilic and botryoid intracytoplasmic inclusion bodies in follicular epithelium are pathognomonic for circovirus (more commonly seen in pigeons than psittacine birds), inclusions in cloacal bursa epithelium and macrophages with circovirus are characterized as semicircles, circles, or paracrystalline arrays of 14–16 nm viral particles.

## OTHER LABORATORY TESTS
**IBDV**: Molecular detection of the viral VP2 gene using rt-PCR. Sequence analysis of VP2 gene to identify the IBDV genotype. Virus isolation in chicken embryos or chicken embryo fibroblast cell cultures is possible but not necessary.
**ARV**: Viral isolation or rt-PCR from affected tissue, tendon, or synovial fluid for definitive diagnosis. ELISA can diagnose reovirus infection and virus exposure, but results are not definitive. Virus neutralization assays can be used to detect type-specific antibodies.
**DEV**: Viral isolation from liver, spleen, or kidney tissues, conventional or quantitative real-time PCR. Serology has little diagnostic value.
**Avian circovirus**: PCR of feces, feather dander, or blood. Biopsy of affected feather follicles showing basophilic intracytoplasmic inclusion. PCR may detect infection in birds that are clinically healthy. PCR analysis can also be used for environmental testing due to the stability of the virus. Histopathology may show intracytoplasmic inclusions in feathers, bursa, thymus, liver, or other organs.

## IMAGING
Endoscopic evaluation of the cloacal bursa may be performed. Targeted biopsies of any identified lesions may be collected using an endoscopic biopsy forceps. Survey radiographs are often normal, but may have changes should there be secondary infections affecting the gastrointestinal tract or other organs.

## DIAGNOSTIC PROCEDURES
N/A

## PATHOLOGIC FINDINGS
N/A

 TREATMENT

## APPROPRIATE HEALTH CARE
The degree of nursing care needed is dependent on severity of disease.

## NURSING CARE
Non-debilitated patients with mild lesions or symptoms may be treated on an outpatient basis if hydrated and eating well on their own, but should be kept isolated. Supportive care may be needed for anorexic, dehydrated, and/or debilitated patients, including fluids (SQ, IV, or IO), easily digestible nutrition, including gavage feeding in cases of inappetence, gastroprotectant medications in cases of GI ulceration and hemorrhage, antimicrobial and/or antimycotic medications as indicated to treat any concurrent secondary infections, and heat support for birds experiencing weight loss or negative energy balance.

## ACTIVITY
Most birds with this condition may be allowed to determine their own level of activity.

## DIET
Although dietary improvements may be needed, changes should be gradual and deferred until the patient has recovered.

## CLIENT EDUCATION
Clients should be educated on disinfection protocols of contaminated areas and appropriate biosecurity practices. Infectious disease testing and quarantine of new birds should be performed prior to introduction into the home, aviary, or flock. Avoid contact with wild, free-flying birds. Clients should also be educated on nutritional requirements for their particular species. Any underlying husbandry deficiencies should be addressed.

## SURGICAL CONSIDERATIONS
Bursectomy can lead to very low levels of antibodies in their blood, however has minimal effect on cell-mediated immune responses. Bursectomized birds are more susceptible to bacterial infections, but not to intracellular bacterial infection. See also Definition section.

 MEDICATIONS

## DRUG(S) OF CHOICE
Analgesia may be used when inappetence or dysphagia is present, including meloxicam 0.5–1 mg/kg PO q12h. Gastroprotectant medications are useful when GI ulceration is present, including famotidine (0.5 mg/kg PO q12–24h), omeprazole (0.5–1 mg/kg PO q12–24h), sucralfate 30 mg/kg PO q8–12h, and/or barium 20 ml/kg PO q24h. Bacterial—appropriate antibiotic therapy based on culture and sensitivity. Mycotic—appropriate antimycotic therapy based on culture and sensitivity. Parasitic—appropriate antiparasitic therapy based on parasite identification.

IBDV—successful specific treatment has not been reported; treatment of secondary infections if present. ARV—successful specific treatment has not been reported; treatment of secondary infections if present. Duck enteritis virus—successful specific treatment has not been reported; treatment of secondary infections if present. Avian circovirus—successful specific treatment has not been reported; treatment of secondary infections if present.

## CONTRAINDICATIONS
Caution with use of NSAIDs with GI ulceration.

## PRECAUTIONS
Fenbendazole can cause toxicity in a number of species, including pigeons and doves, vultures, storks, cockatiels, and lories. Nystatin should not be given in cases of suspected GI ulceration, as this may result in absorption-dependent toxicity. A fecal cytology or fecal occult blood test may help to identify this issue, particularly in patients with anemia.

## POSSIBLE INTERACTIONS
N/A

## ALTERNATIVE DRUGS
N/A

 FOLLOW-UP

## PATIENT MONITORING
If inappetence, anorexia, dehydration, or significant weight loss occurs, hospitalize patient for supportive care and treatment, and obtain appropriate diagnostics. In cases of severe debilitation, severe morbidity, and highly contagious infection, humane euthanasia should be considered.

## PREVENTION/AVOIDANCE
Commercially available vaccines are available for IBDV, ARVs, and DEV. Birds should be fed a species-appropriate high-quality, nutritionally sound diet. Owners should observe good hygiene, and housing, nest boxes, food, and water supply should be carefully kept as clean as possible. Flock biosecurity measures should be observed.

## POSSIBLE COMPLICATIONS
See Pathophysiology and Systems Affected sections.

## EXPECTED COURSE AND PROGNOSIS
Prognosis is typically guarded for birds with necrosis, damage, or atrophy of the bursa due to the decreased B cell (humoral) immune response and lymphocyte depletion. There is no treatment for viral infections that cause

bursal disease. For stress related causes, husbandry and diet can be modified to prevent further damage. IBDV has flock morbidity typically at 100% and mortality ranging from 5% to > 60%. High levels of maternal antibodies can minimize early infection. Vaccination of breeder flocks one or more times during the growing period is recommended, first with a live vaccine and again before egg production with an inactivated vaccine to control this disease. Birds with debilitating signs of viral arthritis, such as lameness and poor mobility affecting ability to reach food/water, should be euthanized. ARV is a well-established cause of viral arthritis, but not all ARVs cause viral arthritis. Prevention of clinical signs depends on serotype-specific immune response through vaccination. There is no treatment for DEV, which has a mortality rate of 5–100%. Recovered birds can become latently infected carriers and may shed the virus periodically. Immunization of breeders and ducklings with live attenuated vaccines can be performed in available countries. Birds with circovirus can range from peracute severe infection to subclinical infection and can live anywhere from months to years after diagnosis. Death is typically due to immunosuppression and secondary infection. Circovirus-positive birds should be isolated due to the contagious nature of this disease, and strict hygiene practices should be followed. New birds should be tested for this disease and quarantine prior to introduction into an aviary.

## MISCELLANEOUS

### ASSOCIATED CONDITIONS
Secondary bacterial, mycotic, and parasitic infections are often found concurrently with disease of the bursa due to suppression of the immune system.

### AGE-RELATED FACTORS
See Signalment section.

### ZOONOTIC POTENTIAL
The bursal conditions discussed in this chapter are not considered infectious to humans. However, it is possible for secondary bacterial, mycotic, parasitic, or other viral infections to be contracted with zoonotic potential.

### FERTILITY/BREEDING
Vertical transmission can occur with ARVs and PBFDV. Egg production in laying hens can decrease with immune suppression.

### SYNONYMS
IBDV: Gumboro disease, infectious bursitis, infectious avian nephrosis.

### SEE ALSO
Circovirus (Psittacines)
Circoviruses (Non-Psittacine Birds)
Herpesvirus (Columbid Herpesvirus 1, in Pigeons and Raptors)
Herpesvirus (Duck Viral Enteritis)
Herpesvirus (Passerine Birds)
Herpesvirus (Psittacid Herpesviruses)
Reoviruses
Respiratory Distress

### ABBREVIATIONS
ARV—avian reovirus
DEV—duck enteritis virus
GI—gastrointestinal
IBD—infectious bursal disease
IBDV—infectious bursal disease virus
NSAIDs—non-steroidal anti-inflammatory drugs
PBFDV—psittacine beak and feather disease virus
PCR—polymerase chain reaction
PiCV—pigeon circovirus
rt-PCR—reverse transcriptase polymerase chain reaction

### INTERNET RESOURCES
Banda, A. (2022). Duck viral enteritis. *MSD Veterinary Manual*: https://www.merckvetmanual.com/poultry/duck-viral-enteritis/duck-viral-enteritis
Blakey, J. (2023). Infectious bursal disease in poultry. *MSD Veterinary Manual*: https://www.merckvetmanual.com/poultry/infectious-bursal-disease/infectious-bursal-disease-in-poultry
Cornell Wildlife Health Lab. Avian reovirus: https://cwhl.vet.cornell.edu/disease/avian-reovirus#collapse9
Hoppes, S.M. (2022). Viral diseases of pet birds. *MSD Veterinary Manual*: https://www.merckvetmanual.com/exotic-and-laboratory-animals/pet-birds/viral-diseases-of-pet-birds#v3305817

Michigan Department of Natural Resources. Duck virus enteritis: https://www.michigan.gov/dnr/managing-resources/wildlife/wildlife-disease/wdm/duck-virus-enteritis
Nicholds, J., Sellers, H.S. (2022). Viral arthritis in poultry. *MSD Veterinary Manual*: https://www.merckvetmanual.com/poultry/viral-arthritis/viral-arthritis-in-poultry
Tabler, T., Wells, J. (2018). Infectious bursal disease (gumboro) in backyard chickens. Mississippi State University Extension Service: http://extension.msstate.edu/publications/infectious-bursal-disease-gumboro-backyard-chickens
World Organisation for Animal Health: www.woah.org

*Suggested Reading*
Choi, Y.R., Kim, S.W., Ke, S., et al. (2022). Avian reoviruses from wild birds exhibit pathogenicity to specific pathogen free chicken by footpad route. *Frontiers in Veterinary Science*, 9:844903.
Dey, S., Pathak, D.C., Ramamurthy, N., et al. (2019). Infectious bursal disease virus in chickens: prevalence, impact, and management strategies. *Veterinary Medicine (Auckland, N.Z.)* 10:85–97.
Gyimesi, Z.S. (2015). Columbiformes. In: *Fowler's Zoo and Wild Animal Medicine*, Vol. 8, (ed. R.E. Miller, M. Fowler), 164–171. St. Louis, MO: Elsevier.
Pendl, H., Tizard, I. (2015). Immunology. In: *Current Therapy In Avian Medicine and Surgery* (ed. B.L. Speer BL), 401–402, 419–421. St. Louis, MO: Elsevier.
Taylor, W.M. (2015). Clinical significance of the avian cloaca: interrelationships with the kidneys and the hindgut. In: *Current Therapy In Avian Medicine and Surgery*, (ed. B.L. Speer BL), 334–335. St. Louis, MO: Elsevier.
Xu, A., Sun, L., Tu, K., et al. (2021). Experimental co-infection of variant infectious bursal disease virus and fowl adenovirus serotype 4 increases mortality and reduces immune response in chickens. *Veterinary Research*, 52:61.

**Authors**: Hannah Attarian, DVM, and Anthony Pilny, DVM, DABVP (Avian)

# CAMPYLOBACTERIOSIS

## BASICS

### DEFINITION
Campylobacteriosis is caused by infection with bacteria from the genus *Campylobacter*, with *Campylobacter jejuni* being most commonly associated with infection.

### PATHOPHYSIOLOGY
Most birds infected with *Campylobacter* are carriers, which are infected, asymptomatic shedders. Clinical disease, such as subacute or chronic hepatitis, can occur, but often, factors such as parasitic or other infections likely predispose the bird to clinical disease.

### SYSTEMS AFFECTED
**Gastrointestinal**: Hemorrhagic enteritis; diarrhea, sometimes with yellow staining.
**Hepatobiliary**: Subacute to chronic hepatitis.
**Non-specific**: Lethargy, anorexia, emaciation.

### GENETICS
All bird species can serve as competent reservoirs for this thermophilic organism.

### INCIDENCE/PREVALENCE
Prevalence varies with species but is generally high in poultry, crows, and gulls. One study found that 25.2% of galliformes, 12.9% of anseriformes, 8.3% of columbiformes, and only one of 179 psittaciformes examined on necropsy were positive for *C. jejuni* (Yohasundram et al.). Another study found a relatively high prevalence in crows (23%) and gulls (25%; Keller et al.).

### GEOGRAPHIC DISTRIBUTION
*Campylobacter* has worldwide distribution.

### SIGNALMENT
All avian species.

### SIGNS

#### General Comments
Most avian species are asymptomatic reservoirs of *Campylobacter*.

#### Historical Findings
Possible exposure to feces of poultry or wild birds. Weight loss, diarrhea, decreased appetite.

#### Physical Examination Findings
Poor body condition. Diarrhea, which might include blood or changes in color of urates to yellow or green.

### CAUSES
Campylobacteriosis is caused by infection with *Campylobacter* sp., most frequently *C. jejuni*.

### RISK FACTORS
Although many birds are infected with *Campylobacter*, few develop clinical disease. Birds that develop clinical disease, such as enteritis or hepatitis, often will have other predisposing factors such as infection with other agents.

## DIAGNOSIS

### DIFFERENTIAL DIAGNOSIS
Other causes of enteritis, diarrhea, or hepatitis such as *Salmonella*, *Escherichia coli*, *Yersinia* spp.

### CBC/BIOCHEMISTRY/URINALYSIS
Asymptomatic patients are unlikely to have any changes. Animals with enteritis diarrhea may have indications of dehydration such as an increased total protein or packed cell volume. Animals with hepatitis may have elevated aspartate aminotransferase and bile acids or decreased albumin and protein.

### OTHER LABORATORY TESTS
A sample of feces or tissue should be submitted for culture to isolate the organism. The diagnostic laboratory should be notified of suspected *Campylobacter* as an etiologic agent because special procedures are needed for growth. Whole genome sequencing is used in investigations to determine the source of an outbreak.

### IMAGING
Radiography may show an enlarged liver if hepatitis is present, but a sample must be collected for culture to determine the etiology of infection.

### DIAGNOSTIC PROCEDURES
Collection of feces or a tissue sample for culture will be needed to definitively diagnose campylobacteriosis. A fine-needle aspirate may be needed to collect a sample from the liver. Samples from affected tissues can be collected at necropsy.

### PATHOLOGIC FINDINGS
The liver may be enlarged, pale, or greenish in color and often congested. Hemorrhage may be present. Enteritis can also be present. Diffuse inflammation may be present.

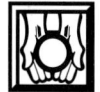

## TREATMENT

### APPROPRIATE HEALTH CARE
Most infected animals are asymptomatic and require no treatment. Treatment for those with clinical disease is described below.

### NURSING CARE
Nutritional support, including fluids, will help correct dehydration associated with diarrhea and weight loss.

### ACTIVITY
Movement of the animal should be limited to reduce fecal contamination, which could lead to exposure of other animals or humans to *Campylobacter*.

### DIET
Although appetite may be decreased, oral intake of normal food and fluids is acceptable.

### CLIENT EDUCATION
*Campylobacter* is zoonotic, and owners must take precautions to eliminate exposure to themselves, other humans, and other animals. Hand washing and cleaning and disinfection of contaminated areas and equipment are essential. Most human infections are associated with consumption of poultry meat.

### SURGICAL CONSIDERATIONS
N/A

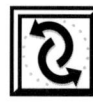

## MEDICATIONS

### DRUG(S) OF CHOICE
Treatment should be based on culture and sensitivity of the organism; asymptomatic patients are unlikely to be identified and treated. Oral erythromycin may be used to treat poultry at a dose of 10–30 mg/kg for 4 days or psittacines at 30–40 mg/kg. Azithromycin is currently used to treat infections in humans.

### CONTRAINDICATIONS
Antibiotics that have not been shown to be appropriate based on culture and sensitivity.

### PRECAUTIONS
*Campylobacter* can develop antibiotic resistance. Fluoroquinolones should not be used in poultry.

### POSSIBLE INTERACTIONS
N/A

### ALTERNATIVE DRUGS
N/A

## FOLLOW-UP

### PATIENT MONITORING
Fecal output and consistency should be monitored and will return to normal typically within 1 week. Attitude should also improve with fluid administration. Plasma biochemistry can be repeated to determine if indicators of hepatitis are improving.

### PREVENTION/AVOIDANCE
Avoid exposure to *Campylobacter* by keeping environments clean and disinfected and purchasing food from reputable sources;

C

wildlife should be excluded from contact with pets or livestock.

## POSSIBLE COMPLICATIONS
Humans can become sick with campylobacteriosis.

## EXPECTED COURSE AND PROGNOSIS
Most animals will not experience clinical disease from infection; those that develop hepatitis have a guarded prognosis and can suffer significant mortality in flock situations.

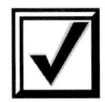 **MISCELLANEOUS**

## ASSOCIATED CONDITIONS
N/A

## AGE-RELATED FACTORS
Young animals may be more likely to develop severe clinical disease.

## ZOONOTIC POTENTIAL
There are approximately 1.5 million cases of human campylobacteriosis in the United States annually. Most of these cases are foodborne, particularly involving consumption of poultry meat and unpasteurized milk, but a smaller number can be due to animal exposure.

## FERTILITY/BREEDING
N/A

## SYNONYMS
N/A

## SEE ALSO
Colibacillosis
Diarrhea
Emaciation
Liver Disease
Pasteurellosis
Salmonellosis

## ABBREVIATIONS
N/A

## INTERNET RESOURCES
Centers for Disease Control and Prevention. (2021). *Campylobacter* (campylobacteriosis): https://www.cdc.gov/campylobacter
Centers for Disease Control and Prevention. (2023). Keeping pets healthy keeps people healthy too: http://www.cdc.gov/healthypets
US Department of Agriculture, Animal and Plant Health Inspection Service. (2023). Defend the flock program: http://healthy birds.aphis.usda.gov
Uzal, F. (2023). Enteric campylobacteriosis in animals. *Merck Veterinary Manual*: http://www.merckmanuals.com/vet/digestive_system/enteric_campylobacteriosis/overview_of_enteric_campylobacteriosis.html
Zhang, Q. (2023). Campylobacteriosis in birds. *Merck Veterinary Manual*: http://www.merckmanuals.com/vet/poultry/avian_campylobacter_infection/overview_of_avian_campylobacter_infection.html

*Suggested Reading*
Keller, J.I., Shriver, W.G., Waldenstrom, J. et al. (2011). Prevalence of *Campylobacter* in wild birds of the mid-Atlantic region, USA. *Journal of Wildlife Diseases*, 47:750–754.
Lin, J. (2009). Novel approaches for *Campylobacter* control in poultry. *Foodborne Pathogens and Disease*, 6:755–765.
Yogasundram, K., Shane, S.M., Harrington, K.S. (1989). Prevalence of *Campylobacter jejuni* in selected domestic and wild birds in Louisiana. *Avian Diseases*, 33:664–667.
**Author**: Marcy J. Souza, DVM, MPH, MPPA, DABVP (Emeritus, Avian), DACVPM

# CANDIDIASIS

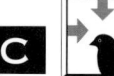

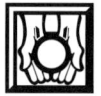

## BASICS

### DEFINITION
Candidiasis is a common yeast infection reported in many species of birds. It is caused by *Candida* spp. with *Candida albicans* being most commonly reported. Other *Candida* sp. have recently been reported as advanced molecular methods for species identification such as PCR and next-generation DNA sequencing become more readily available. *C. albicans* prevalence is followed by *Candida glabrata*, *Candida kefyr*, *Candida lambica*, and *Candida parapsilosis*. Candidiasis is commonly diagnosed in psittacine birds, pigeons and doves, poultry, raptors, and waterfowl, but can cause disease in any bird species. Juvenile birds are most commonly affected. Adult birds can be affected at any age as well. Stress, malnutrition and immunosuppression are key factors. Rarely, infection can be seen even in adult birds without any apparent predisposing factors. Candidiasis is an opportunistic infection and candida spores can be part of normal gastrointestinal flora in apparently healthy birds. Clinical disease occurs with overgrowth, vitamin A deficiency, spoiled feed source, or secondary to primary damage to the mucosal membrane integrity. Infection is usually restricted to the upper GI tract. The oropharynx and the esophagus are primarily affected, but infection can settle in all parts of the digestive system, as well as the choana and the upper respiratory system. Rare involvement of other organ systems occurs.

### PATHOPHYSIOLOGY
Overgrowth of budding candida yeasts on the surface of the GI mucosal membrane results in thickening of the mucosal membrane. Invasion into the deeper cell layer results in protuberant ulcer formations and can lead to compromise or dysfunction of the affected organ. Crop stasis, anorexia, and regurgitation are the most common signs.

### SYSTEMS AFFECTED
**GI**: Oropharynx, esophagus/crop are most commonly affected. Lower GI tract infection in more severe chronic cases.
**Respiratory**: Choana, infraorbital sinus are frequently involved. Parabronchial pneumonia in severe disseminated cases.
**Skin**: Rare, usually in immunocompromised birds.
**Cardiovascular**: Rare, myocarditis in severe disseminated cases.
**Nervous**: Rare, in severe disseminated cases.
**Ophthalmic**: Rare.
**Reproductive**: Rare.

### GENETICS
N/A

### INCIDENCE/PREVALENCE
All *Candida* spp. have worldwide distribution and are considered part of normal GI flora in both captive and free range birds. However, *C. albicans* is the predominant isolate worldwide. Other common isolates include *C. glabrata*, *C. kefyr*, *C. lambica*, and *C. parapsilosis*, *Candida tropicalis*, *Candida hemicola*. *Candida kusei* has been reported in Australia. In one study in healthy cockatiels, *Candida* spp. isolates were found in 65%, with *C. albicans* representing 32% of the isolates. In waterfowl with esophageal mycosis, *C. albicans* was isolated from 43.1%, followed by *C. kefyr* and *C. lambica*. In a recent study in Galliformes, Anseriformes, Psittaciformes, Passeriformes, and Columbiformes with suspected mycosis, candidiasis was in 25%, and *C. albicans* comprised 14.3% of the cases.

### GEOGRAPHIC DISTRIBUTION
Worldwide.

### SIGNALMENT
**Species**: In psittacine birds, cockatiels, lovebirds and budgerigars are over represented. Also common in Passerines, Columbiformes, raptors, waterfowl and backyard poultry.
**Mean age and range**: All ages are susceptible but juvenile birds are highly susceptible.
**Predominant sex**: No sex predilections.

### SIGNS

#### General Comments
Signs are indicative of the organ affected. It can be just one clinical sign in the case of an isolated lesion, or severe systemic illness in the case of disseminated GI, respiratory or other organ system infection.

#### Historical Findings
Anorexia, regurgitation, weight loss, exercise intolerance, coughing and sneezing.

#### Physical Examination Findings
Nasal discharge, coughing and sneezing, crop stasis, halitosis, tachypnea and labored breathing, stomatitis (oral white plaques), melena/hematochezia, partially digested stool.

### CAUSES
*Candida* spp.

### RISK FACTORS
Hand feeding (psittacine birds). Young age. Stress: Overcrowding, raptors used for falconry, and backyard poultry are commonly affected due to inevitable increased stress levels. Malnutrition from rancid feed, vitamin A deficiency. Immunosuppression. Poor environmental hygiene. Concurrent disease (trichomoniasis, poxvirus, other). Prolonged antibiotic therapy. Feather destructive behavior. Chronic skin infection. Cockatiels can harbor mixed population of *Candida* spp. in their GI tract and can disseminate the organisms into the environment.

## DIAGNOSIS

### DIFFERENTIAL DIAGNOSIS
Vitamin A deficiency (common in psittacines). Capillariasis (common in non-psittacines), mycobacteriosis, chlamydiosis, trichomoniasis, macrorhabdiosis. Pox virus infection in the relevant species. Stomatitis, ingluvitis, esophagitis, gastroenteritis of other etiology.

### CBC/BIOCHEMISTRY/URINALYSIS
Usually unremarkable. Fibrinogen can be elevated.

### OTHER LABORATORY TESTS
Cytology from an affected lesion will show numerous budding yeasts and possibly pseudohyphae alongside inflammatory cells and bacteria. Crop cytology is especially useful. Gram stains are both effective in demonstrating infection on fecal or crop samples. C/S. PCR may be used to identify specific *Candida* sp. in cases of refractory infection or resistance. Histopathology.

### IMAGING
Whole-body radiographs may demonstrate signs that are compatible with ileus such as distended crop, gas filled loops of bowel. Delayed GI tract emptying time can be demonstrated with contrast barium radiographs or fluoroscopy. Skull radiographs are generally not useful in demonstrating sinusitis.

### DIAGNOSTIC PROCEDURES
Sinus flush and ingluvial lavage or swabbing can aid in collecting samples for cytology and culture and molecular testing (PCR, next-generation DNA sequencing). Endoscopy can be used to evaluate the thickened and inflamed crop, proventriculus and ventriculus. "Turkish towel" is a term used to describe the appearance of the esophagitis/ingluvitis caused by candidiasis.

### PATHOLOGIC FINDINGS
Thickened and ulcerative mucosal membrane with abundant yeasts, budding or forming pseudohyphae accompanied by necrosis and granulomatous inflammation.

## TREATMENT

### APPROPRIATE HEALTH CARE
In the individual patients, health care should be aimed at a specific affected system but also at alleviating underlying risk factors that contribute to the pathogenicity of candidiasis, such as: stress, overcrowding, and poor nutritional hygiene.

## NURSING CARE
Outpatient care is sufficient in most cases. Fluid therapy and nutritional support may be needed in debilitated patients.

## ACTIVITY
N/A

## DIET
Nutritional support may be necessary with patients that suffer anorexia or weight loss. Vitamin A supplementation may promote healing of the mucosal membranes and will correct possible underlying deficiency.

## CLIENT EDUCATION
Improve hygiene measures and reduce stress.

## SURGICAL CONSIDERATIONS
N/A

# MEDICATIONS
## DRUG(S) OF CHOICE
Nystatin is the drug of choice. It acts on the mucosal membrane surface and does not get absorbed systemically, so it is a safe drug to use compared with other antifungals; 100,000–300,000 IU/kg PO q8–12h for 7–14 days is the recommended regimen. Lower dose preferred. Amphotericin B 100 mg/kg PO q12–24h is another recommended drug as it is not absorbed systemically from the GI tract. Topical treatment: Topical antifungal (miconazole, amphotericin B, terbinafine, enilconazole are some that are available) gels or ointments can be applied directly on oral lesions to aid with systemic therapy. They can be used nasally or as part of a nasochoanal flush q12–24h for 7–10 days. Silver sulfadiazine can be used topically. Emulsion combined with ciprofloxacin is available and well tolerated, and is easy to use in most birds.

## CONTRAINDICATIONS
N/A

## PRECAUTIONS
All drugs require direct contact with the lesion to be effective and are of low risk if there is no systemic absorption. Amphotericin B can be nephrotoxic and should be used to treat persistent infection in well-hydrated patients, and when diffuse systemic ulcerative disease is not suspected, to avoid systemic absorption.

## POSSIBLE INTERACTIONS
N/A

## ALTERNATIVE DRUGS
Azoles—systemic use should be spared for severe infection where systemic infection is suspected or as a treatment against resistant strains. Azoles should not be used when severe liver disease is suspected as they may cause anorexia and elevated liver enzymes. Fluconazole 5–10 mg/kg q12h PO, 10 mg/kg q24h PO (cockatiels), higher dose of 20 mg/kg q48h PO has also been reported in psittacines. Itraconazole 5–10 mg/kg q24h PO (lower dose recommended), dosing can be divided q12h. Voriconazole 10–20 mg/kg q24h PO. Medicated water may be used in a flock situation when it is impractical to treat the individual bird. Fluconazole 100 mg/L drinking water for 8 days. Recent research has suggested that Chinese herbal medicine may be an effective treatment against *C. glabrata* infection in poultry.

# FOLLOW-UP
## PATIENT MONITORING
N/A

## PREVENTION/AVOIDANCE
N/A

## POSSIBLE COMPLICATIONS
Failure to thrive in cases of infected juvenile birds.

## EXPECTED COURSE AND PROGNOSIS
Follow-up examination and crop/oral cytology preparations and fecal cytology evaluation is recommended after 10–14 days. Prognosis is good.

# MISCELLANEOUS
## ASSOCIATED CONDITIONS
N/A

## AGE-RELATED FACTORS
N/A

## ZOONOTIC POTENTIAL
*Candida* spp. are abundant in the environment. However, cockatiels have been reported to be environmental asymptomatic shedders and can pose potential risk to humans, especially if immunocompromised. Close genetic relation has been shown between *C. albicans* isolated from humans and chickens.

## FERTILITY/BREEDING
N/A

## SYNONYMS
Sour crop, thrush, Turkish towel.

## SEE ALSO
Aspergillosis
Diarrhea
Flagellate Enteritis
Ileus (Functional Gastrointestinal, Crop Stasis)
*Macrorhabdus ornithogaster*
Nutritional Imbalances
Oral Plaques
Poxvirus
Regurgitation and Vomiting
Sick-Bird Syndrome
Trichomoniasis
Undigested Food in Droppings
Urate and Fecal Discoloration

## ABBREVIATIONS
C/S—culture and sensitivity
GI—gastrointestinal
PCR—polymerase chain reaction

## INTERNET RESOURCES
Association of Avian Veterinarians: www.aav.org
Merck & Co. *MSD Manuals*: www.merckmanuals.com
National Library of Medicine: www.ncbi.nlm.nih.gov

*Suggested Reading*
Domán, M., Makrai, L., Lengyel, G., et al. (2021). Molecular diversity and genetic relatedness of *Candida albicans* isolates from birds in Hungary. *Mycopathologia*, 186:237–244.
Domán, M., Makrai, L., Bali, K., et al. (2020). Unexpected diversity of yeast species in esophageal mycosis of waterfowls. *Avian Diseases*, 64:532–535.
Sidrim, J.J., Maia DC, Brilhante RS, et al. (2010). Candida species isolated from the gastrointestinal tract of cockatiels (*Nymphicus hollandicus*): In vitro antifungal susceptibility profile and phospholipase activity. *Veterinary Microbiology*, 145:324–328.
Talazadeh, F., Ghorbanpoor, M., Shahriyari, A. (2022). Candidiasis in birds (Galliformes, Anseriformes, Psittaciformes, Passeriformes, and Columbiformes): A focus on antifungal susceptibility pattern of *Candida albicans* and non-albicans isolates in avian clinical specimens. *Topics in Companion Animal Medicine*, 46:100598.
Zhang, S., Zhao, Q., Xue, W., et al. C. (2021). The isolation and identification of *Candida glabrata* from avian species and a study of the antibacterial activities of Chinese herbal medicine in vitro. *Poultry Science*, 100:101003.
**Author:** Shachar Malka, DVM, DABVP (Avian), DACEPM

# CAPTURE MYOPATHY (EXERTIONAL RHABDOMYOLYSIS)

## BASICS

### DEFINITION
Capture myopathy (CM) is a non-infectious metabolic disease of animals that occurs as a result of muscle damage following extreme exertion, struggling or stress to that animal. CM is commonly seen in situations of chemical immobilization, capture, restraint, and or transport, or may result secondary to other diseases or encounters in a wild environment. It is associated with a poor prognosis, and thus a high morbidity and mortality. Clinically, the key features of the disease include a metabolic acidosis, muscle necrosis, and myoglobinuria

### PATHOPHYSIOLOGY
The pathogenesis of CM has been described as having three key contributing components: the perception of fear, sympathetic nervous and adrenal system stimulation, and muscular activity. CM occurs as a result of an alteration of blood flow to the tissues and subsequently an exhaustion of the normal aerobic energy stores, especially those within the skeletal muscle. Once the ATP stores in the muscles has been exhausted, there is a decrease in the delivery of oxygen and nutrients to the muscles, and increase in the lactic acid production, and an inadequate removal of the cellular waste products that are produced. As the muscles undergo this damage, necrosis occurs and they release their intracellular contents, which includes creatine kinase and myoglobin, into the blood stream. Despite the initial commonalities that occur to result in CM, the results of this breakdown can then lead to one of four primary CM syndromes (capture shock syndrome, ataxic myoglobinuric syndrome, ruptured muscle syndrome, delayed peracute syndrome). Even within these syndromes, CM is on a continuum and there may be overlap within each of these syndromes within a single patient. The release of these products into the bloodstream requires processing, and when myoglobin reaches the kidneys for breakdown, it can result in tubular necrosis and renal failure.

### SYSTEMS AFFECTED
Musculoskeletal, cardiac, renal. CM can be differentiated from other forms of rhabdomyolysis as a result of the pathophysiology causing negative effects on both the skeletal and cardiac muscle following muscular exertion and high levels of stress.

### GENETICS
N/A

### INCIDENCE/PREVALENCE
Varies depending on the scenario with which the bird is presented. Many iatrogenic circumstances, such as overexertion, disturbance, excessive handling, transportation, and shock, can all contribute to an increased incidence of disease.

### GEOGRAPHIC DISTRIBUTION
While a specific geographic region is not implicated in CM, environments with extremes in ambient temperature, rain, and elevated humidity have demonstrated increased incidence of CM. Additionally, the presence of challenging terrain, such as steep hills, mountains, or rocky underfooting, or water hazards can also increase CM incidence.

### SIGNALMENT
Any prey species can be susceptible to CM. Within the avian taxa, the long-legged wading birds appear to be highly susceptible, likely a result of the struggle and exertion that occurs prior to capture, and the placement in restraint devices after capture.

### SIGNS

#### Historical Findings
The history of a bird with CM will be highly suspected based on the history and clinical presentation of the patient. Most birds will have a history of a recent chase, difficult capture, or prolonged transportation, or some combination of these. A complete necropsy is required to confirm a diagnosis. Additionally, a complete and thorough physical examination and assessment for other disease processes is necessary to aid in a diagnosis.

#### Physical Examination Findings
Avian patients that experience CM can present in various ways depending on the species, the individual, and the circumstances of the incident.
**Capture shock syndrome**: Occurrence: 1–6 hours post capture. Physical examination may detect depression or altered mentation, hyperpnea and/or tachypnea, tachycardia, hyperthermia, and weak and thready pulses.
**Ataxic myoglobinuric syndrome**: Occurrence: several hours to days post capture. Physical examination may detect ataxia, ranging from mild to severe, and torticollis.
**Ruptured muscle syndrome**: Occurrence: 24–48 hours post capture. Physical examination may detect weakness in the pelvic limbs and hyperflexion of the hock as a result of gastrocnemius rupture.
**Delayed peracute syndrome**: Occurrence: 24 hours post capture. On distant examination, these animals will appear normal, but when placed in a stressful situation such as capture, will attempt escape, stop abruptly, and then die shortly thereafter.

### CAUSES
CM can be distinguished from other causes of rhabdomyolysis due to the dual effect on both skeletal and cardiac muscle. CM is a complex and multifactorial disease process with the underlying reason behind its cause not fully understood or known.

### RISK FACTORS
There are many risk factors that have been implicated as predisposing or contributing factors to the incidence of CM. Often the mnemonic "SECONDS" is used, which describes species, environment, capture-related, other diseases, nutrition, drugs, and signalment as factors that may increase the predisposition or risk of CM.

#### Species
In general, prey species are considered to be at a higher risk of CM. Long-legged wading birds are particularly predisposed to CM.

#### Environment
Temperature, humidity, and terrain can all influence the incidence of CM.

#### Capture-Related
There are many capture-related risk factors that can contribute to an increased incidence of CM. Predisposing factors include high-speed chases; extended durations of exertion without rest periods; handling for prolonged periods of time; prolonged restraint; struggling during restraint, especially when held in abnormal positions; crating; transportation; excessive fear and stimulus, especially over a period of time. A compounding factor associated with CM is injuries that occur in the process of capture.

#### Other Diseases
The presence of an underlying infectious or non-infectious disease also has potential to increase the incidence of CM. For example, any disease process that can result in anemia, including severe parasitic infestations, can result in compounding factors that result in increased incidence of CM.

#### Nutrition
Specific nutrient deficiency scenarios, including vitamin E and selenium can predispose avian species to CM. Additionally, it is suspected that premigratory birds consuming food at an elevated nutrition plane and carrying additional fat stores may be at a higher risk. It is also theorized that the provision of food, water, and nutrients such as vitamin E and selenium during or after transport may help to mitigate the incidence of CM in these animals.

#### Drugs
There are certain drugs and drug combinations that have been implicated in the incidence of rhabodomyolysis in humans, including opioids, a commonly used drug class in avian medicine. It is well documented that the administration of opioids in certain species can result in excitation, hyperactivity, and hyperthermia, and when these are combined with the additional risk factors in the patient, the incidence of CM may be elevated. Additionally, any drugs that can lead to excitation, spontaneous or spastic

## (CONTINUED) CAPTURE MYOPATHY (EXERTIONAL RHABDOMYOLYSIS)

movement, muscle rigidity, elevation in body temperature, and elevation in catecholamines can all play a role in contributing to CM in the avian patient.

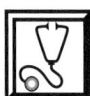

# DIAGNOSIS

### DIFFERENTIAL DIAGNOSIS
White-muscle disease associated with vitamin E and selenium deficiency. Plant toxicities (e.g. *Cassia occidentalis*, *Cassia obtusifolia*, and *Karwinskia humboldtiana*), malignant hyperthermia, hypocalcemia, early tetanus, myositis.

### CBC/BIOCHEMISTRY/URINALYSIS
The most common changes on routine biochemistry include extreme elevations in CK and AST. Both these biochemical parameters are indicators of muscle damage. If measured, aldolase, LDH, and hydroxybutyrate dehydrogenase will also be elevated as a result of muscle cell lysis. Additional changes that can be detected include elevations in myoglobin, uric acid, potassium, and urea. Hypo- and hypercalcemia have both been reported due to alterations in calcium metabolism, with additional elevations in serum phosphate. Metabolic lactic acidosis has also been described in cases of CM.

### OTHER LABORATORY TESTS
Hematology: The presence of a stress leukogram may be documented in the avian patient. Additionally, persistent elevations in leukocyte count, even upon resolution of CM clinical signs have also been reported in avian species. Other hematological changes are not well described in CM patients.

### IMAGING
Although overall imaging does not provide substantial benefit to avian patients with CM, in humans, certain imaging modalities do help to determine the degree of renal changes and muscular changes. MRI has been shown to be extremely useful in human patients with exertional myopathy with the ability to detect swelling of the kidneys, alterations in corticomedullary definition, and changes in the renal hypointensity. Additionally, MRI allowed for detection of the muscles specifically affected by CM, demonstrating increased signal intensity of on T2-weighted and STIR sequences and decreased signal intensity on T1-weighted sequences. MRI may not be a particularly feasible option in most avian patients with CM, but even ultrasound has potential utility to demonstrate changes in the affected muscles including disorganization of the orientation of the muscle fibers, presence of a ground glass image, fascial thickening, and anechoic areas.

### DIAGNOSTIC PROCEDURES
Typically, aside from routine hematology and biochemistry, blood gas analysis, with or without imaging, combined with a history highly suspicious of CM, additional diagnostic procedures are not required.

### PATHOLOGIC FINDINGS
The presence of muscle damage may be detected on gross necropsy or based on histopathology, even if no clinical signs have been detected at the time of postmortem. However, typically at the time of necropsy, severe muscle alterations are detected. The presence of pathological changes in the skeletal muscles is one of the most prominent changes that will be detected on gross necropsy examination of the patient. Often, whole muscle bellies may be affected, and though bilateral changes are detected, they are often asymmetric in nature.

# TREATMENT

### APPROPRIATE HEALTH CARE
Unfortunately, treatment of CM is generally unrewarding. Treatment focuses on aggressive supportive care, but is often associated with many challenges, especially in wild animals, where the stress of treatment and handling combined with the cost of intensive therapy can be limiting.

### NURSING CARE
There are a multitude of nursing care options that can be used when treating CM patients.
**Analgesia**: The provision of analgesia can provide significant benefit to avian patients with CM due to the severe muscle pain that is invoked with the disease. Additionally, patients in severe pain become severely anxious and distressed, resulting in worsening of clinical signs and disease, compounding the difficulty of treatment. Multiple analgesic options can be considered including NSAIDs (provided that renal status is appropriate), opioids, and gabapentin.
**Dantrolene sodium**: Dantrolene sodium is a drug used in racehorses with exercise-induced exertional myopathy. The drug works by suppressing the release of calcium from the sarcoplasmic reticulum. While there are no reports of dantrolene administration in CM patients, the mechanism of action combined with successful use in horses and other species lends promise to its utility in avian CM patients.
**Muscle relaxants**: The use of centrally acting muscle relaxants including the drug class of benzodiazepines (diazepam, midazolam) can provide substantial utility in reducing muscle spasms that are associated with CM. Additionally, these drugs have a sedative effect, which can aid in reducing the distress associated with CM. Methocarbamol, which also acts centrally for muscle relaxation can also provide utility in CM cases and was used in a case of successful treatment in rhea.
**Nutritional supplementation**: The use of vitamin E and selenium supplements has been advocated for prevention of CM, although the true efficacy has been debated. Avian species have been successfully treated with and without the use of vitamin E and selenium.
**Hyperbaric oxygen**: Hyperbaric oxygen has been used in humans with rhabdomyolysis but has largely not been accessible in veterinary medicine.
**Sodium bicarbonate**: Sodium bicarbonate can be useful to counteract the acidemia that occurs as a result of CM.
**Fluid therapy**: Ideally, provision of a balanced electrolyte intravenous solution should be used to help manage the many biochemical effects of CM, including metabolic acidosis, hyperkalemia, dehydration, and myoglobinuria.
**Nutritional support**: In avian patients with CM, it can be challenging for the individual to meet their required nutritional needs. If patients are underconditioned, have additional deficiencies, or weight loss, these are noted to be negative prognostic indicators; however, appropriate supplementation of nutrition can have a significant impact on successful treatment of CM.
**Physical therapy**: Physical therapy is a vital component in the treatment of CM and has demonstrated improvement in muscle coordination, strength, and function in multiple avian species. In recumbent or severely compromised avian patients, the use of slings can allow for gradual return to weight bearing; additionally, water baths can be used for wading birds with CM.

### ACTIVITY
Patients with CM should be allowed a slow and controlled return to activity.

### DIET
As indicated, nutritional support is critical in patients with CM and should be provided in the form of high quality, species appropriate food, and potential for gavage feeding if the patient cannot meet their nutritional needs on their own.

### CLIENT EDUCATION
N/A

### SURGICAL CONSIDERATIONS
N/A

C

## MEDICATIONS

### DRUG(S) OF CHOICE
Analgesia—opioids, NSAIDs, gabapentin. Muscle relaxants—benzodiazepines, methocarbamol. Dantrolene sodium. Sodium bicarbonate.

### CONTRAINDICATIONS
N/A

### PRECAUTIONS
Caution should be taken when handling any CM avian patient due to concerns for additional stress and anxiety that can exacerbate clinical signs of CM.

### POSSIBLE INTERACTIONS
N/A

### ALTERNATIVE DRUGS
N/A

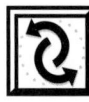

## FOLLOW-UP

### PATIENT MONITORING
Each patient should be monitored closely for progression of clinical signs associated with CM. In cases of worsening and uncontrollable pain, quality of life and humane euthanasia should be considered.

### PREVENTION/AVOIDANCE
The best preventative measure that can be taken to avoid CM is to ensure that the avian patient being captured has limited external stressors. Prevention of CM does depend on the species being captured and thus, the method of capture. Additionally, understanding the purpose of the capture and where it will occur is critical to ensuring a successful outcome for the avian patient. During capture, close attention should be paid to the temperature, humidity, and terrain, and if the conditions are not optimal, capture should be delayed if at all possible. All procedures and handling should be carried out by experienced personnel and should be kept as brief and minimally stressful as possible. Whenever possible, training and desensitization should be used to reduce the incidence of CM. If immobilizing drugs are necessary for the patient, they should have characteristics of a rapid onset and recovery, and methods that ease delivery. Additionally, the volume of drug administered should be as small as possible.

### POSSIBLE COMPLICATIONS
Rhabdomyolysis, renal dysfunction to renal failure, capture-induced cardiomyopathy, cardiac fibrillation, sudden death.

### EXPECTED COURSE AND PROGNOSIS
Currently, no therapeutic approach guarantees successful recovery from CM. Typically, once clinical signs of capture myopathy are present, the avian patient is considered to have a poor prognosis for recovery.

## MISCELLANEOUS

### ASSOCIATED CONDITIONS
Low body condition in chronic cases. Cardiac lesions with resultant exercise intolerance to failure. Renal injury to failure.

### AGE-RELATED FACTORS
Very young and very elderly animals appear to have a higher predisposition to CM.

### ZOONOTIC POTENTIAL
N/A

### FERTILITY/BREEDING
N/A

### SYNONYMS
Exertional rhabdomyolysis, muscular dystrophy, white muscle disease, overstraining disease, spastic paresis, stress myopathy, transport myopathy, muscle necrosis, idiopathic necrosis.

### SEE ALSO
N/A

### ABBREVIATIONS
AST— aspartate aminotransferase
ATP—adenosine triphosphate
CK— creatine kinase
CM—capture myopathy
LDH—lactate dehydrogenase
MRI—magnetic resonance imaging
NSAIDs—non-steroidal anti-inflammatory drugs
STIR—short tau inversion recovery

### INTERNET RESOURCES
N/A

*Suggested Reading*
Businga N, Langenberg J, Carlson L. (2007). Successful treatment of capture myopathy in three wild greater sandhill cranes. *Journal of Avian Medicine and Surgery*, 21:294–298.
Paterson, J. (2014). Capture myopathy. In: *Zoo Animal and Wildlife Immobilization and Anesthesia*, 2nd edn. (ed. G. West, D. Heard, N. Caulkett), 171–179. Ames, IA: Wiley.
Rogers, D., Battley, P., Sparrow, J., et al. (2004). Treatment of capture myopathy in shorebirds: a successful trial in northwestern Australia. *Journal of Field Ornithology*, 75:157–164.
Williams, E., Thorne, E. (1996). Exertional myopathy. In: *Noninfectious Diseases of Wildlife*, 2nd edn. (ed. A. Fairbrother, L. Locke, G. Hoff), 181–193. Ames, IA: Iowa State Universtiy Press.
**Author:** Sara Gardhouse, DVM, DABVP (ECM), DACZM

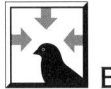

## BASICS

### DEFINITION
Color changes of the skin and cere are variations of normal pigmentation due to a disease process.

### PATHOPHYSIOLOGY
The pathophysiology of color changes of the skin and cere varies depending upon the underlying condition. Etiologies include hormonal influences, bruising/edema (trauma), neoplastic (melanoma, sarcomas, hemangioma/hemangiosarcoma, and mast cell tumors), or inflammatory changes (thermal trauma, infectious, or neoplastic causes).

### SYSTEMS AFFECTED
Skin.

### GENETICS
N/A

### INCIDENCE/PREVALENCE
Varies with the underlying cause.

### GEOGRAPHIC DISTRIBUTION
N/A

### SIGNALMENT
**Species**: Brown hypertrophy of the cere is most common in budgerigars.
**Mean age and range**: Brown hypertrophy of the cere occurs in mostly older budgerigars. Crop burns are generally found in young birds being hand fed.
**Predominant sex**: None.

### SIGNS
#### Historical Findings
The owner reports changes in the color of the skin.

#### Physical Examination Findings
**Cere**: The cere shows dark brown hypertrophy, hyperkeratosis, and hyperplasia, sometimes with occlusion of the nares, rather than the normal pink or tan in a female budgerigar and blue in a male budgerigar.
**Crop**: The skin covering the crop shows variable color changes ranging from erythematous to dark or black. An ulcer may form in the crop, allowing the contents to spill onto the surface of the feathers covering the crop.
**Toes**: The skin on the extremities, usually toes, may vary from pale to erythematous and edematous to dark or black. In severe cases, skin or toes may slough.
**Eyelid margins**: The skin at the eyelid margins and conjunctiva shows discrete erythematous macules that then become brown to black papules, then vesicles that erode and crust. In some species, the only findings are hyperpigmented macules.

**Abdomen**: The featherless tracts of skin over the abdomen show petechia or ecchymoses. Raised blacked to reddish nodules.

### CAUSES
**Cere**: Brown hypertrophy of the cere in budgerigar hens is caused by increased estrogen levels and may be related to high-fat diets. In male budgerigars, the change is related to a testicular (Sertoli cell) tumor producing estrogen.
**Crop**: Crop burns are caused by thermal damage from hand-feeding food that is too hot.
**Toes**: Frostbite or other thermal injury caused by exposure to low or high temperatures is often seen in birds housed outside during winter months or birds housed inside, resulting in thermal burns from landing on stoves or heaters.
**Eyelid margins**: Avian cutaneous poxvirus (*see* Poxvirus).
**Abdomen**: Trauma-causing hematomas or edema. Pigmented mass relating to neoplastic processes (melanomas, mast cells, dermal carcinomas).

### RISK FACTORS
Hand feeding is a risk factor for crop burns. Housing birds outside in cold climates or inside with excess to stoves and heaters are risk factors for thermal trauma.

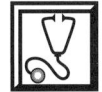

## DIAGNOSIS

### DIFFERENTIAL DIAGNOSIS
Brown hypertrophy of the cere—*Knemidocoptes* spp. mites. Crop burn—foreign body penetration. Frostbite/thermal burn—ulcerative pododermatitis, photosensitization, contact dermatitis, constricted toe.

### CBC/BIOCHEMISTRY/URINALYSIS
N/A

### OTHER LABORATORY TESTS
N/A

### IMAGING
N/A

### DIAGNOSTIC PROCEDURES
These conditions are often diagnosed based only on history and physical examination.

### PATHOLOGIC FINDINGS
Brown hypertrophy of the cere—hyperkeratosis, and hyperplasia of the cere. Thermal trauma—histopathology shows coagulative necrosis with a peripheral inflammatory infiltrate of heterophils and macrophages and a well-demarcated inflammatory margin between unaffected and necrotic tissue. Pigmented mass—histopathology shows neoplastic processes (melanomas, mast cells, dermal carcinomas).

Dermal hematomas or edema—hemorrhage, dilated vessels, and neovascularization or fluid accumulation.

## TREATMENT

### APPROPRIATE HEALTH CARE
**Brown hypertrophy of the cere**: In budgerigar hens, no treatment is necessary apart from manual removal of any hyperkeratosis occluding the nares. In male budgerigars, the gonadal tumor is generally considered difficult to due to the size of the gonads and the location of large vessels. Deslorelin implants and other GnRH agonists have been used to reduce clinical signs.
**Crop burns**: Full-thickness crop burns are life threatening, and aggressive therapy is needed. Stabilize the bird and initiate fluid therapy and appropriate antibiotic therapy for secondary bacterial infections. Monitor the patient for several days as the full extent of the burn might not be evident upon initial examination. Once the extent of the burn is identified, anesthetize the bird for surgical debridement of the necrotic tissue. Close the crop and overlying skin separately. Bandage the surgical site during the initial healing stages and use an Elizabethan collar or similar protective device if the bird damages the surgical site.
**Thermal trauma**: Stabilize the bird and initiate fluid therapy, analgesics, appropriate wound care, and prophylactic antibiotic therapy for secondary bacterial infections. Monitor the patient for several days as the full extent of the thermal trauma might not be evident upon initial examination. Once the extent of the trauma is identified, anesthetize the bird for surgical debridement of the necrotic tissue. Bandage the surgical site during the initial healing stages and use an Elizabethan collar or similar protective device if the bird damages the surgical site.
**Pigmented dermal mass**: Biopsy mass for histological results. Obtain surgical margins. Radiation or palliative therapy, depending on severity. Stage and look for signs of metastasis. See chapters on neoplasia.
**Dermal hematomas**: Investigate the underlying cause (region of hematoma can help to pinpoint injury); frank hemorrhage requires immediate attention. Provide analgesia and supportive care. Bruising will turn a greenish color 2–3 days after the traumatic event due to the presence of biliverdin. If multiple ecchymotic areas are present, possible clotting disorders or significant inflammation should be investigated.

**C**

### NURSING CARE

Nursing care varies depending on the presentation. Nursing care may be particularly helpful in cases of burns and frostbite.

### ACTIVITY

Activity should be limited when dermal trauma is suspected.

### DIET

Appropriate formulated diet for the species.

### CLIENT EDUCATION

Crop burns—educate hand feeder in proper hand feeding formula heating and temperature testing protocols, including not using a microwave, which may create hot spots in the food. Thermal trauma—educate clients on proper housing requirements during cold weather and safety tips to reduce incidents with stove tops and heaters.

### SURGICAL CONSIDERATIONS

N/A

### MEDICATIONS

### DRUG(S) OF CHOICE

Antibiotics may be indicated in cases of crop burns and trauma. Peripheral vasodilators such as pentoxifylline or isoxsuprine can be considered to manage edema in cases of frostbite and burns. Analgesia should be provided in cases of thermal or dermal trauma.

### CONTRAINDICATIONS

N/A

### PRECAUTIONS

N/A

### POSSIBLE INTERACTIONS

N/A

### ALTERNATIVE DRUGS

N/A

### FOLLOW-UP

### PATIENT MONITORING

N/A

### PREVENTION/AVOIDANCE

Crop burns—avoid hand feeding baby birds with too hot food. Thermal trauma—house birds in appropriate temperatures to avoid thermal damage due to cold weather.

### POSSIBLE COMPLICATIONS

Secondary infection is possible in the case of crop burns and frostbite.

### EXPECTED COURSE AND PROGNOSIS

Brown hypertrophy of the cere—good prognosis for budgerigar hens, guarded to poor long-term prognosis for male budgerigars. Possible treatment with testicular tumors include deslorelin implants or surgical gonad removal (surgical options have moderate to high risk due to the gonad's size and approximation to large vessels). Crop burns and thermal or dermal trauma—severe cases have a poor prognosis if substantial tissue damage is involved. Crop burns detected early have a good to guarded prognosis if the patient is stabilized early, secondary infections are managed, and adequate nutrition is provided. Pigmented tumors—prognosis depends on neoplastic type and aggressiveness. Usually, most avian neoplasias are locally invasive. If surgical margins are obtained, then a good prognosis with a low chance of reoccurrence. If margins are not obtained, or there are signs of metastasis, prognosis is poor (see also chapters on neoplasia).

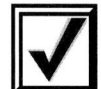

### MISCELLANEOUS

### ASSOCIATED CONDITIONS

N/A

### AGE-RELATED FACTORS

N/A

### ZOONOTIC POTENTIAL

N/A

### FERTILITY/BREEDING

N/A

### SYNONYMS

N/A

### SEE ALSO

Ectoparasites
Feather-Damaging and Self-Injurious Behavior
Feather Disorders
Nutritional Imbalances
Rhinitis and Sinusitis

### ABBREVIATIONS

GnRH—gonadotropin-releasing hormone

### INTERNET RESOURCES

N/A

*Suggested Reading*

Girling, S. (2006). Dermatology of birds. In: *Skin Diseases of Exotic Pets* (ed. S. Patterson), 3–14. Oxford: Blackwell Science.

Schmidt, R.E., Reavill, D.R., Phalen, D.N (2015). Integument. In: *Pathology of Pet and Aviary Birds*, 2nd edn., 237–262. Hoboken, NJ: Wiley.

Straub, J., Zenker, I. (2013). First experience in the hormonal treatment of Sertoli cell tumors in budgerigars (*Melopsittacus undulatus*) with absorbable extended-release GnRH chips (Suprelorin®). In: *Proceedings from the International Conference on Avian, Herpetological & Exotic Mammal Medicine, Wiesbaden, April 20–26.* pp. 299–300.

**Author:** Rodney W. Schnellbacher, DVM, DACZM

**Acknowledgements:** updated from chapter previously authored by Thomas M. Edling, DVM, MSpVM, MPH and Heide M. Newton, DVM, DACVD

C

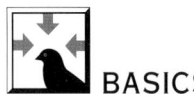

# BASICS

## DEFINITION
*Chlamydia psittaci* is an obligate intracellular Gram-negative bacteria. Other *Chlamydia* spp. have been identified in birds, including *Chlamydia buteonis* and *Chlamydia avium*. At least eight serovars and nine genotypes of *C. psittaci* are described. While the organism is not stable in the environment, it can remain infectious for at least 1 month if present within organic matter (dirty cages, fecal material). Asymptomatic carriers are common, and the organism is only shed intermittently. Stress may increase shedding of *C. psittaci*; this includes physiologic (egg laying) and environmental stresses.

## PATHOPHYSIOLOGY
*C. psittaci* is shed in oculonasal discharge and feces (varies by species) and is transmitted by inhalation of aerosolized secretions or fecal material. Duration of shedding can vary by strain and by host. The elementary body is the pathogen's infectious stage. Elementary bodies attach to and enter the host cells, where they develop into non-infectious reticulate bodies within the phagosomes of the host cell. These reticulate bodies multiply and enlarge, and after several intermediate forms will transform back to elementary bodies, which then rupture out of the cell. Respiratory epithelial cells are affected first. The organism then spreads hematogenously to the reticuloendothelial system.

## SYSTEMS AFFECTED
**Respiratory**: Upper respiratory signs, air sacculitis, pneumonia.
**Ophthalmic**: Secondary to upper respiratory disease.
**GI**: Enteritis.
**Hemic/lymphatic/immune**: Splenomegaly as a result of reticuloendothelial cell infection.
**Hepatobiliary**: Hepatitis.

## GENETICS
N/A

## INCIDENCE/PREVALENCE
Variable, depending on species.

## GEOGRAPHIC DISTRIBUTION
Worldwide distribution.

## SIGNALMENT
*C. psittaci* has been isolated from over 460 species of birds. It is most often diagnosed in psittacines, with cockatiels and budgerigars the most frequently infected. Pigeons and doves have a higher rate of infection than other pet non-psittacine birds. Younger birds appear to be more susceptible to clinical disease. Juvenile raptors, especially red-tailed hawks, seem to present with *C. buteonis* infection most commonly.

## SIGNS

### General Comments
Incubation period is 3 days to several weeks. Acute and chronic illness reported. Some birds may be asymptomatic carriers, and infection can occur despite no known exposure.

### Historical Findings
Lethargy and depression, sneezing, fluffed feathers, anorexia, abnormal urates (green), diarrhea, death (adult or neonate), reproductive losses.

### Physical Examination Findings
Ocular discharge, conjunctivitis, nasal discharge, depression, dyspnea, biliverdinuria, diarrhea, emaciation, dehydration.

## CAUSES
Bacterial infection with *Chlamydia* spp.

## RISK FACTORS
Immunosuppression is a risk factor for development of clinical signs in an infected patient. This can result from stresses such as shipping, crowding, poor sanitation and husbandry, breeding, or other illnesses. Disease transmission is facilitated by close spacing of cages (including stacked cages) and poor sanitation practices. Birds that travel to settings where other birds will be in close quarters are at increased risk of exposure. This includes bird shows, fairs, bird fanciers' meetings, boarding facilities, veterinary facilities, and bird stores.

# DIAGNOSIS

## DIFFERENTIAL DIAGNOSIS
Given the non-specific clinical signs, numerous diseases can mimic chlamydiosis. Specific testing is required to reach a diagnosis. Common rule-outs include other bacterial causes of rhinitis and keratoconjunctivitis, as well as ocular trauma, herpesviral infection, paramyxoviral infection, and avian influenza.

## CBC/BIOCHEMISTRY/URINALYSIS
Leukocytosis, with heterophilia and monocytosis, is commonly seen. The leukocytosis is often severe, with a WBC count of 2–3 times normal or more possible. A non-regenerative mild anemia may be seen in chronic cases.

## OTHER LABORATORY TESTS
**Culture**: Considered the gold standard, but specialized shipping and laboratory methods are required. Culture is not always the most practical option. Preferred specimens include combined swabs of the conjunctiva, choana, and cloaca, or liver biopsy samples in live patients; and samples of liver and spleen from necropsy specimens. If feces are submitted, a pooled sample should be collected over 3–5 days.
**Serology**: Useful in detecting exposure to the organism, but a single titer may not be sufficient for definitive diagnosis; it is considered a probable case if there is a single elevated titer with appropriate clinical signs or other laboratory findings. Paired samples demonstrating a four-fold titer increase over a 2-week period are preferred for definitive diagnosis. False negatives may be seen with acute or antibiotic therapy initiated before sample collection. The titer can remain elevated despite successful treatment. Methods include EBA (highest early in infection), IFA, and CF (more sensitive than agglutination methods).
**Antigen detection**: May be performed by IFA, PCR, or in situ hybridization. False negatives are possible due to intermittent shedding or insufficient numbers of organism in the sample. Results should be interpreted in light of other clinical and laboratory findings. PCR testing of combined conjunctival, choanal, and cloacal swabs or blood samples can be used to detect the DNA of *C. psittaci*. There can be differences between results from different laboratories, as PCR primers and amplification techniques will vary. The test cannot determine if the detected organisms are viable or not, and thus can only identify probable cases. IFA can be used to identify *C. psittaci* within a tissue sample or impression smear, but false positives may be seen due to cross-reactivity with other antigens. Detection of the organism by in situ hybridization is preferred for fixed tissues.

## IMAGING

### Radiographic Findings
Hepatomegaly and splenomegaly are commonly present.

### Ultrasonography
Hepatomegaly may also be appreciable by coelomic ultrasound. The spleen is not ordinarily readily identified on ultrasound, but it may be seen if it is enlarged.

## DIAGNOSTIC PROCEDURES
Biopsy of the liver or spleen may demonstrate the suspected presence of the organism by either IFA or staining (Gimenez, Macchiavello); confirmation requires in situ hybridization, organism isolation, or electron microscopy.

## PATHOLOGIC FINDINGS
Gross necropsy findings may include keratoconjunctivitis, rhinitis and nasal discharge, serositis with yellow exudate,

## CHLAMYDIOSIS                                    (CONTINUED)

pneumonia, air sacculitis, hepatomegaly, and splenomegaly. However, there are no pathognomonic findings that lead to confirmation of chlamydiosis. Pericarditis and tracheitis have been reported in turkeys and waterfowl. Enteritis may be noted in psittacines. Histologically, basophilic inclusion bodies may be noted, as well as basophilic and lymphocytic infiltrates within affected organs, and necrosis. Chromatic staining or IFA can be performed to identify possible chlamydial organisms, but infection should be confirmed by in situ hybridization, organism isolation, or electron microscopy.

### ■ TREATMENT

#### APPROPRIATE HEALTH CARE
Confirmed or probable cases should be immediately isolated from other birds and treated. Humans providing care to affected birds should use appropriate PPE (gloves, masks of N95 rating or higher; surgical masks may not be adequate).

#### NURSING CARE
Appropriate nursing care depends on the severity of the bird's clinical signs. Fluid and nutritional support should be provided as needed. Birds with respiratory signs or dyspnea may benefit from oxygen therapy.

#### ACTIVITY
Activity should be limited as the patient's condition dictates (for example, a weak bird should only be given low perches if at all). Contact with humans should be limited to the smallest number possible, and those people should wear appropriate PPE.

#### DIET
Avoid calcium-rich foods and other items (eg. cuttlebones, mineral blocks), as the gastrointestinal absorption of tetracyclines (e.g. doxycycline) is inhibited by calcium.

#### CLIENT EDUCATION
It is very important that the client be made aware of the zoonotic risks of chlamydiosis, and instructed on proper hygiene and quarantine procedures to be used. The client should be advised to consult their physician immediately regarding any indicated testing or treatment for themselves, especially if they develop symptoms consistent with influenza or respiratory disease. In some localities, this disease is reportable in birds. Clients must continue the full course of antibiotic treatment, even if clinical signs have resolved.

#### SURGICAL CONSIDERATIONS
N/A

### MEDICATIONS

#### DRUG(S) OF CHOICE
Doxycycline is the preferred drug for treating avian chlamydiosis. Oral dosage varies by species: Cockatiels—25–35 mg/kg q24h; Senegal parrots, Amazons— 25–50 mg/kg q24h; African grey parrots, blue and gold macaws, Goffin's cockatoos—25 mg/kg q24h. A long-acting injectable doxycycline (Vibravenos®, Pfizer Animal Health) may also be used at 75–100 mg/kg IM every 5–7 days for the first 4 weeks, then every 5 days for the remainder of the treatment period. This drug is not commercially available in the USA but may be imported in small quantities. Doxycycline-medicated feed has been found effective in budgerigars and cockatiels. Doxycycline-medicated water has been used with success in some species (not budgerigars)—cockatiels 200–400 mg/l; Goffin's cockatoos 400–600 mg/l; grey parrots 800 mg/l. The optimal duration of treatment has not been determined. Traditionally, 45 days has been recommended, but recent data suggest shorter courses of treatment (21–30 days) may be effective.

#### CONTRAINDICATIONS
N/A

#### PRECAUTIONS
If administered prior to sample collection, even a single dose of doxycycline and enrofloxacin can both cause the bird to stop shedding *C. psittaci*, leading to a false negative result by PCR. If possible, samples should be collected prior to treatment if *C. psittaci* is considered a differential diagnosis.

#### POSSIBLE INTERACTIONS
N/A

#### ALTERNATIVE DRUGS
Azithromycin 40 mg/kg PO q48h for 21 days has been shown to be effective in eliminating infection in cockatiels. Injectable oxytetracycline (Liquamycin® LA-200®, Zoetis) has been used at a dose of 75 mg/kg every 3 days. This drug causes injection site irritation and ideally should be used only short term until oral medications can be used (e.g. inappetence, regurgitation).

### FOLLOW-UP

#### PATIENT MONITORING
Body weight and appetite should be monitored thoughout the course of treatment. If abnormalities were detected on the CBC or the biochemical profile, these

should be rechecked while the bird is under treatment; the timing will depend on the severity of the initial changes and the bird's clinical status. Infected birds should be retested by PCR 2 and 4 weeks after completing treatment, especially if a shorter treatment course is pursued.

#### PREVENTION/AVOIDANCE
Avoid acquiring birds that appear to be ill. Testing and quarantine of all new birds, and quarantine those that are ill or have left and returned to the home or aviary (e.g. bird shows, fairs, and other settings where they may in in close proximity to other birds). Isolate sick birds from other birds in the home. Handle them after healthy birds, use PPE, disinfect cages daily, avoid drafts or air currents in the room, moisten bedding before cleaning and mop the floor frequently. Test all birds prior to boarding. Husbandry measures include leaving an adequate distance between cages to present transfer of organic materials, avoidance of stacking cages, solid barriers between adjoining cages, wire-bottomed cages, and substrates that do not easily form dusts, daily cleaning of cages and bowls, and disinfecting cages between occupants.

#### POSSIBLE COMPLICATIONS
Human zoonosis is possible. In some locations, avian chlamydiosis is a reportable disease; consult your state veterinarian's office. Reinfection is possible, necessitating a thorough cleaning and disinfection of the bird's environment. Contact with untested or untreated birds should be avoided.

#### EXPECTED COURSE AND PROGNOSIS
The prognosis is generally good, provided that timely treatment is provided. Individuals in whom disease is more severe or for whom diagnosis and treatment were delayed may experience worse clinical outcomes such as chronic air sacculitis and fibrosis, chronic hepatitis or fibrosis, or death.

### MISCELLANEOUS

#### AGE-RELATED FACTORS
N/A

#### ZOONOTIC POTENTIAL
Humans may become infected with *C. psittaci*, resulting in influenza-like symptoms or other respiratory ailments. Those at highest risk include young children, elderly persons, and immunocompromised individuals. The client should be advised to consult their physician immediately should they develop these symptoms, and alert their physician that

they have been exposed to a confirmed or suspected case of avian chlamydiosis. Psittacosis is a nationally notifiable disease in humans. If a necropsy is performed, PPE should be worn. If possible, the necropsy should be performed within a fume hood; alternatively, the bird's body may be wetted with a solution of detergent and water to avoid aerosolization of infectious agents.

## FERTILITY/BREEDING
As immunosuppression and stress can contribute to an individual developing chlamydiosis, breeding birds are susceptible to disease. Birds with chlamydiosis should not be bred until the infection has cleared. It is recommended that breeding pairs both be tested for *Chlamydia* prior to breeding. Breeding stress may also lead to increased shedding, putting the hatchlings at risk of infection.

## SYNONYMS
Psittacosis, ornithosis (humans), parrot fever (humans).

## SEE ALSO
Atherosclerosis
Liver Disease

## ABBREVIATIONS
CBC—complete blood count
CF—complement fixation
EBA—elementary body agglutination
GI—gastrointestinal
IFA—immunofluorescence assay
PCR—polymerase chain reaction
PPE—personal protective equipment
WBC—white blood cell

## INTERNET RESOURCES
Forbes, N. (2008). Avian chlamydiosis. *LafeberVet*: https://lafeber.com/vet/avian-chlamydiosis
National Associationof State Public Health Veterinarians. Psittacosis and chlamydiosis compendium and resources: http://www.nasphv.org/documentsCompendiaPsittacosis.html

## Suggested Reading
Balsamo, G., Maxted, A.M., Midla, J.W., et al. (2017). Compendium of measures to control *Chlamydia psittaci* infection among humans (psittacosis) and pet birds (avian chlamydiosis). *Journal of Avian Medicine and Surgery*, 31:262–282.
Guzman, D.S.M., Diaz-Figueroa, O., Tully, T. Jr., et al. (2010). Evaluating 21-day doxycycline and azithromycin treatments for experimental *Chlamydophila psittaci* infection in cockatiels (*Nymphicus hollandicus*). *Journal of Avian Medicine and Surgery*, 24:35–45.
Knittler, M.R., Sachse, K. (2015). *Chlamydia psittaci*: Update on an underestimated zoonotic agent. *Pathogens and Disease*, 73:1–15.
Seibert, B., Keel, M.L., Kelly, T.R., et al. (2021). *Chlamydia buteonis* in birds of prey presented to California wildlife rehabilitation facilities. *Public Library of Science One*, 16:e0258500.
Stokes, H.S., Berg, M.L., Bennett, A.T.D. (2021). A review of chlamydial infections in wild birds. *Pathogens*, 10:948.
**Author**: Kristin M. Sinclair, DVM, DABVP (Avian Practice, Exotic Companion Mammal Practice)

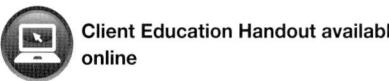 **Client Education Handout available online**

# CHRONIC EGG LAYING

C

## BASICS

### DEFINITION
Chronic and excessive egg laying without regard to clutch number, size, and nesting behaviors. This continuous laying occurs without the presence of a bonded mate or outside of a breeding season. It is considered a maladaptive behavior disorder where birds do not cease laying to brood or when a desired number is reached for the species.

### PATHOPHYSIOLOGY
Chronic egg laying is a commonly seen disorder in clinical avian practice. Most birds continue to lay regardless of clutch size, nest sites, or presence of a mate. Egg production is a normal process in domestic laying hens; however, calcium, vitamin, and protein depletion frequently occurs. Oviductal and uterine muscle atony can develop and lead to complications such as egg binding and egg malformation. Lack of enough vitamin D3 and depletion of vitamin E and selenium can also occur.

### SYSTEMS AFFECTED
**Reproductive**: Fatigue and exhaustion, risk of egg retention leading to egg binding. Other ovarian and uterine disorders may also be associated with chronic laying.
**Endocrine/metabolic**: Calcium depletion and electrolyte imbalances can develop leading to life-threatening conditions. Elevations of lipids can lead to strokes. Presence of an egg can lead to transient elevation of uric acid from renal parenchymal compression.
**Behavioral**: Hens will act broody and try to nest, may hide, and can show aggression while protecting eggs.
**GI**: Hens typically retain feces while nesting.
**Integument**: Feather destructive behavior may result from chronic unaltered hormonal state and stress.

### GENETICS
Some species may have a genetic predisposition for chronic and uncontrolled egg laying. It is particularly common in cockatiels, budgies, and lovebirds.

### INCIDENCE/PREVALENCE
Chronic egg laying is a common problem in single female bird households. More commonly seen in smaller avian species, and most prevalent in cockatiels. Females housed with other females or male birds can also be chronic egg layers.

### GEOGRAPHIC DISTRIBUTION
N/A

### SIGNALMENT
**Species**: Most commonly seen in cockatiels, finches, canaries, and lovebirds.
**Mean age and range**: Sexually mature hens (age of maturity varies widely among species); some species may not start laying until later in life.
**Predominant sex**: Occurs only in females of egg-laying age.

### SIGNS
#### General Comments
Observation of excessive egg production without pause between clutches and disregard of number of eggs already laid.

#### Historical Findings
Constant production of eggs. Mate relationship with member of the household or another bird. Broody behaviors may include hiding, paper shredding, nesting in spaces, and being cage aggressive. Hens may sit on or nest inanimate objects. Hens may spend a lot of time at the bottom of their cage. Some eggs may be misshapen or thin shelled. Sudden and unexpected death is possible, especially in the smaller species.

#### Physical Examination Findings
Normal to no abnormal findings are possible. Abnormal coelomic palpation is consistent with reproductive tract enlargement. Weight gain. Sometimes a palpable egg is present in the caudal coelomic cavity. Pubic bones are typically spread apart. Vent enlargement, engorgement, or a flaccid appearance. Abdominal wall herniation may occur. In some cases, pathologic fractures can occur secondary to calcium depletion. Hens may be obese, underweight, or normal body condition. Sudden death.

### CAUSES
**Behavioral anomaly**: Lack of ability to rear chicks to delay next egg laying cycle. People or toys and mirrors may simulate a mate stimulus to lay eggs. Presence of nest site, box, or materials can contribute to chronic egg laying.
**Disease of captivity**: Lack of normal stimuli for breeding and egg laying, such as length of daylight, food availability, temperature. Lack of true nest sites, building, and entire process of rearing through weaning.

### RISK FACTORS
Poor nutritional state or incomplete diets lacking enough vitamins and calcium may lead to long term complications. Absence of additional and enough calcium supplementation may lead to complications. Not seeking veterinary care or advice on methods to decrease or stop egg laying.

## DIAGNOSIS

### DIFFERENTIAL DIAGNOSIS
Pathologic fractures may be indirectly related and secondary to osteoporosis and calcium depletion. Coelomic distention with mass effect may be from an egg, organomegaly, ascites, neoplasia, or hernia.

### CBC/BIOCHEMISTRY/URINALYSIS
Hypercalcemia is a normal finding in an egg-laying hen. Calcium concentrations in the normal reference range indicate a calcium deficiency in an actively laying bird. Hypercholesterolemia is a common finding during egg production. Hyperglobulinemia may be seen as a physiologic response while the hen is producing eggs. Hyperuricemia can be seen with egg compression and space occupation. Hypertriglyceridemia is seen during times of egg production. Mild anemia and mild leukocytosis may be seen in chronically reproductive female birds.

### OTHER LABORATORY TESTS
Protein electrophoresis may show hyperglobulinemia in egg-laying birds characterized as a marked monoclonal increase in the betaglobulin fraction. Ionized calcium levels may provide a more exact measure of calcium status, but levels are frequently normal as it is the protein-bound calcium that is elevated in reproductive females.

### IMAGING
#### Radiographic Findings
Radiology is useful to confirm presence of a shelled egg. Polyostotic hyperostosis or osteomyelosclerosis of the long bones due to medullary ossification is common. The presence of an egg and enlarged reproductive tract create space occupation and difficulty interpreting radiographs. Pathologic fracture/metabolic bone disease may be evident as decreased overall bone opacity with obvious fractures, especially of the long bones. Increased soft-tissue opacity in the mid to caudal coelomic cavity representing reproductive tract enlargement. Oviductal impaction with egg remnants may be present.

#### Ultrasonography
Ultrasonography may be useful to fully evaluate the coelomic cavity.

### DIAGNOSTIC PROCEDURES
N/A

### PATHOLOGIC FINDINGS
Only if there is disease associated with chronic egg laying such as ascites, ectopic egg

C

production, or yolk-associated coelomitis. Metritis may occur but is often relative to chronic laying.

# TREATMENT

## APPROPRIATE HEALTH CARE
Only needed if there are secondary complications to the chronic egg laying. Health care varies based on clinical findings.

## NURSING CARE
Only needed if complications develop such as egg binding.

## ACTIVITY
No change is required and exercise and flight should be encouraged.

## DIET
Appropriate calcium supplementation is mandatory, sometimes in several forms. Transition to a diet that includes pelleted foods and calcium rich supplements. Vitamin supplements that include omega fatty acids and Vitamins D3 and Vitamin E.

## CLIENT EDUCATION
Clients should be educated that egg formation and laying is a normal process in birds, but chronic or excessive laying is not and that steps need to be taken to reduce egg production. Alteration of environmental stimuli, decreased photoperiod, alteration of nest sites, toys, and other inanimate objects that may be sexually stimulating and decreased physical stimulation from humans/mates. Encourage a flock relationship rather than with one person. Relocation of cage, redecoration, distraction techniques including boarding or taking the bird on a trip may be useful. Avoid any stimulatory petting or feeding. Any eggs should be left in an attempt to have the hen sit for periods of time where egg laying will temporarily cease. Remove male/other birds if present and related to increased egg-laying behavior. Hormonal therapy with leuprolide acetate and deslorelin implants should be discussed with clients as a means to decrease or stop egg production. Periodic laying by healthy birds throughout the year can be acceptable and tolerated.

## SURGICAL CONSIDERATIONS
Salpinghysterectomy may be required in patients with chronic egg laying or undesirable behavioral changes secondary to chronic hormonal states. This is a complicated procedure that should only be performed by skilled avian veterinarians. Medical or surgical repair of fractures may be warranted.

# MEDICATIONS

## DRUG(S) OF CHOICE
Leuprolide acetate, a long-acting GnRH analog used to prevent ovulation and egg production. Doses vary: 700–800 µg/kg IM for birds < 300 g, 500 µg/kg IM for birds ≥ 300 g q21–30d. Calcium gluconate (10%) injectable 50–100 mg/kg SQ, IM (diluted); for hypocalcemia, dilute 1:1 with sterile water for injections. Calcium glubionate 25–100 mg/kg PO q24h; daily oral calcium supplementation for hypocalcemia. Deslorelin implants may be surgically placed for prolonged control or arrest of egg laying q2–6m depending on response.

## CONTRAINDICATIONS
Use of medroxyprogesterone acetate, levonorgestrel, hCG, testosterone, and tamoxifen are associated with risk of severe adverse effects.

## PRECAUTIONS
N/A

## POSSIBLE INTERACTIONS
N/A

## ALTERNATIVE DRUGS
N/A

# FOLLOW-UP

## PATIENT MONITORING
Extensive client communication, education, and review of effects of behavioral modification. Periodic blood tests, including biochemistry profile, to monitor plasma calcium levels.

## PREVENTION/AVOIDANCE
Discourage further egg laying for the season by reducing the photoperiod to no more than 8 hours per day. Cover the cage at night to ensure quiet rest. Keep the hen separate from any mate or perceived mates. Reduce foods high in fat and overall quantity of food. Removal of nests and nesting material may help. Leuprolide acetate can be administered monthly, seasonally or when the hen is exhibiting reproductive behavior, to prevent ovulation and egg laying. A deslorelin implant can also be administered and may last for several months. Avoidance could only occur by not having female pet birds or in hens that have undergone successful salpingohysterectomy.

## POSSIBLE COMPLICATIONS
Egg binding with inability to pass an egg; this can be life threatening. Egg yolk coelomitis may develop from ectopic

ovulation leading to ascites, peritonitis, sepsis, and death. Chronic hypocalcemia, osteoporosis, and pathologic fractures can develop without proper nutrition, calcium supplements, and appropriate care. Chronic internal ovulation and reproductive-associated ascites may occur following salpingohysterectomy depending on individuals and species.

## EXPECTED COURSE AND PROGNOSIS
Cessation of egg laying or decreased number of eggs laid for extended periods of time is highly recommended. Prognosis is good if egg laying can be prevented or slowed. Prognosis is guarded in any hen that continues to lay excessively.

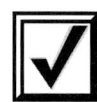

# MISCELLANEOUS

## ASSOCIATED CONDITIONS
Egg binding, oviductal prolapse, lameness, fractures, ectopic egg production.

## AGE-RELATED FACTORS
Any sexually mature bird can lay eggs. Some species, such as sun conures (sun parakeets), may begin egg laying later in life and continue to lay long term.

## ZOONOTIC POTENTIAL
None.

## FERTILITY/BREEDING
In some cases, allowing normal breeding and rearing of chicks may be the only method to stop or delay chronic egg laying but is undesirable for most pet owners and should be discouraged.

## SYNONYMS
N/A

## SEE ALSO
Atherosclerosis
Cloacal Diseases
Cloacal Prolapse
Coelomic Distension
Dyslipidemia/Hyperlipidemia
Dystocia and Egg Binding
Egg Abnormalities
Egg Yolk and Reproductive Coelomitis
Feather-Damaging and Self-Injurious Behavior
Hernia/Pseudohernia
Hypocalcemia and Hypomagnesemia
Lameness
Metabolic Bone Disease
Neoplasia (Reproductive)
Nutritional Imbalances
Ovarian Diseases
Oviductal Diseases

## CHRONIC EGG LAYING

Polyostotic Hyperostosis/Osteomyelosclerosis
Problem Behaviors: Aggression, Biting and Screaming
Regurgitation and Vomiting
Sick-Bird Syndrome

### ABBREVIATIONS
GnRH—gonadotropin-releasing hormone
hCG—human chorionic gonadotropin

### INTERNET RESOURCES
Pollock, C. (2014). Chronic egg laying. *LafeberVet*: https://lafeber.com/vet/chronic-egg-laying

*Suggested Reading*
Bowles, H.L. (2006). Evaluating and treating the reproductive system. In: *Clinical Avian Medicine*, Vol. 2 (ed. G. Harrison, T. Lightfoot), 519–540. Palm Beach, FL: Spix Publishing.
Bowles, H.L. (2002). Reproductive diseases of pet bird species. *Veterinary Clinics of North America. Exotic Animal Practice*, 5:489–506.
Hadley T., (2010) Management of common psittacine reproductive disorders in clinical practice. *Veterinary Clinics of North America. Exotic Animal Practice*, 13:429–438.

Kirchgessner M. (2013) Chronic egg laying. In: *Clinical Veterinary Advisor Birds and Exotic Pets.* (ed. J. Mayer J. and T. Donnely), 164–165. St. Louis, MO: Elsevier Saunders.
Pollock, C.G., Orosz, S.E. (2002). Avian reproductive anatomy, physiology and endocrinology. *Veterinary Clinics of North America. Exotic Animal Practice*, 5:441–474.
**Author**: Anthony A Pilny, DVM, DABVP (Avian)

 **Client Education Handout available online**

# BASICS

## DEFINITION
Viruses within Circoviridae are small, non-enveloped, single-stranded DNA. Of the 11 species of circovirus, PBFDV is the only one identified in parrots. Within PBFDV, there are various viral strains that vary in antigenicity and therefore affect the clinical presentation.

## PATHOPHYSIOLOGY
All strains infect the host destroying cells in the immune system, resulting in immune suppression and increased susceptibility to other infectious agents. One strain variation identified has been shown to affect myeloid and/or erythroid precursors leading to pancytopenia and or anemia. PBFDV has a tropism for growing epithelial cells, resulting in the classic dysplastic changes in growing feathers, rhinotheca (keratin of the upper bill), gnathotheca (keratin of the lower bill) and nails.

## SYSTEMS AFFECTED
**Skin**: progressive, multifocal, feather dystrophy, delayed molt, keratin dystrophy, and fragility.
**Hemic/lymphatic/immune**: immune suppression resulting in one or more secondary infections. The presence of anemia with or without pancytopenia in PBFDV is strain dependent.

## GENETICS
N/A

## INCIDENCE/PREVALENCE
PBFDV infection is found in many species of captive and wild parrots, it is overrepresented in Old World species, particularly those from Africa and the Indo-Pacific regions. Cockatiels and New World parrots seem to be relatively resistant to the development of this disease.

## GEOGRAPHIC DISTRIBUTION
Worldwide. Psittacine circovirus likely originated from Australian Psittaciformes.

## SIGNALMENT
Disease can occur at any age but is most common in fledglings and birds under 1 year old.

## SIGNS

### General Comments
Acute and chronic disease stages have been defined. The clinical presentations in each stage differ markedly and are based on the age and condition of the bird at the time of transmission as well as on the species. In all stages of disease, immunosuppression at various levels will occur.

### Historical Findings
Acute infections that lead to severe depression, anemia, hepatic necrosis, and death are most often seen in nestling or fledgling parrots. Edema of the wing tips and associated pain has also been reported. This stage is often identified in grey parrots. Feather loss and dystrophies are more common in Australasian species, while African species are less likely to show these signs. Beak dystrophies are mainly seen in fledgling cockatoos. Chronic disease is defined by an emersion of clinical signs at any age. When this occurs, it is likely the bird was a survivor of the acute stage of infection. Chronic progressive feather and keratin dystrophy with each subsequent molt are classically the first recognized signs. Although feather loss often becomes diffuse and permanent, lesions can be localized to the remiges and or rectrices. Keratin abnormalities of the beak and nails often present after feather abnormalities have appeared. These individuals may be chronic shedders of psittacine circoviruses. As the viral infection leads to immunosuppression, a variety of secondary infections are common, in particular candidiasis and aspergillosis. Co-infection with other viruses, in particular avian polyomavirus, is also common in some species.

### Physical Examination Findings
Visual feather abnormalities often include shortened lengths, fault lines across the vane, thickened/retained feather sheaths, hemorrhage within the calamus, annular constriction of the calamus or curling. Affected feathers may fall out prematurely. Findings can vary based on feather type and location. Powder down is the first affected feather type in cockatoos and grey parrots. Keratin overgrowth with fracturing of the rhinotheca and gnathotheca and separation of the gnathotheca from the oral mucosa.

## CAUSES
PBFDV. Feather and beak lesions are caused by virus growth in the developing feather and the germinal cells of the rhamphotheca. Damages the bursa of Fabricius and the thymus as well as circulating cells of the immune system, causing immune suppression and secondary infections.

## RISK FACTORS
Poor quarantining and screening procedure for new birds coming into a collection.

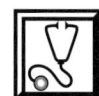

# DIAGNOSIS

## DIFFERENTIAL DIAGNOSIS
The pattern and type of feather disease and signalment are important in differential diagnosis. It is thought that birds engaging in feather destructive and/or automutilatory behaviors will typically have normal feathers that they cannot reach (on their head and neck) whereas birds infected with PBFDV will have a generalized feather disease. Anecdote confirms that cockatoos use their feet to reach and remove feathers from the head and should be considered when applying this line of thinking. Inappropriate husbandry and nutrition can lead to feather changes in young parrots that may be reminiscent of those associated with PBFD. Feather coloration changes have many etiologies and are not pathognomonic for PBFD. Avian polyomavirus infections in nestling budgerigars often will result in identical signs to that of PBFDV infection and can only be differentiated with PCR-based diagnostics or histopathology. Keratin abnormalities of the beak and nails can also be caused by chronic liver disease, beak malocclusion, and in some instances can be self-inflicted secondary to repetitive trauma or behavioral stereotypies. Neoplasia and bacterial and fungal infections of the beak can also result in abnormal keratin development and growth. The disease is generally considered less likely in adult birds, cockatiels, and neotropical parrots. However, infection with clinical signs is still possible in these species.

## CBC/BIOCHEMISTRY/URINALYSIS
Owing to the immunosuppressive effects of all viruses within the Circoviridae family, hematologic and biochemical findings will vary based on the presence or absence of comorbidities. Anemia, leukopenia, thrombocytopenia, pancytopenia and/or elevations in liver function markers may be seen in the acute form of PBFDV. EPH data from chronically affected parrots regularly reports low serum protein characterized by hypo-prealbuminemia and hypo-gammaglobulinemia.

## OTHER LABORATORY TESTS
Commercial PCR assays are available for detecting circovirus via blood, newly erupted feathers, and tissues. The circovirus species-appropriate PCR assay should be used to achieve the best chance at diagnosis. Clinical juvenile birds tend to be persistently viremic until death. Hemagglutination inhibition may be useful.

## IMAGING
In acute cases, an enlargement of the hepatic silhouette may be observed. Although imaging is not directly helpful in the diagnosis of Circoviridae infections, because of the high prevalence of comorbidities in these patients, full diagnostic workups including imaging in clinically ill patients are supported.

C

## CIRCOVIRUS (PSITTACINES)

### DIAGNOSTIC PROCEDURES
Feather and skin biopsies have been used to verify PBFDV infections in parrots with feather dysplasia. In situ hybridization can be used.

### PATHOLOGIC FINDINGS
Disease is best identified in the bursa of Fabricius, feather follicles, spleen, esophagus, and crop. Pathologic findings are dependent on the disease stage. These include but are not limited to: (1) Basophilic intracytoplasmic inclusions within macrophages commonly identified within the feather pulp, thymic, and bursal tissue. These inclusions are occasionally seen in the Kuppfer cells of the liver and spleen. (2) Hepatic congestion and multifocal necrosis. (3) Multifocal epithelial necrosis, hyperplasia, and hyperkeratosis. (4) Bursal and thymic atrophy and necrosis. (5) Necrosis of the oral epithelium and crop in severe cases.

## TREATMENT

### APPROPRIATE HEALTH CARE
The infection is generally fatal. Supportive care may be helpful. Identifying and treating comorbidities, reduction of stress, and feeding a high-quality diet may prolong chronically infected individuals. Whole-blood transfusions of pancytopenic birds can be tried. Interferons have also been used, but efficacy is questionable.

### NURSING CARE
N/A

### ACTIVITY
N/A

### DIET
N/A

### CLIENT EDUCATION
PBFDV-positive birds are a source of infection to the other birds in the owner's home. Disinfection can be challenging due to the non-enveloped nature of this virus and the massive shedding through feather danders. Peroxide compounds (Virkon® S, DuPont) have been shown to be helpful in decontamination.

### SURGICAL CONSIDERATIONS
N/A

## MEDICATIONS

### DRUG(S) OF CHOICE
No drugs change the impact of any strains within PBFDV.

### CONTRAINDICATIONS
N/A

### PRECAUTIONS
N/A

### POSSIBLE INTERACTIONS
N/A

### ALTERNATIVE DRUGS
N/A

## FOLLOW-UP

### PATIENT MONITORING
N/A

### PREVENTION/AVOIDANCE
All susceptible birds should be tested after purchase and prior to or during quarantine, depending on the context.

### POSSIBLE COMPLICATIONS
Increased susceptibility to other infectious diseases.

### EXPECTED COURSE AND PROGNOSIS
There is the potential for some individuals to make a full recovery and no longer shed the virus, but the infection is most often fatal. This has been reported in both ecelctus parrots and lorikeets. In patients with significant beak and feather abnormalities, proper and potentially adaptive husbandry may improve longevity. Death often occurs secondary to difficulty eating or other infectious comorbidities.

## MISCELLANEOUS

### ASSOCIATED CONDITIONS
See above.

### AGE-RELATED FACTORS
Fledglings and juvenile birds are more susceptible.

### ZOONOTIC POTENTIAL
N/A

### FERTILITY/BREEDING
N/A

### SYNONYMS
Psittacine circovirus, psittacine beak and feather disease

### SEE ALSO
Anemia
Beak Malocclusion (Lateral Beak Deformity)
Beak Malocclusion (Mandibular Prognathism)
Beak Injuries
Feather-Damaging and Self-Injurious Behavior
Feather Disorders
Polyomavirus

### ABBREVIATIONS
EPH—protein electrophoresis
PBFD— psittacine beak and feather disease
PCR—polymerase chain reaction

### INTERNET RESOURCES
N/A

*Suggested Reading*
Raidal, S.R. (2012). Avian circovirus and polyomavirus diseases. In: *Fowler's Zoo and Wild Animal Medicine Current Therapy*, Volume 7 (ed. R.E. Miller), 297–303. St. Louis, MO: Elsevier.
Ritchie, B.W. (1995). *Avian Viruses: Function and Control*. Lake Worth, FL: Wingers Publishing.
Sarker, S., Ghorashi, S.A., Forwood, J.K., et al. (2014). Phylogeny of beak and feather disease virus in cockatoos demonstrates host generalism and multiple-variant infections within Psittaciformes. *Virology*, 460–461:72–82.
Speer. *Current Therapy in Avian Medicine and Surgery*. St. Louis, MO: Elsevier. 2016.
Swayne, D.E. (2013). Chicken infectious anemia virus and other circovirus infections. In: *Diseases of Poultry* 13th edn. (ed. D.E. Swayne), 247–288. Ames, IA: Wiley.
**Author**: Bianca Murphy, DVM, DABVP (Avian)

# CIRCOVIRUSES (NON-PSITTACINE BIRDS)

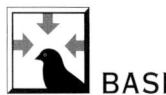

## BASICS

### DEFINITION
The circovirus family comprises a group of small, non-enveloped, single-stranded DNA viruses that infect a wide range of mammalian and avian hosts. This chapter describes circoviruses in non-psittacine species. In birds, circoviruses result in either asymptomatic infection or cause keratin abnormalities and disease secondary to immunosuppression through attacks on the lymphoid centers of the immune-naïve nestlings and juveniles; adults are often asymptomatic.

### PATHOPHYSIOLOGY
Avian circovirus particles are environmentally stable and spread through feather dander, crop secretions, and stools; however, vertical transmission has been reported with CAV and suggested with PiCV. Once infection occurs, the host's lymphoid immune centers and rapidly growing epithelial cells are attacked resulting in immune suppression (increasing susceptibility to other infectious agents) and feather dystrophy. LDCV tropism is limited to growing feathers and the manifested dystrophy is similar to that of PBFD.

### SYSTEMS AFFECTED
**Hemic/lymphatic/immune**: (PiCV, CaCV, GoCV, GuCV, CAV) immune suppression resulting in one or more secondary infections. Severe anemia (CAV).
**Skin/exocrine**: (LDCV, FiCV, DuCV, GoCV) abnormalities with growing feathers and feather follicles.
**Musculoskeletal**: (PiCV) Poor performance.
**Hepatobiliary**: (CaCV, FiCV) cholestasis, hepatic necrosis.
**Neurologic**: (GuCV) recumbency and paralysis.
**Respiratory**: (PiCV, GoCV, FiCV) respiratory distress.
**Gastrointestinal**: (OCV, PiCV) enteritis, diarrhea.

### GENETICS
N/A

### INCIDENCE/PREVALENCE
Unknown as infections are often subclinical or latent. Of the non-psittacine forms identified, only PiCV, LDCV, and GuCV are known to infect wild populations.

### GEOGRAPHIC DISTRIBUTION
These viruses are found worldwide.

### SIGNALMENT
**PiCV**: Domestic and feral rock pigeons; nestlings and juvenile birds (4 weeks to 1 year of age).
**GoCV**: Domestic geese; juvenile birds.

**CaCV**: Domestic canaries; adults and nestlings.
**FiCV**: Gouldian (*Chloebia gouldiae*) and Zebra (*Poephila guttata*) finches; adults and young birds.
**DuCV**: Domestic ducks, especially muscovy, pekin, and mallards; ducklings 3–4 weeks of age are most susceptible.
**CAV**: Domestic chickens, 2–3 weeks of age.
**LDCV**: Senegal doves (*Spilopelia senegalensis*) of Australia only. Mean age and range unreported.
**GuCV**: Ring-billed (*Larus delawarensis*) and black-headed (*Larus ridibundus*) gulls, with a single reported case in a kelp gull (*Larus dominicanus*); juveniles.
**OCV**: Captive ostrich chicks.
These viruses have no sex predilection.

### SIGNS
**PiCV**: High morbidity and mortality of young birds, ill thrift, poor performance. PiCV is immunosuppressive and thus signs are caused by secondary infectious agents. Pharyngitis, rhinitis and conjunctivitis, anorexia, diarrhea, weight loss, depression, dyspnea, death.
**GoCV**: High morbidity and mortality of young birds. Runting and stunting syndrome, anorexia, weight loss, depression, dyspnea, feather abnormalities, death.
**CaCV**: High morbidity and mortality of young birds. Coelomic enlargement. Gallbladder congestion visible through the skin as a "black spot." Pinpoint muscular hemorrhages. Feather abnormalities. Death.
**FiCV**: High morbidity and mortality in adult and young birds. Lethargy, anorexia, feather abnormalities, dyspnea, sinusitis/rhinitis, death.
**DuCV**: Stunting syndrome, ill thrift, poor growth. Feather abnormalities (especially over dorsum), feather shaft hemorrhage.
**CAV**: Morbidity and mortality in chicks 2–3 weeks of age. Anorexia/hypoxia. General malaise, pallor. Poor vaccine response to infectious agents.
**LDCV**: Feather abnormalities resembling PBFD.
**GuCV**: Morbidity and mortality outbreaks especially in groups of juveniles. General malaise, recumbency, and paralysis. Secondary infections (especially aspergillosis and *Riemerella anatipestifer*). Death.
**Ostrich CV**: Ill thrift or "fading chick syndrome" in young birds. General malaise, weight loss, anorexia/hypoxia, diarrhea, death.

### CAUSES
Nine genera of non-psittacine circoviruses (PiCV, GoCV, CaCV, FiCV, DuCV, CAV, LDCV, GuCV, OCV) have been shown to cause disease in birds. The signs associated

with infection depend on the organ targeted by the virus and the host's immune response.

### RISK FACTORS
Risk factors are not well described in the literature for most types of non-psittacine circoviruses. PiCV is common in domestic and wild pigeons and it is thus difficult or impossible to keep out of a loft. CAV occurs in flocks that are not vaccinated.

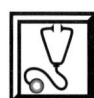

## DIAGNOSIS

### DIFFERENTIAL DIAGNOSIS
Risk factors are not well described in the literature for most types of non-psittacine circoviruses. For many birds, clinical signs are related to immune suppression and secondary conditions. PiCV: Circovirus-like incisions have been seen in wood pigeons. LDCV: Dermatosis of other origin, feather trauma from cat attack.

### CBC/BIOCHEMISTRY/URINALYSIS
These tests, while important to establish a minimum data based and evaluate health status, are not helpful in identifying infected individuals (e.g. bloodwork does not correlate with histopathological findings in PiCV-infected squabs). Exception: Anemia is seen in chickens affected with CAV.

### OTHER LABORATORY TESTS
PCR assays may be used on tissue samples, especially the bursa of Fabricius and other lymphoid tissue of young birds and growing feather follicles in those birds with feather changes. The spleen and liver are particularly important organs to test with FiCV. Commercially available PCR tests for PiCV are obtainable for blood and tissue samples. OCV has been demonstrated within embryo and chick tissues using PCR, Southern blot, and in situ hybridization. In cases where inclusion bodies are not see in classical tissue samples, but for which circovirus is still suspected, consider electron microscopy and/or nucleic acid probes for diagnosis.

### IMAGING
While it is important to establish a minimum data base and evaluate health status, imaging is not reported to be helpful in identifying infected individuals.

### DIAGNOSTIC PROCEDURES
Feather biopsies have been used to verify circovirus infections with LDCV.

### PATHOLOGIC FINDINGS
While not always present, inclusion bodies (botryoid, basophilic intracytoplasmic) found within commonly affected issues (bursa of Fabricius and other lymphoid tissue, growing feather follicles) are pathognomonic for avian

circovirus. Infiltrated tissues (e.g. lymphoid and bone marrow) may be atrophied and carry varying degrees of necrosis. Other tissue abnormalities concurrently found are often attributed to concurrent infection, disease, and immune suppression. Uniquely, canaries infected with CaCV are found to have macroscopic, pinpoint muscle hemorrhages, an enlarged coelom, necrosis of oral epithelium, and a congested gallbladder visible through the skin, hence the nickname "black spot disease." Hemorrhage along feather follicles shafts are seen with DuCV. Inclusion bodies have not been found in ostrich tissue samples for OCV; however, it is unknown whether the bursae samples were evaluated.

## TREATMENT

### APPROPRIATE HEALTH CARE
There are no reported definitive treatments which greatly alter the course of circovirus infection. Depending on species and practicality, generalized supportive care measures may be provided based on assessment (e.g. heat, fluids, assist feedings, and as needed broad-spectrum antibiotics) and concurrent morbidities.

### NURSING CARE
N/A

### ACTIVITY
N/A

### DIET
N/A

### CLIENT EDUCATION
These birds are a source of infection to other birds.

### SURGICAL CONSIDERATIONS
N/A

## MEDICATIONS

### DRUG(S) OF CHOICE
There are no treatments for these viruses.

### CONTRAINDICATIONS
N/A

### PRECAUTIONS
N/A

### POSSIBLE INTERACTIONS
N/A

### ALTERNATIVE DRUGS
N/A

## FOLLOW-UP

### PATIENT MONITORING
N/A

### PREVENTION/AVOIDANCE
Virus particles (shed in one or a combination of stool, feather dander, and crop secretions) are highly stable and very resistant to chemical inactivation and environmental degradation. Maximizing hygiene and husbandry to reduce morbidity are paramount where possible, as prevention and control may be impossible.

### POSSIBLE COMPLICATIONS
Increased susceptibility to other infectious diseases.

### EXPECTED COURSE AND PROGNOSIS
Morbidity and mortality is increased, especially in young birds, but varies based on circovirus type. Recovery may be seen, even in squabs with moderate to severe bursal damage.

## MISCELLANEOUS

### ASSOCIATED CONDITIONS
See above.

### AGE-RELATED FACTORS
N/A

### ZOONOTIC POTENTIAL
N/A

### FERTILITY/BREEDING
N/A

### SYNONYMS
**PiCV:** Young pigeon disease; Columbid circovirus (separate from LDCV)
**CAV:** Anaemia–dermatis syndrome; blue wing disease; infectious anaemia, haemorrhagic syndrome
**OCV:** Fading chick syndrome
**CaCV:** Black spot disease

### SEE ALSO
N/A

### ABBREVIATIONS
CaCV—canary circovirus
DuCV—duck circovirus
FiCV—finch circovirus
GoCV—goose circovirus
GuCV—gull circovirus
LDCV—laughing dove circovirus
OCV—ostrich circovirus
PBFD—psittacine beak and feather disease
PCR—polymerase chain reaction
PiCV—pigeon circovirus

### INTERNET RESOURCES
N/A

*Suggested Reading*
Paré, J.A., Robert, N. (2007). Circovirus. In: *Infectious Diseases of Wild Birds* (ed. N.J. Thomas, C.T. Atkinson), 194–205. Ames, IA: Blackwell.
Raidal SR. (2011). Avian circovirus and polyomavirus diseases. In: *Fowler's Zoo and Wild Animal Medicine Current Therapy* (ed. R.E. Miller RE, M.E. Fowler), 297–303. St. Louis, MO: Saunders.
Todd, D. (2000). Circoviruses: immunosuppressive threats to avian species: A review. *Avian Pathology*, 29:373–394.
Woods, L.W., Latimer, K.S. (2000). Circovirus infection of nonpsittacine birds. *Journal of Avian Medicine and Surgery*, 14:154–163.
**Author:** Julia Shakeri, DVM, DABVP (Avian Practice)

# BASICS

## DEFINITION
Cloacal diseases include any disease that directly or indirectly involves or affects the cloaca. Cloacal prolapse is discussed in a separate chapter in this text.

## PATHOPHYSIOLOGY

### Anatomy of the Avian Cloaca and Vent
The cloaca is the collection chamber for the final products from the GI (feces), urologic (urine and urates), and genital (eggs, sperm) tracts in birds. The cloaca comprises three compartments (from cranial to caudal): (1) The coprodeum (the largest compartment), which communicates with the distal colon; (2) the urodeum (the smallest compartment), which communicates with the distal ureters and oviduct(s) or vas deferens; (3) the proctodeum, which opens to the outside of the body through the vent (Figure 1). These compartments are separated by sphincter-like folds. The bursa of Fabricius, an immune organ, is associated with the dorsal wall of the proctodeum and is largest in juvenile birds. The vent is the external opening to the cloaca and is comprised of dorsal and ventral lips at the mucocutaneous junction. The vent is controlled by several muscles including the cloacal sphincter muscle.

### Diseases
**Cloacitis**: Inflammation of the cloaca can be associated with primary or secondary bacterial, viral, mycotic, or parasitic infections. Foreign body granulomas have been reported but are rare in birds.

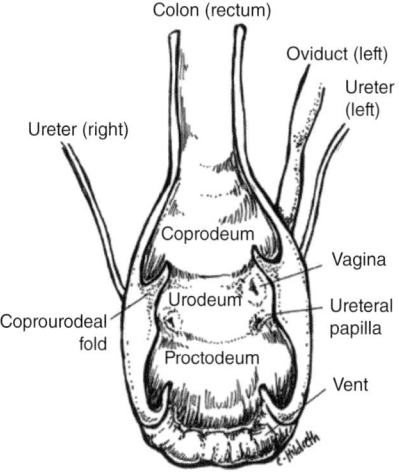

Figure 1.

Diagram of the avian cloaca and associated anatomic structures.

Cloacal inflammation can also be cause by mechanical irritation associated with excessive self-stimulatory sexual behavior. Cloacal inflammation can also be associated with neoplasia and other diseases.

**Trauma**: Traumatic injury to the cloaca can result from dystocia, blunt force trauma, and other causes.

**Neoplasia**: PsHV-1, the etiologic agent of Pacheco's disease, is also associated with cloacal mucosal adenomatous polyps ("papillomas") and adenocarcinomas, particularly in neotropical psittacine species such as Amazon parrots. Cloacal adenocarcinomas are locally invasive and have potential for vascular invasion and distant metastasis. Other reported neoplasms involving the avian cloaca include squamous cell carcinoma, fibrosarcoma, lipoma, liposarcoma, lymphoma, hemangioma, hemangiosarcoma, and oviductal leiomyosarcoma.

**Atony**: Cloacal atony can result from spinal disease, peripheral neuropathy, behavioral fecal retention, and other causes. Cloacal atony can result in cloacal distension, megacloaca, and cloacal dysbiosis.

**Obstruction**: Obstruction of the cloaca can be caused by cloacal uric acid (urates) or fecal concretions (cloacoliths), granulomatous or neoplastic masses, or retained eggs. In most cases, the underlying pathogenesis of cloacolithiasis is unknown.

## SYSTEMS AFFECTED
GI: Infection, inflammation, obstruction, neoplasia, prolapse, dilatation, atony, trauma. Reproductive: Obstruction, prolapse. Renal/urologic: Obstruction.

## GENETICS
None known.

## INCIDENCE/PREVALENCE
A prevalence of cloacal disease of 3.8% (43/1137) in a study cohort of psittacine birds was reported in one recent retrospective study.

## GEOGRAPHIC DISTRIBUTION
N/A

## SIGNALMENT
**Species**: Cloacitis and cloacal neoplasia—adenomatous polyps are more common in neotropical psittacine species such as Amazon parrots and macaws than in other psittacine species. Obstructive diseases of the cloaca—cloacoliths are relatively uncommon in birds in general but have been most often described in budgerigars, macaws, grey parrots, Amazon parrots, and raptors.
**Mean age and range**: Variable.
**Predominant sex**: Cloacal disease is more common in female birds.

## SIGNS

### Historical Findings
Changes in body posture, tenesmus, hematochezia, diarrhea, flatulence, malodorous droppings, decreased fecal production, presence of blood, urates, or feces on the feathers or skin surrounding the vent or on the beak, self-inflicted feather damage around the vent, cloacal prolapse, and signs of generalized illness such as decreased appetite and lethargy.

### Physical Examination Findings
Examination findings are frequently consistent with historical findings. The vent can be slightly everted manually in larger psittacine birds with gentle manipulation for visual inspection of the distal cloacal mucosa. A lubricated swab or gloved finger (if the bird is large enough) can be carefully inserted into the cloacal lumen for further examination. A speculum or otoscope can also be used to visually inspect the cloacal lumen, but the field of view is generally limited. Cloacoliths can often be palpated through the cloacal wall. Irregular, cobblestone-like cloacal mucosal lesions that bleed easily are characteristic of adenomatous polyps ("papillomas"). Polyps may be internally confined or may be prolapsed. Diluted acetic acid (vinegar) can be applied to the cloacal mucosa to further evaluate for polypoid changes.

## CAUSES

### Cloacitis
**Bacterial**: *Escherichia coli*, *Clostridium* spp. (e.g. *Clostridium tertium*), *Mycobacterium* spp.
**Viral**: PsHV-1.
**Mycotic**: *Candida albicans*, *Trichosporon begielli*, *Aspergillus* spp.
**Parasitic**: *Cryptosporidium* avian genotype V, *Giardia* spp.; helminths—Coccidia.
**Other**: Foreign body granuloma, inflammation associated with excessive self-stimulatory sexual behavior, other cloacal diseases.

### Trauma
Blunt force trauma, dystocia, other.

### Neoplasia
Adenomatous polyp associated with PsHV-1 ("papilloma"), adenocarcinoma, squamous cell carcinoma, lymphoma, lipoma, liposarcoma, oviductal leiomyosarcoma.

### Atony
Spinal disease, peripheral neuropathy, excessive egg laying, dystocia, behavioral fecal retention.

### Obstruction
Cloacolithiasis, dystocia, neoplasia, granulomatous disease, vent or cloacal stricture.

## RISK FACTORS
**Cloacitis**: Concurrent cloacal or intestinal diseases, dysbiosis.
**Trauma**: Chronic egg laying (risk factor for dystocia).

## CLOACAL DISEASES (CONTINUED)

C

**Neoplasia**: Infection with PsHV-1 for adenomatous polyps or cloacal adenocarcinoma.

**Atony**: Spinal disease, excessive egg laying.

**Obstruction**: Concurrent viral infection (e.g. PsHV-1), other concurrent cloacal disease, behavioral fecal retention, chronic dehydration, nutritional disorders such as hypovitaminosis A (resulting in epithelial squamous metaplasia).

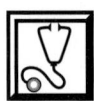

# DIAGNOSIS

## DIFFERENTIAL DIAGNOSIS

Intracoelomic diseases (e.g. peritonitis), spinal disease, reproductive tract disease, urologic tract disease.

## CBC/BIOCHEMISTRY/URINALYSIS

Hematologic and plasma biochemistry findings are usually within normal reference intervals for birds with cloacal disease. Inflammatory diseases may be associated with a leukocytosis and heterophilia. Excessive blood loss may result in a regenerative anemia. Bilateral ureteral obstruction may result in hyperuricemia or azotemia. Urinalysis may be helpful in differentiating urologic tract diseases.

## OTHER LABORATORY TESTS

Cytology using modified Wright–Giemsa stains can be performed on cloacal swabs or feces to evaluate the cellular population of the cloaca. Gram stain and aerobic or anaerobic bacterial or fungal cultures can be performed on cloacal swabs or fecal samples to further characterize the cloacal microflora. Mineral analysis can be performed on extracted cloacoliths.

## IMAGING

### Radiographic Findings

Survey and contrast radiography: Dilation of the intestinal tract can be associated with cloacal obstructive diseases. Cloacoliths can occasionally be identified radiographically. Contrast GI radiography can be useful to evaluate for filling defects, dilation, and changes in motility. Contrast media can also be instilled directly into the cloacal lumen for contrast radiography.

### Ultrasonography

Ultrasonography can be helpful to assess intraluminal cloacal disease such as cloacal neoplasia and intussusception. Instillation of warm saline or water into the cloacal lumen is often helpful in visualizing the cloacal wall and lumen.

### Advanced Imaging

**Fluoroscopy**: Fluoroscopy can be useful to evaluate for filling defects, dilation, and abnormal changes in motility.

**CT**: Can be used to further evaluate the avian cloaca. Intravenous iodinated contrast (e.g. iohexol) can be beneficial in further characterizing the cloaca as well as the distal ureters and other associated structures and in the identification of any vascularized mass(es).

## DIAGNOSTIC PROCEDURES

Masses identified by visual inspection can be surgically biopsied for histopathology and other diagnostic testing (e.g. culture, special stains). A ventral cloacotomy is occasionally required for complete surgical access. Endoscopic evaluation by infusion cloacoscopy can be helpful in visualizing the cloacal lumen and wall to evaluate for the presence of pathology and for the collection of biopsy samples. Caution is warranted with biopsy collection to prevent inadvertent full thickness perforation of the cloacal wall. Cloacoliths can often be visualized endoscopically. Endoscopic fragmentation and removal of cloacoliths has been described in birds.

## PATHOLOGIC FINDINGS

**Cloacitis**: Affected tissues may appear red, ulcerated, thickened or edematous, and may bleed easily. Histologic findings include ulceration, inflammation, fibrosis, and variable presence of etiologic agents such as bacteria, yeasts, and fungi.

**Trauma**: Traumatic injury is frequently associated with acute hemorrhage and ecchymosis.

**Neoplasia**: Adenomatous polyps are often raised or ulcerated, irregular, and thickened, and may have a cobblestone appearance on gross exam. Other neoplasms may be evident as visible or palpable masses within the cloaca or prolapsed through the vent opening. Histopathology is generally diagnostic for cloacal neoplasia.

**Obstruction**: Grossly visible cloacal obstructions include cloacoliths, eggs, granulomas, or neoplasms.

# TREATMENT

## APPROPRIATE HEALTH CARE

Treatment must be specific to the underlying cause to be successful. Mild disease can be treated as an outpatient, more moderate to severe disease generally requires hospitalization for inpatient nursing care.

**Cloacitis**: Bacterial cloacitis is generally treated with antibiotics, ideally based on results from microbiologic culture and sensitivity. Mycotic cloacitis is treated with appropriate antifungal agents. Parasitic infections are treated with appropriate antiparasitic agents.

**Trauma**: Tears involving the cloacal wall can sometimes be surgically repaired. Supportive care measures are taken to manage associated pathology such as soft tissue edema and hematomas.

**Neoplasia**: Surgical excision, electrosurgery, silver nitrate cautery, cryosurgery, laser surgery, cloacoscopic diode laser ablation, and mucosal stripping have been described for the treatment of adenomatous polyps and other cloacal neoplasms in birds. In most cases, adenomatous polyps are confined to the proctodeum. A cloacotomy may be necessary for maximum visualization and surgical access to the cloaca.

**Atony**: Treatment of cloacal atony involves treating any underlying primary neurologic condition and promoting frequent defecation through mechanical cloacal evacuation or behavioral training.

**Obstruction**: Cloacoliths can be manually, endoscopically, or surgically fragmented and extracted.

## NURSING CARE

Supportive care includes analgesic therapy, fluid and nutritional support, and appropriate antimicrobial therapy when indicated.

## ACTIVITY

Activity should be restricted for birds with cloacal disease apart from cloacal atony, as activity may promote increased frequency of defecation.

## DIET

For birds with excessive cloacal distension and fecal retention, dietary items with excessive simple sugars, starches, and fats should be avoided to reduce the risk of cloacal dysbiosis.

## CLIENT EDUCATION

Clients should be educated on the normal components of a bird's droppings (feces, urates, urine) and monitor for abnormal findings in the droppings (e.g. fresh blood, mucus, absence of feces). If the cloacal disease is associated with excessive self-stimulatory sexual behavior, the client should be educated on appropriate husbandry and physical interaction with their pet bird.

## SURGICAL CONSIDERATIONS

None apart from cloacotomy for improved access to the cloacal lumen for inspection and sample collection.

# MEDICATIONS

## DRUG(S) OF CHOICE

Appropriate antibiotics should be used for primary and secondary bacterial infections, ideally based on results of culture and sensitivity testing. Metronidazole and clindamycin are often effective for clostridial cloacitis. Fluoroquinolones are often effective for infections with *E. coli*. Appropriate antifungal or antiparasitic agents should be used for mycotic and parasitic infections. Analgesics such as NSAIDs, opioids, tramadol, gabapentin, and local anesthetics should be considered as needed. Chemotherapy may be effective in some cases of cloacal neoplasia. Hormonal agents such as long-acting GnRH analogs (e.g. leuprolide acetate, deslorelin acetate) can be considered if excessive self-stimulatory sexual behavior is present and refractory to other methods of control.

## CONTRAINDICATIONS
None specific to cloacal diseases.

## PRECAUTIONS
None specific to cloacal diseases.

## POSSIBLE INTERACTIONS
None specific to cloacal diseases.

## ALTERNATIVE DRUGS
N/A

 FOLLOW-UP

## PATIENT MONITORING
Patients with cloacal disease should be closely monitored based on the nature of their disease. Patients should be examined at least every few months during and after treatment. Repeat testing such as fecal or cloacal swab, Gram stain or culture, and radiographs should be considered based on the nature of each case.

## PREVENTION/AVOIDANCE
If the cloacal disease is associated with excessive self-stimulatory sexual behavior, the client should be educated on the proper care and husbandry and physical interaction for their pet bird.

## POSSIBLE COMPLICATIONS
Vent and/or cloacal stricture is a potential complication following cloacotomy and chronic cloacal disease.

## EXPECTED COURSE AND PROGNOSIS
**Cloacitis**: The prognosis is fair to excellent for most bacterial, mycotic, and parasitic causes of cloacitis.
**Trauma**: The prognosis is dependent upon the severity of trauma and the anatomic structures involved.

**Neoplasia**: The prognosis for cloacal neoplasia is fair to guarded or poor depending upon the underlying cause, extent of disease, response to therapy, and presence of complicating diseases. Vent or cloacal stricture can result from adenomatous polyps associated with PsHV-1 infection and/or secondary to surgical debulking.
**Atony**: The prognosis for cloacal atony is fair to guarded depending on the underlying cause and how well cloacal distension and dysbiosis are managed.
**Obstruction**: The prognosis for cloacolithiasis is fair to excellent if the cloacolith can be removed, although recurrence has been reported.

 MISCELLANEOUS

## ASSOCIATED CONDITIONS
Papillomatosis, dystocia, salpingitis, excessive self-stimulatory sexual behavior, trauma, bile duct or pancreatic adenocarcinoma associated with PsHV-1 infection.

## AGE-RELATED FACTORS
Variable.

## ZOONOTIC POTENTIAL
None.

## FERTILITY/BREEDING
Birds with confirmed or suspected infection with PsHV-1 should not be bred.

## SYNONYMS
N/A

## SEE ALSO
Chronic Egg Laying
Cloacal Prolapse
Clostridiosis
Colibacillosis
Cryptosporidiosis
Diarrhea
Dystocia and Egg Binding
Enteritis and Gastritis
Flagellate Enteritis
Helminthiasis (Gastrointestinal)
Herpesvirus (Psittacids)
Infertility
Neoplasia (Gastrointestinal and Hepatic)
Neoplasia (Reproductive)
Oviductal Diseases
Urate and Fecal Discoloration

## ABBREVIATIONS
CT—computed tomography
GI—gastrointestinal
GnRH—gonadotropin-releasing hormone
NSAIDs—non-steroidal anti-inflammatory drugs
PsHV-1—psittacid herpesvirus 1

## INTERNET RESOURCES
N/A

*Suggested Reading*
Curtiss, J.B., Leone, A.M., Wellehan, J.F., et al. (2015). Renal and cloacal cryptosporidiosis (*Cryptosporidium* avian genotype V) in a major Mitchell's cockatoo (*Lophochroa leadbeateri*). *Journal of Zoo and Wildlife Medicine*, 46:934–937.
Evans, E.E., Mitchell, M.A., Whittington, J.K., et al. (2014). Measuring the level of agreement between cloacal Gram's stains and bacterial cultures in Hispaniolan Amazon parrots (*Amazona ventralis*). *Journal of Avian Medicine and Surgery*, 28:290–296.
Gelis, S. (2008). Evaluating and treating the gastrointestinal system. In: *Clinical Avian Medicine* (ed. G.J. Harrison, T.L. Lightfoot), Vol. 1, 411–440. Palm Beach, FL: Spix Publishing.
Gill, K.S., Helmer, P.J. (2020). Cloacal diseases in companion parrots: A retrospective study of 43 cases (2012–2018). *Journal of Avian Medicine and Surgery*, 34:364–370.
Graham, J.E., Tell, L.A., Lamm, M.G., et al. (2004). Megacloaca in a Moluccan cockatoo (*Cacatua moluccensis*). *Journal of Avian Medicine and Surgery*, 18:41–49.
Lee, A., Lennox, A., Reavill, D. (2014). Diseases of the cloaca: A review of 712 cloacal biopsies. *Proceedings of the Association of Avian Veterinarians Annual Conference*, pp. 51–60.
Lumeij, J.T. (1994). Gastroenterology. In: *Avian Medicine: Principles and Application* (ed. B. Ritchie, G.J. Harrison, L. Harrison), 509–512. Lake Worth, FL: Wingers.
Mission, M.B. (2021). Surgery of the avian gastrointestinal tract. In: *Surgery of Exotic Pets* (ed. R.A. Bennett, G.W. Pye), 175–189. Hoboken, NJ: Wiley.
**Author**: Lauren V. Powers, DVM, DABVP (Avian Practice), DABVP (Exotic Companion Mammal Practice)

 **Client Education Handout available online**

# CLOACAL PROLAPSE

C

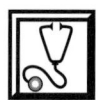

## BASICS

### DEFINITION
Cloacal prolapse is defined as a condition in which internal tissues are intermittently or persistently prolapsed beyond the natural opening to the vent. Cloacal prolapse can be a transient and physiologically normal condition (e.g. associated with normal oviposition in female birds) or a pathologic (transient or persistent) condition.

### PATHOPHYSIOLOGY
Prolapse of the cloaca wall is most often associated with excessive straining associated with undesired behaviors such as excessive self-stimulatory sexual behavior. However, cloacal wall prolapse can also occur with diseases directly or indirectly involving the cloaca. Prolapses can also be associated with the left uterus (shell gland, distal female reproductive tract) or oviduct (proximal female reproductive tract), colon, small intestines, phallus (in species that possess them), or granulomatous or neoplastic masses.

### SYSTEMS AFFECTED
**Gastrointestinal**: Prolapse, infection, inflammation, obstruction, neoplasia, atony, intusussception, herniation, dilation.
**Reproductive**: Prolapse, dystocia, neoplasia, torsion, obstruction.
**Renal/urologic**: Urolithiasis, obstruction.

### GENETICS
N/A

### INCIDENCE/PREVALENCE
In one recent retrospective clinical report, 3.8% (43/1137) of all birds in the study cohort had cloacal disease, 28/43 (65.1%) of which had prolapse of the cloaca wall, 11/43 (25.6%) had oviductal prolapse, and 2/43 (4.7%) had prolapse of gastrointestinal tissues.

### GEOGRAPHIC DISTRIBUTION
N/A

### SIGNALMENT
**Species**: Prolapse of the cloaca wall and prolapse of gastrointestinal tract tissues are more frequent in cockatoos than in other psittacine species.
**Mean age and range**: Variable.
**Predominant sex**: In a recent report, 19/28 (67.9%) of cases of cloacal wall prolapse were female. Prolapse of the left shell gland (uterus) and oviduct only occurs in female birds.

### SIGNS
#### Historical Findings
The primary historical finding associated with cloacal prolapse is the visible intermittent or persistent presence of prolapsed tissues extending beyond the natural vent opening. However, prolapsed tissues may not be readily visible or otherwise apparent to clients. Other historical findings may include changes in body posture, increased respiratory rate and effort, tenesmus, hematochezia, diarrhea, flatulence, malodorous feces, decreased fecal production, excessive grooming or other self-inflicted feather damage around the vent, presence of blood or urofeces on the feathers or skin surrounding the vent or on the beak, as well as signs of generalized illness such as decreased appetite and lethargy.

#### Physical Examination Findings
Examination findings are often consistent with historical findings. The size of a cloacal prolapse varies widely from a few millimeters of cloacal wall to often large portions of the gastrointestinal or genital tract. The area around a prolapse should be carefully probed and inspected to identify the anatomic structures and relative position. Prolapsed cloacal wall is generally smooth unless affected by adenomatous polyp formation. The ureteral openings can often be observed along the lateral walls of a prolapsed urodeal wall, identified by the passage of urates and urine. Prolapsed left shell gland (uterine) and/or oviductal tissues arise from the left side of the cloaca (urodeum) and will often have pink longitudinal striations that can help differentiate them from other tissues such as the colon. Prolapsed colonic tissues lack longitudinal folds and are generally centrally located within the cloaca. Intestinal prolapses, intussusceptions, and herniations are difficult to differentiate from colonic prolapses. Palpation of the coelom may identify the presence of solid masses or fluid.

### CAUSES
**Cloacal wall prolapse**: Excessive self-stimulatory sexual behavior, cloacitis (bacterial, viral, mycotic, parasitic), cloacal neoplasia (eg. adenomatous polyps associated with PsHV-1 infection, adenocarcinoma), cloacolithiasis, trauma, ureterolithiasis, cloacal atony, spinal disease, pudendal nerve trauma or neuritis, peripheral neuropathy.
**Shell gland (uterine) and oviductal prolapse**: Dystocia, delayed oviposition (egg binding), chronic egg laying, oviductal inertia/exhaustion, salpingitis, oviductal neoplasia, excessive self-stimulatory sexual behavior, trauma.
**Colonic prolapse**: Colitis, colonic neoplasia, cloacitis, intestinal obstruction, colonic intussusception, intestinal parasitism, granulomatous disease (e.g. mycobacteriosis), megacolon, excessive self-stimulatory sexual behavior.
**Small intestinal prolapse**: Enteritis, intestinal obstruction, trauma, intestinal intussusception, cloacal wall necrosis with intestinal herniation.
**Phallus prolapse**: Excessive sexual activity, balanitis.

### RISK FACTORS
Excessive self-stimulatory sexual behavior, chronic egg laying, obesity, inactivity, malnutrition.

## DIAGNOSIS

### DIFFERENTIAL DIAGNOSIS
Coelomic wall hernia, pericloacal neoplasia.

### CBC/BIOCHEMISTRY/URINALYSIS
Hematologic and plasma biochemistry findings are usually within normal reference intervals for birds with cloacal prolapse. Inflammation may be associated with a leukocytosis and heterophilia. Bilateral ureteral obstruction may result in hyperuricemia or azotemia.

### OTHER LABORATORY TESTS
Cytology can be performed on cloacal swabs or feces to evaluate the cellular population of the cloaca. Gram stain and aerobic or anaerobic bacterial or fungal cultures can be performed on cloacal swabs or fecal samples to further characterize the cloacal microflora. Mineral analysis can be performed on extracted cloacoliths and ureteroliths.

### IMAGING
#### Radiographic Findings
Survey radiographs are recommended in all cases of cloacal prolapse to further evaluate for underlying disease. Shelled eggs or collapsed mineralized shell material may be visible in the area of the left oviduct and/or shell gland (uterus). Dilation of the distal intestinal tract can be associated with intestinal obstructive diseases. Cloacoliths and ureteroliths can occasionally be identified radiographically. Contrast GI radiography and contrast fluoroscopy can be useful to evaluate for filling defects, dilation, and changes in GI motility.

#### Ultrasonography
Coelomic ultrasonography can be helpful to assess for intracoelomic disease including the presence of free fluid (ascites) and masses. Ultrasonography is also useful to evaluate for the presence of egg or egg material as well as for ureterolithiasis. However, air naturally present within the caudal thoracic and abdominal air sacs often interferes with full evaluation of the urologic tract by ultrasound.

### DIAGNOSTIC PROCEDURES
Surgical biopsy and histopathology of prolapsed masses and tissues should be performed when indicated, based on the

appearance of prolapsed tissues and the presumed or suspected underlying cause. Cloacoscopy is indicated for visual inspection of the cloacal lumen and wall and can be useful for the collection of biopsy specimens. Caution is warranted with biopsy collection to prevent unintentional full thickness perforation of the cloacal wall.

### PATHOLOGIC FINDINGS
Prolapsed tissue can usually be identified by gross appearance. Histopathology on biopsy specimens collected from prolapsed tissues and masses may be unremarkable or demonstrate pathologic changes such as inflammation or neoplasia.

## TREATMENT
### APPROPRIATE HEALTH CARE
Birds with cloacal prolapse should be stabilized and administered appropriate analgesic therapy and other supportive care measures. Viable prolapsed tissues should be returned to their normal anatomic location when possible after inspection and diagnostic sample collection (when indicated). If a shelled egg is present within a prolapsed left shell gland (uterus) or oviduct, it should be carefully removed prior to reduction of the prolapse. In certain cases, manual reduction with return to a normal anatomic location may not be possible without surgical intervention. But, when possible, viable prolapsed tissues should be gently aseptically cleansed, lubricated, and then manually returned to their normal anatomic position using sterile lubricated swabs or gloved fingers. Application of a sugar solution (e.g. 50% dextrose) may be helpful in reducing soft tissue swelling prior to reduction. Heavy sedation (e.g. midazolam, butorphanol) or general anesthesia is often indicated when attempting to reduce a cloacal prolapse. In cases where the prolapse cannot be immediately reduced, or if the prolapsed tissues are non-viable, the prolapsed tissues should be kept clean and lubricated until further treatment can be performed. Treatment must be aimed at the underlying cause to be successful. Mild cases of cloacal prolapse can be treated on an outpatient basis, but more severe cases of cloacal prolapse and debilitated birds generally require hospitalization for inpatient nursing care.

### NURSING CARE
Supportive care includes analgesic therapy, fluid and nutritional support, and appropriate antimicrobial therapy.

### ACTIVITY
Activity should be restricted for birds with cloacal prolapse.

### DIET
Dietary items with excessive simple sugars, starches, and fats should be reduced or eliminated in overconditioned birds, birds that demonstrate excessive self-stimulatory sexual behavior, and birds with cloacal disease that are prone to dysbiosis.

### CLIENT EDUCATION
If the cloacal prolapse is associated with excessive self-stimulatory sexual behavior, the client should be educated on appropriate husbandry and physical interaction with their pet bird. All nesting material should be removed and birds should be prevented from accessing perceived nesting sites.

### SURGICAL CONSIDERATIONS
Prolapsed cloacal masses such as adenomatous polyps can be surgically debulked or excised using one of several described methods such as surgical excision (with or without cloacotomy), electrocautery, chemical cauterization, cryotherapy, or "mucosal stripping." Otherwise, viable prolapsed tissues should be cleansed and returned to their normal anatomic position when possible and medically appropriate.

#### *Retention Sutures*
Once the prolapse has been reduced, sutures can be placed transversely across the vent opening to prevent immediate recurrence. Typically, one full-thickness suture is placed on either side of the vent opening, incorporating the dorsal and ventral vent lips, at about one-third of the way across the vent opening on each side. The sutures must be placed close enough to each other to prevent reprolapse but far enough apart to allow the normal passage of urofeces. Purse-string sutures are not recommended in birds. Sutures are generally removed after 2–3 weeks. Retention sutures alone are inadequate in the long-term prevention of chronic cloacal wall prolapse recurrence.

#### *Long-Term Surgical Options for Chronic Cloacal Wall Prolapse*
Chronic self-stimulatory sexual behavior often results in the mechanical stretching of the vent, vent sphincter muscle and other muscles, and the cloaca itself, resulting in irreversible vent and cloacal flaccidity. Diseases such as cloacal atony associated with spinal disease can also result in an excessively dilated and flaccid cloaca. The risk of cloacal wall prolapse recurrence is high in these cases. Reconstructive surgery (i.e. cloacopexy, ventplasty) may be indicated in an attempt to prevent prolapse recurrence. Recurrence is possible with any reconstructive surgical technique and clients must be prepared for this possibility.
**Cloacopexy**: Rib and incisional cloacopexy techniques have been described. Intestinal entrapment has been reported with rib

cloacopexy. Adhesion formation is also a potential postoperative complication for cloacopexy.
**Ventplasty**: Ventplasty permanently reduces the size of the vent opening. Ventplasty involves trimming and closure of one or more sections of the vent margin. The most common ventplasty technique described consists of trimming away a thin strip of epithelial tissue at the mucocutaneous junction of the vent on either side and the reapposition of mucosa to mucosa and skin to skin, cranial to caudal, such that the new vent opening is approximately one-third the width of the original vent opening and wide enough for at least one cotton-tipped applicator to pass through. An asymmetrical ventplasty technique for the management of chronic recurrent cloacal wall prolapse after previous surgical failure has been reported in five psittacine birds with good surgical success.
**Colopexy**: Incisional colopexy has been described for the treatment of colonic prolapse in a sulfur-crested cockatoo. Colopexy may be less likely to result in intestinal entrapment than cloacopexy.
**Salpingohysterectomy**: In some cases of prolapse of the left oviduct and/or shell gland (uterus), salpingohysterectomy may be indicated if the prolapsed tissues are non-viable, neoplastic, and/or if the prolapse cannot be resolved with more conservative techniques.

## MEDICATIONS
### DRUG(S) OF CHOICE
Analgesics such as NSAIDs (e.g. meloxicam), opioids (e.g. butorphanol), gabapentin, tramadol, and local anesthetics should be part of the clinical management plan for cloacal prolapse. Appropriate antibiotics should be used for primary and secondary bacterial infections based on results of culture and sensitivity testing. Appropriate antifungal or antiparasitic agents should be used for mycotic and parasitic infections. Hormonal agents such as long-acting GnRH analogs (eg. leuprolide acetate, deslorelin acetate) can be considered if excessive sexual stimulation is present and cannot be effectively managed through behavioral, environmental, and dietary modification alone.

### CONTRAINDICATIONS
None specific to cloacal prolapse.

### PRECAUTIONS
None specific to cloacal prolapse.

### POSSIBLE INTERACTIONS
None specific to cloacal prolapse.

## CLOACAL PROLAPSE          (CONTINUED)

### ALTERNATIVE DRUGS

Melatonin stimulates the production of GnIH in birds, thereby inhibiting GnRH, and may be helpful in reducing undesired self-stimulatory sexual behaviors. Alternative therapeutics should be combined with a customized behavioral and dietary modification plan and pharmacologic treatment when indicated.

## FOLLOW-UP

### PATIENT MONITORING

Patients with cloacal prolapse should be closely monitored based on the nature of their disease. Patients should be examined at least every few months during and after treatment.

### PREVENTION/AVOIDANCE

If the cloacal prolapse is associated with excessive self-stimulating sexual behavior, the client should be educated on the proper care and husbandry and physical interaction for their pet bird.

### POSSIBLE COMPLICATIONS

Chronic cloacal wall prolapse can result in necrosis of the cloacal wall and intestinal herniation, indirect prolapse, and strangulation. Direct intestinal prolapse can also result in strangulation and necrosis of the bowel. Potential complications of cloacopexy and ventplasty include dehiscence of the surgical sites(s), which may result in peritonitis, and vent or cloacal stricture.

### EXPECTED COURSE AND PROGNOSIS

The prognosis for cloacal prolapse due to behavioral causes is fair to guarded, as often the underlying behavior is difficult to manage and control and recurrence and complications are common. In one recent retrospective report, 7/11 (64%) of oviductal prolapses survived to discharge and 5 (45%) had no recurrence when rechecked, whereas neither of the 2 birds with gastrointestinal prolapsed survived to discharge.

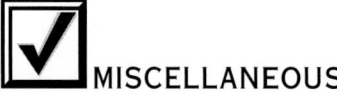

## MISCELLANEOUS

### ASSOCIATED CONDITIONS

Egg binding (delayed oviposition), salpingitis, excessive self-stimulatory sexual behavior, "papillomatosis," bile duct or pancreatic adenocarcinoma associated with PsHV-1 infection.

### AGE-RELATED FACTORS

Variable.

### ZOONOTIC POTENTIAL

N/A

### FERTILITY/BREEDING

Female birds with shell gland (uterine) or oviductal prolapse and male birds with phallus prolapse should be rested or retired from breeding.

### SYNONYMS

N/A

### SEE ALSO

Chronic Egg Laying
Clostridiosis
Colibacillosis
Diarrhea
Dystocia and Egg Binding
Enteritis and Gastritis
Flagellate Enteritis
Helminthiasis (Gastrointestinal)
Herpesviruses (Psittacids)
Neoplasia (Gastrointestinal and Hepatic)
Neoplasia (Reproductive)
Oviductal Diseases
Phallus Prolapse and Diseases

### ABBREVIATIONS

GI—gastrointestinal
GnIH—gonadotropin inhibitory hormone
GnRH—gonadotropin-releasing hormone
NSAIDs—non-steroidal anti-inflammatory drugs
PsHV-1—psittacid herpesvirus 1

### INTERNET RESOURCES

N/A

*Suggested Reading*
Cococcetta, C., Binanti, D, Matteucci, G., et al. (2020). Antemortem diagnosis and surgical management of a rectum intussusception and cloacal wall prolapse in a hybrid falcon (*F. cherrug* x *F. peregrinus*) associated with bacterial enteritis. *Journal of Exotic Pet Medicine*, 33:10–13.
Dutton, T.A., Forbes, N.A., Carrasco, D.C. (2016). Cloacal prolapse in raptors: Review of 16 cases. *Journal of Avian Medicine and Surgery*, 30:133–140.
Lennox, A., Lee, A. (2018). Cloacal, uterine, and rectal prolapse. In: *BSAVA Manual of Avian Practice A Foundation Manual* (ed. J. Chitty, D. Monks), 358–365. Gloucester, UK: British Small Animal Veterinary Association.
Mission, M.B. (2021). Surgery of the avian gastrointestinal tract. In: *Surgery of Exotic Pets* (ed. R.A. Bennett, G.W. Pye), 175–189. Hoboken, NJ: Wiley.
Radlinsky, M.G., Carpenter, J.W., Mison, M.B., et al. (2004). Colonic entrapment after cloacopexy in two psittacine birds. *Journal of Avian Medicine and Surgery*, 18:175–182.
van Zeeland, Y.R.A., Schoemaker, N.J., van Sluijs, F.J. (2014). Incisional colopexy for treatment of chronic, recurrent colocloacal prolapse in a sulphur-crested cockatoo (*Cacatua galerita*). *Veterinary Surgery*, 43: 882–887.
Zaheer, O., Beaufrère, H., Jajou, S., et al. (2020). Asymmetrical cloacoplasty for the treatment of chronic cloacal prolapse in psittaciformes: A case series. *Journal of Avian Medicine and Surgery*, 34:172–180.

**Author**: Lauren V Powers, DVM, DABVP (Avian Practice), DABVP (Exotic Companion Mammal Practice)

 **Client Education Handout available online**

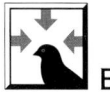

# BASICS

## DEFINITION
Avian clostridiosis caused by *Clostridioides* spp. (formerly *Clostridium*) refers to enteric disease, commonly with secondary cholangiohepatitis, and is not to be confused with botulism, which is caused by *Clostridium botulinum*. *Clostridia* are anaerobic Gram-positive spore-forming bacilli. They can produce a large number of toxins that are known to cause gas gangrene in affected tissues. However avian clostridiosis commonly refers to the necrotic enterocolitis form. *Clostridium perfringens* and *Clostridium difficile* are the most commonly described genera in all avian species, but other species such as *Clostridium sordellii*, *Clostridium tertium* and *Clostridium colinum* have been described. *C. colinum* is considered to be the predominant pathogen in ulcerative enteritis in quails. Clostridiosis has been described in a wide range of captive or free-range avian species that are commonly presented for veterinary care including backyard poultry, quails, psittacine birds, raptors, and waterfowl, but is most researched in the domestic chicken (broilers). Clostridiosis can cause acute or peracute necrotizing enterocolitis that leads to a high mortality rate or chronic enterocolitis with lower mortality but with significant morbidity, depending on the avian species that is affected. It has long been thought that the wide range of endotoxins produced by *Clostridia* and used to classify different strains are responsible for their pathogenicity. Thus, *C. perfringens* type A and *C. difficile* type A were considered highly pathogenic and specific diagnostic tests were designed to detect the specific toxinogenic strains. Recent evidence establishes that a newly described toxin, necrotic enteritis B-like toxin (NetB), and various other factors are responsible for the necrotic enteritis form of the disease, while alpha toxin has been proved to mediate the gas gangrene disease. Other factors include preceding coccidial infection in chickens and nectar diet in Lories and lorikeets. *Clostridia* are opportunistic pathogens and can be found in the GI tract and in fecal samples of healthy raptors and ground dwelling birds, such as poultry and waterfowl, but are considered an abnormal finding in psittacine birds. *C. difficile* is ubiquitous in the environment and has a wide host range. *C. difficile* infection is the most common cause of antibiotic-associated diarrhea and one of the common infections in humans, and animals are an important reservoir for *C. difficile* causing human diseases. In a recent study, wild griffon vultures were postulated to be spreading highly antibiotic resistant strains of *C. difficile* from the pig carcasses they were feeding on.

## PATHOPHYSIOLOGY
In infections caused by *C. perfringens*, NetB toxin, a member of a beta pore-forming toxin family, causes cell rounding and lysis of the intestinal epithelial cells. The gene for its production is upregulated only when there is a high density population of the bacteria. Such high clostridial population is enabled by a high polysaccharide diet and by concurrent coccidial infection (*Eimeria* spp.). The *Eimeria* parasites kill epithelial cells and induce leakage of proteins that are necessary for the enhanced colonization by *Clostridia*. The mucin secreted in response to the *Eimeria* infection serves as a preferred growth substrate for *Clostridia*. The massive inflammatory response, including heterophils, lymphocytes, and plasma cells, produces ulcerative necrotic enteritis and in many cases invades the biliary system, resulting in severe cholangiohepatitis.

## SYSTEMS AFFECTED
**Gastrointestinal**: Necrotic enteritis is the most common form. Colitis, megacolon and cloacitis are seen in psittacines (cockatoos, lories) and raptors.
**Hepatobiliary**: Cholangiohepatitis occurs in chronic or subclinical cases that allow colonization of the liver through the bile duct.
**Renal**: In systemic end-stage disease, sepsis.

## GENETICS
N/A

## INCIDENCE/PREVALENCE
All *Clostridia* spp. are distributed worldwide and found in soil. Subclinical infection with chronic diarrhea has been described in all affected species from broilers to cockatoos. This allows persistent flock infection, as many birds in a flock situation remain untreated.

## GEOGRAPHIC DISTRIBUTION
Worldwide.

## SIGNALMENT
**Species:** Described in many species. Cockatoos and Lories are considered predisposed among psittacine birds, but clostridiosis has been reported in many species of parrots. Raptors are considered unsusceptible and infection is rare. Disease is very common in commercial flocks (i.e. broilers or quails).
**Mean age and range:** Juvenile birds are more susceptible. In broiler chickens, clostridiosis usually occurs at 4 weeks after hatching. In cockatoos, the disease is commonly secondary to other factors and occurs in sexually mature birds. Hand-fed psittacine birds are predisposed.
**Predominant sex:** Higher predilection in phallus-containing birds, such as Anseriformes and Struthioniformes (ostrich, emu, etc.), should prolapse occur.

## SIGNS
### General Comments
Clinical signs can differ in accordance with the affected species or the form of the disease. For example, in cockatoos with chronic cloacitis, diarrhea or feather damaging behavior may be the only signs. In raptors, lories, or chickens, peracute disease may result in death with no preceding clinical signs. Acute or chronic disease can manifest in severe diarrhea among other signs.

### Historical Findings
Poor digestion resulting in weight loss or poor weight gain in flocks. Diarrhea, anorexia and weakness. Malodorous feces is very common among psittacine birds. Feather picking. Prolapsed cloaca. Bloody stool. Regurgitation.

### Physical Examination Findings
Good body condition score in acute/peracute infection. Lethargy. Weight loss in chronic infections. Prolapsed cloaca (psittacine birds, ostrich, waterfowl). Hematochezia. Malodorous feces. Retained feces. Soiled vent. Feather destructive behavior (psittacines).

## CAUSES
*Clostridia* spp.

## RISK FACTORS
**Nutritional**: A high polysaccharide diet is proposed as an important factor in promoting the proliferation of *C. perfringens*. Nectarivorous species, such as lories and lorikeets, are highly susceptible. In falconry raptors, meat storage techniques have been implicated to be a contributing factor in the proliferation of *C. perfringens*, as has hand-feeding practice used in rearing young psittacine birds.
**Stress and immunosuppression**: Stress has been shown to alter the intestinal flora and to elevate the risk for necrotizing enteritis.
**Cloacal diseases**: Cloacal prolapse, enterolith, impaction. Egg binding. Other: Chronic salpingitis. Intestinal/cloacal neoplasia. Papillomatosis. Behavioral—owner-induced masturbatory behavior, delayed defecation behavior (psittacine species). Concurrent coccidiosis (poultry). Cloacal/colonic atony. Toxicosis (especially zinc or lead).

## DIAGNOSIS

### DIFFERENTIAL DIAGNOSIS
Coccidiosis, papillomatosis, megacolon, other infectious enteritis (viral, bacterial, parasitic, fungal), toxicosis, neoplastic or inflammatory disease.

### CBC/BIOCHEMISTRY/URINALYSIS
Complete blood count may show leukocytosis with heterophilia and monocytosis. In acute infection, leukopenia may occur, because of massive intraluminal leukocytosis. Anemia may be present in subclinical or chronic infections. Elevated liver enzymes may be seen.

### OTHER LABORATORY TESTS
Fecal Gram-stained cytology is very typical of the large Gram-positive sporulated bacilli; however, sporulating bacilli are not always seen in cases of clostridial enteritis. Spore-forming bacteria can be seen in small numbers in the feces from healthy raptors or ground-dwelling birds but should always be considered abnormal in psittacine species. Definitive diagnosis can be obtained by anaerobic culture/sensitivity. However, *Clostridia* organisms are fastidious and may result in false negative culture. PCR is now available for specific strains or at the genus level. Serum immunoassays targeting *C. perfringines* and *C. difficile* toxins can result in false negative results.

### IMAGING
Coelomic radiographs of gas-filled loops of bowel, megacolon and megacloaca are compatible with clostridiosis. Hepatomegaly may also be present.

### DIAGNOSTIC PROCEDURES
N/A

### PATHOLOGIC FINDINGS
Gross lesions of severe cases are usually restricted to the small intestines and/or the colon and cloaca, but can also be present in other organs such as liver and kidney. The intestines are usually thin walled and gas filled. The necrotic enteritis is characterized by extensive ulcerative necrosis covered with bile-stained pseudomembrane, while mild subclinical cases may have multiple smaller ulcers. Microscopic examination typically shows a strong inflammatory reaction, with heterophils and lymphocytic plasmacytic infiltration. This is different than gas gangrene caused by alpha toxin that usually lacks the microscopic inflammatory reaction. There is a clear demarcation line between viable and necrotic tissue. Large Gram-positive rods are associated with the area of necrosis. The liver may be enlarged with signs of cholangiostasis and hepatitis.

## TREATMENT

### APPROPRIATE HEALTH CARE
Treatment should be targeted to remove or alter any underlying condition that may have served as a predisposing factor in the development of clostridiosis. Remove cloacal impactions, treat egg binding, correct cloacal prolapse, etc. Reduce stress. Improve hygiene measures when feed is suspected as a source of infection (falconry, hand-reared psittacines and lorikeets).

### NURSING CARE
Fluid and nutritional support are necessary in debilitated patients.

### ACTIVITY
N/A

### DIET
Avoid high polysaccharide diets.

### CLIENT EDUCATION
N/A

### SURGICAL CONSIDERATIONS
In psittacine birds, especially cockatoos, with recurrent infections secondary to recurrent cloacal prolapse or chronically dystrophic cloaca, surgical modification of the cloacal lesion may be necessary.

## MEDICATIONS

### DRUG(S) OF CHOICE
Pharmacological treatment is composed of antibiotics against anaerobic bacteria and GI protectants. GI promotility drugs are usually not necessary. Metronidazole or penicillins are usually the drugs of choice, macrolides can be used as well: Metronidazole 20–50 mg/kg PO q12h for 10–14 days; amoxicillin/clavulanate 125 mg/kg PO q12h for 10–14 days; azithromycin 10–30 mg/kg PO q24h for 10–14 days.

### CONTRAINDICATIONS
N/A

### PRECAUTIONS
N/A

### POSSIBLE INTERACTIONS
N/A

### ALTERNATIVE DRUGS
Other antibiotics that are effective against anaerobic bacteria can be used.

## FOLLOW-UP

### PATIENT MONITORING
Repeated fecal Gram stains can be reviewed to confirm resolution of the infection once antibiotic therapy is completed.

### PREVENTION/AVOIDANCE
Avoid sexual stimulation in psittacine species. Implement excellent hygienic feeding practice.

### POSSIBLE COMPLICATIONS
Decreased meat and egg production in commercial flocks.

### EXPECTED COURSE AND PROGNOSIS
In mild and subclinical cases that are treated early, the prognosis is good. However, subclinical infection in a flock situation usually becomes chronic. Recurrent clostridiosis is common in psittacines that suffer from chronic cloacal dysfunction. In acute clinical infections, mortality tends to be high in all avian species.

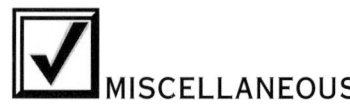

## MISCELLANEOUS

### ASSOCIATED CONDITIONS
Coccidiosis, cloacal prolapse, cloacitis.

### AGE-RELATED FACTORS
Juvenile birds are more susceptible.

### ZOONOTIC POTENTIAL
Cross-infection between humans and avian species with clostridiosis has not been reported. However, humans are susceptible to clostridiosis and good hygiene standards are preventive.

### FERTILITY/BREEDING
N/A

### SYNONYMS
Necrotic enteritis, quail disease

### SEE ALSO
Botulism
Cloacal Disease
Cloacal Prolapse
Coccidiosis (Intestinal)
Coccidiosis (Systemic)
Dehydration
Dystocia and Egg Binding
Emaciation
Herpesvirus (Columbid Herpesvirus 1 in Pigeons and Raptors)
Herpesvirus (Duck Viral Enteritis)
Ileus (Functional Gastrointestinal, Crop Stasis)
Neurologic (Non-Traumatic Diseases)
Oviductal Diseases
Phallus Prolapse and Diseases
Sepsis
Toxicosis (Heavy Metals)
Urate and Fecal Discoloration

### ABBREVIATIONS
GI—gastrointestinal
NetB—necrotic enteritis B-like toxin
PCR—polymerase chain reaction

## INTERNET RESOURCES

Association of Avian Veterinarians: www.aav.org
Merck & Co. MSD Manuals:
www.merckmanuals.com
National Library of Medicine: https://www.
ncbi.nlm.nih.gov

*Suggested Reading*

Moono, P., Foster, N.F., Hampson, D.J.,
et al. (2016). *Clostridium difficile* infection
in production animals and avian species:
A review. *Foodborne Pathogens and Diseases*,
13:647–655.

Sevilla, E., Marín, C., Delgado-Blas, J.F., et al.
(2020). Wild griffon vultures (*Gyps fulvus*) fed
at supplementary feeding stations: Potential
carriers of pig pathogens and pig-derived
antimicrobial resistance? *Transboundary and
Emerging Diseases*, 67:1295–1305.

Timbermont, L., Haesebrouck, F., Ducatelle,
R., Van Immerseel, F. (2011). Necrotic
enteritis in broilers: An updated review on
the pathogenesis. *Avian Pathology*, 40:
341–347.

Van Immerseel, F., Rood, J.I., Moore, R.J.,
Titball, R.W. (2009). Rethinking our
understanding of the pathogenesis of
necrotic enteritis in chickens. *Trends in
Microbiology*, 17:32–36.

**Author:** Shachar Malka, DVM, DABVP
(Avian), DACEPM

# COAGULOPATHIES AND COAGULATION

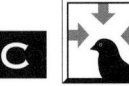

## BASICS

### DEFINITION
Coagulation is a vital physiological defense mechanism against hemorrhage whereby blood changes from a liquid to a gel, forming a clot and initiating wound healing. It involves both cellular components, primarily thrombocytes and cells of the vasculature, and biochemical components including coagulation factors of the intrinsic, extrinsic pathways, and common pathways. These pathways are activated by protein signals triggered by vascular damage and inflammation. The initial coagulation event is followed by fibrinolysis, which clears the clot and restores blood circulation.

### PATHOPHYSIOLOGY
Coagulopathies can stem from either thrombocytopenia, abnormal cellular function (e.g. NSAID induced), or deficiencies in coagulation factors.

### THROMBOCYTOPENIA
Lack of production by the bone marrow, increased consumption (DIC), loss (marked blood loss) or destruction (immune mediated) could all result in thrombocytopenia. DIC is the most common cause of true thrombocytopenia in birds, with many reports secondary to a variety of bacterial and viral infections. Spurious result: Clot formation and/or thrombocyte clumping during collection is extremely common, particularly if blood is collected in heparin (compared with EDTA), and particularly if venipuncture was challenging. Blood smears should always be checked for the presence of thrombocyte clumps, as clumping can lead to an underestimation of the thrombocyte count if only those that are individually scattered are counted. In addition, blood, including thrombocytes, may be diluted by anticoagulant, such as when needles or syringes are preheparinized but an insufficient volume of blood is obtained for the volume of heparin already in the needle/syringe.

### COAGULATION FACTOR DEFICIENCY
Lack of production, which can be inherited or acquired, or increased consumption (DIC). The most frequently reported coagulopathies in birds are toxin-induced (e.g. AR, sulfonamide antibiotics, roxarsone), DIC, nutritional deficiencies, and hepatic failure (which is most often secondary to viral diseases, toxins such as aflatoxins and other mycotoxins, and fatty liver hemorrhagic syndrome in laying hens). Inherited coagulation factor deficiencies are rare in birds. As described for thrombocytopenia,

spurious results secondary to clotting in the tube should be a top differential when interpreting prolonged coagulation times.

### UNCLEAR PATHOGENESIS
**Conure bleeding syndrome**: An uncommon and potentially fatal syndrome whereby conures present with bleeding, often from the mouth and respiratory tract. This has been reported typically in young birds but some older birds are also affected without gender predilection. The cause is still unknown but liver disease secondary to inadequate diet (calcium, vitamin K and vitamin D) has been implicated.
**PSGAGs**: Implicated in cases of fatal hemorrhage in several species of birds. The mechanism of action is not clear but direct anticoagulant action of PSGAGs is suspected.
**Hypervitaminosis E-associated coagulopathy** in pink-backed pelicans (*Pelecanus rufescens*). Several pelicans from a zoo died in a case series and other pelicans responded to vitamin K treatment. A possible mechanism of interference of alpha-tocopherol metabolites with vitamin K was suggested.

### ANTICOAGULANT RODENTICIDES
ARs inhibit vitamin K1–2,3-epoxide reductase, which impairs vitamin K metabolism. Second-generation ARs include brodifacoum, bromadiolone, chlorophacinone, difenacoum, difethialone, and diphacinone. These drugs are longer lasting, with greater affinity for their target, and are long-lasting in the environment. Exposure can occur following direct ingestion of bait or, more likely, through ingestion of animals that have ingested bait through hunting (birds of prey) or scavenging. Toxicity varies by species and raptors, particularly owls, appear more sensitive than other birds.

### DISSEMINATED INTRAVASCULAR COAGULATION
Infectious agents implicated in DIC in birds include bacteria, particularly Gram-negative bacteria, and viruses, which may directly cause DIC or may predispose the patient to development of secondary bacterial and fungal infections: *Erysipelothrix rhusiopathiae*, *Escherichia coli*, *Salmonella gallinarum* and *Salmonella pullorum*, *Streptococcus zooepidemicus*, avian herpesviruses, eastern equine encephalitis, highly pathogenic avian influenza, infectious bursal disease, polyomavirus, reovirus.

### SYSTEMS AFFECTED
Coagulopathies can affect many systems, which may be due to local effects of petechiation/hematomas or due to the

ensuing anemia and decreased oxygen-carrying capacity. In addition, the primary cause for the bleeding disorder may cause clinical signs beyond the bleeding diathesis.
**Hemic/lymphatic/immune**: Depending on the cause and severity of the bleeding disorder, one may observe anemia secondary to blood loss, multiple cytopenias (including a leukopenia and/or lack of regeneration in the erythrocytes) if the thrombocytopenia is due to bone marrow disease.
**Skin/exocrine**: Petechiation and hematomas may be visible upon examination of the skin. There may be bleeding from new feather follicles.
**Neurologic**: Hemorrhaging within the spinal cord, brain, or cranium may lead to clinical signs (e.g. ataxia, obtundation) depending on the location and extent of the bleed.
**Reproductive**: Necropsy or endoscopy may reveal bloody vitellogenic follicles or reproductive tract.
**Ophthalmic**: Hyphema and hemorrhage in sclera and orbital cavities may be noted.
**Pulmonary/GI**: Hemorrhage from the respiratory tract may lead to epistaxis or blood in the mouth. Melena or frank blood may be noted in feces if there is bleeding in the upper and lower GI tract, respectively.

### GENETICS
Inherited bleeding disorders are uncommonly reported in birds.

### INCIDENCE/PREVALENCE
Coagulopathy in general is under reported due to lack of available diagnostic testing and the large blood volumes required for testing, which makes this unlikely to be used in small birds, particularly one with a history of bleeding. The incidence is expected to vary widely based on a number of factors including the species, diets and habitat which affect the likelihood of exposure to certain pathogens and toxins. Many studies have documented a high prevalence of anticoagulant exposure in wild birds of prey in the range of 50–90% in North America, but also in Europe.

### GEOGRAPHIC DISTRIBUTION
Bleeding disorders can occur anywhere.

### SIGNALMENT
Signalment varies depending on the cause.

### SIGNS
In general, small hemorrhage such as petechiation is due to thrombocyte deficiency or dysfunction while larger haemorrhage, such as hematoma, is more likely to be due to coagulation factor deficiency. Hemorrhage: petechiation, hematoma formation, hyphema, epistaxis, oral bleeding, melena, or bloody stool. Clinical signs of blood loss or anemia such as pale mucus membranes, lethargy, hypovolemic shock. Other clinical

signs associated with the cause of the bleeding disorder (e.g. other clinical signs of an infection agent or toxin). There may not be any clinical signs.

## CAUSES

Vitamin K deficient diet: The first coagulopathy described in chicks in 1935. Sulfa drugs disrupt flora and decrease absorption of vitamin K. Documented in poultry fed antibiotics for increased production, but may occur in any species. Other iatrogenic causes (polysulfated glycosaminoglycans). Anticoagulant rodenticides. Hepatic failure, which can be secondary to toxins (including chronic and acute mycotoxins, rapeseed), hepatic lipidosis, hemochromatosis, infectious agents (including chlamydiosis, mycobacteriosis, polyomavirus, adenovirus), and neoplasia. DIC: Acquired syndrome characterized by disseminated intravascular activation of coagulation secondary to vasculitis, and a number of infectious agents (see above). Lack of production by the bone marrow, including viral causes (e.g. circovirus) and hemic neoplasia causing myelophthisis.

## RISK FACTORS

Depend on the mechanism for the bleeding disorder.

## DIAGNOSIS

### DIFFERENTIAL DIAGNOSIS

See above.

### CBC/BIOCHEMISTRY/URINALYSIS

#### Complete Blood Count

**Thrombocytes**: The normal thrombocyte count in birds is usually around 20,000–30,000 thrombocytes/µl, however, species-specific reference intervals often do not include thrombocytes and many hematology laboratories do not provide thrombocyte counts. Examination of blood smears to look for thrombocyte clumps and estimate the thrombocyte counts are therefore necessary.
**Erythrocytes**: An anemia (low hemoglobin concentration, low erythrocyte count, packed cell volume and/or hematocrit) may also be evident on CBC, accompanied by a hypoproteinemia if the anemia is due to blood loss.
**Abnormal cells**: May be present if there is a hemic neoplasm present.

#### Biochemistry Profile

Hypoproteinemia secondary to blood loss or liver failure. Increased hepatic enzyme activity or bile acids secondary to hypoxia (due to anemia) or hepatocellular damage.

#### Urinalysis

Hematuria, if bleeding in the urinary tract, or possibly due to contamination of urine with blood from the reproductive or gastrointestinal tract.

### OTHER LABORATORY TESTS

Numerous studies have described coagulation testing in birds. Most assays required blood collection into 3.2% or 3.8% sodium citrate (blue top) at the ratio of one part citrate to nine parts whole blood. Whole blood should be centrifuged to separate plasma within 30 minutes. Plasma can be frozen; however, since freeze–thaw cycles can affect the results, using fresh plasma is recommended.

#### Activated Clotting Time

Point of care test performed in clinic using a tube with appropriate ratio of diatomaceous earth at 98.6°F (37°C). Screens for deficiencies/abnormal function of the coagulation factors involved in the contact activation (intrinsic) pathway and common pathway [factors VIII, IX, V, X, II (thrombin) and I (fibrinogen)]. This is not as sensitive as PT but can be done in house (quick turnaround time, inexpensive). Normal results in birds are typically < 120 seconds with some species-specific variation. Coagulation factor deficiencies lead to prolonged times.

#### Prothrombin Time

Performed using thromboplastin/calcium reagent. Screens for deficiencies/abnormal function of the coagulation factors involved in the tissue activation (extrinsic) and common pathways [factors VII, V, X, II (thrombin), I (fibrinogen)]. Requires avian-specific reagent for diagnostic analysis, which is, to the author's knowledge, not yet commercially available. When avian specific reagent is used, reference intervals are commonly 9–15 seconds in the adult bird. Younger birds commonly have extended PT.

#### Russell Viper Venom Time

Russell viper venom directly activates factor X, and thereby the common pathway [factor V, II (thrombin), I (fibrinogen)]. This test can be found in human diagnostic laboratories as it is used in the diagnosis of lupus. Requires 0.5–1 ml serum and volume may preclude use in smaller birds. Should be validated on a species-specific basis. Normal times in pigeons are < 200 seconds.

#### Activate Partial Thromboplastin Time

Typically not used in birds due to lack of reagent.

#### Fibrinogen

Heat precipitation technique using two hematocrit tubes, one unheated and one heated to 132.8°F (56°C) for 3 minutes. Two measured total solids values, obtained using a refractometer, are subtracted providing

fibrinogen estimated. Hypofibrinogenemia can be an indicator of DIC or liver failure, however, since fibrinogen is also an acute-phase protein and increases with inflammation; the resulting fibrinogen levels in patients with bleeding disorders are variable.

#### Dynamic Viscoelastic Coagulometry

Thromboelastography is a method of testing the efficiency of blood coagulation. More common tests of blood coagulation include PT and aPTT, which measure coagulation factor function, but TEG also can assess platelet function, clot strength, and fibrinolysis, which these other tests cannot. TEG normals have been described in chickens and Hispaniolan Amazon parrots. Because few facilities have the ability to perform TEG, this modality is not yet readily available to practitioners.

#### Other Coagulometers

Other point of care coagulometers are available, such as the ROTEM® (Tem Innovations GmbH, Munich, Germany) thromboelastometer and the Sonoclot® (Sienco Inc., Boulder, CO) analyzer. Some refence values are available for these tests in some species of birds, mainly birds of prey.

### IMAGING

Radiographs may be warranted as part of a standard work up to rule out differentials such as trauma, neoplasia/granulomas/organomegaly, but otherwise does not typically aid in diagnosis of the etiology of the coagulopathy.

### DIAGNOSTIC PROCEDURES

Surgical or endoscopic intervention for diagnosis or therapy should be approached cautiously due to risk of overt hemorrhage.

### PATHOLOGIC FINDINGS

Hemorrhage (petechiation, hematomas) into cavities, organs, musculature, under the skin etc.

## TREATMENT

### APPROPRIATE HEALTH CARE

Treatment must be specific to the underlying cause to be successful. Hospitalization for inpatient nursing care is generally required.

### NURSING CARE

Gentle handling with soft blanket and pads is warranted to prevent hematoma formation. Optimal treatment of severe hemorrhage from anticoagulant rodenticide toxicosis is transfusion of whole blood to replace both red blood cells and clotting factors. Although heterologous (different species) and homologous (same species) blood transfusions have been described, homologous are recommended due to short survival time of

**C**

heterologous red blood cells and possible acute immune reaction.

## ACTIVITY
The patient's activity should be restricted in a padded cage and possibly in the dark or with hoods to decrease self-trauma.

## DIET
Vitamin $K_1$ (phylloquinone) is regularly administered orally (0.13 mg/kg) to poultry as part of basic nutrition to prevent vitamin K deficiency, with documented decreased PT in comparison with controls. This may be considered in conure bleeding syndrome or unexplained coagulopathy.

## CLIENT EDUCATION
Typically with either hepatic disease or DIC there are underlying conditions that must be treated to resolve the condition.

## SURGICAL CONSIDERATIONS
To be avoided if possible.

## MEDICATIONS
### DRUG(S) OF CHOICE
Injectable or oral vitamin $K_1$ (phytonadione) is recommended for coagulopathies due to hypovitaminosis K, induced by rodenticide, nutritional deficiency, or antibiotic administration. If marked liver disease is suspected, pretreatment with vitamin K for 24–48 hours prior to biopsy could be considered. Reported dosage ranges are 0.2–2.2 mg/kg SC q4–8h, although higher doses (2.5 mg/kg SC) q12h until hemostasis has been achieved have also been reported (Murray, 2011). Doses are similar but delivered IM according to Carpenter's formulary. Oral treatment with vitamin $K_1$ (not $K_3$) from 1–5 mg/kg is possible in birds but anticoagulant treatment dosages have not been validated with pharmacokinetic trials. The K vitamins are essential cofactors for microsomal vitamin K-dependent carboxylases, which catalyze posttranslational conversion of glutamyl residues to gamma carboxyglutamyl residues in mature proteins. Vitamin K hydroquinone is the active cofactor form required by factors II, VII, IX, and X for clot formation. Vitamin K hydroquinone is recycled by vitamin K reductase. This is the enzyme that is inhibited by the coumarin anticoagulants. A 5 mg/kg vitamin K administration at the time of 10 mg/kg warfarin administration resulted in no change in PT in dosed animals. This indicates that vitamin K is an effective therapy. Vitamin $K_3$ (menadione) has not been effective against high doses of dicoumarol-type anticoagulants.

## CONTRAINDICATIONS
Heparin, NSAIDs, vitamin $K_3$ (ineffective due to its delayed onset of action).

## PRECAUTIONS
Anaphylactic reactions to injectable Vitamin K have been reported in mammals and are possible in birds though rare.

## POSSIBLE INTERACTIONS
N/A

## ALTERNATIVE DRUGS
N/A

## FOLLOW-UP
### PATIENT MONITORING
Vitamin K therapy is typically instituted for extended periods in birds with rodenticide intoxication as PT assays may not be available. Consider that half-life of brodifacoum in the liver is > 300 days. Therapy may be discontinued when the PT has returned to normal.

### PREVENTION/AVOIDANCE
Supervise birds at all times when out of their enclosure to limit the risk of exposure to toxins. Birds with previously noted bleeding issues (i.e. conure bleeding syndrome) should have precautions taken to minimize risk during future venipunctures (i.e. use medial metatarsal veins only, so that a pressure wrap can be applied). If jugular venipuncture is required, consider premedication with vitamin K for 2–3 days prior to event.

### POSSIBLE COMPLICATIONS
Obtaining blood samples may result in life threatening situations.

### EXPECTED COURSE AND PROGNOSIS
**DIC:** Prognosis is guarded to poor and based on resolution of the underlying condition.
**AR:** Owing to the extended half-life of many ARs, the patient may clot normally during therapy and proceed to hemorrhage when vitamin K therapy is discontinued. Owners should monitor this closely.

## MISCELLANEOUS
### ASSOCIATED CONDITIONS
N/A

### AGE-RELATED FACTORS
N/A

### ZOONOTIC POTENTIAL
Dependent upon underlying disease.

### FERTILITY/BREEDING
Coagulopathy may result in abnormal oviposition and decreased chick survivability.

### SYNONYMS
Hemostasis, clotting or bleeding disorder, bleeding diathesis

### SEE ALSO
Anemia
Liver Disease
Hemorrhage
Sick-Bird Syndrome
Toxicosis (Anticoagulant Rodenticide)
Toxicosis (Heavy Metals)
Trauma

### ABBREVIATIONS
aPTT—activated partial thromboplastin time
AR—anticoagulant rodenticide
CBC—complete blood count
DIC—disseminated intravascular coagulation
EDTA—ethylenediaminetetraacetic acid
GI—gastrointestinal
NSAIDs—non-steroidal anti-inflammatory drugs
PSGAG—polysulfated glycosaminoglycan
PT—prothrombin time
RVV—Russell viper venom time
TEG—thromboelastography

### INTERNET RESOURCES
Cornell University College of Veterinary Medicine. eClinPath: https://eclinpath.com

*Suggested Reading*
Anderson, K., Garner, M.M., Reed, H.H. et al. (2013). Hemorrhagic diathesis in avian species following intramuscular administration of polysulfated glycosaminoglycan. *Journal of Zoo and Wildlife Medicine* 44:93–99.
Campbell, T., Grant, K. (2022). *Exotic Animal Hematology and Cytology*. Hoboken, NJ: Wiley.
Gentry, P.A. (2004). The comparative aspects of blood coagulation. *Veterinary Journal* 168:238–251.
Murray, M. (2011). Anticoagulant rodenticide exposure and toxicosis in four species of birds of prey presented to a wildlife clinic in Massachusetts, 2006–2010. *Journal of Zoo and Wildlife Medicine* 42:88–97.
Russel, K.E., Heatley, J.J. (2022). Avian hemostatis. In: *Schalm's Veterinary Hematology* (ed. M.B. Brooks, K.E. Harr, D.M. Seelig, et al.), 865–874. Hoboken, NJ: Wiley.
**Author:** Melanie Ammersbach, DVM, DACVP (Clin Path)
**Acknowledgements:** The author would like to acknowledge Dr. Kendal Harr, DVM, DACVP, who wrote the chapter in the previous edition of this book, upon which this chapter was built.

# COCCIDIOSIS (INTESTINAL)

## BASICS

### DEFINITION
Coccidiosis is a clinical intestinal disease caused by coccidians, which are nonmotile protozoal parasites, most commonly of the species *Eimeria*, *Caryospora*, and *Isospora*. Coccidiasis is the presence of coccidians in the intestines without clinical disease. Coccidia in avian species tend to be host specific and, while subclinical disease may be more common, many coccidian species do not cause clinical disease. *Eimeria* species tend to be the primary intestinal pathogens of avian species, and are most problematic in farmed birds (e.g. chickens, turkeys, ducks) raised commercially and in confinement, as well as zoo and pet bird species. Subclinical coccidiosis in the poultry industry is associated with major economic losses due to poor weight gain, stunted growth, reduced production, and high morbidity and mortality. Seven species of *Eimeria* (*Eimeria acervulina*, *Eimeria brunetti*, *Eimeria maxima*, *Eimeria mitis*, *Eimeria necatrix*, *Eimeria praecox*, and *Eimeria tenella*) are recognized as infecting chickens. Coccidian infections, while common and frequently subclinical, do not generally cause disease in free-ranging birds.

### PATHOPHYSIOLOGY
Most coccidians have a direct life cycle, in which infected birds shed non-infective oocysts (sporont) in feces. Oocysts sporulate within 48 hours and become infective (sporocysts containing infective sporozoites). Susceptible birds ingest infective oocysts during feeding or drinking, the sporocysts walls break in the ventriculus, and the sporozoites invade intestinal epithelial cells. Within the intestines, oocysts may undergo several stages of development before becoming sexually mature male and female parasites. Mature female coccidia release non-infective oocysts into the environment through the feces and the direct life cycle continues. The life cycle is complete in 4–8 days in most psittacine and poultry species, and 7–14 days in some free-ranging bird species. In most cases, birds infected with coccidia will develop immunity and recover, although reinfection is common. The presence of disease depends on number of host intestinal epithelial cells invaded and the host immune status. Severely infected birds may die acutely. Intestinal tissue damage can result in anorexia, diminished nutrient absorption, melena or passing of frank blood, anemia, dehydration, and immune compromise of the intestines leading to secondary bacterial and/or fungal infections.

### SYSTEMS AFFECTED
Small and large intestines are affected; damage to intestinal epithelial cells and intestinal villi disrupts normal function.

### GENETICS
In commercial poultry, there is some evidence that certain genetic lines may have greater resistance to specific coccidial species infection compared with others, but this has not been systematically evaluated. In non-monocultured species, there is no known genetic basis for intestinal coccidiosis.

### INCIDENCE/PREVALENCE
The exact incidence and prevalence are currently unknown. The presence of coccidia in the gastrointestinal tracts of many avian species is common, but mere presence is not always associated with disease. Most free-ranging birds are likely infected, and farmed avian species are commonly infected and are more likely to exhibit clinical signs.

### GEOGRAPHIC DISTRIBUTION
Coccidia are found worldwide, and any avian species are susceptible. Crowding will exacerbate the spread of the parasite, likely leading to disease. This is typical of commercial poultry operations.

### SIGNALMENT
**Species**: All avian species are potentially susceptible to infection.
**Mean age and range**: All ages are susceptible; in poultry, younger birds are considered to be at greater risk of morbidity and mortality.
**Predominant sex**: Both sexes are susceptible.

### SIGNS
Frequently, birds are asymptomatic and subclinical. Clinical signs may range from nothing to one or more of lethargy, fluffed feathers, anorexia, weight loss, crop stasis, diarrhea (watery, hemorrhagic, tarry), and death. Frank blood in droppings is a common finding in poultry. Decreased egg production can be observed in breeding or laying birds.

### CAUSES
Direct exposure to oocysts in the environment, and ingestion via fecal–oral route of transmission.

### RISK FACTORS
Exposure to coccidian parasites. Inadequate biosecurity protocols and poor hygiene of both personnel and equipment. Sanitization plays a major role in reducing the dissemination of the parasite. Pest control is important for dissemination of the parasites by decreasing the presence of rodents and insects. Overcrowding, especially in avian species used for food production or maintained in pet stores and aviculture. Heavily raced pigeons are also predisposed. Stress may exacerbate infection. In free-ranging birds, stress can predispose to

epizootics; typically associated with staging areas during spring migration. In commercial poultry operations, other vaccines, such as those used to prevent infectious bursal disease virus or Newcastle disease virus, may cause immunosuppression, and exacerbate coccidial disease manifestations.

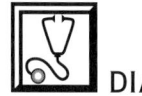

## DIAGNOSIS

### DIFFERENTIAL DIAGNOSIS
Coccidiosis should be included as a differential diagnosis for any bird with diarrhea and/or hematochezia. Bacterial or fungal enteritis. Mycobacterial enteritis. Gastrointestinal nematodiasis. Cryptosporidiosis.

### CBC/BIOCHEMISTRY/URINALYSIS
Most commonly, there are no hematologic abnormalities with intestinal coccidiosis, with the exception of anemia in severe cases. Non-specific changes associated with dehydration and emaciation, which might include increased hematocrit and decreased electrolytes.

### OTHER LABORATORY TESTS
Microscopic fecal examination is the most common method for detecting coccidia.

### IMAGING
In pet birds, radiographic and CT images may indicate thickened intestinal walls secondary to inflammation, but this would not be considered specific to coccidial infection.

### DIAGNOSTIC PROCEDURES
Finding oocysts in a fecal float and direct smear are the diagnostic methods of choice. However, routine fecal exams in avian species without clinical signs may be positive for coccidia. In these cases, some veterinarians choose to treat based on quantification of coccidia on the fecal smear of float, and taking in consideration of context (zoo exhibit, chicken flock, canary aviary, racing pigeons, etc.). This empirical approach is at the discretion of the individual veterinarian. In cases of death prior to antemortem diagnosis, a necropsy will be required with identification of coccidian on an intestinal scraping and/or histopathologic evidence of intestinal epithelial invasion by coccidian. Endoscopy and biopsy—in larger bird species in which an endoscope can be passed into the small intestine, a biopsy of the intestinal mucosa may be useful. In chickens, quantitative real-time PCR of fecal samples has been demonstrated to identify the DNA of some, but not all, *Eimeria* spp. Research into next-generation sequencing of *Eimeria* spp. is currently being conducted, which

should help to identify species-specific coccidia in commercial poultry.

## PATHOLOGIC FINDINGS

### Gross Lesions
Most commonly, hemorrhagic enteritis of the small intestine is observed, but location of lesions can vary with species of coccidian, avian species, and severity of infection.

### Histopathologic Lesions
Depending on the coccidian species, parasite load, and GI organ site of infection, coccidiosis can result in a range of pathologic conditions, including mild enteritis, mild-to-moderate inflammation of the intestinal wall with pinpoint hemorrhages and mucosal sloughing, complete intestinal villar destruction resulting in extensive hemorrhage, necrosis, and death. Typically, schizonts are observed in the intestinal epithelial cells along with merozoites, infiltrating neutrophils and eosinophils.

## TREATMENT

### APPROPRIATE HEALTH CARE
Most birds can be treated as outpatients; critically ill birds may need hospitalization and more intensive supportive care. In flock situations, water-based anticoccidial treatments are commonly instituted.

### NURSING CARE
For pet birds, supportive care may be necessary due to fluid/blood loss associated with diarrhea and/or hematochezia and fecal occult blood. Fluid support of crystalloid fluid (e.g. lactated Ringer's solution, 0.9% saline, Normosol®, Hospira, Inc., Lake Forest, IL) replacement is standard of care; administered either subcutaneously (40–60 ml/kg depending on level of dehydration) or via IV catheter in emergency situations. Any individual bird should be maintained in a warm environment, which may include and incubator or heat lamp.

### ACTIVITY
N/A

### DIET
Recently, there is interest in adding certain elements to the diet in commercial poultry operations to change the microbiome of chickens, as well as altering the composition of droppings, which may or may not maintain viable coccidia in the environment. For example, probiotics reportedly reduce the numbers of pathogenic microorganisms in the gastrointestinal tract while simultaneously enhancing the beneficial microbial flora leading to a reduction in intestinal lesions, improved growth performance, and less morbidity and mortality.

## CLIENT EDUCATION
Since treatment generally entails oral administration of medication, either directly or indirectly through medicated feed and water, the client must be instructed about methods of administration.

## SURGICAL CONSIDERATIONS
N/A

## MEDICATIONS

### DRUG(S) OF CHOICE

#### General Comment
Drug resistance to anticoccidial medications is a constant concern, particularly in flock medicine.

#### Medications for Individual Patients
**Amprolium**: Chickens 25 mg/kg PO q24h; typically treat for 5 days; pigeons 25 mg/kg PO q24h, typical treat for 5 days; raptors 30 mg/kg PO q24h x 5 days.
**Clazuril**: Most species 5–10 mg/kg PO q24h for 3 days, off 2 days, then on 3 days.
**Diclazuril**: 10 mg/kg PO q12h every other day for 6 doses; some resistant *Eimeria* sp.
**Ponazuril**: Indian peafowl 20–40 mg/kg PO once for at least 8 days; most species 10–20 mg/kg PO, repeat in 10–14 days.
**Sulfadimethoxine**: Most species 25 mg/kg PO q12h for 5–7 days; raptors, psittacines 50 mg/kg PO q24h x 5 days, then off 3 days, then on 5 days.
**Sulfaquinoxaline**: Lories, pigeons 100 mg/kg PO q24h for 3 days, then off 2 days, then on 3 days.
**Toltrazuril**: Budgerigars, raptors 7–10 mg/kg PO q24h for 2–3 days; pigeons 20–35 mg/kg PO once.
**Trimethoprim/sulfamethoxazole**: Most species 30–50 mg/kg PO q12–24h.

#### Medications for Monocultured Flocks and Aviculture (Food and Water Based)
**Amprolium**: Most species, including chickens, passerines, budgerigars 50–100 mg/l drinking water for 5–7 days; pigeons 200 mg/l drinking water for 5–7 days; poultry 575 mg/l drinking water (using 9.6% solution) for 5–7 days; poultry, cranes 115–232 mg/kg feed for 5–7 days.
**Decoquinate**: Poultry 20–40 mg/kg feed q5–7d.
**Diclazuril**: Poultry 5–10 mg/l drinking water for 5–7 days; 1 mg/kg feed for 5–7 days.
**Dintolamide**: Poultry 40–187 mg/kg feed.
Monensin: Poultry gamebirds, cranes 70–100 mg/kg feed.
**Sulfachlorpyridazine**: Passerines, pigeons 300 mg/l drinking water for 5 days, off 3 days, on 5 days and repeat multiple times;

cockatiels, budgerigars 400 mg/l drinking water for 30 days.
**Sulfadimethoxine**: Poultry, pigeons 250–500 mg/l drinking water for 5 days.
**Sulfadimethoxine/ormetoprim**: Poultry, game birds 10 mg kg feed or 320–525 mg/l drinking water.
**Sulfaquinoxaline**: Poultry, pigeons 250–500 mg/l drinking water for 6 days, then off 2 days, then on 6 days.
**Toltrazuril**: Psittacines 2–5 mg/l drinking water for 2 days, repeat in 14–21 days; waterfowl: 12.5 mg/l drinking water for 2 days; poultry 25 mg/kg drinking water for 2 days; passerines 75 mg/l drinking water for 2 days/week for 4 weeks; pigeons 75 mg/l drinking water for 5 days.
**Trimethoprim/sulfamethoxazole**: Poultry, pigeons 320–525 mg/l drinking water.

### CONTRAINDICATIONS
N/A

### PRECAUTIONS
There are now several drug resistant strains of Coccidia in the world, especially in avian monoculture facilities.

### POSSIBLE INTERACTIONS
N/A

### ALTERNATIVE DRUGS
Outside the United States and Europe, there is great interest in feeding a variety of plant extracts, such as tannins, garlic, herbal mixtures (e.g. *Echinacea*, *Glycyrrhiza*), plant-derived essential oils (e.g. extracts from spices and other plants), and predatory fungi species (larvicidal and ovicidal fungi).

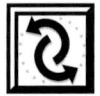

## FOLLOW-UP

### PATIENT MONITORING
Fecal float and fecal direct smears 1–2 weeks post treatment. Hematochezia and fecal occult blood should be controlled after treatment.

### PREVENTION/AVOIDANCE
Vaccines are used in poultry operations, but not in individual pet birds. Live attenuated and non-attenuated vaccines are available, with the goal of producing subclinical coccidiosis, which have proven to be most effective. However, this approach can is associated with decreased performance and increased bacterial enteritis in poultry operations. In addition, the use of live vaccines can contribute large numbers of oocysts accumulating in chicken litter, resulting in higher levels of exposure and both subclinical and clinical disease. Recombinant vaccines are being studied but have the disadvantage of not yet being able to

elicit a broad spectrum of protective immune responses as the live or live-attenuated vaccines.

## POSSIBLE COMPLICATIONS
The primary complication associated with treatment is that the bird(s) may become lifelong carriers of coccidia and having the potential to continue to infect other birds.

## EXPECTED COURSE AND PROGNOSIS
With appropriate treatment, the prognosis for eliminating clinical signs (e.g. diarrhea, hematochezia) is good. However, completely eliminating the organisms from the patient, and the environment, may contribute to constant reinfection, particularly in poultry operations and aviaries.

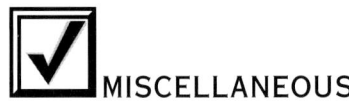 MISCELLANEOUS

## ASSOCIATED CONDITIONS
Any disease process or vaccine that can contribute to immunocompromise in the bird or birds may increase the likelihood that coccidia in the environment will become invasive to the intestinal tract.

## AGE-RELATED FACTORS
Younger birds in commercial poultry operations are considered more susceptible to infection with coccidia in addition to increased morbidity and mortality.

## ZOONOTIC POTENTIAL
N/A

## FERTILITY/BREEDING
N/A

## SYNONYMS
N/A

## SEE ALSO
Clostridiosis
Coccidiosis (systemic)
Colibacillosis
Enteritis and Gastritis
Flagellate Enteritis
Foreign Bodies (Gastrointestinal)
Helminthiasis (Gastrointestinal)
Ileus (Functional Gastrointestinal, Crop Stasis)
Neoplasia (Gastrointestinal and Hepatic)

## ABBREVIATIONS
CT—computed tomography
GI—gastrointestinal
PCR—polymerase chain reaction

## INTERNET RESOURCES
For detailed information related to coccidian in free-ranging birds, see Cole, R.A., Friend, M. (1999). Parasites and Parasitic Diseases. (Field Manual of Wildlife Diseases). *Other Publications in Zoonotics and Wildlife Disease*, 15: https://digitalcommons.unl.edu/cgi/viewcontent.cgi?article=1014&context=zoonoticspub
For information about poultry coccidiosis, see Gerhold, R.W. (2023). Coccidiosis in poultry. *MSD Veterinary Manual*: http://www.merckmanuals.com/vet/poultry/coccidiosis/overview_of_coccidiosis_in_poultry.html

*Suggested Reading*
Alnassan, A.A., Kotsch, M., Shehata, A.A., et al. (2014). Necrotic enteritis in chickens: development of a straightforward disease model system. *Veterinary Record*, 174:555–561.

Doneley, R.J.T. (2009). Bacterial and parasitic diseases of parrots. *Veterinary Clinics of North America. Exotic Animal Practice*, 12:417–432.
Dorrestein, G.M. (2009). Bacterial and parasitic diseases of passerines. *Veterinary Clinics of North America. Exotic Animal Practice*, 12:433–451.
Guzman, D.S,-M., Beaufrère, H., et al. (2023). Birds. In: *Carpenter's Exotic Animal Formulary* (ed. J.W. Carpenter, C.A. Harms), 223–274. St. Louis, MO: Elsevier.
Harlin, R., Wade, L. (2009). Bacterial and parasitic diseases of Columbiformes. *Veterinary Clinics of North America. Exotic Animal Practice*, 12:453–473.
Lee, Y., Lu, M., Lillehoj, H.S. (2022). Coccidiosis: recent progress in host immunity and alternatives to antibiotic strategies. *Vaccines*, 10:215.
Mohsin, M., Abbas, R.Z., Yin, G., et al. (2021). Probiotics as therapeutic, antioxidant and immunomodulatory agents against poultry coccidiosis. *World's Poultry Science Journal*, 77:331–345.
Shirley, M.W., Lillehoj, H.S. (2012). The long view: a selective review of 40 years of coccidiosis research. *Avian Pathology*, 41:111–121.
Snyder, R.P., Guerin, M.T., Hargis, B.M., et al. (2021). Exploiting digital droplet PCR and next generation sequencing technologies to determine the relative abundance of individual Eimeria species in a DNA sample. *Veterinary Parasitology*, 296:109443.

**Author**: Kurt K. Sladky, MS, DVM, DACZM, DECZM (Zoo Health Management & Herpetology)

# COCCIDIOSIS (SYSTEMIC)

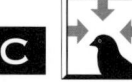

# BASICS

## DEFINITION
Systemic coccidiosis is caused by an extraintestinal infection with specific species of coccidia, generally in the genera *Eimeria*, *Isospora*, and *Caryospora*. Historically, the genus *Atoxoplasma* was thought to be a cause; however, this coccidium has recently been determined to be indistinct from *Isospora*. The infective coccidians are host, tissue, and cell-specific and complete their development in both the GI tract and extraintestinally. Infections cause significant morbidity and mortality, especially in passerines. In cranes, this disease is called disseminated visceral coccidiosis.

## PATHOPHYSIOLOGY
The life cycle is direct. The bird ingests the sporulated oocysts lying in its environment. Transovarian transmission may also be possible. Oocysts undergo schizogony (merogony; asexual phase) in the intestine. If the schizonts produced are deep in the intestinal mucosa, they may damage the mucosa when they divide, causing enteritis. After schizogony, they differentiate into micro and macro gametocytes, which fuse to form the zygote (gametogony or sexual phase, which is non-pathogenic). An oocyst wall forms around the zygote as it develops and matures. The oocysts are released into the intestinal lumen and passed with the feces onto the ground, where they sporulate under favorable conditions of moisture and temperature. In cases of systemic coccidiosis, the asexual phases occur both intra- and extraintestinally; however, the sexual phase takes place only in the intestines. The basic host response in systemic coccidiosis to coccidian development in the tissues is granulomatous inflammation. This change is primarily because of the infiltration of phagocytic mononuclear cells laden with developing asexual stages of coccidia in the organs and tissues. The consequent rupture of the host cells initiates a necrotizing lymphohistiocytic inflammation.

## SYSTEMS AFFECTED
**Gastrointestinal**: Diarrhea, enteritis, edema of the duodenum and jejunum.
**Musculoskeletal**: Emaciation, severe pectoral muscle atrophy, pectoral muscle myositis, weight loss.
**Behavioral**: Severe depression, ruffling of feathers, grouped birds huddle together.
**Hemic/lymphatic/immune**: Invasion of mononuclear cells with zoites, splenitis, severe leukocytosis.
**Hepatobiliary**: Hepatitis, "thick liver disease."
**Respiratory**: Bronchopneumonia.
**Renal/urologic**: Nephritis.
**Cardiovascular**: Myocarditis.
**Nervous**: Generalized neurologic signs, weakness.
**Endocrine/metabolic**: Pancreatitis.
**Skin**: Dermatitis.

## GENETICS
N/A

## INCIDENCE/PREVALENCE
Not uncommon. More prevalent in captive birds due to stress, husbandry conditions, and overcrowding. Reported in numerous families/orders of birds, including Passeriformes, Anseriformes, Apterygiformes, Gruiformes, Sphenisciformes, Procellariiformes, Pelecaniformes, and raptors (uncommon).

## GEOGRAPHIC DISTRIBUTION
This disease has been seen in both captive and wild birds all over the world.

## SIGNALMENT
This disease has been seen in both captive and wild birds all over the world.

## SIGNS

### General Comments
May be asymptomatic. May not show any abnormalities until stressed.

### Historical Findings
Significant stressor in recent history (such as transport, recent hatching), or chronic or concurrent disease process. Onset of clinical signs is usually acute.

### Physical Examination Findings
Diarrhea, sometimes greenish in color; can also be mucoid or mucosanguinous. Weight loss/emaciation; seen commonly as severe pectoral muscle atrophy. Lethargy. Weakness. Inappetence. Wet tail feathers, vent. Cloacal swelling. Coelomic distention associated with hepatomegaly. Ruffled feathers. Huddling with other birds. Dyspnea, associated with bronchopneumonia. Leg weakness and/or tendency to tip forward with renal coccidiosis. Non-specific neurologic signs. Small, white, raised nodules in the oral cavity. Acute death.

## CAUSES
Infection with *Eimeria* sp., such as *Eimeria reichenowi* and *Eimeria gruis* in cranes, *Eimeria tenella*, *Eimeria maxima*, and *Eimeria necatrix* in chickens, *Eimeria adenoides* in turkeys, *Eimeria gaviae* in the common loon, *Eimeria boschadis* in the mallard duck, *Eimeria christianseni* in the mute swan, *Eimeria somaterie* in the common eider, or *Eimeria columbarum* and *Eimeria labbeana* in the domestic pigeon. Mixed infections are not uncommon in pigeons and chickens. *Eimeria apteryxii* causes renal coccidiosis in North Island brown kiwi, rowi, and southern brown kiwi. Infection with *Isospora* sp., such

as *Isospora michaelbakeri* in sparrows, *Isospora canaria* (*serini*) in canaries, *Isospora robini* in American robins, *Isospora gryphoni* in American goldfinches, *Isospora picoflavae* in northern yellow-shafted flicker, *Isospora lunara* in finches, or *Isospora superbusi* or *Isospora greineri* in superb starlings. Novel isospora species causing infection include *Isospora tristum* n. sp. in common mynah and *Isospora zimmermani* n. sp. in barn swallows. *Isospora serini* was formerly referred to as *Atoxoplasma* or *Lankesterella* infection (uncommon) with *Eimeria* and *Caryospora* in raptors.

## RISK FACTORS
Poor husbandry, overcrowding, neonatal status, immunosuppression or concurrent infection, and/or environmental stressor(s).

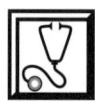

# DIAGNOSIS

## DIFFERENTIAL DIAGNOSIS
Lead poisoning, botulism, trichomoniasis, candidiasis, tuberculosis (mycobacteriosis), aspergillosis, paratuberculosis, avian cholera, duck viral enteritis, other protozoal infections (leukocytozoon, sarcocystis, toxoplasma), erysipelas, campylobacteriosis, salmonellosis, mycotoxins, phytotoxins, neoplasia.

## CBC/BIOCHEMISTRY/URINALYSIS
Possible hemoconcentration secondary to dehydration. Possible anemia due to blood loss in feces, if any is present. Possible elevations in liver enzymes if liver is affected. Possible elevation in uric acid if kidneys are affected. May not see any hematologic abnormalities. Merozoites may be seen in the cytoplasm of mononuclear cells on blood smear.

## OTHER LABORATORY TESTS
Fecal direct smear and/or flotation to look for the presence of coccidia. Feces are best collected from the affected bird(s) in the afternoon (2–6 p.m.) due to oocyst shedding rhythms. It is possible for birds to have systemic coccidiosis without shedding oocysts in the feces. PCR is the diagnostic of choice, and can be run on blood or feces antemortem, or tissues postmortem. For fecal analysis, it is recommended to collect and pool feces for 5 consecutive days. DNA sequencing on feces is also a preferred diagnostic.

## IMAGING

### Radiographic Findings
Consider the use of dental radiography or mammography in very small patients. May demonstrate the presence of masses in the thoracic and/or coelomic cavities; rule out granulomas vs. neoplasia vs. other. May

demonstrate asymmetry of the hepatic silhouette; rule out hepatomegaly, splenomegaly, neoplasia, other. May locate a metal foreign body; important in ruling out heavy metal toxicosis as a differential diagnosis. Whole-body radiographs to identify any abnormalities seen, which may provide information in cases that are showing non-specific clinical signs of illness.

### Ultrasonography
Results limited depending on the size of the bird. May reveal organ enlargement and/or architectural changes. May reveal discrete masses. May reveal thickened bowel walls.

## DIAGNOSTIC PROCEDURES
Fine-needle aspirate and cytology of masses located vs. biopsy and histopathology. Exploratory coeliotomy. Impression smears of major organs can show mononuclear cells with zoites in cytoplasm. Necropsy, especially if there is a flock of potentially exposed birds.

## PATHOLOGIC FINDINGS
### Gross
Grayish-white nodules (granulomas) disseminated throughout many organs and tissues, reportedly seen on the surface and parenchyma of the liver, lung, spleen, kidneys, heart, adventitia of the blood vessels (including the carotid and femoral arteries), serosa and mucosa of the esophagus, proventriculus, ventriculus, intestines, cloaca, the mesentery and parietal peritoneum, submucosa of the trachea and main bronchi, epimysium and parenchyma of pectoral and cervical muscles, and subcutaneous tissues of the thoracic and cervical regions. Mottling of the liver and hepatomegaly; may see yellow-orange color to liver. Congestion and enlargement of the spleen. Hyperemia of the duodenal mucosa. Lung consolidation. Frothy material in the trachea. Distention of the bowels. Duodenum and jejunum creamy white in color with walls 4–5 times thickened. Kidneys grossly swollen with white pinpoint foci of urates and cellular debris.

### Histopathology
Granulomas composed of inflammatory cells surrounded by a thin fibrous capsule with cellular infiltrate including macrophages, lymphocytes, plasma cells, and few heterophils. Numerous pale basophilic, round to oval uninucleated and multinucleated bodies, 5–10 μm in diameter scattered throughout the granulomas. Developing meronts in the cytoplasm of macrophages. Some granulomas do not contain meronts.
**Liver**: Lymphoid aggregates protruding into the lumen of portal and hepatic veins, sometimes nearly occluding the smaller hepatic veins. Multifocal areas of

granulomatous inflammation. Extensive areas of necrosis.
**Small intestines**: Moderate to severe multifocal infiltration of the lamina propria by macrophages, lymphocytes, and few heterophils with gametogonic stages of coccidia in epithelial lining cells. Developing coccidial stages also found within macrophages in granulomatous infiltrates and in lymphatics or capillaries in the lamina propria and tunica muscularis. Inflammation and mild focal necrosis of the intestinal villi associated with coccidian oocysts and gametocytes in the epithelium. Large numbers of gamonts, oocysts, and meronts, some of which can be large, with large merozoites, present among necrotic intestinal glands.
**Lungs**: Multifocal areas of consolidation, and parabronchi and bronchioles contain a pleocellular exudate. Airways may contain coccidian oocysts similar to those seen in the gut.
**Spleen**: Multifocal areas of granulomatous inflammation. Extensive areas of necrosis.
**Heart**: Multifocal areas of granulomatous inflammation.
**Kidneys**: Multifocal areas of granulomatous inflammation.
**Bursa of Fabricius**: Multifocal areas of granulomatous inflammation.

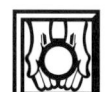

# TREATMENT
## APPROPRIATE HEALTH CARE
Emergency inpatient intensive care management. Birds in a flock should be separated from all birds showing illness immediately.

## NURSING CARE
Subcutaneous fluids can be administered (25–50 ml/kg) q8–12h, or as needed. IV access may be difficult to obtain and maintain depending on the size of the patient; consider IO catheterization if intravascular fluids are needed. In most patients, lactated Ringer's solution or Normosol®-R (Hospira, Inc., Lake Forest, IL) crystalloid fluids are appropriate. Maintenance fluids are estimated at 50–100 ml/kg/day. Consider the addition of dextrose at 2.5–5% to the subcutaneous or IV fluid administration, especially if the bird is inappetent or anorexic. Supplemental oxygen therapy may be warranted depending on clinical signs. Supplemental heat should be provided at all times to hospitalized animals; temperature should be determined by the species that is being treated. Gavage feeding should be considered if the patient will not eat on its own. Strict hygiene should be practiced to decrease the parasite load in the patient's environment and to prevent

cross-contamination between patients. Handling should be kept as minimal as possible to avoid stressing the patient.

## ACTIVITY
Dependent on how clinically affected the patient is. The patient's activity should be limited enough to maintain IV or IO catheter placement and patency and to provide supplemental heat to the patient, if needed. Consideration should also be given to the ability to properly disinfect the patient's environment when deciding how much space a patient should have access to.

## DIET
The patient should continue to eat their normal diet, if possible. If the patient is inappetent or anorexic, consider gavage feeding an appropriate formula twice daily. This may also help in medicating the patient.

## CLIENT EDUCATION
Prevention of this disease should be strongly stressed over reliance on treatment, as true systemic infection with coccidiosis (intracellular stages of life cycle) is untreatable (see Prevention/Avoidance section for details).

## SURGICAL CONSIDERATIONS
There is no surgical treatment for systemic coccidiosis. Anesthetizing a patient with systemic coccidiosis should be performed only when absolutely necessary, as the likelihood of patient death under anesthesia is relatively high.

# MEDICATIONS
## DRUG(S) OF CHOICE
Important to note that medications will treat the intestinal stages (i.e. reduce oocyst shedding), but generally are unable to influence the intracellular or extraintestinal stages; monensin and possibly toltrazuril; however, may also have an effect against extraintestinal parasites. There is increasing resistance to sulfonamides, diclazuril, and amprolium, so these drugs should be used sparingly.
**Anseriformes**: Amprolium 115–235 mg/kg of feed; ponazuril 10–20 mg/kg PO once, repeat in 10–14 days; clazuril 7 mg/kg PO for 3 days, off 2 days, on 3 days; sulfonamides.
**Cranes**: Monensin 99 mg/kg of feed; for treatment or prevention of DVC; ormetoprim-sulfadimethoxine, 0.015% ormetoprim and 0.026% sulfadimethoxine in feed for 3 weeks; trimethoprim/ sulfamethoxazole 16–24 mg/kg daily.
**Passerines**: sulfachlorpyridazine 150–300 mg/l in drinking water for 5 days a

**C**

week for 2–3 weeks, may need to continue cycle for months; sulfadimethoxine 20–50 mg/kg PO twice daily for 3–5 days a week, repeat after 5 days as necessary; sulfadimidine sodium 50–150 mg/kg PO IM twice daily for 3–5 days a week, repeat after 5 days; sulfamethazine 75–185 mg/kg PO daily for 3 days, repeat after 5 days; sulfaquinoxaline 100 mg/kg PO daily for 3 days on, 2 days off, repeat; amprolium 50–100 mg/l in drinking water for 5–7 days, intended for treatment of *Eimeria* sp. and *Isospora* sp.; toltrazuril 12.5 mg/kg PO daily for 2 days, off 5 days, then repeat the 7-day cycle as needed (months); for treatment of atoxoplasmosis/*Isospora* sp. diclazuril 10 mg/kg PO twice daily on days 0, 1, 2, 4, 6, 8, 10, or 5 mg/l in drinking water.

**Raptors**: toltrazuril 10 mg/kg PO daily for 2 doses, then repeat in 2 weeks; sulfadimethoxine, 55 mg/kg PO day 1, then 25 mg/kg PO daily for 10 days; trimethoprim/sulfadiazine 60 mg/kg PO twice daily for 3 days on, 2 days off, repeat; clazuril, 5–10 mg/kg PO daily for 3 days, repeat once or twice with 2 days off; toltrazuril 0.25 ml/kg PO daily for 2 doses; amprolium 30 mg/kg PO daily for 5 doses.

## CONTRAINDICATIONS
Avoid the use of sulfonamides in animals with severe renal or hepatic impairment. Sulfonamides may also be teratogenic.

## PRECAUTIONS
N/A

## POSSIBLE INTERACTIONS
N/A

## ALTERNATIVE DRUGS
Tea tree oil 1% showed similar results when compared to treatment with amprolium in Japanese quail.

## FOLLOW-UP

## PATIENT MONITORING
Fecal flotation and direct smear should be repeated weekly for 4 weeks or until smear and flotations are consistently negative. Patient should be monitored for resolution of

clinical signs and ability to maintain weight and health status without nursing care.

## PREVENTION/AVOIDANCE
Decreasing the concentration of coccidia in the soil or environment is the best way to prevent birds from becoming infected. If possible, birds should be housed on concrete, tile, or other easily cleaned and disinfected artificial flooring, which is cleaned regularly. Suspended wire flooring is another option to help with sanitation. Food and water dishes should be kept off of the ground. Alternatively, if birds are to be housed outdoors, yearly or every third year pen rotation will help to reduce coccidia concentrations in the soil. Stress reduction and prevention of crowding are also of high importance in prevention. Additionally, vaccines have been developed for chickens, which if administered shortly after birth, can provide similar protection for chicks against coccidiosis compared to conventional oral coccidiostats.

## POSSIBLE COMPLICATIONS
Acute death.

## EXPECTED COURSE AND PROGNOSIS
Dependent upon which organ systems are affected and how severely infected the patient is. Prognosis for systemic coccidiosis with organ involvement and/or granuloma formation is grave, despite treatment and nursing care.

## MISCELLANEOUS

## ASSOCIATED CONDITIONS
Secondary infections from parasites, bacteria, viruses, and/or fungi are all commonly seen. There is report of lymphosarcoma development in severely affected gastrointestinal tract of affected American goldfinches, suggesting the possibility of parasite-associated lymphoma.

## AGE-RELATED FACTORS
Neonates are at increased risk of mortality.

## ZOONOTIC POTENTIAL
None.

## FERTILITY/BREEDING
Avoid the use of sulfonamides in reproductive animals as they may be teratogenic.

## SYNONYMS
Disseminated visceral coccidiosis.

## SEE ALSO
Aspergillosis
Botulism
Candidiasis
Campylobacteriosis
Flagellate Enteritis
Hemoparasites/Hematozoans
Mycobacteriosis
Mycotoxicosis
Neoplasia (Gastrointestinal and Hepatic)
Pasteurellosis
Salmonellosis
Sarcocystosis
Toxicosis (Heavy Metals)
Toxoplasmosis

## ABBREVIATIONS
DVC—disseminated visceral coccidiosis
GI—gastrointestinal
PCR—polymerase chain reaction

## INTERNET RESOURCES
N/A

*Suggested Reading*
Carpenter, J.W., Harms, C.A., eds. (2023). *Carpenter's Exotic Animal Formulary*, 6th edn. St. Louis, MO: Elsevier.
Knight, A., Ewen, J.G., Brekke, P., Santure, A.W. (2018). The evolutionary biology, ecology and epidemiology of coccidia of passerine birds. *Advances in Parasitology*, 9:35–60.
Novilla, M.N., Carpenter, J.W. (2004). Pathology and pathogenesis of disseminated visceral coccidiosis in cranes. *Avian Pathology*, 33:275–280.
Speer, B.L., ed. (2016). *Current Therapy in Avian Medicine and Surgery*. St. Louis, MO: Saunders.
Tully TN, Dorrestein GM, Jones AK, eds. (2009). *Handbook of Avian Medicine*, 2nd edn. Woburn, MA: Butterworth-Heinemann.
**Authors**: Alison Jeffrey, DVM, and James W. Carpenter, MS, DVM, DACZM
**Acknowledgements**: Christine T. Higbie, DVM, DACZM

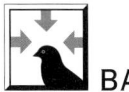

# BASICS

## DEFINITION
Swelling of the coelomic cavity.

## PATHOPHYSIOLOGY
Pathologic distension of the coelom may be due to a space-occupying mass effect, ascites, herniation, or obesity. Note that moderate distension of the coelom associated with egg production can be a normal finding in hens. Additionally, chicks of some species can normally have full and distended coelomic cavities due to prominent gastrointestinal tracts. Organomegaly may be a result of an infectious process, inflammation, congestion, abscessation, or neoplasm. Distension of the gastrointestinal tract can be due to either an obstruction or ileus. Egg binding and dystocia can lead to distension of the reproductive tract. Ascites within a bird's coelomic cavity can be a result of increased vascular hydrostatic pressure, decreased oncotic pressure, leakage of vessels, or a combination of these factors. These conditions are often a sequela of congestive heart failure, hepatopathy, neoplasia, or an inflammatory condition in the coelom.

## SYSTEMS AFFECTED
**Respiratory**: Compression of the air sacs by space-occupying mass effect or fluid can lead to increased respiratory effort.
**Gastrointestinal**: Partial or complete obstruction of intestinal bowel loops by intraluminal mass or compression by an extraluminal mass; intestinal strangulation may occur if bowel loops are caught within a hernia; pancreatitis and hepatopathies can lead to ascites.
**Integument**: Localized plucking of feathers in the coelomic region in response to discomfort from the distension; xanthomas and lipomas can develop on the bird's ventrum in association with obesity; accumulation of feces may occur on the tail feathers if the distension displaces the opening of the vent
**Neuromuscular**: Compression of the ischiatic nerves by coelomic masses can lead to paresis or paralysis of the pelvic limbs.
**Renal**: Damage to the kidneys and hyperuricemia can develop due to compression of renal parenchyma and ureters by a coelomic mass.
**Reproductive**: Egg binding or an impacted oviduct; egg-yolk peritonitis can lead to significant fluid accumulation and adhesion formation.

## GENETICS
N/A

## INCIDENCE/PREVALENCE
Coelomic distension is a common clinical sign for various disease processes, including ascites, organomegaly, ileus, neoplasms, obesity, dystocia, and body wall hernias. Distension of the coelom is a normal finding in hens during periods of reproductive activity and oviposition. Neonatal/juvenile chicks of some species can normally have full and distended coeloms.

## GEOGRAPHIC DISTRIBUTION
N/A

## SIGNALMENT
**Species predilections**: Ovarian neoplasms—cockatiels, chickens; ovarian cysts—cockatiels, budgerigars, canaries; testicular neoplasms—budgerigars, cockatiels; obesity—Amazon parrots, Quaker parrots, budgerigars; xanthomagranulomatosis—eclectus parrots, budgerigars.
**Mean age and range**: Altricial neonate chicks (psittacine, passerines) normally have a full and distended coelom.
**Predominant sex**: Distension from an enlarged reproductive tract (either physiologic or pathologic) occurs in sexually mature hens.

## SIGNS
### Historical Findings
Distended abdomen. Tail bobbing and/or open-mouth breathing. Generalized lethargy and depression; may be on the bottom of the cage. Decreased appetite. Exercise intolerance, trouble flying. May have a history of recent egg-laying. May have a history of straining (either to defecate or to lay an egg).

### Physical Examination Findings
Swollen coelom—may palpate egg, mass, or fluid. Increased respiratory effort, especially after handling. Wide-based stance or drooped wings. Fecal and/or urate accumulation over vent and tail feathers. Exercise intolerance. Anorexia. Lethargic and depressed. Wheezing or crackles auscultated over lungs and caudal air sacs (ascites). Holosystolic heart murmur (cardiomyopathy). Yellow or green urates (hepatopathy).

## CAUSES
**Obesity**: Both intracoelomic and extracoelomic fat may be observed.
**Intracoelomic mass effect**: Enlarged reproductive tract—egg, ovarian cysts, salpingitis, metritis, oophoritis, oviduct impacted with inspissated yolk; hepatomegaly—hepatic lipidosis, hepatitis, chlamydiosis; splenomegaly—chlamydiosis,

hemorrhage or hematomas; obstructed or distended gastrointestinal bowel loops or cloaca—fecalith, cloacal mass, ileus; neoplasia—ovarian, testicular, renal, pancreatic, hepatic, gastrointestinal, lymphoma/lymphosarcoma, lipomas, teratomas; intracoelomic abscesses; granulomas and xanthogranulomatosis.
**Ascites**: Cystic ovarian disease; egg yolk coelomitis or salpingitis; ovarian neoplasia; testicular neoplasia; hepatic cirrhosis; protein-losing nephropathy; protein-losing enteropathy; congestive heart failure; iron storage disease/hemochromatosis; polyomavirus; mycobacteriosis; aspergillosis (granulomatous pneumonia leading to pulmonary hypertension); pancreatitis.
**Body wall herniation**: May contain bowel loops, reproductive tract.

## RISK FACTORS
Chronic egg layers and obese birds are at greater risk for egg binding and body wall herniation. Birds fed a high-fat diet in conjunction with a sedentary lifestyle are prone to obesity and are at risk for hepatic lipidosis, lipoma, and cardiac disease. Ingestion of moldy peanuts and grain may lead to aflatoxicosis which can result in hepatic cirrhosis and ascites. Birds in the Ramphastidae (toucan) and Sturnidae (mynah) families are at greater risk for iron storage disease.

# DIAGNOSIS

## DIFFERENTIAL DIAGNOSIS
**Dyspnea/respiratory distress**: Primary respiratory condition such as pneumonia, sinusitis, or tracheal obstruction; a painful condition; heat exhaustion; cardiac disease.
**Wide-based stance/lameness**: Weakness in the pelvic limbs from either neurologic dysfunction, thromboembolic disease; musculoskeletal injury; generalized weakness.

## CBC/BIOCHEMISTRY/URINALYSIS
Hypercalcemia, hyperglobulinemia, and hypercholesterolemia are normal findings in reproductively active hens. Moderate to severe hypoalbuminemia and decreased A : G ratio if a protein-losing nephropathy or enteropathy, or advanced hepatic disease is present; neonates generally also have lower total protein and plasma albumin levels. Leukocytosis with heterophilia with or without toxic changes is common with coelomitis. May have severe leukocytosis with monocytosis if an infectious disease process such as mycobacteria or chlamydia is involved; a higher white blood cell count

can be a normal finding in juvenile psittacine birds. Elevated bile acids if hepatopathy is present. Hyperlipidemia may be noted in obese birds and birds with hepatic lipidosis.

## OTHER LABORATORY TESTS

Cytologic analysis of fine needle aspirate or aspirated fluid; clear transudates are suggestive of heart failure or hypoproteinemia; exudates are suggestive of an infectious and/or inflammatory process; yolk or lipid globules are often noted with egg-yolk peritonitis; neoplastic cells may be noted with neoplastic effusions. Bacterial culture and sensitivity are highly recommended if purulent material or exudate is aspirated. Histopathology of biopsied masses is used to differentiate between hyperplasia, inflammatory processes, and different types of neoplasms.

## IMAGING

### Radiographic Findings

Distension of the caudal coelom can be visualized on lateral views. Widening of the hepatic silhouette often noted on ventrodorsal views. May have poor serosal detail of the distended coelomic cavity, especially if ascites is present. A GI contrast study with barium may help characterize the coelomic distension and help delineate a mass effect. Shelled eggs may be present in cases of egg binding.

### Ultrasonography

Visualization of the coelomic cavity is enhanced if the coelomic distension is due to ascites or a mass effect. Ultrasound allows for better evaluation of coelomic masses, unshelled eggs, cystic ovaries, distended/thickened intestinal loops, and loops of bowel within hernias. A large heart, large hypoechoic liver, ± ascites are noted in cases of CHF. An echocardiogram may be indicated to evaluate for changes in the heart. Changes associated with hepatic cirrhosis can include small hyperechoic liver with nodular margins, ± ascites due to portal hypertension. Hepatic changes associated with hepatic lipidosis include a large hyperechoic liver.

### Advanced Imaging

Cross-sectional imaging allows for the coelomic cavity to be imaged without superimposition of anatomic structures; CT can also better differentiate tissue type and some masses may contrast enhance.

## DIAGNOSTIC PROCEDURES

If ascites present, centesis of the coelom is both diagnostic and therapeutic. Laparoscopy allows for visualization and biopsy of coelomic masses or organomegaly. Eggs located ectopically within the coelom may also be visualized.

## PATHOLOGIC FINDINGS

Varies with the cause of coelomic distension. Ascites may be noted within one or more of the peritoneal cavities. Fluids may be transudate or exudate. Inspissated egg yolk may be noted within the coelomic cavity with egg yolk peritonitis. Organomegaly or neoplastic masses of the kidney, liver, spleen, pancreas, ovary, oviduct, or testicle may be seen. Adhesions or carcinomatosis may be noted within coelomic cavity. Cardiomegaly with right-sided, left-sided, or biventricular enlargement noted in birds with cardiac disease; atherosclerosis of coronary, pulmonary, and systemic vasculature may also be noted.

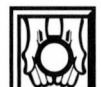

## TREATMENT

### APPROPRIATE HEALTH CARE

Treatment will be dictated by the underlying cause of the coelomic distension. Birds demonstrating significant respiratory compromise from a mass effect or ascites may need to be hospitalized for oxygen supplementation. Hens that are distended due to egg binding may respond to conservative medical management. If there is no response to medical management or if tissue is prolapsed, surgical intervention may be required to remove the egg. Patients with lipomas can be managed conservatively on an outpatient basis with dietary management. However, surgical excision of lipomas may be necessary if conservative medical therapy fails. Control of infection and inflammation needs to be addressed when medically managing cases of egg-yolk peritonitis; salpingohysterectomy and removal of inspissated egg yolk may be required once the patient is stabilized. Cystic ovarian disease, ovarian neoplasia, and testicular neoplasia are rarely treated surgically due to the vascular supply to the gonads; periodic coelomocentesis and medical management with hormone therapy may provide symptomatic treatment. Coelomocentesis helps alleviate pressure on the air sacs; centesis can be repeated as necessary on an outpatient basis. Surgical excision of some neoplasms may alleviate symptoms if metastasis has not already occurred. Phlebotomy (1% of body weight q7d) can be performed in birds with iron storage disease to reduce stored liver iron levels.

### NURSING CARE

Oxygen supplementation should be provided if the patient has respiratory compromise. Nutritional support by gavage feeding if the patient is anorexic or has significant loss in muscle mass. If there is an egg present in the coelom, the hen should be placed in a warm,

humidified incubator to encourage oviposition. Supplemental calcium, pain medications, and parental fluids may be beneficial. Therapeutic coelom centesis is beneficial if ascites is noted.

### ACTIVITY

Minimize stress and activity, since the patient may have limited respiratory capacity.

### DIET

Gavage feed if the patient is not eating. If the patient is obese, reduce calories by limiting foods high in fat and reducing the overall quantity of food. However, make sure that the patient is continuing to eat if hepatic lipidosis is present. Calcium supplementation should be provided for hens that are egg laying to prevent calcium deficiency. Birds susceptible to iron storage disease should be on a specially formulated low iron diet.

### CLIENT EDUCATION

If the patient is obese, foraging activities should be incorporated into the bird's daily routine to encourage exercise to help the bird lose weight. If the patient is laying eggs, the hen should be monitored for prolonged straining, as this can be a sign of egg binding. If ascites is present, centesis of the coelom may need to be repeated as needed to provide relief for dyspnea. If an infectious process is suspected, the patient should be quarantined from other birds. Precautionary measures should be discussed for birds with zoonotic diseases, especially if they are exposed to any immunocompromised people.

### SURGICAL CONSIDERATIONS

Patient may have compromised ability to breathe due to compression of air sacs. Intubation with positive pressure ventilation is strongly recommended if undergoing surgery. If ascites present, extra care must be taken to prevent damaging the air sacs during the surgical approach to minimize the risk of fluid aspiration through the air sacs.

## MEDICATIONS

### DRUG(S) OF CHOICE

An antibiotic may be considered if an infection is suspected and ideally is based on culture and sensitivity results. Meloxicam 1–1.6 mg/kg PO, IM, IV q12h can be administered if an inflammatory process is involved or if the patient appears painful. Treatments will vary greatly depending on the cause of the distension.

**For ascites:** Furosemide 0.1–2 mg/kg PO, SQ, IM, IV q6–24h; diuretic to remove excess fluid in cases of CHF or liver insufficiency.

**For reproductive-related disorders:** Leuprolide acetate 200–800 µg/kg IM q2–6w (for cessation of egg laying as an

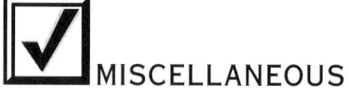

# COELOMIC DISTENSION

adjunct therapy for egg binding), 1500–3500 µg/kg IM q2–4w (for ovarian/testicular tumors), synthetic GnRH agonist. Deslorelin 4.7 mg implant SQ q2–5m, synthetic GnRH agonist; long-term implant. Note that the use of this implant in birds is considered off-label use; as an FDA-indexed drug is prohibited in the United States for use in poultry.
**For congestive heart failure**: Furosemide 1–5 mg/kg IM q2-12 for acute treatment, then 1–10 mg/kg PO q 8–12h for maintenance—diuretic to remove excess fluid in cases of CHF or liver insufficiency. Benazepril HCl 0.25–0.5 mg/kg PO q24h or enalapril 1.25–5 mg/kg PO q12h, ACE inhibitors used in the management of CHF and hypertension. Pimobendan 6–10 mg/kg PO q12h, inodilator (has inotropic and vasodilator effects) used in the management of CHF.
**For iron storage disease**: Deferoxamine 100 mg/kg SQ/IM q24h; iron chelator for birds with ISD.
**For hepatic cirrhosis/fibrosis**: Colchicine 0.02–0.2 mg/kg PO q12–24h; antifibrotic used in the treatment of cirrhosis of the liver.

## CONTRAINDICATIONS
Furosemide is contraindicated in patients with anuria. Deferoxamine should not be used in patients with severe renal failure.

## PRECAUTIONS
Overdose of furosemide can cause dehydration and electrolyte imbalances.

## POSSIBLE INTERACTIONS
Colchicine may cause additive myelosuppression when used in conjunction with medications with bone marrow depressant effects (i.e. antineoplastics, immunosuppressants, chloramphenicol, amphotericin B).

## ALTERNATIVE DRUGS
Hepatoprotective medication such as silymarin may be beneficial if a hepatopathy is suspected. L-carnitine has been used to help reduce obesity and the size of lipomas in budgerigars.

# FOLLOW-UP

## PATIENT MONITORING
Repeat radiographs can be used to evaluate if the coelomic distension is decreasing or increasing in size. If coelomic distension is due to obesity, weight loss through diet restriction and exercise should be gradual and closely monitored with frequent weight checks. Hens with a history of egg binding should be closely monitored during egg-laying season. Administration of a

GnRH agonist can be given seasonally whenever the hen begins to display reproductive behaviors to deter egg laying. An echocardiogram should be repeated on patients with CHF to evaluate the response to heart medications. The patient's uric acid levels should also be monitored every few weeks to months to assess their renal function. Bile acid levels should be monitored every few weeks to months to evaluate hepatic function in patients with suspected hepatopathies. If a salpingohysterectomy is performed for the treatment of reproductive disorders, the patient may be at risk for internal laying and future cases of egg yolk peritonitis. The hen may need preventative doses of a GnRH agonist to prevent further laying.

## PREVENTION/AVOIDANCE
Obesity can be prevented by encouraging foraging behavior and providing a healthy and balanced diet. Owners should not be offering food items high in fat on a regular basis. A GnRH agonist may be administered seasonally to deter egg laying.

## POSSIBLE COMPLICATIONS
Impaired fecal emptying or gastrointestinal obstruction. Cloacal/oviductal prolapse or coelomic wall herniation can occur with excessive straining associated egg binding. Compression of the kidney can lead to renal compromise and/or lameness of the pelvic limbs. Lateral puncture of the coelomic cavity when performing coelomcentesis may result in leakage of fluid directly into the air sac and can result in drowning of the patient. GI obstruction may occur when fecaliths or eggs are lodged in the pelvic canal or if neoplasms originate in the cloaca.

## EXPECTED COURSE AND PROGNOSIS
Prognosis varies with the cause of distension. Prognosis is good if the distension is due to an egg and the hen is healthy. However, if there is prolonged egg binding or there is egg-yolk peritonitis, the prognosis is fair to guarded, depending on if treatment is instituted in a timely manner. Birds with ascites usually have a guarded to poor long-term prognosis as most causes (i.e. CHF, hepatic cirrhosis, ovarian neoplasia) are usually progressive even with treatment. Benign neoplasms such as lipomas have a good prognosis if treatment and diet modification is instituted early; other neoplasms generally have a guarded to poor long-term prognosis. Some testicular and ovarian neoplasms have some response to repeated hormone therapy. Hernias have a good prognosis as long as intestinal bowel loops have not become entrapped and compromised within the hernia.

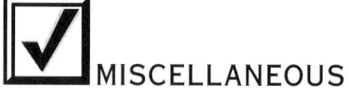

# MISCELLANEOUS

## ASSOCIATED CONDITIONS
Unilateral or bilateral hind limb paresis may be noted if a coelomic mass is compressing the ischiatic nerve. Ileus or an obstructive process of the GI tract may lead to scant fecal production or malodourous feces from bacterial overgrowth.

## AGE-RELATED FACTORS
Altricial neonate and juvenile chicks will normally have a full and distended appearance to their coelom. Congestive heart failure secondary to atherosclerosis usually affects mature, older birds.

## ZOONOTIC POTENTIAL
Though no cases of bird-to-human mycobacteriosis are reported, owners must be advised of the potential zoonotic risk, especially to immunocompromised individuals.

## FERTILITY/BREEDING
If the oviduct is damaged during the course of the egg binding or during treatment, the hen may be predisposed to subsequent cases of egg binding/dystocia.

## SYNONYMS
Abdominal distension (often used to describe, though technically birds do not have an abdomen).

## SEE ALSO
Aspergillosis
Atherosclerosis
Chlamydiosis
Congestive Heart Failure
Dystocia and Egg Binding
Egg Yolk and Reproductive Coelomitis
Hepatic Lipidosis
Iron Storage Disease
Liver Disease
Mycobacteriosis
Neoplasia (Gastrointestinal and Hepatic)
Neoplasia (Lymphoproliferative)
Neoplasia (Renal)
Neoplasia (Reproductive)
Obesity
Appendix 8, Algorithm 5: Coelomic Distension

## ABBREVIATIONS
ACE—angiotensin-converting enzyme
CHF—congestive heart failure
CT—computed tomography
FDA—Food and Drug Administration
GI—gastrointestinal
GnRH—gonadotropin-releasing hormone

## INTERNET RESOURCES
N/A

## COELOMIC DISTENSION                                    (CONTINUED)

*Suggested Reading*

Antinoff, N. (2021). Birds with big bellies: What do I need to know? *ExoticsCon Virtual* 2021 Proceedings.

Donovan, T.A., Garner, M.M., Phalen, D., et al. (2022). Disseminated coelomic xanthogranulomatosis in eclectus parrots (*Eclectus roratus*) and budgerigars (*Melopsitacus undulatus*). *Veterinary Pathology*, 59:143–151.

Taylor, W.M. (2016). Pleura, pericardium, and peritoneum: the coelomic cavities of birds and their relationship to the lung–air sac system. In: *Current Therapy in Avian Medicine and Surgery* (ed. B.L. Speer), 345–362. St. Louis, MO: Elsevier.

Scagnelli, A.M., Tully, T.N. Jr. (2017). Reproductive disorders in parrots. *Veterinary Clinics of North America. Exotic Animal Practice*, 20:485–507.

Sedacca, C.D., Campbell, T.W., Bright, J.M., et al. (2009). Chronic cor pulmonale secondary to pulmonary atherosclerosis in an African grey parrot. *Journal of the American Veterinary Medical Association*, 234:1055–1059.

Keller, K.A., Beaufrère, H., Brandão, J., et al. (2014). Long-term management of ovarian neoplasia in two cockatiels (*Nymphicus hollandicus*). *Journal of Avian Medicine and Surgery*, 27:44–52.

Juan-Sallés, C., Soto, S., Garner, M.M., et al. (2011). Congestive heart failure in 6 African grey parrots (*Psittacus erithacus*). *Veterinary Pathology*, 48:691–697.

Starkey, S.R., Morrisey, J.K., Stewart, J.E., et al. (2008). Pituitary-dependent hyper-adrenocorticism in a cockatoo. *Journal of the American Veterinary Medical Association*, 232:394–398.

**Author**: Sue Chen, DVM, DABVP (Avian)

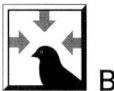
## BASICS

### DEFINITION
*Escherichia coli* are Gram-negative, facultative anaerobic rods and members of the Enterobacteriaceae family. Serotyping is based on three antigens found in the cell wall: somatic antigen O, flagellar antigen H, capsular antigen and the fimbrial or F antigens. *E. coli* is ubiquitous and considered a common intestinal inhabitant of the GI tract in many avian species (especially raptors, pigeons, passerines, and ratites) and has been isolated from the cloaca of clinically normal psittacine species (especially *Cacatua* sp). Isolated *E. coli* may be a pathogen, potential pathogen, commensal or transient flora. Colibacillosis refers to any localized or systemic infection caused entirely or partly by avian pathogenic *E. coli* (APEC) and is often an acute bacterial disease reported in chickens, turkeys and ducks; it is the most common infectious bacterial disease of poultry and infections result in significant economic loss for the poultry industry. It may cause disease in all avian species.

### PATHOPHYSIOLOGY
APEC strains may cause local or systemic infections and are commonly of the O1, O2, and O78 serogroups. Extraintestinal pathogenic *E. coli* (ExPEC) strains cause disease outside the intestinal tract. Most APEC are ExPEC. APEC tend to be less toxigenic than mammalian or human *E. coli*, although pigeons can be a source of shigatoxin-producing *E. coli* strains. The virulence of *E. coli* serotypes and their enterotoxins varies; most are non-pathogenic. Systemic infectious occur when bacteria spread hematogenously from the respiratory system or GI tract. Avian *E. coli* enterotoxins cause diarrhea by hypersecretion of fluids into intestinal lumen. Serotypes of *E. coli* are classified according to the Kauffmann scheme. In most serologic typing schemes, only the O and H antigens are determined.

### SYSTEMS AFFECTED
Avian colibacillosis is a multifaceted syndrome that can affect multiple body systems; the name of disease is often based upon the tissue(s) or organ(s) affected and may manifest as a localized or systemic infection.
**Gastrointestinal**: Ingluvitis, enteritis, coligranuloma, typhlitis.
**Cardiovascular**: Pericarditis, endocarditis, myocarditis.
**Hepatobiliary**: Coligranuloma, hepatitis, perihepatitis cholangitis, cholecystitis, hepatic serositis.

**Hemic/immune**: Thrombi and microthrombi in liver and lungs, splenitis.
**Musculoskeletal**: Arthritis, osteomyelitis, polyserositis, synovitis.
**Neurologic**: Meningitis, meningoencephalitis.
**Special senses**: Labyrinthitis, anterior uveitis, panophthalmitis, hypopyon.
**Renal/urologic**: Glomerulonephritis, polyuria.
**Reproductive**: Infertility, salpingitis, oophoritis, orchitis, epididymitis.
**Respiratory**: Air sacculitis, pneumonia, coligranuloma, sinusitis, tracheitis.
**Skin/exocrine**: Dermatitis, pododermatitis and abscesses.
**Omphalitis/yolk sac infections**: Unretracted yolk sac.

### GENETICS
Genetic resistance or predisposition among companion (psittacine) species is not known. Resistance is variable among genetic lines of poultry (chickens and turkeys).

### INCIDENCE/PREVALENCE
More commonly reported in poultry; however, all birds can suffer from this disease. Young birds more likely to be affected with increased severity of disease. Sporadic reports of disease in species other than poultry. *E. coli* can be isolated from clinically normal psittacines including free-ranging parrot species; considered more common in cockatoos than other psittacines. *E. coli* is not normally found in intestinal tract of passerine species but can be found in the intestinal tract and feces of raptors and pigeons and other free-ranging species.

### GEOGRAPHIC DISTRIBUTION
Worldwide.

### SIGNALMENT
All avian species and ages are susceptible. Clinical disease is most often reported in commercial chicken, turkey, and duck flocks. In poultry, young birds are more frequently affected, and disease severity is greater in younger birds, including embryos. Coliform salpingitis/coelomitis is a common cause of mortality in breeders. Colibacillosis in older birds often manifests as an acute septicemia.

### SIGNS
Clinical signs can be inapparent or non-specific and may vary with age, tissue(s) or organ(s) involved, and concurrent disease. Symptoms include lethargy, depression, dehydration, anorexia, weakness, ruffled feathers, diarrhea, rancid smell to feces, biliverdinuria, respiratory disease, retarded growth, weight loss, lameness, regurgitation, vomiting, moribund, and sudden death. Localized infections have fewer or milder clinical signs than systemic disease.

### CAUSES
*E. coli*, although colibacillosis often occurs concurrently with other diseases. *Escherichia fergusonii* and *Escherichia albertii* have been isolated from birds and may cause disease or are of public health concern.

### RISK FACTORS
Healthy birds are generally resistant to infection. Disease most commonly associated with environmental and host factors. Poor hygiene and fecal contamination of food and water sources, perches, flooring, and environment in general. Mechanical transmission of *E. coli* following fecal contamination of the egg shell or poor hatchery hygiene. Overcrowding. Poor ventilation. Concurrent disease (viral, bacterial, fungal, or parasitic infections; toxin exposure). Immunosuppression. Nutritional deficiencies, maldigestion or malabsorption. Damage to skin or mucosal barriers. Overwhelming exposure due to environmental contamination. Stress.

## DIAGNOSIS

### DIFFERENTIAL DIAGNOSIS
Any number of infectious or inflammatory diseases, or toxicoses can resemble colibacillosis. Hepatic, renal, or pancreatic disease. Bacterial diseases: *Chlamydia psittaci, Salmonella* spp., *Klebsiella* spp., *Pseudomonas* spp., *Proteus* spp., *Pasteurella* spp., *Yersinia* spp., *Clostridium* spp., *Campylobacter* spp., *Aeromonas* spp., *Citrobacter* spp., *Erysipelothrix rhusiopathiae, Vibrio* spp., *Mycoplasma* spp., *Staphylococcus* spp., *Streptococcus* spp., *Enterococcus* spp., *Mycobacterium* spp., *Listeria* spp., *Actinobacillus* sp., *Actinomyces* spp. Parasitic diseases: Coccidiosis (*Isospora* sp., *Eimeria* sp., *Sarcocystis* sp. and *Toxoplasma* sp.), *Trichomonas* spp., *Giardia* sp., *Hexamita* sp., *Histomonas meleagridis, Crytposporium* spp., Hemoparasites (*Hemoproteus* spp., *Plasmodium* spp.), Helminths (*Capillaria* spp., *Ascaridia* spp., *Microtetrameres* spp., *Heterakis* spp., *Cardiofilaria* spp., *Chandlerella* sp., *Syngamus* sp., *Seratospiculum* spp.), Cestodes. Viral diseases: adenovirus, bornavirus, herpesvirus, circovirus, polyomavirus, paramyxovirus, reovirus, West Nile virus. Fungal diseases: aspergillosis, *Macrorhabdus ornithogaster* (avian gastric yeast), *Candida* spp. Neoplasia. Toxicoses: heavy metals (lead GI foreign body and obstruction. Salpingitis, orchitis. Stress. Maldigestion or malabsorption. Septicemia. Trauma. Iatrogenic: anthelmintic, antibiotic therapy.

C

**C**

## CBC/BIOCHEMISTRY/URINALYSIS
Few abnormalities may be noted in your birds due to rapid death. Chemistry abnormalities may indicate which organ or tissues are affected.

## OTHER LABORATORY TESTS
Blood culture.

## IMAGING
N/A

## DIAGNOSTIC PROCEDURES
Diagnosis based upon bacterial culture and identification of *E. coli*. Previous antimicrobial therapy may affect culture results. Isolation of pure culture of *E. coli* from blood (antemortem) or necropsy tissue (bone marrow, heart blood, liver, spleen, visceral lesions) is indicative of primary or secondary colibacillosis. *E. coli* isolates grown on blood and MacConkey agar; avian isolates of *E. coli* are usually non-hemolytic on sheep (5%) blood agar. Addition of Congo red to growth medium may indicate pathogenicity of strain. Pathogenicity of isolates determined using multiplex PCR.

## PATHOLOGIC FINDINGS
Numerous tissues or organs affected.

### Localized Infection
Ingluvitis, coligranuloma, typhlitis, enteritis (mucosal inflammation in small intestine); common in humans and other mammals but not poultry. Omphalitis/yolk sac infection—inflammation of the umbilicus and yolk sacculitis. Coliform cellulitis—sheets of serosanguineous to caseated, fibrinoheterophilic exudate in subcutaneous tissues; associated with skin trauma. Swollen head syndrome—acute to subacute cellulitis of periorbital and adjacent subcutaneous tissues; inflammatory exudate accumulates beneath the skin as a result of *E. coli* infections following upper respiratory viral infections in poultry; portal of entry is the conjunctiva or inflamed mucous membranes of the infraorbital sinuses or nasal cavities. Salpingitis, orchitis, epididymitis.

### Systemic Infection
Colisepticemia—presence of *E. coli* in the blood; associated with many lesions. Polyserositis—inflammation of many serosal surfaces within the coelomic cavity. Granulomatous disease. Pericarditis often associated with myocarditis—serous and serofibrinous exudates accumulate within the pericardial sac, as disease progresses exudate causes adhesion of pericardial sac to epicardium; results in constrictive pericarditis. Vegetative endocarditis. Respiratory colisepticemia—infectious bronchitis virus, Newcastle disease virus, mycoplasmas are common predisposing agents in poultry; lesions in the respiratory tract are found in the trachea, lungs, air sacs (thickened with caseous exudate), and are typical of subacute polyserositis, initial lesions consist of edema and heterophilic inflammation; phagocytes, macrophages and giant cells appear later in course of disease. Hemorrhagic septicemia in turkeys; characterized by circulatory pathology, discoloration of serosal fat, hemorrhage on serosal surfaces, pulmonary edema and hemorrhage, and enlargement of the spleen, liver, and kidneys. Neonatal colisepticemia 24–48 hours post hatch; initial pathologic lesions consist of congested lungs, edematous serous membranes, and splenomegaly. Meningitis/meningoencephalitis—uncommon. Panophthalmitis—uncommon but can be severe; hypopyon and hyphema are seen initially; retinal detachment, retinal atrophy and lysis of lens may occur. Osteoarthritis, osteomyelitis, polyarthritis, synovitis.

## TREATMENT

### APPROPRIATE HEALTH CARE
Stabilize patient and provide nursing care as indicated. Critical patients may not be able to tolerate an extensive clinical examination. Provide appropriate supportive care (nutritional support and fluid therapy) to resolve anorexia, dehydration. Provide appropriate antibiotic therapy based upon culture and sensitivity. Minimize handling of debilitated/critically ill patients.

### NURSING CARE
Specific care depends upon location and severity of disease. Administer warmed crystalloid fluid (PO, SQ, IV or IO) 50–150 ml/kg/day; provide daily maintenance plus half of calculated dehydration deficit and ongoing losses (diarrhea, dehydration, regurgitation, or vomiting) during first 24 hours; repeat during second 24-hour period; route may vary depending upon severity of dehydration. Colloids such as hetastarch may be administered to patient that are hypovolemic and hypoproteinemic; 10–15 ml/kg q8h for 1–4 treatments if indicated; reduce rate of crystalloid administration by half when giving colloids. Debilitated birds should receive fluid therapy to correct dehydration before feeding. Supplemental oxygen as indicated. Nutritional support essential for birds that are anorexic.

### ACTIVITY
Restrict activity to cage rest during hospitalization.

### DIET
Provide appropriate diet for the species affected.

## CLIENT EDUCATION
Since diseases is commonly associated with environmental factors discuss biosecurity, environmental hygiene, overcrowding, stress, air flow, and ventilation with owner to reduce risk and lessen exposure. Eliminate underlying cause in flock situations and control other diseases such as intestinal parasitism. Avoid fecal contamination of eggs. Quarantine all new birds entering the flock or home. Avoid exposure to free-ranging bird such as passerine species. Zoonotic potential.

## SURGICAL CONSIDERATIONS
N/A

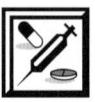

## MEDICATIONS
### DRUG(S) OF CHOICE
Antimicrobial therapy should be based upon culture and susceptibility (MIC) testing of *E. coli* isolates due to increasing resistance of *E. coli* to many antibiotics, including fluroquinolones, aminoglycosides, tetracyclines, trimethoprim/sulfamethoxazole, and chloramphenicol. Some *E. coli* isolates may be multiresistant. Empirical therapy should be instituted pending results of culture and sensitivity. Consult Food Animal Residue Avoidance Databank (FARAD.org) for antibiotic choices when managing backyard flocks; especially prohibited and restricted drug use in food animals.

**Trimethoprim/sulfadiazine**: Psittacines 30 mg/kg PO q8h, 20 mg/kg SQ, IM q12h; raptors 12–60 mg/kg PO q12h; pigeons 60 mg/kg PO q12h, 475–950 mg/l in drinking water; galliformes 107 mg/l in drinking water.

**Trimethoprim/sulfamethoxazole**: Psittacines 40–50 mg/kg q12h, 20 mg/kg PO q12h; raptors 48 mg/kg PO, IM q12h; pigeons 60 mg/kg PO q24h; passerines 10–50 mg/kg PO q24h; most species 100 mg/kg PO q12h; ducks 20–50 mg/kg PO q12h; chickens 50 mg/kg PO q12h; 360–400 mg/l drinking water; geese 400 mg/kg in feed.

**Enrofloxacin**: Psittacines 15 mg/kg PO q12–24h, 30 mg/kg PO, IM q24h, 100–200 mg/l in drinking water; raptors 15 mg/kg PO, IM, IV q24h; pigeons, 20–30 mg/kg PO, SQ, IM q12h, 100–200 mg/l in drinking water; passerines 10–20 mg/kg PO q24h, 200 mg/l in drinking water.

**Ciprofloxacin**: Psittacines 15–20 mg/kg PO, IM q12h; raptors 10–20 mg/kg PO q12h, 50 mg/kg PO q12h; pigeons 5–20 mg/kg PO q12h, 250 mg/l in drinking water; passerines 20–40 mg/kg PO, IV q12h.

**Marbofloxacin**: Most species 5 mg/kg PO q24h; psittacines (blue and gold macaws) 2.5–5.0 mg/kg PO q24h; raptors 10–15 mg/kg PO, IM q12–24h, 2–3 mg/kg IV, IO q24h.

**Amikacin**: Psittacines 10–15 mg/kg IM, IV q8–12h, 10–15 mg/kg IM q12h; raptors 10–15 mg.kg IM q24h; passerines 15–20 mg.kg SQ, IM, IV q8–12h; ring-necked pheasants (pharmacokinetic study) 10 mg/kg SQ, IM q8h for 14 days.

**Chloramphenicol palmitate**: Psittacines 30–50 mg/kg PO q6–8h; raptors 50 mg/kg PO q6–12h; pigeons 25 mg/kg q8h, 250 mg/kg PO q6h; passerines 50–100 mg/kg PO q6–12h, 100–200 mg/l in drinking water.

**Chloramphenicol succinate**: Psittacines 50 mg/kg IM, IV q6–12h; raptors 30 mg/kg IM q8h, 50 mg/kg IM, IV q6–12h; pigeons 60–100 mg/kg IM q8h; passerines 50–80 mg/kg IM q12–24h, 50 mg/kg IM q8–12h.

**Ceftazidime**: Most species 50–100 mg/kg IM, IV q4–8h.

**Cefotaxime**: Psittacines 75–100 mg/kg IM q12h; raptors 75–100 mg/kg IM q12h; pigeons 100 mg/kg IM q8–12h.

**Amoxicillin/clavulanate** (Clavamox®, Zoetis, Parsippany, NJ): Most species 125 mg/kg PO q6h; psittacines 125 mg/kg PO q12h; raptors 125 mg/kg PO q12h; pigeons 125 mg/kg PO q12h; poultry 125 mg/kg PO q8h; chickens (pharmacokinetic study) 125 mg/kg PO q12h, 500 mg/l in drinking water.

**Piperacillin**: Most species 100–200 mg/kg IM, IV q6–12h; psittacines 100 mg/kg IM q12h, psittacines (Amazon parrot) 75–100 mg/kg IM q4–6h; raptors 100 mg/kg IM, IV q8–12h; raptors (red-tailed hawks and great horned owls), 100 mg/kg IM q4–6h; pigeons 100 mg/kg IM, IV q8–12h.

## CONTRAINDICATIONS

Fluoroquinolones are banned in poultry in the USA and many other countries; Cephalosporin use is restricted in chickens and turkeys. Avoid long-term indiscriminate use of antibiotics in flocks or pet birds to prevent development of resistant strains of *E. coli*.

## PRECAUTIONS
N/A

## POSSIBLE INTERACTIONS
N/A

## ALTERNATIVE DRUGS

Alternative methods for control of colibacillosis include prebiotics, probiotics, enzymes, digestive acidifiers, vitamins, immune enhancers, anti-inflammatory drugs, and other antimicrobial products. *Lactobacillus* spp. administration may inhibit colonization of *E. coli* in the intestine. Essential oils and bacteriophage administration may be effective in reducing

mortality associated with *E. coli*. Vitamin E supplementation has been shown to have both prophylactic and therapeutic benefits for *E. coli* infections in poultry.

 FOLLOW-UP

## PATIENT MONITORING

Monitor patient's response to therapy and general behavior. Repeat fecal examination.

## PREVENTION/AVOIDANCE

Quarantine all new additions to flock or pet birds for a minimum of 30 days. Ensure good health and nutritional status of poultry and pet birds. Ensure daily cleanliness of the environment, housing, and cage conditions, and reduce dust. Avoid indiscriminate use of antibiotics in flock and pet birds. Owners should wash hand and take appropriate biosecurity measures before handling healthy birds. Vaccines (live, inactivated, and recombinant) are available for poultry; however, no vaccine product or procedure has demonstrated a high level of efficacy in commercial production, and no product is used widely in the industry at the present time.

## POSSIBLE COMPLICATIONS
N/A

## EXPECTED COURSE AND PROGNOSIS

Prognosis depends upon the severity of disease and tissue(s) or organs(s) affected. Life-threatening infections in young birds; adult birds may have less severe morbidity and mortality. Severe infections carry a poor prognosis.

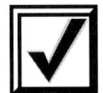 MISCELLANEOUS

## ASSOCIATED CONDITIONS
N/A

## AGE-RELATED FACTORS

Young birds are at greatest risk of infection and septicemia.

## ZOONOTIC POTENTIAL

*E. coli* are present in the intestinal tract of most animals and are shed in feces. Always wash hands after handling. Human infection usually associated with direct animal contact or ingestion of contaminated poultry products. Illness in humans often manifests as an acute gastroenteritis. Children and immunocompromised individuals should not come in contact with patients with diarrhea or handle young poultry. All eggs and poultry products should be refrigerated and prepared according to FDA safety recommendations.

## FERTILITY/BREEDING
N/A

## SYNONYMS

*E. coli* septicemia, colisepticemia, hemorrhagic septicemia, coligranuloma (Hjarrre's disease), Air sac disease (chronic respiratory disease), swollen head syndrome, venereal colibacillosis, coliform cellulitis (inflammatory or infectious process), peritonitis, salpingitis, orchitis, osteomyelitis/synovitis (including turkey osteomyelitis complex), panophthalmitis, omphalitis/yolk sac infection, enteritis.

## SEE ALSO
N/A

## ABBREVIATIONS

APEC—avian pathogenic *E. coli*
ExPEC—extraintestinal pathogenic *E. coli*
FDA—Food and Drug Administration
GI—gastrointestinal
MIC—minimal inhibitory concentration
PCR—polymerase chain reaction

## INTERNET RESOURCES

Nolan, L.K. (2022). Colibacillosis in poultry. *MSD Veterinary Manual*: http://www. merckmanuals.com/vet/poultry/colibacillosis/ overview_of_colibacillosis_in_poultry.html
Food Animal Residue Avoidance Databank (FARAD): farad.org

*Suggested Reading*
Crespo, R., Petritz, O.A. (2022). Backyard poultry, gamebirds, and waterfowl. In: *Carpenter's Exotic Animal Formulary*, 6th edn. (ed. J.W. Carpenter, C.A. Harms), 444–449. St Louis, MO: Elsevier.
Guzman, D.S.M., Beaufrère, H., Welle, K.R., et al. (2022). Birds. In: *Carpenter's Exotic Animal Formulary*, 6th edn. (ed. J.W. Carpenter, C.A. Harms), 222–443. St Louis: Elsevier, pp..
Hidasi, H.W., Neto, J.H., Moraes, D.M.C., et al. (2013). Enterobacterial detection and Escherichia coli antimicrobial resistance in parrots seized from the illegal wildlife trade. *Journal of Zoo and Wildlife Medicine*, 44:1–7.
Koutsianos, D., Athanasiou, L., Mossialos, D., et al. (2020). Colibacillosis in poultry: A disease overview and the new perspectives for its control and prevention. *Journal of the Hellenic Veterinary Medicine Society*, 71:2425–2436.
Morishita, T.Y., Porter, R.E. (2021). Gastrointestinal and hepatic diseases. In: *Backyard Poultry Medicine and Surgery: A guide for veterinary practitioners*, 2nd edn. (ed. C.B. Greenacre, T.Y. Morishita), 289–316. Hoboken, NJ: Wiley.
Nolan, L.K., Vaillancourt, J., Barbieri, N.L., et al. (2020). Colibacillosis. In: *Diseases of Poultry*, 14th edn. (ed. D.E. Swayne), 770–830. Hoboken, NJ: Wiley-Blackwell.

**Author**: Michael P. Jones, DVM, DABVP (Avian)

# CONGESTIVE HEART FAILURE

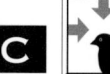

## BASICS

### DEFINITION
Congestive heart failure (CHF) occurs when the heart cannot maintain adequate cardiac output to support blood pressure or fails to empty venous reservoirs, leading to lethargy, depression, weakness, vascular congestion, and fluid transudation. This state is not a primary diagnosis but is the end result of compensatory changes influenced by an underlying primary disease process.

### PATHOPHYSIOLOGY
Heart failure typically results from end-stage structural or functional cardiovascular or pulmonary system abnormalities. It can arise from myocardial failure, valvular insufficiency, ventricular overload, conduction disturbances, or diastolic dysfunction, leading to reduced ventricular ejection or filling.

### SYSTEMS AFFECTED
Cardiovascular, endocrine/metabolic, gastrointestinal, hepatobiliary, nervous/neuromuscular, musculoskeletal, hemic/immune, renal/urologic, respiratory, integumentary, behavorial.

### GENETICS
There is no direct genetic basis specified for heart failure, but some underlying cardiac diseases, like dilated cardiomyopathy in turkeys, may have genetic components. Parrots with congenital cardiac or vascular malformations exhibit an elevated risk.

### INCIDENCE/PREVALENCE
As a significant endpoint in avian cardiovascular pathology, the prevalence of heart failure varies but is particularly observed in poultry and psittacines. The relatively few published studies examining the prevalence of cardiac disease in psittacines have shown a prevalence between 5.2% and 36%. In one postmortem study, 58% of birds with cardiac disease had died of CHF and the remaining 42% had cardiac lesions that were considered incidental and secondary to systemic infectious diseases. Species predisposed to atherosclerotic disease, to include several psittacine species, pigeons, raptors, turkeys, and chickens, may have a higher risk for presenting with CHF.

### GEOGRAPHIC DISTRIBUTION
There is no specific geographic distribution.

### SIGNALMENT
**Species**: All avian species are at risk, with age and presentation contingent upon the underlying pathology.

**Predominant sex**: Overall, there is no specific sex predilection for myocardial disease, except where atherosclerotic disease is an underlying factor; female psittacines are at higher risk than males and the opposite is true in turkeys and chickens.

### SIGNS
#### General Comments
Birds with CHF present most commonly with dyspnea and tachypnea due to air sac compression secondary to a combination of pulmonary edema, ascites, and organomegaly.

#### Historical Findings
Exercise intolerance, falling/collapse, syncope, stroke, seizure, lethargy, dysrexia, dyspnea, tachypnea, coelomic distention.

#### Physical Examination Findings
Tachycardia, arrythmia, murmur, poor pulse quality or deficits, exercise intolerance, tachypnea, dyspnea, harsh lung sounds, cyanosis, pallor, coelomic distention, extension of the liver lobes caudal the sternal margin, peripheral venous congestion, peripheral edema, failure to absorb subcutaneous fluids. Altered mentation, paresis, ataxia, syncope, seizure, blindness, anisocoria, vestibular signs, other neurologic deficits.

### CAUSES
Myocardial diseases. Atherosclerosis. Valvular insufficiency. Arrhythmias. Infectious agents. Nutritional deficiencies. Toxins. Congenital anomalies.

### RISK FACTORS
Variable, contingent on the underlying etiology of heart failure.

## DIAGNOSIS

### DIFFERENTIAL DIAGNOSIS
Differential diagnoses will include other cardiovascular diseases, neurologic diseases, respiratory diseases, or intracoelomic pathology producing similar clinical signs and physical examination findings. As these signs and symptoms may be vague and non-specific, a comprehensive diagnostic workup will be required to identify and characterize cardiovascular disease and rule out other causes.

### CBC/BIOCHEMISTRY/URINALYSIS
CBC and biochemical data are helpful in the determination of the potential primary eitology of CHF, together with the patient's suitability for therapy. Indicators of renal function imparement (elevated uric acid) is a poor prognostic indicator. Elevation of

plasma lipid or cholesterol has yet to be confirmed as predictive for atherosclerotic disease and care should be taken not to overinterpret these data. Elevations in white cell count or devations from normal in the absolute/differential cell counts identified in the CBC data may results in consideration of infectious disease as a primary etiology. A hematocrit should be measured to assess for the presence of erythrocytosis.

### OTHER LABORATORY TESTS
None.

### IMAGING
#### Radiographic Findings
Properly positioned orthogonal ventrodorsal and lateral projections should be obtained to survey for underlying etiology leading to CHF. Common findings consistent with congestive heart failure include cardiomegaly, hepatomegaly, and an increased pulmonary radiodensity with prominent reticular pattern. Cardiac measurement can be performed on the ventrodorsal projection by measuring the cardiac width by the thoracic width, both at their widest point. Dividing cardiac width by thoracic width provides a percentage consistent with heart size which then must be interpreted based on what normal is for that species.

#### Echocardiographic Findings
Echocardiography provides further insight into the potential etiology leading to CHF. In many avian species, this imaging technique can be complicated by the sternal plate and airsacs which limit complete visualization of structures in some cases. Using a standard transcoelomic approach, only two views are available in most birds, a four-chamber view, and an aortic outflow view. Cross-sectional views are not possible with this approach and cardiac measurements cannot be accurately made. Common findings include pericardial effusion, myocardial hypertrophy, valvular insufficiency, chamber dilatation, cardiac or pericardial masses, aneurysmal dilatation.

#### Ultrasonographic Findings
Imaging of the remainder of the coelom can provide helpful data and is recommended to perform in tandem with echocardiography. Findings can include uniform hyperechogenicy of hepatic parenchyma, dilatation of the hepatic veins, coelomic effusion.

### DIAGNOSTIC PROCEDURES
Electrocardiography can help in identifiying arrythmias; however, instrumentation is required for accurate evaluation. Due to the need for patients to be either sedated or anesthetized, this is infrequently performed at

the time of CHF diagnosis. Direct blood pressure evaluation can be obtained but, again, this is proceduraly challenging and requires anesthesia, not ideal for patients with CHF. Indirect blood pressure has been unreliable in avian patients.

## PATHOLOGIC FINDINGS
Gross pathologic findings of CHF may include pericardial effusion, hepatomegaly, splenomegaly, pulmonary edema, ascities,

 TREATMENT

### APPROPRIATE HEALTH CARE
Identification and treatment of the associated lesions and underlying causes.

### NURSING CARE
Stress should be minimized in cardiac patients. Particular care should be exercised during handling and restraint of these patients. Sedation should be considered to minimize stress, exertion, and dyspnea.

### ACTIVITY
Limitations should be individually applied and focused on ensuring easy access to food/water and protection from injury.

### DIET
Diet modifications are not advised in birds with unmanaged CHF. Adjustments to a balanced formulation if needed can be considered once the patient is stable.

### CLIENT EDUCATION
Clients should be taught to watch for signs of decompensation such as tachypnea, dyspnea, lethargy, and/or dysrexia, as these are indications for a repeat examination and adjustments in therapy.

### SURGICAL CONSIDERATIONS
Pericardiocentesis may be used if there is significant pericardial effusion. Endoscopic creation of a pericardial window may be useful for chronic pericarditis. Otherwise, surgical treatment is not practical for the treatment of heart disease in birds.

 MEDICATIONS

### DRUG(S) OF CHOICE
Therapeutic choices are driven by the underlying cause for CHF. As such, other therapeutic agents may be required than those in this list. Dosages can change based on taxonomic order and should be determined based on the lastest versions of exotics formularies or related articles.

Some dose ranges exist only as empirical data. Identification of the primary etiology is critical to the success of management. Diuretics: Furosemide—oral bioavailability is poor and doses should be increased 2–3× that of parenteral dose; spironolactone—not effective as a sole agent. Vasodilators: Enalapril, isoxsuprine, sildenafil. Positive ionotropes: Pimobendan, digoxin. Negative ionotropes: Carvedilol, propranolol.

### CONTRAINDICATIONS
Renal impairment precludes use of loop diuretics as these agents will worsen renal function. If uric acid levels are abnormal, there are minimal effective options for CHF management.

### PRECAUTIONS
Renal function should be evaluated prior to the use of diuretics, as these pharmacologic agents depend on renal function for clearance and will worsen exisiting renal disease. Infectious and congenital causes for CHF exist, albeit rarely, and should be considered as a differential in young parrots with no atherosclerotic lesions. Furosemide via oral administration exhibits poor bioavailability leading to the significant increase in oral dosing in comparison to parenteral options.

### POSSIBLE INTERACTIONS
None.

### ALTERNATIVE DRUGS
N/A

 FOLLOW-UP

### PATIENT MONITORING
Monitoring guidelines are dependent on the severity of clinical signs at the time of diagnosis. In hospital, supplemental oxygen and parenteral diuretic therapy with daily echocardiography until the patient's clinical signs and visible effects of volume overload are controlled are recommended. Outpatient management may be attempted in cases where patients are not oxygen dependent, but success may be limited by this approach. Medication dosing should initially be re-evaluated every 3–4 weeks, followed by q3–6m recheck evaluations where physical examination, echocardiography ± radiography guides the need for changes in therapy. Owners should be monitoring daily for early signs of dyspnea, tachypnea, hyporexia, exercise intolerance, as these are indicators for therapeutic plan adjustment.

### PREVENTION/AVOIDANCE
Prevention of aquired dieseases such as atherosclerosis leading to CHF starts at a young age and is dependent on a balanced diet, exercise regimen, and controlling reproductive activity.

### POSSIBLE COMPLICATIONS
N/A

### EXPECTED COURSE AND PROGNOSIS
Prognosis is variable and can be dependent on the severity of disease at the time of diagnosis.

 MISCELLANEOUS

### ASSOCIATED CONDITIONS
Atherosclerosis, pulmonary hypertension, endocarditis, endocardiosis, myocardial disease, arrhythmia.

### AGE-RELATED FACTORS
All ages are at risk; however, this risk increases with age.

### ZOONOTIC POTENTIAL
None.

### FERTILITY/BREEDING
Patients with cardiovascular disease should not be used for breeding, nor should reproduction be encouraged.

### SYNONYMS
Heart failure.

### SEE ALSO
Atherosclerosis
Coelomic Distension
Myocardial Diseases

### ABBREVIATIONS
CHF—congestive heart failure

### INTERNET RESOURCES
N/A

*Suggested Reading*
Fitzgerald, B.C. (2022). Cardiovascular diseases in pet birds: Therapeutic options and challenges. *Veterinary Clinics of North America: Exotic Animal Practice*, 25:469–501.
Fitzgerald, B.C., Beaufrère, H. (2015). Cardiology. In: *Current Therapy in Avian Medicine and Surgery* (ed. B.L. Speer), 252–328. St. Louis, MO: Elsevier.
**Authors:** Brenna Colleen Fitzgerald, DVM, DABVP (Avian), and Bianca Murphy, DVM, DABVP (Avian)

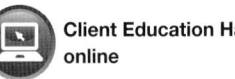 **Client Education Handout available online**

## COXIELLOSIS

 **BASICS**

### DEFINITION
Coxiella is a Gram-negative, obligate intracellular bacteria. *Coxiella burnettii*, the causative organisms for Q-fever, is the sole species currently understood to act pathogenically in humans and ruminants. However, many species of *Coxiella* are known to exist and were previousy considered to be non-pathogenic. When applied to the class Aves, it is these other *Coxiella* species (not *C. burnettii*) that appear to act pathogenically in these animals. Coxiella-like organisms, *Coxiella avium*, or *Candidatus* Coxiella avium have been used to name these organisms in the scientific literature.

### PATHOPHYSIOLOGY
The severity of this disease process varies greatly. Clinical signs ranged from inapparent illness to severe lethargy, weakness, altered mental status, seizures, and death. Timely identification of the organism and successful treatment is challenging and poorly described.

### SYSTEMS AFFECTED
Hepatobiliary, cardiovascular, gastrointestinal, nervous, neuromuscular, respiratory.

### GENETICS
N/A

### INCIDENCE/PREVALENCE
Currently, the prevalence of pathogenic *Coxiella* spp. is still being defined, owing to previous absence of specific screening options for this organism, together with difficulties isolating it in normal culture media affect our true understanding. There are small numbers of reported cases (*n* = 13) in the literature. These include a hawk-headed parrot (*Deroptyus accipitrinus*), a golden-mantled rosella, two cockatiels (*Nymphicus hollandicus*), a canary-winged parakeet (*Brotogeris versicolurus chiriri*), a kakariki (*Cyanoramphus novaezelandiae*), a blue and gold macaw, a rainbow lorikeet (*Trichoglossus moluccanus*), Swainson's lorikeet (*Trichoglossus haematodus moluccanus*), and iris lorikeet (*Psitteuteles iris*), eclectus parrot (*Eclectus roratus*), black-brown barbet (*Psilopogon oorti*), and paradise tanager (*Tangara chilensis*).

### GEOGRAPHIC DISTRIBUTION
Worldwide.

### SIGNALMENT
Cases have been identified in psittacines and a toucan at this time. No breed, age or range prelidictions. No predominant sex.

### SIGNS
#### General Comments
Non-specific clinical signs are regularly reported. Progressive lethargy and decreased interest in vocalization are routinely reported.

#### Historical Findings
Based on current reports, no significant shared history exists.

#### Physical Examination Findings
Abnormalities noted on physical examination are non-specific. Shared exam findings include decreased pectoral muscle mass, coelomic distention secondary to hepato ± splenomegaly, weakness, ataxia.

### CAUSES
*Coxiella* sp. organism (Gram-negative bacteria) also known as Coxiella-like organism, *Coxiella avium* or *Candidatus* Coxiella avium.

### RISK FACTORS
Risk factors for this disease are unclear at this stage. Although some cases had potential exposure to other wild birds, no clear connection has been made. *Coxiella* spp. ares routinely found in ticks and thus there is an outstanding theory that exposure to ticks may result in disease transmission. The infection is also diagnosed in strictly indoor birds.

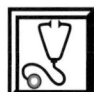 **DIAGNOSIS**

### DIFFERENTIAL DIAGNOSIS
Owing to the non-specific clinical presentation, differentials are very broad. When considering *Coxiella* as a differential, it is important to remember that it is a relatively non-prevalent disease at this time. Identification is aided by hematologic, biochemical, and radiographic study data. Current cases have considered differentials that may cause neurologic symptoms and malaise such as West Nile virus and avian influenza. Diseases that result in hepatomegaly and splenomegaly must also be considered, and often include but are not limited to infectious (mycobacterium, chlamydiosis, polyomavirus, circovirus, paramyxovirus) and neoplastic etiologies.

### CBC/BIOCHEMISTRY/URINALYSIS
Heterophil morphology: Left shift and moderate toxic changes (increased cytoplasmic basophilia and degranulation), moderate leukocytosis, moderate monocytosis.
Chemistry: No abnormalities reported thus far.

### OTHER LABORATORY TESTS
EPH: Hypergammaglobulinemia.

### IMAGING
Properly positioned ventrodorsal and right lateral projections were helpful in all cases. Imaging ranged from plain films to CT studies. Findings in both methodologies included severe splenomegaly and hepatomegaly. Cardiomegally may be noted. In experienced users, ultrasonography coud be useful.

### DIAGNOSTIC PROCEDURES
Histopathology from splenic/liver biopsies is supported in conjunction with further confirmatory tests. Molecular testing can be performed from endoscopic liver and splenic biopsies or a cloacal swab. However, the routes of shedding of the organism are not known. PCR (16S RNA) has been used to confirm *Coxiella* sp. organisms from splenic and liver tissue. This bacterium was confirmed using 16S bacterial PCR and electron microscopy. Real-time PCR (GroEL and DnaK) has routinely identified organisms when present in both liver and splenic tissues. Cloacal, choanal, and conjunctival swabs, together with blood, were briefly investigated with cloacal swabs yielding the most organisms. Therefore, sites other than the spleen/liver may be a fair consideration prior to the pursuit of more invasive sample procedures from the liver and spleen. This does not preclude the need for invasive sampling if results from less invasive methods are negative. This PCR was developed via collaboration with the University of Florida. *Coxiella* cannot be cultured on routine bacteriologic media.

### PATHOLOGIC FINDINGS
Gross necropsy findings regularly included emaciation (decreased pectoral muscle mass), hepatomegaly, and splenomegaly.

#### Cytologic Findings
Mononuclear phagocytes with cytoplasmic vacuoles containing structures consistent with bacteria nucleated cells consisted predominantly of a heterogeneous lymphoid population and hema- topoietic precursors. Lymphoid cells consisted of small and intermediate to large lymphocytes admixed with low to moderate numbers of plasma cells, consistent with a reactive population. In some cases, microscopic intracytoplasmic inclusions were found not only in the liver and spleen, but also in the epicardium, endocardium, pulmonary interstitum, kidney, adrenal and thyroid glands, brain, bursa, and bone marrow.

*Histopathologic Findings*
Lymphohistiocytic and heterophilic splenitis with multifocal thrombosis and necrosis, together with multifocal necrotizing hepatitis and multifocal exocrine pancreas necrosis were regularly present. Some histiocytes within the brain parenchyma and the perivascular cuffs had displaced nuclei and smudged eosinophilic or amphophilic cytoplasmic inclusions that were azurophilic in Gimenez stains, and had a positive PAS reaction. Granulomatous encephalitis and myocarditis were found in the lorikeets and eclectus parrot, respectively. Coxiella-like bacteria within macrophages of the spleen, liver, bone marrow, kidneys, and adrenals, further characterized using 16S bacterial PCR and electron microscopy.

# TREATMENT

## APPROPRIATE HEALTH CARE
Determining the necessity of in patient management and supportive care should be based on each individual's physical examination and clinical signs.

## NURSING CARE
Depending on the severity of clinical signs and physical exam findings, supportive therapies may be beneficial.

## ACTIVITY
Owing to the severity of lethargy and neurologic clinical signs, patients may benefit from alternative housing without high perches and long distances to climb. Easy access to food and water, alongside protection from injury should be ensured.

## DIET
In the reported cases, ensuring proper nutritional support was necessary. Be wary of pursing conversion to formulated diets prior to resolution of any disease process as this adjustment may result in further stress or weight loss in these patients.

## CLIENT EDUCATION
Zoonotic potential is under investigation; proceed with care and thoughtful biosecurity.

## SURGICAL CONSIDERATIONS
N/A

# MEDICATIONS

## DRUG(S) OF CHOICE
Based on treatment suggestions for *C. burnetti*, doxycycline 20 mg/kg PO q12hrs

for 200 days is the considered therapeutic route for identified cases. Azithromycin 40 mg/kg PO q24h may also be tried. Treatment has only been reported in a single case and was successful. Please note that doxycycline dosages can vary based on species. Please refer to the a recent edition of an exotic animal formulary for species-specific dose guidelines.

## CONTRAINDICATIONS
N/A

## PRECAUTIONS
N/A

## POSSIBLE INTERACTIONS
N/A

## ALTERNATIVE DRUGS
No studies have been done to assess efficacy of alternative therapeutics for Avian *Coxiella* spp. Extrapolation from human literature supports potential efficacy of fluorquinolones, together with tetracyclines and some macrolides.

# FOLLOW-UP

## PATIENT MONITORING
To date, few successful treatment have been reported.

## PREVENTION/AVOIDANCE
N/A

## POSSIBLE COMPLICATIONS
Owing to the seemingly advanced nature of this disease process at the time of presentation, death is likely.

## EXPECTED COURSE AND PROGNOSIS
Prognosis current is unclear as information in the scientific literature is scarce and antemortem diagnosis is rare due to the limited availability of commercial PCR for the organism and the low prevalence. However, a high rate of fatalities is reported.

# MISCELLANEOUS

## ASSOCIATED CONDITIONS
N/A

## AGE-RELATED FACTORS
N/A

## ZOONOTIC POTENTIAL
Transmission of avian coxiellosis to people has yet to be documented. However, the similarities of this *Coxiella* sp. to *C. burnetii*

support use of biosecurity measures when dealing with suspected cases.

## FERTILITY/BREEDING
N/A

## SYNONYMS
N/A

## SEE ALSO
Adenovirus
Chlamydiosis
Herpesvirus (Psittacid Herpesviruses)
Liver Disease
Spleen (Diseases of)

## ABBREVIATIONS
CT—computed tomography
EPH—protein electrophoresis
PAS—periodic acid-Schiff
PCR—polymerase chain reaction

## INTERNET RESOURCES
N/A

*Suggested Reading*
Ebani, V.V., Mancianti, F. (2022). Potential Role of Birds in the Epidemiology of *Coxiella burnetii*, Coxiella-like agents and *Hepatozoon* spp. *Pathogens*, 11(3):298.
Flanders, A.J., Speer, B., Reavill, D.R., et al. (2020). Development and validation of 2 probe-hybridization quantitative PCR assays for rapid detection of a pathogenic *Coxiella* species in captive psittacines. *Journal of Veterinary Diagnostic Investigation*, 32:423–428.
Flanders, A.J., Rosenberg, J.F., Bercier, M., et al. (2017). Antemortem diagnosis of coxiellosis in a blue and gold macaw (*Ara ararauna*). *Journal of Avian Medicine and Surgery.*, 31:364–372.
Kabakchiev, C., Beaufrère, H., Knight, B., et al. (2016). Coxiella-like infection in juvenile Eclectus parrot (*Eclectus roratus*): Diagnosis and management. *Proceedings, ExoticsCon*, 311.
Needle, D.B., Agnew, D.W., Bradway, D.S., et al.. (2020). Avian coxiellosis in nine psittacine birds, one black-browed barbet, and one paradise tanager. *Avian Pathology*, 49:268–274.
Shivaprasad, H.L., Cadenas, M.B., Diab, S.S. (2008). Coxiella-like infection in psittacines and a toucan. *Avian Diseases*, 52:426–432.
Vapniarsky, N., Barr, B.C., Murphy, B. (2012). Systemic Coxiella-like infection with myocarditis and hepatitis in an eclectus parrot (*Eclectus roratus*). *Veterinary Pathology*, 49:717–722.
**Author**: Bianca Murphy, DVM, DABVP (Avian Practice)

# CROP BURN

 BASICS

## DEFINITION
Crop burn is a colloquial term for thermal injury of the crop resulting in varying degrees of injury, from edema to necrosis and perforation of the crop, subcutaneous tissue, and skin.

## PATHOPHYSIOLOGY
The majority of cases occur in hand-reared chicks where hand-feeding formula is overheated. Manufacturers generally recommend feeding formula at temperatures of 100–106°F (37.7–41.1°C) and recommend the formula temperature be determined with a thermometer. Microwaving formula also creates a risk of "hot spots" within the formula. Injuries can range from mucosal edema and sloughing to necrosis and perforation or fistula formation. Severe burns frequently result in death. Incidences of non-hand-fed birds willingly consuming overheated liquids or food are rare, but could also occur.

## SYSTEMS AFFECTED
Injuries are most commonly seen in the most dependent portion of the crop where formula accumulates. However, burns can also occur in the oral cavity including the tongue, the esophagus, and the non-dependent (cranial) aspects of the crop. Injury and necrosis produce pain and reluctance to eat, leading to weight loss and dehydration, and can lead to secondary infection and sepsis.

## GENETICS
N/A

## INCIDENCE/PREVALENCE
This injury is seen most commonly in non-parent-raised chicks being fed either by commercial or hobby breeders, or by new owners encouraged or desiring to participate in the hand-rearing process. The sale of non-weaned birds is not recommended due to problems with inexperienced feeders, and the ethical concerns associated with imprinting young birds on humans. Crop burns can also occur in non-weaned wild birds.

## GEOGRAPHIC DISTRIBUTION
Crop burns are seen more commonly in areas with a higher concentration of less-experienced or hobby bird breeders, although unweaned birds are sometimes shipped long distances.

## SIGNALMENT
Unweaned birds of any kind, including orphaned wildlife, but this issue appears to be most commonly reported in psittacines. The age of weaning is different for various bird species, with an approximate range of 6–14 weeks for psittacines (e.g. 6 weeks for cockatiels to 14 weeks for larger cockatoos).

## SIGNS

### Historical Findings
For mild crop burns, owners may report a decrease in activity and reluctance to accept hand feeding. The crop area and overlying skin may appear thickened or edematous. The most obvious sign is a scab forming over the crop (which may be concealed by developing feathers depending on the age of the bird), which progresses to a fistula and the appearance of hand-feeding formula leaking from the site soon after feeding.

### Physical Examination Findings
Physical exam findings depend on the extent of the injury and can include lethargy and reduced feeding response, crop thickening, edema, hyperemia, necrosis, and the presence of a fistula. Birds with severe injuries and sepsis can present in shock and moribund.

## CAUSES
Crop burns are caused by the feeding or ingestion of food that is above a safe temperature.

## RISK FACTORS
Any time unweaned birds are not fed by parents, the risk for crop burns exists. This is especially true when hand-feeding individuals are less experienced or not taking extreme care to measure the temperature of the formula before feeding.

 DIAGNOSIS

## DIFFERENTIAL DIAGNOSIS
Crop injury and perforation may be caused by foreign body migration and perforation, and trauma, especially if hand feeders are using a gavage tube to deliver formula instead of allowing the bird to take formula by mouth. This happens occasionally when breeders are attempting to reduce the time it takes to feed multiple birds. Thermal injury to the skin of the crop could happen from exposure to external heat source, such as a heating pad. Bacterial or fungal ingluvitis is also part of the differential diagnosis. Lethargic birds reluctant to eat may be sick from many other causes.

## CBC/BIOCHEMISTRY/URINALYSIS
Complete blood count may often show evidence of inflammation. Birds with sepsis often have highly abnormal leukocyte differentials and morphology. The biochemistry panel often reveals elevation in AST and especially CK, and possibly elevated total protein due to clinical dehydration.

## OTHER LABORATORY TESTS
A cytologic evaluation of a crop swab in birds without obvious evidence of crop burn may show the presence of inflammatory cells and Gram-negative bacteria, sometimes with bacterial phagocytosis. Periodic monitoring of crop swabs may be useful in birds receiving antibiotics to screen for secondary *Candida* sp. overgrowth.

## IMAGING
Standard imaging such as radiography is often not helpful for diagnosis of crop burn.

## DIAGNOSTIC PROCEDURES
In cases where diagnosis is uncertain and the injury is not obvious, ingluvioscopy could be useful to identify lesions and potentially collect biopsy samples.

## PATHOLOGIC FINDINGS
Histopathology of the crop and adjacent soft tissues show changes typical of thermal necrosis, often with secondary bacterial infection.

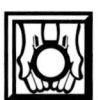 TREATMENT

## APPROPRIATE HEALTH CARE
Initial treatment focuses initially on pain management, correction of fluid deficits and secondary infection, and nutritional support. It is not necessary or advised to surgically address necrosis or fistulas immediately (see Surgical Considerations section).

## NURSING CARE
Fluid requirements are calculated (maintenance plus correction of dehydration, and delivered parentally IV/IO or SQ, as appropriate, or, if the crop is still functional and emptying despite the injury, PO). Nutritional requirements (in the form of volume of hand feeding) are calculated per manufacturer's instructions and fed PO (in many cases, adequate formula can reach the proventriculus despite loss through a fistula). In cases where the crop appears completely non-functional, or loss through the fistula appears extreme, feeding may be accomplished via soft rubber feeding tube directly into the proventriculus. The proventriculus is not able to hold the volume normally delivered into the crop; therefore, in this situation, meals should be smaller and given more frequently. Small frequent liquid meals are fed after crop surgery for 2–3 days before increasing the volume fed per feeding.

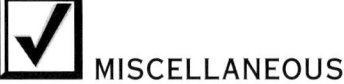
Esophagostomy tubes may be recommended in some birds.

## ACTIVITY
There are no specific activity restrictions for this condition; very sick birds should be hospitalized.

## DIET
Young birds begin accepting larger pieces of food as weaning progresses. However, in the case of crop burns, liquid hand-feeding formula may be best tolerated until the crop heals and weaning can progress. There are several reputable manufacturers of hand-feeding formula. Formulas must be fed as directed by the manufacturer without supplementation of either other foods or vitamins/minerals. Homemade hand-feeding formulas are not recommended.

## CLIENT EDUCATION
Discharge instructions should be thorough and should include steps to take should the bird experience delays in crop emptying, decreases in normal stool production, or other general decline.

## SURGICAL CONSIDERATIONS
Surgery is appropriate for repair of crop necrosis and fistula formation. Surgery is performed when the patient is stable, and fluid deficits, pain, and infection are controlled. Delays in repair, even with larger fistulas, are important to ensure that all injured tissue has declared itself, to avoid additional surgeries. Birds can temporarily tolerate large fistulas as long as nutritional requirements can be met (in most cases, most food enters the proventriculus despite loss from the fistula). General anesthesia is required for crop surgery, with appropriate analgesia and premedication. The skin is separated from the crop, and both debrided to normal-appearing tissue. The crop is sutured separately using monofilament absorbable suture, simple continuous pattern with a second everting layer if desired. Skin is sutured using the same suture and simple interrupted pattern. A collar or bandage may be required to protect the site.

 MEDICATIONS

## DRUG(S) OF CHOICE
Analgesics should include opioids in the acute phases when discomfort is likely more severe. NSAIDs are also useful, and can be continued longer term. Antimicrobials are best selected based on culture and sensitivity, but first-tier antimicrobials appropriate for the specific bird species can be selected empirically. Stress, injury, and antibiotic use may predispose birds to secondary *Candida* ingluvitis. Monitor for yeast via crop cytology; alternatively, some practitioners treat prophylactically.

## CONTRAINDICATIONS
Birds with large crop fistulas may not receive the entire dosage per administration, as drug may be lost through the fistula. In these cases, gavage-tube administration into the esophagus can be considered. Some drugs may be appropriate by injection for short-term use.

## PRECAUTIONS
None.

## POSSIBLE INTERACTIONS
N/A

## ALTERNATIVE DRUGS
N/A

 FOLLOW-UP

## PATIENT MONITORING
Birds should be assessed frequently in the early stages. Important considerations are crop motility (the time the crop takes to empty after the hand-feeding formula is delivered), general condition, and body weight. Birds receiving adequate nutrition pass full, formed stool. Droppings that are small, dry, and dark in color indicate inadequate intake.

## PREVENTION/AVOIDANCE
Anyone hand feeding a bird must be educated on proper feeding temperatures and the importance of measuring the temperature with a thermometer with every feeding.

## POSSIBLE COMPLICATIONS
Severe or untreated crop burns can result in death. Repair of a crop fistula too early may result in the need for additional surgeries as additional injured tissue declares itself.

## EXPECTED COURSE AND PROGNOSIS
Mild to moderate crop burns are treatable and carry a good prognosis. However, severe burns may result in shock, septicemia, and death. Fistulas that are untreated rarely heal and become permanent, severely impacting quality of life.

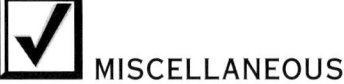 MISCELLANEOUS

## ASSOCIATED CONDITIONS
Crop burns can result in loss of body condition due to inability to take in adequate nutrition, and, in cases of severe injury and secondary infection, sepsis and death.

## AGE-RELATED FACTORS
Most injuries are in young, non-weaned birds, including wild birds.

## ZOONOTIC POTENTIAL
N/A

## FERTILITY/BREEDING
N/A

## SYNONYMS
Thermal ingluvial injury.

## SEE ALSO
Candidiasis
Dehydration
Emaciation
Enteritis and Gastritis
Ileus (Functional Gastrointestinal, Crop Stasis)
Regurgitation And Vomiting

## ABBREVIATIONS
AST—aspartate aminotransferase
CK—creatine kinase
NSAIDs—non-steroidal anti-inflammatory drugs

## INTERNET RESOURCES
Information on proper hand-feeding techniques, including recommended formula temperatures, are available from the manufacturers. Many have detailed information on their company websites.

*Suggested Reading*
Ebisawa, K., Jusuda, S., Nakayama, S., et al. (2022). Effects of rearing methods on feather-damaging behavior and corticosterone metabolite excretion in the peach-face lovebird (*Agapornis roseicollis* Viellot). *Journal of Veterinary Behavior*, 54;28–35.
Mison, M.B., Bennett, R.A. (2022). Surgery of the avian gastrointestinal tract. In: *Surgery of Exotic Animals* (ed. R.A. Bennet, G.W. Pye), 175–189. Ames, IA: Wiley Blackwell.
Van Zeeland, Y.R., Friedman, S.G., Bergman, L. (2016). Behavior. In: *Current Therapy in Avian Medicine and Surgery* (ed. B.L. Speer), 177–251. St. Louis, MO: Elsevier.
**Authors**: Angela M. Lennox, DVM, DABVP (Avian and Exotic Companion Mammal), DECZM (Small Mammal) and Crystal Matt, DVM

C

# CRYPTOCOCCOSIS

## BASICS

### DEFINITION
Cryptococcosis is a yeast infection caused by *Cryptococcosis gatti* or *Cryptococcus neoformans*.

### PATHOPHYSIOLOGY
*Cryptococcus neoformans* is ubiquitous in the environment. It occurs naturally in plant debris, soil and avian droppings; occasionally isolated from fruits, vegetables, dairy products, and the digestive tract of the cockroach. *Cryptococcosis gatti* is difficult to isolate from the environment, being found almost exclusively from leaves, bark and wood collected under the canopies of flowering red river gum (*Euclayptus camaldulensis*) trees. Physiological, ecological and serological differences occur between *C. neoformans* (found in pigeon droppings in cosmopolitan areas) and *C. gattii* (associated with blooming Eucalyptus plants in tropical regions). *C. neoformans* is a saprophytic imperfect yeast which reproduces by budding. A thick, polysaccharide, mucilaginous capsule surrounds perfectly spherical yeast cells. A sexual or perfect state of *C. neoformans* (termed *Filobasidiella neoformans*) is demonstrated by mating the fungus in vitro. *F. neoformans* produces mycelia (hyphae) which give rise to (basidio) spores. *C. neoformans* grows well on various culture media at (77.0–98.6°F (25–37°C) within 48 hours. *C. neoformans* has a distinct biochemical profile, which allows it to be rapidly differentiated from other yeasts and/or bacteria found in bird droppings or sputum from immuonocompromised human patients. One key profile is its ability to synthesize melanin from certain catecholamine precursors via phenoloxidase activity. Birdseed agar, a selective media enriched in catecholamines, facilitates melanin synthesis or pigmentation in *C. neoformans* colonies. A second key profile is the ability to catabolize xanthine, urea, uric acid and creatinine, which are all abundant in avian excreta. *C. neoformans* has been isolated from the feet, beak and GI tract of pigeons. At temperatures above 104°F (40°C) *C. neoformans* is unable to grow in vitro or in vivo in chicken embryos. The core temperature of most birds is 104°F (40°C). Birds are thus believed to be naturally resistant to infection, due to their high core body temperature and the inhibitory effects of normal intestinal flora. Upper respiratory tract infections have been assumed to be more prevalent as a source of initial infection because of the lower temperature. Because *C. neoformans* does not appear to cause clinical infection in pigeons, it has also been hypothesized that pigeons are a mechanical carrier and disseminator in the environment.

### SYSTEMS AFFECTED
Cardiovascular, GI, respiratory, neuromuscular, ocular.

### GENETICS
N/A

### INCIDENCE/PREVALENCE
Cryptococcosis is commonly isolated from pigeon droppings around the world but the prevalence of disease in pigeons is unknown. Pet birds are rarely diagnosed with cryptococcosis. Cryptococcosis organisms have been isolated from pet birds without birds showing signs of clinical disease.

### GEOGRAPHIC DISTRIBUTION
Cryptococcosis organisms have been isolated from pigeons throughout the world. Red river gum trees are concentrated in tropical and subtropical regions where *C. gatti* infections are endemic. *C. gatti* is endemic in rural Australia.

### SIGNALMENT
Birds of any species, age and sex can be diagnosed with cryptococcosis.

### SIGNS
Diarrhea, listlessness, anorexia, weakness, dyspnea and anemia have been reported. If ocular or nasal infection is present, clear nasal discharge and/orbital swelling may be present. If the CNS is involved, inability to fly, listing, paresis, blindness or limberneck of the jaw and neck may occur. Galliforms have a granulomatous form of the disease which affects the lung, spleen liver and GI tract. Gelatinous masses in birds with CNS signs are highly suspect for cryptococcosis.

### CAUSES
*C. neoformans, C. gatii.*

### RISK FACTORS
Pigeons worldwide have been found to be carriers of cryptococcosis. Blooming eucalyptus trees (*E. camaldulensis*) have been associated with outbreaks of cryptococcosis.

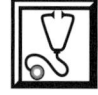

## DIAGNOSIS

### DIFFERENTIAL DIAGNOSIS
The antemortem signs of illness are non-specific, making a list of differential diagnoses expansive. Any condition causing weakness, lethargy, ataxia or anemia should be on the list of clinical differentials.

### CBC/BIOCHEMISTRY/URINALYSIS
Postmortem diagnosis is more common than antemortem diagnosis. Cryptococcosis can be diagnosed on cytology or via culture. If impression smears are made India ink will identify the mucopolysaccharide capsule. Hematoxylin and eosin, PAS, mucicarmine or silver stains can be used for histopathological specimens. Anemia has been reported in infected birds.

### OTHER LABORATORY TESTS
N/A

### IMAGING
N/A

### DIAGNOSTIC PROCEDURES
N/A

### PATHOLOGIC FINDINGS
Cryptococcosis is rarely found antemortem in avian patients.

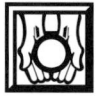

## TREATMENT

### APPROPRIATE HEALTH CARE
The zoonotic nature of cryptococcosis mandates that humane euthanasia be considered in the face of antemortem diagnosis.

### NURSING CARE
N/A

### ACTIVITY
The zoonotic nature of cryptococcosis mandates discussion of strict confinement as human infections are common from the dust of avian excreta.

### DIET
N/A

### CLIENT EDUCATION
Clients should be advised that cryptococcosis is a zoonotic pathogen. Clients who are immunocompromised are at elevated risk of infection.

### SURGICAL CONSIDERATIONS
N/A

## MEDICATIONS

### DRUG(S) OF CHOICE
Amphotericin B and fluconazole

### CONTRAINDICATIONS
N/A

### PRECAUTIONS
N/A

**(CONTINUED)**

**POSSIBLE INTERACTIONS**
N/A

**ALTERNATIVE DRUGS**
N/A

 **FOLLOW-UP**

**PATIENT MONITORING**
N/A

**PREVENTION/AVOIDANCE**
*C. neoformans* is found in pigeon excreta worldwide and is therefore all but impossible to avoid.

**POSSIBLE COMPLICATIONS**
N/A

**EXPECTED COURSE AND PROGNOSIS**
Disseminated cryptococcosis in avian patients is usually not responsive to treatment.

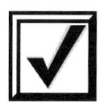 **MISCELLANEOUS**

**ASSOCIATED CONDITIONS**
N/A

**AGE-RELATED FACTORS**
N/A

**ZOONOTIC POTENTIAL**
Cryptococcosis is a zoonotic disease. Isolates of *C. neoformans* measuring 0.6–3.5 µm in diameter have been isolated from aerosols generated from soil and pigeon droppings. Extreme care should be taken when handling birds suspected of carrying the disease, as inhalation is a primary route of infection. Immunocompromised individuals are at greater risk of contracting cryptococcosis. For these reasons, treatment of birds who test positive for cryptococcosis should be well thought out. The possibility of human infection is likely to make treatment for avian cryptococcosis impractical.

**FERTILITY/BREEDING**
N/A

**SYNONYMS**
N/A

**SEE ALSO**
Anemia

**ABBREVIATIONS**
CNS—central nervous system
GI—gastrointestinal
PAS—periodic acid-Schiff

**INTERNET RESOURCES**
N/A

*Suggested Reading*
Chowdhary, A. Randhawa, H.S., Prakash, A., et al. (2012). Environmental prevalence of *Cryptococcus neoformans* and *Cryptococcus gattii* in India: An update. *Critical Reviews in Microbiology*, 38:1–16.
Levitz, S.M. (1991). The ecology of *Cryptococcus neoformans* and the epidemiology of Cryptococcosis. *Reviews of Infectious Diseases*, 13:1163–1169.
Raso, T.F., Werther, K., Miranda, M.J., et al. (2004). Cryptococcosis outbreak in psittacine birds in Brazil. *Medical Mycology*, 42:355–362.
Velasco, M.C. (2000). Candidiasis and cryptococcosis in birds. *Seminars in Avian and Exotic Pet Medicine*, 9:1835–1850.
**Author**: Kemba L Marshall, MPH, DVM, DABVP (Avian)
**Acknowledgements**: The author wishes to acknowledge the teachers, professors and patients who have allowed her to learn and live out the dreams she had as the eight-year-old version of herself.

C

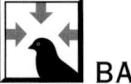

## BASICS

### DEFINITION
Zoonotic parasitic disease caused by *Cryptosporidium* spp. affecting the gastrointestinal tract and occasionally the respiratory, biliary, and urinary tracts causing clinical and subclinical infections in human, mammals, and birds.

### PATHOPHYSIOLOGY
Six species of *Cryptosporidium* in birds: *Cryptosporidium meleagridis, Cryptosporidium baileyi, Cryptosporidium galli, Cryptosporidium avium, Cryptosporidium ornithophilus* and *Cryptosporidium proventriculi* (former avian genotype III) and avian genotypes I, IV, VI–IX, duck genotype, Eurasian woodcock genotype, finch genotype I–III, YS-2017 genotype from owls, and goose genotype I–IV. Other mammalian species have been also recovered from birds such as *Cryptosporidium hominis, Cryptosporidium xiaoi, Cryptosporidium canis, Cryptosporidium muris, Cryptosporidium andersoni, Cryptosporidium parvum* and *Cryptosporidium tyzzeri*. In wild birds, at least six species have been identified (*C. andersoni, C. parvum, C. meleagridis, C. avium, C. baileyi,* and *C. galli*) and five genotypes (goose genotype I, goose genotype II, avian genotype I, avian genotype III, and avian genotype VI). *Cryptosporidium* is an apicomplexan parasite; it has a single-host life cycle with sexual and asexual processes in the intestine of the host. Three developmental stages—meronts, gamonts and oocysts. Oocysts are infectious without having to go through sporulation, allowing autoinfection. Thick-walled oocysts are excreted and can be inhaled or ingested; intracellular but extracytoplasmic establishment. Lesions and the clinical signs are due to mononuclear mucosal inflammation and hyperplasia, mucous production, as well as dysplasia, metaplasia and even neoplasia of glandular elements. Oocysts survive for long time outside the host.

### SYSTEMS AFFECTED
**Respiratory**: Mostly upper but also some lower respiratory signs – sinuses, glottis, trachea, air sacs and lungs.
**Ophthalmic**: Conjunctivitis.
**GI**: Enteritis, mainly proventricular and occasionally ventricular disease in small psittacines and owls.
**Urinary**: Kidneys and ureters.
**Hemolymphatic**: Bursa.

### GENETICS
N/A

### INCIDENCE/PREVALENCE
Unknown global incidence. Commonly overlooked and underreported; high percentage of asymptomatic shedders. Prevalence variation among species, geographical zones, and husbandry (free living, captive kept). In wild birds, 3.96%; prevalence can be 4–40% but commonly varies between 3% and 15%.

### GEOGRAPHIC DISTRIBUTION
*Cryptosporidium* is an ubiquitous microorganism with global distribution.

### SIGNALMENT
**Species**: 16 avian orders and 50 avian species; most reports involve Galliformes (chicken, quail, turkey, peafowl, red grouse), Passeriformes (finches, canaries) and Psittaciformes. *C. baileyi, C. galli* and avian genotype I were found in Passeriformes. *C. bailey, C. avium* and *C. proventriculi* were found in Psittaciformes. *C. proventriculi* was infectious for cockatiels under experimental conditions, but not for budgerigars or chicken. *C. avium* did not infect pheasants but was found in ducks. In chicken, jungle fowl, black-throated finches and Major Mitchell cockatoo manifest with renal disease. In owls, it can manifest with neurologic disease and proventriculitis. *Cryptosporidium*-associated disease in falcons, pigeons, gulls, owls, ostriches, stone curlews, penguins, toucans, and waterfowl.
**Mean age and range**: Generally seen in young birds (especially in chickens, turkey, quail, ostrich, duck, and falcons), but in one study of small psittacine the age range was 8 weeks to 13 years; it is worth mentioning that chronic vomiting in older lovebirds has been seen as a result of gastric neoplasia related to cryptosporidial infection.

### SIGNS
#### General Comments
Findings are generally related to respiratory or gastrointestinal disease but also occasionally renal disease.

#### Historical Findings
Generally seen as isolated cases, but there may be an outbreak of respiratory disease or gastrointestinal disease (quail, turkeys, chickens, stone curlew) or respiratory disease in young falcons.

#### Physical Examination Findings
**Respiratory cases**: Sneezing, nasal discharge, swelling of infraorbital sinuses, coughing, conjunctivitis, dyspnea with open mouth breathing, stridor, swelling of the glottis, weight loss, otitis.

**Gastrointestinal cases**: Depression, weight loss, vomiting, true diarrhea, passage of bulky stools with undigested food/seeds, dehydration, abdominal pain.

### CAUSES
Direct infection with *Cryptosporidium* spp., environmental (indirect) contamination, ingestion of infected prey in raptors.

### RISK FACTORS
Water or soil infestation or inhalation of infectious material or mechanical carriers (cockroaches), poor hygiene, overpopulation, immaturity of immune system (young birds), circoviral infection.

## DIAGNOSIS

### DIFFERENTIAL DIAGNOSIS
**Respiratory disease**: Mycoplasmosis, fowl cholera (pasteurellosis), aspergillosis (brooder pneumonia), infectious bronchitis, infectious laryngotracheitis, avian influenza, avian pox, Newcastle disease, chlamydiosis, trichomoniasis, airsacullitis, aspergillosis.
**GI disease**: Intestinal parasites— coccidiosis, giardiasis, hexamitiasis, histomoniasis, helminthiasis. Macrorhabdosis. Bacterial infection— salmonellosis, colibacillosis, pasteurellosis, *Clostridium colinum* (quail), other *Clostridia*, other bacteria. Fungal infection—candidiasis, aspergillosis. Chlamydiosis. Mycobacteriosis. Viral disease—Newcastle disease, avian influenza, other.

### CBC/BIOCHEMISTRY/URINALYSIS
Non-specific hematological /biochemical abnormalities. Hyperuricemia, hyperphosphatemia and Ca : P imbalance in renal cases. Absolute monocytosis and altered albumin : globulin ratio in owls with neurologic infection. Dehydration, elevation in total protein, hematocrit, white blood cell count in GI or respiratory infection.

### OTHER LABORATORY TESTS
Fecal flotation can reveal the small 2–6 μm oocysts but they can be difficult to find. Fecal direct smears should be done, especially in small psittacines to check for co-infection with other protozoa and *Macrorhabdus* sp. Acid-fast staining of feces can reveal the acid-fast organisms. PCR testing can be performed on fecal or cytological samples. IFA or ELISA analysis of fecal samples is uncommonly performed. Wright's staining of cytological samples (conjunctiva, glottis) may be helpful in identifying the organism. Viral testing

C

(especially circovirus) to check for underlying immunosuppressive disease. C/S of feces or respiratory secretions can be performed. Histopathology of deceased patients.

## IMAGING
Respiratory system endoscopy; airsacculitis with microcystic lesions (falcons) and bronchopneumonia. GI plain radiography; gas in the GI tract and/or thickening of the proventriculus. Filling defect of the proventriculus in contrast radiographs in lovebirds with proventriculitis.

## DIAGNOSTIC PROCEDURES
Cytological and microbiological sampling of infected tissues, such as conjunctiva, sinus lavage flush, tracheal/airsac lesions and proventricular biopsy.

## PATHOLOGIC FINDINGS
**Respiratory disease**: Gross—conjunctivitis, nasal discharge, swollen sinuses, tracheitis, swollen glottis, pneumonia, airsacculitis. Microscopically, excess mucous production, proliferation of mucosa, presence of cryptosporidia.
**GI disease**: Gas and excess liquid in the intestine, thickened proventriculus with excess mucous and liquid, mass in the wall of the proventriculus (lovebirds). Microscopic—presence of *Cryptosporidium* on the surface of the mucosal epithelial cells, the apical surfaces of the mucosal glands, the glandular lumina, along their primary and secondary ducts, mild to moderate mononuclear infiltration of the lamina, mild fibrosis, mucosal hyperplasia, proliferation, and exfoliation, glandular and ductular hyperplasia, dilatation, disorganization or disruption, and necrosis; metaplasia, dysplasia and neoplasia of glandular elements. Birds with concomitant macrorhabdosis more severe lesions.

## TREATMENT

### APPROPRIATE HEALTH CARE
Isolation and regular screening of asymptomatic carriers. Inpatient isolation hospitalization of critical cases. Mild cases managed as outpatients until laboratory results.

### NURSING CARE
In critical care patients, fluid, nutritional, and thermal support. Treatment for secondary bacterial, fungal or macrorhabdial disease might be necessary, depending on clinical judgment or the results of culture and sensitivity.

### ACTIVITY
N/A

## DIET
Birds that become anorectic must be supported with assisted feeding with special formula regimens. For carnivore species (falcons, owls), the prey animals should be tested.

## CLIENT EDUCATION
Given the low recovery rate and the zoonotic potential, euthanasia or treatment effort should be extensively discussed with the owner. Owner should be warned on the treatment longevity (i.e. weeks) with possible unrewarding outcome. Clients should be informed that there is a zoonotic potential as well as a transmission potential among other species. Detailed hygiene instructions should be highlight upon suspicion. Immunocompromised (HIV+) humans and children should avoid close contact with infected birds.

## SURGICAL CONSIDERATIONS
N/A

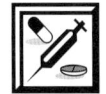

## MEDICATIONS

### DRUG(S) OF CHOICE
Low success treatment rate. Paramomycin alone (100 mg/kg, b.i.d. PO) or with azithromycin has been recommended historically but there are few reports of success. The drug is expensive and difficult to obtain. Falcons treated with paromomycin or azithromycin for respiratory cryptosporidiosis of *C.parvum* or *C. baileyi* did not respond to treatment. Azithromycin (40 mg/kg) eliminated *C. baileyi* oocyst excretion in scops owl. Ponazuril (20 mg/kg, s.i.d. PO) had a dramatic response within 24 hours in cases of respiratory cryptosporidiosis in falcons infected with *C.baileyi*. No pharmacokinetic or pharmacodynamic data exist for its use in birds. Combination of toltrazuril, spiramycin, halofuginone in stone curlews did not reduce the mortality. Use of hyperimmune bovine colostrum and halofuginone, or combination of sulfadiazine/trimethoprim, spiramycin and metronidazole in green iguanas decreased disease and euthanasia rates. Nitazoxanide has been used in humans with cryptosporidiosis, but there no information about its use in birds.

### CONTRAINDICATIONS
N/A

### PRECAUTIONS
Biosecurity/hygiene measures of the owner/ nursing staff.

### POSSIBLE INTERACTIONS
N/A

## ALTERNATIVE DRUGS
New active substances or drug combinations are being investigated in human medicine. The drug clofazimine has been tested in HIV-positive human patients with cryptosporidiosis proved ineffective. Target-based screens identified inhibitors of lysyl-tRNA synthetase, phenylalanyl-tRNA synthetase, methionyl-tRNA synthetase, and calcium-dependent protein kinase 1. Phenotypic screens led to discovery of a phosphatidylinositol 4-kinase inhibitor, the piperazine MMV665917, and the benzoxaborole AN7973, which could in the future lead in cryptosporidiosis treatment. The combination of atorvastatin (20 mg/kg) and nitazoxanide (1000 mg/kg) showed a synergistic effect through reduction of the number of oocysts shed and improvement of the histopathological changes induced by *Cryptosporidium* spp. infection in the small intestine, colon, stomach, and lungs of infected immunosuppressed mice. The combination of secnidazole and nitazoxanide recorded the maximal reduction of *C. parvum* oocyst shedding, endogenous stages count, and intestinal histopathology, regardless of the immune status of the infected mice. Curcumin (4.3 mg/kg/day) reduced and eliminated the *C.parvum* oocysts in BALB/c model of mice.

## FOLLOW-UP

### PATIENT MONITORING
Body weight and appetite recording. Repeated fecal screening (acid-fast stain, PCR). Resolution of underlying/concomitant disease (e.g. aspergillosis).

### PREVENTION/AVOIDANCE
Feeding of infected quail or wild prey to falcons should be avoided. Birds should not be placed in close contact with infected birds. Flock screening to detect asymptomatic carriers. Disinfection of the environment should be performed to decrease or eliminate the presence of the organism (difficult). *Cryptosporidium* oocysts can be managed by heat or chemical disinfection treatment as hydrogen peroxide, sterilization processes using steam, ethylene oxide, chlorine dioxide, ozone, and ultraviolet light, which have been used to sterilize drinking water. Strong bleach or ammonia solution, or steam cleaning might be helpful.

### POSSIBLE COMPLICATIONS
N/A

### EXPECTED COURSE AND PROGNOSIS
The prognosis is guarded to poor, regardless choice of drug therapy and supportive care. Treatment course can be frustrating as it

C

usually presents a waveform pattern of temporary clinical improvement, followed by sudden death.

 **MISCELLANEOUS**

**ASSOCIATED CONDITIONS**
Underlying circoviral or borna viral infection; some patients develop secondary disease colibacillosis. Small psittacines with concurrent macrorhabdosis or intestinal flagellates.

**AGE-RELATED FACTORS**
N/A

**ZOONOTIC POTENTIAL**
The zoonotic rate of cryptosporidiosis showed an annual increase of 13% in USA, while the zoonotic cryptosporidiosis percentage was 5–38% in Asian countries. At least two species of *Cryptosporidium* have been found in both humans and birds (*C. meleagridis* and *C. parvum*). the *C. meleagridis* caused symptoms in an HIV-positive woman in Poland, while in developing countries it is the most prevalent in HIV-positive patients and children. *C. meleagridis* is responsible for 1–4% human infections. Other avian specific (psittacine, finch, falcons) cryptosporidia are so far host specific, so do not currently pose a zoonotic threat.

**FERTILITY/BREEDING**
Breeding, fertility rates, and egg production greatly decrease with cryptosporidial infection.

**SYNONYMS**
N/A

**SEE ALSO**
Aspergillosis
Bordetellosis
Candidiasis
Chlamydiosis
Circovirus (Psittacines)
Circoviruses (Non-Psittacine Birds)
Diarrhea
Enteritis and Gastritis
Flagellate Enteritis
Helminthiasis (Intestinal
*Macrorhabdus ornithogaster*
Mycobacteriosis
Mycoplasmosis
Orthoavulaviruses
Pasteurellosis
Pneumonia
Respiratory Distress
Rhinitis and Sinusitis
Salmonellosis
Trichomoniasis
Undigested Food in Droppings
Urate and Fecal Discoloration
Also individual viral diseases

**ABBREVIATIONS**
C/S—culture and sensitivity
ELISA—enzyme-linked immunosorbent assay
GI—gastrointestinal
HIV—human immunodeficiency virus
IFA—immunofluorescence assay
PCR—polymerase chain reaction

**INTERNET RESOURCES**
N/A

*Suggested Reading*
Azmanis, P., di Somma, A., Pappalardo, L., et al. (2018). First detection of *Cryptosporidium parvum* in falcons (Falconiformes): Diagnosis, molecular sequencing, therapeutic trial and epidemiological assessment of a possible emerging disease in captive falcons. *Veterinary Parasitology*, 252:167–172.
Love, M.S., Choy, R.K. (2021). Emerging treatment options for cryptosporidiosis. *Current Opinion in Infectious Diseases*, 34:455–462.
Ryan, U., Zahedi, A., Feng, Y., Xiao, L. (2021). An update on zoonotic Cryptosporidium species and genotypes in humans. *Animals (Basel)*, 11(11):3307.
Ryan, U.M., Feng, Y., Fayer, R., Xiao, L. (2021). Taxonomy and molecular epidemiology of Cryptosporidium and Giardia: A 50 year perspective (1971–2021). *International Journal for Parasitology*, 51:1099–1119.
Wang, Y., Zhang, K., Chen, Y., et al. (2021). Cryptosporidium and cryptosporidiosis in wild birds: A One Health perspective. *Parasitology Research*, 120:3035–3044.
**Author:** Panagiotis Azmanis DVM, PhD, Dip ECZM (Avian)

# BASICS

## DEFINITION
Dehydration is a loss of body fluids exceeding fluid intake.

## PATHOPHYSIOLOGY
Loss of body fluids leads to both increased blood solute and increased osmolality due to increased sodium levels. Normally, water molecules shift out of cells and into blood to restore the balance between intra- and extracellular spaces. Increased water intake and increased renal water retention serve to restore fluid balance. Dehydration results when restorative mechanisms fail. Severe dehydration can progress to hypovolemia and ultimately to hypovolemic shock.

## SYSTEMS AFFECTED
Circulatory, digestive, urogenital.

## GENETICS
N/A

## INCIDENCE/PREVALENCE
Specific prevalence data are lacking but dehydration can be seen more commonly in hotter months for birds housed in outdoor enclosures, or when only one water bowl or dish is available in a multibird habitat. Dehydration is common with a variety of disease processes.

## GEOGRAPHIC DISTRIBUTION
N/A

## SIGNALMENT
Any avian species of any age/sex can present dehydrated.

## SIGNS
### Historical Findings
Lethargy, depression, anorexia. Firm or smaller than normal stools.

### Physical Examination Findings
Skin tenting. Dry oral mucosa. Dry eyes. Slow refill time of veins once pressure has been released.

## CAUSES
Degenerative/developmental—neonatal crop atony. Anomalous/autoimmune. Metabolic/mechanical—foreign body, impaction, compression of crop, nematodiasis. Nutritional/neoplastic—neoplasia, liver disease, renal disease. Inflammatory/infectious—proventricular dilatation disease, gastritis, septicemia. Traumatic/toxic—gastric ulcer, tube feeding. Blocked water nozzles/empty water dish/competition within enclosure for water dish.

## RISK FACTORS
N/A

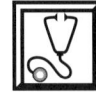

# DIAGNOSIS

## DIFFERENTIAL DIAGNOSIS
N/A

## CBC/BIOCHEMISTRY/URINALYSIS
PCV and TS are used to estimate patient hydration. Measurements should be taken daily to monitor the patient's progress. The author recommends microhematocrit tubes because only the amount of blood collected in the hub of a needle will be required to measure PCV and TS. Plasma electrolytes and osmolality are increased. Bird droppings have three components: feces, uric acid and urates. The fecal portion can be influenced by what the bird is eating and may range in color from brown to green. A suspension of white to cream color flocculent material describes the uric acid and urates. Water and mucus in avian droppings are clear and viscous. Uric acid is the end product of protein metabolism in avian patients. Hepatosynthesis is the primary means of uric acid production. Uric acid is filtered and actively secreted so that 7–16 times as much uric acid is secreted as is filtered. Most secreted uric acid is in the form of an insoluble precipitate. With most uric acid being secreted, blood uric acid levels are unaffected by moderate changes in GFR. During severe dehydration, urine flow is too low move urates through tubules blood uric acid levels are likely to increase. Blood urea concentrations above 10–15 mg/dl are considered elevated for most birds. A notable exception is post prandial uric acid concentrations of carnivorous birds which can be significantly elevated. Birds produce small amounts of urea resulting in low blood concentrations of urea at 1–2 mg/dl. In the hydrated bird, urea is not absorbed but is eliminated through glomerular filtration. Urea is absorbed when birds are dehydrated. Urine specific gravity ranges from 1.005–1.020 g/ml in normal avian patients. Dehydrated birds increase their blood and urine osmolality. The cloaca can absorb water from urine stored there. Urine that moves into the rectum can also have water absorbed into the rectum.

## OTHER LABORATORY TESTS
N/A

## IMAGING
Radiographs may show renal hypoplasia as evidenced by increased air sac diverticulum separating the dorsal renal surface from the ventral synsacrum.

## DIAGNOSTIC PROCEDURES
N/A

## PATHOLOGIC FINDINGS
N/A

# TREATMENT

## APPROPRIATE HEALTH CARE
In addition to treatment of underlying causes of dehydration, both the deficit and maintenance fluids for appropriate hydration should be addressed. Suggested dehydration estimates are: 5% dehydration—subtle skin tenting and loss of elasticity; 10–12% dehydration—pronounced skin tenting, dry eyes and mucous membranes; 12–15% dehydration—skin remains tented, sunken eyes; upper eyelid does not fall back into place once lifted.

## NURSING CARE
For mild dehydration, crystalloids can be administered subcutaneously into the inguinal fold. Severely dehydrated patients and those presenting in hypothermic shock cannot be treated adequately with subcutaneous fluids. For moderate to severe dehydration, IV/IO fluid administration is indicated; oral fluids are not recommended for critically ill patients. The fluid deficit (ml) equals the degree of dehydration (%) multiplied by the patient's body weight in grams. The fluid deficit should be replaced over 12–24 hours in birds without cardiopulmonary compromise and over 24–36 hours if cardiopulmonary compromise exists. Up to 50 ml/kg can be administered as an IV bolus to a bird. In small birds (budgerigars, parakeets and passerines) an IO catheter is more sturdy and practical than an IV catheter. The distal ulna is the preferred site for IO catheterization. A 25-gauge needle can be used for parakeets and budgerigars, while a 27-gauge is recommended for passerines and canaries. Landmarks for correct IO catheter placement are the distal ulna prominence located on the dorsal surface of the ulna just proximal to the carpal joint. Using the non-dominant hand, hold the ulna between the thumb and index finger. With the dominant hand, guide the needle through the bone cortex with a slight twisting motion using the thumb and index finger. The needle should be seated up to the hub. To check correct catheter placement, gently flush a small amount of fluid (0.5–1.0 ml) through the needle. This fluid will be visible and palpable in the basilic vein. If no fluid flows, a bone plug in the needle used to pierce the boney cortex may be present and a new needle of the same or larger gauge may need to be seated. In passerines, the IO catheter can be secured with tape. In larger birds, the catheter can be secured with suture through both the skin and butterfly tape. LRS and other crystalloid solutions are

D

indicated to correct dehydration and the recommended maintenance dose is 50 ml/kg/day. Each 100 ml of LRS contains sodium chloride (0.6 g), sodium lactate (0.31 g), potassium chloride (0.03 g), calcium chloride dehydrate (0.02 g) and water in sufficient quantity. Per liter of LRS, there are 130 mEq sodium, 4 mEq potassium, 3 mEq calcium, 110 mEq chloride, and 28 mEq lactate. Sodium is the major cation of the ECF and functions in the control of water distribution, fluid balance and osmotic pressure. Together with chloride and bicarbonate, sodium regulates the acid–base balance. Potassium, the major cation of ICF, is involved in protein synthesis and carbohydrate utilization, and is important in both muscle contraction and nerve conduction. Chloride, the major ECF anion, also participates in acid–base balance. The cation calcium is involved in bone development, blood clotting, and cardiac/neuromuscular function. Sodium lactate can be oxidized to bicarbonate and/or converted to glycogen.

### ACTIVITY
Hospitalized patients should have restricted activity to prevent not only overexertion but also catheter damage.

### DIET
Fresh vegetables and fruits added to a pelleted diet will increase the patient's water intake.

### CLIENT EDUCATION
Clients should be encouraged to provide multiple water bowls/bottles and also to refill water dishes/bottles daily.

### SURGICAL CONSIDERATIONS
N/A

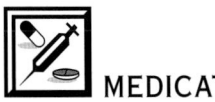 **MEDICATIONS**

### DRUG(S) OF CHOICE
N/A

### CONTRAINDICATIONS
Avoid the use of any potentially nephrotoxic drugs or hypertonic intravenous injections (e.g. radiographic contrast media) in the face of dehydration.

### PRECAUTIONS
N/A

### POSSIBLE INTERACTIONS
N/A

### ALTERNATIVE DRUGS
N/A

 **FOLLOW-UP**

### PATIENT MONITORING
N/A

### PREVENTION/AVOIDANCE
Owners should provide fresh water daily. For birds that soil water with pellets, produce, bedding or excrement, water bottles can be used. Multiple water bowls at multiple levels in the cage may also be used. Water or food dishes should never be placed directly under a perch.

### POSSIBLE COMPLICATIONS
N/A

### EXPECTED COURSE AND PROGNOSIS
Mild dehydration has a better prognosis for being corrected. Moderate and severe dehydration can lead to cell shrinkage, as fluid is pulled out of intracellular spaces and into extracellular spaces. This cell shrinkage can be accompanied with varying degrees of major organ dysfunction, most often affecting the liver and kidneys.

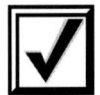 **MISCELLANEOUS**

### ASSOCIATED CONDITIONS
Any problem or disease affecting birds can lead to dehydration. It is important to note that arthritis can lead to dehydration because of the associated pain when moving about the cage to get to the water dish. Visceral and peripheral uric acid deposition may result in severe dehydration and renal dysfunction.

### AGE-RELATED FACTORS
N/A

### ZOONOTIC POTENTIAL
N/A

### FERTILITY/BREEDING
Because dehydration can impact all systems and organs in the body, fertility and breeding can both be negatively impacted due to dehydration.

### SYNONYMS
N/A

### SEE ALSO
Anorexia
Bornaviral Disease (Aquatic Birds)
Bornaviral Disease (Psittaciformes)
Diarrhea
Emaciation
Ileus (Functional Gastrointestinal, Crop Stasis)
Joint Diseases
Lameness
Polydipsea
Polyuria
Regurgitation and Vomiting
Renal Diseases
Sick-Bird Syndrome
Urate and Fecal Discoloration

### ABBREVIATIONS
ECF—extracellular fluid
GFR—glomerular filtration rate
LRS—lactated Ringer's solution
PCV—packed cell volume
TS—total solids

### INTERNET RESOURCES
N/A

*Suggested Reading*
De Matos, R., Morrisey, J.K. (2005). Emergency and critical care of small psittacines and passerines. *Seminars in Avian and Exotic Pet Medicine*, 14:90–105.
Lichtenenberger, M. (2004). Principles of fluid therapy in special species. *Seminars in Avian and Exotic Pet Medicine*, 13:142–153.
Styles D.K., Phalen D.N. (1998). Clinical avian urology. *Seminars in Avian and Exotic Pet Medicine*, 7:104–113.
**Author**: Kemba L. Marshall, MPH, DVM, DABVP (Avian)
**Acknowledgements**: The author wishes to acknowledge the teachers, professors and patients who have allowed her to learn and live out the dreams she had as the eight-year old version of herself.

BASICS

## DEFINITION
Dermatitis is inflammation of the skin. Dermatitis is a non-specific term that encompasses multiple possible clinical presentations and is not a diagnosis or disease. Skin lesions observed in birds with dermatitis can include crusts, scales, hyperkeratosis, lichenification, erosions and ulcerations, nodular thickening and other proliferative changes, erythema, edema, exudate, and pruritus. For details on specific conditions, consult the relevant chapters.

## PATHOPHYSIOLOGY
The pathophysiology of dermatitis varies dependent on the underlying etiology. Characterization of the skin lesions provides a first step to creating a list of differential diagnoses and determining appropriate diagnostics and treatments.

## SYSTEMS AFFECTED
Skin/exocrine—localized, multifocal, or generalized skin lesions may be present. Hemic/lymphatic/immune—blood loss may occur in birds which develop dermatitis as a sequela to self-injurious behavior. Additionally, dermatitis leads to a loss of skin barrier function, which may predispose to (secondary) infections. Dermatitis can involve primary skin disorders, but may also result from underlying systemic diseases, both infectious and non-infectious.

## GENETICS
N/A

## INCIDENCE/PREVALENCE
Varies with the underlying cause but, overall, dermatitis is a common presenting sign in avian species, particularly psittacine birds.

## GEOGRAPHIC DISTRIBUTION
N/A

## SIGNALMENT
**Species**: All avian species are affected, but certain syndromes seem to affect a particular species. Chronic ulcerative dermatitis is a condition that primarily seems to affect (peach-faced) lovebirds (*Agapornis roseicollis*). Grey parrots (*Psittacus erithacus*) seem overrepresented and account for a majority of birds affected with superficial chronic ulterative dermatitis of the ventral wing surface. Amazon parrots (*Amazona* spp.) seem more prone to develop (necrotic) foot dermatitis. Fungal dermatitis (favus) is commonly diagnosed in chickens. Knemidocoptic mange is most commonly reported in budgerigars, finches, and

chickens. Poxvirus infections are commonly noted in chickens, pigeons, passerines, waterfowl, and birds of prey. Cutaneous papillomatosis has been reported in grey parrots, cockatoos, canaries, and finches. Pododermatitis is commonly identified in backyard poultry (chicken, waterfowl), birds of prey, and pet psittacine and passerine birds Photosensitization due to St. John's wort is mostly reported in waterfowl. Lovebird and budgerigar seem over predisposed to polyfolliculitis. Cockatiels have been also affected.
**Mean age and range**: N/A for most causes. Constricted toe is seen in psittacine birds prior to fledging.
**Predominant sex**: None.

## SIGNS
Signs of dermatitis may include one or more of the following. Hyperkeratosis, crusts and/or scales. In case of knemidocoptic mange, the hyperkeratosis is present on the face, cere, feet and/or legs, and often has a honeycombed appearance with small holes. Favus typically presents as white, powdery spots on the comb and feet. Hypovitaminosis A will commonly lead to a dry and flaky skin, hyperkeratosis and scaling, rhinitis, blepharitis, blunting of the choanal papillae, white oral placques and sublingual swelling due to squamous metaplasia of the epithelial surfaces. Erosion or ulceration (defect in or absence of skin) of the skin anywhere on body, including the plantar foot region, (ventral) patagium, axillary region, keel, neck, and uropygial gland region. Erosion or ulceration of the skin is commonly noted in birds with self-injurious behaviors. Nodular thickening or proliferative changes in the skin anywhere on body (including eyelid margins, corner of beak, face, feet, and uropygial gland). Cutaneous or dry pox is characterized by proliferative wartlike lesions on the unfeathered parts such as the beak, eyelids, nostrils, legs, and feet. Papillomatosis also presents as wartlike skin proliferations, which are typically found on the face and feet. Erythema. Swelling or edema. St. John's wort (*Hypericum perforatum*) toxicity leads to photosensitization with subsequent erythema, edema, and pruritus of affected skin on the legs and feet, and may progress to vesicle and bulla formation, serum exudation, ulceration, crust formation, and skin necrosis. In birds with constricted toe syndrome, one or more toes will demonstrate marked swelling and edema of the distal digit, with a thin (< 1 mm) band of constricting tissue encircling its circumference; with time, lesions may become necrotic. Frostbite typically results in

edema of the distal extremities (wing tip). Pruritus, often leading to self-mutilation of the skin. Depending on the underlying cause, lesions may be localized, multifocal, or generalized. Dermatitis can be accompanied with inflammation or infection of the feather follicles, feather-damaging behavior, and/or automutilation.

### General Comments
Lesion type, location, and distribution should be described as specifically as possible. The term "dermatitis" is non-specific and should not be used to describe lesions or as a (differential) diagnosis.

### Historical Findings
Any of the dermatologic signs as listed above may be reported by the owner. History may reveal one of the following predisposing factors. Hypovitaminosis A, bacterial/fungal dermatitis—unbalanced, all-seed diet, or other immunosuppressive conditions. Prior trauma. Pododermatitis—dietary imbalances, suboptimal housing (abrasive surfaces, inappropriate bedding or perches, inadequate hygiene), lack of exercise, medical conditions leading to unilateral weight bearing Poxvirus—outdoor housing, exposure to insect vectors (mosquitos), preventive vaccination, frostbite—exposure to low temperatures (winter months). Constricted toe syndrome—low humidity, entanglement of toes with thin fibers. Photosensitization—exposure to St. John's wort. In case of self-mutilation, a thorough history is warranted to identify potential predisposing factors.

### Physical Examination Findings
One of more of the clinical signs as listed above may be noted on physical examination depending upon the underlying cause. In polyfolliculitis, the affected feathers are often found on the dorsal neck and tail. Several feathers may emerge from one feather shaft. Eventually, fluctuant subcutaneous swellings containing viscid fluid may be observed.

## CAUSES
**Crusts/scales**: *Knemidocoptes* spp. mite infestation. Bacterial dermatitis (e.g. *Staphylococcus aureus*, *Enterobacter cloacae*, *Escherichia coli*). Favus/dermatophytosis (*Trichophyton* spp., *Microsporum gypseum*). Fungal dermatitis (*Aspergillus* spp., *Malassezia* spp., *Mucor* spp., *Candida* spp.). Avian poxvirus. Papillomavirus. Pododermatitis. Hypovitaminosis A, dietary imbalances. Squamous cell carcinoma.
**Erosions and ulcerations**: Ulcerative dermatitis resulting from (self-inflicted) trauma, with or without secondary bacterial

D

or fungal infection. Ulcerative pododermatitis. Avian poxvirus.

**Nodular and/or proliferative changes**: Avian poxvirus. Cutaneous papillomas caused by papillomavirus. Bacterial dermatitis, abscess (e.g. *Mycobacterium* spp., *Nocardia* spp., *E. coli*) Fungal dermatitis (*Cryptococcus* spp., *Aspergillus* spp.). Feather follicle cyst. Neoplasia, including squamous cell carcinoma, basal cell tumor, lipoma, fibrosarcoma, fibroma, lymphosarcoma, melanoma, xanthoma, and uropygial gland tumors.

**Edema**: Photosensitization due to ingestion of St John's wort by waterfowl: St John's wort contains hypericin. Exposure of the skin to direct sunlight allows photons to react with hypericin to create unstable, high-energy molecules. The high-energy molecules create free radicals that increase the permeability of outer cell and lysosomal membranes. This cell membrane damage results in leakage of cellular potassium and cytoplasmic extrusion, and lysosomal membrane damage releases lytic enzymes into the cell. These processes incite inflammation and lead to edema, skin ulceration and necrosis. Constricted toe—no confirmed etiology is known, although low humidity and entanglement with thin fibers have been suggested as contributing factors. Frostbite.

**Pruritus**: Mite infestation—quill or feather mites, blood sucking mites. Bacterial dermatitis. Fungal dermatitis. Hypersensitivity. Contact dermatitis. Non-specific, immune-mediated dermatitis. Hypovitaminosis A, dietary imbalances.

## RISK FACTORS

Vary with the underlying cause. The risk factor for photosensitization is ingestion of St John's wort and exposure to direct sunlight.

# DIAGNOSIS

## DIFFERENTIAL DIAGNOSIS

See Causes section for differential diagnoses of specific skin lesions, and appropriate chapters for additional differential diagnoses for each etiology.

## CBC/BIOCHEMISTRY/URINALYSIS
N/A

## OTHER LABORATORY TESTS
N/A

## IMAGING
N/A

## DIAGNOSTIC PROCEDURES

Cytologic examination of skin lesions (scrapings, tape strip, impression smear, swab, fine-needle aspirate) or feather pulp (feather digest) to diagnose (secondary) bacterial or fungal folliculitis or dermatitis, pox virus, ectoparasites (feather or quill mites, *Knemidocoptes*), neoplasia. C/S of skin lesions and/or feather pulp to diagnose bacterial or fungal dermatitis or folliculitis. Aseptic preparation of the surroundings is required to prevent contamination risk. Next-generation DNA sequencing techniques can also be used to help identify bacterial presence, and generally do so with greater accuracy than traditional culturing methods. Histological evaluation of (paired) skin and feather follicle biopsies can provide a definitive diagnosis of infectious, inflammatory and/or neoplastic skin disease. Intradermal skin testing to diagnose hypersensitivity reactions, allergic skin disease. However, these tests are not reliable in birds due to their thin skin and diminished reaction to histamine. Other diagnostic procedures may apply to diagnose underlying systemic disease.

## PATHOLOGIC FINDINGS

Vary with underlying cause. Photosensitization: Histopathology of skin reveals hyperkeratosis, parakeratosis and edema of the epidermis with areas containing vesicles, crusting and infiltration of polymorphonuclear leukocytes. Hypersensitivity: Histopathology of skin biopsies is non-diagnostic, and reveals perivascular inflammatory cell foci in the dermis and subcutis consisting primarily of mononuclear cells and possibly granulocytes. Traumatic, self-inflicted skin disease: Histopathology reveals superficial dermal scarring with or without inflammation in the affected sites and an absence of inflammation in the unaffected sites.

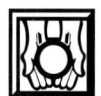

# TREATMENT

## APPROPRIATE HEALTH CARE

Treatment depends on the underlying cause. NSAIDs (e.g. meloxicam) are often beneficial to help alleviate inflammation and pain. Photosensitization—treatment is supportive and starts with removing the bird from access to direct sunlight. Hypersensitivity: Anecdotal evidence supports therapies such as dietary manipulations and essential fatty acid supplementation. There is no direct evidence to support immunotherapy for hypersensitivity in avian species but research is ongoing. Immune-mediated skin disease—use of topical and/or systemic corticosteroids or immune-modulating drugs such as cyclosporine may be considered; caution is warranted with these drugs, given their immunosuppressive effects.

## NURSING CARE

Depends on the cause and general condition of the patient. Protective bandaging may be useful to protect the wound from self-injury and contamination, and promote wound healing. Lesions in areas that are under constant tension, such as the propatagium can be difficult to treat and manage and will require additional use of bandages to temporarily reduce movement and stretching and facilitate healing. Supportive therapy (fluid therapy, assisted feeding) may be warranted in debilitated patients.

## ACTIVITY

Depends on the cause. Immobilization using bandages may be useful, especially if skin lesions are present in areas with a high degree of mobility (e.g. joints).

## DIET

Birds on an all-seed diet may be predisposed to (secondary) infections and hypovitaminosis A; hence, conversion to a balanced (pelleted) diet is advised. Photosensitization: Restrict access to St John's wort. Hypersensitivity: Perform an elimination diet trial as diagnostic test, and cease feeding any foods that are identified as allergens. Essential fatty acid supplementation may be helpful.

## CLIENT EDUCATION

Infectious skin disease is commonly secondary to immunosuppression; hence, optimization of nutrition, husbandry and management are strongly advised. Photosensitization: Restrict access to St John's wort. Owners should be made aware that hypersensitivity in birds is not well understood. Keeping a journal of how their bird reacts to diets, environmental conditions, supplements and treatments is important in managing these cases.

## SURGICAL CONSIDERATIONS
None.

# MEDICATIONS

## DRUG(S) OF CHOICE

NSAIDs (e.g. meloxicam) are often beneficial given their anti-inflammatory and analgesic properties. Photosensitization: Antimicrobial therapy based on C/S, and analgesia, as needed.

## CONTRAINDICATIONS
N/A

## PRECAUTIONS
Topical ointments (e.g. silver sulfadiazine) can be used in birds, but may negatively affect feather quality and waterproofing characteristics. In addition, birds may accidentally ingest the medication while preening, thereby potentially leading to toxicity. Immunosuppressive or immunomodulating drugs may increase the risk for secondary bacterial and/or fungal infections. Appropriate prophylaxis may therefore be indicated. Itraconazole in regular doses has been reported to lead to (hepato)toxicity in grey parrots and should be used with caution in these species. Ivermectin has a relatively narrow safety margin and may potentially induce toxicity in certain species (e.g. finches).

## POSSIBLE INTERACTIONS
N/A

## ALTERNATIVE DRUGS
N/A

## FOLLOW-UP

### PATIENT MONITORING
Depending on the severity and cause, weekly to biweekly rechecks may be advised. Photosensitization, constricted toe, frostbite: Birds should be monitored closely until completely healed. Hypersensitivity: Owners should keep a journal recording how their bird reacts to diets, environmental conditions, supplements and treatments.

### PREVENTION/AVOIDANCE
Eliminate exposure to risk factors and optimize housing, husbandry, and nutrition, where applicable. Vaccination may be possible (e.g. for poxvirus).

### POSSIBLE COMPLICATIONS
Dermatitis and pruritus may predispose to self-injurious behaviors. Secondary bacterial and/or fungal infections are a common sequela to any type of dermatitis or skin trauma. (Severe) skin infections may spread to underlying tissues and/or cause systemic disease (e.g. pododermatitis is known to be a predisposing factor for endocarditis).

## EXPECTED COURSE AND PROGNOSIS
Depends on the ability to identify and eliminate the inciting cause for the dermatitis. Mite infestation, bacterial, and fungal infections generally carry a good prognosis. Photosensitization: The prognosis is good to guarded depending on amount of St John's wort ingested and time in direct sunlight. Hypersensitivity to food has a good prognosis if eliminated from the diet. The prognosis for hypersensitivity to environmental allergens is good to guarded depending on whether the allergen can be identified and controlled.

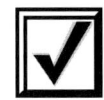
## MISCELLANEOUS

### ASSOCIATED CONDITIONS
N/A

### AGE-RELATED FACTORS
N/A

### ZOONOTIC POTENTIAL
N/A

### FERTILITY/BREEDING
N/A

### SYNONYMS
N/A

### SEE ALSO
Ectoparasites
Feather Cyst
Feather Damaging and Self-Injurious Behavior
Feather Disorders
Hypothermia
Neoplasia (Integument)
Nutritional Imbalances
Papillomatosis (Cutaneous)
Pododermatitis
Poxvirus
Toes and Nails (Diseases of)
Trauma
Xanthoma/Xanthogranulomatosis
Wounds

### ABBREVIATIONS
C/S—culture and sensitivity
NSAIDs—non-steroidal anti-inflammatory drugs

## INTERNET RESOURCES
Barrington, G.M. (2022). Photosensitization in animals. *Merck Veterinary Manual*: http://www.merckmanuals.com/vet/integumentary_system/photosensitization/overview_of_photosensitization.html
Lightfoot, T.L. (2022). Skin and feather disorders of pet birds. *Merck Veterinary Manual*: https://www.merckvetmanual.com/bird-owners/disorders-and-diseases-of-birds/skin-and-feather-disorders-of-pet-birds
Veterian Key. Avian dermatology: https://veteriankey.com/avian-dermatology

*Suggested Reading*
Abou-Zahr, T. (2023). Avian Dermatology. *Veterinary Clinics of North America: Exotic Animal Practice*, 26:327–346.
Carpenter, J.W., Harms, C. (2022). *Exotic Animal Formulary*, 6th edn. St. Louis, MI: Elsevier.
Girling, S. (2006). Dermatology of Birds. In: *Skin Diseases of Exotic Pets* (ed. S. Patterson), 3–14. Oxford, UK: Blackwell Science.
Nett-Mettler, C. (2014). Allergies in birds. In: *Veterinary Allergy* (ed. C. Noli, A. Foster, W. Rosenkrantz), 422–427. Chichester, UK: Wiley.
Schmidt, R.E., Lightfoot, T.L. (2011). Integument. In: *Clinical Avian Medicine* (ed. G. Harrison, T. Lightfoot), Vol. 1, 395–409.
Schmidt, R.E., Reavill, D.R., Phalen, D.N. (2015). Integument. In: *Pathology of Pet and Aviary Birds*, 2nd edn., 237–262. Ames, IA: Wiley.
Worell, A.B. (2013). Dermatological conditions affecting the beak, claws, and feet of captive avian species. *Veterinary Clinics of North America: Exotic Animal Practice*, 16:777–799.

**Author**: Yvonne R. A. van Zeeland, DVM, MVR, PhD, DECZM (Avian, Small Mammal), CPBC, and Nico J. Schoemaker, DVM, PhD, DECZM (Small Mammal, Avian), DABVP (Avian)
**Acknowledgements**: Thomas M. Edling, DVM, MSpVM, MPH, and Heide M. Newton, DVM, DACVD, who wrote the previous version of this topic.

# DIABETES INSIPIDUS

## BASICS

### DEFINITION
Diabetes insipidus (DI) is characterized by the incapacity of the kidney to concentrate the urine, extreme thirst, and the production of large quantities of dilute urine.

### PATHOPHYSIOLOGY
Central DI is the lack of production of AVT, the avian antidiuretic hormone. Nephrogenic DI is the inability of the kidney to respond to AVT.

### SYSTEMS AFFECTED
Endocrine, renal, and central nervous systems.

### GENETICS
Hereditary condition in certain strains of white leghorn chickens. A hereditary form of DI was also diagnosed in a clutch of wild Kākā in New Zealand.

### INCIDENCE/PREVALENCE
Unknown, but DI is uncommonly seen.

### GEOGRAPHIC DISTRIBUTION
N/A

### SIGNALMENT
Central DI has been reported in a grey parrot; it has also been diagnosed in other Psittaciformes. The authors have diagnosed DI in two grey parrots, suggesting that it may be more common in this psittacine species. It is suspected that DI may occur with pituitary neoplasia in budgerigars. Nephrogenic DI has not been reported in Psittaciformes. It is documented as being a hereditary condition in certain strains of white leghorn chickens and has been experimentally induced in quails.

### SIGNS
#### Historical Findings
Severe PU/PD: The degree of PU/PD is usually highly suggestive of DI. Water intake may be as high as 1 l/kg/day. Lethargy, behavioral changes.

#### Physical Examination Findings
Usually no specific clinical signs are seen. Dehydration. Blindness, anisocoria, mydriasis in case of a pituitary mass.

### CAUSES
**Central DI**: Decreased production of AVT by the supraoptic and paraventricular nuclei of the hypothalamus. Decreased release of AVT from the posterior pituitary gland (neurohypophysis)—trauma, neoplasia (e.g. meningioma, pituitary adenoma). PU/PD has been associated in several species (e.g. budgerigars) with an intracranial neoplasia (pituitary adenoma or adenocarcinoma, ependymal tumors). It is possible that these

cases had central DI, but this has not been confirmed. Infection or inflammation. Congenital.
**Nephrogenic DI**: Congenital/hereditary (e.g. white leghorn chickens). Kidney disease (not reported in companion birds). Hypercalcemia.

### RISK FACTORS
Central DI: Unknown, trauma. Nephrogenic DI: Predisposition of white leghorn chickens.

## DIAGNOSIS

### DIFFERENTIAL DIAGNOSIS
**PU/PD**: Behavioral: primary polydipsia—psychogenic polydipsia (published case in a grey parrot, turkeys).
**Other endocrine disease**: Diabetes mellitus, hyperadrenocorticism.
**Diet related**: Diets too rich in salt. Large amount of fruits in the diet (polyuria without polydipsia).
**Organ dysfunction**: Renal failure/medullary washout, Gastroenteritis/cloacitis, cloacal prolapse, severe hepatopathy.
**Infectious diseases**: Paramyxovirus infection in pigeons. Proventricular dilatation disease.
**Toxicosis**: Heavy metal toxicosis, ethylene glycol, aminoglycosides, hypervitaminosis D3.
**Iatrogenic**: Steroids, hormonal therapy. Other: Hypokalemia, hypercalcemia, egg laying, hypoadrenocorticism (not reported in birds).

### CBC/BIOCHEMISTRY/URINALYSIS
Results compatible with dehydration: increased electrolytes (Na, K, Cl), increased hematocrit and increased total solids despite polydipsia. Sodium is particularly high. Mild hyperglycemia may be noted likely due to catecholamine response to hypovolemia. No other abnormalities have been reported in central or nephrogenic DI in birds, but it is reasonable to think that nephrogenic DI could be associated with elevated renal parameters.

### OTHER LABORATORY TESTS
The typically severe PU/PD combined with plasma osmolality measurement and a modified water deprivation test is usually diagnostic. Plasma osmolality: Elevated despite polydipsia (higher than 320 mmol/l in grey parrots). It is suggestive of diabetes insipidus since with psychogenic polydipsia, the plasma osmolality tends to be decreased. UOSM much lower than plasma osmolality (e.g., 40–60 mmol/l). USG can be useful to approximate the urine osmolality; in Hispaniolan Amazon parrots, UOSM = (−57) + 25749(USG-1) with

USG measured with a canine specific gravity scale on a veterinary refractometer.

### IMAGING
**MRI**: Gold standard to investigate central DI—may reveal an intracranial lesion (neoplasia, vascular anomaly). CT is not as sensitive as MRI but could also be useful to identify pituitary lesions.
**Radiographs and coelomic ultrasound**: May be useful in suspected cases of nephrogenic DI to evaluate the size and aspect of the kidneys, but are not sensitive. Avian kidneys are usually not visible on ultrasound without concurrent coelomic distention.
**Coelioscopy**: Gold standard in suspected cases of nephrogenic DI, to visualize the kidneys and perform a biopsy for histology. Histopathology may not confirm nephrogenic diabetes insipidus in the absence of renal lesions.

### DIAGNOSTIC PROCEDURES
**Water deprivation test**: Should be performed in hospital to diagnose diabetes insipidus. Owing to the significant risks of rapid dehydration during a water deprivation test, it is suggested to closely monitor the patient and adapt the water deprivation test to the patient's condition. Plasma and urine osmolality should be measured prior to the procedure. Water is withdrawn from the bird. Plasma and urine osmolalities are measured 1–2 hours after water removal (these tests can be repeated more frequently in larger birds). The bird's weight should be periodically monitored during the procedure and the patient should not lose more than 10% body weight overall. In central and nephrogenic DI, the plasma osmolality rapidly increases and the urine osmolality stays very low. In psychogenic polydyspia, the urine osmolality increases and the plasma osmolality may slightly increase.
**Antidiuretic hormone response test:** Performed to differentiate central DI from nephrogenic DI. Arginine vasopressin (suggested dose: 10–20 µg/kg) or arginine vasotocin (suggested dose 5–10 µg/kg) is administered to the bird (conjunctival, intranasal, or intramuscular). Plasma and urine osmolalities are measured 1–2 hours after the treatment (these tests may be repeated more frequently in larger birds). In central DI, the plasma osmolality should stabilize itself and the urine osmolality should increase. In nephrogenic DI, the bird continues to lose weight, the plasma osmolality continues to increase and the urine osmolality stays very low.

### PATHOLOGIC FINDINGS
Pituitary masses may be seen. Renal lesions may be observed.

# TREATMENT

## APPROPRIATE HEALTH CARE
Birds should have access to water at all time. If dehydrated, fluid therapy may be indicated (subcutaneous or intravenous/intraosseous if the dehydration is severe).

## NURSING CARE
N/A

## ACTIVITY
N/A

## DIET
Central DI: N/A. Nephrogenic DI: If kidney disease is suspected, a prescription diet with good quality proteins could be recommended. A diet low in sodium may be useful.

## CLIENT EDUCATION
Inform the client that the clinical management of the disease is complex, that the treatment is lifelong, that the bird should have unlimited access to water at all time.

## SURGICAL CONSIDERATIONS
N/A

# MEDICATIONS

## DRUG(S) OF CHOICE
**Central DI**: Arginine vasopressin (mammalian hormone) 20 µg/kg b.i.d. Best results intramuscular, but intraconjunctival administration has been reported as well. May also be given intranasal. Only seems to be partially effective in birds. Arginine vasotocin (avian hormone) 0.5–12 µg/kg b.i.d. intranasal or conjunctival. The drug is available from research companies (e.g. Sigma) and needs to be compounded. Has been associated with successful results in a case of central DI in a grey parrot seen by the authors. Start with a lower dose, monitor the progression of the disease and increase the dose if necessary. AVT decreases GFR, mostly in the loopless nephrons, increases water reabsorption through aquaporins in the collective duct, and it may also stimulate water reabsorption in the colon. With severe and long standing polyuria, response to

antidiuretic therapy may be delayed due to renal medullary washout.
**Nephrogenic DI**: Treatment of the underlying cause if possible. Hydrochlorothiazide is a diuretic that has been proven to decrease urine output in human patients with nephrogenic diabetes insipidus. The response may be mild, however.

## CONTRAINDICATIONS
N/A

## PRECAUTIONS
N/A

## POSSIBLE INTERACTIONS
N/A

## ALTERNATIVE DRUGS
N/A

# FOLLOW-UP

## PATIENT MONITORING
Water intake monitoring at home by the owner. Plasma osmolality to monitor treatment efficacy. Urine osmolality to monitor treatment efficacy. Daily water consumption log.

## PREVENTION/AVOIDANCE
N/A

## POSSIBLE COMPLICATIONS
Dehydration and death if no access to water even for a short period.

## EXPECTED COURSE AND PROGNOSIS
Guarded.

# MISCELLANEOUS

## ASSOCIATED CONDITIONS
N/A

## AGE-RELATED FACTORS
N/A

## ZOONOTIC POTENTIAL
N/A

## FERTILITY/BREEDING
N/A

## SYNONYMS
N/A

## SEE ALSO
Bornaviral Disease (Psittaciformes)
Chronic Egg Laying
Cloacal Diseases
Dehydration
Diarrhea
Egg Yolk and Reproductive Coelomitis
Enteritis and Gastritis
Diabetes Mellitus and Hyperglycemia
Liver Disease
Neoplasia (Neurological)
Neurologic (Non-Traumatic Diseases)
Nutritional Imbalances
Orthoavulaviruses
Pancreatic Diseases
Polydipsia
Polyuria
Renal Diseases
Toxicosis (Heavy Metals)
Vitamin D Toxicosis

## ABBREVIATIONS
AVT—arginine vasotocin
CT—computed tomography
DI—diabetes insipidus
GFR—glomerular filtration rate
MRI—magnetic resonance imaging
PD—polydipsia
PU—polyuria
UOSM—urine osmolality
USG—urine specific gravity

## INTERNET RESOURCES
N/A

*Suggested Reading*
Brummermann, M., Braun, E.J. (1995). Renal response of roosters with diabetes insipidus to infusions of arginine vasotocin. *American Journal of Physiology. Regulatory, Integrative and Comparative Physiology*, 269:R57–63.
Lumeij, J.T., Westerhof, I. (1998). The use of the water deprivation test for the diagnosis of apparent psychogenic polydipsia in a socially deprived African grey parrot (*Psittacus erithacus erithacus*). *Avian Pathology*, 17: 875–878.
Starkey, S.R., Wood, C., de Matos, R., et al. (2010). Central diabetes insipidus in an African Grey parrot. *ournal of the American Veterinary Medical Association*, 237:415–419.
**Authors**: Delphine Laniesse, DVM, DVSc, DECZM (Avian), and Hugues Beaufrère, Dr Med Vet, PhD, DABVP (Avian), DECZM (Avian), DACZM

# DIABETES MELLITUS AND HYPERGLYCEMIA

## BASICS

### DEFINITION
Hyperglycemia is defined as an abnormal elevation of serum blood glucose. Although reference ranges may vary between species, hyperglycemia is generally suspected in birds when glucose levels exceed 20 mmol/l (350 mg/dl) and confirmed when > 28 mmol/l (500 mg/dl). Diabetes mellitus (DM) is a disease caused by (i) an inherited or an acquired deficiency in insulin production by the pancreas, (ii) by the ineffectiveness of the insulin produced on target tissues, or (iii) by glucagon excess, which can all result in hyperglycemia and associated clinical signs.

### PATHOPHYSIOLOGY
Hyperglycemia results from DM caused by a defect in insulin secretion (destruction/absence of the Langerhans pancreatic islets), insulin action (insulin resistance), or both of these mechanisms. Action of stress hormones or drugs on insulin and glucose metabolism. The relative importance of glucagon and insulin in avian metabolism and the pathogenesis of DM have been extensively discussed in several avian species. Most studies suggest that avian DM may be caused by an excess of glucagon and not a deficiency of insulin. However, recent cases using validated insulin assays and immunohistochemistry on tissue showed the existence of type 1 DM in some individual birds. When hyperglycemia persists over time, the glucose reabsorption threshold is reached within the kidneys, and glucose will be excreted in the urine. This leads to an increase in urine osmotic pressure, which inhibits the renal reabsorption of water, resulting in polyuria, secondary dehydration, and compensating polydipsia. The lack of insulin or insulin resistance will promote the release of free fatty acids from lipid storage sites as a source of energy, which is converted by the liver into ketone bodies. Ketoacidosis will occur once the body reaches its buffering capacity.

### SYSTEMS AFFECTED
Endocrine/metabolic, renal/urologic, behavioral, gastrointestinal, hemic/lymphatic/immune, Neuromuscular, reproductive.

### GENETICS
Unknown.

### INCIDENCE/PREVALENCE
Stress hyperglycemia is very common. DM is rare.

### GEOGRAPHIC DISTRIBUTION
None.

### SIGNALMENT
Macaws, toucans, cockatiels, and budgerigars seem to be more susceptible. It is more common in adults. No predominant sex.

### SIGNS
#### Historical Findings
Polyuria, polydipsia, polyphagia, weight loss, lethargy, abnormal behavior.

#### Physical Examination Findings
Poor body condition.

### CAUSES
**For moderate hyperglycemia**: Stress and pain. Corticosteroids, medroxyprogesterone. Female reproductive activity/disease.
**For severe hyperglycemia/DM**: Obesity. Inappropriate diet. Pancreatitis. Bacterial (Chlamydia, Gram negative); viral (paramyxovirus 3, herpesvirus, polyomavirus, adenovirus, poxvirus); inflammatory; hemosiderosis; amyloidosis; hypervitaminosis a; secondary to egg-yolk coelomitis; Chronic zinc toxicity. Genetics. Neoplasia. Pancreatectomy.

### RISK FACTORS
Female in reproductive phase. Inappropriate diet (e.g. dog food diet for toucans, highly refined sugar diet for parrots).

## DIAGNOSIS

### DIFFERENTIAL DIAGNOSIS
**PU/PD associated with systemic signs**: Renal disease—heavy metal poisoning; nephritis; nephrotoxicity; gout; urolith; neoplasia; hypercalcemia. Reproductive disease—egg binding. Sepsis. Nutritional—hypovitaminosis A, hypervitaminosis D, excess dietary sodium. Iatrogenic—aminoglycosides; allopurinol; sulfonamides; tetracyclines; cephalosporins; cloacolith.
**PU/PD associated without systemic signs**: Can be physiologic during breeding season. Stress associated with handling, transport, and the environment. High water content of food (fruits). Psychogenic polydipsia.

### CBC/BIOCHEMISTRY/URINALYSIS
Hematology varies with the underlying cause. Biochemistry—increased blood glucose, triglycerides, cholesterol, B-hydroxybutyric acid and hepatic enzymes. Possibly elevated lipase and amylase with pancreatitis. Blood gas analysis for ketoacidosis. Handheld glucometers have been shown to be unreliable

in birds. Use of laboratory analyzer should therefore be favored as much as possible.

### OTHER LABORATORY TESTS
Fructosamines result from an irreversible, nonenzymatic, insulin-independent binding of glucose to serum proteins. This glycosylation reaction occurs throughout the life span of albumin and is proportional to the glucose concentration over that period of time (1–3 weeks in cats and dogs). Because the half life of avian serum proteins is notably lower than in domestic mammals, fructosamines may reflect the blood glucose state of diabetic birds over a shorter period. Fructosamine blood levels in clinically normal psittacine birds were between 113 and 238 μmol/l, and diabetic birds usually have values >300 μmol/l. Urinalysis: Usually not helpful as samples are often contaminated with feces. However, the massive polyuria observed in diabetic birds allows for better separation of the urine from the feces to reduce contamination. Monitoring of glucose and ketones in the urine is not invasive and may be useful in small species like budgerigars. However, interpretation remains questionable. Choanal and cloacal swabs, blood, and feathers for PCR for both *Chlamydia psittaci* and avian polyomavirus, which are noted as potential causes of pancreatitis in birds. Measurement of serum insulin concentration by radioimmunoassay. Measurement of blood zinc levels.

### IMAGING
Radiography and ultrasonography can be useful to rule out other causes of PU/PD.

### DIAGNOSTIC PROCEDURES
Pancreatic biopsy. Liver biopsy in toucans (hemosiderosis).

### PATHOLOGIC FINDINGS
No gross lesions. Hypoplasia, atrophy, and/or vacuolization of islet cells. Inflammation is rare with DM.

## TREATMENT

### APPROPRIATE HEALTH CARE
Diabetic patients generally require emergency inpatient care management as they often present with ketoacidosis.

### NURSING CARE
Aggressive fluid therapy, including correction of any acid–base or electrolyte imbalance (potassium, bicarbonate). Placement in a warm incubator in a low stress environment. Assisted feeding as needed. Control of

concurrent inflammatory and/or infectious diseases.

## ACTIVITY
N/A

## DIET
Low carbohydrate and low-fat diet is generally recommended. However, drastic changes in the diet should be made only when the bird is stable.

## CLIENT EDUCATION
Treatment of DM is difficult and requires multiple adjustments over time. Insulin therapy might require teaching proper IM injection techniques to the clients.

## SURGICAL CONSIDERATIONS
Birds with DM should ideally be stabilized before undergoing a surgery.

 **MEDICATIONS**

## DRUG(S) OF CHOICE
Insulin 0.3–1.3 iu/kg q12h IM, to be adjusted according to the clinical signs and glucose curves. Insulin preparations available to the practitioner are in a constant state of change. Many varieties of insulin that have been used in avian cases in the past are no longer available. Glipizide 0.3–1 mg/kg q12h PO. Highly variable results.

## CONTRAINDICATIONS
Insulin is contraindicated in case of hypoglycemia and severe allergy to bovine, porcine or human insulin proteins. Glipizide is contraindicated in case of severe burns, severe trauma, severe infection, diabetic coma or other hypoglycemic conditions, major surgery, ketosis, ketoacidosis, or other significant acidotic conditions.

## PRECAUTIONS
Insulin should not be injected at the same site every time or lipodystrophic reactions could occur. Insulin overdose can induce hypoglycemia. Glipizide should only be used with extreme caution with untreated endocrine dysfunctions; renal or hepatic function impairment; prolonged vomiting; emaciation or debilitated condition.

## POSSIBLE INTERACTIONS
Insulin has shown interaction in mammals with many drugs including beta blockers, enalapril, diltiazem, MAO inhibitors, fluoxetine, sulfonamides, and corticosteroids. Glipizide has shown interaction in mammals with many drugs including antifungal azoles, beta blockers, chloramphenicol, corticosteroids, MAO inhibitors, and sulfonamides.

## ALTERNATIVE DRUGS
Synthetic somatostatins have been used successfully in one avian case.

 **FOLLOW-UP**

## PATIENT MONITORING
Daily monitoring of clinical signs and body weight. Blood glucose curves. No standard protocol exists for birds. Therefore, blood glucose curves can be done using the clinician judgment, as it is not always possible to draw blood from birds every hour for a prolonged period of time. Fructosamine levels.

## PREVENTION/AVOIDANCE
Feed an appropriate diet for the species. Avoid contact with other birds to diminish the risks of an infectious pancreatitis.

## POSSIBLE COMPLICATIONS
Diabetic ketoacidosis and insulin overdose are life-threatening conditions.

## EXPECTED COURSE AND PROGNOSIS
Prognosis greatly varies with the primary cause, which might never be known. Birds are very unpredictable in their response to insulin therapy. Adjustments of the therapy may take weeks.

 **MISCELLANEOUS**

## ASSOCIATED CONDITIONS
Hemosiderosis in toucans.

## AGE-RELATED FACTORS
N/A

## ZOONOTIC POTENTIAL
N/A

## FERTILITY/BREEDING
Birds with DM might not be breeding actively if not stable.

## SYNONYMS
N/A

## SEE ALSO
Adenoviruses
Ascites
Chlamydiosis
Chronic Egg Laying
Coelomic Distention
Dehydration
Diabetes Insipidus
Diarrhea
Egg Yolk and Reproductive Coelomitis
Hepatic Lipidosis
Herpesvirus (Columbid herpesvirus 1, in Pigeons and Raptors)
Herpesvirus (Duck Viral Enteritis)
Herpesvirus (Passerine Birds)
Herpesvirus (Psittacid Herpesviruses)
Iron Storage Disease
Liver Disease
Neoplasias
Nutritional Imbalances
Obesity
Ocular Lesions
Orthoavulaviruses
Pancreatic Diseases
Polydipsia
Polyuria
Poxvirus
Renal Diseases
Oviductal Diseases
Sick-Bird Syndrome
Urate and Fecal Discoloration

## ABBREVIATIONS
DM—diabetes mellitus
MAO—monoamine oxidase inhibitor
PCR—polymerase chain reaction
PD—polydipsia
PU—polyuria

## INTERNET RESOURCES
N/A

*Suggested Reading*
Desmarchelier, M., Langlois, I. (2008). Diabetes mellitus in a Nanday conure (*Nandayus nenday*). *Journal of Avian Medicine and Surgery*, 22:246–254.
Hazelwood, R.L. (2000). Pancreas. In: *Sturkie's Avian Physiology*, 5th edn. (ed. G.C. Whittow), 539–555. St. Louis, MO: Academic Press.
Lumeij, J.T. (1994). Endocrinology. In: *Avian Medicine: Principles and Application* (ed. B.W. Ritchie, G.J. Harrison, L.R. Harrison), 582–606. Lake Worth, FL: Wingers Publishing.
Oglesbee, B. (1997). Diseases of the endocrine system. In: *Avian Medicine and Surgery* (ed. R.B. Altman, S.L. Clubb, G.M. Dorrestein, K. Quesenberry), 482–488. Philadelphia, PA: Saunders.
Rae, M. (2000). Avian endocrine disorders. In: *Laboratory Medicine: Avian and Exotic Pets* (ed. A.M. Fudge), 76–89. Philadelphia, PA: Saunders.
**Author:** Marion Desmarchelier, DMV, MSc, DACZM, DECZM (Zoo Health Management), DACVB
**Acknowledgements:** Shannon Ferrell, DVM, DABVP (Avian), DACZM

# DIARRHEA

## BASICS

### DEFINITION
Abnormally increased frequency, liquidity and volume of fecal discharge.

### PATHOPHYSIOLOGY
Imbalance of intestinal absorption, secretion, and/or motility. Impaired absorption can result from inflammation (enteritis), maldigestion (PDD, pancreatitis, neoplasia), dietary malassimilation, osmotically active agents (fiber), toxins (heavy metals), and hemorrhage (neoplasia). Increased secretion and motility frequently result from infectious agents (bacterial, parasitic, and viral infections) that stimulate intestinal epithelial cell hypersecretion.

### SYSTEMS AFFECTED
GI; cardiovascular—compromise to collapse with excessive fluid losses; endocrine/metabolic—dehydration, fluid, electrolyte, acid–base abnormalities.

### GENETICS
No specific genetic or breed predisposition.

### INCIDENCE/PREVALENCE
Diarrhea is a relatively common problem encountered in birds.

### GEOGRAPHIC DISTRIBUTION
N/A

### SIGNALMENT
No specific breed, age, or sex predilection.

### SIGNS
#### Historical Findings
Abnormal liquid or unformed stool. Abnormal coloration of stool. Undigested food in stool. Soiled vent feathers. Polyuria/polydipsia. Vomiting. Anorexia. Depression.

#### Physical Examination Findings
Dehydration. Emaciation. Weakness. Soiled vent feathers.

### CAUSES
Bacterial infection—*Campylobacter* spp., *Chlamydia psittaci*, *Escherichia coli*, *Pseudomonas* spp., *Aeromonas* spp., *Salmonella* spp., *Citrobacter* spp. Viral infection—adenovirus, avian polyomavirus, herpesvirus, circovirus, PDD (bornavirus), paramyxovirus. Parasite infection—Coccidia, *Cryptosporidia* spp., *Microsporidia* spp., *Giardia* spp., *Hexamita* spp. Obstruction—foreign bodies, neoplasia, parasites. Metabolic disorders—liver disease (atoxoplasmosis), renal disease. Dietary—changes/intolerance, foods with increased water/fiber content, contaminated food. Maldigestion—pancreatitis, hepatobiliary disease, malabsorption syndrome, intestinal neoplasia, stress, and anorexia. Drugs and toxins—heavy metals (lead, zinc), pesticides, plant toxins.

### RISK FACTORS
Exposure to other birds carrying disease. Abrupt dietary changes. Inappropriate diet. Inappropriate environment (heavy metal exposure from cage, toys, paint).

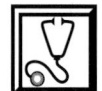

## DIAGNOSIS

### DIFFERENTIAL DIAGNOSIS
Normal stools can be loose, but without increased frequency, discoloration, or undigested food elements. Certain species (e.g. lories) normally have more liquid stools from diet. Polyuria (formed stool with a large volume of surrounding urine) can mimic diarrhea. High volume secretory diarrhea suggests possible infectious etiology. Concomitant neurologic signs suggests possible heavy metal toxicity or toxins.

### CBC/BIOCHEMISTRY/URINALYSIS
Leukocytosis with heterophilia may be seen with gastroenteritis resulting from bacterial infection. Hypochromic, regenerative anemia can be seen with lead toxicity and gastric ulceration/bleeding. Amylase may be elevated with underlying pancreatitis or enteritis (levels are normally higher in avian species). Abnormal renal and/or hepatic laboratory values may indicate additional etiologic causes.

### OTHER LABORATORY TESTS
Gram stains and cultures of fecal, cloacal, crop, and/or proventricular swabs. Cytologic examination of fecal, cloacal, crop, and/or proventricular lavage fluid. Fecal Gram stain for assessment of intestinal flora. Direct fecal examination for protozoal parasite evaluation. Fecal flotation for intestinal parasite examination. Heavy metal testing: Normal lead blood level in birds is < 2.5 ppm. 0.25 ppm is significant when associated with clinical signs; > 0.5 ppm is high regardless of findings. Normal zinc blood level in parrots is < 2.5 ppm. 2.6–3.4 ppm is above normal; 3.5–4.4 ppm is high; > 4.5 ppm is toxic.

### IMAGING
Survey whole-body radiographs may indicate obstruction, foreign body, mass, organomegaly. Contrast radiography or ultrasonography may find mucosal irregularities, thickening of the bowel wall or mass effect. Contrast radiography/fluoroscopy can be used to assess GI motility.

### DIAGNOSTIC PROCEDURES
Endoscopy of the upper GI tract or cloaca can be performed if evidence of masses. Removal of foreign bodies, biopsy/impression smears of abnormal masses or other organs (e.g. kidney, liver) if indicated.

### PATHOLOGIC FINDINGS
Evidence of enteritis (mucosal inflammation and damage/ulceration) should be present in mucosal biopsies from patients with infectious diarrhea.

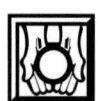

## TREATMENT

### APPROPRIATE HEALTH CARE
Treatment must be specific to the underlying cause to be successful. Mild disease (dietary modifications, mild infections) can be treated as an outpatient, more moderate to severe disease (infection, chronic disease, toxins) generally require hospitalization for parenteral therapy and fluid management.

### NURSING CARE
Administer warmed crystalloid fluids SQ, IV, IO (100–150 ml/kg/day maintenance plus dehydration and deficit correction) at a rate of 10–25 ml/kg over a 5-minute period or at a continuous rate of 100 ml/kg/q24h. Increase environmental temperature to 85–90°F (29–32°C). Provide a humidified environment by placing warm moist towels in the incubator. Nutritional support is required in most cases.

### ACTIVITY
Patients should be rested in a quiet environment to minimize additional stressors.

### DIET
Dependent on the underlying cause and patient ability to consume food. Diets developed for recovery and nutritional support designed to provide easily digestible nutrients and high energy. Gavage/tube feeding formula (20–30 m./kg q6–12h).

### CLIENT EDUCATION
Review of proper dietary requirements. Review of sources of heavy metal toxicity, when indicated. Care for additional birds in the home, especially for infectious diarrhea.

### SURGICAL CONSIDERATIONS
Exploratory endoscopy and other surgical procedures should only be pursued if there is evidence of obstruction/mass. For heavy-metal foreign bodies, patients should be stabilized and on chelation therapy before any surgical procedure is attempted. Surgical removal of objects from the gastrointestinal

tract can be done endoscopically (or with magnets for metals), but proventriculotomy or enterotomy procedures may be necessary if other attempts to remove foreign objects fail.

## MEDICATIONS

### DRUG(S) OF CHOICE
Appropriate antimicrobial therapy based on culture and sensitivity and suitable diagnostic testing. Appropriate antiparasitic medication based on culture and sensitivity. Chelation therapy, if indicated.

### CONTRAINDICATIONS
Cathartics may cause diarrhea and are contraindicated in birds that present with diarrhea, dehydration, and hypovolemia.

### PRECAUTIONS
Use caution when initiating antibiotic therapy unless bacterial infection is suspected from initial diagnostic testing, as this may worsen diarrhea or cause anorexia.

### POSSIBLE INTERACTIONS
D-penicillamine should not be given if lead is present in the gastrointestinal tract (increases absorption of heavy metal particles).

### ALTERNATIVE DRUGS
Sucralfate (25 mg/kg PO q8h)—esophageal, crop, and gastrointestinal protectant. Kaolin/pectin (2 ml/kg PO q6–12h)—intestinal protectant, antidiarrheal. Bismuth subsalicylate (1–2 ml/kg PO q12h)—intestinal protectant, antidiarrheal. Cimetidine (5 mg/kg PO, IM q8–12h)—proventriculitis, gastric ulceration.

## FOLLOW-UP

### PATIENT MONITORING
Monitor hydration status and weight on a daily basis while hospitalized. Monitor eating habits and/or response to gavage/tube feeding. Monitor stool volume, consistency, color, and odor as a response to treatment. Repeat CBC and plasma chemistry panel to monitor treatment response and recovery approximately one week following initiation

of treatment. If parasites and/or microorganisms are the primary cause of diarrhea, retest for treatment response and status of infection following completion of treatment.

### PREVENTION/AVOIDANCE
Provide an appropriate fresh diet and clean (filtered) drinking water. Reduce environmental stress and sources of toxin exposure. Quarantine all new birds and those that have been exposed to other avian species for a minimum of 30 days.

### POSSIBLE COMPLICATIONS
Diarrhea may worsen/persist following treatment due to severe infection, continued environmental exposure, additional stressors and exposures, and multifactorial disease.

### EXPECTED COURSE AND PROGNOSIS
Acute cases with a diagnosed treatable cause have a good prognosis toward complete resolution. Chronic cases in sick patients have a more guarded prognosis. For severe diarrhea in patients with untreatable conditions (e.g. circovirus, PDD) the prognosis is eventually grave despite apparent recovery of the acute event.

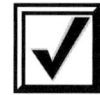

## MISCELLANEOUS

### ASSOCIATED CONDITIONS
Dehydration, hypovolemic cardiovascular and renal failure. Septicemia. Anorexia, cachexia. Anemia, hypoalbuminemia.

### AGE-RELATED FACTORS
N/A

### ZOONOTIC POTENTIAL
*Chlamydia psittaci*, *Giardia*, *Salmonellosis* sp.

### FERTILITY/BREEDING
N/A

### SYNONYMS
Pasty vent

### SEE ALSO
Bornaviral Disease (Aquatic Birds)
Bornaviral Disease (Psittaciformes)
Cloacal Diseases
Enteritis and Gastritis
Flagellate Enteritis

Foreign Body (Gastrointestinal)
Helminthiasis (Gastrointestinal)
Liver Disease
Polyuria
Renal Diseases
Sick-Bird Syndrome
Toxicosis (Heavy Metals)
Undigested Food In Droppings
Urate and Fecal Discoloration
Appendix 8, Algorithm 2: Diarrhea

### ABBREVIATIONS
CBC—complete blood count
GI—gastrointestinal
PDD—proventricular dilatation disease

### INTERNET RESOURCES
LafeberVet (resource for exotic animal veterinary professionals): https://lafeber.com/vet

*Suggested Reading*
Bauck, L. (2000). Abnormal droppings. In: *Manual of Avian Medicine* (ed. G.H. Olsen, S.E. Orosz, S.E.), 62–70. St Louis, MO: Mosby.
Gelis, S. (2006). Evaluating and treating the gastrointestinal system. In: *Clinical Avian Medicine* (ed. G.J. Harrison, T.L. Lightfoot), 411–440. Palm Beach, FL: Spix Publishing.
Hadley, T.L. (2005). Disorders of the psittacine gastrointestinal tract. *Veterinary Clinics of North America. Exotic Animal Practice*, 8:329–349.
Jones, M.P., Pollock, C.G. (2000). Supportive care and shock. In: *Manual of Avian Medicine* (ed. G.H. Olsen, S.E. Orosz, S.E.), 17–46. St Louis, MO: Mosby.
Monks, D. (2005). Gastrointestinal disease. In: *BSAVA Manual of Psittacine Birds*, 2nd edn. (ed. N. Harcourt-Brown, J. Chitty), 180–190. Quedgeley, UK: British Small Animal Veterinary Association.
Oglesbee, B.L. (1997). Differential diagnosis. In: *Avian Medicine and Surgery* (ed. R.B. Altman, S.L. Clubb, G.M. Dorrestein, K. Queensberry), 225–226. Philadelphia, PA: Saunders.
**Author**: Rodney Schnellbacher DVM, ACZM
**Acknowledgements**: updated from first edition chapter authored by Julie DeCubellis, DVM, MS

# DISCOSPONDYLITIS

## BASICS

### DEFINITION
Discospondylitis is a primary infection of the cartilaginous vertebral end plates, with secondary involvement of the intervertebral disc and adjacent bone of the vertebral body (epiphyses). It is important to distinguish this disease from other vertebral infections, including spondylitis. Spondylitis, or vertebral body osteomyelitis, is an infection of the vertebral body. Although considered a distinct entity, spondylitis frequently coexists with discospondylitis. In poultry, enterococcal spondylitis is an emerging disease causing epidemic spinal infections.

### PATHOPHYSIOLOGY
The pathophysiology of discospondylitis in birds is unclear. Hematogenous spread from an underlying source of infection is considered the most likely cause of endogenous infection. Direct extension of infection from paravertebral tissue secondary to a migrating foreign body is reported in dogs but has not been reported in birds. Iatrogenic infection is also not reported in birds, as spinal surgery is much less commonly performed compared with humans and dogs. Traumatic and infectious lesions of the vertebral column, including discospondylitis, are most commonly reported in the free thoracic vertebrae (FTV) of birds. A singular FTV is present in the trunk of most bird species. This is most commonly the penultimate thoracic vertebra, located between the notarium cranially and the synsacrum caudally, and is considered a weak point within the vertebral column. Suggested causes for the increased prevalence of disease at this location include increased mechanical stress at this point due to a lever effect between the notarium and synsacrum, increased vascularization, and microtrauma. Neurologic dysfunction may result in cases of discospondylitis from severe proliferation of fibrous tissue and bone at the site of infection and inflammation. In rare cases, collapse of the intervertebral space and/ or pathologic vertebral fracture may also occur resulting in spinal cord compression. Transmission of pathogenic *Enterococcus cecorum*, the cause of enterococcal spondylitis of poultry, is through the fecal–oral route. Intestinal colonization and subsequent bacteremia occur as early as the first week of life. Spread to and infection of the FTV occurs at 3 weeks. Although initially suspected, clinical intestinal disease is not required to allow bacteremia. The source of the infection in poultry is unclear as the bacterium is not detected in the environment prior to or following the growing period and vertical transmission has not been demonstrated.

### SYSTEMS AFFECTED
Musculoskeletal, nervous, neuromuscular.

### GENETICS
There is no genetic basis for discospondylitis. Higher susceptibility of broilers to enterococcal spondylitis secondary to genetic selection is suspected.

### INCIDENCE/PREVALENCE
Prevalence of discospondylitis in birds is unknown but suspected to be very low, based on the few confirmed reports. Spondylitis (vertebral body osteomyelitis) is more commonly reported in birds, especially poultry. Prevalence of greater than 5% has been reported in broiler flocks.

### GEOGRAPHIC DISTRIBUTION
No geographic distribution has been reported for discospondylitis. Enterococcal spondylitis has a worldwide distribution with outbreaks reported in Europe, South Africa, Iran, Brazil, Canada, and the USA.

### SIGNALMENT
**Species**: Confirmed cases of discospondylitis have been reported in a white stork (*Ciconia ciconia*), yellow-eyed penguin (*Megadyptes antipodes*), black-footed penguin (*Spheniscus demersus*), and greater flamingo (*Phoenicopterus roseus*). Penguins are predisposed to nontraumatic spinal disorders and may also be at increased risk of discospondylitis; however, this has not been confirmed. Clinical signs and radiographic lesions consistent with discospondylitis have been reported in a peregrine falcon (*Falco peregrinus*); however, vertebral osteomyelitis was considered more likely, based on the young age and kyphotic angulation of the spine. It is suspected that vertebral osteomyelitis may have been confused with vertebral physitis in this case. A case of multicentric septic osteomyelitis and arthritis was reported in a gyrfalcon (*Falco rusticolus*), with radiographic and histopathologic lesions also supportive of discospondylitis. Spondylitis is commonly reported in poultry and less commonly in birds of prey and psittacine birds.
**Breed predilections**: None reported for discospondylitis. Enterococcal spondylitis affects broilers and broiler breeders.
**Mean age and range**: Due to the low number of reported avian cases of discospondylitis, conclusions regarding the common signalment for this disease are limited. No common age pattern has been identified. Ages of the reported cases were 8 months, 1 year, 22 years, and unknown. The peregrine falcon with similar lesions was 6 weeks of age, and the gyrfalcon was 2 years old. Enterococcal spondylitis affects young broilers with clinical signs starting between 1 and 18 weeks of age but most commonly reported between 5 and 8 weeks.

**Predominant sex**: No sex predilection exists for discospondylitis in birds. Enterococcal spondylitis in chicken predominantly affects males; females are rarely affected.

### SIGNS
#### Historical Findings
Clinical signs of discospondylitis may be vague and associated with general malaise, including lethargy, hyporexia or anorexia, and weight loss. Alterations in posture and gait are often the first symptoms reported by caregivers. Gait change may range from mild lameness to paralysis and immobility. Patients are commonly found in ventral or sternal recumbency or sitting back on their hocks. Inability to ambulate to food and water can lead to dehydration, starvation, emaciation, and death.

#### Physical Examination Findings
Birds affected with discospondylitis often have an altered postural stance and lumbosacral kyphosis or, less commonly, scoliosis. Neurologic function may be normal or neurologic deficits may be present, including motor dysfunction of the limbs caudal to the lesion (paraparesis or paralysis), proprioceptive deficits, decreased withdrawal reflex, and decreased patellar reflex. Affected birds may rest in sternal recumbency or sit back on their hocks and tail. Ataxia characterized by severe imbalance, tiptoe walking, and difficulty standing upright have been reported. Spinal pain is reported and may present as the patient biting over the affected area or increased pain response during palpation of the spine. Poultry affected by spondylitis most commonly exhibit lameness, symmetrical hind limb paresis or paralysis, kyphosis of the spine at the level of the free thoracic vertebra, and arching of the back. Sitting back on the hocks with cranial extension of the legs is considered a classic symptom associated with this disease. In severe cases, birds may also be sternally or laterally recumbent with an inability to walk. Weight loss and reduced growth rates are commonly reported due to inability to move to food.

### CAUSES
*Staphylococcus aureus* and *Staphylococcus intermedius* are the most commonly isolated pathogens in humans and dogs, although several bacterial and fungal organisms have been reported. Bacterial organisms associated with discospondylitis in avian species include *Serratia marcescens* (a Gram-negative bacillus in the Enterobacteriaceae family) and *S. aureus*. *Corynebacterium amycolatum* was suspected in one case of a free-ranging yellow-eyed penguin based on a flock history of stomatitis but was not isolated from the vertebral lesion. In poultry, pathogenic *Enterococcus cecorum* is the causative agent of

enterococcal spondylitis. This Gram-positive bacterial coccus was previously named *Streptococcus cecorum* and was reclassified in 1989. Pathogenic *E. cecorum* is phenotypically and genetically distinct from commensal isolates. Other bacterial causes of spondylitis in birds include *Enterococcus faecalis*, *Enterococcus durans*, *Enterococcus hirae*, *Staphylococcus* spp., and *Escherichia coli*. Mycotic spondylitis, caused by *Aspergillus* spp. and *Mucor* spp. infection, has also been reported in birds. There have been no reports of mycotic discospondylitis in birds.

## RISK FACTORS
Spinal trauma, especially after collision in wild birds, may predispose to discospondylitis due to transient bacteremia or, less likely, primary microbial inoculation. In humans and dogs, advanced age and concurrent infections (especially of the urogenital and respiratory tracts) are reported as risk factors for discospondylitis. These risk factors have not been confirmed in avian patients. Proposed risk factors for enterococcal spondylitis of broilers include restricted use of antibiotic feed additives, use of growth promotors, and increased prevalence of concurrent infections.

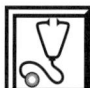

# DIAGNOSIS

## DIFFERENTIAL DIAGNOSIS
Spondylitis (vertebral osteomyelitis or vertebral osteoarthritis), spinal trauma, spondylolisthesis ("kinky back"), intervertebral disc extrusion, scoliosis, fibrocartilaginous embolism, congenital deformity, neoplasia (of the spinal cord, vertebral column, gonad, or kidney), viral infection (avian influenza, bornavirus, Newcastle disease virus, West Nile virus, equine encephalitis virus, Marek's disease), meningitis, gangliosidosis/lysosomal storage disease, avian vacuolar myelinopathy, avian ganglioneuritis, heavy-metal toxicity, botulism, organophosphate and carbamate toxicosis, tick paralysis, rhabdomyolysis,

## CBC/BIOCHEMISTRY/URINALYSIS
The most commonly reported blood work changes include leukocytosis and elevated plasma proteins with hypoalbuminemia and hyperglobulinemia, suggesting inflammation and infection. Both heterophilia and heteropenia have been reported in avian species with confirmed discospondylitis. A mild non-regenerative anemia was diagnosed in one case.

## OTHER LABORATORY TESTS
Bacteriologic culture and sensitivity is recommended to help determine the causative agent and guide therapy. In dogs

with discospondylitis, 45–75% will have a positive blood culture. Blood culture was used in a case of discospondylitis in a greater flamingo and can be considered if bone culture is deemed too risky.

## IMAGING
### Radiographic Findings
Diagnosis of discospondylitis is often based on radiographic findings. However, radiographs may be normal early in the disease process for patients with discospondylitis. In a white stork with confirmed discospondylitis, radiographic lesions were not evident until 4 weeks post-spinal trauma. This is similar to reports in humans with discospondylitis, where radiographic changes may not appear until 2 weeks to several months after the onset of infection. In birds, lesions of the FTV are most commonly reported and include erosion or lysis of the end plates, collapse of the disc space with adjacent sclerosis, and irregular proliferative bony changes. Disc spaces may later appear widened due to secondary lysis of adjacent bone. In severe cases, compression and instability of the vertebral bodies may be evident. Discospondylitis can be differentiated from vertebral osteomyelitis on radiographs by specific involvement of the disc space and adjacent vertebral end plates. Myelography via the atlanto-occipital space has been used in birds for the diagnosis of spinal-cord disease but is considered riskier as the cerebellomedullary cistern can be quite small and overlies a large venous plexus.

**CT**: More sensitive for the diagnosis of discospondylitis and can detect inflammation of paravertebral tissues not apparent on radiographic analysis. Findings on CT can include sclerotic vertebral body end plates, end plate lysis, and presence of granulomatous tissue. Vertebral canal narrowing and spinal cord compression may also be observed. CT can be used for initial diagnosis as well as monitoring of disease progression and therapeutic response.

**MRI**: Has the potential to detect the presence of discospondylitis before the development of substantial end plate osteolysis. Early lesions on MRI may include edema, reactive vascular tissue, and hyperemia. MRI is the preferred diagnostic imaging modality for spinal infections in humans, due to the capacity for early detection; however, use of MRI for the diagnosis of avian discospondylitis has not been reported.

**Thermographic imaging**: Allowed noninvasive localization of spondylitis lesions in a bufflehead duckling (*Bucephala albeola*) prior to palpable or visible spinal changes.

## DIAGNOSTIC PROCEDURES
Percutaneous fine needle aspiration using fluoroscopic or CT guidance is recommended for definitive diagnosis of the underlying cause. Samples should be submitted for bacterial and fungal culture. In humans, microbial culture via needle aspirates yields microbial growth in approximately 58% of cases. Open surgical biopsy is also reported in other species but may have a higher risk of complications in avian patients.

## PATHOLOGIC FINDINGS
On gross evaluation of birds with discospondylitis, affected vertebral bodies contain necrotic end plates and granulomatous bony lesions. The articular ends of the vertebral bodies may be abscessed. Medullary bone is replaced with thick fibrovascular tissue in chronic disease. Histopathologic analysis will reveal effacement of the vertebral body end plates and replacement by fragmented necrotic cartilage. Inflammatory infiltrates are present with extensive viable and degenerate heterophils, macrophages, multinucleated giant cells, lymphocytes, histiocytes, osteoclasts, and plasma cells. Intralesional bacteria or fungi may be present. In enterococcal spondylitis, the FTV (T4) and adjacent vertebral bodies of the notarium or synsacrum are necrotic. A large, firm swelling is present on the ventral surface of the spine at the level of the articulating thoracic vertebra and contains tan to yellow caseonecrotic material characterized by yellow to gray, granular and friable exudate surrounded by a thick white fibrous connective tissue capsule on cross-section. There is increased size of the vertebral body, resulting in narrowing of the overlying spinal canal and secondary compression of the spinal cord. On histopathologic analysis, bone is replaced by a central amalgam of necrotic tissue, inflammatory exudate (including fibrin, hemorrhage, and heterophils), and connective tissue. The inflammatory mass results in stenosis of the vertebral column and compression of the spinal cord, as seen grossly. Gram-positive bacterial colonies are often associated with osseous and cartilaginous sequestra located within the exudate.

# TREATMENT

## APPROPRIATE HEALTH CARE
As in humans and dogs, avian patients with severe neurologic deficits should be hospitalized for intravenous therapy. Cases with mild symptoms may be managed on an outpatient basis.

**D**

## NURSING CARE
Physiotherapy, including walking with support, passive range of motion exercises, and swimming (if indicated for the species affected), is recommended.

## ACTIVITY
Cage rest is recommended for patient with discospondylitis to reduce pain and prevent pathologic fractures or luxations of the vertebral bodies.

## DIET
Fluid therapy and nutritional support are recommended in cases where patients are not eating and drinking on their own.

## CLIENT EDUCATION
N/A

## SURGICAL CONSIDERATIONS
Surgical intervention has not been reported for avian discospondylitis. Surgery may be considered for open biopsy if there is no response to initial therapy or for decompression of the spinal cord if substantial neurologic deficits are present with compression of the spinal cord confirmed on imaging and in cases refractory to appropriate medical therapy. However, surgical debridement may result in severe complications, including loss of function to thin cortices of the bones that compose the avian vertebral column.

## MEDICATIONS

### DRUG(S) OF CHOICE
Long-term antimicrobial therapy (6 weeks to several months) against the causative organism based on culture of the lesion or blood is recommended. Since *Staphylococcus* spp. are most commonly isolated in humans and dogs and have also been isolated from birds with discospondylitis and spondylitis, treatment with a betalactam antibiotic is recommended in cases where a causative agent has not been identified. A first-generation cephalosporin (e.g. cephalexin 35–50 mg/kg IM or PO q6h) or amoxicillin potentiated with clavulanic acid 125 mg/kg PO q8h is recommended. However, it should be noted that resistance to cephalosporins by *Staphylococcus* spp. may be as high as 18% in dogs and 30% in humans. Therefore, use of a first-generation cephalosporin drug alone may not effectively control the infection. Alternatively, a betalactam antibiotic combined with an aminoglycoside or fluoroquinolone can be prescribed. Although

multiple antibiotics have shown efficacy against the commonly reported bacterial causes of discospondylitis and spondylitis, it is difficult to achieve adequate antibiotic concentrations in the vertebral column, and this may contribute to treatment failure. Avian species reported to be affected by discospondylitis are also highly susceptible to aspergillosis. Antifungal medication, such as voriconazole 12–18 mg/kg PO q8-12h or itraconazole 5–10 mg/kg PO q12h, can be considered as a preventative even if fungal culture is negative. Anti-inflammatory and analgesic medications are also indicated. Meloxicam 0.5–1 mg/kg IM or PO q12h is most commonly reported in avian patients with discospondylitis. The use of gabapentin has also been reported.

### CONTRAINDICATIONS
Steroids are contraindicated as they may cause immunosuppression and worsened infection.

### PRECAUTIONS
N/A

### POSSIBLE INTERACTIONS
N/A

### ALTERNATIVE DRUGS
N/A

## FOLLOW-UP

### PATIENT MONITORING
Treatment should be continued until there is no radiographic evidence of active disease. Reported markers of radiographic quiescence in other species include the absence of a lytic focus and smoothing, followed by loss of sclerotic margins, around the lytic focus or replacement by bridging of the affected vertebrae.

### PREVENTION/AVOIDANCE
N/A

### POSSIBLE COMPLICATIONS
Permanent neurologic deficits may occur in patients secondary to severe proliferative lesions at the site of infection, collapse of the intervertebral space, or pathologic vertebral fractures. Death may occur secondary to systemic spread of infection or starvation.

### EXPECTED COURSE AND PROGNOSIS
Prognosis for discospondylitis in avian species is poor compared with humans and dogs. All reported cases died or were euthanized due to lack of response to therapy. Spondylitis of poultry is also associated with a poor prognosis with average mortality at slaughter of 7–8% (reports as high as 35%).

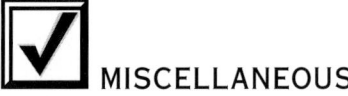

## MISCELLANEOUS

### ASSOCIATED CONDITIONS
N/A

### AGE-RELATED FACTORS
N/A

### ZOONOTIC POTENTIAL
N/A

### FERTILITY/BREEDING
N/A

### SYNONYMS
Diskospondylitis. Enterococcal spondylitis may be referred to as epidemic infectious spinal necrosis, vertebral osteoarthritis or VOA, or "kinky back" (also used to describe a developmental disease of chickens called spondylolisthesis).

### SEE ALSO
Marek's Disease
Neoplasia (Neurological)
Neurologic (Non-Traumatic Diseases)
Neurologic (Trauma)

### ABBREVIATIONS
CT—computed tomography
FTV—free thoracic vertebra
MRI—magnetic resonance imaging

### INTERNET RESOURCES
Boulianne, M. (ed.) (2013). *Avian Disease Manual*, 7th edn. American Association of Avian Pathologists: https://aaap.memberclicks.net/avian-disease-manual-old-edition

*Suggested Reading*
Bergen, D.J., Gartrell, B.D. (2010). Discospondylitis in a yellow-eyed penguin (*Megadyptes antipodes*). *Journal of Avian Medicine and Surgery*, 24:58–63.
Braga, J.F.V., Martins, N.R.S., Ecco, R. (2018). Vertebral osteomyelitis in broilers: a review. *Brazilian Journal of Poultry Science*, 20:605–616.
Field, C.L., Beaufrère, H., Wakamatsu, N., et al. (2012). Discospondylitis caused by *Staphylococcus aureus* in an African black-footed penguin (*Spheniscus demersus*). *Journal of Avian Medicine and Surgery*, 24:232–238.
Poeta, P., Sargo, R.F., Valente, J.M., et al. (2016). Serratia marcescens discospondylitis in a white stork (*Ciconia ciconia*). *SOJ Microbiology & Infectious Diseases*, 4:1–5.
Xie, S., Shuang-Li, G., De Busscher, V., Hsu, C. (2020). What is your neurologic diagnosis? *Journal of the American Veterinary Medical Association*, 257:703–706.

**Author**: Brynn McCleery, DVM, DABVP (Avian Practice)

# BASICS

## DEFINITION
Dyslipidemia are abnormalities in the plasma lipid profile, usually an increase in one or several lipid fractions caused by disturbances in lipid metabolism. Most commonly recognized are elevations in plasma cholesterol, VLDL cholesterol, LDL cholesterol, non-HDL cholesterol, and triglycerides. The benefits of high HDL cholesterol in birds, as it is the case in mammals, is unknown and elevated HDL cholesterol is often seen in dyslipidemic psittacine birds, albeit to a lesser degree than non-HDL cholesterol. A shift in HDL/LDL ratio is frequently seen in dyslipidemic birds. Other dyslipidemia characterized in humans but of unknown occurrence and significance in birds include, among others, decrease in HDL cholesterol, raised lipoprotein (a), raised apoB, increased ratio apoB/apoA1, increased ratio non-HDL/HDL, raised "small, dense" LDL, and increased LDL particle numbers. LDL and HDL subfractions are also present but their characterization and diagnostic values have been poorly investigated in birds.

## PATHOPHYSIOLOGY
Dyslipidemia in birds is presumably caused by disturbances in normal lipid metabolism associated with inadequate nutrition, captive lifestyle, dysregulated vitellogenesis, and possibly other species and individual risk factors. Dyslipidemia is a presumed risk factor or comorbid condition to atherosclerosis, hepatic lipidosis, hepatic diseases, pancreatic diseases, xanthomatous lesions, obesity, adipocytic tumors, and possibly others. However, the association has not been confirmed in most instances. Birds are also suspected to develop a similar metabolic syndrome as described in mammals, but this has not been investigated. Avian lipid metabolism has marked differences from mammals. Birds have a larger ability to store fat, a poorly developed lymphatic system, lipogenesis is mostly restricted to the liver (include adipose tissue in mammals), portomicrons instead of chylomicrons, HDL is the predominant cholesterol type in healthy birds (vs. LDL in humans), and different apolipoproteins are present.

## SYSTEMS AFFECTED
Hepatic, adipose.

## GENETICS
Restricted ovulator (RO) chicken—mutation in the VLDL receptor gene. Experimentally inbred laboratory strains of quails and pigeons have higher cholesterol than other breeds. Genetic factors may play a role in some individuals. In mammals, deficient LDL receptor, enzymes, or apolipoproteins are the causes of various familial dyslipidemias.

## INCIDENCE/PREVALENCE
Unknown, but suspected to be prevalent in Quaker parrots and older psittacine birds.

## GEOGRAPHIC DISTRIBUTION
N/A

## SIGNALMENT
**Species**: All birds are susceptible to dyslipidemia. Among psittaciformes, Quaker parrots seem particularly susceptible. Amazon parrots, grey parrots, and cockatiels seem to have slightly higher cholesterol than other psittacine species. Psittacine birds adapted to high-fat diet (e.g. macaws, palm cockatoos) are expected to show a lower susceptibility to dyslipidemia. Female birds undergoing vitellogenesis have lipidemic changes that may be characterized as dyslipidemic when chronic.
**Mean age and range**: Any age may be affected but older psittacine birds may be more susceptible. In mammals, plasma lipid fractions increase with age.
**Predominant sex**: Both, but female birds are prone to dyslipidemia due to physiologic or abnormal vitellogenesis.

## SIGNS
Signs are related to the causes or consequences of altered lipid metabolism or associated conditions (see corresponding sections) and may include reproductive signs—ascites, reproductive behavior, chronic egg laying, feather damaging behavior; cutaneous signs—cutaneous xanthomatosis, cutaneous adipocytic tumors (e.g. lipomas); neurological signs—central neurological signs caused by lipid emboli or carotid atherosclerosis; cardiovascular signs due to atherosclerosis—congestive heart failure, ataxia, hind limb weakness, dyspnea; hepatic signs—abdominal distention, gastrointestinal signs. Nonspecific signs include lethargy, depression, decreased appetite, overweight, obesity.

## CAUSES
**Vitellogenesis in female birds**: This may be physiological but is often maladaptive in captive psittacine birds, and is associated with inappropriate chronic reproductive stimulation. Under estrogen stimulation, the liver produces two very-low density lipoproteins, vitellogenin and VLDLy.
**Diet**: An inappropriate diet may contribute to the development of dyslipidemia and other diseases Excessive dietary intake. Postprandial hyperlipidemia. High fat and multideficient diet, typically all-seed diet in granivorous/frugivorous birds. Animal products containing animal saturated fat and cholesterol (egg, meat) in granivorous/frugivorous birds. Overreliance on day-old chicks in certain susceptible raptors (controversial). Inappropriate prey items for certain birds of prey and possibly others (e.g. rats and day-old chicks for insectivorous or piscivorous birds). Lack of lipotropic factors that promote lipid catabolism such as methionine, choline, and vitamin Bs. Lack of physical activity, obesity.
**Hepatobiliary disease**: May lead to changes in plasma lipid fractions as the liver is the source of cholesterol, lipid, and apolipoprotein synthesis. In particular, biliary obstruction often results in elevated plasma cholesterol.
**Pancreatitis**: Has been shown to be associated with dyslipidemia in mammals.
**Endocrine diseases**: Hypothyroidism is not well characterized in birds but is a prominent cause of hypercholesterolemia in companion mammals. Diabetes mellitus is an important cause of dyslipidemia in human patients but this association is not well characterized in birds, especially since diabetes mellitus is not common in birds.
Certain drugs may alter some lipid fractions such as steroids, progestins, thiazides, β-blockers, triazole antifungals, and cyclosporine. Second hand smoke in pet birds may also contribute to dyslipidemic disorders. Inflammation is associated with a decrease in HDL cholesterol in mammals.

## RISK FACTORS
See Causes section.

# DIAGNOSIS

## DIFFERENTIAL DIAGNOSIS
Laboratory errors. Physiological female reproductive activity. See Causes section.

## CBC/BIOCHEMISTRY/URINALYSIS
Plasma lipemia may lead to an elevation in total solids and may interfere with some biochemical assays.

## OTHER LABORATORY TESTS
Various lipoprotein assays are used in mammals to measure the different lipoprotein fractions but most have not been properly validated in the different avian species. Some laboratory tests may not be accurate for measuring cholesterol fractions in birds. It is recommended that birds are fasted prior to measurement, as some lipid fractions may greatly increase after a meal. Selected methods classically used for cholesterol fraction/lipoprotein determinations areas follows.
**Ultracentrifugation**: Gold standard, but laboratory intensive method and classically not commercially available. Plasma lipoproteins are separated according to their

D

density by a series of centrifugal steps using density gradient (salt solutions) at relative centrifugal fields of 200–300,000 G. Then cholesterol is measured in each fraction. Density limits have not been published for parrot plasma but have been used in pigeons. Modified techniques using different compounds to generate density gradients have been described.

**Laboratory analyzers**: Enzymatic and precipitation colorimetric assays are classically used to measure the total cholesterol, the HDL cholesterol, and the triglycerides. In a standard laboratory analyzer, direct LDL measurement and indirect LDL estimation are typically unreliable in birds. For instance, the Friedewald formula has been shown to be unreliable in Quaker parrots. HDL is generally reliable and can be used to calculate the non-HDL cholesterol, which encompasses all atherogenic lipoproteins. Hypertriglyceridemia may interfere with HDL and other lipoprotein measurements.

**Electrophoresis**: Lipoproteins can be separated in a single operation but this has not been validated in birds. Electrophoretic techniques have been used in research in birds, including Quaker parrots. High-resolution polyacrylamide gel electrophoresis (Lipoprint®, Quantimetrix, Redondo Beach, CA) has been used in several species of birds.

**Magnetic resonance spectroscopy**: Not described in birds. Gel permeation high-performance liquid chromatography (Liposearch®, GP-HPLC Systems, Japan) has been used to characterize lipoproteins in Quaker parrots. Lipidomics using mass spectrometry has been used in parrots to study and characterize dyslipidemia.

## IMAGING
Dyslipidemia has classically been associated with atherosclerosis and hepatic lipidosis. As such, hepatomegaly may be observed on radiographs. Please consult the Atherosclerosis chapter for specific diagnostic findings on vascular imaging.

## DIAGNOSTIC PROCEDURES
N/A

## PATHOLOGIC FINDINGS
Histopathologic lesions that may be concurrent with dyslipidemia include hepatopathies, xanthomatous lesions, and atherosclerosis.

## TREATMENT
### APPROPRIATE HEALTH CARE
Decreasing reproductive stimuli in pet birds may be beneficial.

## NURSING CARE
Supportive care.

## ACTIVITY
Activity level should be as high as possible. Opportunities for increased activity may be scarce in captivity but caretakers should be encouraged to promote physical exercise with flying, playgrounds, and foraging setups.

## DIET
The provision of a balanced diet supplemented with fruits and vegetables is probably the most important aspect of the treatment in captive parrots. Decreasing the overall amount of food may be beneficial, especially in overconditioned birds. Discontinue the feeding of animal products to psittacine birds. Non-animal items do not contain any cholesterol. Switch to a pelletized diet if the bird is on an all-seed diet. Low-fat pelletized diet (e.g. Roudybush® Low Fat Maintenance, Woodland, CA) may be beneficial in some cases. Some species are adapted to consume higher fat diet than others (e.g. macaws, palm cockatoos). Omega-3 fatty acids may help. They can be provided, among other items, with flaxseeds, walnuts, flaxseed oil, and fish oil. In birds of prey, day-old chicks should probably be limited or avoided in certain species such as gyrfalcons, insectivorous species, and kites.

## CLIENT EDUCATION
Inform the clients about proper diet for respective species, the need for adequate physical exercise, and how to reduce reproductive stimulation in females.

## SURGICAL CONSIDERATIONS
N/A

## MEDICATIONS
### DRUG(S) OF CHOICE
Only limited information is available for most drugs listed below. Most is empirical and pharmacological information has rarely been obtained in birds. For treatment of heart failure, please see corresponding section. Statins: Lipid lowering agents, which are competitive inhibitors of the HMG-CoA reductase enzyme in hepatic cholesterol synthesis. Pharmacokinetic studies on rosuvastatin in Amazon parrots failed to reach therapeutic concentrations at 10–25 mg/kg. Atorvastatin at 20 mg/kg PO q12–24h can be recommended in Amazon parrots and cockatiels based on pharmacokinetic studies. Atorvastatin at 20 mg/kg PO q12h for 2 weeks in Quaker parrots and atorvastatin at 10 mg/kg PO q12h in Amazon parrots did not lead to

significant decrease in blood lipids. Additional pharmacological studies on statins are ongoing. Other statins of interest include simvastatin, lovastatin, pravastatin, and fluvastatin. Should not be taken while feeding grapefruits and concurrently with azole antifungals. Statins also have non-lipid effects such as beneficial properties on endothelial function, vascular inflammation, immune modulation, oxidative stress, thrombosis, and plaque stabilization. Fibrates: Hypolipidemic drugs, which are agonists of the PPARα that stimulates β-oxidation of fatty acids. Fibrates mainly cause a decrease in blood triglycerides. Gemfibrozil and fenofibrate. No pharmacokinetic information are available in companion birds. Other lipid lowering agents include cholesterol absorption inhibitors (ezetimibe) and nicotinic acid. GnRH agonists (leuprolide acetate, subcutaneous deslorelin implant) may be given to decrease reproductive hyperlipidemia and as part of the treatment of reproductive conditions.

### CONTRAINDICATIONS
N/A

### PRECAUTIONS
N/A

### POSSIBLE INTERACTIONS
The combination of statins with fibrates may increase the risk of rhabdomyolysis. Some statins (e.g. atorvastatin) interact with drugs metabolized through the cytochrome P450 pathway, such as azole antifungals. Grapefruits should not be fed to birds receiving statins; this may increase plasma levels.

### ALTERNATIVE DRUGS
N/A

## FOLLOW-UP
### PATIENT MONITORING
Blood cholesterol and lipoproteins should be monitored on a regular basis. Peak effects of statins may not be evident for several weeks.

### PREVENTION/AVOIDANCE
See Diet and Activity sections. Reduction of captive reproductive stimuli for female birds.

### POSSIBLE COMPLICATIONS
Atherosclerotic diseases. Obesity. Diabetes mellitus. Hepatic lipidosis. Xanthomatosis, xanthomas. Adipocytic tumors. Endogenous lipid pneumonia. Corneal lipid deposits.

### EXPECTED COURSE AND PROGNOSIS
N/A

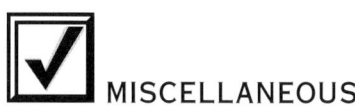

## MISCELLANEOUS

### ASSOCIATED CONDITIONS
Atherosclerosis, obesity, diabetes mellitus, hepatic lipidosis, xanthomatosis, xanthomas, adipocytic tumors.

### AGE-RELATED FACTORS
Plasma lipid levels may increase with age.

### ZOONOTIC POTENTIAL
N/A

### FERTILITY/BREEDING
Plasma cholesterol and lipids increase with reproductive activity; increase is expected with physiological vitellogenesis in female breeding birds.

### SYNONYMS
N/A

### SEE ALSO
Atherosclerosis
Chronic Egg Laying
Hepatic Lipidosis
Neoplasia (Integument)

Nutritional Imbalances
Obesity
Pancreatic Diseases
Xanthoma/Xanthogranulomatosis

### ABBREVIATIONS
apoA1—apolipoprotein A1
apoB—apolipoprotein B
GnRH—gonadotropin-releasing hormone
HDL—high-density lipoprotein
HMG-CoA—3-hydroxy-3-methylglutaryl coenzyme A
LDL—low-density lipoprotein
PPAR—peroxisome proliferator-activated receptor
VLDL—very-low-density lipoprotein

### INTERNET RESOURCES
N/A

*Suggested Reading*
Beaufrère, H (2022). Blood lipid diagnostics in psittacine birds. *Veterinary Clinics of North America. Exotic Animal Practice*, 25:697–712.
Beaufrère, H., Wood D. (2023). Comparison of lipoprotein analysis using gel-permeation high-performance liquid chromatography and a biochemistry analyzer in normlipidemic and dyslipidemic Quaker parrots (*Myiopsitta monachus*). *Journal of Avian Medicine and Surgery*, 36:345–355.
Beaufrère, H. (2013). Atherosclerosis: Comparative pathogenesis, lipoprotein metabolism and avian and exotic companion mammal models. *Journal of Exotic Pet Medicine*, 22:320–335.
Facon, C., Beaufrère, H., Gaborit, C., et al. (2014). Cluster of atherosclerosis in a captive population of black kites (*Milvus migrans* subsp.) in France and effect of nutrition on the plasma lipidogram. *Avian Diseases*, 58:176–182.
Petzinger, C., Bauer, J. (2013). Dietary considerations for atherosclerosis in avian species commonly presented in clinical practice. *Journal of Exotic Pet Medicine*, 22:358–365.

**Author**: Hugues Beaufrère, DVM, PhD, Dipl ACZM, Dipl ABVP (Avian), Dipl ECZM (Avian)

# DYSTOCIA AND EGG BINDING

## BASICS

### DEFINITION
Egg binding is the delay in the passage of an egg through the reproductive tract. Normal transit time through the reproductive tract varies between species and even among individuals but is generally between 24 and 48 hours for most companion pet species. Dystocia is when the egg is stuck and unable to pass through the reproductive tract.

### PATHOPHYSIOLOGY
Egg binding is a commonly seen obstetric disorder in clinical practice. Delayed transit of the egg puts the hen at risk for dystocia. Delayed or failure of an egg to pass can be caused by anatomic issues with the reproductive tract and/or issues with the egg being oversized, malformed, or abnormally positioned. Dysfunction of the oviduct can be a result of inflammation or infection, damage to the oviductal wall, inertia secondary to calcium deficiency, torsions, and the presence of a persistent right oviduct. Masses of the reproductive tract, cloaca, or other coelomic organs can compress the lumen of the oviduct, thus obstructing the passage of an egg. Chronic egg laying results in the physical exhaustion of the reproductive tract and depletion of body stores of calcium. Subsequently, oviductal muscle atony develops and results in delayed oviposition. Chronic straining and muscle atony can lead to prolapses of the cloaca and/or oviduct which may or may not contain the stuck egg. The distal uterus, vagina, and vaginal–cloacal junction are the most common areas for dystocia. Musculoskeletal deformities of the pelvic canal, either congenital or acquired after injury, can physically obstruct the passage of an egg.

### SYSTEMS AFFECTED
**Reproductive**: Prolonged straining can result in a prolapsed oviduct or the cloaca. Pressure necrosis or tear of the oviduct wall may occur.
**Respiratory**: Increased respiratory effort can be seen due to compression of the air sacs by the space-occupying egg and enlarged reproductive tract.
**GI**: Hen may not be able to defecate if the egg is obstructing the cloaca.
**Renal**: Damage to the kidney can develop due to compression of renal parenchyma by the retained egg. Hyperuricemia can occur if the egg is obstructing the cloaca or compressing the ureters.
**Neuromuscular**: Unilateral or bilateral paresis or paralysis of the pelvic limbs can result from compression of the ischiatic nerve by the retained egg.
**Integument**: Localized plucking of feathers of the caudal ventrum or over the back may occur in response to discomfort from the retained egg.

### GENETICS
Some breed lines may have a genetic predisposition for egg binding/dystocia.

### INCIDENCE/PREVALENCE
Common, especially in smaller species and hens that are chronic egg layers. Higher incidence is noted when birds breed out of their natural season or are first-time egg producers.

### GEOGRAPHIC DISTRIBUTION
N/A

### SIGNALMENT
**Species predilections**: Cockatiels, budgerigars, lovebirds, finches, canaries, cockatoos, and Amazon parrots have increased risk for egg binding and dystocia.
**Mean age and range**: Hens of egg-producing age (sexual maturity varies between species).
**Predominant sex**: Females of reproductive age.

### SIGNS

#### Historical Findings
Hen may be a novice egg layer. For experienced hens, there may be recent egg laying with a sudden cessation of egg production. Recently laid eggs may be abnormally sized, misshapen, thin-shelled, or unshelled. Signs of nesting behavior, such as shredding paper, seeking dark places, or being cage protective may be noted at home. Hen may have a wide-based stance or be actively straining to pass the egg. Changes in fecal production and character may be noted including scant to no fecal production or blood in the droppings. Feces and urates may have adhered to the tail/vent. Increased respiratory effort (i.e. tail-bobbing, open-mouth breathing) may be noted, especially after increased activity such as flying. A decreased appetite, lethargy, and generalized weakness may be noted. The cloaca or oviduct may be prolapsed with chronic straining; egg(s) may be adhered within the prolapsed tissue. Lameness of one or both pelvic limbs may be noted. Sudden death is not uncommon, especially in smaller species such as finches and canaries.

#### Physical Examination Findings
A normally shelled egg is typically palpable in caudal coelom; however, eggs that are soft-shelled, shell-less, or located cranially in the oviduct may not be palpable on coelomic palpation. Unproductive straining or "winking" of the vent may be noted; the vent may also be flaccid. Wide-based stance and dyspnea may be noted due to coelomic distension. Feces and urates may have accumulated on the vent and tail feathers. Hematochezia may be noted. Blood may also stain the vent. Severe and continued straining can present with cloacal or oviductal prolapse, with or without an egg adhered within the prolapsed tissue. Hen may be obese, thin, or of normal body condition. Unilateral or bilateral hind-limb weakness or paresis; feet may feel cold; the patient may present in sternal recumbency due to weakness in the legs. Severe lethargy and generalized weakness can be noted in patients with prolonged dystocia.

### CAUSES
**Reproductive**: Chronic egg laying (common); oversized, malformed, or abnormally positioned eggs (common); salpingitis or metritis; oviductal torsion; tears or damage to the oviduct; adhesions of the oviduct; persistent cystic right oviduct.
**Metabolic**: Calcium deficiency (metabolic or nutritional)—common; vitamin E deficiency; selenium deficiency.
**Neoplasia**: Neoplasia of the reproductive tract, cloaca, or other coelomic organs.
**Other**: Secondary to systemic disease; stress; musculoskeletal deformities of the pelvic canal (congenital or acquired); genetic predisposition; obesity; malnutrition; breeding out of natural season.

### RISK FACTORS
Previous episodes of egg binding or dystocia may result in damage to the oviduct. An all-seed diet predisposes the hen to calcium deficiency and obesity. Chronic egg laying, often due to environmental cues such as prolonged exposure to daylight, presence of a mate or perceived mate (e.g. owner or toy), and access to nesting material or nesting site. Untreated chronic egg-laying leads to the depletion of calcium stores, which can result in thin or unshelled eggs and muscle atony.

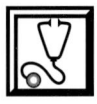

## DIAGNOSIS

### DIFFERENTIAL DIAGNOSIS
**Coelomic distension**: Ascites; egg-yolk coelomitis; impacted oviduct; body-wall hernias; organomegaly, neoplasia, abscesses, or granulomas of any of the coelomic organs.
**Straining**: Gastroenteritis, fecaliths, or constipation; cloacal masses; uroliths.
**Dyspnea**: Pneumonia, sinusitis, or tracheal obstruction; pain; heat exhaustion; cardiac

disease; space-occupying masses or fluid in the coelomic cavity.

**Pelvic limb lameness or paresis**: Traumatic injury to pelvic limbs or spine; pododermatitis; osteomyelitis; lead toxicity; intramedullary or compressive spinal neoplasia; lumbosacral plexus compression secondary renal or ovarian neoplasms; claudication secondary to atherosclerosis.

## CBC/BIOCHEMISTRY/URINALYSIS
Marked hypercalcemia is a normal finding in egg-laying birds as they are mobilizing calcium for shell production. A calcium level in normal reference ranges may be indicative of a relative calcium deficiency. Hypercholesterolemia and hyperglobulinemia are normal findings in an ovulating hen. Leukocytosis characterized by a relative heterophilia is not uncommon in egg-laying birds. Muscle tissue damage may lead to elevated aspartate aminotransferase and creatine phosphokinase levels. Uric acid levels may be elevated if the retained egg is preventing the passage of urates due to compression of the ureters or blockage of the cloaca.

## OTHER LABORATORY TESTS
Hyperglobulinemia may be noted on EPH in egg-laying birds. It is characterized by marked monoclonal increases in the betaglobulin fraction caused by selective increases in transferrin. Aerobic culture or gram stain of the oviduct may be indicated to rule out an infection of the reproductive tract. Swabs of the cloaca more likely reflect bacterial populations of the proctodeum, urodeum, or coprodeum instead of the microflora of the oviduct.

## IMAGING
### Radiographic Findings
Orthogonal radiographs are useful in determining the size, location, position, and number of eggs present in the oviduct. Radiographs can also help evaluate if the egg is thin-shelled, shell-less, or malformed. Polyostotic hyperostosis (osteomyelosclerosis) of the long bones provides a calcium reserve for the formation of eggshells and is a normal finding in an egg-laying bird. Hens that are calcium-depleted have normal or osteopenic bone density. An active reproductive tract is seen as increased soft-tissue opacity in the mid-to-caudal region of the dorsal coelom on lateral radiographs and causes a widening of the hepatic silhouette on ventrodorsal radiographs.

### Ultrasonography
Nonmineralized eggs (i.e. soft-shelled, unshelled eggs) that are not visible on radiographs can be evaluated by ultrasonography. The extraoviductal location

of ectopic eggs can be confirmed by the egg's independent position from the oviduct.

## DIAGNOSTIC PROCEDURES
Endoscopy may be used in larger birds to visualize the lumen of the oviduct to assess for torsion or masses. Additionally, eggs located ectopically within the coelom may be visualized by laparoscopy.

## PATHOLOGIC FINDINGS
Salpingitis and metritis, either as the cause or secondary to the egg binding, may be noted. An ectopic egg may result if an egg is retropulsed back up the oviduct or through a tear in the oviduct wall into the coelomic cavity.

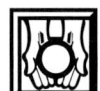 TREATMENT

### APPROPRIATE HEALTH CARE
Hens that exhibit mild clinical signs for 24 hours or less often respond to medical management alone but should be carefully monitored for worsening of clinical signs. For hens straining for over 24–48 hours or demonstrating severe clinical symptoms, earlier surgical intervention may be necessary.

### NURSING CARE
In many cases, stabilization with supportive measures should be attempted first to give the hen the opportunity to lay the egg. Hens should be kept in a humidified incubator warmed up to 85–90°F (29.4–32.2°C) that is ideally in a quiet and low-light setting to minimize stress. Fluid supplementation should be provided via subcutaneous and/or oral administration to help keep the hen properly hydrated. Pain should be managed with analgesics and anti-inflammatory medication. Calcium supplementation is beneficial if calcium deficiency is suspected. Antibiotics are not usually warranted but may be necessary if an underlying infectious process or traumatized tissue is noted.

### ACTIVITY
Minimize stress and activity by keeping the hen in a quiet and low-light setting (i.e. incubator or cage that is partially covered with a towel).

### DIET
If not eating or producing feces, the hen may need to be gavage fed a critical care formula for nutritional support. Calcium supplementation is especially important for hens that have been on nutritionally deficient all-seed diets. Layer or breeder-type rations are formulated with higher calcium content and should be used for egg-laying chickens and waterfowl.

## CLIENT EDUCATION
To give the reproductive tract an opportunity to heal after a bout of egg binding/dystocia, owners should discourage further egg laying for the rest of the season. Reduce photoperiod to no more than 8–10 hours per day by covering the cage at night. Eliminate inappropriate petting over the hen's dorsum. Separate hen from mates or perceived mates. Reduce high-calorie foods as well as the overall quantity of food. Remove access to nests and nesting material. Move the cage to an unfamiliar environment. Seed-based diets are often deficient in important nutrients and can lead to calcium deficiency in egg-laying hens. A good formulated pelleted diet and/or calcium supplementation should be used. Layer rations should be used if available. Leuprolide acetate or deslorelin can be administered to prevent further egg laying that season.

## SURGICAL CONSIDERATIONS
If the egg is caudal enough in the oviduct, manual extraction through the cloaca can be attempted. To facilitate removal, percloacal (transcloacal) ovocentesis and collapse of the eggshell may be necessary in some cases. Percutaneous (transcoelomic) ovocentesis can be used for eggs that cannot be visualized through the cloacal opening; however, it has a higher risk for damage to the oviduct with subsequent tears and adhesion formation. Salpingohysterectomy can be performed to remove the oviduct and egg. This is a technically challenging procedure and should be performed by veterinarians familiar with avian reproductive anatomy. A salpingotomy can be performed to remove the egg if the egg-laying potential of the hen needs to be preserved. Compromised ability to breathe due to compression of air sacs by egg and enlarged reproductive tract. Intubation with positive pressure ventilation is strongly recommended if undergoing surgery. Placement of an intraosseous catheter may be difficult due to medullary bone formation in the ulna and tibiotarsal bones. If the hen is stable and the surgery can be delayed, presurgical administration of leuprolide acetate 1–2 weeks prior can help reduce the size and vascularity of the reproductive tract. Administration of leuprolide acetate also will decrease the bone density of the long bones allowing for easier placement of an intraosseous catheter.

 MEDICATIONS

### DRUG(S) OF CHOICE
**Calcium supplementation**: Calcium gluconate (10%) 50–100 mg/kg SQ, IM (diluted); for hypocalcemia; dilute 1 : 1 with saline or sterile water for injections.

# DYSTOCIA AND EGG BINDING　　(CONTINUED)

**Pain management**: Meloxicam 1–1.6 mg/kg PO, IM q12–24h. NSAIDs. Butorphanol tartrate 1–5 mg/kg q2–3h PRN IM, IV; opioid agonist-antagonist for pain management.

**Hormone therapy**: Leuprolide acetate 100–1200 μg/kg IM q2–4 weeks; long-acting synthetic GnRH analog used to prevent ovulation. Deslorelin 4.7 mg implant SQ; GnRH superagonist (note: deslorelin is an FDA indexed product in the United States and thus its use is prohibited in poultry). Oxytocin: 3–5 iu/kg IM, hormone for induction of smooth muscle contraction (see also Contraindications and Precautions sections). Equivocal response in birds. PGE$_2$ gel 0.02–0.1 mg/kg topically to uterovaginal sphincter; causes relaxation of the uterovaginal sphincter and oviductal contractions.

**Antibiotics**: If an infection is present; ideally to be based on culture and sensitivity.

## CONTRAINDICATIONS
Use of oxytocin is contraindicated if the uterovaginal sphincter is not dilated and if adhesions or uterine masses are present.

## PRECAUTIONS
Oxytocin should be preceded by calcium administration; must check that uterovaginal sphincter is open, otherwise rupture of shell gland or reverse peristalsis may occur; also contraindicated in cases of adhesions and uterine masses.

## POSSIBLE INTERACTIONS
Pregnant women and asthmatics should avoid handling PGE$_2$; gloves should be worn when administering this medication.

## ALTERNATIVE DRUGS
Acupuncture and chiropractic adjustments have been described as adjunct integrative therapies. Homeopathic remedies include calcarea carbonica, kali carbonicum, and pulsatilla pratensis.

 **FOLLOW-UP**

## PATIENT MONITORING
Repeat radiographs to assess if the egg has progressed down the oviduct with medical management. Repeat films can be taken several days later if the patient is stable. However, if the hen is declining the films should be taken earlier to see if surgical intervention is required.

## PREVENTION/AVOIDANCE
Discourage further egg laying for the season—reduce the photoperiod to no more than 8–10 hours per day by covering the cage at night, keep the hen separate from any mate or perceived mates, reduce foods high in fat and overall quantity of food, and remove nests and nesting material. Leuprolide acetate or deslorelin can be administered seasonally or when the hen is exhibiting reproductive behavior to prevent ovulation and egg formation. A deslorelin implant may have longer-lasting effects (deslorelin is an indexed drug in the USA and thus its use is prohibited in poultry).

## POSSIBLE COMPLICATIONS
Ectopic eggs may result if reverse peristalsis or rupture of the oviduct occurs. Prolonged straining can result in prolapse of the oviduct or cloaca. Multiple eggs may be present in the oviduct if the hen continues to ovulate despite the presence of an egg already in the oviduct. Hens that have undergone salpingohysterectomy may be at risk for internal ovulation and subsequent egg yolk peritonitis. Certain species (e.g. ducks) appear to be at higher risk. Measures to discourage reproductive behavior should be implemented. Complications from ovocentesis and egg implosion include retained shell fragments, oviductal/cloacal damage, hemorrhage, coelomitis/salpingitis.

## EXPECTED COURSE AND PROGNOSIS
Prognosis is good if the hen is otherwise in good health and supportive care is instituted early in the course of the disease. Some cases of egg binding/dystocia can be prolonged (i.e. weeks to months) without any outward clinical signs of illness. Though not ill, these hens are unlikely to pass their egg without surgical intervention and are at risk for additional issues such as multiple eggs in the oviduct, ectopic eggs, and egg yolk peritonitis. Prognosis is fair to guarded if the health status of the hen is compromised or if the egg binding is secondary to an ongoing disease process. Eggs that are not palpable on physical examination and retained higher up in the oviduct require more invasive treatment, such as percutaneous implosion of the egg or salpingohysterectomy, both of which are higher-risk procedures. Damage to the oviduct predisposes the hen to future bouts of egg binding/dystocia.

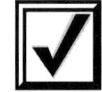 **MISCELLANEOUS**

## ASSOCIATED CONDITIONS
Ectopic eggs, oviductal or uterine prolapse, coelomic distension, lameness.

## AGE-RELATED FACTORS
First-time layers and older birds may have increased risk.

## ZOONOTIC POTENTIAL
N/A

## FERTILITY/BREEDING
If the oviduct is damaged during the course of the egg binding or during treatment, the hen may be predisposed to subsequent cases of egg binding and dystocia.

## SYNONYMS
Egg retention

## SEE ALSO
Chronic Egg Laying
Cloacal Disease
Cloacal Prolapse
Coelomic Distention
Egg Yolk and Reproductive Coelomitis
Lameness
Neurologic (Non-Traumatic Diseases)
Nutritional Imbalances
Ovarian Diseases
Oviductal Diseases
Polyostotic Hyperostosis/
Osteomyelosclerosis
Appendix 8, Algorithm 6: Egg Binding

## ABBREVIATIONS
EPH—protein electrophoresis
FDA—Food and Drug Administration
GI—gastrointestinal
GnRH—gonadotropin-releasing hormone
NSAIDs—non-steroidal anti-inflammatory drugs
PGE—prostaglandin E$_2$

## INTERNET RESOURCES
Pollock, C. (2012). Reproductive emergencies in birds. *LafeberVet*: https://lafeber.com/vet/reproductive-emergencies

*Suggested Reading*
Scagnelli, A.M., Tully, T.N. Jr. (2017). Reproductive disorders in parrots. *Veterinary Clinics of North America. Exotic Animal Practice*, 20:485–507.
Abou-Zahr, T., Carrasco, D.C., Jones, S.J., et al. (2019). Percloacal ovocentesis in the treatment of avian egg binding: Review of 20 cases. *Journal of Avian Medicine and Surgery*, 33:251–257.
Antinoff, N. (2021). Birds with big bellies: What do I need to know? *ExoticsCon Virtual 2021 Proceedings*.
Petritz, O.A. (2016). Clinical applications and considerations for the use of GnRH agonists. In: *Current Therapy in Avian Medicine and Surgery* (ed. B.L. Speer BL), . 446–454 St. Louis, MO: Elsevier.
Bowles, H.L. (2006). Evaluating and treating the reproductive system. In: *Clinical Avian Medicine*, Vol. II (ed. G.J. Harrison, T.L. Lightfoot), 519–539. Palm Beach, FL: Spix Publishing.

**Author**: Sue Chen, DVM, Dipl. ABVP (Avian)

# EASTERN AND WESTERN EQUINE ENCEPHALITIS VIRUSES (EEV/WEEV)

## BASICS

### DEFINITION
Eastern and Western equine encephalitis viruses (EEEV/WEEV) are RNA arboviruses in the family Togaviridae, and the genus *Alphavirus*. They are transmitted by female mosquitoes, and cause neurological disease and potentially death in multiple bird species, horses, humans, and certain other individual mammal species. WEEV is much less common in humans and has a much lower mortality rate and a high probability of being subclinical in humans. There has been evidence of submergence of WEEV, perhaps due to ecologic factors, which may explain the reduction in prevalence in the Western USA. Only EEEV lineage 1 is meant when EEEV is discussed further in this chapter.

### PATHOPHYSIOLOGY
The mosquito *Culiseta melanura* is the primary vector species. It is a mosquito species that spreads EEEV between birds. Horses and humans (perhaps pet and zoo birds?) infected by EEEV are bitten by "bridge" mosquito species such as *Aedes* spp., *Coquillettidia* spp., and *Culex* spp. For WEEV, the primary mosquito vector is *Culex tarsalis*, but *Aedes* spp. and the tick *Dermacentor andersoni* can also serve as vectors.

### SYSTEMS AFFECTED
Nervous, musculoskeletal, GI, endocrine/metabolic, respiratory, reproductive.

### GENETICS
None reported.

### INCIDENCE/PREVALENCE
Seasonal patterns occur based upon mosquito activity. Usually seen in late spring and summer in USA but may become more year round due to climate change. Exposure and transmission in overwintering regions is an issue. Drought may contribute to severity. Areas where there is no aggressive mosquito mitigation. The infection in the individual bird is usually acute and lasts up to a week, with a very high but short viremic period. There also appears to be periodic "spikes." Likely similar patterns emerge based upon a myriad of factors that occur in birds. However, isolated cases outside mosquito season have been documented in birds. Incubation period is 5–14 days for WEEV and 4–10 days for EEEV (rarely up to 21 days) in birds. Some birds become detectably viremic 1 day post inoculation.

While most clinical birds progress rapidly or improve, there has been a subset with clinical signs for weeks to months.

### GEOGRAPHIC DISTRIBUTION
Regionality is one differentiation between these viruses, with EEEV mostly in upper Midwest/Northeast/Southeast United States and the Caribbean regions (group/lineage I—humans, birds, horses) and WEEV mostly west of the Mississippi River. Both can be found down into Central and South America (EEEV group/lineages IIA, IIB, III, and IV, now called Madariaga virus in horses); WEEV is found worldwide.

### SIGNALMENT
**Species**: All bird species are likely reservoirs, amplifiers, and infection sources for dead end hosts; most cases are likely subclinical. Species most likely to be clinical include Ratites (emus, cassowaries) and certain gallinaceous groups (chukar partridges, turkeys, pheasants), whooping cranes. Reptiles and amphibians are also known reservoirs.
**Mean age and range**: Young of the year may be more susceptible.
**Predominant sex**: None.

### SIGNS
#### Historical Findings
Any history of neurological signs or acute systemic signs in highly susceptible species.

#### Physical Examination Findings
Both WEEV and EEEV manifest similarly clinically, if WEEV manifests at all. As birds are the reservoir species, non-clinical presentation is most likely for WEEV in birds with certain species exceptions.
**Nervous**: altered mentation, neurologic abnormalities, seizures, paresis, paralysis, ataxia, abnormal neck movements (S curvature), reluctance to stand, side step when does stand for balance.
**Behavioral**: Depression.
**Musculoskeletal**: Some crossover with nervous system descriptions.
**GI**: Anorexia, watery diarrhea, severe hematochezia, emesis of blood-stained ingesta.
**Endocrine/metabolic**: Hyperthermia in mammals.
**Respiratory**: Hyperpneic when roused.
**Reproductive**: Drop in egg production in poultry.
**General**: Death is likely most common sign in birds, weight loss.

### CAUSES
WNV.

### RISK FACTORS
Immunosuppression, age, species predilection, lack of previous exposure, drought, poor regional mosquito mitigation, ± lack of vaccination.

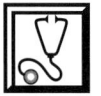

## DIAGNOSIS

### DIFFERENTIAL DIAGNOSIS
Other arboviruses (WNV, St. Louis encephalitis, LaCrosse, Powassan, Buggy Creek), trauma, heavy-metal toxicity, bacterial meningitis, fungal meningitis, protozoal meningitis, baylisascariasis, hepatoencephalopathy, neoplasia, other toxins, vascular disease (stroke, aneurysm, atherosclerosis), avian vacuolar myelinopathy, nutritional deficiency or excess (vitamin E, B6, B12 deficiencies).

### CBC/BIOCHEMISTRY/URINALYSIS
Not much information on this in birds, since death is common if clinical. In cassowaries, leukocytosis, hyperuricemia, abnormally high liver enzyme activities, and hyper-β globulinemia, which was indicative of acute inflammation, have been noted.

### OTHER LABORATORY TESTS
EEEV-specific IgM antibody in serum or CSF samples, and confirmed by neutralizing antibody testing of acute and convalescent phase serum specimens. Brain, spinal cord, and other tissues may also be collected from necropsied animals and tested. Only a few state public health laboratories conduct EEEV/WEEV testing and require BSL-3 conditions. It is recommended to reach out to the CDC Infectious Diseases Laboratories for guidance on testing (https://www.cdc.gov/laboratory/specimen-submission/form.html).

### IMAGING
Only useful to rule out other etiologies.

### DIAGNOSTIC PROCEDURES
N/A

### PATHOLOGIC FINDINGS
Gross lesions are usually non-specific. In an emu with WEEV, marked congestion of the meninges, brain, liver, spleen, kidney, and mesenteric blood vessels. The small intestinal content was scanty and mucoid. Congestion of brain and meninges may be seen as well as ecchymotic hemorrhages due to antemortem trauma. In cassowary chicks with EEEV, coelomitis and evidence of diarrhea. Histologic lesions in EEEV are typical of encephalitis, which include severe

# EASTERN AND WESTERN EQUINE ENCEPHALITIS VIRUSES (EEV/WEEV)

gliosis with necrosis of the neuropil in the cerebrum and through the corona radiating to the thalamus and perivascular cuffing throughout the mid and hindbrain, and cervical spinal cord. In the cassowary chicks with EEEV, encephalitis, vasculitis, hepatitis, nephritis, and splenitis were frequent noted. In WEEV, encephalitis, vasculitis, hepatitis, nephritis, and splenitis may be noted. In the emu case, multifocal, moderate, mixed lymphocytic, histiocytic, and heterophilic meningitis with blood vessels of the meninges and neuropil markedly dilated and congested. A moderate increase in oligodendroglia and neuronal satellitosis were seen in the mid and caudal brain stem. Scattered groups of distended empty axonal spaces and rarely axonal degeneration was observed in the neuropil.

## TREATMENT

### APPROPRIATE HEALTH CARE
Patients should be isolated separately from other susceptible avian species. Debilitated patients may not be able to thermoregulate and would benefit from placement into a heated ICU with oxygen supplemented or in larger patients a cage with added subfloor heating or heat lamp.

### NURSING CARE
Much of this care is based upon West Nile virus treatment recommendations, owing to the high caseload and management of that disease. The bird may need to be stabilized to keep from thrashing and self-traumatizing, regurgitating, and aspirating. Large birds may benefit from hay bales or a sling. Smaller birds may require towels and removal from a wire cage to prevent falls. Padding may be needed to minimize pressure sores or rub wounds. Consider a tail feather protector. Some may swallow with orally placed food; others require supportive feeding or esophageal tube placement. Patients who are not eating need to have caloric supplementation with one of the commercial powdered/liquid enteric formulations per label instructions. If the patient is dehydrated, supplemental fluid administration is warranted. Warm fluids to 100–103°F (37.8–39.4°C), 50–60 ml/kg q24h subcutaneously. An IV or IO catheter may be placed in severely debilitated patients with 10 ml/kg slow bolus over 5–10 minutes. Regular cleaning/plucking of fecal/urate contaminated feathers should be assessed. Cold laser therapy to minimize edema and ligament contracture may be warranted.

### ACTIVITY
Minimize exposure to sound, light, and tactile stimulation early on. However, over time, increasing exposure to stimulus seems to encourage the bird to help with management. If the patient is not standing on its own, initiate physical therapy.

### DIET
Assisted nutritional support is usually required early on and essential for the extended temporal component of recovery from this disease. Watch closely, especially early on, for aspiration from regurgitation.

### CLIENT EDUCATION
Birds clinically affected by EEEV/WEEV may recover over a few weeks, but most severely affected cases carry a guarded prognosis and require a commitment of supportive care for 45–90 days.

### SURGICAL CONSIDERATIONS
Potential placement of feeding tubes.

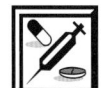

## MEDICATIONS

### DRUG(S) OF CHOICE
Most treatments are supplemental. Broad-spectrum or synergistic use of antimicrobials may be helpful but do not address the primary problem. The use of anti-inflammatories such as NSAIDs, corticosteroids, and/or IV DMSO may also be warranted. In cases of seizures or disorientation, IM/IN midazolam may help in the short term and gabapentin may be useful to consider. Maropitant as an appetite stimulant could be another tool. For birds previously and currently on a good balanced diet, vitamin E injections to prevent captive capture myopathy are generally not needed or helpful.

### CONTRAINDICATIONS
Remember that if bird is considered a food animal or wildlife being released that could enter the human food chain, all applicable laws should be considered and severely limit the use of medications.

### PRECAUTIONS
Despite previous mention, it is important to remember that corticosteroids are 4–8 times more potent in birds compared with mammals, so repeated use should be carefully evaluated. They also likely suppress the immune system, which may or not be helpful.

### POSSIBLE INTERACTIONS
N/A

### ALTERNATIVE DRUGS
N/A

## FOLLOW-UP

### PATIENT MONITORING
Follow-up serology may help track; repeat CBC and chemistries may help monitor for organ failure, hydration issues, and secondary infections.

### PREVENTION/AVOIDANCE
Mosquito control measures should be implemented: Screened housing, fans, avoiding stagnant water, larvicides, and stocking mosquito fish in ponds. Insect repellents create toxicity concerns with birds and are *not* recommended at this time. Isolate infected individuals and quarantine new animals. Currently, there are a number of vaccines developed for use in horses available in the USA. The challenge is one's comfort level (safety?) of using a product that has other equine vaccines in it, as they are often part of a combination vaccine. A WNV may be added to these combination products. Several current products have all three arbovirus components and equine tetanus toxoid in it, as the closest to arbovirus vaccine only. Zoological facilities in areas of concern vaccinate sensitive avian species (mostly Ratites) with these vaccines. Extra-label use of vaccines or use of vaccines that have not been adequately assessed in the target animal (i.e. controlled challenge studies) should be done with caution and should not be assumed to be protective. Seroconversion studies using this product in birds have not occurred, to the author's knowledge. WNV does not persist for long periods outside the host. Bleach, most disinfectants, aldehydes, ethanol, moist and dry heat, as well as drying, are sufficient for general cleaning.

### POSSIBLE COMPLICATIONS
Death can occur.

### EXPECTED COURSE AND PROGNOSIS
Most cases in birds are subclinical, excepting certain species. As death is the most common presenting sign in clinically affected birds, it should be considered at best a guarded prognosis in clinical birds.

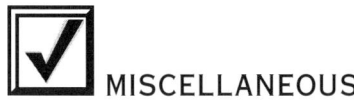

## MISCELLANEOUS

**ASSOCIATED CONDITIONS**
N/A

**AGE-RELATED FACTORS**
Juvenile birds may be more susceptible (cassowary chick dieoff); however, naïve geriatric birds may also be at risk.

**ZOONOTIC POTENTIAL**
Generally, not considered a direct zoonotic disease because of the mosquito involvement; however, there is risk during handling tissues and fluids, inhalation, mucous membrane contact, open cuts and puncture wounds from a needle stick or contaminated equipment. Gloves should be worn when handling suspect animals and bedding.

**FERTILITY/BREEDING**
Decreased egg production in poultry.

**SYNONYMS**
Triple E, sleeping sickness.

**SEE ALSO**
Atherosclerosis
Liver Disease
Neurologic (Non-Traumatic Diseases)
Neurologic (Trauma)
Nutritional Imbalances
Ocular Lesions
Seizures
Toxicosis (Heavy Metals)
Trauma
Neoplasia (Neurologic)
West Nile Virus

**ABBREVIATIONS**
BSL-3—biosecurity level 3
CSF—cerebrospinal fluid
DMSO—dimethyl sulfoxide
EEE—eastern equine encephalitis
GI—gastrointestinal
ICU—intensive care unit
IgM—immunoglobulin M
NSAIDs—nonsteroidal anti-inflammatory drugs
VEEV—Venezuelan equine encephalitis virus
WEEV—western equine encephalitis virus
WNV—West Nile virus

**INTERNET RESOURCES**
Centers for Disease Control and Prevention. Eastern equine encephalitis virus: https://www.cdc.gov/easternequineencephalitis/index.html
Wikipedia. Eastern equine encephalitis: https://en.wikipedia.org/wiki/Eastern_equine_encephalitis
Wikipedia. Western equine encephalitis: https://en.wikipedia.org/wiki/Western_equine_encephalitis_virus

*Suggested Reading*
Bergren, N.A., Haller, S., Rossi, S.L., et al. (2020). "Submergence" of Western equine encephalitis virus: Evidence of positive selection argues against genetic drift and fitness reductions. *PLoS Pathogogy*, 16:e1008102.
Borkowski, R. (2018). Western equine encephalitis virus (WEEV). In: *Infectious Disease Manual 2023*, 716–719. American Association of Zoo Veterinarians.
Guthrie, A., Citino, S., Rooker, L., et al. (2016). Eastern equine encephalomyelitis virus infection in six captive southern cassowaries (*Casuarius casuarius*). *Journal of the American Veterinary Medical Association*, 249:319–324.
Thompson, K. (2023). Eastern equine encephalitis virus (EEEV). In: *Infectious Disease Manual 2023*, 712–715. American Association of Zoo Veterinarians.
Randolph, K.D., Vanhooser, S.L., Hoffman, M. (1994). Western equine encephalitis virus in emus in Oklahoma. *Journal of Veterinary Diagnostic Investigation*, 6: 492–493.
**Author**: Eric Klaphake, DVM, DACZM

# ECTOPARASITES (MITES)

## BASICS

### DEFINITION
Mites or Acari are tiny arthropods that are related to ticks. Based on the classification schemes described by Zhang (2011) and Krantz and Walter (2009), mites are classified into two major groups, the superorder Parasitiformes (Anactinotrichida) and the superorder Acariformes (Actinotrichida).
The Parasitiformes are further subdivided into four orders: Holothyrida (a small group of scavenging mites native to former Gondwana landmasses), Ixodida (ticks), Mesostigmata (a large order of predatory and parasitic mites), and the Opilioacarida (a small group of large, long-legged segmented mites). The Acariformes can be divided into two main clades: the Sarcoptiformes and the Trombidiformes. Members of the orders Ixodida, Mesostigmata, Trombidiformes, and Sarcoptiformes are the main causes of health problems in animals. Many types of mites can inhabit a bird's feathers, quills, skin, subcutaneous tissue, and respiratory tracts. Of these, the blood-sucking or red mites (*Dermanyssus gallinae*), northern fowl mite (*Ornithonyssus sylviarum*), feather and quill mites (Syringophilidae, *Protolichus* spp. *Dubininia* spp.), and mites of the genus *Knemidocoptes* are the most common and clinically relevant.

### PATHOPHYSIOLOGY
Mites live on the skin and/or feathers, where they can cause direct irritation with resultant dermatitis, hyperkeratosis, and feather lesions. In severe cases, birds are irritable and can develop anemia. Northern fowl mites and red mites are the most common mites in poultry; the Northern fowl mite spends its entire lifecycle on the birds, whereas red mites live in cracks and crevices in the environment and only emerge and attack the birds at night. *Knemidocoptes* are burrowing mites that might present with long incubation and asymptomatic carriers, but can cause severe disfiguring dermatitis and thickening of the skin if the infestation is not readily identified and treated. Feather and quill mites live between the barbs on the ventral surface of feathers, or in the quills, where they feed on quill secretions, feather pitch, and skin debris. The exception are the Syringophilid mites, which penetrate the quill and suck tissue fluid. Feather and quill mites are host specific, and spend their entire lifecycle is spent on the bird. They generally only cause problems in large numbers.

### SYSTEMS AFFECTED
**Integument**: Dermatitis—up to severe infection and abscess formation, scabs, dandruff, hyperkeratosis, overgrowth, and disfiguration of the beak, loss of toes, feather damage.
**Hemolymphatic**: Blood loss and anemia in certain species.
**Reproductive**: Reduced egg production.
**Orthopedic**: Severe *Knemidokoptes* infestations of the legs and feet (podoknemidocoptiasis) may lead to lameness because of ankylosis of the hock and other joints, necrosis and sloughing of the toes, swollen nail beds and twisted nails.

### GENETICS
Because knemidokoptic mange is seemingly more common in inbred birds, a genetic predisposition or selective immunosuppression has been suggested but is not proven.

### INCIDENCE/PREVALENCE
Incidence is dependent on a number of factors; some mites cause common and serious problems in pigeons, poultry, and nestlings of many species in aviary settings; *Knemidokoptes* in budgerigars and poultry is often seen, but does not appear to be highly contagious. Red mites are a common problem in chicken flocks, particularly with warm and moist weather conditions.
The northern fowl mite is less common than *Dermanyssus*, but can cause significant problems in backyard poultry.

### GEOGRAPHIC DISTRIBUTION
Worldwide; different species have different distribution.

### SIGNALMENT
**Species**: Mites are found in essentially all classes of birds. Feather and quill mites are species and site specific, while red mites are not host specific. Those of the most importance or the most recognized are mentioned here, together with the parasites that affect them. Poultry: red mite (*D. gallinae*), northern fowl mite (*O. sylvarium*), *Knemidokoptes mutans*, *Knemidokoptes gallinae*, and several other mites. Budgerigars, and sometimes canaries, finches: *Knemidokoptes pilae*, feather mites (*Protolichus lunula*, *Dubininia melopsittaci*). Gray-cheeked parakeets and, rarely, in Amazon parrots: sarcoptic mite, *Myialges* spp. Canaries and finches: *D. gallinae* and *O. sylvarium*, *K. pilae*, *Knemidokoptes jamaicensis*, quill mites, epidermotic mites. Pigeons: feather mites (*Megninia columbae* and *Falculifer rostratus*), *K. mutans* (leg mange).
**Mean age and range**: All ages are susceptible, but young birds, especially nestlings, are most susceptible to morbidity and mortality.

Immune-compromised and stressed birds are more likely to be affected.
**Predominant sex**: Both sexes are susceptible.

### SIGNS

#### General Comments
Clinical signs are related to the presence of parasites and their effect on skin and feathers. In severe infestations with blood-sucking mites, anemia and death can occur, especially in nestlings.

#### Historical Findings
With red mites and northern fowl mites, flocks may present with a history of pruritus, restlessness, death of nestlings, reduction of egg production, identification of mites or their droppings in or around birds or on eggs. With knemidokoptic mites, birds present with scaly, crusty, gray to tan lesions on unfeathered skin, especially the legs, feet, and around the beak, eyelids, and periocular areas, and are usually noticeably pruritic. With feather and quill mites, birds may present with pruritus, restlessness and unkempt, ruffled, dull feathers that may break easily. Irritation and pruritus may lead to loss of production in poultry.

#### Physical Examination Findings
Pruritus, restlessness, feet tripping. Presence of ectoparasites on skin, feathers (except for red mites). Dermatitis and associated lesions including flakiness, redness, sores and scabs. *Knemidokoptes*—honeycomb-like hyperkeratotic lesions on the base and commissure of the beak, cere, cloaca, legs, feet. Severe infestations can lead to horny protuberances and distorted growth of the beak (especially the upper mandible) if the germinal layer of the beak is affected. Lameness can be seen in advanced cases where the legs and feet are affected. Feather and quill mites—feather abnormalities including broken feathers, holes in feathers, lines in feathers, hemorrhagic areas in the quills. Red mites, northern fowl mite—depression, anemia.

### CAUSES
See Signalment section.

### RISK FACTORS
Risk factors for developing ectoparasites are mostly related to the exposure to infested animals or materials. Mixing of domestic birds with wild populations can result in the spread of parasite infections. Overcrowding of birds increases the risk or the spread of external parasites. *Knemidokoptes* infestation might be more common in immunocompromised animals. Red mite infestations may become especially problematic during the warmer months of the year.

E

# DIAGNOSIS

## DIFFERENTIAL DIAGNOSIS
Dermatitis and/or folliculitis due to other causes, such as poxvirus, papillomavirus, PBFD (circovirus), bacterial infections, dermatophytosis, other ectoparasites. Feather destructive behavior due to other causes. Brown cere hypertrophy (in budgerigars). Other causes for anemia (e.g. blood loss due to trauma, chronic infections, blood parasites, hemolytic anemia).

## CBC/BIOCHEMISTRY/URINALYSIS
Findings are non-specific, although anemia may be noted in some cases.

## OTHER LABORATORY TESTS
Skin scrapings. Macroscopic and microscopic examination of feather preparations (feather digest).

## IMAGING
N/A

## DIAGNOSTIC PROCEDURES
Direct microscopic examination of parasites. Fecal examination will occasionally show adults or eggs of mites (due to ingestion by the host). Knemidokoptic mange—microscopic examination of skin scrapings prepared with potassium hydroxide. Feather and quill mites—microscopic examination of feathers, feather digest or acetate tape preparations. Red mites—examination of nest boxes and other area around caging to look for mites and excrement. Placing a white cloth under the birds or using commercial mite sticky traps might help to discover mites.

## PATHOLOGIC FINDINGS
Honeycomb-like hyperkeratotic and acanthotic lesions of the beak, cere, legs, and sometimes other areas, as well as beak abnormalities with *Knemidokoptes* infestations. Most other infestations cause skin inflammation, with erythema, dandruff, hyperkeratosis, scabbing, ulceration, and bleeding. Presence of parasites. Feather lesions such as fraying or holes in the feathers may also result from damage caused by feather mites and featherlings. Red mites (*Dermanyssus*) as well as Northern mites (*Ornithonyssus*) normally cause only little cutaneous signs but some irritation, but restlessness, anemia, and debilitation will occur.

# TREATMENT

## APPROPRIATE HEALTH CARE
Most patients with ectoparasites can be treated as outpatients. Treatment of the environment may be needed to achieve adequate ectoparasite control.

## NURSING CARE
Generally not needed, unless severe infestation and significantly debilitated bird.

## ACTIVITY
N/A

## DIET
N/A

## CLIENT EDUCATION
Proper administration of medications as well as their adverse effects should be explained. In flock situations, various husbandry and management practices should be outlined. Treatment of the environment may be needed to achieve adequate ectoparasite control. Certain mites may have zoonotic potential.

## SURGICAL CONSIDERATIONS
N/A

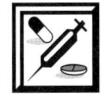

# MEDICATIONS

## DRUG(S) OF CHOICE
Ivermectin is used for most ectoparasitic infestations, especially those involving *Knemidokoptes* spp. Dosage is 0.2–0.4 mg/kg, which can be difficult to administer in small species. Ivermectin can be given PO, by gavage, topically, or IM. Ivermectin can be diluted in propylene glycol; it should be properly mixed to achieve a uniform concentration. Alternatively, the injectable formula can be freshly mixed with tap water. Note that the formulation does not mix well with saline. Moxidectin can be used as an alternative to ivermectin at 0.2 mg/kg PO or by gavage. It can also be used topically in budgerigars 1 mg/bird. Fipronil 3 mg/kg and selamectin 25 mg/kg can be used topically to treat feather and quill mites. Permethrin can be used topically in poultry species to treat ectoparasitic infections. Examples of products that contain permethrin that can be used in poultry include Prozap® Garden and Poultry Dust (Neogen, Lansing, MI) and Permectrin® II (Elanco US Inc., Greenfield, IN); these products have 0-day meat or egg withdrawal times. If non-authorised drugs such as ivermectin or fipronil are used in poultry, withdrawal times and legal regulation in respect to food-producing species need to be considered. Fluralaner (Exzolt®, MSD Animal Health, Rahway, NJ) is licensed for laying chicken at a dosage of 0.5 mg/kg PO or via drinking water. It has shown to be highly effective against red mites and empirically also against *Knemidokoptes* mites. Diatomaceous earth can be used in poultry houses and is helpful to manage internal and external parasites. In a recent study, hens with access to dust baths containing either diatomaceous earth, kaolin clay, or sulphur had a reduction in ectoparasites by 80–100% after 1 week when compared with hens not provided dust baths. Further regular replacement of bedding and nesting material helps suppressing parasites infestation.

## CONTRAINDICATIONS
Although carbaryl 5% powder (Sevin® dust, Garden Tech, Palatine, IL) or sprays have historically been used for treatment of ectoparasites in avian species, carbaryl is regulated by the EPA and has a zero-tolerance policy for use in poultry/food animals.

## PRECAUTIONS
Ivermectin needs to be carefully mixed and administered and should be kept away from exposure to light. Single treatments against mites are not always effective, and repeated dosing may be needed according to the lifecycles of the parasite in question.

## POSSIBLE INTERACTIONS
N/A

## ALTERNATIVE DRUGS
Paraffin oil and mineral oil have been applied to *Knemidokoptes* lesions to suffocate the mites; it also helps to soften some of the larger and more disfiguring lesions. Petroleum jelly or marigold ointment can also be used; care should be taken not to grease legs and feathers with an overload of ointment. Depending on secondary symptoms such as severe dermatitis, additional skin care measures are needed, which may include supportive vitamin A application as well as anti-inflammatory and/or anti-infective drugs.

# FOLLOW-UP

## PATIENT MONITORING
Patients with ectoparasites should be examined at regular intervals for the presence of parasites and retreated if necessary.

## PREVENTION/AVOIDANCE
Treatment of the premises with insecticidal sprays and/or powders should be performed as needed. Cleaning and disinfection of nest boxes and other materials should be done prior to breeding season.

## POSSIBLE COMPLICATIONS
Decreased egg production. Loss of toes or beak tissue can occur in advanced. *Knemidokoptes* cases in budgerigars and finches.

## EXPECTED COURSE AND PROGNOSIS
Ectoparasites generally respond well to treatment; prognosis should be good, except in cases where there is overcrowding or

# ECTOPARASITES (MITES) (CONTINUED)

contaminated premises that have not been properly cleaned and/or treated. *Knemidokoptes* in finches does not always respond as well as in budgerigars, perhaps due to secondary bacterial infection. In chickens, *Knemidokoptes* is often advanced so that treatment can be more time consuming and work intense; further legal regulations for laying chicken need to be considered. Severe red mite infestations may lead to significant morbidity and mortality, especially among nestlings.

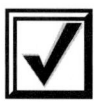 MISCELLANEOUS

## ASSOCIATED CONDITIONS
N/A

## AGE-RELATED FACTORS
Blood-sucking mites cause more significant disease in nestling birds.

## ZOONOTIC POTENTIAL
There have been numerous reports of humans that have been bitten by red mites in heavily invested collections.

## FERTILITY/BREEDING
Breeding, fertility rates, and egg production could decrease, particularly in poultry that are heavily parasitized.

## SYNONYMS
*Knemidokoptes* in budgerigars—scaly face and leg mite. *K. mutans* in chickens—scaly leg mite. *K. gallinae* in chickens—depluming mite or itch mite. *Knemidokoptes* in finches—tassle foot.

## SEE ALSO
Air Sac Mites
Cere and Skin Color Change
Circovirus (Psittacines)
Circoviruses (Non-Psittacine Birds)
Dermatitis
Feather Disorders
Toes and Nails (Diseases of)
Toxicosis (Environmental/Pesticides)

## ABBREVIATIONS
PBFD—psittacine beak and feather disease

## INTERNET RESOURCES
Murillo, A.C. (2022). Mites of poultry. *Merck Veterinary Manual*: http://www.merckmanuals.com/vet/poultry/ectoparasites/mites_of_poultry.html
There are numerous other websites that contain extensive information about poultry ectoparasites.

## Suggested Reading
Chitty, J. (2009). Avian ectoparasites. In: *Proceedings of the AAVAC Annual Conference*, Adelaide, Australia, 77–83.

Clyde, C.I., Patton, S. (2000). Parasitism of caged birds. In: *Manual of Avian Medicine* (ed. G.H. Olsen, S.E. Orosz), 424–448. St. Louis, MO: Elsevier.

Doneley, R.J.T. (2009). Bacterial and parasitic disease of parrots. *Veterinary Clinics of North America: Exotic Animal Practice*, 2:423–431.

Krantz, G.W., Walter, D.E. (2009). *A Manual of Acarology*, 3rd edn. Lubbock, TX: Texas Tech University Press.

Reavill, D.R., Schmidt, R.E., Phalen, D.N. (2015). Integument. In: *Pathology of Pet and Aviary Birds*, 2nd edn., 237–262. Ames, IA: Wiley.

Schmidt, R.E., Lightfoot, T.L. (2011). Integument. In: *Clinical Avian Medicine* (ed. G. Harrison, T. Lightfoot), Vol. 1, 395–409.

Zhang, Z.Q. (2011). Animal biodiversity: An outline of higher-level classification and survey of taxonomic richness. *Zootaxa*, 3148:1–237.

**Authors**: Petra Zsivanovits, DrMedVet, DECZM (Avian), and Yvonne R. A. van Zeeland, DVM, MVR, PhD, DECZM (Avian, Small Mammal)

# ECTOPARASITES (TICKS, LICE, DIPTERANS)

## BASICS

### DEFINITION
Ectoparasites of birds are arthropods (insects and arachnids) that live on or in the skin and feathers. They are represented by acarids, which include the mites (sucking and biting) and ticks (hard and soft), and the insects (lice, mosquitos, flies, and bedbugs). Various different ectoparasites can infest birds, although apart from mites, they are not very commonly encountered in private practice. Insects mostly cause problems in case of severe infestations, and play a significant role in the transmission of other infectious diseases.

### PATHOPHYSIOLOGY
External parasites live on the skin and/or feathers, where they can cause direct irritation with resultant dermatitis and feather lesions. Severe infestations may cause irritation, restlessness and anemia, particularly in nestlings and young birds. Arthropods, such as mosquitoes, ticks, flies, fleas, and lice commonly serve as vectors and can transmit infectious diseases either actively or passively (e.g. poxvirus, hemoprotozoa).

### SYSTEMS AFFECTED
**Integument**: Dermatitis, scabs, dandruff, scales, hyperkeratosis, pruritus.
**Behavior**: Irritation, restlessness.
**Hemolymphatic**: Blood loss and anemia in certain species, transmission of blood parasites (e.g. *Plasmodium, Haemoproteus, Leucocytozoon*), viruses (e.g. arbovirus, poxvirus), and bacteria (*Borrelia* spp.).
**Reproductive**: Reduced egg production.
**Nervous system**: Tick paralysis, encephalitis.

### GENETICS
N/A

### INCIDENCE/PREVALENCE
Ectoparasite infestations with ticks, lice, bedbugs (*Cimex lectularius*), fleas (e.g. *Echidnophaga gallinacea*), blackflies, hippoboscid flies, midges, and mosquitos may occur in birds, but are not as common as mite infestations in captive birds. Incidence can vary, for example by geographical region, month of year, and species involved. Some ectoparasites are quite common and can cause serious problems in pigeons, poultry and nestlings of many species in an aviary setting.

### GEOGRAPHIC DISTRIBUTION
Worldwide; distribution varies depending on the ectoparasite involved.

### SIGNALMENT
**Species**: Ectoparasites are found in essentially all classes of birds; the most common and those of greatest importance are listed here. Ostrich—lice (*Struthioliperirus struthionis*),

ticks (*Argus persicus*). Birds of prey—ticks, hippoboscid flies (birds of prey), sticktight flea (*Echidnophaga gallinacea*). Chicken—European chick flea (*Ceratophyllus gallinae*), sticktight flea, ticks, hippoboscid flies, myiasis due to larvae of Calliphoridae (Blowflies, e.g. *Calliphora*—bluebottle and *Lucilia*—greenbottle). Canaries and finches—quill mites, epidermotic mites, lice. Pigeons: lice—*Columbicola columbae* (wings), *Campanulotes bidentatus* (tail), *Menopon latum* (body), sticktight flea, ticks (*Argus reflexus*), bedbugs, hippoboscid flies. Psittacine birds (import)—sticktight flea (*E. gallinacea*).
**Mean age and range**: All ages are susceptible, but young birds, especially nestlings, are most susceptible to morbidity and mortality. Immune-compromised and stressed birds are more likely to be affected.
**Predominant sex**: Both sexes are susceptible.

### SIGNS

#### General Comments
Clinical signs are primarily related to the presence of parasites and their effect on skin and feathers. In severe cases, anemia, debilitation, and death can occur, especially in nestlings. Clinical signs may result from other infectious diseases that are transmitted by insect vectors. Birds infected with ticks may present extremely sick or collapsed with an extensive haemorrhagic swelling of the face or head. In absence of tickborne pathogens, it is likely that these signs are the result from tick saliva toxin or a hypersensitivity reaction.

#### Historical Findings
Large numbers of fleas, lice, flies, or mosquitos may result in irritation, pruritus, restlessness, death of nestlings, reduced egg production (in poultry flocks). Myiasis is commonly seen during the warmer months of the year in debilitated birds or birds with (infected) wounds. Swelling and erythema associated with ticks, usually on the unfeathered portions of the head, but can also affect other parts of the body. Birds may present with collapse or general malaise. Presence of ectoparasites in large numbers usually indicates suboptimal housing conditions or severe debilitation.

#### Physical Examination Findings
Direct visualization of the ectoparasite, eggs, larvae, or nymphs on the skin or feathers, or in case of myiasis, in wounds. Dermatitis and associated lesions including flakiness, hyperkeratosis, erythema/redness, swelling, sores, and scabs. Feather damage. Pruritus, irritation, restlessness. Depression, collapse, anemia.

### CAUSES
See Signalment section.

### RISK FACTORS
Risk factors for developing ectoparasites are mostly related to the exposure to infested animals or materials. Mixing of domestic birds with wild populations can result in the spread of parasite infections. Overcrowding of birds increases the risk or the spread of external parasites. Suboptimal housing conditions, debilitation or immunocompromise may predispose to clinical problems.

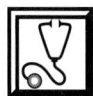

## DIAGNOSIS

### DIFFERENTIAL DIAGNOSIS
Dermatitis and/or folliculitis due to other causes: poxvirus, papillomavirus, dermatophytosis, bacterial dermatitis, PBFD (circovirus), mites. Feather destructive behavior due to other causes. Other causes for anemia (e.g. blood loss due to trauma, chronic infections, blood parasites, hemolytic anemia).

### CBC/BIOCHEMISTRY/URINALYSIS
Findings are non-specific, although anemia may be noted in some cases.

### OTHER LABORATORY TESTS
Microscopic or macroscopic examination of feather samples or acetate tape preparations. Cytology of blood smears may reveal presence of hemoparasites (transmitted by insect vectors).

### IMAGING
N/A

### DIAGNOSTIC PROCEDURES
Direct microscopic examination of parasites. Skin scrapings or acetate tape preparations. Sampling of feathers for preparations. Fecal examination will occasionally show adults or eggs of lice (due to ingestion by the host). Examination of nest boxes and other area around caging to look for ectoparasites, their eggs or excrement.

### PATHOLOGIC FINDINGS
Ectoparasite infestations can cause skin inflammation, with erythema, scaling, hyperkeratosis, scabbing, ulceration, and bleeding. Ectoparasites, their eggs, larvae, or nymphs may be directly visualized. Feather damage feathers may result from lice infestations.

## TREATMENT

### APPROPRIATE HEALTH CARE
Most patients with ectoparasites can be treated as outpatients. Treatment of the environment may be needed to achieve adequate ectoparasite control. Myiasis—cleaning and removal of larvae and eggs.

E

# ECTOPARASITES (TICKS, LICE, DIPTERANS) (CONTINUED)

Treatment of underlying conditions. Wound management and treatment of (secondary) infections. Application of diluted ivermectin sprayed onto contaminated tissue and/or systemic dosing of ivermectin. Monitoring for presence of infectious diseases transmitted by insect or arthropod vectors may be warranted. Manual removal and treatment of ticks with ivermectin. Tick reactions should be treated as an emergency requiring aggressive therapy with fluids, broad-spectrum antibiosis, and short-acting corticosteroids (e.g. dexamethasone).

## NURSING CARE
Generally not needed, unless severe infestation and significantly debilitated bird. Aggressive therapy with fluids and broad-spectrum antibiosis is needed for birds with tick reactions.

## ACTIVITY
N/A

## DIET
N/A

## CLIENT EDUCATION
Proper administration of medications, as well as their adverse effects, should be explained. In flock situations, various husbandry and management practices should be outlined. Treatment of the environment may be needed to achieve adequate ectoparasite control. Risk of transmission of infectious diseases by insect vectors should be explained.

## SURGICAL CONSIDERATIONS
N/A

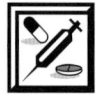

## MEDICATIONS
### DRUG(S) OF CHOICE
Ivermectin is used for treatment of burrowing mites, *Dermanyssus, Ornithonyssus,* myiasis. Apply IM, PO, or topically at a dose of 0.2–0.4 mg/kg. Moxidectin—similar to ivermectin; can be used at a dose of 0.2 mg/kg, PO, or by gavage. Selamectin can be used topically to treat ectoparasites in birds. Fipronil is used for feather/quill mites, lice, fleas, *Dermanyssus* and *Ornithonyssus,* ticks, and hippoboscid flies. Prophylaxis against biting flies. Apply spray (3 mg/kg) to cotton wool and subsequently apply to back of the head, under the wings, and at the base of the tail. Repeat every 2–4 weeks. For biting fly prophylaxis, apply to bare skin weekly or (for falconry birds) whenever flown in risk areas. Permethrin is used for treatment of feather/quill mites, lice, fleas, and hippoboscid flies. Powder applied through plumage, repeated every 2–3 weeks. Piperonil butoxide/pyrethrin has the same efficacy as

permethrin. Apply through plumage and repeat every 10–21 days. Environmental control is achieved with antiparasitics such as Indorex® spray (permethrin, pyriproxyfen; Virbac, Carros, France), Duramitex® (Malathion, dilute 0.93% and paint/spray on perches; Harkers, Bury St Edmunds, UK), Zodiac+ (methoprene/permethrin; Wellmark International, Schaumburg, IL).

## CONTRAINDICATIONS
Although carbaryl 5% powder (Sevin® dust, Garden Tech, Palatine, IL) or sprays have historically been used for treatment of ectoparasites in avian species, carbaryl is regulated by the US Environmental Protection Agency and has a zero-tolerance policy for use in poultry/food animals. Products available for sandfly control in dogs are not currently recommended for use on birds.

## PRECAUTIONS
Ivermectin must be carefully mixed and administered and should be kept away from exposure to light. Caution is warranted when using ivermectin in small passerines (finches) as toxicity has been reported. Environmental sprays should preferably be used in absence of birds to prevent toxicity. When using fipronil, soaking of the bird should be avoided to prevent hypothermia. Single treatments against ectoparasites may not be sufficient, with repeated dosing required according to the lifecycles of the ectoparasite in question.

## POSSIBLE INTERACTIONS
N/A

## ALTERNATIVE DRUGS
Depending on secondary symptoms such as severe dermatitis, additional skin care measures may need to be taken, including supportive vitamin A application as well as anti-inflammatory and/or anti-infective drugs.

## FOLLOW-UP
### PATIENT MONITORING
Patients with ectoparasites should be examined at regular intervals for the presence of parasites and retreated if necessary.

### PREVENTION/AVOIDANCE
Treatment of the premises with insecticidal sprays and/or powders should be performed as needed. Cleaning and disinfection of nest boxes and other materials should be done prior to breeding season. Mosquito netting and covering larger open water containers might be useful to protect aviaries. Avoid bringing ticks into the aviary areas, flying birds in risk areas, and/or use preventive antiparasitics if at increased risk for exposure.

## POSSIBLE COMPLICATIONS
Decreased egg production. Secondary infections due to vector potential of some ectoparasites.

## EXPECTED COURSE AND PROGNOSIS
Ectoparasites generally respond well to treatment; prognosis should be good except in cases where there is overcrowding or contaminated premises that have not been properly cleaned and/or treated. Tick reaction: Monks et al. (2006) describes a therapeutic success rate of 75% following aggressive therapy.

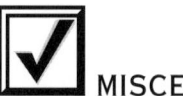

## MISCELLANEOUS
### ASSOCIATED CONDITIONS
Some species can act as vectors for blood-borne diseases such as tularemia, encephalitis, spirochetosis (borreliosis), piroplasmosis, anaplasmosis, dirofilariasis, rickettsial diseases, leucocytozoonosis, and viral diseases such as West Nile, Usutu, Herpes or Poxvirus.

### AGE-RELATED FACTORS
N/A

### ZOONOTIC POTENTIAL
There have been reports of humans becoming bitten by argassid ticks. The sticktight flea might act as a vector for human (murine) typhus. Some pigeon mites and bedbugs associated with pigeons and chickens have been shown to bite humans.

### FERTILITY/BREEDING
Breeding, fertility rates, and egg production could decrease, particularly in poultry that are heavily parasitized.

### SYNONYMS
Myiasis, flystrike.

### SEE ALSO
Air Sac Mites
Cere and Skin Color Change
Circoviruses
Dermatitis
Feather Disorders
Toxicosis (Environmental/Pesticides)
Toes and Nails (Diseases of)

### ABBREVIATIONS
PBFD—psittacine beak and feather disease

### INTERNET RESOURCES
Murillo, A.C. (2022). Mites of poultry. *Merck Veterinary Manual*: http://www.merckmanuals.com/vet/poultry/ectoparasites/lice_of_poultry.html
There are numerous other websites that contain extensive information about poultry ectoparasites.

*Suggested Reading*

Clyde, C.I., Patton, S. (2000). Parasitism of caged birds. In: *Manual of Avian Medicine* (ed. G.H. Olsen, S.E. Orosz), 424–448. St. Louis, MO: Elsevier.

Cole, B.H. (1997). Appendix 7: Parasitic Diseases of Birds: Arthropod Ectoparasites. In: *Avian Medicine and Surgery*, 2nd edn., Ames, IA: Wiley-Blackwell.

Doneley, R.J.T. (2009). Bacterial and parasitic disease of parrots. *Veterinary Clinics of North America: Exotic Animal Practice*, 2:423–431.

Hunkle, N.C., Corrigan, R.M. (2019). External parasites and poultry pests. In: *Diseases of Poultry*, 14th edn. (ed. D.E. Swayne, M. Boulianne, C.M. Logue, et al.), 1135–1156. Ames, IA: Wiley.

Monks, D., Fisher, M., Forbes, N.A. (2006). *Ixodes frontalis* and avian tick-related syndrome in the United Kingdom. *Journal of Small Animal Practice*, 47:451–455.

Philips, J.R. (1990). What's bugging your birds? Avian parasitic arthropods. *Wildlife Rehabilitation*, 8:155.

Reavill, D.R., Schmidt, R.E., Phalen, D.N. (2015). Integument. In: *Pathology of Pet and Aviary Birds*, 2nd edn., 237–262. Ames, IA: Wiley.

Smith, V.S. (2001). Avian louse phylogeny (Phiraptera: Ischnocera): A cladistic based morphology. *Zoological Journal of the Linnean Society*, 132:81–144.

**Authors**: Dr Petra Zsivanovits DECZM (Avian), and Yvonne R.A. van Zeeland, DVM, MVR, PhD, DECZM (Avian, Small Mammal)

**E**

# EGG ABNORMALITIES

 BASICS

## DEFINITION
The abnormal bird's egg may be abnormal in shape, color, density, or size based on the shell, and/or have abnormal development of internal contents. Here, we will refer to all species of female birds with the term "hen", rather than just the domestic chicken. Failure of the egg to hatch, or dead in shell is a common concern when reproduction rather than egg production for food is desired. We focus on that known for parrot eggs, but in many cases only generalities observed from production species can be provided.

## PATHOPHYSIOLOGY
Factors affecting the creation, formation, passage, and development of the egg can be divided into (1) External factors—nutrition, incubation, husbandry, toxic exposure, environmental condition and (2) Bird endogenous factors—behavior, genetics, age, neoplasia. Infectious disease can affect the embryo/egg from creation to after deposition. Infectious diseases may be introduced during egg formation or may enter through the shell after laying. Egg abnormalities are intimately connected with and can signal ill health in the hen.

## SYSTEMS AFFECTED
Reproductive: Most commonly affected system based on the finding of the abnormal egg. Although endocrine/metabolic, musculoskeletal and behavioral systems may also be affected within the hen and cock.

## GENETICS
Genetically incompatible pairs can result in lack of production of offspring or the production of birds/embryos with undesirable traits including excessive egg death, excessive malposition, splay leg, heart deformities.

## INCIDENCE/PREVALENCE
Females of every avian species can be affected, but males also contribute to fertility, genetics, and can introduce infectious disease.

## GEOGRAPHIC DISTRIBUTION
Worldwide.

## SIGNALMENT
**Species**: All birds.
**Breed predilections**: Increased incidence may occur in birds based on selective breeding for excessive egg production (e.g. laying poultry hen). Parrots, particularly cockatiels and grey parrots may lay eggs excessively and may be more prone to egg abnormalities. In zoos and among breeders of rare species, species that may have undergone genetic bottlenecks may have an increased incidence of abnormal eggs.
**Mean age and range**: Reproductive maturity to senility for the species.
**Sex**: Only female.

## SIGNS
### Historical Findings
Lack of egg production, "broodiness", nest building behaviors. Unexpected or excessive egg production, inability to rise or walk, muscular weakness. Abnormally shaped, colored, sized, or shelled eggs for the species. Lack of hatching eggs, eggshells with blood, bile staining or cracks apparent. Deformed embryos at hatch including exposed yolk sacs, weakened chicks, or chicks that die shortly after hatching.

### Physical Examination Findings
May be limited or none. An egg-shaped mass in the caudal coelom, coelomic distension with fluid, or coelomic herniation may be present. Vent laxity. Weakness of the rear limbs and inability to stand may occur with excessive egg production. Externally normal eggs may still have internal abnormalities to include embryo position or formation, signs of bacterial or fungal infection, or abnormal yolk or membrane structures.

## CAUSES
Nutrition, Incubation, Husbandy, Toxic Exposure, Genetics, Trauma, Infectious Disease

## RISK FACTORS
Female sex, Increased age, Species bred for high egg production, Improper husbandry, malnutrition, Toxin exposure

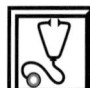 DIAGNOSIS

## DIFFERENTIAL DIAGNOSIS
Differentail diagnoses for the abnormal egg are many. The DAMNITVP scheme provides an overview of likely differentials for egg abnormalities (not an exhaustive list):

**D:** Degenerative of the uterus in the older hen can result in smaller thin shelled eggs or reduced production of eggs.

**M:** Metabolic diseases with nutritional secondary hyperparathyroidism likely the most common; can affect egg production and egg quality; and are therefore associated with egg and embryo malformation.

**N:** Neoplasia of the hen or nutritional deficiency or toxicity of the hen are commonly associated with lack of egg production, abnormal egg production or malformed feti or hatchlings.

**I:** Infectious disease (bacterial, viral or fungal) can be transmitted from the hen, or within the incubator; iatrogenic—use of any oil or many types of antibiotic upon or within the egg can cause embryo death; inherited/congenital/genetic—lack of genetic diversity can result in malformed feti and abnormal eggs.

**T:** Traumatic—trauma to the hen or the egg can cause visible egg shell abnormalities or embryo death; toxic—many antibiotics and many other substances such as disinfectants or even the relatively inert mineral oil can result in embryo malformation or death.

**V:** Vascular—early embryonic death; vascular disease per se appears uncommon as a cause of egg abnormalities, but atherosclerosis may be more common in aged nonreproductively active female birds.

**P:** Parasites can cause abnormal eggs to include parasite inclusion within the egg.

## CBC/BIOCHEMISTRY/URINALYSIS
N/A for egg.

## OTHER LABORATORY TESTS
**Cytology**: Useful for assessment of bacterial or fungal elements inside the egg.
**Culture/PCR**: Detection of specific viral, bacterial, or fungal pathogens within the egg, especially those which are difficult to culture. Can be done on initial egg opening during necropsy or in the live egg. Bacteriological sampling of the intact egg can be performed by drilling a small hole over the air cell, approach as determined by candling, and inserting a swab or a sterilized rigid endoscope. Prior to drilling the shell is cleaned over the drill site using F10®Sc (Health & Hygiene Pty., SA) at a 1: 250 dilution. The hole can be sealed using a tiny quantity of paraffin wax.
**Histopathology**: Assessment of embryo tissues. Yolk removal from the embryo is recommended prior to formalin fixation.
**Fertility test**: Egg fertility may be assessed based on gross observation of an embryo or microscopic or histologic examination of the membranes for evidence of gastrula formation or sperm penetration of the pertinent membranes. Sperm samples can be microscopically evaluated for motility, shape of sperm and tail, and relative quantity of sperm in sample.

## IMAGING
### Candling
Classical and most often used technique to image eggs; can be used to determine embryo viability and to determine entry into the egg for necropsy. A bright, preferably cool, light is shone through the egg in a dark room or darkened container to visualize structures within the egg. Generally, begun about 7–10 days post lay (junction of first and second trimesters) to assess fertility. Before this stage, the movement and temperature fluctuations associated with candling may cause embryonic mortality. After this point, can be done as often as q48h to assess continued embryo growth; once weekly usually sufficient in healthy embryos.

Very early blood vessels can be detected and small cracks and other defects in the shell can be noted and repaired. Observation of early embryonic death (appears as a blood ring) allows removal of dead eggs from nest or incubator to minimize possible bacterial growth in the dead egg. This technique can define and mark the air cell to assess draw down, the approach for entering the egg needed for an assisted hatch or necropsy and confirm embryo death prior to necropsy. Not as useful in thick-shelled, pigmented eggs such as those of cranes, bustards, ostrich, or condors. Once the embryo is large and near to hatch, candling will only show there is a chick, not its viability, unless one sees movement.

### Candling to assess egg viability and stage the embryo

The normal egg has good shell condition and blood vessels radiate from the blastodisc uniformly to resemble a spider. The air cell occurs at the blunt end. Blood vessels in the healthy psittacine are visible beginning at 5–7 days. The infertile egg lacks blood vessels, although a blastodisc may be present. The stages of fertile egg death in chronological order, are early embryonic death (EED), mid-incubation death and prehatching, hatching or late incubation death. Visualization of a blood ring or crescent due to vessel break down and the diffusion of extravascular blood into the embryonic membranes indicates EED. Among parots, EED is the second most common period of embryonic death and appears more common in cockatoos. Causes of EED include improper handling, storage, and incubation parameters, genetics, eggborne infection, contamination, and breeding stock disease or nutritional deficiency. Mid-incubation death is rare. Candling can reveal a darkening of the vessels

around the embryo as the blood supply recedes and lack of an air cell. Improper incubation (most common), nutritional deficiencies, lethal genes, eggborne infections, toxic exposure are associated with midterm egg deaths. Late incubation death is the most common time of egg death in Psittaciformes with incidence of up to 26% in cockatoos. These deaths commonly occur based on improper position, or low incubator humidity (Table 1).

### Digital egg monitor

The Egg Buddy (Avitronics, Truro, UK), a digital egg monitor which uses infrared beams to assess blood flow of the embryo, best assessses viability of the chick in the last third of incubation, and of thick-shelled and dark pigmented eggs. Misclassification of very early or very late embryos as dead with this egg monitor is possible.

### Other Imaging

**Radiography**: Determining embryo presence and positioning/ malposition in species with thick shelled large eggs.

**Endoscopy**: Determining embryo position and for assisted hatch in larger species. Entry point for endoscope is over the air cell, usually in the wide end of the egg. Use candling to identify the air cell location. Take care not to addle the egg (jarring of the developing embryo to the extent that death is caused).

**Digital image capture**: Recommended during egg necropsy for review of embryo position.

**Ultrasound**: Identification of developing follicles and locating eggs in the oviduct.

## DIAGNOSTIC PROCEDURES

### Egg Necropsy

For all egg necropsies, data collected and recorded should include: Egg identifiers— parents, nest/cage, species, date of necropsy, date egg laid, date of egg collection, original

weight of egg at laying; egg measures— weight, length, diameter; external appearance, abnormalities; candling appearance—note position of air cell, abnormalities, stage of development of embryo; breakout appearance, abnormalities, stage of development of embryo; malposition of embryo – if present; samples collected.

### Egg necropsy procedure(s)

(1) External egg examination and measurements. (2) Candling provides egg/ embryonic stage, and access route. (3) Break out: Culture, cytology samples; embryo position observation and staging; gross necropsy abnormalities documentation; collection of histopathology samples. Locate the air cell at the round or blunt end of the egg. After candling and initial egg measures, opening the egg through the air cell with sharp blunt scissors or a large gauge needle is termed "break out". Next examine the internal shell membranes and expose internal contents. Record location, color and size of albumen, yolk, and allantois, note abnormal colors, odor and the circulatory tree. If no chick is present, continue opening via small fragment removal though the air cell until the remaining contents can be poured into a sterile container. Samples to consider: Bacterial, fungal culture, Gram stain, other cytology of external and internal egg membranes, embryo yolk sac, and umbilicus. Yolk samples to assess nutitional staus of the hen. Albumen and shell samples to assess toxicology.

### Embryo Staging and Position

If an embryo is evident, incise elliptically parallel to the long axis to create an egg on the half shell. View and draw or image the chick to determine the embryonic stage and positioning. Although embryonic staging has been determined for some parrots determining the eggmester (EED, mid or

### Table 1

| Malpositions of the embryo. | | | |
|---|---|---|---|
| *Malposition* | *Description* | *Outcome* | *Common Cause* |
| **1** | Head between thighs. Failure to lift, turn head R in last trimester | Lethal | High incubation temperature |
| **2** | Head at small end of egg, chick upside down | 50% lethal, assist hatch | Incubator egg position, low temperature |
| **3** | Head under left wing, rotates head left (not right). Body rotated on egg long axis | Usually lethal | Incubator egg position, temperature, parent malnutrition |
| **4** | Beak (maxilla egg tooth) away from air cell | Slightly low hatchability | Incubator position |
| **5** | Feet over head | Usually lethal | Embryo cannot kick/rotate for hatching |
| **6** | Head over R wing. Head in same plane as wing (psittacines) | Slightly low hatchability | Parent malnutrition |
| **7** | Embryo crossways in egg, often have other defects | Fatal | Small embryos, spherical eggs |
| **Correct** | Head at large end near air cell, head tucked under R wing upside down (most birds) | | |
| | Head at large end near air cell, head at level of R wing (parrots, shorter neck, large head) | | |

prehatch) of death has more diagnostic utility. The normal classical position of the avian embryo has the head at large end, with the bill pointed toward the air cell and tucked upside down under the R wing (Table 1). However, the shorter thicker neck of the parrot chick means the bill lies close to the wing tip, not underneath. Incidence of malpositions > 1–2% triggers diagnostic investigation. Causes of malposition include incorrect egg position in incubation, improper egg turning frequency and angle, incorrect incubator temperature or humidity, and excessive movement, vibration, or damage and infection during incubation.

*Embryo evaluation*
Obtain samples for culture, voriology or toxicology of the abnormal chick, umbilicus, yolk, or liver if gross abnormalities are observed. Should the date of incubation be known, chick growth measurements may also be collected at this stage. After removal of the yolk, embryo fragility then dictates placing the entire body in formalin, after slitting abdominal wall and the back of the head for best formalin permeation.

## PATHOLOGIC FINDINGS
**External**: Abnormal shape or size of egg for the species. Parrot eggs are white, relatively small and have little difference between the blunt and narrow ends. Lack of pip, crack or crush injuries, shell unevenness and corrugated appearance, presence of blood, albumen or yolk on shell, external egg opportunist predators: ants, maggots, flies, or other insects.
**Internal**: Odor, lack of normal structure; free floating untethered yolk. Infected egg/embryo (bacteria or fungus) may have a coagulated yolk, hemorrhages, or a foul odor.

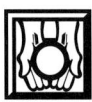

## TREATMENT
### APPROPRIATE HEALTH CARE
Cracks in the eggshell may be secondary to trauma from the parent, trauma from hatchling, or a result of an egg having either inappropriate calcium, phosphorous or protein content. Large cracks or breaks are often terminal, based on egg membrane compromise / pathogen entry. Repair small cracks with white glue, tissue glue or paraffin wax or seal tiny cracks with nail varnish. Seal bite or nail punctures, or other large defects with tissue paper plus glue or parafilm or paraffin, beeswax, and tissue glue. Use the minimum quantity of repair material necessary as coating large surface areas of the egg compromises gas and water exchange through the shell. Avoid use of organic compounds, as excess application may result in embry compromise due to entry of these compounds into the egg.

## NURSING CARE
Ensure appropriate incubation parameters and monitoring of egg weight loss. Appropriate relative humidity and temperature for the species should be known and the egg should lose weight appropriately during the incubation process.

## ACTIVITY
Unless trauma is suspected, activity of hens laying abnormal eggs should not be changed. Abnormal living eggs should be incubated separately from normal eggs to avoid spread of infectious disease. Monitor abnormal live eggs more often than normal eggs (q2–3d) to assist the developing embryo.

## DIET
The diet of the egg is the diet of the hen.

## CLIENT EDUCATION
Multiple egg necropsies and a detailed history are necessary to facilitate diagnosis. History should include records of incubation, parental health, and reproductive history. Incubation records should include temperature, humidity and natural light access for natural incubation. Parental genetics, age, diet, nutrition, and feed additives should be known. Review egg handling practices (incubation, handling, cleaning and observations) with the owner. Record location, nest identification, activities, behavior of nearby birds, and identify the egg collector. Provide egg handling and assessment protocols to egg collectors to assure collection of viable or nonviable eggs, dependent upon the programmatic goals.

## SURGICAL CONSIDERATIONS
None

## MEDICATIONS
### DRUG(S) OF CHOICE
As all antibiotics have potential to negatively affect embryonic growth and development, avoidance of antibiotic use within or upon the developing egg or for the hen producing an egg is preferred.

### CONTRAINDICATIONS
Egg bound birds/eggs should not have exposure to oil of any kind including mineral oil, which may block egg pores and stop transpiration resulting in rapid embryonic death. Use only water-based lubricant in the event of difficulty in passing of an abnormal egg. Antibiotics are to be used with caution should the egg be presumed or desired to be viable (see Drugs of Choice section).

### PRECAUTIONS
Antibiotics may cause embryo malformations and death. Use with caution and only as necessary and indicated based on cytology or

culture findings from the current or previous eggs from the same hen or husbandry conditions.

### POSSIBLE INTERACTIONS
N/A

### ALTERNATIVE DRUGS
N/A

## FOLLOW-UP
### PATIENT MONITORING
Monitor chicks after hatching, as some early deaths in hatched chicks can be related to abnormal incubation or hatching. Monitor eggs based on candling.

### PREVENTION/AVOIDANCE
Review and constantly improve nutrition, husbandry, and hygiene and maintain aviary records of each paired bird's source and parentage. Vaccinate parent birds for preventable diseases. Completely breakdown, disinfect incubators at least once yearly. Remove and disinfect nest boxes or discard after the breeding season is complete. Continued egg assessment for breeding health should include regular egg candling, and submission of all dead eggs for necropsy to determine cause of egg failure and make changes as informed by necropsy findings.

### POSSIBLE COMPLICATIONS
The production of abnormal eggs may signal irreparable damage to the reproductive tract based on infection or neoplastic process in some hens, necessitating salpingectomy. Salpingectomy has a poor survival rate. Early diagnosis and reproductive tract removal is key to continued life for affected birds; continued breeding will not be possible for some hens.

### EXPECTED COURSE AND PROGNOSIS
The survival rate for most abnormal eggs is poor. The course of disease in the hen after production of an abnormal egg is highly variable and depends upon cause, which may range from the soft-shelled egg or corrugated egg from poor nutrition and husbandry, which is relatively easily corrected (improve diet, stop dog chasing hens) with minimal after effects, and has fair prognosis. Infectious disease of the egg has an intermediate prognosis and may depend on improving hygiene, egg or hen treatment and the determination of the infectious agent. Some viral infections may not kill the hen but will results in continued poor quality egg production and or poor doing hatchlings that take inordinate amounts of care to survive to adult hood. Neoplastic or serious infectious disease/sepsis can eventually result in death (grave prognosis).

# MISCELLANEOUS

## ASSOCIATED CONDITIONS
Abnormal egg production is associated with infectious disease/metabolic derangement of the hen. Fatty liver syndrome, cage layer fatigue and egg yolk stroke are all consequences of a malfunctioning reproductive system that can affect many organs (liver, musculoskeletal, nervous).

## AGE-RELATED FACTORS
Older hens may be more prone to neoplastic reproductive disease; however, viral infection, secondary or primary bacterial infection, and or sepsis may also be present in any hen producing an abnormal egg. Older hens are also more likely to lay small, deformed, or soft-shelled eggs during the normal advancing senescence of the reproductive tract.

## ZOONOTIC POTENTIAL
Pathogens of abnormal eggs with zoonotic potential include: *Salmonella* spp., *E. coli*, *Staphylococcus* spp. (anthropozoonosis) *Chlamydia* spp., influenza, Newcastle disease/avian paramyxovirus, and *Aspergillus* spp.

## FERTILITY/BREEDING
Hens that consistently lay abnormal eggs are not good candidates for breeding.

## SYNONYMS
Failure to hatch, dead in shell, soft-shelled egg, deformed egg.

## SEE ALSO
Dystocia and Egg Binding

## ABBREVIATIONS
EED—early embryonic death
PCR—polymerase chain reaction

## INTERNET RESOURCES
Pollock, C. (2008). Egg necropsy form. *LafeberVet*: https://lafeber.com/vet/egg-necropsy-form

*Suggested Reading*
Abbott, U.K., Brice, A.T., Cutler, B.A., Millam, J.R. (1991). Embryonic Development of the Cockatiel (*Nymphicus hollandicus*). *Journal of the Association of Avian Veterinarians*, 5:207–209.
Bucher, T.L. (1983). Parrot eggs, embryos, and nestlings: patterns and energetics of growth and development. *Physiological Zoology*, 56:465–483.
Clubb, S., Phillips, A. (1992). Psittacine Embryonic Mortality. In *Psittacine Aviculture: Perspectives, Techniques, and Research* (ed. R.M. Schubot, K.J. Clubb, S.L. Clubb), ch. 10. Loxahatchee, FL: Avicultural Breeding and Research Center.
Carril, J., Tambussi, C.P. (2015). Development of the superaltricial monk parakeet (Aves, Psittaciformes): embryo staging, growth, and heterochronies. *Anatomical Record*, 298:1836–1847.
Deeming, D.C. (2002). *Avian Incubation: Behaviour, Environment and Evolution*. Oxford, UK: Oxford University Press.
Delany, M.E., Tell, L.A., Millam, J.R., Preisler, D.M. (1999). Photographic candling analysis of the embryonic development of orange-winged Amazon parrots (*Amazona amazonica*). *Journal of Avian Medicine and Surgery*, 13:116–123.
Garcês, A., Pires, I. (2020). Necropsy in eggs. In: *Necropsy Techniques for Examining Wildlife Samples*, 172–177. Singapore: Bentham Science Publishers.
Olsen, G.H. (2000). Embryological considerations. In: *Manual of Avian Medicine* (ed. G.H. Olsen, S.E. Orosz), 189–212. St. Louis, MO: Mosby.
**Authors**: J. Jill Heatley, DVM, MS, DABVP (Avian, Reptilian, Amphibian), DACZM, and Glenn H. Olsen, DVM, MS, PhD
**Acknowledgements**: We thank John Chitty, MRCVS for his contributions to multiple Egg Diagnosis Masterclasses and Wetlabs of the Proceedings of Association of Avian Veterinarians Symposium. Any use of trade, product, or firm names is for descriptive purposes only and does not imply endorsement by the US Government.

# EGG YOLK AND REPRODUCTIVE COELOMITIS

## BASICS

### DEFINITION
The presence of egg yolk material within the coelomic cavity outside of the reproductive tract. It can encompass egg-related peritonitis, ectopic ovulation-associated coelomitis and septic coelomitis.

### PATHOPHYSIOLOGY
Egg yolk coelomitis is a commonly seen reproductive disorder in pet birds. An ovulated follicle (yolk) fails to enter the reproductive tract, inducing an inflammatory response, peritonitis, and secondary bacterial infection. Ascites, organ inflammation, and fibrinous peritonitis can result. Yolk coelomitis causes ascites, which causes dyspnea from fluid space occupation. Yolk coelomitis can be life threatening.

### SYSTEMS AFFECTED
**Reproductive**: Ovulated yolks do not enter the reproductive tract and are free in the coelomic cavity.
**Respiratory**: Dyspnea, increased respiratory effort, or distress occur from fluid accumulation or space occupation decreasing air sac space.
**Endocrine/metabolic**: Ovulating hens typically show hypercalcemia, hyperglobulinemia, and elevated lipids in the blood stream.

### GENETICS
Not definitively known, although it is speculated that it may be a hereditary condition and certain color mutations of psittacine birds may be predisposed.

### INCIDENCE/PREVALENCE
There are no scientific data based on large scale studies; however, the condition could develop in any female bird. Most commonly seen in smaller species, typically cockatiels.

### GEOGRAPHIC DISTRIBUTION
N/A

### SIGNALMENT
**Species predilections**: Cockatiels, budgerigars, waterfowl.
**Mean age and range**: Sexually mature hens of egg producing age (varies greatly between species).
**Predominant sex**: Only affects females past egg-laying age.

### SIGNS
*General Comments*
Clinical signs may be vague and non-specific, such as lethargy and inappetance, or directly attributable to development of peritonitis, ascites, and coelomic distension. Birds may have varying degrees of yolk peritonitis and be unaffected and still show typical clinical signs and physical examination findings.

*Historical Findings*
Bird may have a reproductive history that includes past or chronic egg laying. Recent egg laying or recent cessation of egg laying are commonly seen; birds may still be exhibiting hormonal behaviors. Owners may report loss of appetite, staying at the bottom of the cage, and increased sleeping. Non-specific signs, such as loss of appetite/anorexia, weakness, depression/lethargy, fluffed feathers, and decreased to absent vocalizations are reported. Sudden death.

*Physical Examination Findings*
Coelomic distension is the most common exam finding. Ascites is typically identified as both the cause of distension and dyspnea. Dyspnea/hyperpnea are observed due to space occupation with fluid or organ enlargement and air sac compression and may become worse with handling. Lethargy and depression may be noted. Wide-based stance is sometimes seen. Enlarged, flaccid vent can be seen. Hen may be obese, thin, or normal body condition.

### CAUSES
**Reproductive**: Aberrant reproductive behavior. Chronic or excessive egg laying. Abnormal ovulation. Cystic ovarian disease. Oviductal and ovarian granulomas. Reproductive tract diseases, such as salpingitis, metritis, oviductal rupture, and neoplasia.
**Other**: Genetic predisposition. Obesity. Lack of exercise. Stress.

### RISK FACTORS
Only female birds can develop the condition. Uncontrolled excessive egg laying resulting from prolonged daylight, lack of sleep, presence of real or perceived mate, and nest sites.

## DIAGNOSIS

### DIFFERENTIAL DIAGNOSIS
Coelomic distension—ascites secondary to hepatic disease, cardiac disease, and neoplasia. Fluid within the uterus, uterine torsion, gastrointestinal distention, ovarian cyst, organomegaly. Abdominal wall herniation. Coelomic bacterial infection, abscessation of the coelomic organs. Dyspnea secondary to primary respiratory disease, tissue space occupation, pain/discomfort. Radiographs will aid in determination. Neoplasia of the reproductive tract or other organs.

### CBC/BIOCHEMISTRY/URINALYSIS
Leukocytosis with heterophilia is commonly seen on the complete blood count. Hypercalcemia is a normal finding in an egg-laying hen; values within normal reference ranges indicate deficiency. Elevated hepatic enzyme activity from reactivity or related to egg production. Hyperuricemia may be associated

with reproductive tract enlargement or previous egg laying. Lipemic plasma is seen clinically with elevated lipids related to egg production.

### OTHER LABORATORY TESTS
Hyperglobulinemia may be noted on protein electrophoresis. Coelomocentesis for fluid analysis and cytologic examination to obtain a definitive diagnosis. Aspirated fluid can be stained and evaluated in-house for the presence of protein globules indicative of egg yolk. Cholesterol within aspirated fluid may also be measured and compared with plasma cholesterol. Culture and sensitivity testing of coelomic fluid samples may aid in treatment.

### IMAGING
*Radiographic Findings*
Polyostotic hyperostosis is typically seen as increased ossification of the long bones relating to calcium storage in the hormonally active hen. Radiography is also useful to determine the presence of a shelled egg(s). Decreased overall detail from ascites can preclude a diagnosis so fluid removal is recommended before radiographs are obtained. Contrast radiography is useful and may show a space occupying mass and organ displacement.

*Abdominal/Coelomic Ultrasonography*
Ultrasound will show coelomic fluid, ovarian cysts/follicles, and masses. Ultrasonography is useful for ruling out other disease, such as tumors, reproductive tract torsions, and any other concurrent disease conditions.

*Advanced Imaging*
CT will show organ enlargement or presence of organ disease, especially ovarian or uterine.

### DIAGNOSTIC PROCEDURES
Sample collection (coelomocentesis) for cytologic analysis is diagnostic showing a septic exudate with yolk globules. Endoscopy may be used in larger birds to visualize the oviduct to assess for torsion or masses. Additionally, eggs located ectopically within the coelom may be seen. Coelioscopy should use a midline approach into the intestinoperitoneal cavity within the fluid and lateral approaches through the air sac system should not be used due to likely aspiration of fluids into the lungs.

### PATHOLOGIC FINDINGS
Ascites secondary to peritonitis. Fibrinous peritonitis. Organomegaly. Visible yolk material in the coelomic cavity. Presence of an egg(s) in the reproductive tract.

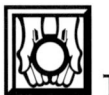

## TREATMENT

### APPROPRIATE HEALTH CARE
Treatment varies based on severity, as some patients will resorb the yolk without

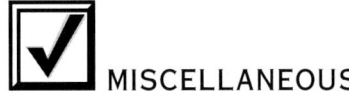

complication. Outpatient treatment with home care instructions may be warranted in stable patients. Hospitalization is needed in patients that are anorexic, severely dyspneic, or showing severe clinical signs. Surgery consisting of a salpingohysterectomy may be indicated in patients with chronic reproductive disease.

### NURSING CARE
Hen should be kept in a humidified incubator warmed up to 90°F (32°C); ideally in a quiet area to minimize stress. Fluid supplementation—parental fluids (e.g. subcutaneous); oral fluids though gavage tube as feedings. Pain management with analgesics and anti-inflammatory medications. Broad-spectrum antibiotics when infection is suspected. Supportive care should include coelomocentesis as indicated. Hormonal treatment with leuprolide acetate or deslorelin acetate implants may help some patients. Some patients may benefit from short-term oxygen therapy.

### ACTIVITY
Patients should be cage rested and monitored for appetite and levels of dyspnea.

### DIET
No changes should be made until the patient has recovered, at which time needed improvements can be addressed. Hospitalized patients will require assisted feedings with clinical care or hand-rearing formula. Transition to a diet that includes formulated pellets and calcium supplementation after recovery.

### CLIENT EDUCATION
Clients should understand some patients have a guarded prognosis. Attempts to prevent or decrease further egg laying are encouraged. Reduction of photoperiod, increase sleep time, removal of nests and nesting materials, and reduction in sexual stimulation by a perceived mate is recommended. Hormonal therapy with leuprolide acetate or deslorelin acetate implants may be warranted.

### SURGICAL CONSIDERATIONS
Dehydrated and anorexic patients need appropriate preanesthetic care. Compromised ability to breathe due to compression of air sacs by egg and enlarged reproductive tract. Intubation with positive pressure ventilation is strongly recommended. Patients with ascites are at increased risk of anesthetic complications should they be placed under anesthesia.

## MEDICATIONS
### DRUG(S) OF CHOICE
Antibiotic therapy should be based on culture and sensitivity results; however, antibiotics such as fluoroquinolones (enrofloxacin 15 mg/kg PO q12h) or

potentiated penicillins (amoxicillin with clavulanic acid 125 mg/kg q8–12h), can be initiated. Analgesics such as butorphanol (1–4 mg/kg IM q2–4h to PRN) are needed during initial treatment. Anti-inflammatories such as meloxicam (0.5–2 mg/kg PO, IM q12–24h) are useful and should be continued for at least 5 days after diagnosis. GnRH agonists such as leuprolide acetate (100–1200 µg/kg IM q3–4w) and deslorelin acetate implants are helpful in both short- and long-term management. Note that doses vary widely with this medication.

### CONTRAINDICATIONS
Coelioscopy through lateral approaches are contraindicated as fluid will gain access to the air sac/lung system.

### PRECAUTIONS
Birds should be restrained in a physiologic upright position as other positions may lead to acute decompensation.

### POSSIBLE INTERACTIONS
N/A

### ALTERNATIVE DRUGS
Various antibiotics may be useful, and may be chosen based on culture and sensitivity testing. Deslorelin acetate implants can be used for long-term prevention of ovulation and egg laying. Holistic therapies can be recommended by specialized veterinarians as adjunct therapy.

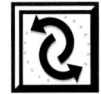

## FOLLOW-UP
### PATIENT MONITORING
Physical examination to determine degree of ascites accumulation and recurrence pattern. Coelomocentesis may be required periodically until the condition resolves.

### PREVENTION/AVOIDANCE
Owners should take steps to discourage and/or minimize egg laying. Treatment with leuprolide acetate injections or a deslorelin acetate implant to prevent ovulation and egg laying.

### POSSIBLE COMPLICATIONS
Sepsis can occur from bacterial translocation and fluid accumulation. Adhesions may result from fibrinous peritonitis. Hens that have undergone salpingohysterectomy may still be at risk for developing yolk associated coelomitis. Sudden death.

### EXPECTED COURSE AND PROGNOSIS
Patients diagnosed quickly have a good prognosis with appropriate medical care and owner compliance. Prognosis is guarded in all patients that present with severe dyspnea. Patients who survive surgery have an excellent prognosis.

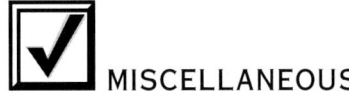

## MISCELLANEOUS
### ASSOCIATED CONDITIONS
Ectopic eggs, adhesion formation, reproductive neoplasia, salpingitis, oophoritis.

### AGE-RELATED FACTORS
N/A

### ZOONOTIC POTENTIAL
N/A

### FERTILITY/BREEDING
Although this can be a random occurrence, birds who experience recurrences should not be used for breeding.

### SYNONYMS
Egg yolk peritonitis.

### SEE ALSO
Atherosclerosis
Chronic Egg Laying
Cloacal Diseases
Coelomic Distention
Dyslipidemia/Hyperlipidemia
Dystocia and Egg Binding
Hypocalcemia and Hypomagnesemia
Lameness
Metabolic Bone Disease
Neoplasia (Reproductive)
Nutritional Imbalances
Polyostotic Hyperostosis/
Osteomyelosclerosis
Ovarian Diseases
Oviductal Diseases
Problem Behaviors: Aggression, Biting and Screaming
Regurgitation and Vomiting
Respiratory Distress
Sick-Bird Syndrome

### ABBREVIATIONS
GnRH—gonadotropin-releasing hormone

### INTERNET RESOURCES
Pollock, C. (2012). Reproductive emergencies in birds. *LafeberVet*: https://lafeber.com/vet/reproductive-emergencies

*Suggested Reading*
Bowles, H.L. (2006). Evaluating and treating the reproductive system. In: *Clinical Avian Medicine*, Vol 2 (ed. G. Harrison, T. Lightfoot), 519–540. Palm Beach, FL: Spix Publishing.
Bowles, H.L. (2002). Reproductive diseases of pet bird species. *Veterinary Clinics of North America. Exotic Animal Practice*, 5:489–506.
Pollock, C.G., Orosz, S.E. (2002). Avian reproductive anatomy, physiology and endocrinology. *Veterinary Clinics of North America. Exotic Animal Practice*, 5:441–474.
Scagnelli A., Tully T. (2017). Reproductive disorders in parrots. *Veterinary Clinics of North America. Exotic Animal Practice*, 20:485–507.
**Author**: Anthony A Pilny, DVM, DABVP (Avian)

# ELECTROCUTION

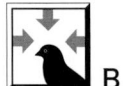

## BASICS

### DEFINITION
Electrocution refers to the severe injury or death of a bird that occurs when an electric current passes through the body.

### PATHOPHYSIOLOGY
Electrocution occurs when a bird makes contact with two pieces of electrical equipment or electricity and a grounded object. The most common scenario where this is observed involves raptors with electrical lines; however, other avian species in the wild, as well as in captivity, can also experience electrocution. Other possible causes of electrocution include lightning, altercations with power cords, and faulty electric circuits.

### SYSTEMS AFFECTED
**Integument**: Feather and skin burns can occur and range from a small to large area affected.
**Musculoskeletal**: Limb fractures are reported in cases of electrocution where muscular contractions occur due to the electrical current that is produced. Traumatic amputations associated with electrocution have been described in avian species.
**Visceral injury**: Ruptured viscera and thermal damage of the internal organs can occur with electrocution. Often, the damage to the internal organs is more extensive than the visible external wounds and burns. Separation of the dermal and muscular layers is common.
**Ocular**: Cataract formation secondary to electrical injury has been reported in a great horned owl.
**Oral**: Electrical burns can be seen in the mouth as a result of pet birds chewing on electrical cords.
**Secondary injuries**: Associated with falls following execution are also commonly reported and may include liver fractures, orthopedic injuries, and contusions. Evidence of hemorrhage including hemocoelom, and hemopericardium can also be detected as a result of vascular tears. Commonly cardiac or respiratory arrest is the outcome resulting in death. The passage of the current through the heart results in ventricular fibrillation and the central nervous system involved affects the respiratory and other vital centers.

### GENETICS
N/A

### INCIDENCE/PREVALENCE
**Raptors**: A retrospective studying evaluating electrical injuries in raptors found that 417 of 2810 (14.8%) raptors submitted over a 15-year time frame had electrocution reported as the cause of death.
**Psittacines**: Although rarely reported, electrical burns in the mouth have been documented in psittacines that chew on household electrical cords and wires.

### GEOGRAPHIC DISTRIBUTION
Power lines are a significant cause of avian mortality in the USA, with an estimated 0.9–11.6 million birds per year. With ongoing proliferation of the electrical infrastructure, the continued conservation threat that electrical lines pose to avian species continues.

### SIGNALMENT
Any bird can be afflicted by electrical injury, but large terrestrial and wetland birds, and smaller, fast-flying species are prone to collision with overhead wires associated with power infrastructure. Among the avian groups, cranes, bustards, flamingos, waterfowl, shorebirds, gamebirds, and falcons are most frequently affected. In the USA, eagles, Buteo hawks, and large owls appear to be most commonly affected, with the golden eagle (*Aquila chrysaetos*) being the most common.

### SIGNS

#### Historical Findings
The history of a bird that has been electrocuted may only be suggestive based on the history and clinical presentation. Although some birds found below power lines may have sustained an electrical injury, it is not the only cause. A complete necropsy is required to confirm a diagnosis of electrocution. Additionally, the findings associated with electrical injury may be challenging to detect on cursory examination and a complete and thorough physical examination is necessary.

#### Physical Examination Findings
Avian patients that experience electrocution may survive the initial injury and recover or may die a later time from complications that occur. The most common physical examination is evidence of electrical burns and singed feathers. The scent of burnt feathers or skin is also often detected on presentation. Death can occur as a result of electrocution and is thought to result from direct passage of the current through the cardiac and/or respiratory centers in the brain, or directly through the heart, causing cardiopulmonary failure.

### CAUSES
Throughout the world, there are over 65 million miles of medium-high voltage power lines with an increasing network growth each year. It is well documented that overhead wires, especially commercial power lines, are a risk to any flighted avian species and that electrocution is a possible consequence of collision with the power lines.

### RISK FACTORS
Species, body size, habitat, young age, power line configuration, wet weather.

## DIAGNOSIS

### DIFFERENTIAL DIAGNOSIS
Trauma (collision, gunshot), toxicity (lead, zinc, other), chemical burn, infectious disease, rhabdomyolysis (capture myopathy).

### CBC/BIOCHEMISTRY/URINALYSIS
Although not well documented in avian species, electrocution can result in rhabdomyolysis and myoglobinuria in human patients. Resultantly, it could be expected that levels of myoglobin would be elevated in the serum and the urine portion of avian droppings. Additionally, creatine kinase levels can be extremely elevated as a result of the massive muscle damage that occurs with electrical injury. If rhabdomyolysis is present, elevations in uric acid may also be detected in situations of acute renal failure.

### OTHER LABORATORY TESTS
In the majority of cases, electrocution burns can be detected on physical examination; however, if they are small and difficult to detect, the use of a dissecting microscope to perform an examination of the skin and feathers can be used to help to differentiate between burned feathers and skin compared to dirty tissue.

### IMAGING
Small foci of metal deposition may occur in cases of electrocution at the areas of the contact points between the tissue anions and the metallic ions from the electrical source or as a result of arcing. Uncommonly, this metallization of the skin may be detected on radiographs or CT. In general, radiographs are more useful to rule out other causes of disease including gunshot, lead ingestion, or fractures as a result of trauma.

### DIAGNOSTIC PROCEDURES
Thermography has been demonstrated to be a useful, non-invasive modality to detect and assess electrocution injuries in birds. In birds that have undergone electrocution, thermography demonstrates asymmetrical temperature distribution, with the injured tissues demonstrating cooler thermal patterns compared to the healthy tissues. In some cases, this is not only a useful diagnostic tool, but can also be used to monitor the progress of an injured tissue, and help to determine if treatments being administered are effective,

E

and what the prognosis might be for that patient.

## PATHOLOGIC FINDINGS

Though the histopathologic findings of electrical injury are not well described in birds, it has been well described in humans. In humans, evidence of intraepidermal separation, coagulation necrosis, and nuclear elongation are the most common features noted on histopathologic examination, but are still not pathognomonic. It is important to distinguish thermal burns from electrical burns, which also requires histopathologic evaluation. Electrocution injuries are typically multifocal, have more than one external wound (indicating an entrance and an exit point), and high greater depth of damage compared with flame burns. In addition to a greater depth of damage, electrocution injury may also demonstrate little surface injury compared with a thermal burn. Delayed lesions in humans also demonstrate necrosis of the vascular tunica media resulting in ruptured of damaged vessels and thrombosis.

## TREATMENT

### APPROPRIATE HEALTH CARE

Treatment of electrocution cases presents challenges as a result of the large amount of unseen tissue damage that can occur. Euthanasia may be warranted in severe cases of prolonged recumbency, multiple fractures, or severe muscle injuries.

### NURSING CARE

Supportive care with wound management, antibiotics for secondary infections, appropriate analgesia, as well as nutritional support and fluid support are all critical to the management of these cases.

### ACTIVITY

Activity should be restricted to allow for healing to occur.

### DIET

N/A

### CLIENT EDUCATION

Clients with psittacines or other pet birds should be counseled to prevent access to any electrical wires that could be chewed and result in electrocution.

## SURGICAL CONSIDERATIONS

Limb amputation may need to be considered in severe situations, once tissue has declared itself.

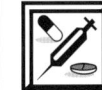

## MEDICATIONS

### DRUG(S) OF CHOICE

Antibiotics, analgesia—opioid, NSAIDs, topical therapy for wounds.

### CONTRAINDICATIONS

N/A

### PRECAUTIONS

Fracture stabilization may be indicated. Caution with handling the electrical injury patient prior to stabilization.

### POSSIBLE INTERACTIONS

N/A

### ALTERNATIVE DRUGS

In cases of distal limb injury, pentoxifylline or other vascular promoting drugs can be considered to increase blood flow to ischemic tissues and improve tissue oxygenation.

## FOLLOW-UP

### PATIENT MONITORING

Each patient should be monitored closely for progression of wounds associated with the electrical injury.

### PREVENTION/AVOIDANCE

The challenge of raptor and other avian electrocutions, particularly those that occur as a result of manmade electrical structures is ongoing, and is unlikely to be resolved in the near or distant future. However, appropriate documentation of these incidences may help to spread awareness of these incidences and in the future serve as a mechanism for prevention of future deaths. In the scenario of pet avian patients, 'bird proofing' of the household to ensure that birds do not have access to electrical cords is appropriate.

### POSSIBLE COMPLICATIONS

Secondary infection, secondary amputation of the affected limbs, delayed vascular necrosis and rupture, cardiac and respiratory arrest, death.

## EXPECTED COURSE AND PROGNOSIS

Prognosis is highly variable and depends on the extent of tissue damage and necrosis.

## MISCELLANEOUS

### ASSOCIATED CONDITIONS

Rhabdomyolysis

### AGE-RELATED FACTORS

N/A

### ZOONOTIC POTENTIAL

N/A

### FERTILITY/BREEDING

N/A

### SYNONYMS

N/A

### SEE ALSO

Trauma

### ABBREVIATIONS

CT—computed tomography
NSAIDs—non-steroidal anti-inflammatory drugs

### INTERNET RESOURCES

N/A

*Suggested Reading*
Kagan, R.A. (2016). Electrocution of raptors on power lines: A review of necropsy methods and findings. *Veterinary Pathology*, 53:1030–1036.
Loss, S.R., Will, T., Marra, P.P. (2014). Refining estimates of bird collision and electrocution mortality at power lines in the United States. *PLoS One*, 9(7):e101565.
Melero, M., González, F., Nicolás, O., et al. (2013). Detection and assessment of electrocution in endangered raptors by infrared thermography. *BMC Veterinary Research*, 9:149.
Saukko, P., Knight, B. (2004). Electrical fatalities. In: *Knight's Forensic Pathology*, 4th edn. (ed. P. Saukko, B. Knight) 325–338. Boca Raton, CA: CRC Press.
Üzün, I., Akyildiz, E., Inanici, M.A. (2008). Histopathological differentiation of skin lesions caused by electrocution, flame burns and abrasion. *Forensic Science International*, 178:157–161.
**Author:** Sara Gardhouse, DVM, DABVP (ECM), DACZM

## EMACIATION

# BASICS

## DEFINITION
Starvation is the prolonged absence of nutrition, the physiologic result of starvation is emaciation. Patients can become emaciated as a result of malnutrition. Malnutrition is defined as any disorder with unbalanced or inadequate nutrition associated with nutritional deficiencies or excess. Malnutrition leads to immunocompromise, altered drug metabolism and lower rates of tissue synthesis and repair. This condition is defined as the loss of body fat and muscle as a result of severe malnourishment or starvation.

## PATHOPHYSIOLOGY
During starvation, normal blood glucose is maintained by increasing hepatic glycogenolysis, increasing gluconeogenesis, and decreasing glycogen stores. Animals decrease blood insulin concentrations and increase blood glucagon concentrations. Glucose is the initial, primary fuel source for the central nervous system, bone marrow, and injured tissue. In the absence of nutrition intake, glycogen stores are rapidly depleted within 24 hours of a fast. New glucose is derived from gluconeogenesis via the breakdown of protein from organs like the liver and also muscle tissue. In the second phase of starvation, lipids from adipose tissue stores are used. Once hepatic glycogen stores and adipose tissue are depleted, amino acids become the energy source for gluconeogenesis in the third phase of starvation. Muscle catabolism releases glucogenic amino acids, pyruvate and lactic acid for energy production in the liver. Amino acids are obtained from the breakdown of skeletal muscle and visceral proteins. Eventually, the liver uses immunoglobulins and lymphokines as a protein source for energy, compromising immune function. Severe fatigue accompanies emaciation due to a severe depletion of muscle mass, together with most vitamins, minerals, and glucose required for homeostasis.

## SYSTEMS AFFECTED
Cardiovascular, digestive, neuromuscular.

## GENETICS
No genetic associations exist.

## INCIDENCE/PREVALENCE
Specific prevalence data are lacking but emaciation can be seen in nestlings of first-time parents who are not feeding appropriately. Emaciation can also be seen in adult, injured raptors that are unable to hunt and young-of-the-year raptors who are not skilled hunters. A range of chronic diseases may also lead to emaciation such as infectious

(e.g. avian bornavirus, mycobacteriosis, aspergillosis) and non-infectious dieases (e.g. renal disease, gastrointestinal diseases, neoplasia).

## GEOGRAPHIC DISTRIBUTION
N/A

## SIGNALMENT
Birds of any species, age and sex can present with emaciation.

## SIGNS
### General Comments
Ravenous or no appetite, scant fecal output, chronic gastrointestinal signs. All seed diets where only hulls are left in the food bowl and foods that are allowed to become moldy or rancid in outdoor enclosures are frequently noted in cases of emaciation. Birds of prey may become emaciated as a result of decreased prey availability and/or extreme weather conditions. Raptors are tolerant of acute food deprivation for various amounts of time. Larger species are more tolerant than smaller species.

### Historical Findings
Lethargy, depression, anorexia, decreased vocalization/energy, smaller than normal stools, undigested seeds in stools.

### Physical Examination Findings
Loss of muscle around the keel, muscle wasting, extreme weight loss, decreased/absent grip, inability to fly and/or sit upright.

## CAUSES
Degenerative/developmental—neonatal crop atony. Anomalous/autoimmune. Metabolic/mechanical—foreign body, impaction, compression of crop, nematodiasis or other internal parasites. Nutritional/neoplastic—cancer cachexia, neoplastic conditions, liver disease, and renal disease. Inflammatory/infectious—proventricular dilation syndrome, macrorhabdus, gastritis, septicemia, papilloma virus, rancid hand-feeding formula/produce, coccidiosis, giardiasis. Traumatic/toxic—lead poisoning, gastric ulcer, aggressive gavage feeding, thermal trauma due to overheated (microwaved) hand-feeding formula, trauma (i.e. vehicular/gunshot) that renders birds flightless or unable to hunt.

## RISK FACTORS
Fledgling birds being hand fed, birds housed in outdoor aviaries, young raptors that have not learned to hunt prey successfully.

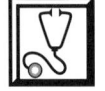

# DIAGNOSIS

## DIFFERENTIAL DIAGNOSIS
Critical illness where birds are in a hypermetabolic state and unable to take in

adequate nutrition, eventually becoming hypoglycemic and acidotic.

## CBC/BIOCHEMISTRY/URINALYSIS
Hypophosphatemia, hypokalemia, hypomagnesemia, hypoglycemia, hypoproteinemia, acidosis.

## OTHER LABORATORY TESTS
Anemia may be present.

## IMAGING
N/A

## DIAGNOSTIC PROCEDURES
N/A

## PATHOLOGIC FINDINGS
Atrophied pectoral musculature with minimal adipose stores (lack of coelomic and cardiac fat).

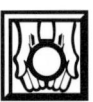

# TREATMENT

## APPROPRIATE HEALTH CARE
Emaciation can often occur with dehydration so appropriate care addresses both fluid and nutritional requirements. Emaciated patients are often dehydrated with concurrent slowed digestion times, so fluid imbalances should be addressed first.

## NURSING CARE
Fluid deficits should be corrected before supplemental, enteral nutrition is offered. The author uses EmerAid® (Lafeber Co., Cornell, IL) for parental nutritional support of critically ill psittacine patients. When critically ill patients are being treated, gavage/tube feeding should always be done last and the patient placed immediately back in its cage. Regurgitation and resultant aspiration pneumonia are always risks associated with gavage feeding. It is always better to feed small amounts frequently (2–4 times daily) as opposed to overfilling the crop.

### To Determine Daily Nutritional Support
(1) Calculate basal metabolic rate: Non-passerine kcal/day = $73.5 \times kg^{0.734}$; passerine: kcal/day = $114.8 \times kg^{0.726}$.
(2) Calculate maintenance requirements as $1.5 \times$ BMR; adjust maintenance requirements for stress, represented by the following multiples of maintenance energy requirements: Starvation 0.5–0.7, elective surgery 1.0–1.2, mild trauma 1.0–1.2, severe trauma 1.1–2.0, growth 1.5–3.0, sepsis 1.2–7.5, burns 1.2–2.0, head injuries 1.0–2.0; kcal/day ÷ kcal/ml formula = amount of formula (ml) required per day.

### Administration
Once the enteral diet has been prepared appropriately for the species in question, the bird should be restrained upright by an assistant. The assistant gently straightens the

neck so that the esophagus is also straightened and tube passage facilitated. The feeder should palpate the crop (when present) at the thoracic inlet to be sure it is empty prior to introducing the tube. Starting from the bird's left, direct the tube toward the right and down into the crop. When properly placed, the tube goes easily and should never be forced. Ball-tipped tubes will displace feathers and can be seen in place through the skin of the neck. Tube feeding should be done in a slow and steady pace. If food is seen swelling at the back of the throat, the procedure should be halted immediately and the bird put down right away. Although tube feeding is a common practice in avian and exotic practices, it should never be done hurriedly or haphazardly. The patient's safety must take top priority at all times.

### Birds of Prey
Determine minimum daily nutritional support required by calculating BMR = $K(W^{0.75})$ is one formula that can be used, where K = amount of kilocalories required for 24 hours (78 kcal for birds of prey) and W represents the weight of the bird in kg. Fresh water should be available to convalescing patients at all times. Intravenous fluid therapy is recommended for patients unable to sit upright in cages or drink normally from a dish. As small amounts of prey are reintroduced to the diet; 1 g of prey fed can be roughly approximated to 1 kcal. Allometric scaling (determination of daily MEC), is similar to the BMR in determining the daily caloric patient needs. For emaciated birds of prey, appropriate supplemental diets include, among others, EmerAid® Carnivore (Lafeber Co., Cornell, IL). Enteral diets should be diluted with an isotonic electrolyte solution and warmed. Never use a microwave to warm enteral diets because of the risk of varying "pockets" of warmth in the food, which can lead to esophageal and crop thermal injury. Initially, 3% of the bird's body weight in grams should be offered in milliliters of enteral diet. If tolerated, the volume of the enteral diet can be increased; do not exceed 5% of the patient's body weight. If the enteral diet is being well tolerated and the patient is gaining weight, whole prey items void of casting material (fur/feathers) can be offered in small, frequent amounts so that of the MEC is fed in 3–4 feedings and held down. Feedings of MEC should be increased by of the MEC daily until the bird is eating 2 × MEC to promote weight gain. If the bird is passing normal feces and gaining weight, casting material can be reintroduced at this point.

## ACTIVITY
Hospitalized patients should have exercise restrictions not only to allow patients time to regain their strength but also to protect indwelling catheters.

## DIET
Compared with parenteral nutrition, human research has concluded that enteral nutrition is associated with reduced costs, better nutritional outcomes, improved wound healing and less mucosal permeability.

### Nutritional Support
**Probiotics**: Probiotics are exogenous bacteria that are introduced into the microbiome of the colon. Known also as a direct fed microbial, probiotics provide beneficial properties to the host. This has been best studied in poultry production medicine. Increased cytokine production, structural modulation and immune modulation account for the positive effects in the intestinal mucosa. These effects combine to prevent pathogenic infections. *Bacillus subtilis* has been shown to increase villus height and structure of the crypts. Increased structure of GI tract crypts and villus height improves nutrient absorption and digestion. Cellular homeostasis is maintained and pathogenic bacteria are deterred by tight junctions secondary to structural modulation.
**Prebiotics**: Prebiotics are non-digestible food stuffs that selectively stimulate the growth and/or activity of a limited number of bacteria in the colon. Effects of prebiotics include stimulated absorption of minerals to improve bone mineralization by increasing the availability of zinc, magnesium, iron and calcium. Non-digestible carbohydrates like oligo and polysaccharides, select peptides, proteins and lipids are prebiotics and not digested in the proximal GI tract. In the caecum, these food ingredients provide energy, metabolic substrates, and essential nutrients for endogenous bacteria.

## CLIENT EDUCATION
Clients should be encouraged to provide food daily and completely discard old food as opposed to adding new food on top of old food.

## SURGICAL CONSIDERATIONS
N/A

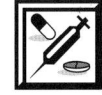

## MEDICATIONS
### DRUG(S) OF CHOICE
N/A

### CONTRAINDICATIONS
N/A

### PRECAUTIONS
N/A

### POSSIBLE INTERACTIONS
N/A

### ALTERNATIVE DRUGS
N/A

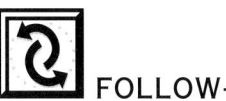

## FOLLOW-UP
### PATIENT MONITORING
Both gram and human baby scales are inexpensive and can easily be fitted with a perch to obtain patient weights daily. During initial recovery, patients are expected to stop losing weight and then weight should steadily increase. The patient's attitude and fecal output should be monitored daily as well. Fecal exams should be done to rule out intestinal parasitism.

### PREVENTION/AVOIDANCE
For psittacine birds at home, owners should be encouraged to monitor food intake by completely changing out foodstuffs daily.

### POSSIBLE COMPLICATIONS
N/A

### EXPECTED COURSE AND PROGNOSIS
If an underlying cause is identified and treatable the prognosis is good to excellent. Neoplasias typically do not have a favorable prognosis.

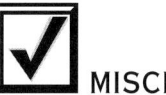

## MISCELLANEOUS
### ASSOCIATED CONDITIONS
**Refeeding syndrome**: In human medicine, refeeding syndrome affects malnourished patients receiving enteral or parenteral nutrition. During starvation, people use protein and fat as opposed to carbohydrates for their main energy sources. Refeeding syndrome is characterized by fluid and electrolyte shifts that occur following increased insulin and decreased glucagon secretion in response to suddenly available glucose. During this time, the body switches from a catabolic to anabolic state. Overfeeding, excessive carbohydrate feeding, and excessive fat administration have all been associated with negative outcomes in human patients.
**Glucagon**: Birds are shown to have lower insulin and higher glucagon levels than mammals. Glucagon appears to be the main hormone regulating avian glucose metabolism. Carnivorous birds have lower insulin levels than chickens. For these reasons direct correlations cannot be made between nutritional support requirements of humans and birds of prey. Pertinent similarities between human patients and birds of prey are however apparent. Chronically malnourished patient support must be done methodically. Supplemental heat and fluid therapy are the first order of business in the avian patients' supportive care needs. Once fluid deficits

have been addressed over 12–24 hours, small volumes of easily digestible food should be offered over multiple (3–4) feedings per day. Thiamine (1–2 mg/kg) containing B vitamin complexes may be a beneficial supplement to improve patient metabolism.

## AGE-RELATED FACTORS
Young raptors that have not learned to hunt prey successfully may be more susceptible to emaciation as well as those facing harsh winter conditions.

## ZOONOTIC POTENTIAL
Emaciation does not have zoonotic potential.

## FERTILITY/BREEDING
Because emaciation can impact all systems and organs in the body, fertility and breeding can be negatively impacted.

## SYNONYMS
Starvation, malnutrition.

## SEE ALSO
Anemia
Anorexia
Dehydration
Ileus (Functional Gastrointestinal, Crop Stasis)
Nutritional Imbalances

## ABBREVIATIONS
BMR—basal metabolic rate
GI—gastrointestinal
MEC—minimum energy cost

## INTERNET RESOURCES
N/A

*Suggested Reading*
Abd El-Hack, M.E., El-Saddony, M.T Shafi M.E., et al. (2020). Probiotics in poultry feed: A comprehensive review. *Journal of Animal Physiology and Animal Nutrition*, 104:1835–1850.
Choudhari A., Shinde S., Ramteke B.N. (2008). Prebiotics and probiotics as health promoter. *Veterinary World*, 2:59–61.
Murray, M. (2014). Raptor gastroenterology. *Veterinary Clinics of North America. Exotic Animal Practice*, 17:211–234.
Orosz, S. (2013). Critical care nutrition for exotic animals, *Journal of Exotic Pet Medicine*, 22:163–177.
Tully, T.N. (2000). Psittacine therapeutics, *Veterinary Clinics of North America. Exotic Animal Practice*, 3:59–90.

**Author:** Kemba L Marshall, MPH, DVM, DABVP (Avian)

**Acknowledgements:** The author wishes to acknowledge the teachers, professors and patients who have allowed her to learn and live out the dreams she had as the eight-year-old version of herself.

# BASICS

## DEFINITION
Gastritis and enteritis are common conditions in pet birds. Sometimes they are part of a more systemic condition, and other times they are isolated problems. Gastritis is any inflammatory condition of the stomach. In birds, there are two sections of the stomach: the proventriculus or glandular stomach, and the ventriculus or gizzard, which is the muscular stomach. Enteritis is any inflammatory condition of the intestines. Typhlitis is inflammation of the ceca. Many pet birds lack ceca, but typhlitis may occur in species where ceca are present.

## PATHOPHYSIOLOGY
Gastritis and enteritis are caused by a wide array of infectious agents. Their pathophysiology varies somewhat, but generally involves some degree of inflammatory cell infiltrate and various degrees of tissue damage to the mucosa, villi, or crypt cells. In some cases, inflammation can occur without infectious agents being present. PDD is a common clinical condition involving the stomach. However, strictly speaking, the disease involves neuritis rather than the stomach itself; the splanchnic ganglia and nerves are usually involved, causing poor gastric tone. In some cases, secondary infections are caused by alterations in motility caused by foreign bodies, papillomas, or other mechanical obstructions.

## SYSTEMS AFFECTED
Behavioral changes involving the appetite, such as anorexia, hyporexia, or polyphagia, can occur with gastritis or enteritis. Cardiovascular changes may include hypovolemia in severe cases. Hepatobiliary infection may occur secondary to enteritis, either via the biliary tree, portal circulation, or septicemia. Musculoskeletal signs may include weight loss and weakness. Feathers may be matted around the vent of the bird and there may be a generally unkempt appearance of the feathers.

## GENETICS
There does not appear to be a genetic component to enteritis and gastritis.

## INCIDENCE/PREVALENCE
Since they are broad categories of disease, enteritis and gastritis are common. Specific diseases vary in their prevalence.

## GEOGRAPHIC DISTRIBUTION
Avian enteritis and gastritis are worldwide conditions. Individual diseases have more variation in their distribution.

## SIGNALMENT
All birds of all ages are susceptible to some forms of gastritis or enteritis. Individual diseases have more specific predilections. For example, *Macrorhabdus* infections are common in budgerigars. Candidiasis is most common in young birds, while mycobacteriosis is most common in older birds.

## SIGNS
### General Comments
Diarrhea is the most common sign associated with enteritis. It should be distinguished from polyuria, which is common with many other conditions. Melena may occur with enteritis or gastritis, and suggests a severe and erosive condition. Hematochezia may occur with enteritis of the more aborad intestines. It can also occur with cloacal disorders. Fetid fecal odor may occur with some types of enteritis or gastritis. This is especially common with clostridial enteritis. Mucus-laden stools may occur, especially with lower intestinal inflammation. Matting of the vent area with feces or urates will be commonly seen with these conditions. Coelomic pain or discomfort may occur. This often presents as very vague signs of malaise and anorexia. Undigested grains or seeds may be passed in cases of gastritis. Generally, grains are not released from the ventriculus until they are ground to a fine particle size. Passage of whole grains is a sign of dysfunction of the ventriculus. Although not consistently seen, vomiting may occur with gastritis. If ingesta backs up into the crop, regurgitation may occur. Dehydration and weight loss can occur due to the loss of fluids and nutrients.

### Historical Findings
Many of the signs of enteritis and gastritis are readily evident to the owner. Regurgitation, vomiting, diarrhea, and fetid fecal odor are all relatively obvious signs. Weight loss can be easily missed by owners. Anorexia or polyphagia may be noted by astute owners.

### Physical Examination Findings
The physical examination should include inspection of the droppings. This may reveal loose stools, melena, hematochezia, strong odor to the feces, undigested grains or other changes to the fecal portion of the droppings. The crop may be thickened or fluctuant on palpation. Fecal or urate matting of the pericloacal feathers may be found. Loss of muscle mass, poor feather condition, or other signs of poor nutrition may be noted.

## CAUSES
PDD caused by avian bornavirus should be mentioned here. However, strictly speaking this is neuritis rather than a true gastritis. Mycobacteriosis can occur anywhere in the GI tract and systemically. In birds, the GI tract is the most common entry site for the organism. Chlamydiosis can result in some gastritis or enteritis, but is not commonly a prominent feature of the disease. Gram-negative bacteria, including *Salmonella* spp., *Escherichia coli*, *Yersinia pseudotuberculosis*, and others can be either primary or opportunistic infections of the stomach or intestines. *Clostridium* spp. commonly infect the intestinal tract. Depending on the strain and the host, the disease can be mild (loose, fetid feces), to extremely severe (hemorrhagic enteritis). *Campylobacter* spp. can cause enteritis and occurs most commonly in passerine species. *Macrorhabdus ornithogaster* or avian gastric yeast is one of the most common causes of gastritis in small species of birds. Candidiasis is a common gastric and intestinal infection. Although it usually causes little inflammation, it is still considered gastritis or enteritis, depending on the site of infection. Coccidiosis is common in some non-psittacine species, but is uncommon in most pet species. It is a concern for backyard poultry, and some zoo or aviary birds. Giardiasis is somewhat common in budgerigars, but rare in other pet species. *Giardia psittaci* is the causative organism. Spironucleosis is common in cockatiels and a few nonpsittacine birds. Ascarids, *Capillaria* spp., *Heterakis gallinarum* (cecal worm), and other helminth parasites can affect the stomach and intestines. Heavy metal ingestion can cause erosive changes in the stomach that often result in secondary inflammation.

## RISK FACTORS
Poor sanitation increases transmission of parasites and primary pathogens, as well as increasing exposure to opportunistic pathogens. In particular, food and water sanitation is critical. The use of moist, high carbohydrate diets, such as lory nectar diets or hand-feeding formula, promotes bacterial growth. Immunocompromise resulting from underlying viral diseases, such as PBFD, stress, and poor nutrition allows opportunists to cause disease. Conditions promoting fecal retention, such as egg laying, cloacal prolapse, or cloacal papilloma, often result in secondary enteritis. High population density increases contact with primary infectious agents.

# DIAGNOSIS

## DIFFERENTIAL DIAGNOSIS
Since both enteritis and gastritis are categories of disease, most differentials include etiologies of these conditions. However, there are a few disorders that have similar signs without inflammation of the

E

GI tract. Such conditions may include hepatic disease, neoplasia, or dietary indiscretion.

## CBC/BIOCHEMISTRY/URINALYSIS
Hematology can vary from normal to having severe leukocytosis, depending on the etiology of the condition. Mycobacteriosis often results in dramatic leukocytosis. Dehydration may result in slight elevations in the hematocrit. GI bleeding or chronic inflammation can result in anemia. Chemistry changes also vary substantially. If there is significant muscle wasting, CK, AST, and uric acid may have mild to moderate elevations. Protein can be elevated if there is dehydration, or can be reduced if there is protein loss in the GI tract. Other chemistries are not likely to be substantially altered, unless there is involvement of other organs in the disease process.

## OTHER LABORATORY TESTS
A variety of other diagnostic tests may aid in the diagnosis of gastritis and enteritis. Addition of iodine or Sudan stain to the feces can reveal undigested starches (amylorrhea) or fats (steatorrhea), respectively, suggesting maldigestion. Simple tests may reveal cellular changes or organisms that may shed light on the etiology. Direct saline preparations of feces or other GI samples may help to identify flagellates, *Macrorhabdus* yeasts, or other distinctive organisms. Gram-stained preparations of the same samples help to delineate the flora further. Culture can help further identify specific bacteria and determine their antimicrobial susceptibility. Microbiome testing can identify organisms that may not grow on routine cultures. Other tests that may be performed on feces or other GI samples include special stains (e.g. acid fast), and PCR tests for a variety of viral, bacterial, fungal, or parasitic agents.

## IMAGING
### Radiographic Findings
Since palpation is often very limited in birds, imaging is critical to developing a full evaluation of the GI tract. Radiography is helpful in identifying anatomic changes in the GI tract. Survey radiographs are often adequate for evaluation, but contrast studies can be used when needed to improve identification of the GI tract. Fluoroscopy can give real-time information on the motility of the GI tract when used with contrast.

### Ultrasonography
Ultrasound is often limited by artifacts caused by the air sac system of birds. However, if there is coelomic effusion or swelling, better views may be obtained.

### Advanced Imaging
Advanced imaging techniques such as plain or contrast CT can give very detailed information about anatomical changes which can suggest particular etiologies. For example,

thickening of the proventricular or enteric walls can suggest infiltrative diseases such as mycobacteriosis.

## DIAGNOSTIC PROCEDURES
Although a diagnosis can frequently be gained by simpler diagnostic samples, collection of gastric washes, either with or without the use of an endoscope, may be indicated in some cases. Histopathology of the stomach or intestine are infrequently performed antemortem because of the high morbidity and mortality of such procedures.

## PATHOLOGIC FINDINGS
Since this is a spectrum of diseases, the pathologic findings can be highly variable. However, inflammation of the intestine, proventriculus, or ventriculus is how these diseases are defined. Grossly, this may be represented by thickened walls, edema, hyperemia, distension, hemorrhage, erosions, or ulcers.

 # TREATMENT

## APPROPRIATE HEALTH CARE
Severely affected patients may require hospitalization for stabilization of their condition. Indications for hospitalization include anorexia, vomiting or regurgitation, severe fluid loss, secondary aspiration pneumonia, or other life-threatening conditions. If there are advanced treatments required that the owner is unable to perform, inpatient care may be advisable until the owner can be instructed to do them or they are no longer required. Outpatient care is appropriate for more mildly affected patients with treatments that are within the comfort level of the caregiver.

## NURSING CARE
In all but the mildest cases, fluid therapy is appropriate. The degree of dehydration should be estimated and that deficit should be added to the maintenance levels. Crystalloid fluids will be sufficient in mild to moderate cases. The route of administration depends on perfusion and the tolerance of the gastrointestinal tract. Routes of administering fluids include IV, IO, SQ, and crop gavage. Severely affected patients, and those that have low protein levels, may benefit from colloids, which must be given IV or IO. Nutritional support can prove challenging in these cases, as the alimentary tract may not tolerate regular food. Although parenteral nutrition can be used for a short time, alimentation should start early. The use of antiemetic drugs can be used to facilitate this. Small, frequent feedings are tolerated best. While balanced nutrition is important, the diet

may have to be simplified when the GI tract is distressed. In the short term, calories and protein can be provided by a simple rice or oatmeal baby cereal diet. As the GI tract heals, more complex dietary components can be added.

## ACTIVITY
While there is no reason to specifically restrict activity, some birds may benefit from added warmth, so a smaller hospital cage with supplemental heat is often appropriate. Additionally, having a small enclosure where food and water are readily accessible will benefit many sick birds.

## DIET
Prolonged fasting is not practical or advisable for most birds. Brief withholding of oral fluids and food may be indicated for patients that are vomiting or regurgitating. When returning to oral fluids and food consumption, it should be done gradually. For less severe conditions, dietary modifications may require extensive modification or none at all, dependent on the etiology of the condition and the current diet of the patient. The long-term goal is to have a nutritionally balanced diet that is tolerated by the GI tract of the bird, and that promotes a healthy and balanced microbial flora. The use of soft, moist, high-carbohydrate foods tends to promote extensive bacterial and yeast growth that occasionally result in GI disease. If these dietary components are deemed essential to the diet of the bird, they should be offered for only brief periods of time. Mycobacterial infections and other conditions that result in weight loss or malabsorption may necessitate an increase in caloric intake.

## CLIENT EDUCATION
Clients should be educated about any potentially zoonotic diseases, such as mycobacteriosis, salmonellosis, and others. Sanitation is often a factor in the development of these diseases, and clients should be taught appropriate sanitation procedures.

## SURGICAL CONSIDERATIONS
Gastritis and enteritis are generally treated medically. However, there are certain surgical procedures that may facilitate diagnosis or treatment. Endoscope-assisted gastric lavage may be performed, often in conjunction with a crop incision and biopsy, to gain a diagnosis and aid in the treatment of gastric conditions. The placement of feeding tubes can facilitate oral treatments and alimentation in selected cases. Generally, esophagostomy tubes are most applicable for this purpose. However, if temporarily bypassing the proventriculus and ventriculus would be beneficial for the patient, a duodenostomy tube can placed.

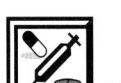 **MEDICATIONS**

### DRUG(S) OF CHOICE

Because of the wide variety of diseases included in this category, there are potentially hundreds of drugs that could be appropriate for treatments. In addition, dosages vary between species of birds. Individual treatment recommendations for all the diseases in this category would be beyond the scope of this chapter. However some generalizations can be made. Eliminate pathogens and restore the microflora balance in the GI tract. Antimicrobial or antiparasitic drugs should be used to treat birds with GI bacterial, fungal, protozoal, or helminth infections. Mycobacterial infections require multiple concurrent antibiotics. Many birds have mixed infections and may require combination therapies. It is important to consider anaerobes such as clostridium that may not be recognized on standard cultures as potential pathogens. In some cases, probiotics can help restore appropriate microbial flora. Although species-specific strains are most likely to be effective, they are not widely available. Protect the GI mucosa from further damage. Histamine-2 blockers such as ranitidine can be used to reduce acid damage to the stomach and small intestine. Adsorbents such as bismuth subsalicylate, kaolin, or similar products coat the mucosa and absorb bacterial toxins. Cholestyramine may absorb bacterial toxins more effectively. Sucralfate adheres to exposed submucosal tissues and provide a protective layer. Control of inflammation should proceed carefully as many systemic anti-inflammatory drugs can predispose to gastric erosions and ulcers. Bismuth subsalicylate can topically treat the intestine. NSAIDs may be used carefully, especially when there is nonspecific inflammation without GI bleeding. Corticosteroids should generally be avoided.

### CONTRAINDICATIONS

There are no specific contraindications for this category of disease.

### PRECAUTIONS

As described, NSAIDs should be used cautiously and only after the patient has had hydration and perfusion restored.

### POSSIBLE INTERACTIONS

As many drugs have GI signs as potential adverse effects, it can be difficult to monitor for adverse effects.

### ALTERNATIVE DRUGS

As there are numerous drugs in each category of therapy, this should not prove to be an issue.

 **FOLLOW-UP**

### PATIENT MONITORING

During hospitalization, weight, appetite, regurgitation or vomiting, and fecal quality should all be monitored. Once stable and sustaining weight with voluntary intake, the patient can be discharged. Follow-up timing depends upon the chronicity of the condition. Often rechecks should be scheduled at 1- to 4-week intervals. Parameters to be monitored include physical examination, weight, stool quality and appetite. Any non-invasive laboratory findings that contributed to the diagnosis should be followed until they return to normal. Repeating more invasive diagnostics may be indicated in some cases, but should be weighed against the risks involved.

### PREVENTION/AVOIDANCE

As a diverse collection of disorders, only general steps can be recommended. Exposure to infectious agents should be minimized by quarantine, sanitation, food safety measures, and other general management procedures. Maintenance of a healthy immune system should be promoted by proper nutrition, stress reduction, and provision of an appropriate habitat.

### POSSIBLE COMPLICATIONS

Dehydration and weight loss are common sequelae of gastritis and enteritis. Ascending infections to the liver can occur through the biliary tree. Bacteremia and septicemia can occur when the GI mucosa is compromised. The liver and kidneys can become infected first because of the hepatic and renal portal systems, respectively. Protein-losing enteropathies can lead to hypoproteinemia. GI hemorrhage can result in hypovolemic shock or anemia. Anemia can be either regenerative or non-regenerative, depending on the severity and chronicity.

### EXPECTED COURSE AND PROGNOSIS

There is a wide range in the ways that these diseases may progress. Some will be transient and self-limiting. Others may be acute and fatal. Still others can be chronic, some causing minimal to mild clinical signs, while others insidiously cause severe tissue damage, ultimately leading to death. Likewise, the prognosis varies from excellent to grave.

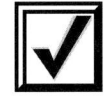 **MISCELLANEOUS**

### ASSOCIATED CONDITIONS

N/A

### AGE-RELATED FACTORS

N/A

### ZOONOTIC POTENTIAL

Some diseases within this category are zoonotic. These include mycobacteriosis, chlamydiosis, salmonellosis, and some strains of other bacteria.

### FERTILITY/BREEDING

N/A

### SYNONYMS

N/A

### SEE ALSO

Anorexia
Bornaviral Disease (Aquatic Birds)
Bornaviral Disease (Psittaciformes)
Campylobacteriosis
Candidiasis
Cloacal Diseases
Clostridiosis
Dehydration
Diarrhea
Emaciation
Flagellate Enteritis
Helminthiasis (Intestinal)
*Macrorhabdus ornithogaster*
Mycobacteriosis
Polyuria
Regurgitation and Vomiting
Trichomoniasis
Undigested Food in Droppings
Urate and Fecal Discoloration

### ABBREVIATIONS

AST—aspartate aminotransferase
CK—creatine kinase
CT—computed tomography
GI—gastrointestinal
NSAIDs—non-steroidal anti-inflammatory drugs
PBFD—psittacine beak and feather disease
PCR—polymerase chain reaction
PDD—proventricular dilatation disease

### INTERNET RESOURCES

N/A

*Suggested Reading*
Welle, K.R. (2016). Gastrointestinal system. In: *Current Therapy in Exotic Pet Practice* (ed. M.A. Mitchell, T.N. Tully Jr), 229–276. St. Louis MO: Elsevier.
Denbow, D.M. (2000). Gastrointestinal anatomy and physiology In: *Sturkie's Avian Physiology*, 5th edn. (ed. G.C. Whittow), 299–325. San Diego, CA: Academic Press.
Girling, S. (2004). Diseases of the digestive tract of psittacine birds. *In Practice*, 26:146–153.
Hadley, T.L. (2005). Disorders of the psittacine gastrointestinal tract. *Veterinary Clinics of North America. Exotic Animal Practice*, 8:329–349.

**Author**: Kenneth R. Welle DVM, DABVP (Avian)

**E**

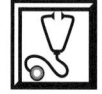

# BASICS

## DEFINITION
A smooth "lump" or "swelling" filled with white, caseous material, which results from the inability of a feather to erupt from the feather follicle (comparable to an ingrown hair in humans).

## PATHOPHYSIOLOGY
Feather cysts often develop as a result of the inability of a feather to break through the skin surface. While the feather continues to grow, it curls up within the follicle and degenerates to a caseous mass. Cysts may continue to grow slowly until they eventually rupture. Secondary infections or hemorrhage may occur.

## SYSTEMS AFFECTED
**Skin/exocrine**: Usually affects the feather follicles of the wing, pectoral or scapular (back) feather tracts; secondary infections may occur.
**Behavioral**: Cysts may irritate, thereby resulting in feather-damaging behavior or automutilation.
**Musculoskeletal**: Large cysts that are present on the wings may result in drooping of the wing and tripping over the wing. These cysts or large cysts on the body may also interfere with flying.
**Hemic**: Trauma to the cyst may result in severe bleeding and subsequent anemia.

## GENETICS
In canaries, the condition is believed to be hereditary, as it is typically seen in "soft-feathered" or "type" breeds. The exact mode of inheritance is unknown.

## INCIDENCE/PREVALENCE
A true incidence is unknown but the condition is commonly seen in canaries and less so in other bird species.

## GEOGRAPHIC DISTRIBUTION
N/A

## SIGNALMENT
**Species**: Commonly seen in soft-feathered canary breeds (e.g. Norwich and Gloucester are prone). Feather cysts are occasionally also seen in other bird species, including budgerigars and other psittacine birds, pigeons, chickens, and birds of prey.
**Mean age and predominant sex**: No age or sex predilection has been reported, but the condition is generally not seen before the first molt.

## SIGNS
### Historical Findings
A slowly growing, white-to-yellowish mass or lump on the body or wings. May develop following a normal molt. Other signs reported by the owner may include inability

to fly, drooping of the wing, and/or feather-damaging behavior or self-mutilation in the region of the affected feather, resulting in skin damage and/or hemorrhage.

### Physical Examination Findings
Feather cysts present as an oval or elongated swelling of the feather follicle with accumulation of dry, concentrically layered, yellow-white material (keratin). Although cysts may occur on any part of the body, they are often found on the wing, back, or pectoral region. One or multiple cysts may be present at a time. Secondary hemorrhage and/or infection may be present. In addition, feather damaging or automutilation of the skin with secondary ulceration and crust formation may be visible. Birds may present with a wing droop or inability to fly if the mass is large.

## CAUSES
Multiple etiologic factors may be involved including one or more of the following. Hereditary factors—particularly in soft-feathered canary breeds. Trauma—damage to the feather follicle resulting in abnormal growth, either iatrogenic or by the bird itself (e.g. due to feather-damaging behavior). Nutritional deficiencies, particularly hypovitaminosis A or amino acid deficiencies. Viral (e.g. PBFD, polyomavirus), bacterial and parasitic infections may potentially influence the occurrence of these cysts Any other condition that interferes with the normal growth and development of a feather.

## RISK FACTORS
N/A

# DIAGNOSIS

## DIFFERENTIAL DIAGNOSIS
Any disorder resulting in the formation of a "mass" or "lump" may be considered in the differential diagnosis of feather cysts. Abscesses or tumorous growths such as xanthomas and lipomas may resemble feather cysts in outer appearance, although cysts generally have a more firm consistency and a layered appearance (when incised). Fine-needle aspirates or excisional biopsies may help to differentiate between feather cysts and other masses.

## CBC/BIOCHEMISTRY/URINALYSIS
N/A

## OTHER LABORATORY TESTS
N/A

## IMAGING
N/A

## DIAGNOSTIC PROCEDURES
Diagnosis is usually made based on the gross morphological appearance of the lump. Fine-needle aspiration or excisional biopsies

can be performed to obtain a definite diagnosis. Cytologic findings are variable, dependent on chronicity of the lesion: early stages may reveal marked numbers of erythrocytes and erythrophagocytosis, whereas chronic stages are often characterized by presence of mixed-cell inflammation with a marked amount of debris, feather fragments, and occasional multinucleated giant cells. In case (secondary) infection is suspected, cyst material can be submitted for C/S testing.

## PATHOLOGIC FINDINGS
Grossly, feather cysts present as a round or elongated white-yellow mass in the skin. Upon incising the mass, the concentrically layered structure of keratin material becomes apparent. Histologically, the mass consists of an outer layer of proliferated stratified squamous epithelium that lines the keratinaceous material of the deformed feather. In case of secondary infection, inflammatory cells and micro-organisms may be present.

# TREATMENT

## APPROPRIATE HEALTH CARE
Treatment of choice consists of removal of the affected feather follicle(s) by excision. Other options include lancing and subsequent curettage and marsupialization or fulguration using radio cautery or laser. These techniques, however, frequently result in recurrence or damage to the adjacent feather follicles. A tourniquet may be used to aid in hemostasis when removing feather cysts on the wing. Cysts are excised, with wounds usually left open to heal by secondary intent. Take care not to damage any adjacent follicles or their blood supply during the procedure, as this may result in formation of new cysts. Hemorrhage is preferably controlled using ligatures rather than radiocautery, as radiocautery can damage adjacent follicles or their blood supply. Feather cysts of the tail may require amputation of the pygostyle. Feather cysts on the body are generally easy to remove using an elliptical or fusiform excision, followed by primary closure of the skin. If multiple cysts are present, removal of the whole feather tract may be considered. In older birds or birds that do not seem to experience any discomfort of the cyst, treatment may not be necessary.

## NURSING CARE
Stabilize any patient that is critical prior to initiating the surgery. Provide appropriate fluid therapy (SQ, IV, IO) prior to, during and after the procedure. After removal of the cyst, bandages (e.g. figure-of-eight bandage

and/or body wrap) may be considered to prevent movement at the surgery site, provide extra hemostasis and protect the wound from contamination or mutilation by the bird. The use of Elizabethan collars, ponchos, or socks may be indicated in birds that pick at the surgical site. The surgical wound is commonly allowed to heal by secondary intention. Once adjacent feathers begin to regrow, debris may be removed on a daily basis using cotton swabs or warm sterile saline flushes.

## ACTIVITY
Birds in which a feather cyst has been removed from the wing may benefit from flight restraint for the first days to a week post-surgery (until the wound has sufficiently healed).

## DIET
In the event that malnourishment is suspected to play a role in the development of a feather cyst, dietary corrections are advised.

## CLIENT EDUCATION
Owners need to be informed about the heritable nature of this condition in canaries and should be aware that cysts commonly recur.

## SURGICAL CONSIDERATIONS
Provide fluids and appropriate nutritional support to any patient with substantial blood loss and stabilize first prior to performing the surgery. Also provide adequate fluid support (SQ, IV, IO) throughout the procedure and maintain proper hemostasis, particularly in smaller birds.

# MEDICATIONS

## DRUG(S) OF CHOICE
Treatment is surgical. Additional pain relief (e.g. NSAIDs) and/or appropriate antibiotics (preferably based on results from C/S testing) are indicated in case of concurrent inflammation and secondary infections.

## CONTRAINDICATIONS
N/A

## PRECAUTIONS
N/A

## POSSIBLE INTERACTIONS
N/A

## ALTERNATIVE DRUGS
N/A

# FOLLOW-UP

## PATIENT MONITORING
Recommend regular check-ups of the bird (e.g. every 6–12 months) to detect new growing cysts in an early stage.

## PREVENTION/AVOIDANCE
N/A

## POSSIBLE COMPLICATIONS
Excessive hemorrhage (e.g. from trauma, self-mutilation, or during surgical excision). Secondary infections of the cysts, particularly when the skin surface is damaged. Automutilation and/or poor wound healing following surgical excision.

## EXPECTED COURSE AND PROGNOSIS
Prognosis is usually good following complete surgical excision. However, recurrence is common, particularly in birds in which a genetic background is suspected.

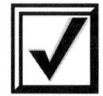

# MISCELLANEOUS

## ASSOCIATED CONDITIONS
Feather-damaging birds may develop one or multiple cysts as a result of chronic trauma to the feather follicles.

## AGE-RELATED FACTORS
N/A

## ZOONOTIC POTENTIAL
N/A

## FERTILITY/BREEDING
Although it is advisable not to breed with affected canaries, show standards accept these types of breeds and award prizes to birds

prone to developing feather cysts, thereby resulting in persistence of this condition in the population.

## SYNONYMS
Feather follicle cyst, feather folliculoma, plumafolliculoma.

## SEE ALSO
Cere and Skin Color Changes
Dermatitis
Feather Damaging and Self-Injurious Behavior
Feather Disorders
Neoplasia (Integument)
Xanthoma/Xanthogranulomatosis

## ABBREVIATIONS
C/S—culture and sensitivity
NSAIDs—nonsteroidal anti-inflammatory drugs
PBFD—psittacine beak and feather disease

## INTERNET RESOURCES
N/A

*Suggested Reading*
Bauck, L. (1987). Radical surgery for the treatment of feather cysts in the canary. *AAV Today*, 1:200–201.
Bennett, R.A., Harrison, G.J. (1997). Soft tissue surgery. In: *Avian Medicine: Principles and Application* (ed. B.W. Ritchie, G.J. Harrison, L.R. Harrison), 1096–1196. Lake Worth, FL: Wingers Publishing.
Fraser, M. (2006). Skin diseases and treatment of caged birds. In: *Skin Diseases of Exotic Pets* (ed. S. Patterson), 22–47. Ames, IA: Blackwell Science.
Harrison, G.J. (2003). Microsurgical procedure for feather cyst removal in a citron-crested cockatoo (*Cacatua sulphurea citrinocristata*). *Journal of Avian Medicine and Surgery*, 17:86–90.
Wheeldon, E.B., Culbertson, M.R. (1982). Feather folliculoma in the canary (*Serinus canarius*). *Veterinary Pathology*, 19:204–206.
**Authors**: Yvonne R. A. van Zeeland, DVM, MVR, PhD, DECZM (Avian, Small Mammal), and Nico J. Schoemaker, DVM, PhD, DECZM (Small Mammal, Avian)

# FEATHER-DAMAGING AND SELF-INJURIOUS BEHAVIOR

F

 **BASICS**

## DEFINITION

Self-injurious behavior includes all behavior in which the bird damages its own tissues, typically by using its beak. In case of feather-damaging behavior, the self-inflicted damage is directed to the feathers and can involve chewing, biting, plucking, and/or fraying of coverts, down feathers, remiges, and rectrices. Typically, the feathers of the head and crest remain unaffected, as these are inaccessible to the bird's beak. In case of self-mutilation or automutilation, the skin and/or deeper structures are also affected. While automutilation and feather-damaging behavior are both classified among self-injurious behaviors and some overlap in causes may exist, the behaviors should be considered as two separate entities.

## PATHOPHYSIOLOGY

In general, three underlying pathophysiological mechanisms should be taken into consideration for self-injurious behavior: (1) Maladaptive behavior, resulting from attempts of the animal to cope with a suboptimal or inadequate environment, which is lacking the appropriate stimuli needed and/or in which aversive stimuli or stressors are present. (2) Malfunctional behavior, resulting from an abnormal psychology, brain development, or altered neurochemistry, which may have developed as a result of the bird's living conditions, particularly in early life. (3) Behavior performed to alleviate pain, pruritus, irritation, or other type of discomfort resulting from an underlying medical (physical) problem.

## SYSTEMS AFFECTED

**Behavioral**: Birds may spend more time on preening and/or preen more intensively, which results in damaged feathers and/or skin; other problem behaviors including anxiety and fear-related behavior, excessive vocalization, sexual behavior, or abnormal repetitive behaviors (such as stereotypic behavior) may also be seen.
**Skin/exocrine**: Feathers may be pulled and/or frayed resulting in generalized or patchy alopecia in areas that are accessible to the bird's beak. Covert and/or down feathers are the main target, although remiges and/or rectrices may be targeted as well. Skin damage and/or (secondary) infections may also be present.
**Endocrine/metabolic**: Metabolic needs may be increased due to lack of insulation and decreased thermoregulatory abilities.
**Hemic/lymphatic/immune**: Blood loss may occur in birds with self-injurious behavior.

## GENETICS

Genetic factors are thought to be involved because of species predilections. Results of a study in feather-damaging Amazon parrots demonstrated high heritability estimates, thereby supporting the hypothesis that a genetic basis may indeed exist.

## INCIDENCE/PREVALENCE

Feather-damaging behavior is estimated to occur in 10–15% of captive parrots.

## GEOGRAPHIC DISTRIBUTION

N/A

## SIGNALMENT

**Species predilections**: Although feather-damaging behavior may occur in any parrot species, grey parrots (*Psittacus erithacus*), Eclectus parrots (*Eclectus roratus*), cockatoos (*Cacatua* spp.) and conures (*Pyrrhura* spp.) appear particularly prone. The condition is seemingly less common in budgerigars (*Melopsittacus* spp.). Aside from parrots, the condition may also be observed in other bird species, including birds of prey, of which the Harris hawk (*Parabuteo unicinctus*) is noted as a highly susceptible species. Similar to feather-damaging behavior, automutilation can occur in any species, but specific species predilections have been associated with specific mutilation syndromes. For example, (ventral) propatagial mutilation is commonly observed in grey parrots; sternal mutilation is commonly seen in cockatoos, particularly the umbrella (*Cacatua alba*), rose-breasted (*Eolophus roseicapilla*), and Moluccan cockatoo (*Cacatua moluccencis*); wing-tip mutilation is common in cockatiels (*Nymphicus hollandicus*); lovebirds (*Agapornis* spp.) are predisposed to axillary and tail-base mutilation; and Amazon parrots (*Amazona* spp.) and monk parakeets (*Myiopsitta monachus*) are prone to mutilate the feet and neck or chest.
**Mean age and range**: Although feather-damaging behavior may occur at any age, it has been suggested that the age of onset lies around the time when parrots become sexually mature. With increasing age, the likelihood of a parrot displaying feather-damaging behavior also increases.
**Predominant sex**: Feather-damaging may occur both in male and female parrots, with a suggested predilection for the female sex.

## SIGNS

### General Comments

Feather-damaging behavior is usually self-inflicted, but in some cases it can be directed to cage mates or nestlings. Severity of self-injurious behavior may vary from mild or localized feather damage or alopecia to severe forms with generalized feather damage, alopecia and/or self-mutilation.

### Historical Findings

The most noticeable sign in birds with feather-damaging or self-injurious behavior is the presence of featherless areas and/or skin damage. Owners may note the bird plucking, biting or pulling its feathers or damaging its skin, but the behavior may be difficult to distinguish from normal preening and may also occur when the owner is not present. Extensive history taking is needed to identify potential underlying medical and/or behavioral causes, and should include information about the self-injurious behavior (onset, duration, clinical course, conditions under which it occurs), possible other behavior or medical problems, and the bird's general condition, as well as a detailed description of the bird's living environment (e.g. housing, enrichment, nutrition) and prior history (incl. rearing conditions).

### Physical Examination Findings

Presence of featherless areas and/or damage to the feathers (fraying, chewing) and/or skin. Feathers are mainly plucked in the easy accessible regions of the neck, chest, flank, inner thigh, and ventral wing surface; feathers of the head and crest are typically unaffected as these are inaccessible to the bird's beak. Contour and down feathers are usually affected, but some birds may also damage the tail and flight feathers. In some birds with skin damage, secondary infections and/or hemorrhage may be present. Location, extent, and type of feather and/or skin damage, as well as any other abnormalities found during the physical examination should be noted, as these may provide clues towards the potential underlying cause, thereby emphasizing the importance of conducting a thorough and systematic hands-on examination.

## CAUSES

Numerous causes for feather damaging and/or automutilation have been reported. However, a definitive causation is not always clear or unambiguous. In essence, any disease or condition causing pain, pruritis or other type of discomfort could initiate self-injurious behavior.
**Underlying medical conditions**: Some medical underlying diseases leading to self-injurious behavior include ecto- and endoparasites (e.g. *Knemidocoptes*, feather or quill mites, lice, *Giardia*, *Spironucleus*, protozoal infection, particularly in cockatiels); bacterial or fungal dermatitis and/or folliculitis (including *Staphylococcus*, *Aspergillus*, *Candida*, *Malassezia* spp.); viral infections such as polyomavirus, PBFD (circovirus) and bornavirus; infectious skin and/or feather disease (bacterial, fungal, viral). Skin neoplasia (e.g. xanthoma, lipoma, squamous cell carcinoma). Nutritional deficiencies (e.g. hypovitaminosis A) and/or dietary imbalances. Low humidity levels, lack of

bathing opportunities. Airborne, topical, and/or ingested toxins, including cigarette smoke, scented candles, air fresheners, hand lotions and creams, heavy-metal ingestion (e.g. lead, zinc). Hypersensitivity, skin allergy. Systemic diseases such as chlamydiosis, avian ganglioneuritis. Internal disease involving the respiratory tract (e.g. air sacculitis, pneumonia), liver (e.g. hepatitis), gastrointestinal tract (e.g. colic, gastroenteritis), cardiovascular system (e.g. atherosclerosis, cardiomyopathy), or urogenital tract (e.g. renomegaly, cystic ovaries, egg binding). Endocrine and/or metabolic conditions (e.g. hypothyroidism, diabetes mellitus, hypocalcemia). Orthopedic disorders (e.g. osteosarcoma, fracture, osteomyelitis) or conditions associated with neuropathic pain. Improper wing trim or (iatrogenic) trauma.

**Socioenvironmental factors**: Can contribute to the development and persistence of self-injurious behaviors. Examples include social isolation or overcrowding. Imprinting on humans, inappropriate social interaction with humans leading to sexual arousal and possibly frustration, especially if a mate is lacking (often cyclic or seasonal changes occurring). Inability to perform species-typical behaviors (most notably feeding and foraging activities), resulting in redirected feather-damaging behavior. Lack of mental and cognitive stimulation, resulting in boredom, especially for the more intelligent species. Small cage or poor cage design that limits the parrot's ability to move around and/or fly. Sudden changes to the environment, lack of predictability and/or controllability of the environment. Sleep deprivation, abnormal photoperiod. Exposure to aversive stimuli or other stressful conditions leading to (chronic) stress and anxiety (feather-damaging behavior can serve as a coping mechanism, resulting in dearousal). Poor socialization at a young age, leading to generalized fear and phobias. Traumatic events. Responses of the caregiver that may inadvertently reinforce the behavior, especially in attention seeking birds.

**Neurobiological factors**: May also contribute to the onset and perpetuation of self-injurious behaviors. This may include both hormones (e.g. corticosterone, sex hormones) and neurotransmitters (e.g. dopamine, serotonin, endorphins), which affect and alter the animal's physiology and brain function. Neurotransmitter changes in particular have been associated with development of abnormal repetitive behaviors that can be compared to obsessive–compulsive or impulsive disorders in humans.

## RISK FACTORS
Feather-damaging and self-injurious behaviors are generally regarded as multifactorial disorders that may be influenced by a number of medical, genetic, neurobiologic, and/or socioenvironmental factors. Any type of

disease causing pain, discomfort, irritation, or pruritus may result in onset of feather-damaging behavior and automutilation. Early living conditions, particularly hand rearing, inadequate socialization, and deprivement may predispose the bird to develop feather-damaging behavior. Lack of an appropriate living environment (particularly lack of foraging opportunities) and/or presence of stressors, both in early life and present living conditions, may influence the onset of abnormal behavior. Self-injurious behavior may unintentionally be reinforced by the owner, as their responses may be rewarding the bird. Neurotransmitter (e.g. serotonin, dopamine, endorphin) deficiencies and/or excesses may play a role in the onset and/or maintenance of the self-injurious behavior, although little is currently known about the underlying neuropathophysiologic mechanisms.

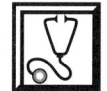

## DIAGNOSIS

### DIFFERENTIAL DIAGNOSIS
Feather-damaging behavior should be distinguished from other causes of alopecia or feather loss, including normal molt and/or apteria (not recognized by an inexperienced owner), cage mate plucking (excessive allopreening), (iatrogenic) trauma, feather loss due to parasitism or bacterial, mycotic or viral infections, and plucking related to normal brooding behavior (bird preparing a brood patch). In addition, causes for lack of feather growth (e.g. hypothyroidism, malnutrition, PBFD) should be ruled out. A thorough behavioral and medical workup are needed to identify any and all underlying causes and contributing factors to the self-injurious behavior. Medical underlying causes are highly suspected in birds with automutilation. Dependent on the location, certain causes may be more or less likely (e.g. peripheral arterial disease is highly likely in case of mutilation of the propatagium, chest area, legs or feet, whereas renal, spinal, or uropygial problems are more commonly associated with tail-base mutilation). In case the self-injurious behavior is more likely to originate from a psychological cause (e.g. stress, anxiety or boredom due to a suboptimal environment, attention-seeking behavior), effort should be made to identify the potential underlying triggers (antecedents) and reinforcing factors (consequences) that may have contributed to the onset and maintenance of the behavior.

### CBC/BIOCHEMISTRY/URINALYSIS
Leukocytosis, heterophilia, and/or monocytosis may be seen in case of (secondary) infections. In case of blood loss,

hematocrit values may be decreased. Plasma CK values may be elevated. Depending on the underlying cause, other abnormalities may be noted.

### OTHER LABORATORY TESTS
Fecal examination (including wet mount and flotation, hemacolor, or Gram stain); for example, for diagnosis of *Giardia*, *Spironucleus*, other endoparasites, dysbacteriosis, or yeast infections (e.g. *Macrohabdus ornithogaster, Candida albicans*). PCR testing for specific pathogens on full blood (circovirus) or cloacal swab (polyomavirus, avian bornavirus, *Chlamydia psittaci*). Serology testing for avian bornavirus, *C. psittaci*. Heavy-metal screening for lead or zinc toxicosis. TSH stimulation tests for hypothyroidism (if feather growth is absent).

### IMAGING
Whole-body radiographs and (contrast-enhanced) CT may be useful to identify various underlying causes including heavy-metal intoxication, reproductive disorders (e.g. egg binding), hepato-, spleno- or renomegaly, PDD, pneumonia, air sacculitis, neoplastic conditions, musculoskeletal disease (e.g. osteoarthritis, osteomyelitis, fractures, osteosarcoma), and peripheral arterial disease (atherosclerosis). Ultrasound may be indicated to rule out or diagnose hepatomegaly, reproductive disorders (e.g. egg peritonitis, cystic ovary), neoplastic conditions, cardiac disease, ascites.

### DIAGNOSTIC PROCEDURES
Additional diagnostic tests that may be useful to diagnose underlying medical conditions include cytologic examination of skin lesions (scrapings, tape strip, impression smear, swab, fine-needle aspirate) or feather pulp (feather digest) to diagnose (secondary) bacterial or fungal folliculitis or dermatitis, pox virus, ectoparasites (feather or quill mites, *Knemidocoptes*), neoplasia. C/S of skin lesions and/or feather pulp to diagnose bacterial or fungal dermatitis or folliculitis. Aseptic preparation of the surroundings is required to prevent contamination risk. Next-generation DNA sequencing techniques can also be used to help identify bacterial presence, and generally do so with greater accuracy than traditional culturing methods. Histopathology of (paired) skin and/or feather follicle biopsy samples to diagnose a variety of infectious, inflammatory and/or neoplastic skin diseases (e.g. PBFD, polyomavirus, bacterial and fungal folliculitis, quill mite infestation, xanthomatosis, squamous cell carcinoma, feather follicle cysts). Intradermal skin testing to diagnose hypersensitivity reactions, allergic skin disease; however, these tests are

not reliable in birds due to their thin skin and diminished reaction to histamine. Endoscopy (e.g. to diagnose air sacculitis, hepato- or nephropathy, splenomegaly, pancreatic disorders, reproductive disease).

## PATHOLOGIC FINDINGS

Gross pathological findings of patchy or generalized alopecia, or feather damage with or without skin damage and/or secondary infections, with the head typically remaining unaffected. Histopathology may help to distinguish between inflammatory and traumatic (self-inflicted) skin disease. Inflammatory skin disease is characterized by presence of perivascular inflammation in the superficial or deep dermis of clinically affected and unaffected sites (i.e. outside of the reach of the bird's beak). Traumatic skin disease is characterized by superficial dermal scarring, ± inflammation in the affected sites and an absence of inflammation in the unaffected sites. Any inflammatory cells typically include lymphocytes and occasionally plasma cells, histiocytes, and granulocytes.

## TREATMENT

### APPROPRIATE HEALTH CARE

Address medical conditions appropriately, if present. In case of mutilation of the skin and/or deeper structures, mechanical barriers such as Elizabethan collars, neck braces, "ponchos," "jackets," "vests," or bandages can be used. These are, however, merely symptomatic and may cause additional stress. Always select the least intrusive option that is effective, as this will help to minimize stress, physical discomfort, and possible harm and injury in the long-term. Self-inflicted wounds often require open-wound management and healing by secondary intent. Multimodal analgesia is often warranted in patients with automutilation to alleviate pain and prevent long-term potentiation (which can lead to worsening and perpetuation of the behavior). Correct the diet and/or modify the bird's housing and living conditions to address any environmental factors that may be involved. Promote a more stimulating and appropriate environment by means of increasing the size of the enclosure, taking the bird outdoors and/or providing ultraviolet B lighting, providing social contact, (chewing) toys, puzzle feeders, and other forms of environmental enrichment. In particular, foraging enrichment has been shown to effectively reduce feather-damaging behavior. Training and behavior modification techniques, such as desensitization, counter-conditioning, and

differential reinforcement of alternate (desired) behaviors may be employed to alter the behavior of the bird and provide the bird a mentally stimulating challenge or task. Local application of foul-tasting substances is controversial, as these may result in deterioration. In (secondary) skin infections, the use of appropriate antibiosis (preferably based on results of a culture and sensitivity testing) and/or NSAIDs may be considered. Drug therapy with psychoactive, mood-altering drugs may be warranted in cases that are refractory to treatment with enrichment and/or behavior modification (see Medication). In case of mutilation of a single extremity, amputation may be considered in refractory cases.

### NURSING CARE

In case of severe skin damage, wound management followed by placement of a protective wound dressing and/or "jacket" or "poncho" to prevent the bird from further mutilating itself is indicated. In case of (severe) blood loss, fluid therapy and/or blood transfusions may be considered.

### ACTIVITY

Promote the bird's species-typical behaviors and provide the bird with sufficient exercise and mental challenge to satiate its needs.

### DIET

Nutrition of the bird should be optimized to correct for any potential deficiencies or excesses which may exacerbate the behavior. If fed a seed mixture exclusively, owners should be advised to convert the bird to a balanced (pelleted) diet. Omega-3 fatty 0.1–0.2 ml/kg PO q12–24h can be added to the diet, as these have anti-inflammatory properties and can help to alleviate dry skin. Provide the bird with mental and/or physical challenges by offering the food in a puzzle feeder, hiding, and/or mixing it with inedible items. Larger-sized food particles and/or treats (e.g. walnuts, pine cones) may also promote the bird's foraging activities.

### CLIENT EDUCATION

Provide the bird with adequate nutrition and a low-stress, stimulating environment in which it is able to display its species-typical behaviors. To create a stimulating environment, various types of enrichment may be offered to the bird, which stimulate the bird's senses and provide a physical and mental challenge. Particularly, chewing toys, puzzle feeders, and other types of foraging enrichment promote the bird's natural behavior and can help to satiate the behavioral need to forage while providing a good distraction from the self-injurious behavior. Create awareness that the owner may (unintentionally) be reinforcing the behavior by paying attention to the bird when it is displaying the self-injurious

behavior in an attempt to distract the bird or getting it to stop plucking or biting its skin and/or feathers. Emphasize that there is no quick-fix solution to this condition: it will require time, effort, and lots of patience to successfully redirect and resolve self-injurious behavior. Create awareness that once a bird is a chronic plucker or mutilator, the condition may be challenging to treat, with relapses occurring frequently.

### SURGICAL CONSIDERATIONS

Amputation of a wing or leg may be considered in severe, refractory automutilation, if mutilation is limited to that particular area. Adequate precautions should be taken to avoid (continued) mutilation at the surgical site.

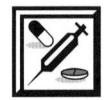

## MEDICATIONS

### DRUG(S) OF CHOICE

In refractory cases, and as an adjunct therapy to a behavior modification plan, pharmacologic intervention using psychoactive, mood-altering drugs may be considered. Of these, clomipramine seems the best investigated, but other options include dopamine antagonists (e.g. haloperidol), opiate receptor antagonists (e.g. naloxone, naltrexone), tricyclic antidepressants (e.g. amitriptylline, clomipramine, doxepin), serotonergic reuptake inhibitors (e.g. fluoxetine, paroxetine), benzodiazepines (e.g. alprazolam, clonazepam, diazepam, lorazepam), anxiolytic drugs (e.g. buspirone). Hormone therapy using GnRH agonists (e.g. deslorelin implants and leuprolide acetate) may be indicated when feather-damaging behavior is suspected to be sexual or hormonally related. Multimodal analgesia is warranted in patients that inflict damage to the skin or deeper structures, and may include the use of NSAIDs (e.g. meloxicam, carprofen, robenacoxib), gabapentin, opioids (e.g. butorphanol), tramadol, and other analgesics. In case of underlying medical conditions and/or secondary infections, other types of medication may need to be given.

### CONTRAINDICATIONS

Corticosteroids are generally contraindicated due to their immunosuppressive effects.

### PRECAUTIONS

Since limited information is available on the use of psychoactive, mood-altering drugs in birds, these preparations should be used with caution and titrated carefully to effect while also monitoring closely for any adverse effects. Many of these drugs may take several weeks to take effect and should be gradually weaned off to prevent withdrawal symptoms from occurring.

# (CONTINUED) FEATHER-DAMAGING AND SELF-INJURIOUS BEHAVIOR

## POSSIBLE INTERACTIONS
Interactions between psychoactive drugs are common and may potentially be hazardous. Simultaneous use should, therefore, be avoided. When switching from one drug to another, the bird should first be fully weaned off of one drug prior to starting the new drug, to reduce the risk of undesired adverse effects.

## ALTERNATIVE DRUGS
N/A

 FOLLOW-UP

## PATIENT MONITORING
Regular rechecks are recommended. As it may take at least 3–4 weeks for feathers to regrow once they are pulled, monthly to bimonthly rechecks seem appropriate, unless the condition is severe and/or worsens (in which case, more frequent rechecks may be scheduled). During rechecks, a detailed inspection of the plumage and skin condition is warranted, in which photographs and/or periodic scoring of plumage condition (using specifically designed feather scoring systems) can serve as meaningful tools to help monitor changes in the behavior as it is commonly difficult to observe changes in the behavior directly. Owners are advised to keep a log and document when the feather-damaging behavior occurs, which may help to identify possible underlying causes. In case of (secondary) infections or underlying medical conditions, a CBC and/or biochemistry may be performed to monitor changes in the bird's health status. If psychoactive drugs are used, owners are instructed to monitor their bird carefully for potential adverse effects and to contact their veterinarian immediately when adverse effects are suspected or observed.

## PREVENTION/AVOIDANCE
Provide the bird with a stimulating, low-stress living environment and adequate nutrition. Particularly, the provision of (novel) enrichment, training and exercise (e.g. taking the bird outside for walks) may help to create and maintain a stimulating and controllable environment that allows the bird to perform its species-specific behaviors and make its own decisions, while simultaneously preventing the development of feather damaging and other problem behaviors. Hand rearing of young birds should be avoided, as this may increase the risks of the bird developing developing feather damaging and other problem behavior later in life.

## POSSIBLE COMPLICATIONS
Severe feather loss may lead to a compromise of thermoregulatory abilities, and may affect the bird's metabolic needs and immune system, thereby resulting in increased susceptibility to disease. Hemorrhage. Secondary infections, particularly if skin damage is present.

## EXPECTED COURSE AND PROGNOSIS
Feather damaging and automutilation are challenging conditions to treat, with recurrence and relapses commonly occurring, especially if one is unable to identify and eliminate the underlying cause. However, even if an underlying cause is successfully identified and treated, self-injurious behavior may perpetuate as a result of other, reinforcing factors. Prognosis is therefore often considered guarded, with chances of a successful outcome decreasing once the condition becomes more chronic and ritualized. Hence, early intervention is recommended to increase the changes of a successful outcome.

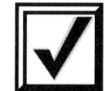 MISCELLANEOUS

## ASSOCIATED CONDITIONS
Birds with feather-damaging behavior may also display other forms of abnormal repetitive behavior, such as stereotypic behaviors (e.g. circling, tumbling, tongue playing, head bobbing, or twirling). Automutilation is commonly associated with an underlying medical condition.

## AGE-RELATED FACTORS
N/A

## ZOONOTIC POTENTIAL
N/A

## FERTILITY/BREEDING
Since genetic factors cannot be excluded, breeding with feather-damaging birds is best avoided.

## SYNONYMS
Feather picking, feather plucking, feather pulling, feather destructive behavior, pterotillomania, self-mutilation, automutilation.

## SEE ALSO
Cere and Skin Color Changes
Circovirus
Dermatitis
Ectoparasites
Feather Disorders
Flagellate (Intestinal)
Nutritional Imbalances
Problem Behaviors
Appendix 8, Algorithm 12: Feather-Damaging Behavior

## ABBREVIATIONS
C/S—culture and sensitivity
CK—creatine kinase
CT—computed tomography
GnRH—gonadotropin-releasing hormone
PBFD—psittacine beak and feather disease
PCR—polymerase chain reaction
PDD—proventricular dilatation disease
TSH—thyroid-stimulating hormone

## INTERNET RESOURCES
World Parrot Trust Reference Library. Behaviour and training: http://www.parrots.org/index.php/referencelibrary/behaviourandenviroenrich
Behavior Works: http://www.behaviorworks.org
Super Bird Creations. Make your own bird toys: https://makeyourownbirdtoys.com

*Suggested Reading*
Fluck, A., Enderlein, D., Piepenbring, A., et al. (2019). Correlation of avian bornavirus-specific antibodies and viral ribonucleic acid shedding with neurological signs and feather-damaging behaviour in psittacine birds. *Veterinary Record*, 184:476.
Jenkins, J.R. (2001). Feather picking and self-mutilation in psittacine birds. *Veterinary Clinics of North America: Exotic Animal Practice*, 4:651–667.
Nett, C.S., Tully, T.N. (2003). Anatomy, clinical presentation and diagnostic approach to feather-picking pet birds. *Compendium on Continuing Education for the Practicing Veterinarian*, 25:206–219.
Orosz, S.E. (2006). Diagnostic work-up of suspected behavioural disorders. In: *Manual of Parrot Behavior* (ed. A.U. Luescher), 195–210. Oxford, UK: Blackwell.
Rubinstein, J., Lightfoot, T.L. (2012). Feather loss and feather destructive behavior in pet birds. *Journal of Exotic Pet Medicine*, 21:219–234.
Seibert, L.M. (2006). Feather-picking disorder in pet birds. In: *Manual of Parrot Behavior* (ee. A.U. Luescher), 255–265. Oxford, UK: Blackwell.
van Zeeland, Y.R.A. (2018). Medication for behavior modification in birds. *Veterinary Clinics of North America: Exotic Animal Practice*, 21:115–149.
van Zeeland, Y.R.A., Friedman, S.G., Bergman, L. (2016). Behavior. In: *Current Therapy in Avian Medicine and Surgery* (ed. B.L. Speer), 531–549. Elsevier, St. Louis, MO.
van Zeeland, Y.R.A., Spruit, B.M., Rodenburg, T.D., et al. (2009). Feather damaging behaviour in parrots: a review with consideration of comparative aspects. *Applied Animal Behaviour Science*, 121:75–95.

**Authors**: Yvonne R. A. van Zeeland, DVM, MVR, PhD, DECZM (Avian, Small Mammal), and Nico Schoemaker, DVM, PhD, DECZM (Small Mammal, Avian)

 **Client Education Handout available online**

# FEATHER DISORDERS

## BASICS

### DEFINITION
Feather dystrophy is characterized by the formation of abnormally shaped feathers, which may be present as a localized or generalized disorder. Feather discoloration is a change of the normal coloration of a feather, which may involve only part of the feather (e.g. spots) or the feather as a whole, and can be limited to a single or a few feathers, or more extensive, involving multiple feathers or the entire plumage.

### PATHOPHYSIOLOGY
Abnormal growth of dystrophic feathers is the result of (in)direct damage to the feather follicle, follicular collar, or developing feathers. Feathers derive their coloration from pigments (melanins, porphyrins, and carotenoids) and/or structural conditions of the feather that modify or separate the components of white light (e.g. Tyndall effect, iridescence). Lack of certain nutrients that serve as a precursor for the aforementioned pigments, as well as conditions affecting the feather structure can result in a feather color change.

### SYSTEMS AFFECTED
Skin/exocrine—one or multiple abnormally formed or shaped feathers and/or follicles (feather dystrophy) or abnormally colored feathers. Feather dystrophy and/or discoloration does not affect any organ system itself, but underlying conditions that affect the structure or color of a feather may affect other organ systems. See Polyomavirus and Circovirus chapters for their respective effects on the hepatobiliary, hemic/lymphatic/immune and/or renal/urologic system. Additionally, organ dysfunction and metabolic conditions (e.g. hypothyroidism) can negatively affect feather quality.

### GENETICS
Feather duster disease is a feather dystrophic condition that occurs in English show budgerigars (*Melopsittacus undulatus*) and is caused by a recessive gene. Straw feather disease is an unusual, lethal disorder in canaries (*Serinus canaria*), whereby the feathers fail to emerge from the feather sheath and the barbs and barbules fail to develop. In lutino cockatiels, a bald patch is often present behind the crest feathers, which is believed to have a sex-linked genetic origin. A hereditary decrease in the number of feathers, resulting in partial or complete featherlessness, is also noted in other domesticated species of birds, including canaries, finches, chickens, pigeons, and waterfowl. Genetic mutations may result

in change of color of the feathers. Generalized color mutations, such as lutinos, are bred specifically for the show.

### INCIDENCE/PREVALENCE
Feather duster disease, straw feather disease, and porcupine feathers are rare conditions. With proper management in breeding facilities, the incidence of circovirus and polyomavirus infections has decreased considerably throughout the past decade. With proper nutrition, the incidence of feather discoloration should be minimal.

### GEOGRAPHIC DISTRIBUTION
N/A

### SIGNALMENT
Feather duster disease is seen in English show budgerigars during the development of the first feathers. Straw feather disease affects canaries. Porcupine feathers, which resemble straw feather disease in canaries, have been reported in Japanese quail and in homer and fantail pigeons. Feather dystrophy due to polyomavirus infections is commonly seen in smaller psittacines (particularly budgerigars, lovebirds) during the development of the first feathers, from the age of 10 days onwards. Baldness of the crown of the head, behind the crest, is typically recognized in lutino cockatiels. Stress lines are commonly noted in young birds and may be associated with illness or a change in diet, or disruption of the feeding schedule during weaning. Feather dystrophy due to circovirus infections are seen in all psittacine breeds up to the age of 3 years. Australasian species are most prone, followed by African and then South American species. Feather discoloration can occur in all birds, regardless of the species, age, or sex. Species that are known to require carotenoids in their diet to obtain a normal plumage color include flamingos and specific color-bred canaries. If white birds (such as ducks) are fed carotenoids, their plumage color may change.

### SIGNS
In feather duster disease, the feathers continue to grow, resulting in extremely long, curly feathers covering the entire body of the budgerigar. Porcupine feathers and feathers from birds affected with straw feather disease have a straw-like appearance and resemble porcupine quills due to a failure of the barbs/barbules to develop or uncoil (the shaft of the feather generally appears normal). Stress lines are translucent lines across the vane of a feather, oriented perpendicular to the shaft, which represent segmental dysplasia that occurred due to a brief period of dysfunction in the epidermal collar from which the feather arises. See Polyomavirus chapter for

the feather dystrophic signs seen in birds infected with this virus. See Circovirus (Psittacines) chapter for the progressive feather dystrophic signs seen in birds infected with this virus. Feather discoloration: any discoloration from the normal plumage color (e.g. red feathers in the normal gray plumage of African grey parrots, yellow discoloration of feathers in Amazon parrots, overall/generalized dull plumage due to lack of carotenoid diet in canaries).

### CAUSES
Multiple etiologic factors may be involved in feather dystrophy. Hereditary—in budgerigars with feather duster disease. Trauma—damage to the feather follicle resulting in abnormal growth, either iatrogenic or by the bird itself (e.g. due to plucking). Viral (e.g. PBFD, polyomavirus, West Nile virus in raptors). Corticosteroid release in relation to stressful events (e.g. transport, restraint, nutritional deficiencies, food deprivation, or environmental stressors) during feather growth Any other condition that interferes with the normal growth and development of a feather (e.g. nutritional deficiency, liver disease). Multiple etiologic factors may be involved in feather discoloration. Nutritional deficiencies (i.e. carotenoids, nonheme iron, tyrosine, copper, choline, lysine, methionine and/or riboflavin). Hereditary—genetic mutations. Inflammation—early circovirus infection. Metabolic disease—liver disease, hypothyroidism, neoplasia (e.g. pituitary tumor). Intoxication—chronic lead toxicosis, drug administration (e.g. thyroxine, fenbendazole). Localized color changes involving single or a few feathers are most likely the result of a localized inflammatory process or trauma that affected the growing feather or its follicle during its development.

### RISK FACTORS
N/A

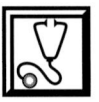

## DIAGNOSIS

### DIFFERENTIAL DIAGNOSIS
N/A

### CBC/BIOCHEMISTRY/URINALYSIS
Liver enzymes and bile acids may be elevated in birds with feather changes related to liver disease (e.g. hepatic lipidosis). Supporting evidence for hypothyroidism includes elevated cholesterol, triglycerides, liver enzymes, and a mild non-regenerative anemia. A TSH-stimulation test, resulting in a < 2- to 3-fold increase in T4 levels 4–6 hours after administration of TSH (1 U/kg IM)

is considered diagnostic for hypothyroidism. Lead and zinc levels may be determined if heavy metal toxicosis is suspected.

## OTHER LABORATORY TESTS
Testing for specific pathogens (circovirus, polyomavirus) may be indicated to determine whether these viruses are involved in feather dystrophy.

## IMAGING
N/A

## DIAGNOSTIC PROCEDURES
Histological evaluation of a feather follicle biopsy will provide the most accurate diagnosis for the cause of feather dystrophy. Diagnostic procedures for specific diseases which may cause feather dystrophy and/or discoloration are described under the specific conditions.

## PATHOLOGIC FINDINGS
Histologic findings of feather follicle biopsies from birds infected with circovirus and polyomavirus infections are described under these specific topics.

# TREATMENT

## APPROPRIATE HEALTH CARE
Treatment should be aimed at eliminating the underlying cause. Treatment options for the specific diseases that may lead to feather dystrophy and/or feather discoloration can be found under the specific topics.

## NURSING CARE
N/A

## ACTIVITY
N/A

## DIET
When malnutrition is suspected as a cause for the feather discoloration, conversion to a complete, pelleted diet is advised, which may result in feather color reverting back to normal after a subsequent molt. In some birds, a second molt may be necessary for the full plumage to return to normal.

## CLIENT EDUCATION
Owners need to be informed about heritability of feather duster disease and straw feather disease, as well as the need to provide supportive care to these birds. The infectious nature of circovirus and polyomavirus infections (i.e. avoid contact with other birds, especially neonates and juveniles). The necessity of feeding a complete, pelleted diet.

## SURGICAL CONSIDERATIONS
N/A

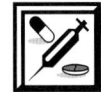

# MEDICATIONS

## DRUG(S) OF CHOICE
Suppletion with levothyroxine will help to resolve the clinical signs in birds diagnosed with hypothyroidism.

## CONTRAINDICATIONS
N/A

## PRECAUTIONS
N/A

## POSSIBLE INTERACTIONS
N/A

## ALTERNATIVE DRUGS
N/A

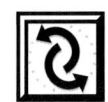

# FOLLOW-UP

## PATIENT MONITORING
Budgerigars with feather duster disease are not able to fly and may have difficulty eating. Euthanasia should be advised, although some owners prefer providing supportive care. To monitor the effect of nutritional treatment of feather discoloration, a recheck after at least one molt is needed.

## PREVENTION/AVOIDANCE
To prevent dissemination of feather duster or straw feather disease, do not breed with the parents or siblings of affected birds. Use a closed aviary concept to prevent birds from contracting infection with circovirus and/or polyomavirus infections. Feed birds a well-balanced (pelleted) diet to prevent feather discoloration due to malnutrition.

## POSSIBLE COMPLICATIONS
Birds with feather duster disease may have difficulty eating and are, therefore, at risk of starvation. Birds with circovirus infections are prone to develop secondary infections due to the associated immune suppression.

## EXPECTED COURSE AND PROGNOSIS
The prognosis for birds with feather duster disease and circovirus infections is unfavorable. Feather regrowth may occur in small psittacines infected with polyomavirus. After correction of the diet, feather discoloration will generally return to normal after one (or two) molts.

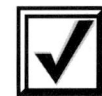

# MISCELLANEOUS

## ASSOCIATED CONDITIONS
Conditions associated with circovirus and polyomavirus infections and nutritional deficiencies can be found in the relevant chapters.

## AGE-RELATED FACTORS
Feather duster disease, circovirus and polyomavirus infections are diagnosed at an early age.

## ZOONOTIC POTENTIAL
N/A

## FERTILITY/BREEDING
It is advised not to breed with the parents or siblings of budgerigars with feather duster disease, nor with canaries affected with straw feather disease. It is advised to (temporarily) stop breeding during an outbreak of polyomavirus infections in small psittacines.

## SYNONYMS
Budgerigars with feather dystrophy due to circovirus or polyomavirus infections—French moult; runners; hoppers, creepers; budgerigar fledgling disease. Feather duster disease—chrysanthemum disease.

## SEE ALSO
Cere and Skin, Color Changes
Circovirus (Psittacines)
Dermatitis
Ectoparasites (Mites)
Ectoparasites (Ticks, Lice, Dipterans)
Feather Cyst
Feather-Damaging Behavior
Nutritional Imbalances
Polyomavirus

## ABBREVIATIONS
PBFD—psittacine beak and feather disease
TSH—thyroid-stimulating hormone

## INTERNET RESOURCES
Birds Online. Feather duster budgies: http://www.birds-online.de/gesundheit/gesgefieder/featherduster_en.htm

*Suggested Reading*
Cooper, J.E., Harrison, G.J. (1997). Dermatology. In: *Avian Medicine: Principles and Application* (ed. B.W. Ritchie, G.J. Harrison, L.R. Harrison), 607–639. Lake Worth, FL: Wingers Publishing.
Doneley, R. (2016). Diseases of the skin and feathers. In: *Avian Medicine and Surgery in Practice: Companion and aviary birds*, 2nd edn., 163–187. Boca Raton, FL: CRC Press.
Harrison, G.J., McDonald, D. (2006). Nutritional disorders. In: *Clinical Avian Medicine* (ed. G.J. Harrison, T.L. Lightfoot), 108–140. Palm Beach, FL: Spix Publishing.
Pass, D.A. (1995). Normal anatomy of the avian skin and feathers. *Seminars in Avian Exotic Pet Medicine*, 4:52–160.
Price-Waldman, R., Stoddard, M.C. (2021). Avian coloration genetics: recent advances and emerging questions. *Journal of Heredity*, 112:395–416.

F

F

Roudybush, T. (1986). Growth, signs of deficiency, and weaning in cockatiels fed deficient diets. *Proceedings of the Annual Meeting of the Association of Avian Veterinarians*, Miami, FL, 333–340.

Sarker, S., Forwood, J.K., Raidal, S.R. (2020). Beak and feather disease virus: biology and resultant disease. *WikiJournal of Science*, 3:1–5.
van Zeeland, Y.R.A., Schoemaker, N.J. (2014). Plumage disorders in psittacine birds – part 1: Feather abnormalities.

*European Journal of Companion Animal Practice*, 24:34–47.
**Authors**: Nico Schoemaker, DVM, PhD, DECZM (Small Mammal, Avian), and Yvonne R. A. van Zeeland, DVM, MVR, PhD, DECZM (Avian, Small Mammal)

# BASICS

## DEFINITION
Enteritis is defined as inflammation of the small intestine. There are several flagellated protozoa that infect birds. Those that cause intestinal disease are limited to *Giardia* spp., *Spironucleus* (*Hexamita*) spp., and *Cochlosoma* spp. While *Trichomonas* spp. and other trichomonads, as well as *Histomonas meleagridis*, cause significant problems in a variety of birds, they do not generally cause enteritis and are not covered in this chapter.

## PATHOPHYSIOLOGY
There is generally a direct fecal–oral life cycle for all these parasites. Infectious organisms are ingested and establish themselves in the intestines, where the parasites multiply by binary fission. These cause enteritis with resultant clinical signs and possible dermatologic manifestations; there may be malabsorption of nutrients and fat-soluble vitamins, which can cause complications. Secondary bacterial and/or yeast infections can occur also.

## SYSTEMS AFFECTED
**GI:** Small intestinal lesions and dysfunction.
**Integument:** Pruritus and feather/skin lesions secondary to some flagellate infections such as *Giardia psittaci*.

## GENETICS
N/A

## INCIDENCE/PREVALENCE
Not well documented. Many studies are done to determine the prevalence of these organisms in wild populations, but the finding of the organism does not equate with evidence of disease. Giardiasis is most common in budgerigars, with many asymptomatic carriers; nestlings die at 10–28 days; *Spironucleus* spp. infections in turkeys are not as common as they were several decades ago; *Spironucleus columbae* has been associated with morbidity and mortality in pigeons within the first year of life; *Spironucleus meleagridis* (formerly *Hexamita meleagridis*) associated with GI disease and mortality in psittacine birds including cockatiels, 8/83 juvenile cockatiels submitted for necropsy demonstrated a protozoal flagellate enteropathy consistent with spironucleosis; cochlosomiasis is reported sporadically and appears to be more common in cockatiels in Australia.

## GEOGRAPHIC DISTRIBUTION
These parasites are all likely to be found worldwide.

## SIGNALMENT
**Species:** *Giardia* spp. including *G. psittaci* in budgerigars, cockatiels, lovebirds, rarely other parrots, finches, great blue herons, raptors, waterfowl, poultry, and toucans. *Spironucleus* spp. in pigeons (*S. columbae*), turkeys (*S. meleagridis*), budgerigars, cockatiels, Australian king parrots, splendid grass parakeets, cranes, pheasant, quail, chukar partridge, peafowl. *Cochlosoma* spp. in finches, especially Gouldians, cockatiels.
**Mean age and range:** All ages are susceptible, but young birds, especially nestlings, are most susceptible to morbidity and mortality. Adult carriers are extremely common with most of these parasites. Cochlosomiasis is seen mostly in finches from 10 days to 6 weeks of age.
**Predominant sex:** Both sexes are susceptible.

## SIGNS

### General Comments
Clinical signs are related to the enteritis caused by these organisms; disease is generally seen in young animals.

### Historical Findings
Flock problem usually in aviaries. Disease outbreaks in nestlings mostly. *S. columbae* in pigeons seen in young squabs in spring and summer. Cochlosomiasis in finches is most commonly seen as a result of fostering under Bengalese finches. There is a 10–100% mortality in budgerigars. Occasional outbreaks occur after introduction of new birds, but often will occur in a closed flock after stressors such as moulting, breeding.

### Physical Examination Findings
**Giardiasis:** Chronic to intermittent watery, whitish diarrhea. Malodorous mucoid stools. Nestlings caked with feces. Listlessness. Weak. Depression. Poor feathering. Ruffled feathers. Anorexia. Distended crop, rarely vomiting and regurgitation. Weight loss and emaciation. Neonatal mortality. Parents may look normal. Feather picking can be seen in cockatiels—ferociously pluck from wings, flanks, legs—often screaming while doing so.
***Spironucleus* spp:** Chronic, often intractable diarrhea—copious, foamy, malodorous, yellow or intensely green. Dehydration. Weight loss and emaciation. Young birds may die; older birds do not. Poults/squabs at first nervous and active, but later listless and huddled, then convulsions and death.
**Cochlosomiasis:** Diarrhea—moist bulky droppings. Weight loss and emaciation. Shivering due to dehydration and hypothermia. Debilitation. Difficulties with moulting. Death. Feather picking in cockatiels.

## CAUSES
**Giardiasis:** In budgerigars, the organism appears to be *G. psittaci*, but it is unclear as to which species of *Giardia* inhabit and/or cause disease in which species of bird.
**Cochlosoma spp:** *S. meleagridis* causes disease in turkeys and psittacines such as budgerigars and cockatiels. It is not yet clear whether there are strain differences between cockatiels and other avian species such as turkeys.

## RISK FACTORS
Raising Australian finches under society finches puts them at risk for cochlosomiasis. Overcrowding and stress is a risk factor for all of these infections. Mixing species (peafowl with turkeys) increases the risk of spironucleosis. Adding new stock to a closed population is a risk.

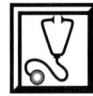

# DIAGNOSIS

## DIFFERENTIAL DIAGNOSIS
Any causes of enteritis, depending on the species. Bacterial, such as *Escherichia coli*, *Salmonella* spp. clostridial infection, *Campylobacter* sp., yersiniosis, mycobacteriosis, other Gram-negative organisms. Other protozoal diseases such as coccidiosis and cryptosporidiosis. Macrorhabdosis. Viral diseases (many) in pigeons, adenovirus, paramyxovirus.

## CBC/BIOCHEMISTRY/URINALYSIS
Usually not performed, but eosinophilia has been found in cockatiels and budgerigars with giardiasis; hypoproteinemia can result from malabsorption.

## OTHER LABORATORY TESTS
Diagnosis is by identification of the organism in fecal samples or scrapings from the intestines of a fresh carcass. Saline wet mounts of fresh feces are best—within 10 minutes of voiding if possible; adding iodine might help in identifying *Giardia*; warming the saline might be helpful for *Spironucleus* spp. Shedding is often intermittent and it might be necessary to perform multiple fecal smears. *Giardia* and *Spironucleus* spp. trophozoites can be identified by their size and shape and characteristic movement; sometimes *Giardia* cysts can be seen on direct smears but are hard to identify. Fecal trichrome staining— several stools are collected over a 3-day period and stored in polyvinyl alcohol or 10% formalin and stained with a fecal trichrome stain. Zinc sulfate centrifugation technique—*Giardia* cysts can often be seen. Fecal cytology—Wright's/Giemsa/Dif-Quik

F

# FLAGELLATE ENTERITIS (CONTINUED)

staining may reveal *Spironucleus* spp. or other organisms. Gram staining may demonstrate *Giardia* trophozoites. Molecular testing (PCR and ELISA) may be useful but may not be readily available.

## IMAGING
If radiographs are performed, it is unlikely to help in the diagnosis, but could help to rule out other problems. Gas-filled intestines might be seen.

## DIAGNOSTIC PROCEDURES
Collection of feces, cloacal contents or intestinal scrapings.

## PATHOLOGIC FINDINGS
**Giardiasis:** Sometimes no lesions. Distended small intestine with excessive fluid and mucous and/or yellowish creamy material. Histologically, a mononuclear inflammatory infiltrate; organisms found in mucous between the villi, villar atrophy.
**Spironucleosis:** Severe catarrhal enteritis in young birds. Watery intestinal contents with large numbers of organisms seen on microscopic examination of material from the crypts. Atony and distension, especially in the upper small intestine. Small ulcerative lesions in ileum and rectum have been noted. Secondary bacterial infections or other concurrent such as *Macrorhabdus ornithogaster*, are commonly seen.
**Cochlosomiasis:** Typical postmortem lesions are not well described, but likely similar to the other flagellates.

# TREATMENT
## APPROPRIATE HEALTH CARE
Patients that are critical need to be hospitalized and treated accordingly; patients that are not critical can be treated as outpatients.

## NURSING CARE
Nursing care can be done in the sicker patients, including providing thermal and nutritional support and fluid therapy. In flock situations, this might be impractical.

## ACTIVITY
N/A

## DIET
N/A

## CLIENT EDUCATION
Proper administration of medications should be explained. Hygiene and husbandry and management practices need to be outlined in the case of flock and aviary situations.

## SURGICAL CONSIDERATIONS
N/A

# MEDICATIONS
## DRUG(S) OF CHOICE
Several drugs of the nitroimidazole class are suggested for these diseases; dosages and response will vary. Metronidazole in water for 5 days or individual treatment at 25 mg/kg PO q12h or 50 mg/kg q24h for 5–10 days. Ronidazole 2.5–20 mg/kg PO. Carnidazole 20 mg/kg PO. Fenbendazole 50 mg/kg PO q24h for 3 days. Ipronidazole doses range from 125–250 mg/l water. For cochlosomiasis in finches, ronidazole at 400 mg/kg egg food and 400 mg/l drinking water for 5 days. After a pause of 2 days, the regimen is repeated.

## CONTRAINDICATIONS
N/A

## PRECAUTIONS
Dimetridazole—if exceeding 100 mg/l for 5 days, torticollis can be a sign of toxicosis. Metronidazole can cause toxicosis in finches. Ronidazole toxicity (neurologic signs and/or death) reported in society and Lady Gouldian finches that were accidentally overdosed with ronidazole at 4200 mg/l. Fenbendazole can be toxic to cockatiels, pigeons and doves, lorries, storks, Old World vultures, and other birds. Use with caution or at lower dosages.

## POSSIBLE INTERACTIONS
N/A

## ALTERNATIVE DRUGS
Treat secondary bacterial infections with antibiotics or as based upon results of culture and sensitivity.

# FOLLOW-UP
## PATIENT MONITORING
Patients with intestinal flagellate infections should be evaluated at regular intervals. Physical examination of affected flocks and individuals as well as repeated fecal examinations should be performed as needed.

## PREVENTION/AVOIDANCE
Environmental hygiene, such as thorough cage cleaning to remove organic debris, disinfecting with quaternary ammonium compounds or 10% bleach, keeping aviaries dry to reduce the number of infectious cysts; insect control, prevent overcrowding (low stocking density), elevate food and water dishes, use floor grates. Isolate and quarantine all new birds as well as any infected birds. For spironucleosis, consider removing carrier birds, separate older stock from poults, exclude other avian host species from poultry flock. For cochlosomiasis, avoid fostering Australian finches under Bengalese (society) finches.

## POSSIBLE COMPLICATIONS
Secondary bacterial infections should be suspected in cases where antiprotozoal treatment seems to be inadequate. Reinfection is common also.

## EXPECTED COURSE AND PROGNOSIS
Untreated nestlings will often die, with a variable degree of mortality; recovered birds can remain as carriers. Giardiasis appears to be more treatable than cochlosomiasis and spironucleosis.

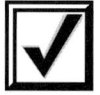

# MISCELLANEOUS
## ASSOCIATED CONDITIONS
There can be secondary bacterial and/or yeast infections associated with any of these diseases; cockatiels can have a secondary pruritus and associated feather picking disorder; it has been speculated that there is a malabsorption of fat soluble vitamins, with potential vitamin E deficiency and muscle weakness in cockatiels.

## AGE-RELATED FACTORS
The very young are most affected in all of these protozoal diseases; parents/adults are often asymptomatic carriers.

## ZOONOTIC POTENTIAL
It is unclear as to whether there is spread of *Giardia* from birds to humans. It is poorly documented, and it remains to be determined.

## FERTILITY/BREEDING
N/A

## SYNONYMS
N/A

## SEE ALSO
Cere and Skin Color Changes
Diarrhea
Feather Damaging Behavior/Self-Injurious Behavior
Gastritis and Enteritis
Helminthiasis (Gastrointestinal)
Nutritional Imbalances
Problem Behaviors: Aggression, Biting and Screaming

Trichomoniasis
Undigested Food in Droppings
Urate and Fecal Discoloration

## ABBREVIATIONS
ELISA—enzyme-linked immunosorbent assay
GI—gastrointestinal
PCR—polymerase chain reaction

## INTERNET RESOURCES
For more information, searches on VIN, PubMed and other veterinary medical search engines will reveal much useful information.

*Suggested Reading*
Brandão, J., Beaufrère, H. (2013). Clinical update and treatment of selected infectious gastrointestinal diseases in avian species. *Journal of Exotic Pet Medicine*, 22:101–117.

Clyde, C.I., Patton, S. (2000). Parasitism of Caged Birds. In: *Manual of Avian Medicine* (ed. G.H. Olsen, S.E. Orosz), 424–448. St Louis, MO: Mosby.
Doneley, R.J.T. (2009). Bacterial and parasitic disease of parrots. *Veterinary Clinics of North America. Exotic Animal Practice*, 12:423–431.
Langlois, I. (2021). Medical causes of feather damaging behavior. *Veterinary Clinics of North America. Exotic Animal Practice* 24:119–152.
Levy, M.G., Powers L.V., Gore K.C., Marr H.S. (2015). *Spironucleus meleagridis*, an enteric diplomonad protozoan of cockatiels (*Nymphicus hollandicus*): Preliminary molecular characterization and association with clinical disease. *Veterinary Parasitology*, 208: 169–173.

Patton, S. (2000). Avian parasite testing. In: *Laboratory Medicine–Avian and Exotic Pets* (ed. A.M. Fudge), 147–156. Philadelphia, PA: Saunders.
Reuschel M., Pantchev N., Vrhovec M.G., et al. (2020). Occurrence and molecular typing of Giardia psittaci in parakeets in germany: A case study. *Avian Diseases* 64: 228–233.
Schmidt R.E., Reavill D.R., Phalen D.N. (2015). Gastrointestinal system and pancreas. In: *Pathology of Pet and Aviary Birds* (ed. R.E. Schmidt D.R. Reavill, D.N. Phalen), 55–94. Ames, IA: Wiley.

**Author**: João Brandão, LMV, MS, DECZM (Avian), DACZM
**Acknowledgements**: updated from the first edition chapter authored by George Messenger.

F

# FOREIGN BODIES (GASTROINTESTINAL)

## BASICS

### DEFINITION
Gastrointestinal foreign bodies are relatively common in captive birds. Both indoor and outdoor birds are at risk of ingesting foreign material. Outdoor housed non-psittacine birds are more likely to ingest sand, rocks, bedding, plant material, and large metallic objects such as screws, coins, and wires. Of the indoor pet psittacine birds, young cockatoos seem to be at a greater risk of foreign object ingestion. Small conures of any age with fleece sleeping huts are at risk for fiber impactions. While any household item has the potential to become a foreign body, commonly ingested items include pieces of cage toys, cage hardware, grit, perches, and bedding. Flighted pet birds may chew ledges, woodwork, and other objects in the vicinity where they land and perch. Old paint may contain lead.

### PATHOPHYSIOLOGY
Not all foreign ingested material results in disease. Clinical signs and disease state are based on size, amount, and type of material ingested, location within the GI tract, and potential toxicity of the foreign matter. Small pieces of non-toxic material may pass through the GI tract without consequence. Ingested toxic material containing lead or zinc can lead to a systemic illness unrelated to particle size. Ingested wires, although uncommon, can lead to traumatic gastritis and perforation and may additionally contain toxic metals. Gastric impaction may also occur with repeated ingestions of foreign materials.

### SYSTEMS AFFECTED
**GI**: Irritation, ulceration, perforations, partial or full obstruction, decreased motility/crop stasis, gastric impaction, peritonitis, pancreatitis.
**Hemic**: Anemia (lead/zinc).
**Renal**: Hemoglobinuria (lead).
**Nervous**: Seizures, paresis (lead).

### GENETICS
N/A

### INCIDENCE/PREVALENCE
Ingestion of foreign material is relatively common in indoor pet birds. Of the outdoor birds, ratites on sand are at high risk for sand impaction. Waterfowl risks include lead sinkers and hooks in fishing areas. Backyard poultry pets can pick up metal objects, plastic, glass, small rocks, or overeat straw bedding.

### GEOGRAPHIC DISTRIBUTION
There is no geographic distribution unique to the development of foreign bodies; however, lead-associated objects are most likely seen in older urban dwellings where lead-based paint exists (lead was outlawed in paint in the early 1970s).

### SIGNALMENT
**Species**: Psittacines (cockatoos, baby birds), galliformes, ratites, waterfowl, some scavenger birds.
**Mean age and range**: All ages susceptible but young cockatoos overrepresented in the literature, and recently, conures with fleece sleeping sacs.
**Predominant sex**: Both sexes at risk.

### SIGNS

#### General Comments
Signs of illness are generally nonspecific "sick bird." Signs of GI stasis or obstructions (regurgitation, vomiting, coelomic distention, diarrhea) may also be observed.

#### Historical Findings
Anorexia, lethargy, fluffed feathers, diarrhea, vomiting, decreased vocalizations, not perching, falling, seizures, behavior changes. Some birds regurgitate.

#### Physical Examination Findings
Some birds have no physical examination abnormalities. Weakness. Dehydration. Weight loss. Crop stasis. Crop impaction. Melena. Hemoglobinuria (lead). Anemia. Paresis in limbs.

### CAUSES
N/A

### RISK FACTORS
Uncaged and unsupervised pet birds are at risk. Caged birds with inappropriate toys, fleece sleeping huts, sandpaper or cement perches, overexposure to grit, access to bedding like corncob or sand. Older urban environments are more likely to have lead-based paint. Birds foraging on the ground such as chickens, some waterfowl, and ratites can be indiscriminate eaters.

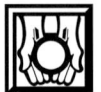

## DIAGNOSIS

### DIFFERENTIAL DIAGNOSIS
Proventricular dilatation disease (avian bornavirus). Renal disease. Liver disease. Neoplasia (proventricular/esophageal, thoracic inlet). Thyroid tumor (for crop stasis/regurgitation.) Epilepsy (lead toxicosis and seizures). Fungal ventriculitis (especially in *Eclectus*). GI parasitism (outdoor aviaries).

### CBC/BIOCHEMISTRY/URINALYSIS
Depending on foreign material ingested potential findings include: hyperuricemia, anemia, elevated liver enzymes, and hematuria. GI obstruction may also lead to severe electrolytic and acid–base disorders.

### OTHER LABORATORY TESTS
Metal toxicity best diagnosed by specific toxin blood testing—lead (whole blood), zinc (plasma).

### IMAGING

#### Radiographic Findings
Whole-body radiographs taken in lateral and ventrodorsal projections enable visualization and location of foreign material. Metallic foreign bodies are usually still in the GI tract at time of presentation but can pass out in feces or be absorbed. Mineral-based gravel and grit are readily visible but radiolucent material such as bedding, fibers, string, wood, or plastic may require contrast studies using barium sulfate or iohexol to visualize. Sick patients unable to tolerate sedated radiographs can have a standing dorsoventral film to rule out metal pieces. GI contrast fluoroscopy can be performed in the unsedated bird to evaluate motility of the GI tract. Dilation and low motility of the GI tract is suggestive for, but not diagnostic of proventricular dilatation disease.

#### Ultrasonography
Whole body CT is helpful especially for concurrent diseases but is not always readily available.

### DIAGNOSTIC PROCEDURES
Endoscopic examination (ingluvioscopy or gastroscopy using either a rigid or flexible endoscope) for identification and removal of proventricular or ventricular foreign bodies.

### PATHOLOGIC FINDINGS
Zinc toxicity can result in acute sloughing of the koilin layer of the ventriculus. Zinc also causes acute hemolytic anemia and necrotizing pancreatitis. Lead toxicity can be challenging to diagnose via necropsy so in suspect cases take radiographs of the carcass to evaluate for metal ingestion. Backyard poultry pets often have a variety of foreign material types in the gizzard, some can be incidental. Obstruction will lead to GI distension.

## TREATMENT

### APPROPRIATE HEALTH CARE
Pet birds that are sick from ingesting a foreign body need to be treated as inpatients until stable. Some birds require

## (CONTINUED)        FOREIGN BODIES (GASTROINTESTINAL)

F

surgery or endoscopy but will need to be stabilized before prolonged anesthetic procedures.

### NURSING CARE
Birds with foreign body disease are usually painful and dehydrated. Parenteral analgesics and fluid therapy are indicated. LRS maintenance dose is 50 ml/kg divided q8–12h but needs to be increased if diarrhea, vomiting, or hemoglobinuria from lead toxicity. Other fluids may be selected or fluid additives added depending on hypovolemic status and acid–base and electrolytic imbalances. If using injectable chelation therapy (e.g., calcium EDTA), do not give in same location as LRS as subcutaneous chelation may occur. Do not use NSAIDs in cases with potential gastric erosions or ulcers. Parenteral butorphanol at 1–5 mg/kg IM q1–4h or hydromorphone/buprenorphine depending on species can be used in most cases but can result in transient dose-dependent sedation. Indoor pet birds need warm, quiet, dark incubator without a perch if weak. Nutritional support will vary depending on function of the GI tract. Gavage feeding is generally needed in sick birds that are not regurgitating. Use antibiotics if compromise of the GI tract is suspected (ulceration, perforation, melena).

### ACTIVITY
Sick birds should be confined with limited activity and no flying and no perch. Remove water bowls if ataxic or seizuring.

### DIET
Bird should be NPO if crop stasis, obstructed, impacted, or perforated in the GI tract. Sick birds benefit from gavage feedings of an enteral diet until able to resume normal diet. Use an easy to absorb enteral formula such as EmerAid® (Lafeber, Cornell, IL). Baby bird powdered hand-feeding formulas can also be used.

### CLIENT EDUCATION
It is beneficial to inspect the cage where the bird may have picked up foreign material. Have the owner remove sandpaper, grit, inappropriate bedding like fleece sleeping huts, and toys as needed. Clients need to assess premises if lead exposure took place indoors. Outdoor areas also need to be inspected. Some owners may also use metal detectors to detect and remove potential items that could be swallowed by ground-dwelling birds such as ratites and backyard poultry.

### SURGICAL CONSIDERATIONS
Small particles can often pass the GI tract unassisted or with the use of laxatives/lubricants. Foreign objects that are not amenable to endoscopic retrieval must be removed surgically. Foreign objects and impactions in the crop can be easily and safely removed with an ingluviotomy. Surgery of the proventriculus and ventriculus carries a much greater risk and deserves careful consideration. Complications include leakage at the incision site, peritonitis and dehiscence. Proventriculomtomy is best performed using a left lateral approach. Using this approach, the ventriculus can also be accessed through an incision over the isthmus. An alternative approach is through a ventral coeliotomy incision that can be extended laterally along the keel. Using this approach, the ventriculus is incised over the thin elliptical muscles. For ventricular foreign bodies that require surgical removal, this author prefers the ventral approach.

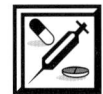 MEDICATIONS

### DRUG(S) OF CHOICE
Small particles in the lower GI tract can be treated with laxatives (cat hairball type, lactulose, or Epsom salts/magnesium sulfate) or lubricants (mineral oil/peanut butter). Magnesium sulfate is used when there is still lead in the GI tract to bind and decrease absorption (500–1000 mg/kg PO q12–24h for 1–3 days). Patients with lead or zinc toxicity are best treated with parenteral chelation using calcium EDTA (calcium disodium versenate/ededate calcium disodium) at 30–35 mg/kg SQ q12h, in saline only (not LRS) to decrease pain at injection site. Direct IM injections are given at home if hospitalization is not possible. For enteral therapy in stable birds, use oral preparations of DMSA or succimer at 30 mg/kg PO q12h for 7–21 days. Birds with gastric ulcers should be treated with sucralfate suspension (1 ml/kg PO q8h) and metoclopramide 1–2 mg/kg IM q8–12h). Antiemetic drugs include metoclopramide (1–2 mg/kg PO, SQ, IM) and maropitant (1 mg/kg SQ, IM).

### CONTRAINDICATIONS
N/A

### PRECAUTIONS
Do not use NSAIDs like meloxicam or carprofen in patients with gastric foreign bodies, melena, or hemoglobinuria.

### POSSIBLE INTERACTIONS
Do not give calcium EDTA chelation therapy in fluid pocket with LRS to avoid chelation in the subcutis and decreased bioavailability.

### ALTERNATIVE DRUGS
For the treatment of heavy metal or zinc toxicity, penicillamine can be used in most species at 50 mg/kg PO q24h for 1–6 weeks once stable or after treatment with calcium EDTA.

 FOLLOW-UP

### PATIENT MONITORING
Repeat radiographs to evaluate location or elimination of foreign material as needed. Droppings can also be checked for the presence of foreign material. In birds with toxic blood levels of lead or zinc, follow-up blood testing is generally recommended after the cessation of chelation therapy. Chelation can cause a transiently high metal level as the toxin is being eliminated from the bloodstream.

### PREVENTION/AVOIDANCE
Pet birds should not be unsupervised in the household, and should be caged when owners are away. Environmental clean-up for outdoor housed birds.

### POSSIBLE COMPLICATIONS
Perforations from sharp metallic objects are possible. Seizures from heavy metal toxicity. Intestinal obstructions and death. Renal failure from severe acute hemoglobinuria.

### EXPECTED COURSE AND PROGNOSIS
Most patients with small pieces of foreign material pass them without complications. Lead and zinc toxic patients often survive and recover well if diagnosed early and appropriately treated. Birds that require surgical intervention of the lower GI tract carry a more guarded prognosis.

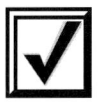 MISCELLANEOUS

### ASSOCIATED CONDITIONS
N/A

### AGE-RELATED FACTORS
Young birds may be more prone to foreign body ingestion.

### ZOONOTIC POTENTIAL
N/A

### FERTILITY/BREEDING
N/A

### SYNONYMS
N/A

### SEE ALSO
Anemia
Aspiration
Bornaviral Disease
Coelomic Distention
Enteritis and Gastritis
Helminthiasis (Gastrointestinal)
Ileus (Functional, Crop Stasis)
Regurgitation and Vomiting
Sick-Bird Syndrome
Toxicosis (Heavy Metals)

# FOREIGN BODIES (GASTROINTESTINAL)

## ABBREVIATIONS

CT—computed tomography
DMSA—2,3 dimercaptosuccinic acid
EDTA—ethylenediaminetetraacetic acid
GI—gastrointestinal
LRS—lactated Ringer's solution
NSAIDs—non-steroidal anti-inflammatory drugs

## INTERNET RESOURCES

Pollock, C. (2012). Heavy metal poisoning in birds. Lafebervet.com: https://lafeber.com/vet/heavy-metal-poisoning-in-birds

*Suggested Reading*

Cotton, R., Divers, S. (2017). Endoscopic removal of gastrointestinal foreign bodies in two african grey parrots (*Psittacus erithacus*) and a hyacinth macaw (*Anodorhynchus hyacinthinus*). *Journal of Avian Medicine and Surgery*, 31:335–343.

Hoefer, H.L. (2005). Management of gastrointestinal tract foreign bodies in pet birds. *Exotic DVM*, 7.3:4–27.

Hoefer H.L., Levitan, D. (2013). Perforating foreign body in the ventriculus of an umbrella cockatoo (Cacatua alba). *Journal of Avian Medicine and Surgery*, 27:128–135.

Lamb, S. (2019). Obstruction by fibrous foreign object ingestion in two green-cheeked conures (*Pyrrhura molinae*) and a jenday conure (*Aratinga jandaya*). *Journal of Exotic Pet Medicine* 31:127–132.

Lupu, C., Robins, S. (2009). Comparison of treatment protocols for removing metallic foreign objects from the ventriculus of budgerigars (*Melopsittacus undulatus*). *Journal of Avian Medicine and Surgery*, 23:186–193.

Mison, M., Bennett, R.A. (2022). Surgery of the avian gastrointestinal tract. In: *Surgery of Exotic Animals*, 175–189. Hoboken, NJ: Wiley.

**Author**: Heidi L. Hoefer, DVM, DABVP (Avian)

F

BASICS

## DEFINITION
Fracture is the complete or partial disruption of the integrity of bone. Can be further classified as a closed fracture (absence of a wound communicating with deeper tissue and bone) or an open fracture (presence of a wound communicating with deeper tissue and bone). Can be described based on fracture characteristics (e.g. transverse, oblique, comminuted) and fracture location (e.g. proximal, distal, articular).

## PATHOPHYSIOLOGY
The majority of fractures in birds, particularly free-living birds, are of traumatic etiology. Pathologic conditions that weaken bone, such as nutritional secondary hyperparathyroidism and neoplasia, can be causal factors but are not the focus of this chapter.

## SYSTEMS AFFECTED
Musculoskeletal. Skin—if fracture/luxation is open. Neuromuscular: Injury to nerves can accompany fractures and luxations. Cardiovascular: Generalized trauma can result in signs of shock.

## GENETICS
None.

## INCIDENCE/PREVALENCE
Unknown; however, traumatic injuries and resulting fractures are seen commonly in free-living birds of prey admitted to wildlife clinics or rehabilitation centers.

## GEOGRAPHIC DISTRIBUTION
None.

## SIGNALMENT
N/A

## SIGNS
### General Comments
The signs associated with traumatic fractures and luxations can be similar if the fracture is close to a joint. In these cases, the two can only be distinguished by careful palpation of the anesthetized bird and properly positioned, orthogonal view radiographs. Signs of generalized trauma may be present in birds suffering fractures. The overall status of the bird must be addressed along with the fracture.

### Historical Findings
Free-living birds are often found in or on the side of a road due to having collided with a motor vehicle. Captive or pet birds may have a witnessed event of flying into an object, such as a window, becoming entangled, being stepped on, or being attacked by another animal.

### Physical Examination Findings
Wing droop or lameness. Inability to fly in the absence of a wing droop can occur. Swelling. Bruising. If complete fracture—palpable sharp bone fragments and discontinuity of bone cortices. Laceration of skin if fracture is open.

## CAUSES
Motor vehicle collision (free-living birds). Collision with an object such as a window. Gunshot injuries (free-living birds). Attack by other animals. Crushing injuries. Entanglement.

## RISK FACTORS
In pet birds, allowing unsupervised and unrestricted access to the home environment increases the chances of accidental traumatic injury.

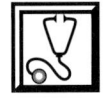 DIAGNOSIS

## DIFFERENTIAL DIAGNOSIS
Soft tissue injury. Sprain or strain.

## CBC/BIOCHEMISTRY/URINALYSIS
N/A

## OTHER LABORATORY TESTS
N/A

## IMAGING
Radiography is generally sufficient for diagnosing fractures. Although there may be cases in which advanced imaging such as CT may be beneficial, given the adequacy of standard radiographs in the majority of cases, CT is not routinely indicated for the diagnosis of fractures. Fractures are usually readily visualized on properly positioned, orthogonal view radiographs, although incomplete fractures may be less obvious. Soft-tissue swelling is often present with both fractures. It is beneficial to obtain whole-body radiographs in birds that have suffered trauma, rather than focusing on the area of injury, to rule out concurrent injuries. General anesthesia or sedation is usually necessary to obtain diagnostic orthogonal view radiographs; however, the bird's overall condition must first be considered and addressed.

## DIAGNOSTIC PROCEDURES
N/A

## PATHOLOGIC FINDINGS
N/A

 TREATMENT

## APPROPRIATE HEALTH CARE
Inpatient medical management—appropriate therapy for concurrent traumatic injuries; temporary stabilization of fracture. Surgical management once patient is stable—necessary for best prognosis for some fractures. Outpatient medical management once the fracture is stabilized either surgically or through external coaptation.

## NURSING CARE
Fluid therapy is indicated in patients suffering from generalized trauma. Temporary bandaging of the affected bone(s) is indicated to prevent further soft-tissue trauma, to prevent closed fractures from becoming open, and to increase patient comfort level. Injuries of the wing distal to the elbow can be immobilized with a figure-of-eight bandage. Injuries proximal to the elbow or involving the elements of the pectoral girdle (coracoid, clavicle, and scapula) can be immobilized with a figure-of-eight bandage, together with a body wrap. Injuries of the leg distal to the hock can be immobilized by taping the tarsometatarsus to the tibiotarsus with the hock in flexion. Injuries proximal to the hock can be immobilized via this type of bandage with the leg also wrapped against the body. Some fractures can be successfully managed and carry a good prognosis for full return to function when treated with bandaging alone. Examples include midshaft fractures of the ulna if the radius is intact, fractures of the bones of the pectoral girdle, and tarsometatarsal fractures in birds weighing < 100 g. In birds weighing < 50 g, such as passerines, bandaging and/or cage rest may be the only realistic treatment options in some cases due to the small size of the patient. Wound care is indicated for open fractures.

## ACTIVITY
Patient activity should be restricted throughout the duration of treatment and gradually increased after surgical fixation or external coaptation is removed.

## DIET
N/A

## CLIENT EDUCATION
If return to flight or normal ambulation is imperative, owners should be counseled regarding treatment options that carry the best prognosis for restoration of full function. Owners should be made aware that certain injuries, such as articular fractures that are not easily reduced, carry a poor to grave prognosis for return to full function and may result in degenerative joint disease over time. Owners should be informed of the monitoring and follow-up care that will be required during the course of management. For birds in which mobility may be permanently impaired due to the injury, owners should be counseled regarding modification of housing to accommodate the bird's needs.

F

## FRACTURES

### SURGICAL CONSIDERATIONS

Successful management of orthopedic injuries in birds requires knowledge of avian anatomy and bone healing, together with the characteristics of avian bone and of the avian patient as a whole. Orthopedic repair in birds should not be undertaken without careful study of techniques and careful consideration of the needs of the individual bird. The references listed at the end of this chapter provide comprehensive information on avian orthopedics and will help guide clinicians' decision making regarding specific fracture management. Best course of treatment is always determined on an individual basis. Factors to consider include patient size, the type and location of the fracture, the need for full return to function, the proximity of a fracture to a joint, the surgical experience level of the clinician, and the availability of orthopedic referral services. Avian practitioners who refer patients for surgical repair should be prepared to provide guidance to the surgeon regarding the factors that differentiate orthopedic surgery in birds from that in mammals if the surgeon has limited experience with birds. Open fractures are common in birds due to the lack of soft tissue coverage over the distal limbs; however, open fractures can have a good prognosis if treated promptly and appropriately. Some avian bones are pneumatic. Which bones are pneumatic varies among species. The humerus is commonly pneumatic, as well as the femur in many species. Irrigation of these bones during triage of open fractures or during surgical repair must be performed very cautiously to avoid introducing irrigation solutions into the connecting air sacs. Avian cortices are very thin. This characteristic can affect the ability of the bone to hold hardware. The high calcium content of avian bones makes them brittle and prone to fissures. The ideal fixation device is lightweight and entirely removable. Owing to the small size of many avian patients, heavy fixation devices will result in discomfort and morbidity. In free-living birds intended for release, all hardware should be completely removed in most cases. An external skeletal fixator with an intramedullary pin incorporated into the connecting bar (ESF-IM pin tie-in, or tie-in fixator) has been used successfully in many long-bone fractures in multiple species of birds. The small size of many birds (e.g. passerines) and the fact that the bones of the wing are non-weightbearing are considerations affecting the choice of appropriate stabilization or repair. Bone healing in otherwise healthy birds receiving appropriate nutrition occurs rapidly. Clinical union can be complete in as little as 3 weeks and rarely requires longer than 6 weeks.

### MEDICATIONS

#### DRUG(S) OF CHOICE

Analgesics—pain management is of the utmost importance in emergent patients and throughout the course of treatment. Opiods can be used in initial stages of treatment as well as peri- and postoperatively. NSAIDs can be used postoperatively and during the course of management. Opioids, tramadol, or gabapentin can be combined with NSAIDs for multimodal analgesia. Antibiotics—indicated perioperatively for open fractures, and generally for the duration of time an ESF-IM pin tie-in is in place. Amoxicillin-clavulanic acid and ceftiofur crystalline free acid are appropriate empiric choices. If infection is present or suspected, culture and sensitivity should guide antibiotic selection. Antifungals should be considered prophylactically for species at higher risk of respiratory aspergillosis secondary to antibiotic therapy and for species of free-living birds at higher risk due to the stress of being held in captivity for treatment and rehabilitation.

#### CONTRAINDICATIONS

Consult the Food Animal Residue Avoidance Databank (FARAD.org) for antibiotic choices when managing backyard flocks or wild birds considered to be major or minor food animals.

#### PRECAUTIONS

NSAIDs—avoid or use with caution in hypovolemic patients and in patients with hepatic or renal impairment.

#### POSSIBLE INTERACTIONS

N/A

#### ALTERNATIVE DRUGS

N/A

### FOLLOW-UP

#### PATIENT MONITORING

Radiographic monitoring should be performed every 7–10 days during the course of treatment to monitor healing. For fractures managed with external coaptation, bandage changes should also be performed every 7–10 days. Appropriate therapy for and monitoring of wounds associated with open fractures must be performed. For fractures managed with external coaptation, initial wound care may necessitate more frequent bandage changes. Clinical union by formation of fibrous callus, which may not be visible on radiographs, precedes bony callus formation. Palpation of a firm callus at the fracture site despite lack of visible callus on radiographs indicates appropriate healing. Inspection and cleaning of pin sites in patients with external skeletal fixators should be performed daily by owners for pet birds, if possible. Free-living birds in a rehabilitation setting should be examined in hand at least weekly, but daily handling is best avoided, if possible, to decrease patient stress level. In free-living birds, full return to function is a requirement for releasing the bird back to its natural habitat. Birds must be flight tested, observed for normal flight or locomotion/perching ability, and flight conditioned in a flight cage of appropriate size for the species.

#### PREVENTION/AVOIDANCE

Modification of the home environment may be necessary for pet birds that incurred an injury via an accident in the home.

#### POSSIBLE COMPLICATIONS

Decreased range of motion in joints secondary to bandaging—reversible in most cases following removal of bandage. In birds with leg fractures, the contralateral foot may develop bumblefoot if weight bearing is not restored to the injured leg during or following treatment. Degenerative joint disease and loss of range of motion with articular fractures. Malunion or permanent decreased range of motion resulting in inability to fly or chronic lameness. Nonunion. Osteomyeltitis or soft tissue infection.

#### EXPECTED COURSE AND PROGNOSIS

Highly variable and dependent on injury, selected course of treatment, and need for full function. If return to full function is not required, prognosis is for healing and acceptable outcome for most orthopedic injuries with appropriate treatment is good. For free-living birds requiring full function, prognosis for many orthopedic injuries can be also good if appropriate management and flight reconditioning is provided. Prognosis for healing is poor for chronic fractures. Prognosis for full return to function is poor for articular fractures that are not easily reduced.

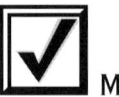

### MISCELLANEOUS

#### ASSOCIATED CONDITIONS

N/A

#### AGE-RELATED FACTORS

None.

#### ZOONOTIC POTENTIAL

None.

**F**

## FERTILITY/BREEDING
N/A

## SYNONYMS
N/A

## SEE ALSO
Air Sac Rupture
Angular Limb Deformity (Splay Leg)
Arthritis
Lameness
Metabolic Bone Disease
Pododermatitis
Trauma
Wounds (Including Bite Wounds, Predator Attacks)

## ABBREVIATIONS
CT—computed tomography
ESF-IM—external skeletal fixator intramedullary
NSAIDs—non-steroidal anti-inflammatory drugs

## INTERNET RESOURCES
Food Animal Residue Avoidance Databank. US Food Animal Species Classifications: http://www.farad.org/us-food-animals.html

*Suggested Reading*
Beaufrère, H. (2009). A review of biomechanic and aerodynamic considerations of the avian thoracic limb. *Journal of Avian Medicine and Surgery*, 23:173–185.
Harcourt-Brown, N.H. (2005). Orthopaedic and beak surgery. In: *BSAVA Manual of Psittacine Birds* (ed. N. Harcourt-Brown, J. Chitty), 120–135. Gloucester, UK: British Small Animal Veterinary Association.
Helmer, P., Redig, P. (2006). Surgical resolution of orthopedic disorders. In: *Clinical Avian Medicine* (ed. G.J. Harrison, T.L. Lightfoot), 761–774. Palm Beach, FL: Spix Publishing.
Orosz, S.E., Ensley, P.K., Haynes, C.J. (1992). *Avian Surgical Anatomy: Thoracic and Pelvic Limbs*. Philadelphia, PA: Saunders.
Redig, P.T., Ponder, J. (2016). Orthopedic Surgery. In: *Avian Medicine*, 3rd edn. (ed. J. Saymour), 312–358. St. Louis, MO: Elsevier.

**Author**: Maureen Murray, DVM, DABVP (Avian)

# HEAT STROKE

## BASICS

### DEFINITION
Heat stroke results when the body's cooling mechanisms are unable to control the rising temperature. In birds, this occurs when the body has a water deficit resulting from evaporative cooling.

### PATHOPHYSIOLOGY
In response to hyperthermia, vasodilation occurs to increase blood flow to the non-feathered skin and upper respiratory tract, which results in an increase in the bird's surface temperature. Evaporative cooling also occurs, resulting in extracellular fluid loss and subsequent dehydration, hypovolemia, and hyperosmolarity, leading to heat stroke.

### SYSTEMS AFFECTED
Heat stroke has systemic effects including hypotension, brain hypoxia and neuronal dysfunction, and cellular fatigue. Birds do not have sweat glands.

### GENETICS
N/A

### INCIDENCE/PREVALENCE
Long-term exposure (hours) to heat stress may lead to heat stroke.

### GEOGRAPHIC DISTRIBUTION
Any country where high temperatures and heat waves occur.

### SIGNALMENT
Any bird exposed to increased air temperatures, indoor or outdoor.

### SIGNS
Hyperthermia—panting with decreased tidal volume, increased heart rate, increased surface temperature, holding wings away from body. Progress to ataxia, seizure, coma with heat stroke.

### CAUSES
When the air temperature is higher than the thermal neutrality zone for the bird—about 60–75°F (30–35°C) for most species. This zone may be higher in passerines and tropical species and lower in arctic species and poultry. Above this zone, the resting metabolic rate increases significantly, and the core body temperature can increase, resulting in evaporative water loss and dehydration.

### RISK FACTORS
Increased avian mortality risk from lethal dehydration during heat waves. Smaller species (10–42 g) are at greater risk when the air temperature is higher than their body temperature, as they can lose more than 5%

of their body weight per hour from evaporative cooling. Birds kept outdoors on a hot day are at increased risk. Placing in incubator without thermostat. Heat support during anesthesia without monitoring core body temperature. Underlying dehydration.

## DIAGNOSIS

### DIFFERENTIAL DIAGNOSIS
Panting, increased heart rate—pneumonia, tracheal irritation, trauma, stenosis, pain. Holding wings away from body, ataxia, seizure, coma—heavy metal toxicity, avian bornavirus, mycotoxin, Marek's disease in poultry, etc.

### CBC/BIOCHEMISTRY/URINALYSIS
Budgerigars exposed to heat had a decreased hematocrit, with a significant increase in heterophils and decrease in lymphocytes. The number of basophils remained stable. May see increased PCV/TS and increased osmolarity from dehydration.

### OTHER LABORATORY TESTS
N/A

### IMAGING
*Radiographic Findings*
Could see pulmonary congestion.

*Ultrasonography*
Could see hyperechoic liver on imaging.

*Advanced Imaging*
CT: Could see pulmonary congestion and reduced Hounsfield units in the liver.

### DIAGNOSTIC PROCEDURES
N/A

### PATHOLOGIC FINDINGS
A study looking at organ histopathology in Australian desert birds after heat exposure reported pulmonary congestion, interstitial and pulmonary hemorrhage, micro- and macrovesicular hepatocellular vacuolation, and congestion of the kidneys and gastrointestinal tract.

## TREATMENT

### APPROPRIATE HEALTH CARE
Cutaneous evaporation is highly efficient at heat dissipation. Cool and rehydrate patient.

### NURSING CARE
Attempt to reduce temperature: place feet and legs into cool water, wet feathers down to the skin with water or alcohol, consider

instilling a small amount of cool water into cloaca if heat stroke. Provide room temperature crystalloid fluids 50–150 ml/kg/day SQ maintenance and correct dehydration. Consider IV or IO Plasmalyte-A® (Baxter Healthcare, Deerfield, IL) if in shock, fluid boluses of 10–15 ml/kg. Oxygen support if persistent respiratory signs after cooling. Crop feeding 2–3 times a day if anorexic following recovery.

### ACTIVITY
Keep activity and stress levels down to prevent further temperature increase until patient is stable and normothermic.

### DIET
Once normothermic and stable, offer regular diet. If anorexic, gavage feed parrot hand feeding formula, such as Hagen Tropican® Hand-Feeding Formula (Rolf C. Hagen Inc., Mandsield, MA), or Mazuri® Hand Feeding Formula (Mazuri Exotic Animal Nutrition, St. Louis, MO): 35 ml/kg crop volume.

### CLIENT EDUCATION
Inform clients that hyperthermia and heat stroke can occur in birds kept outdoors on very hot days even if they are inactive and fully shaded. Discuss poor prognosis when birds present with heat stroke.

### SURGICAL CONSIDERATIONS
N/A

## MEDICATIONS

### DRUG(S) OF CHOICE
NSAIDs to reduce hyperthermia—meloxicam 1 mg/kg IV/IM/SQ/PO q12h.

### CONTRAINDICATIONS
Drug doses are based on select psittacine species. Doses for specific species should be verified (e.g. Columbiformes, meloxicam 2 mg/kg PO q12h). Hypertonic saline without subsequent isotonic fluids in a dehydrated patient. Heated subcutaneous fluids or further heat support.

### PRECAUTIONS
Although renal disease with standard meloxicam doses has not been reported in psittacine, it is recommended to rehydrate prior to use to avoid renal injury.

### POSSIBLE INTERACTIONS
N/A

### ALTERNATIVE DRUGS
Hepatoprotectants such as silymarin can be considered for birds with hepatic lipidosis. Antibiotics can be considered in birds with

pulmonary hemorrhage. Furosemide 0.15–2 mg/kg IM, SQ if pulmonary edema present. Midazolam 2 mg/kg IM/IV/IO if seizure activity.

## FOLLOW-UP

### PATIENT MONITORING
Monitor birds closely in heated enclosures and account for species ecology prior to setting temperatures. For example, Arctic species and birds housed outdoors may have a lower heat tolerance threshold. Following hyperthermia or heat stroke event, monitor hydration (ulnar vein refill time, eyelid skin tent, tenacity of oral saliva, PCV/TS). Monitor pulmonary and GI signs, respiratory rate and effort, as well as fecal hemoccult in psittacines for GI bleeding. To check for neurologic deficits, perform serial neurologic exams to assess response to treatment.

### PREVENTION/AVOIDANCE
Migrating sea ducks use their legs as heat dumping organs and allow for heat dissipation during swimming. Consider providing pool of water for waterfowl maintained indoors. Monitor patient when thermal support provided and ensure that they are well hydrated prior to heat support. Provide unlimited access to water for evaporative cooling and provide relief from heat when outdoors.

### POSSIBLE COMPLICATIONS
Death. Renal tubular damage leading to elevated uric acid and gout. Secondary bacterial or fungal infection from pulmonary congestion and hemorrhage. If the patient survives, could require monitoring and management of hepatic lipidosis.

### EXPECTED COURSE AND PROGNOSIS
In poultry, recovery has occurred when hyperthermia remains below 44.5°C but results in death beyond this temperature. Temperature tolerance is based on the species and their ecology. Once heat stroke develops, it is suspected to have poor prognosis. Data on recovery are lacking in psittacine species.

## MISCELLANEOUS

### ASSOCIATED CONDITIONS
Dehydration

### AGE-RELATED FACTORS
N/A

### ZOONOTIC POTENTIAL
N/A

### FERTILITY/BREEDING
N/A

### SYNONYMS
Hyperthermia

### SEE ALSO
Dehydration
Hypotension/hypovolemia

### ABBREVIATIONS
GI—gastrointestinal
PCV—packed cell volume
TS—total solids

### INTERNET RESOURCES
N/A

*Suggested Reading*
Conradie, S.R., Woodborne, S.M., Wolf, B.O., et al. (2020). Avian mortality risk during heat waves will increase greatly in arid Australia during the 21st century. *Conservation Physiology*, 8: coaa048.
Guillemette, M., Polymeropoulos, E.T., Portugal, S.J., et al. (2017). It takes times to be cool: on the relationship between hyperthermia and body cooling in a migrating seaduck. *Frontiers in Physiology*, 8:532.
McKechnie, A.E., Whitfield, M.C., Smit, B., et al. (2016). Avian thermoregulation in the heat: efficient evaporative cooling allows for extreme heat tolerance in four southern hemisphere columbids. *Journal of Experimental Biology*, 219:2145–2155.
Quesenberry, K.E., Hillyer, E.V. (1994). Supportive care and emergency therapy. In: *Avian Medicine: Principles and applications* (ed. B.W. Ritchie, G.J. Harrison, L.R. Harrison), 382–416. Lake Worth, FL: Wingers Publishing.
Xie, S., Woolford, L., McWhorter, T.L. (2020). Organ histopathology and hematological changes associated with heat exposure in Australian desert birds. *Journal of Avian Medicine and Surgery*, 34:41–51.
Yahav, S. (2015). Regulation of body temperature: Strategies and mechanisms. In: *Sturkie's Avian Physiology* 6th edn. (ed. C.G. Scanes), 869–905. St. Louis, MO: Academic Press.

**Author**: Trinita Barboza DVM, DVSc, DACZM

H

# HELMINTHIASIS (BODY CAVITY AND CARDIOVASCULAR)

## BASICS

### DEFINITION

Helminths inhabiting avian body cavities and the cardiovascular system are not as common as gastrointestinal parasites. Although many are non-pathogenic, in specific situations, with several species, morbidity and mortality can occur. These helminths are a diverse group that includes the trematodes schistosomes and the nematodes filaroids, *Avioserpens*, and *Eustrongylides*. Avian schistosomes, such as *Trichobilharzia*, are digenean trematodes inhabiting the circulatory system of their definite avian host, most commonly waterfowl. They can be divided into visceral or nasal species depending on their predilection sites. Aquatic mollusks are the intermediate hosts. Filarioids are nematodes inhabiting the tissues and body cavities. They involve a hematophagous invertebrate intermediate host ingesting the highly specialized first-stage bloodborne larvae called microfilariae. In most cases, filarioid nematodes are non-pathogenic in birds. However, the adult forms of some species have been consistently associated with clinical disease, such as *Chandlerella quiscali* causing encephalitis in emus, or *Splendidofilaria eurycerca* affecting the hearts of swans and geese. Microfilariae are very rarely pathogenic, but can occasionally cause local inflammation when outside of the blood vessels, in their walls, or even create a mechanical obstruction to the blood flow when present in large numbers in the vessels. Avioserpensosis comprises infections of the subcutaneous tissues of waterbirds caused by the nematodes of the genus *Avioserpens*. These parasites produce swellings in the submandibular areas and limbs of ducks and other waterfowl, causing morbidity and sometimes mortality.

### PATHOPHYSIOLOGY

**Schistosomes**: Clinical signs and lesions are related to the presence of adults in the intestinal and portal veins, egg release in the intestines, and migration of larvae throughout the CNS.
**Filarioids**: Most are non-pathogenic. However, specific parasites at the adult stage have caused severe inflammatory reactions in various organs of sensitive species. In rare occasions, high burden of microfilariae in the blood vessels of an organ (e.g. lungs) can contribute to morbidity and mortality.
**Eustrongylides**: Larval stages contained in fish are ingested by the avian host and will perforate the stomach wall, causing severe tubular fibrinous to fibrous peritonitis.
**Avioserpensosis**: Larval stages are ingested and will molt in the avian host body cavity, then migrate to the subcutaneous tissues via the air

sacs to become adults. The adult forms will create nodules and swellings that can interfere with swallowing, breathing, and swimming.

### SYSTEMS AFFECTED

GI, nervous, cardiovascular, skin/exocrine, respiratory, hemic/lymphatic/immune, hepatobiliary, musculoskeletal.

### GENETICS

N/A

### INCIDENCE/PREVALENCE

**Schistosomes, filaroids**: Not a major cause of mortality and morbidity.
**Eustrongylides**: Major cause of mortality in nestling wading birds.
**Avioserpensosis**: Rare cause of mortality.

### GEOGRAPHIC DISTRIBUTION

Worldwide. Schistosomes—freshwater habitats in all temperate and tropical regions of the world. Filaroids—varies with the geographical and seasonal distribution of the hematogenous invertebrate vector (intermediate host).

### SIGNALMENT

**Species**: Schistosomes: Waterfowl and passerine birds. Filaroids have been reported in almost all avian families. *Eustrongylides*—Ardeidae (*Eustrongylides ignotus*) and mergansers (*Eustrongylides tubifex*). Avioserpensosis is found in domestic ducks and geese, and less commonly, other water birds.
**Mean age and range**: Schistosomes—mortality may be higher in chicks based on experimental infections. Filaroids—unknown. *Eustrongylides* and avioserpensiosis—mortality is higher in chicks.
**Predominant sex**: No known sex predilection.

### SIGNS

#### General Comments

Most infections are asymptomatic or associated with non-specific signs such as lethargy.

#### Historical Findings

Possible exposure to a water snail (schistosomes), hematogenous invertebrate vector (filaroids), fish (*Eustrongylides*), copepod or paratenic host (avioserpensosis).

#### Physical Examination Findings

**Schistosomes**: Weight loss, lethargy, lameness, respiratory distress, mucoid blood-flecked feces, neurological signs.
**Filaroids**: Mostly non-pathogenic, except weight loss and acute depression with *Sarconema eurycerca* (Anatidae); joint swelling and lameness with *Pelecitus* (Psittaciformes, grebes, coots), feather loss with *Eulimdana clava* (pigeons), neurologic signs with *Chandlerella quiscali* (emus).
**Eustrongylides**: Ataxia, lethargy, emaciation, pale mucous membres, regurgitations, neurologic signs.

**Avioserpensosis**: Swelling of the throat causing swallowing difficulties, anorexia, growth retardation, lethargy, asphyxiation, swelling of the hocks causing swimming problems.

### CAUSES

**Schistosomes**: Cercariae present in contaminated water infect their host by attaching to the skin or by being ingested, then migrating to blood vessels.
**Filarioids**: Infestation of the avian host by third-stage larvae through a puncture wound from the hematogenous arthropod vector, then develop into fourth and fifth larval stage then adults with various body locations.
**Eustrongylides**: Ingestion of a fish containing larval stages.
**Avioserpensis**: Ingestion of copepods or paratenic host containing larval stages.

### RISK FACTORS

**Schistosome**: Presence of snails in the water of the habitat; translocation to new habitats.
**Filarioids**: Presence of infected hematogenous arthropod vector in the environment; morbidity and mortality is higher in birds that were already compromised.
**Eustrongylides**: Eutrophication of foraging sites.

## DIAGNOSIS

### DIFFERENTIAL DIAGNOSIS

As clinical signs are non-specific, differential diagnosis is extensive and includes atherosclerosis, other infectious diseases, trauma, malnutrition, metabolic disturbances, and neoplasia. Most species are non-pathogenic. Exclude other potential causes before considering helminthiasis. *Eustrongylides* lesions should be differentiated from ascaroid nematodes or foreign body perforation. Avioserpensosis lesions should be differentiated from abscess, foreign bodies, neoplasia, cysts, or other parasitic nodules.

### CBC/BIOCHEMISTRY/URINALYSIS

**Schistosomes**: Leukocytosis with heterophilia and monocytosis.
**Filarioids**: Microfilariae on the blood smears.
**Eustrongylides**: Anemia and eosinophilia.

### OTHER LABORATORY TESTS

**Schistosomes**: Smear of nasal mucosa, fecal examination.
**Filarioids**: Buffy coat microscopic wet mount; skin biopsies (for subcutaneous species).
**Eustrongylides**: Fecal examination.
**Avioserpensosis**: As adults are ovoviviparous, larvae are directly released into the environment. Adult identification in the nodules is diagnostic.

### IMAGING

For *Eustrongylides*, the typical tortuous tract can sometimes be visible on radiographs.

## DIAGNOSTIC PROCEDURES

Finding adult worm at necropsy is key to identify the species. *Eustrongylides*: Manual palpation of the tortuous tracts, laparoscopy.

## PATHOLOGIC FINDINGS

**Schizotomes**: Obliterative endophlebitis (adults in intestinal and portal veins), enteritis (egg release), inflammation in various systems (CNS, subcutaneous tissue, lungs, nasal cavity, linked to larval migration), hemorrhages (nasal cavity, lungs).

**Filarioids**: Presence of the adult worms in various locations causing chronic inflammation such as in the walls of pulmonary arteries in American crows (*Splendidofilaria caperata*), cardiomegaly, myocardial hemorrhage, inflammation and necrosis in Anatidae (*Sarconema eurycerca*), swellings and nodules in legs and feet and tenosynovitis in Psittaciformes (*Pelecitus* spp.), encephalitis in farmed emus (*C. quiscali*).

**Eustrongylides**: Adhesions, protruding nodules and penetrating tubules on intestines, liver, air sacs, proventriculus, abdominal wall, pericardium, etc. Fibrinous peritonitis.

**Avioserpensosis**: Swellings and nodules in the neck and hocks can be small to very large and fibrous. Secondary bacterial infections can occur.

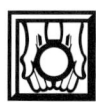

## TREATMENT

### APPROPRIATE HEALTH CARE

Filarioids: No intervention is generally preferred unless clinical signs are obviously related to the presence of these parasites, which remains rare.

### NURSING CARE

Supportive care.

### ACTIVITY

N/A

### DIET

N/A

### CLIENT EDUCATION

N/A

### SURGICAL CONSIDERATIONS

N/A

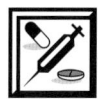

## MEDICATIONS

### DRUG(S) OF CHOICE

**Schistosomes**: Praziquantel (high doses, 200 mg/duck q24h for 3 days).

**Filarioids**: Fenbendazole, levamisole, or menbendazole have been suggested to treat psittacine birds. Ivermectin has been successfully used in emus to prevent clinical signs.

**Eustrongylides** and **aviosperensosis**: No reported treatment.

### CONTRAINDICATIONS

N/A

### PRECAUTIONS

Filaroids and *Eustrongylides*: Drugs killing adult worms may lead to marked local inflammatory reactions that are more severe than the original immune reaction to the presence of the parasite.

### POSSIBLE INTERACTIONS

N/A

### ALTERNATIVE DRUGS

None reported.

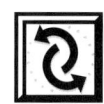

## FOLLOW-UP

### PATIENT MONITORING

Filarioids: Assess the presence of microfilaria on a blood smear.

### PREVENTION/AVOIDANCE

**Schistosomes**: Control of snails in the environment.

**Filarioids**: Control hematogenous arthropod vectors.

**Avioserpensosis**: Provide ducklings and goslings with uncontamined food and water, as well as preventing contact with paratenic hosts.

### POSSIBLE COMPLICATIONS

Schistosomes: Multifocal inflammation can cause mortality in some cases.

### EXPECTED COURSE AND PROGNOSIS

**Schistosomes**: Highly variable depending on the host immune reaction and the species involved.

**Filarioids**: Most species are non-pathogenic, but with pathogenic species, clinical course is usually slow and can lead to chronic infestation.

**Eustrongylides**: Prognosis highly variable with the species and age of infection, can cause epizootic episodes.

**Avioserpensosis**: Bacterial secondary infection and impaired food ingestion can lead to death.

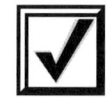

## MISCELLANEOUS

### ASSOCIATED CONDITIONS

None.

### AGE-RELATED FACTORS

Chicks are more sensitive to *Eustrongylides* and avioserpensosis infestation.

### ZOONOTIC POTENTIAL

**Schistosomes**: Responsible for a dermatitis called swimmer's itch (pruritus, possible secondary bacterial infections).

**Filarioids and avioserpensosis**: None known.

**Eustrongylides**: Humans can get infected and die by eating raw fish (rare).

### FERTILITY/BREEDING

No reported effects.

### SYNONYMS

N/A

### SEE ALSO

Anemia
Anorexia
Diarrhea
Enteritis and Gastritis
Liver Disease
Neural Larva Migrans
Neurologic (Non-Traumatic Diseases)
Neurologic (Trauma)
Regurgitation and Vomiting
Seizures
Sick-Bird Syndrome

### ABBREVIATIONS

CNS—central nervous system

### INTERNET RESOURCES

Centers for Disease Control and Prevention. Cercarial dermatitis: https://www.cdc.gov/dpdx/cercarialdermatitis/index.html

*Suggested Reading*
Ahmed, M.S., Khalafalla, R.E., Al-Brakati, A., et al. (2020). Descriptive pathological study of avian schistosomes infection in whooper swans (*Cygnus cygnus*) in Japan. *Animals*, 10: 2361.
Atkinson, C.T., Thomas, N.J., Hunter, D.B. (eds.). (2008). *Parasitic Diseases of Wild Birds*. Ames, IA: Wiley-Blackwell [pp. 246–260, 289–315, 384–387, 439–462].
Larrat, S., Dallaire, A.D., Lair, S. (2012). Emaciation and larval filarioid nematode infection in boreal owls (*Aegolius funereus*). *Avian Pathology*, 41: 345–349.
Law, J.M., Tully, T.N., Stewart, T.B. (1993). Verminous encephalitis apparently caused by the filarioid nematode *Chandlerella quiscali* in emus (*Dromaius novaehollandiae*). *Avian Diseases*, 37: 597–601.

**Author**: Marion Desmarchelier, DMV, MSc, DACZM, DECZM (Zoo Health Management), DACVB
**Acknowledgements**: Shannon Ferrell, DVM, DABVP (Avian), DACZM

H

# HELMINTHIASIS (GASTROINTESTINAL)

## BASICS

### DEFINITION
Gastrointestinal helminthiasis includes any macroparasitic disease in birds in which parasitic worms known as helminths infect the GI tract. The four major groups of helminths include nematodes (roundworm-like), cestodes (tapeworms), trematodes (flukes), and acanthocephalans (horny- or spiny-headed worms).

### PATHOPHYSIOLOGY
Transmission of these organisms is either direct, by ingestion of embryonated eggs, or indirect, by ingestion of an intermediate host. The intermediate host varies according to the parasite species; for example, cestodes require an intermediate host such as pillbugs, cockroaches, beetles, flies, etc. The life cycle begins once the parasite is inside the host, generally with the attachment of the larva to the mucosa. Damage occurs through direct irritation and/or blood loss; parasites can also cause obstruction of the GI tract in heavy parasitic burdens.

### SYSTEMS AFFECTED
**GI**: Helminth parasites can be found throughout the GI tract, from the oral cavity to the intestines.
**Hepatobiliary**: Trematodes may infect the liver and bile and pancreatic ducts.

### GENETICS
N/A

### INCIDENCE/PREVALENCE
Gastrointestinal parasites are commonly found in free-ranging and captive wild birds but also in domestic species, mainly animals with access to the outside. Although infestations are often subclinical, it is estimated that 10% of helminths cause significant disease in birds. Nematodes are the most significant in number of species and in economic impact. Of species found in poultry, *Ascaridia galli*, *Heterakis gallinarum*, *Capillaria* sp., and *Raillietina* sp. are the most common helminths in chicken populations. Chickens housed in backyard and free-range systems have higher prevelances (> 80%) than chickens housed in cage production settings (approximately 60%). Waterfowl is one of the vertebrate groups with the greatest diversity of parasites, potentially due to their natural history, diversity of dietary habits, migratory and seasonal patterns. Nematodes are particularly a problem in wild-caught birds or those housed in planted aviaries that favor the parasite's life cycle.

### GEOGRAPHIC DISTRIBUTION
Helminth parasites are seen in birds worldwide. Some parasites are more common in certain parts of the world, most likely as a result of the presence of the intermediate hosts.

### SIGNALMENT
**Species**: More prevalent in wild birds or birds with access to the outside, but all species of birds can develop GI helminthiasis. Some examples are chickens—over 100 species of parasites seen; Anseriformes—over 800 species of helminths seen; ostriches— *Libyostrongylus douglassi*; pigeons—ascarids most common, *Capillaria* spp., *Dispharynx spiralis* (proventriculus), *Ornithostrongylus* spp. (proventriculus), *Tetrameres* spp., tapeworms, trematodes; parrots—ascarids, *Capillaria* spp., tapeworms; insectivorous finches—cestodes.
**Mean age and range**: Highly variable.
**Predominant sex**: Both sexes are susceptible.

### SIGNS

#### General Comments
Signs and findings include those that may be seen in conjunction with this condition and those that occur concurrently as a result of the inciting problem. Subclinical infections are not uncommon and presence of GI helminths does not imply active disease.

#### Historical Findings
There are many possible historical findings in association with this condition depending on the specific disorder. Animals with outside access, animals with chronic weight loss, stunted growth may be more likely to have GI helminths.

#### Physical Examination Findings
Lethargy. Poor condition. General debilitation. Diarrhea. Undigested seed in droppings. Vomiting. Weight loss. Death in some species with some parasites. Anorexia, dysphagia, crop mass, head flicking and anemia in capillariasis of the upper GI tract. In Anseriformes with *Sphaeridiotrema globulus*—bloody cloacal discharge, wing droop, death in 5–6 days, chronic enteritis possible, weight loss, lameness.

### CAUSES
There are thousands of species of helminth parasites in avian hosts. Some of the more common or important parasites are listed here. Ascarids—especially young raptors, budgerigars, cockatiels, princess parrots, Australian grass parakeets, chickens. Capillarids—raptors, pigeons, pheasant, vulturine guinea fowl. Cestodes— insectivorous finches, parrots of wild origin, especially grey and eclectus parrots, and

cockatoos—*Raillietaenia*, *Choanataenia*, *Gastronemia*, *Idiogenes*, and *Amoebataenia*. *Dispharynx nasuta*—wild game birds, pigeons, passerines. *Libyostrongylus douglassi* (ostrich)—proventricular worms. *Amidostomum* spp.—Anseriformes. *Eustrongylides ignotus*—herons and egrets— proventricular worms. *Tetrameres* spp.— ducks, chickens, pigeons, aquatic birds—proventricular worms. Trematodes— especially *Sphaeridiotrema globulus* in water birds—scaup, mallards.

### RISK FACTORS
Helminths are more commonly seen in birds housed in cages with access to the ground, outdoor aviaries or flocks that interact with wild birds, and in wild-caught birds. Presence of intermediate hosts. Parasites will be seen more frequently in situations where there are poor hygienic conditions, such as inadequately maintained pigeon lofts and chicken coops. Planted aviary and zoo situations are harder to clean and, therefore, birds can become reinfected by ingesting ova and intermediate hosts. Addition of new animals to the flock may introduce novel parasites to the population.

## DIAGNOSIS

### DIFFERENTIAL DIAGNOSIS
Bacterial infections of the GI tract— salmonellosis, Gram-negative infections, *Enterococcus* spp., clostridial infection. Flagellate enteritis. Candidiasis. Cryptosporidiosis. Chlamydiosis. Macrorhabdosis. Mycobacteriosis. Viral infections—adenovirus, paramyxovirus, reovirus, coronavirus, rotavirus, herpesvirus, bornavirus, and more. GI neoplasia. Numerous other diseases that result in poor body condition and weight loss.

### CBC/BIOCHEMISTRY/URINALYSIS
Although not well documented, eosinophilia might be present with parasitism; leukocytosis with heterophilia might be seen in cases where there is significant inflammation; certain organisms tend to cause anemia; hypoproteinemia could result from malabsorption. Liver involvement, as in the case of trematodiasis, could result in elevated bile acids and liver enzymes.

### OTHER LABORATORY TESTS
Fecal flotation. Direct smears with or without saline. Intestinal or proventricular scrapings on necropsy. Other tests to check for concurrent bacterial or viral infection, such as fecal Gram staining, fecal acid-fast

stain and other stains, culture and sensitivity, PCR—*Cryptosporidium* spp., viral diseases.

## IMAGING
Imaging is not generally carried out, but in cases of GI parasitism where there are no fecal sample results or the results are negative, radiographs might be performed; findings would be non-specific and would not necessarily be helpful except to rule out some other disorders. Contrast studies may be beneficial to identify partial or complete obstructions caused by a heavy parasitic burden, or changes to the intestinal surface and filling. Ultrasound may be helpful to evaluate specific areas of the GI tract and/or, in some cases, presence of obstructions caused by parasites.

## DIAGNOSTIC PROCEDURES
N/A

## PATHOLOGIC FINDINGS
In general, pathological findings are confined to the GI tract, from the mouth to the ceca. There are varying degrees of inflammation, thickening of the intestinal walls, epithelial hyperplasia, ulceration, necrosis, sloughing, hemorrhage, or plaque-like lesions, and occasional perforation of the stomach or intestinal wall, depending upon the parasite and the location. In all cases, there are accumulations of the parasites, either in the lumen or imbedded in the wall of the intestine. Depending on the parasite and the location in the body, various lesions are found. Examples include *Sphaeridiotrema globulus*—fibrinohemorrhagic ulcerative enteritis in the lower small intestine in scaup, canvasback long-tailed ducks, swans and mallards. Roundworms—intestinal blockage can occur. *Tetrameres* spp.—raspberry-like appearance of the stomach of pigeons. *Dispharynx* and *Ornithostrongylus* in pigeons—severe proventricular hemorrhage. *Capillaria* spp.—oral and/or crop inflammatory masses, diphtheritic oral lesions, hemorrhagic inflammation around commissures of beak.

## TREATMENT

### APPROPRIATE HEALTH CARE
Patients that are critical need to be hospitalized for work-up and treatment. Patients that are unthrifty and are diagnosed with parasitism at the time of the office visit can be treated as outpatients.

### NURSING CARE
Supportive care must be done in the sicker patients. This might include providing warmth, fluid therapy, nutritional support/gavage feeding and fluid therapy.

## ACTIVITY
N/A

## DIET
N/A

## CLIENT EDUCATION
Proper administration of medications should be explained. For poultry, provide appropriate withdrawal times. Discuss control of intermediate hosts and reduction of risk factors for reinfection.

## SURGICAL CONSIDERATIONS
N/A

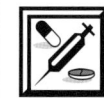

## MEDICATIONS

### DRUG(S) OF CHOICE
It is difficult to draw conclusions about the proper use of anthelmintics for all birds, due to the wide variety of species and types of parasites involved. Medications that are commonly used in mammals are generally safe and effective in birds, including ivermectin, moxidectin, pyrantel pamoate, levamisole and praziquantel. Fenbendazole is one of the most commonly used antihelminthic drug but can cause toxicity in multiple species such as pigeons, pelicans, storks, and Old World vultures. Examples of specific and general dosages that are suggested for some conditions are:

**Anseriformes**: For cestodes—praziquantel 10–20 mg/kg PO; repeat in 10–14 days. For roundworms, gizzard worms, stomach worms—ivermectin 200 µg/kg PO once. Acanthocephalans in Anseriformes—thiabendazole.

**Parrots**: For tapeworms—praziquantel 8 mg/kg IM, PO and fenbendazole.

**Pigeons**: For ascarids, *Capillaria*, *Tetrameres*, strongyles, fenbendazole 10–12 mg/kg PO q24h for 3 days (in one publication, 8/12 pigeons died with signs of fenbendazole toxicity after 30 mg/kg PO q24h for 5 days). For nematodes, including ascarids, pyrantel pamoate 25 mg/kg PO; repeat in 14 days. Best for all nematodes, excellent for *Capillaria* spp. and *Tetrameres* spp., but less effective for ascarids, ivermectin 200 µg/kg PO, SQ, IM. For cestodes, praziquantel 10–30 mg/kg PO; repeat in 10–14 days. *Capillaria* (difficult to eradicate): Fenbendazole 100 mg/kg once or 25 mg/kg daily for 5 days, repeat in 14 days. Toxicity to fenbendazole has been reported in many species such as pigeons and pelicans; oxfendazole 10 mg/kg, levamisole 40 mg/kg (narrow safety margin); repeat in 14 days; moxidectin 20 µg/kg, ivermectin 200 µg/kg.

**Finches**: For gizzard worms, 80 mg levamisole or 50 mg fenbendazole/l of drinking water for three days.

**Chickens and turkeys**: Use licensed products such as hygromycin B and fenbendazole according to label instructions. Meat and/or egg withdrawal times vary with products.

### CONTRAINDICATIONS
Consult Food Animal Residue Avoidance Databank (FARAD.org) for drug choices when managing backyard flocks.

### PRECAUTIONS
Fenbendazole can cause toxicosis in a number of species, including pigeons and doves, vultures, storks, among others. This can manifest as bone marrow suppression and direct intestinal tract cell damage in affected species. Fenbendazole should not be administered to poultry during molt, because it may interfere with feather regrowth. Ivermectin needs to be diluted properly. It is best to dilute in propylene glycol and is sensitive to light.

### POSSIBLE INTERACTIONS
Hygromycin B is a cholinesterase inhibitor, and treated birds should not be exposed to other cholinesterase inhibitors (drugs, insecticides, pesticides, or chemicals) within 3 days before or after treatment.

### ALTERNATIVE DRUGS
The use of diatomaceous earth supplemented at 2% in feed and fed continuously lowers numbers of *Heterakis* and *Capillaria* in chickens.

## FOLLOW-UP

### PATIENT MONITORING
All patients should be monitored for signs of toxicity during treatment. Follow-up examinations, including fecal examinations and/or further deworming should be performed as clinical experience dictates.

### PREVENTION/AVOIDANCE
Control is achieved by preventing access to fecal matter, and fecal-contaminated food and water. If this is not feasible, regular deworming (every 2–3 months) may be necessary. Deworm pigeons prior to the racing and breeding season. Environmental control to prevent access to insects (or other intermediate hosts) and feces is essential. Insect control is essential to prevent cestode reinfestation. Removal of earthworms should ideally be done. Pigeon lofts must be thoroughly cleaned regularly.

### POSSIBLE COMPLICATIONS
Secondary bacterial infections can occur with some of these parasites.

H

## HELMINTHIASIS (GASTROINTESTINAL)    (CONTINUED)

### EXPECTED COURSE AND PROGNOSIS

Many cases of parasitism in birds are seen in wildlife, zoo, and aviary birds. Therefore, detection is not necessarily done until the bird has died. In cases of flock parasitism, once a diagnosis is made, most parasites can be quite effectively treated.

 **MISCELLANEOUS**

### ASSOCIATED CONDITIONS

There could be secondary bacterial infections with some of these parasites. In chickens, *Heterakis gallinarum* is commonly a carrier of *Histomonas meleagridis* also. Neurologic impairment may be caused by aberrant migration of the raccoon roundworm, *Baylisascaris procyonis*, into the central nervous system of avian species which can serve as an intermediate host.

### AGE-RELATED FACTORS

Young or immunocompromised birds are more likely to suffer the effects of helminth parasitism.

### ZOONOTIC POTENTIAL

Although proven zoonotic transmission of helminths from birds to humans is underreported, there are avian helminth parasites that can also cause disease in humans.

### FERTILITY/BREEDING

Birds that are seriously ill have a decreased potential for reproduction. Heavy parasitism of several types can result in a drop in egg production in poultry.

### SYNONYMS

N/A

### SEE ALSO

Anemia
Bornaviral Diseases
Diarrhea
Emaciation
Enteritis and Gastritis
Liver Disease
Oral Plaques
Regurgitation and Vomiting
Undigested Food in Droppings
Urate and Fecal Discoloration
Sick-Bird Syndrome

### ABBREVIATIONS

GI—gastrointestinal
PCR—polymerase chain reaction

### INTERNET RESOURCES

Hauck, R. (2024). Helminthiasis in poultry (nematode and cestode infestations). *MSD Veterinary Manual*: http://www.merckmanuals.com/vet/poultry/helminthiasis/overview_of_helminthiasis_in_poultry.html
For a list of approved drugs for poultry: www.fda.gov

### Suggested Reading

Brandão, J., Beaufrère, H. (2013). Clinical update and treatment of selected infectious gastrointestinal diseases in avian species. *Journal of Exotic Pet Medicine* 22:101–117.

Clyde, C.I., Patton, S. (2000). Parasitism of caged birds. In: *Manual of Avian Medicine* (ed. G.H. Olsen, S.E. Orosz), 424–448. St Louis, MO: Mosby.

Doneley R.J.T. (2009). Bacterial and parasitic disease of parrots. *Veterinary Clinics of North America. Exotic Animal Practice*, 12:423–431.

Mathison B.A., Pritt B.S. (2018). A systematic overview of zoonotic helminth infections in North America. *Laboratory Medicine* 49(4):e61–e93.

Patton, S. (2000). Avian parasite testing. In: *Laboratory Medicine–Avian and Exotic Pets* (ed. A.M. Fudge), 147–156. Philadelphia, PA: Saunders.

Schmidt R.E., Reavill D.R., Phalen D.N. (2015). Gastrointestinal system and pancreas. In: *Pathology of Pet and Aviary Birds* (ed. R.E. Schmidt, D.R. Reavill, D.N. Phalen), 55–94. Ames, IA: Wiley.

Shifaw A., Feyera T., Walkden-Brown S.W., et al. (2021). Global and regional prevalence of helminth infection in chickens over time: a systematic review and meta-analysis. *Poultry Science* 100:101082.

**Author**: João Brandão, LMV, MS, DECZM (Avian), DACZM

**Acknowledgements**: updated from chapter in first edition authored by George Messenger.

## BASICS

### DEFINITION
Respiratory helminthiasis is any macroparasitic disease in birds in which any part of the respiratory tract is infected with parasitic worms known as helminths. These parasites are further classified as nematodes (roundworm-like), trematodes (flatworms), leeches, and schistosomes (blood flukes).

### PATHOPHYSIOLOGY
Transmission is either direct, by ingestion of embryonated eggs, or indirect, by ingestion of an intermediate host, depending on the parasite species. While capable of a direct life cycle, some species of tracheal worms rely heavily on earthworms as a transport or intermediate host; they also use multiple paratenic hosts (slugs, ants, beetles, many other invertebrates). Intermediate hosts are required for infection with spirurid nematodes (air sac worms), filarioid nematodes, and schistosomes (specifically snails). While leeches feed on birds, they do not need to otherwise infect them or any other host to complete their lifecycle. Except for leeches, once inside the host, the life cycle begins with the hatching of larva in the GI tract followed by migration through the body (either directly or through the blood stream) to the target area of the respiratory tract. Illness occurs through direct irritation/damage of respiratory tissues and/or along migratory tissue paths, predisposing to secondary infection, respiratory difficulties, and/or blood loss; parasites can also cause mechanical obstruction of the airway(s) through direct blockage or secondary to tissue swelling and damage.

### SYSTEMS AFFECTED
The degree and combination of systems affected varies based on helminthic type, host species, and age.
**Respiratory**: Helminth parasites can be found throughout the respiratory tract, from the upper (nasal cavity and trachea) to lower airways (air sacs and bronchi/parabronchi of the lungs).
**Hemic/lymphatic/immune**: Secondary infections related to direct or indirect damage by the parasite.
**GI**: Helminth parasites can be found throughout the GI tract, from the oral cavity to the intestines.
**Cardiovascular**: Blood vessels are a common migratory path; microfilaria of filarioid nematodes and schistosomes are commonly found in blood vessels. Hemorrhage.

**Musculoskeletal**: Weight loss/underconditioned.
**Behavioural**: Head shaking.
**Nervous**: Nasal schistosomes can migrate through the CNS.
**Reproductive**: Decreased breeding.
**Skin/Exocrine**: Unkept feathers.

### GENETICS
N/A

### INCIDENCE/PREVALENCE
The true incidence of respiratory helminthiasis is difficult to assess, especially in wild avian populations, as the absence of clinical signs with many infestations makes detection of infected individuals difficult. Leeches: The incident of infections peak in spring and summer when leeches seek out hosts and reproduce; opportunistic feeding in ice-free wetlands may occur during winter. Trematodes: Outbreaks of illness and death are seen in domestic ducks, geese, and zoological species housed on sources of water shared with wild waterfowl (reservoirs, natural wetlands, ponds). Schistosomes: Mortality is typically low, with outbreaks in wildlife populations; domestic waterfowl are exposed through shared water sources. Nematodes *Syngamus* and *Cyathostoma*: Clinical illness with infection is uncommon in wild populations.

### GEOGRAPHIC DISTRIBUTION
Worldwide. Depends on helminth species.

### SIGNALMENT
Species: See Causes section.

### SIGNS
#### General Comments
Signs and findings include those that may be seen in conjunction with this condition and those that occur concurrently as a result of the inciting problem.

#### Historical Findings
There are many possible historical findings in association with this condition depending on the specific disorder. Dyspnea. Signs of chronic illness. Poor doers.

#### Physical Examination Findings
Non-specific general malaise. Weight loss. Dyspnea, sometimes with "gaping"/gasping and outstretched necks and open mouths. Head shaking/flicking. Coughing. Ill-thrift. Anorexia/hyporexia. Adipsia/hypodipsia. Neurologic abnormalities with nasal schistosomes species. Death in some species, depending on level of compromise. Less likely to breed.

### CAUSES
There are many of species of respiratory helminth parasites in avian hosts. Some of the more common or important parasites are

listed here. Tracheal nematodes: *Syngamus* spp.—wild and range-reared fowl (turkeys, chickens, pheasants), perching birds (finches, canaries); less common in waterfowl, herons, storks, pelicans, woodpeckers; *Cyathostoma* spp.—especially waterfowl and other water birds. Air sac (spirurid) nematodes (*Serratospiculum* spp.)—mainly falcons. Filarioid nematodes: *Parochoncerca, Splendidofilaria, Chandlerella, Aproctella* spp. Trematodes (flatworms, air sac flukes)—snail kites (*Rostrhamus sociabilis*), tropical zoo birds. Leeches—especially waterfowl. Schistosomes (blood flukes): Migratory waterbirds including shorebirds and especially waterfowl.

### RISK FACTORS
*Syngamus* spp.—ground- or invertebrate-feeding birds. Predatory birds may become infected by consuming infected rodents or birds. Confined rearing. Gouldian finches often symptomatic with subclinical or asymptomatic infections in other finch species and canaries. Trematodes: Snail feeding birds. Leeches: Waterbirds that reside in lakes or rivers, especially that feed under moist vegetation. Schistosomes: Waterbirds residing in all temperate and tropical freshwater habitats (coincides with the presence of snail intermediate host). Confined rearing, increased density, and poor hygiene are also predisposing factors.

## DIAGNOSIS

### DIFFERENTIAL DIAGNOSIS
Vary based on species of bird and environment—captive vs. wild. Bacterial, fungal, or viral infections of the respiratory tract. Inhaled irritants and toxins. Oral toxins (avocado). Foreign body. Aberrant migration of GI nematodes. Trauma. Numerous other diseases that result in respiratory distress, head-shaking/yawning, poor body condition, and weight loss.

### CBC/BIOCHEMISTRY/URINALYSIS
Findings are not commonly documented, but in theory eosinophilia might be present with parasitism; leukocytosis with heterophilia might be seen in cases where there is significant inflammation; certain organisms tend to cause anemia.

### OTHER LABORATORY TESTS
Nasal swab cytology. Fecal flotation or sedimentation. Direct smears with or without saline. Transillumination of the trachea in canaries/finches may demonstrate mites

H

within trachea. Necropsy evaluation. Histopathology. Other tests to check for concurrent bacterial, fungal, or viral infection.

## IMAGING

Imaging is often carried out as part of baseline diagnostics (radiographs) or advanced evaluation (CT, endoscopy) in cases showing clinical signs of illness, including respiratory concerns. Findings are often non-specific (unless directly visualized such as with endoscopy) and would not necessarily be helpful to rule in or out parasites without tissue and other testing but would help in the determination of concurrent illness and lesion localization.

## DIAGNOSTIC PROCEDURES

Histopathology, necropsy.

## PATHOLOGIC FINDINGS

Depending on the parasite and location in the body, various lesions are found. In general, pathologic findings are confined to the respiratory tract, from the nasal passages to the air sacs. There are varying degrees of inflammation, thickening of respiratory tissues, necrosis, hemorrhage, edema, and airway obstruction.

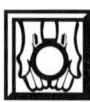

# TREATMENT

## APPROPRIATE HEALTH CARE

Patients that are critical need to be hospitalized for workup and treatment. Patients that are in respiratory distress and are diagnosed with parasitism at the time of the office visit may require oxygen and in hospital care prior to electing outpatient care options.

## NURSING CARE

Supportive care is indicated with sicker patients. This might include providing oxygen, warmth, fluid therapy, nutritional support/gavage feeding and fluid therapy.

## ACTIVITY

If dyspnea or exercise intolerance is seen, as practical, activities should be restricted in captive or rehab avians.

## DIET

N/A

## CLIENT EDUCATION

Proper administration of medications should be explained. For poultry, provide appropriate withdrawal times. Discuss control of intermediate hosts and reduction of risk factors for transmission and reinfection.

## SURGICAL CONSIDERATIONS

Avian species in severe respiratory distress related to primary tracheal obstruction may benefit from air sac cannulation.

# MEDICATIONS

## DRUG(S) OF CHOICE

It is difficult to draw conclusions about the proper use of anthelmintics for all birds, due to the wide variety of species and types of parasites involved. Medications that are commonly used in mammals are generally safe and effective in birds, including ivermectin, selamectin, and praziquantel. The author suggests consulting an exotic/zoological animal drug formulary. Trematodes—praziquantel 10–20 mg/kg PO, repeat in 10–14 days. Nematodes—ivermectin 0.2 mg/kg PO, SQ, topically over right jugular, IM once every 2 weeks for 3 doses, Flock treatment of finches/canaries 0.8–1 mg/l in drinking water; selamectin 23–92 mg/kg topically, dosed anecdotally once then every 2 weeks for 3 doses or once in 2 weeks, then 30 days later. Leeches—ivermectin 0.2–2 mg/kg PO, SQ, topically on skin, IM, once then in 7–14 days. Schistosomes—snail elimination is paramount. Individual birds can be treated with praziquantel baits for dabbling ducks (200 mg/duck for 3 days) or via injection (necessary for *Mergus merganser*, 200 mg/kg once). While difficult, effective treatment of wild avian populations is possible.

## CONTRAINDICATIONS

Consult the Food Animal Residue Avoidance Databank (FARAD.org) for drug choices when managing backyard flocks. Consult additional formulary resources for more information on species specific dosing and drug toxicities.

## PRECAUTIONS

Praziquantel is toxic to canaries and finches. Ivermectin must be diluted properly. It is best to dilute in propylene glycol and is sensitive to light. Fenbendazole is toxic in a number of species such as pigeons.

## POSSIBLE INTERACTIONS

N/A

## ALTERNATIVE DRUGS

Anecdotal reports of light dusting with a topical organophosphate carbaryl 5% (Sevin® Dust, GardenTech, Palatine, IL) has been suggested, but toxicity is a concern.

# FOLLOW-UP

## PATIENT MONITORING

All patients should be monitored for signs of toxicity during treatment. Follow-up examinations, including fecal examinations and/or further deworming, should be performed as clinical experience dictates.

## PREVENTION/AVOIDANCE

Control is achieved by preventing access to intermediate hosts, fecal matter, and fecal-contaminated food and water.

## POSSIBLE COMPLICATIONS

Severe and life-threatening respiratory distress and secondary bacterial and fungal infections can occur with some of these parasites.

## EXPECTED COURSE AND PROGNOSIS

Many cases of parasitism in birds are seen in wildlife, zoo, and aviary birds. They are thus not necessarily detected until the bird has died. In cases of flock parasitism, once a diagnosis is made, many parasites can be treated, but environmental factors related to exposure need to be addressed to prevent reinfection.

# MISCELLANEOUS

## ASSOCIATED CONDITIONS

There may be associated secondary bacterial or fungal infections with some of these parasites.

## AGE-RELATED FACTORS

Young or immunocompromised birds would be more likely to suffer the effects of helminth parasitism.

## ZOONOTIC POTENTIAL

Cercarial dermatitis (Swimmer's itch) is associated with the cutaneous penetration of cercaria of avian schistosomes into the skin of humans.

## FERTILITY/BREEDING

Birds that are seriously ill have a decreased potential for reproduction.

## SYNONYMS

N/A

## SEE ALSO

Air Sac Mites
Arrhythmias
Ascites
Aspergillosis
Aspiration Pneumonia
Avian Influenza
Chlamydiosis
Congestive Heart Failure
Cryptosporidiosis
Helminthiasis (Gastrointestinal)
Mycoplasmosis
Myocardial Diseases
Neural larva migrans
Orthoavulaviruses
Pericardial Effusion/Diseases
Pneumonia
Poxvirus

Respiratory Distress
Rhinitis/Sinusitis
Sarcocystosis
Sick-Bird Syndrome
Toxicosis (Airborne)
Toxicosis (Environmental, Pesticides)
Toxicosis (Ingested)
Tracheal Disease and Syringeal Disease
Trauma
Trichomoniasis

### ABBREVIATIONS

CNS—central nervous system
GI—gastrointestinal

### INTERNET RESOURCES

Merck & Co., Inc. *MSD Veterinary Manual*:
Merckvetmanual.com

*Suggested Reading*

Atkinson, C.T., Thomas, N.J., Hunter, D.B.
(2008). *Parasitic Diseases of Wild Birds*.
Ames, IA: Wiley-Blackwell.
Delaski, K.M., Nelson, S., Dronen, N.O.,
et al. (2015). Detection and management
of airs sac trematodes (*Szidatitrema*
species) in captive multispecies avian
exhibits. *Journal of Avian Medicine and
Surgery*, 29:345–353.

Speer, B.L. (ed.). (2016). *Current Therapy in
Avian Medicine and Surgery*. St. Louis, MO:
Elsevier.
Harrison, G.J., Lightfoot, T.L. (eds.). (2006).
*Clinical Avian Medicine*. Palm Beach, FL:
Spix Publishing.

**Author**: Julia Shakeri, DVM, DABVP (Avian
Practice)

H

# HEMOPARASITES

 **BASICS**

## DEFINITION
Infectious organisms, typically protozoans or helminths, that have life stages in the blood of an avian host.

## PATHOPHYSIOLOGY
### Lifecycle of Plasmodium
An infected vector (typically a *Culex* spp. mosquito) bites an uninfected bird; parasite sporozoites are passed into the bird's blood and via the bloodstream reach the liver; in the liver, the sporozoites develop into pre-erythrocytic schizonts, which then become merozoites; merozoites enter erythrocytes and develop into macrogametocytes (female), microgametocytes (male), or segments (schizonts). Schizonts divide in erythrocytes (intra-erythrocytytic merogony) indefinitely until the bird dies or the bird's immune system responds, so there is potential for persistence of infection with frequent relapses. Second-generation and subsequent generation exoerythrocytic schizonts can be seen in tissues other than the liver. Birds typically undergo an acute phase of infection where parasitemia increases steadily to a peak at 6–12 days after infection, then the host immune system begins to bring the infection under control; chronic infection then persists for the life of the bird, with recurrence of clinical disease possible.

### Lifecycle of Haemoproteus
A vector (typically a midge or hippoboscid) ingests gametocytes in RBCs of an infected bird; inside the insect vector the parasites migrate from the insect's GI tract to the bloodstream, then to the salivary glands as sporozoites; sporozoites are injected into the bloodstream of a new bird when the insect feeds; sporozoites migrate from the bird's bloodstream into endothelial cells of various tissues (lung, liver, bone marrow, spleen) where they develop into schizonts; each schizont contains many merozoites that are released into the bloodstream when the endothelial cell dies; merozoites in the bloodstream enter RBCs to become gametocytes. Gametocytes in a bird's RBCs can become infective in as little as 7 days after they enter the bird's RBCs; parasitemia in a host bird peaks at 10–21 days after infection and falls rapidly within 7 days to a low intensity.

### Lifecycle of Leukocytozoon
A vector (typically a black fly) ingests gametocyte-containing blood from an infected bird; gametocytes develop into

sporozoites inside the fly; the fly injects sporozoites into the bloodstream of a new bird; sporozoites travel from the bloodstream of the new bird to invade endothelial and parenchymal cells of various tissues, such as liver, heart and kidney; sporozoites develop into schizonts, which then rupture and release merozoites that infect RBCs and leukocytes. Alternatively, released merozoites may be ingested by macrophages to become megaloschizonts in tissues such as the liver, lung and kidney, and from that point the megaloschizonts may release merozoites that develop into gametocytes.

### Species
Possible clinical signs due to direct blood-cell effects such as anemia: *Plasmodium* spp., *Aegyptianella* spp., Leukocytozoon spp. (not common). Possible clinical signs due to multiorgan and muscle tissue destruction as parasites progress through life cycle stages: *Plasmodium* spp., *Leukocytozoon* spp., *Atoxoplasma* spp., *Haemoproteus* spp. (unusual). Transmitted via mosquitoes (*Culex* spp., *Mansonia crassipes*, *Aedeomyia squamipennis*), *Plasmodium* spp., some *Trypanosoma* spp. Transmitted via hippoboscid flies: Some *Haemoproteus* spp., some *Trypanosoma* spp. Transmitted via biting midges (ceratopogonids, *Culicoides* spp.), most *Haemoproteus* spp., *Leukocytozoon caulleryi*. Transmitted via black flies (simuliids): most *Leukocytozoon* spp., some *Trypanosoma* spp. Transmitted via mites, ticks, fleas or other arthropods: some *Trypanosoma* spp., *Hepatozoon* spp., *Babesia* spp., *Aegyptianella* spp., *Borrelia anserina*. Transmitted via ingestion of sporulated oocysts (feces-contaminated water or food): *Atoxoplasma* spp.

## SYSTEMS AFFECTED
**Behavioral**: Lethargy and weakness are seen in symptomatic infections of most avian hemoparasites.
**Cardiovascular**: Hemolytic anemia—*Plasmodium* spp., *Aegyptianella* spp., *Haemoproteus* spp.(unusual), *Leukocytozoon* spp. (unusual), *Bor. anserina*. Lymphocytosis, leukocytosis—*Plasmodium* spp., *Leukocytozoon* spp. (unusual).
**Hemic/lymphatic/immune**: Spleen—*Atoxoplasma* spp., *Leukocytozoon* spp.
**Hepatobiliary**: Liver—*Plasmodium* spp., *Atoxoplasma* spp., *Leukocytozoon* spp.
**Nervous**: Central nervous system signs—*Plasmodium* spp., *Leukocytozoon* spp.
**Neuromuscular**: Loss of balance, lameness or reluctance to move in Galliformes—*Plasmodium* spp.
**Respiratory**: Lungs—*Atoxoplasma* spp.

## GENETICS
N/A

## INCIDENCE/PREVALENCE
Prevalence of *Atoxoplasma* spp. can approach 100% in some passerine collections. *Haemoproteus* spp. are the most common blood parasite genus in birds. *Haemoproteus* spp., *Leukocytozoon* spp. and *Plasmodium* spp. are relatively common in wild birds. Seasonality of parasitemia generally coincides with vector prevalence.

## GEOGRAPHIC DISTRIBUTION
*Aegyptianella* spp. usually affect birds of tropical or subtropical climates. *Haemoproteus* spp. are distributed worldwide in temperate, tropical and subtropical climates. *Plasmodium* spp. and *Leukocytozoon* spp. are found in all zoogeographic regions except Antarctica (lack of mosquito vectors).

## SIGNALMENT
Species: *Atoxoplasma* spp. are especially pathogenic in small passerines, especially the families Fringillidae and Sturnidae. *Aegyptianella pullorum* affects Galliformes (chickens, turkeys) and Anseriformes (ducks, geese). *Trypanosoma* spp. usually affect passerines, Galliformes, waterfowl and pigeons. *B. anserina* usually affects Galliformes or waterfowl. *Haemoproteus* spp. are found in many species, especially passerines, Strigiformes and Columbiformes. *Plasmodium* spp. have been found in birds from nearly all avian orders (not yet reported in Struthioniformes, Coliiformes, or Trogoniformes). *Plasmodium relictum* has been found in natural infections of birds of at least 70 avian families. *Plasmodium* spp. appears to be especially pathogenic in penguins, small passerines, Galliformes (chickens, turkeys) and Anseriformes (ducks, geese). *Leukocytozoon* infections have been most often reported in passerines, Galliformes and Coraciiformes, but appear most pathogenic in Anseriformes (ducks, geese, swans), Galliformes (chickens), Columbiformes, and less commonly in Falconiformes. *Leukocytozoon simondi* is especially pathogenic in ducks and geese, and *L. caulleryi* is especially pathogenic in chickens in Asia. *Aegyptianella* spp. have been reported in many species including Galliformes, pigeons, crows, Anseriformes, ratites, falcons, passerines and psittacines. *A. pullorum* is pathogenic in chickens.
**Mean age and range**: Atoxoplasmosis is usually a disease of young birds, particularly fledglings, and adults are usually asymptomatic.
**Predominant sex**: None.

(CONTINUED)

## SIGNS

### General Comments
Most avian hemoparasites are of little clinical significance; however, many types of avian hemoparasites can become pathologic under stressful conditions (e.g. captivity, breeding season, migration), when they infect a host species that is out of its natural ecosystem (e.g. captivity), or when vector species invade new geographic areas (e.g. due to climate change).

### Historical Findings
Lethargy, listlessness—*Plasmodium* spp., *Leukocytozoon* spp., *Babesia shortti*, *Haemoproteus* spp. (unusual), *Leukocytozoon* spp. (unusual), *Bor. anserina*. Labored breathing—*Leukocytozoon simondi* (unusual). Central nervous system signs (ataxia, convulsions)—*Plasmodium* spp., *Leukocytozoon* spp. Diarrhea—*L. simondi* (unusual), *Aegyptianella pullorum*. Erratic flight or other neurologic signs, vomiting—*Leukocytozoon toddi*. Loss of balance, lameness or reluctance to move in galliformes—*Plasmodium* spp. Acute death—*L. simondi* in juveniles.

### Physical Examination Findings
Weight loss—*Haemoproteus* spp., *Leukocytozoon* spp. Pale mucous membranes—*Plasmodium* spp., *Bab. shortti*, *Haemoproteus* spp. (unusual), *Leukocytozoon* spp. (unusual). Jaundice—*Aegyptianella* spp., *Bab. shortti*. Typically asymptomatic—*Trypanosoma* spp., *Hepatozoon* spp., most *Babesia* spp., *Haemoproteus* spp., *Leukocytozoon* spp., *Trypanosoma* spp., microfilaria of filarial nematodes.

## CAUSES
See Pathophysiology section.

## RISK FACTORS
Likelihood of clinical signs due to avian hemoparasites increases with seasonal changes in photoperiod, increased vector prevalence, increased reproductive activity, and exposure to predators. Likelihood of clinical signs is inversely correlated with host immunocompetence.

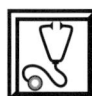

# DIAGNOSIS

## DIFFERENTIAL DIAGNOSIS
Most avian hemoparasites are differentiated using their appearance in blood smears. Multiple genera of hemoparasites may be present in the same patient. Numerous other nonparasitic etiologies exist for the nonspecific clinical signs of lethargy and weight loss.

## CBC/BIOCHEMISTRY/URINALYSIS
**Parasites inside RBCs**: *Haemoproteus* spp.—elongate pigmented gametocyte, usually alongside or wrapping around rather than deforming the RBC nucleus. The degree of parasitemia can be used as a gauge of general immunocompetence of the host (inverse correlation). *Plasmodium* spp.—usually a round pigmented gametocyte, trophozoite or schizont that may displace the RBC nucleus, but may be elongate and not displace the RBC nucleus. In contrast to *Haemoproteus* spp., *Plasmodium* can show schizogony in RBCs and endothelial cells of various organs, gametocytes can displace the RBC nucleus, and parasite stages can be seen within thrombocytes and leukocytes as well as in RBCs. *Leukocytozoon* spp.—a gametocyte is sometimes round but is typically large, elongate, with wispy ends, and without pigmented granules; may distort the infected host cell so much that the cell's original identification is difficult. *Aegyptianella* spp.—tiny nonpigmented vacuole appearance in RBCs. *Babesia* spp.—nonpigmented white vacuole.
**Parasites inside white blood cells**: *Hepatozoon* spp.—in monocytes or lymphocytes. *Atoxoplasma* spp.—a single merozoite or a meront in monocytes or lymphocytes, causing an indentation in the cell's nucleus. *Leukocytozoon* spp. *Plasmodium* spp.
**Parasites inside thrombocytes**: *Plasmodium* spp.
**Extracellular parasites**: *Haemoproteus* spp. (if several hours elapsed between blood collection and smear preparation), *Trypanosoma* spp. (long, flagellated, with an undulating membrane), microfilaria of filarial nematodes, *Bor. anserina* (spirochete with loose spirals).
**Hemoglobinuria**: *Plasmodium* spp.
**Elevation of AST or ALT**: *Leukocytozoon* spp. (unusual), *Atoxoplasma* spp., *Haemoproteus* spp., *Plasmodium* spp.
**Hypoalbuminemia**: Plasmodium spp.
**Hypergammaglobulinemia, therefore hyperproteinemia**: *Plasmodium* spp.
**Anemia**: *Plasmodium* spp., *Aegyptianella* spp., *Haemoproteus* spp. (unusual), *Leukocytozoon* spp. (unusual), *Bor. anserina*, *Aegyptianella* spp.
**Lymphocytosis, leukocytosis**: *Plasmodium* spp., *Leukocytozoon* spp. (unusual), *Haemoproteus* spp.

## OTHER LABORATORY TESTS
Buffy coat smear, looking for parasites amongst white blood cells from a centrifuged hematocrit tube of whole blood—especially used for *Atoxoplasma* spp. and *Trypanosoma* spp. PCR of tissues or whole blood. Fecal direct smear and centrifugation/flotation with Sheather's sugar solution sometimes used for *Atoxoplasma* spp. The oocysts of organism cannot be differentiated in this manner from typical enteric species of *Isospora* (two sporocysts containing four sporozoites each); however, the relative prevalence of *Atoxoplasma* versus enteric *Isospora* in some avian species is so disproportionate that the finding of oocysts in feces is diagnostic for *Atoxoplasma*. However, there is no correlation between presence of *Atoxoplasma* oocysts in feces and the presence of mononuclear merozoites in the same bird at the same time. Increased intensity of green color (biliverdin) in feces. Several serological tests (agar gel precipitation, counter-immunoelectrophoresis, immunofluorescence, ELISA, immunoblot analysis, latex agglutination) have been developed for *L. caulleryi*, but not for other *Leukocytozoon* spp.

## IMAGING
N/A

## DIAGNOSTIC PROCEDURES
See blood analysis recommendations.

## PATHOLOGIC FINDINGS
Splenomegaly: *Atoxoplasma* spp., *Haemoproteus* spp., *Plasmodium* spp., *Leukocytozoon* spp., *Aegyptianella* spp., *Bor. anserina*. Hepatomegaly: *Atoxoplasma* spp., *Haemoproteus* spp., *Plasmodium* spp., *Leukocytozoon* spp., *Aegyptianella* spp., *Bor. anserina*. Hepatic necrosis: *Atoxoplasma* spp., *Haemoproteus* spp., *Leukocytozoon* spp., *Aegyptianella* spp. Renal necrosis: *Aegyptianella* spp. Lung lesions: *Haemoproteus* spp. Muscle necrosis (white or hemorrhagic streaks): *Haemoproteus* spp. Atoxoplasmosis: also may see necrotic foci in spleen and/or heart; pancreatic edema and/or hemorrhage; fluid accumulation in intestines; ascites. Impression smears of spleen, liver or lung can be used to detect *Atoxoplasma* spp. sporozoites. *Atoxoplasma* can be confirmed in infected tissues via PCR.

# TREATMENT

## APPROPRIATE HEALTH CARE
See Medications section.

## NURSING CARE
If a patient is symptomatic, general supportive care should be provided (nutrition, hydration, appropriate temperature, calm environment).

## ACTIVITY
See Nursing Care section.

## DIET
See Nursing Care section.

## CLIENT EDUCATION
Chronic infection with some avian hemoparasites (e.g. *Haemoproteus*) may stimulate immunity to reinfection with homologous parasites of the same species, so treatment may be elected against in cases of asymptomatic

infection. However, immunosuppression due to stress or other factors may cause recrudescence of parasitemia and clinical signs.

## SURGICAL CONSIDERATIONS
N/A

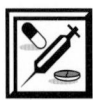

## MEDICATIONS

### DRUG(S) OF CHOICE
*Atoxoplasma* spp.—reported treatment options include: Sulfachloropyrazine in drinking water at a dosage of 300 ppm (1 g 30% powder per 1 l drinking water). If sulfachlorpyrazine is used, a vitamin B6 supplement should be given during the treatment (not available in the USA); sulfachloropyridazine in drinking water at a dosage of 300 ppm. If sulfachlorpyridazine is used, a vitamin $B_{12}$ supplement should be given during the treatment (not available in the USA); toltrazuril 12.5 mg/kg PO q24h for 14 days; ponazuril 20 mg/kg PO q24h 7–10 days. *Haemoproteus* spp.—reported treatment options include atebrine, plasmochin, chloroquine sulfate, quinacrine, primaquine, mefloquine, buparvaquone, pyrimethamine, pyrimethamine-sulfadoxine combinations, and tetracyclines. *Plasmodium* spp.—reported treatment options include chloroquine phosphate, primaquine phosphate, pyrimethamine-sulfadoxine combinations, mefloquine, sulfamonomethoxine, sulfachloropyrazine, doxycycline, halofuginone and atovaquone/proguanil combinations. *Leukocytozoon* spp.—reported treatment options include pyrimethamine, pyrimethamine-sulfamonomethoxine in combination, clopidol, atebrine, trimethoprim-sulfamethoxazole combination, melarsomine, and primaquine. *Aegyptianella* spp.—doxycycline, tetracyclines. *Bab. shortti* in Falconiformes—imidocarb dipropionate 5–13 mg/kg IM q7days for 2–3 weeks.

### CONTRAINDICATIONS
N/A

### PRECAUTIONS
N/A

### POSSIBLE INTERACTIONS
N/A

### ALTERNATIVE DRUGS
N/A

## FOLLOW-UP

### PATIENT MONITORING
See blood analysis in CBC/Biochemistry/Urinalysis section.

### PREVENTION/AVOIDANCE
Two vaccines were developed for *Plasmodium relictum*; both provided protection for penguins and canaries against natural infection, but immunity was short-lived in canaries and immunity waned to that of unvaccinated control birds when challenged with mosquito vectors a year later. Two vaccines have been developed for protection of chickens against *L. caulleryi*. Frequent replacement of drinking water, bathing bowls and enclosure substrate to prevent ingestion of sporulated oocysts—*Atoxoplasma* spp. Protection from flying insect vectors with screening—*Plasmodium* spp., some *Trypanosoma* spp., *Haemoproteus* spp., *Leukocytozoon* spp. Protection from tick vectors with use of acaricides—some *Trypanosoma* spp., *Hepatozoon* spp., *Babesia* spp., *Aegyptianella* spp. Absolute prevention of infection may be counterproductive for protection from some hemoparasite-induced diseases, as birds naïve to infection are much more likely to experience morbidity and mortality if subsequently infected.

### POSSIBLE COMPLICATIONS
N/A

### EXPECTED COURSE AND PROGNOSIS
Atoxoplasmosis is often a diagnosis made postmortem. Most other hemoparasites are either asymptomatic, or their numbers are able to be reduced in the host with appropriate medications.

## MISCELLANEOUS

### ASSOCIATED CONDITIONS
N/A

### AGE-RELATED FACTORS
N/A

### ZOONOTIC POTENTIAL
None.

### FERTILITY/BREEDING
N/A

### SYNONYMS
The term "malaria" is most accurately associated with *Plasmodium* spp., but some older literature uses the word "malaria" to refer to *Haemoproteus* spp. infections. Haemoproteosis, hematozoan disease, haemosporidian disease, blood parasite disease, Bangkok hemorrhagic disease (*L. caulleryi*), "going light" (*Atoxoplasma* spp.) in passerines, "black spot disease" (*Atoxoplasma* spp.—due to liver visible through body wall). Note, some older reports of *Lankesterella* infection may have been actually due to *Atoxoplasma* spp.

## SEE ALSO
Anemia
Coagulopathies and Coagulation
Coccidiosis (Systemic)
Ectoparasites
Emaciation
Hemorrhage
Liver Disease
Sick-Bird Syndrome

## ABBREVIATIONS
ALT—alanine aminotransferase
AST—aspartate aminotransferase
ELISA—enzyme-linked immunosorbent assay
GI—gastrointestinal
PCR—polymerase chain reaction
RBC—red blood cell

## INTERNET RESOURCES
Norton, T.M., Greiner, E., Latimer, K. Little, S.E. (2007). Medical protocols recommended by the US Bali Mynah SSP. American Association of Zoo Veterinarians: https://www.aazv.org/page/547
VanWettere, A.J. (2022). Blood borne organisms in poultry. *Merck Veterinary Manual*: https://www.msdvetmanual.com/poultry/bloodborne-organisms/bloodborne-organisms-in-poultry

*Suggested Reading*
Atkinson, C.T., Thomas, N.J., Hunter, D.B. (eds). (2008). *Parasitic Diseases of Wild Birds*. Hoboken, NJ: Wiley. [Relevant chapters include: 2: Haemoproteus, by Carter T. Atkinson. 3: Avian Malaria, by Carter T. Atkinson. 4: Leukocytozoonosis, by Donald J. Forrester and Ellis C. Greiner. 5: Isospora, Atoxoplasma and Sarcocystis, by Ellis C. Greiner.]
Campbell, T.W. (2012). Hematology of birds. In: *Veterinary Hematology and Clinical Chemistry*, 2nd edn. (ed. M.A. Thrall, G., Weiser, R. Allison, T.W. Campbell), 262–266. Hoboken, NJ: Wiley.
Peirce, M.A. (2000). Hematozoa. In: *Avian Medicine* (ed. J. Samour), 245–252. London: Mosby.
Remple, J.D. (2004). Intracellular hematozoa of raptors: a review and update. *Journal of Avian Medicine and Surgery*, 28:75–88.
Valkiunas, G. (2004). *Avian Malaria Parasites and Other Haemosporidia*. Boca Raton, FL: CRC Press.
**Author**: Rodney W. Schnellbacher, DVM, DACZM
**Acknowledgements**: updated from first edition chapter authored by Lisa Harrenstien, DVM, DACZM

# BASICS

## DEFINITION
Hemmorrhage is the loss of blood from the vascular space into surrounding tissues or from body surfaces.

## PATHOPHYSIOLOGY
Hemorrhage can be acute or chronic in nature. Chronic anemia develops more rapidly than mammals. RBC lifespan is 28–45 days. Clotting occurs via extrinsic clotting and thromboplastin. TBV is approximately 4.8–10% of body weight, based on species. Only 1% of the bird's weight is recommended for blood work (i.e. 1 ml blood/100 g body weight). Clinical signs of hemorrhage result from one of two mechanisms: (1) Blood loss from damaged or diseased vessels, resulting from trauma or surgery; secondary to infectious, inflammatory, or neoplastic processes that cause vessel erosion and infiltration. (2) Bleeding diatheses of defects of normal hemostatic processes. Failure of platelet plug formation and coagulopathies. Birds have a predisposition for haemorrhage: Loose attachments to SQ tissues; relatively high blood pressure; skin fragility. Birds can withstand a greater percentage of blood loss than mammals. The LD50 of blood loss in ducks (*Anas platyrhynchas*) was 60% of their TBV. Tachycardia is not noted until 25–45% of TBV is lost. Birds are better able to maintain MAP and stroke volume independent of peripheral vascular tone. Theory for the adaptation is the absence of an autonomic response, mobilization of immature erythrocytes and rapid extravascular fluid resorption from skeletal muscle.

## SYSTEMS AFFECTED
**Cardiovascular**: Anemia, hypotension, heart murmur, increased cardiac output.
**Integument/musculoskeletal**: Weakness, decreased palor, bruising, petechia.
**Hepatobiliary**: Liver and splenic enlargement.
**Metabolic**: Change in function due to hypoxia.
**Ophthalmic**: Pale conjunctiva, uveitis, glaucoma.
**Respiratory**: Dyspnea, tachypnea.

## GENETICS
N/A

## INCIDENCE/PREVALENCE
N/A

## GEOGRAPHIC DISTRIBUTION
Most causes of hemorrhage have no geographic distribution. Herpesvirus is mostly associated with South American parrots. Sarcocystosis: Most of USA, especially Gulf coast. Worldwide distribution: Adenovirus of turkeys, colibacillosis, *M. ornithogaster*, paramyxovirus, polyomavirus.

## SIGNALMENT
Species: All avian species can be affected. Bleeding diathesis of conures is more commonly found in blue-crowned, peach-fronted, orange-fronted and Patagonian species. Budgerigars—*Macrorhabdus ornithogaster*, neoplasia, hepatic lipidosis. IPD—macaws, Amazon parrots, conures and hawk head parrots. Polyomavirus is more common in neonatal budgerigars less than 15 days of age. Quakers—Quaker mutilation syndrome. Adenovirus of turkeys. Amazon parrots—hepatic lipidosis. Mynah, toucan, birds of paradise, tanager—hemochromatosis. African grey parrots—anxiety.

## SIGNS

### General Comments
Vascular injury is the most common cause of hemorrhage.

### Historical Findings
Non-specific signs such as weakness, lethargy, anorexia, and death. Recent history of trauma or surgery. Respiratory changes. Multiple members of a flock are affected in infectious and toxicologic diseases.

### Physical Examination Findings
Abdominal distention. Blood in urates or stool. Cloacal haemorrhage. Cold distal extremities. Collapse. Death. Depression/lethargy. Ecchymosis, green discoloration in later stages. Epistaxis. Hematuria secondary to renal neoplasia or toxicities. Hemoptysis. Hyphema. Hypovolemia. Melena. Pale mucus membranes. Petechiation. Puncture wounds. Recumbency. Retinal Hemorrhage. Solid masses. Tachycardia or Bradycardia. Tachypnea. Shock. Compensatory phase (first stage): Typical exam findings of tachycardia and hypertension. This is typically seen with blood loss of less than 20% of TBV. Early decompensatory phase (second stage): Decreased blood flow to the kidneys, GI tract, skin, and muscles. Typical exam findings include tachycardia, ± hypothermia, normal to decreased blood pressure, pale mucous membranes, prolonged CRT, cool limbs, and depression. This phase typically occurs with blood loss > 25–30% TBV. Decompensatory phase (final stage): Typical exam finding include bradycardia,

hypothermia, hypotension, pale mucous membranes, and absent CRT, occurs > 30% of TBV.

## CAUSES
**Aneurysm**: Aneurysm, aortic rupture of turkey, emu, and ostrich.
**Behavioral/Self Mutilation**: Anxiety, attention-seeking behavior, boredom, compulsion disorders, displacement behaviors, overcrowding, pain.
**Coagulopathy**: Anticoagulant rodenticides, DIC, color mutation in cockatiels—factor deficiency, liver disease, hepatic lipidosis, thrombocytopenia.
**Environmental**: Aerosols, cigarette smoke, improper humidity.
**Iatrogenic**: Aggressive nail or wing trims, blood oversampling, laceration of blood vessels during venipuncture, recent surgery, failure to use proper hemostatic techniques.
**Idiopathic**: Bleeding diathesis of conures, self mutilation of *Agapornis* spp.
**Infectious**: Bacterial dermatitis—cockatiel mutilation syndrome, hemorrhagic septicemia of turkeys, MRSA, pneumonia, sarcocystosis, *Staphylococcus* spp.; GI—parasites, *Giardia*, PMV-3 GI hemorrhage, psittacine herpesvirus 1, 2 (IPD), adenovirus (GI hemorrhage in turkeys), *M. orthinogaster*, polyomavirus—neonatal budgerigars are especially susceptible to GI haemorrhage; respiratory—pneumonia, hemoptysis poultry: IBDV, Gallid herpesvirus 1, avian influenza, fowl poxvirus, *Mycoplasma galliseptica*, NVD, infectious bronchitis, fowl adenovirus.
**Metabolic**: Cardiovascular—microvascular hemorrhage from hypertension, anemia, or hyperviscosity; GI disease—enteritis/gastritis, GI foreign bodies, pancreatitis and pancreatitic neoplasia, ulcers; genitourinary disease—cloacal papillomas primary or secondary to IPD, cloacal/uterine prolapse, cloacitis, cloacoliths, egg binding, salpingitis, metritis, pain from organ enlargement, phallic prolapse.
**Neoplasia**: Hemorrhage of affected organ, xanthoma, lipoma.
**Nutritional deficiencies**: Diet deficient in vitamin K, malnutrition leading to squamous metaplasia, bleeding diathesis of conures (possible), starvation, fatty liver hemorrhagic syndrome (chickens).
**Trauma**: Bite wounds from inter-mate or cage-mate aggression, broken blood feather, cannibalism, chemical exposure, electrical shock, power line trauma, flying into stationary objects, gunshot wounds, predators/interaction other pets, recent fall, aggressive wing trim, cardiac disease, neuromuscular disease, night fright, vehicular and windmill trauma.

H

**Toxicity:** Anticoagulant rodenticides, estrogen, heavy metal, medications (NSAIDs, clopidogrel, sulfonamindes, heparin, warfarin, plasma expanders, estrogens, cytotoxic drugs), sulfa-containing drugs in gallinaceous birds.

## RISK FACTORS
Coagulation disorders.

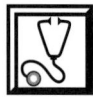

# DIAGNOSIS

## DIFFERENTIAL DIAGNOSIS
Respiratory or cardiovascular disease. Other causes of shock. Hemolytic anemia. Impaired erythrocyte production.

## CBC/BIOCHEMISTRY/URINALYSIS
Caution in birds with excessive hemorrhage. Only 1% of the bird's weight is recommended for blood work (i.e. 1 ml blood/100 g body weight) so all blood loss from hemorrhage and bruising must be taken into account. Biochemistry panel: Liver enzyme abnormalities (elevated bile acids, AST, LDH, GGT, ALT), GGT elevations in IPD with subsequent bile duct carcinoma; other non-specific laboratory abnormalities maybe noted; trauma may also show elevation in CK and potassium; uric acid elevation in renal disease. Hemogram: Anemia—typically defined a as PCV< 35%, however normals can vary with different species. PCV will normalize in 2–7 days after acute blood loss. Hemogram will show a non-regenerative in acute hemorrhage (< 2 days). Hemogram may show signs of regeneration between 2 and 7 days. Polychromasia, reticulocytosis, macrocytosis, anisocytosis. Polychromasia is noted in mallard ducks 12 hours post-hemorrhagic event. Decreased hemoglobin levels. Hypoproteinemia. Thrombocytopenia secondary to consumption; non-budgerigar parrots with polyomavirus. Urinalysis— hematuria, hyaline casts.

## OTHER LABORATORY TESTS
Coagulation: Prothrombin time measurement 9–15 seconds in adult birds, increased in younger birds. ACT normally < 120 seconds. Fecal: Occult blood, parasitism/*Giardia*. Thromboelastography has been described in some avian species, including poultry and Hispaniolan Amazon parrots (limited availability). Fluid cytology: Erythrocytes, phagocytosis of erythrocytes, iron pigment, or hemosiderin. Blood pressure measurement to assess cardiovascular status and detect hypotension or hypertension. Culture and PCR for various disorders. Intradermal skin testing for allergies. Heavy metal elevations.

## IMAGING
Radiographs may show changes depending on the cause. Loss of serosal detail due to coelomic effusion, hepatomegaly/ microhepatica, other evidence of trauma, mass effect, metallic densities, microcardia, enlargement of reproductive structures. Endoscopy to evaluate abdominal masses, the upper GI tract, cloacal or reproductive disorders.

## DIAGNOSTIC PROCEDURES
N/A

## PATHOLOGIC FINDINGS
**Peracute**: Findings may be limited to generalized GI with superficial hematomas, hemarthrosis, body cavity hemorrhages, and/or GI blood.
**Acute**: Above findings, as well as hemorrhages within various tissues, phagocytized erythrocytes on cytology or histology.
**Chronic**: Above findings, as well as erythrocyte proliferation in the bone marrow, hepatic sinusoids, and splenic red pulp; accumulations of hemosiderin on histology.

# TREATMENT

## APPROPRIATE HEALTH CARE
Outpatient medical management is possible if the hemorrhage is minimal and the laceration/abrasion is small. Inpatient medical management: Address active haemorrhage. Compression or pressure wrap application—apply compression for 30–60 seconds, avoid compression of the keel. Bleeding nail: Silver nitrate or potassium permanganate application on a bleeding nail or cautery. Removal of broken blood feather. Note: Although pulling a blood feather is commonly recommended, this can result in damage to the feather follicle. Hemostatic matrix. Electrocautery. Emergency surgery as indicated. Identify and correct underlying metabolic disease and treat accordingly.

## NURSING CARE
Minimize stress by placing in a quiet area with minimum traffic. Place in warm, humid environment (85–90°F [29.4–32.2°C] and 70% humidity), unless there is evidence of head trauma. Dyspneic birds place in incubator with 78–85% oxygen supplementation at 5 l/minute. Stop access to feathers in self/mutilation cases with a collar designed for birds, wraps or bandaging.

## ACTIVITY
Restrict activity until PCV normalizes or after surgical recovery. Place in a smaller cage and restrict flight.

## DIET
Nutritional support via gavage feeding for anorexic patients. Gavage 5% of body weight initially and slowly increase up to 8–10% to avoid aspiration. Crop emptying can take 2–4 hours. Rehydrate prior to starting nutritional support. Change all birds to a nutritionally complete diet.

## CLIENT EDUCATION
Debilitated birds have a poor prognosis despite treatment. Heavy metal toxicosis: Identify sources of heavy metals. Discuss behavior modification for self-mutilation, behavioral disorders and cage-aggressive mates. Cage modification for high fall-risk birds and overcrowding. Environmental enrichment.

## SURGICAL CONSIDERATIONS
Surgery may be necessary if bleeding cannot be stopped with pressure. Prior to surgery, patients with hypotension, excessive blood loss or hypovolemic shock should be stabilized. Electrocautery should be used to minimize blood loss. Imping for birds that fall due to excessive wing trims. Endoscopic or surgical removal of foreign bodies, bleeding masses, or uncontrolled internal haemorrhage.

# MEDICATIONS

## DRUG(S) OF CHOICE
*Fluid Therapy*
Warm fluids to 100–104°F (37.8–40°C). SQ or PO indicated for mild levels of blood loss. Crystalloids should be sufficient. SQ—place up to 10 ml/kg in each SQ injection site; use the inguinal web, intrascapular, and axillary areas; LRS absorbs well. IO/IV indicated for moderate levels of blood loss, surgery or hypothermia. Allow for rapid administration and dissemination—IV 22- to 26-gauge catheter in jugular, basophilic, ulnar, or medial metatarsal, vein; may be difficult in birds < 100 g. IO catheter—distal ulna or proximal tibiotarsus. Confirm placement with radiographs, Higher risk of infection and joint complications; 80% of fluid deficit should be replaced over 6–8 hours in acute loss and over 12–24 hours in chronic loss. Consider adding a colloid (3–5 ml/kg), especially if hypotensive or hypovolemic. Plasmalyte A closest to avian plasma. Management of hypovolemic shock or PCV < 20%: Replace via IO/IV catheter, assess blood pressure, heart rate, mucous membranes, and CRT to assess response to treatment. Repeat fluid boluses until the blood pressure is > 90 mmHg. Replacing

H

1–2% body weight will increase PCV 2–5%. Perform whole-blood transfusion in anemic patients with TP < 1 mg/dL. Treatment choices: Transfusion—use an 18-μm blood filter; calculate the patient's TBV (4.8–10% of body weight depending on species); replace 10–20% of the blood volume IV/IO over 1–5 minutes in decompensatory shock, otherwise 1 ml/kg/hour over 15 minutes, then rest over 2–4 hours. Homologous transfusion is ideal transfusion method.

### Crossmatching
**Major crossmatch**: Donor erythrocytes/recipient serum.
**Minor crossmatch**: Donor serum/recipient erythrocytes. Perform for second transfusion. Perform for first transfusion for chickens. Anticoagulant CPDA 0.1 ml/0.9 ml blood (first choice), heparin 2 IU/ml blood. Blood cannot be stored; half-life 6–11 days.

### Heterologous Transfusion
Best to use bird of same genus and crossmatch (major and minor). Monitor for viral disease or blood parasite infection transfer; half-life 1/2–4.5 days. Monitor for fluid overload and transfusion reactions. More common in repeat transfusions or heterologous transfusions. Hypertonic saline 3 ml/kg over 10 minutes ± hetastarch 3–5 ml/kg—use as a last choice. Oxyglobin (5 ml/kg) IV/IO slowly over 1 minute, repeat every 15 minutes (manufacturing currently discontinued). Once stable, place on crystalloids for maintenance, deficits, and ongoing losses. If there is no response to above treatments, check blood gases, PCV/total protein and ECG. If hypoglycemic, give 50% dextrose 50–100 mg/kg IV slowly to effect. Dilute 1:1 with 0.9% saline. Additional medications may be needed based on the disease process. Pain management: Psychotropic drugs, antibiotics, erythropoietin/iron dextran, vitamin K, B vitamins.

### CONTRAINDICATIONS
Hypotonic fluids are contraindicated in birds with salt glands. SQ or PO fluids contraindicated in hypovolemia, hypothermia, and shock due to peripheral vasoconstriction. Hypertonic fluids and colloids, fluids containing > 2.5% dextrose contraindicated in brown pelicans and turkey vultures. LRS contraindicated for rapid effusion. IO catheter contraindicated in the ulna of Cathartiformes. Colloid contraindicated in coagulopathy, congestive heart failure, renal disease, pneumonia. Avoid drugs with anticoagulant of anti-platelet effects (NSAIDs, clopidogrel, sulfonamindes, heparin, warfarin, plasma expanders, estrogens, and cytotoxic drugs). Adequan (PSGAG) hss been associated with fatal hemorrhage/bleeding diathesis in multiple avian species.

### PRECAUTIONS
Indirect blood pressure measurement does not always correlate with direct arterial measurement; but it can provide information of blood pressure trends.

### POSSIBLE INTERACTIONS
N/A

### ALTERNATIVE DRUGS
N/A

 **FOLLOW-UP**

### PATIENT MONITORING
Monitor for cessation of active bleeding and petechiation formation. Stabilization/normalization of hematocrit/PCV and total solids. Typically occurs within 2–7 days. Hemorrhagic/hypovolemic shock—resolution of tachycardia, bradycardia, hyper or hypertension. Normalization of PCV/TS typically occurs within 3–6 days. Monitor PCV/TS daily in the acute phase and CBC routinely. Blood pressure—perform serial measurements until normalized.

### PREVENTION/AVOIDANCE
Remove access to heavy metals. Perform proper and routine wing trimming if needed (may not apply to all cases). Discuss risk of unsupervised interaction with another animal or unsupervised activity. Provide proper enclosures for birds to prevent injury. Avoid airborne perfumes/odors and topical products around birds with feather damaging behavior.

### POSSIBLE COMPLICATIONS
N/A

### EXPECTED COURSE AND PROGNOSIS
Severe anemia can lead to death. Depends on the following: Initial stabilization and correction of hemorrhagic shock; ability to identify and control active haemorrhage; minimization of trauma.

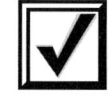 **MISCELLANEOUS**

### ASSOCIATED CONDITIONS
N/A

### AGE-RELATED FACTORS
Young chicks and geriatric birds are more prone to a poor prognosis.

### ZOONOTIC POTENTIAL
N/A

### FERTILITY/BREEDING
N/A

### SYNONYMS
Bleeding diathesis, conure bleeding syndrome.

### SEE ALSO
Adenoviruses
Anemia
Beak Malocclusion
Cloacal Diseases
Colibacillosis
Coagulopathies and Coagulation
Enteritis and Gastritis
Feather Cyst
Feather Damaging and Self-Injurious Behavior
Fractures
Helminthiasis (Gastrointestinal)
Hemoparasites
Herpesvirus (Duck Viral Enteritis)
Liver Disease
*Macrorhabdus ornithogaster*
Neoplasia (Gastrointestinal and Hepatic)
Neoplasia (Lymphoproliferative)
Neoplasia (Reproductive)
Nutritional Imbalances
Orthoavulaviruses
Pancreatic Diseases
Phallus Prolapse and Diseases
Pneumonia
Polyomavirus
Problem Behaviors: Aggression, Biting and Screaming
Regurgitation and Vomiting
Renal Diseases
Sarcocystosis
Sick-bird Syndrome
Toe and Nail Diseases
Toxicosis (Anticoagulant Rodenticide)
Toxicity (Heavy Metals)
Trauma
Urate and Fecal Discoloration
Uropygial Gland Diseases
Wounds (Including Bite Wounds, Predator Attacks)

### ABBREVIATIONS
ACT—activated coagulation time
ALT—alanine transverse
AST—aspartate aminotransferase
CBC—Complete Blood Count
CK—creatine kinase
CPDA—citrate phosphate dextrose adenine
CRT—capillary refill time
CT—computer tomography
DIC—disseminated intravascular coagulation
ECG—electrocardiogram
EEE/WEE—Easter/wEstern Equine encephalomyelitis
GGT—gamma-glutamyl transferase
GI—gastrointestinal
IBDV—infectious bursal disease
IPD—internal papilloma disease
LD50—amount of blood loss required to cause mortality 50% of the patients
LDH—lactate dehydrogenase

# HEMORRHAGE

LRS—lactated Ringer's solution
MAP—mean arterial pressure
MRSA—methicillin-resistant *Staphylococcus aureus*
NSAIDs—non-steroidal anti-inflammatory drugs
PCR—polymerase chain reaction
PCV—packed cell volume
PMV—paramyxovirus
PSGAG—polysulfated glycosaminoglycan
NDV—Newcastle disease virus
NSAIDs—non-steroidal anti-inflammatory drugs
RBC—red blood cell

TBV—total blood volume
TS—total solids

## INTERNET RESOURCES
N/A

*Suggested Reading*
Fordham, M., Roberts, B.K. (eds.). (2016). Emergency and critical care [special issue]. *Veterinary Clinics of North America: Exotic Animal Practice*. 19(2):1–14.
Lennox, A. (2013). Avian Critical Care. *Avian Critical Care. Proceedings BSAVC.* Gloucester, UK: British Small Animal Veterinary Association.

Lichtenberger, M., Orcutt, C., Cray, C. et al. (2009). Comparison of fluid types for resuscitation after acute blood loss in mallard ducks (*Anas platyrhynchos*). *Journal of Veterinary Emergency and Critical Care*, 19:467–472.

**Author**: Erika Cervasio, DVM, DABVP (Avian, Canine, Feline)

**Acknowledgements**: Heather W. Barron, DVM, DABVP (Avian); Rebecca Duerr, DVM, MPVM, PhD; Angela Lennox, DVM, DABVP (Avian); Marla Lichtenberger DVM, DACVECC; Kristin Vyhnal DVM, MS, DACVP.

# BASICS

## DEFINITION
Excessive accumulation of lipids, mainly triglycerides within the liver, resulting in hepatic dysfunction, liver failure, and death.

## PATHOPHYSIOLOGY
Disruption in lipid homeostasis, characterized by imbalances in hepatic lipid accumulation, transportation, and metabolism, leading to excessive hepatic lipid accumulation/storage. Altered lipid metabolism and accumulation can result from increased intake (high-fat diets, obesity), increased lipogenesis (endocrine, stress), reduced transport of lipids from the liver (nutritional deficiencies), and decreased fatty acid oxidation. Intrahepatic lipid accumulation causes impaired cellular function and cholestasis, ultimately leading to hepatic failure.

## SYSTEMS AFFECTED
Hepatobiliary. Gastrointestinal. Skin/exocrine. Hemic/lymphatic. Immune (coagulopathy in advanced disease). Nervous (advanced disease).

## GENETICS
N/A

## INCIDENCE/PREVALENCE
Relatively common problem encountered in caged birds. Well-known disease in fattening turkeys. Egg-laying chickens, associated with vitellogenesis. Male quaker parrots have a higher prevalence of hepatic lipidosis than other psittacine species. However, this finding may be specific to the species, as females from other avian species with chronic reproductive activity might have a higher prevalence of hepatic lipidosis than males. Reported in grey parrots, barred owls, and common mynas.

## GEOGRAPHIC DISTRIBUTION
N/A

## SIGNALMENT
More common in Amazon parrots, cockatoos (especially galah cockatoos), budgerigars, lorikeets, quaker parrots, and poultry. Reproductively active females. Male quaker parrots.

## SIGNS

### Historical Findings
Nonspecific sickness. Anorexia and/or regurgitation. Polyuria/polydipsia. Dyspnea. Green stools. Biliverdinuria.

### Physical Examination Findings
Slightly overweight to obese. Lethargy and weakness, encephalopathy (rare, end stage). Dehydration. Poor feather condition (pigment changes, stress bars, feather picking). Abnormal and discolored nails, overgrown rhinotheca with degenerative keratin changes (especially budgerigars). Dyspnea (from hepatic enlargement and/or intracoelomic fat). Abdominal distension (hepatic enlargement and/or ascites). Palpable hepatic enlargement. Polyuria, diarrhea, regurgitation, and/or vomiting. Increased biliverdin green pigment in urine and stool (from cholestasis). Melena or bloody droppings (end-stage coagulopathy).

## CAUSES
Can be multifactorial; avian lipid metabolism is complex and incompletely understood. Imbalance of lipid intake, endogeneous lipid production, and lipid metabolism. Increased lipid intake—high-fat, low-protein diets (seed based), overfeeding, excessive high-energy intake in neonates (cockatoos, macaws). Increased lipid production—hormonal lipogenesis (estrogens during egg laying, hormone-sensitive lipase in diabetes mellitus), drug-induced lipogenesis (corticosteroids, pesticides), and peripheral lipolysis (catecholamines in stress, thyroxine with thyroid dysfunction, but not seen with rapid weight loss). Impaired lipid metabolism—multinutrient-deficient diets, including essential fatty acids (linoleic acid), sulfur amino acids (choline, methionine, cysteine), lipotrophic factors (L-carnitine), and vitamins (biotin, vitamins $B_1$, $B_2$, $B_6$, and $B_{12}$, E, and folic acid).

## RISK FACTORS
Inappropriate diet and overfeeding. Restricted exercise, sedentary lifestyle. Obesity. Chronic stress. Thyroid disease. Genetic predisposition. Reproductive activity in females, associated with vitellogenesis, egg production, and blood estradiol concentration, as estrogens can enhance hepatic lipogenesis.

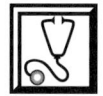

# DIAGNOSIS

## DIFFERENTIAL DIAGNOSIS
Hepatic lipidosis must be distinguished from other causes of hepatomegaly. Vascular congestion (passive congestion, portal hypertension in cardiovascular disease). Toxin-induced (mycotoxins such as aflatoxins, plants, pesticides, heavy metals, environmental toxins). Drug-induced (e.g. antifungals, volatile anesthetics, some antibiotics, corticosteroids, vitamin A). Hepatic masses (vascular anomalies, neoplasia or metastases). Storage or breakdown product accumulation (amyloidosis—rare in psittacines; iron storage disease—especially in lorikeets, Sturnidae, and Ramphastidae). Infectious hepatitis—bacterial (*Chlamydia psittaci*, *Mycobacteria* spp., Gram-negative hepatitis), viral (polyomavirus, herpesvirus, adenovirus, reovirus), and parasitic (trematodes, protozoa).

## CBC/BIOCHEMISTRY/URINALYSIS
Mild CBC changes (mild non-regenerative anemia, leukocytosis, or leukopenia) vs. inflammatory hepatopathies. Evidence of hepatocellular damage: AST elevation—Not consistently elevated in lipidosis, may be normal in advanced disease. Should always be interpreted with CK. GLDH—liver-specific mitochondrial enzyme increased with severe damage. Evidence of impaired hepatocellular function. Bile acids may be moderate to highly elevated (high sensitivity and specificity). Decreased synthetic function results in low total protein, albumin, coagulation factors, uric acid. Evidence of altered lipid metabolism. Lipemic serum (can interfere with biochemical testing), suspected association with dyslipidemia. Hypertrygliceridemia and hypercholesterolemia. Other findings: hypoglycemia (impaired gluconeogenesis, starvation, diabetes, chronic disease); hypokalemia (vomiting/regurgitation, polyuria).

## OTHER LABORATORY TESTS
Infectious hepatitis studies should be negative. Coagulation studies will be abnormal in advanced disease.

## IMAGING
CT—hepatic attenuation measured in Hounsfield's units could be valuable, but avian-specific values for hepatic lipidosis have not been studied. Radiographs demonstrate hepatic enlargement with compression of air sacs and over inflation of more cranial air sacs. Ascites may be present but without evidence of cardiomegaly. Ultrasonography should document an enlarged liver with smooth contours and diffuse hyperechoic parenchymal alteration. Increased visceral fat deposits and/or atherosclerosis may also be present.

## DIAGNOSTIC PROCEDURES
Endoscopic visualization of the liver by lateral (from caudal thoracic air sac into peritoneal cavity) or direct ventral approach will find an enlarged, rounded liver with pale to mottled yellow-tan parenchyma. Ultrasound-guided FNA of the liver in a study in Amazon parrots showed low hepatocyte yield due to hemodilution; however, samples were adequate for determining vacuolation as seen in hepatic lipidosis.

## PATHOLOGIC FINDINGS
Definitive diagnosis of hepatic lipidosis requires a liver biopsy in a stable patient (severe lipidosis/metabolic crisis is a

contraindication). Ultrasound-guided FNA of the liver may show evidence of vacuolation if hepatic lipidosis is present. Histopathology documents vacuolization and degenerative changes of hepatocytes, with areas of parenchymal destruction and inflammation. Overall prognosis correlated to severity of histopathology.

## TREATMENT

### APPROPRIATE HEALTH CARE
Stabilize and improve patient's physical condition and nutritional status. Treat secondary conditions that may be causing hepatic lipidosis. Formulate a plan for gradual weight loss (including increased activity) and improved nutrition. Limit stressors.

### NURSING CARE
Supportive care with administration of warmed fluids (avoid lactate and high glucose/dextrose infusions) (50–150 ml/kg/day maintenance plus dehydration deficit correction). Provide a warm incubator, including oxygen if dyspneic or depressed. Nutritional support and dietary changes are required.

### ACTIVITY
Sick patients should be rested in a quiet environment to minimize additional stressors. Once stabilized, activity should be increased as part of a weight loss program.

### DIET
Nutritional management/supplementation is critical for treatment; nutritional therapy should be species specific. Well-balanced diet—formulated diets with correct quantities of fresh fruits and vegetables facilitate management, supplemental vitamins can be added. Increased high-quality protein content to reduce hepatic lipid accumulation (unless concern for hepatic encephalopathy) using a recovery or neonatal psittacine formula such as Recovery Formula (Harrison's, Brentwood, TN; crude protein 35%); Exact (Kaytee, Chilton, WI; crude protein 22%); Juvenile hand-feeding formula, (Harrison's, Brentwood, TN; crude protein 26%). Match intake with resting energy needs (to inhibit peripheral lipolysis) but avoid excessive caloric intake. Gavage feeding may be necessary to restore nutritional balance in anorectic birds.

### CLIENT EDUCATION
Hepatic lipidosis is most often the result of chronic nutritional problems. Provide a dietary and nutritional supplementation plan according to the species. Discuss ways to increase activity (enrichment, flight, etc.).

### SURGICAL CONSIDERATIONS
Liver biopsy should only be performed in a stable patient without evidence of metabolic crisis, coagulopathy, or hepatic vascular congestion. Ascitic fluid should not be removed (protein reservoir) unless there is dyspnea or it is needed for diagnostic purposes.

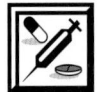

## MEDICATIONS

### DRUG(S) OF CHOICE
Managing hepatic lipidosis can be challenging, requiring a focus on addressing the underlying cause. Currently, there is limited evidence-based information regarding its treatment, and medications are often used on an empirical basis targeting specific clinical signs. Nutritional supplementation—vitamins (especially B complex, E, $K_1$, and biotin), essential amino acids, and lipotrophic factors (choline and methionine, 40–50 mg/kg q24h). Nausea should be treated with antiemetic drugs (metoclopramide, 0.5 mg/kg q12h; maropitant citrate 1 mg/kg SQ q24h). Severe hypoproteinemia may require supplementation to increase colloid oncotic pressure (hetastarch, 10–15 ml/kg/d IV or 5 ml/kg bolus). If present, hepatic encephalopathy can be managed with lactulose 150–650 mg/kg q12h. Estrogen-induced lipidosis from chronic egg laying can be suppressed with leuprolide acetate 100–1250 µg/kg IM q14d) or deslorelin implants (q2–6 m depending on response).

### CONTRAINDICATIONS
Avoid protein supplementation if there is concern for hepatic encephalopathy.

### PRECAUTIONS
Anabolic steroids inhibit bile flow and may increase the risk of hepatic lipidosis (shown in cats). Anabolic steroids and glucocorticoids also have an inhibitory influence on beta-oxidation. Tetracyclines (e.g. doxycycline) have lipogenic effects on hepatocytes in mammals and should be used with caution in birds with hepatic lipidosis.

### POSSIBLE INTERACTIONS
N/A

### ALTERNATIVE DRUGS
L-carnitine (100–250 mg/kg q24h) is a component of the mitochondrial membrane and is necessary for beta-oxidation. Although regularly used in feline hepatic lipidosis, its efficacy is debated. Antioxidant agents may be helpful in preventing hepatocellular oxidative stress and stabilizing membranes. NAC and SAMe 15–20 mg/kd q24h are glutathione precursors, sources of sulfur-containing amino acids, and may assist in hepatocyte lipid metabolism. SAMe is also a precursor of L-carnitine. Ursodeoxycholic acid 15 mg/kg q24h has cytoprotective, anti-inflammatory, antioxidant (via glutathione), and anti-fibrotic effects on hepatocytes. It is used to treat human and feline cholestatic disorders, but it is not useful for ameliorating triglyceride accumulation. Atorvastatin 10–20 mg/kg PO q12h. Statin drugs are the most effective class of hypolipidemic and anti-atherosclerotic drugs, further information is needed regarding the efficacy for hepatic lipidosis treatment.

## FOLLOW-UP

### PATIENT MONITORING
Assess progression of dietary changes and gradual weight loss at regular rechecks until stable. Reassess hepatic function/damage by hepatic biochemistry monitoring at rechecks. A recheck biopsy may be indicated after completion of therapy.

### PREVENTION/AVOIDANCE
Initiate a nutritionally balanced pelletized diet, avoiding excessive energy intake. Avoid excessive seed intake. Encourage exercise and play. Minimize stressors. Suppress chronic egg laying. Monitor for signs of hepatic disturbance.

### POSSIBLE COMPLICATIONS
Failure to correct diet and weight management can lead to worsening hepatic lipidosis with risk of death from liver failure and/or encephalopathy.

### EXPECTED COURSE AND PROGNOSIS
Hepatic lipidosis is a chronic disease and, following initiation of treatment and modifications, takes time to reverse. After resolution of any acute crisis with a guarded prognosis, outcome is dependent on the severity of lipidosis at presentation and the ability to maintain dietary and other changes to correct the underlying predisposing factors.

## MISCELLANEOUS

### ASSOCIATED CONDITIONS
Obesity, atherosclerosis, neurologic signs, diabetes mellitus, dyspnea, weakness.

### AGE-RELATED FACTORS
N/A

### ZOONOTIC POTENTIAL
N/A

### FERTILITY/BREEDING
Chronic egg laying and estrogenic influence can cause hepatic lipidosis.

(CONTINUED)

## SYNONYMS
Fatty liver syndrome, hepatic steatosis, fatty infiltration of the liver.

## SEE ALSO
Ascites
Atherosclerosis
Beak Malocclusion (Mandibular Prognathism)
Beak Malocclusion (Lateral Beak Deformity)
Chronic Egg Laying
Coagulopathies
Coelomic Distention
Dyslipidemia
Egg Yolk and Reproductive Coelomitis
Hemorrhage
Iron Storage Disease
Liver Disease
Neoplasia (Integument)
Nutritional Imbalances
Obesity
Pancreatic Diseases
Seizure
Sick Bird Syndrome
Thyroid Diseases
Toe and Nail Diseases
Undigested Food in Droppings

## ABBREVIATIONS
AST—aspartate aminotransferase
CBC—complete blood count
CK—creatine kinase
CT—computed tomography
FNA—fine-needle aspiration
GLDH—glutamate dehydrogenase
NAC—N-acetylcysteine
SAMe—S-adenosyl-methionine

## INTERNET RESOURCES
N/A

*Suggested Reading*
Abd El-Wahab, A., Chuppava, B., Dimitri, R., Visscher, C. (2021). Hepatic lipidosis in fattening turkeys: A review. *German Journal of Veterinary Research*, 1:48–66.
Beaufrère, H., Reavill, D., Heatley, J., Susta, L. (2019). Lipid-related lesions in quaker parrots (*Myiopsitta monachus*). *Veterinary Pathology*, 56:282–288.
Grunkemeyer, V.L. (2010). Advanced diagnostic approaches and current management of avian hepatic disorders. *Veterinary Clinics of North America: Exotic Animal Practice*, 13:413–427.
Lumeij, J. (1994). Hepatology. In: *Avian Medicine: Principles and Application* (ed. B.W. Ritchie, G.J. Harrison, L.R. Harrison), 522–537. Lake Worth, FL: Wingers Publishing.
**Author**: Mariana Sosa-Higareda, DVM

H

# HERNIA/PSEUDOHERNIA

## BASICS

### DEFINITION
Hernia is a defect in the coelomic wall with viscera or fat protruding through into a hernial sac. Pseudohernia is a thinning and distension of the entire coelomic wall without protrusion of coelomic organs through a hernial ring.

### PATHOPHYSIOLOGY
**Hernia**: Coelomic hernias have been reported secondary to trauma, organomegaly, and mass effect in the coelomic cavity. In turkey poults, umbilical hernias have been reported with bacterial infection and inflammation of the hernial ring, as well as congenital hernias. **Pseudohernia**: In females, suspected to be from high estrogen levels causing oviductal and follicular enlargement and possible hepatic lipidosis resulting in tension on the coelomic wall and ventral midline thinning of the aponeurosis. Coelomic wall muscle atony from alteration in calcium metabolism in chronic egg laying birds may also occur. Pseudohernia has also been described secondary to obesity and space-occupying coelomic masses.

### SYSTEMS AFFECTED
Dependent on the organs herniated, GI tract or oviduct obstruction and strangulation. If underlying organomegaly or mass effect, could have respiratory signs secondary to compression of air sacs, pelvic limb paralysis from compression of ischiatic nerve, elevated uric acid from renal parenchymal compression, or obstruction of ureters. Feather plucking over hernia or pseudohernia secondary to discomfort.

### GENETICS
N/A

### INCIDENCE/PREVALENCE
More than 19 publications or pseudohernias and hernias. Imaging or surgery is required to distinguish the two. No current information on incidence or prevalence.

### GEOGRAPHIC DISTRIBUTION
N/A

### SIGNALMENT
**Hernia**: Any species, sex, or age. Young turkey poults.
**Pseudohernia**: Female sex, species predilection in cockatoos (*Cacatua* species) and budgerigars (*Melopsittacus undulatus*).

### SIGNS
Respiratory signs (increased effort, tail bobbing), lethargy, fluffed, straining to defecate or lay eggs. GI signs including anorexia and fecal matting below vent, feather destructive behavior over hernia or pseudohernia, and exercise intolerance. Suspected cases have a pot-bellied appearance or protrusion of the coelomic cavity beyond coelomic distension.

### CAUSES
See risk factors.

### RISK FACTORS
**Hernia**: Trauma, congenital, organomegaly, or space-occupying coelomic mass resulting in straining, pressure, and herniation of coelomic wall.
**Pseudohernia**: Chronic hyperestrogenism, ovarian cysts, chronic egg laying, and oviductal enlargement, obesity with increased visceral fat (high-fat diet with sedentary lifestyle), or organomegaly (e.g. hepatic lipidosis).

## DIAGNOSIS

### DIFFERENTIAL DIAGNOSIS
Extra coelomic mass effect—lipoma or other subcutaneous tumor, cyst, anasarca. Coelomic space-occupying mass—lipoma, cyst, abscess/granuloma, neoplasia, effusion. Organomegaly causing space occupying displacement—hepatomegaly, oviductal impaction, egg bound, renomegaly. Respiratory signs from other coelomic disease (e.g. effusion), primary respiratory disease (ex. Teflon toxicity, pneumonia).

### CBC/BIOCHEMISTRY/URINALYSIS
No pathognomonic changes. Chronic reproductively active females with pseudohernias may have elevated calcium and globulins. Traumatic hernia may have elevated CK, AST, LDH from muscle damage.

### OTHER LABORATORY TESTS
Chromogen-based fecal occult test to detect gastrointestinal bleeding from herniation—false positive with consumption of high citrus fruits and animal products.

### IMAGING

#### Radiographic Findings
Coelomic distension visible on lateral view and widening of the hepatic silhouette on ventrodorsal view. Barium-swallow contrast radiography to help delineate GI tract.

#### Ultrasonography
Coelomic ultrasound to visualize if organs are within a hernia sac or coelomic cavity. Evaluation for organ enlargement such as ovarian cysts and oviductal enlargement or coelomic masses.

#### Advanced Imaging
Contrast enhanced CT to visualize organs and their location in the coelomic cavity without superimposition. Measurement of liver density though Hounsfield units for hepatic lipidosis.

### DIAGNOSTIC PROCEDURES
N/A

### PATHOLOGIC FINDINGS
Coelomic distension. Hernia: Traumatic—hemorrhage, hematoma, muscle damage, fibrosis or adhesions, herniated organ congestion and strangulation, organomegaly from fat or neoplastic infiltrate, mass effect from neoplasia, abscess, granuloma. Pseudohernia: Possible oviductal and follicular enlargement, hepatic lipidosis, abdominal fat accumulation; thinning and longitudinal splitting between coelomic muscle fibers.

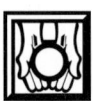

## TREATMENT

### APPROPRIATE HEALTH CARE
**Hernia**: stabilize, provide analgesia and nursing care as indicated. Minimize handling if critically ill.
**Pseudohernia**: May have reduced tolerance of stress due to compression of air sacs; minimize handling. If stable, outpatient management with dietary and exercise modifications. Surgical repair if indicated. Hormonal therapy for cystic ovaries and oviductal enlargement.

### NURSING CARE
Oxygen support if respiratory compromise from mass effect or coelomic distension. General supportive care for anorexia and dehydration: crystalloids (SQ, IV, IO) 50–150 ml/kg/day maintenance and correct dehydration, crop feeding 2–3 times/day.

### ACTIVITY
**Hernia**: Minimize activity until healed from surgical repair.
**Pseudohernia**: Limit activity if patient in respiratory distress. If clinically stable for outpatient management, advise daily activity and foraging to encourage weight loss.

### DIET
If on high caloric seed diet with table scraps, transition to pelleted diet supplemented with vegetables and some fruit. If obese and consuming large quantities of diet, reduce caloric intake. If anorexic, gavage feed parrot hand feeding formula such as Hagen Tropican® Hand-Feeding Formula (Rolf C. Hagen Inc., Mandsield, MA) or Mazuri® Handfeeding Formula (Mazuri Exotic Animal Nutrition, St. Louis, MO) 35 ml/kg crop volume.

### CLIENT EDUCATION
100% of diet should be offered though foraging to meet behavioral needs, as well as to encourage activity. Daily exercise should

be encouraged for weight management. Recommend bird room or control over locomotion (flight, ability to climb and run) for welfare.

## SURGICAL CONSIDERATIONS

**Herniorrhaphy**: Excision of the hernia sac and ring and simple closure if a traumatic or congenital hernia. If a mass is causing compression of air sacs or coelomic organs without metastasis, consider excision prior to coelomic closure. Coelomic surgery with metastatic disease is not indicated.

**Pseudohernia**: Coelomic wall repair if pseudohernia is affecting mobility and quality of life. Surgical repair considered unnecessary if no clinical signs are present due to repair resulting in compression of air sacs and tension on the coelomic wall, which has reduced muscle strength. Space-occupying oviduct can be removed (salpingohysterectomy) if significant compression of air sacs with surgical repair. Ovariectomy in adult birds is not recommended due to close association of vasculature. Surgical approach—elliptical incision to remove a portion of body wall. A prolene mesh can be secured through attachment to the pubis and 8th rib bilaterally, as well as the sternum, to reinforce the pseudohernia. Intubation with positive pressure ventilation advised for respiratory compromise from air sac compression.

## MEDICATIONS

### DRUG(S) OF CHOICE

**Hernia**: Meloxicam (1 mg/kg PO, IM, IV q12h), butorphanol (2 mg/kg IM, IV q2h) in parrots and chickens, hydromorphone (0.1–0.6 mg/kg IM q6h) or buprenorphine (0.1–0.6 mg/kg IM q6h) in raptors for pain.

**Pseudohernia**: GnRH agonist to down regulate and shrink reproductive tract through negative feedback. Can be used for ovarian cysts and reproductive neoplasm. Leuprolide acetate (100–1500 ug/kg IM q2–3 weeks). Deslorelin 4.7 or 9.4 mg SQ implant q3m.

### CONTRAINDICATIONS

Drug doses are based on select psittacine and raptor species. Doses for specific species should be verified (e.g. Columbiformes, meloxicam 2 mg/kg PO q12h). GnRH agonists in chickens due to food animal status.

### PRECAUTIONS

Follow meat and egg withdrawal times for medications used in chickens.

### POSSIBLE INTERACTIONS

N/A

### ALTERNATIVE DRUGS

Hepatoprotectants such as silymarin can be considered for birds with hepatic lipidosis and L-carnitine for those with lipomas.

## FOLLOW-UP

### PATIENT MONITORING

If sent home with a diet and weight loss recommendations, clients should routinely weigh their birds to ensure gradual weight loss. 14-day incision check after hernia or pseudohernia repair. Routine GnRH agonist treatment to prevent internal ovulation for birds that underwent salpingohysterectomy.

### PREVENTION/AVOIDANCE

Pesudohernia: Appropriate husbandry and handling of the bird can avoid chronic reproductive disorders such as being raised by its parents, avoid bonding with one owner, foraging, pelleted diets for parrots, environmental control for exercise and locomotion, and avoidance of sexually stimulating behavior such as hand feeing and petting below the neck. Once the condition has developed, routine GnRH agonists to downregulate the reproductive system.

### POSSIBLE COMPLICATIONS

**Hernia**: Reherniation if underlying disorder was not corrected (e.g. persistent straining, progressive mass effect or organomegaly).

**Pseudohernia**: Surgical reduction may result in respiratory distress due to compression of air sacs, compression of kidneys/ureters resulting in renal compromise, or compression of the ischiatic nerve resulting in pelvic limb paralysis. Salpingohysterectomy with incorrect GnRH agonist interval may lead to internal ovulation and egg-yolk coelomitis. Incisional or mesh infection/granulomas.

### EXPECTED COURSE AND PROGNOSIS

**Hernia**: Good prognosis if herniated organ has not become strangulated. Complete resolution following surgical repair is expected.

**Pseudohernia**: Good prognosis with long term husbandry modifications and weight loss prior to surgery.

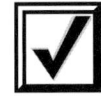

## MISCELLANEOUS

### ASSOCIATED CONDITIONS

**Hernia**: Herniation of intestines could result in ileus or obstruction leading to hematochezia, tenesmus, straining, and fecal matting.

**Pseudohernia**: Vent and tail base fecal matting may be present, feather loss or destructive behavior and ulceration of the pendulous coelomic cavity may occur.

### AGE-RELATED FACTORS

Pesudohernias are more likely to occur in older sexually mature female birds due to chronic estrogen exposure.

### ZOONOTIC POTENTIAL

Low zoonotic risk if mass effect causing hernia is from mycobacteria.

### FERTILITY/BREEDING

Herniation of oviduct or pseudohernia may result in salpingohysterectomy removing future reproductive ability.

### SYNONYMS

Abdominal hernia or pseudohernia

### SEE ALSO

Hepatic Lipidosis
Obesity
Ovarian Diseases
Neoplasia (Gastrointestinal and Hepatic)
Neoplasia (Reproductive)

### ABBREVIATIONS

AST—asparate aminotransferase
CK—creatine kinase
CT—computed-tomography
GI—gastrointestinal
GnRH—gonadotropin-releasing hormone
LDH—lactate dehydrogenase

### INTERNET RESOURCES

N/A

*Suggested Reading*

Barboza, T.K., Beaufrère, H., Chalmers, H. (2018). True coelomic hernia and herniorrhaphy in a yellow-crowned Amazon parrot (*Amazona ochrocephala*). *Journal of Avian Medicine and Surgery*, 32:221–225.

Forbes, N.A. (2016). Soft tissue surgery. In *Avian Medicine*. 3rd edn. (ed. J. Samour), 294–311. St. Louis, MO: Elsevier.

Kailey, A., Brandao, J., Mans, C. (2018). Lateral body wall herniation involving the oviduct in two psittacine birds. *Journal of Avian Medicine and Surgery*, 32:328–335.

Langlois, I., Jones, M.P. (2001). Ventral abdominal hernia associated with hepatic lipidosis in a Red Lory (*Eos bornea*). *Journal of Avian Medicine and Surgery*, 15:216–222.

Taylor, W.M. (2016). Pleura, pericardium, and peritoneum: The coelomic cavities of birds and their relationship to the lung-air sac system. In Current Therapy In *Avian Medicine and Surgery* (ed. B.L. Speer), 345–361. St. Louis, MO: Elsevier.

**Author**: Trinita Barboza DVM, DVSc, DACZM

H

# HERPESVIRUS (COLUMBID HERPESVIRUS 1 IN PIGEONS AND RAPTORS)

## BASICS

### DEFINITION
Enveloped DNA virus, classified in the *Mardivirus* genus, subfamily Alphaherpesvirinae, family Herpesviridae. First described in 1940. Isolated from pigeons and birds of prey. Pigeons are generally considered to be the primary host and are often responsible for spreading the virus to other species.

### PATHOPHYSIOLOGY
Viral infection leads to multifocal visceral necrosis, particularly in the liver and spleen. Upper respiratory tract and upper GI tract inflammation/ulceration may also be seen.

### SYSTEMS AFFECTED
Hepatobiliary, hemic/lymphatic/immune (spleen, bone marrow), GI (including pancreas), respiratory (upper respiratory tract), renal/urologic.

### GENETICS
Racing or fancy breeds of pigeons are anecdotally suggested to be predisposed.

### INCIDENCE/PREVALENCE
The prevalence of subclinical infection has consistently been found to be high in wild and feral pigeons in different parts of the world, with reported prevalence as high as 50–70%. Environmental survival time of this virus is unknown, but other alphaherpesviruses (such as Marek's disease) may remain infectious for 8 months at 71.6–77°F (22–25°C) and 3 years at 39.2°F (4°C).

### GEOGRAPHIC DISTRIBUTION
Distributed world-wide in free-ranging pigeons.

### SIGNALMENT
**Pigeons**: Squabs of either sex between 10 and 16 weeks of age are clinically affected. Adults that survive infection are typically asymptomatic unless immunocompromised.
**Birds of prey**: Any age/sex. Fatal disease, with mortality approaching 100%. Species predilections—falcons, owls, eagles, hawks, and buzzards.

### SIGNS
**Pigeons**: Depression, anorexia, conjunctivitis, diarrhea, neurologic abnormalities, rhinitis, oral/pharyngeal ulceration, dyspnea, or completely asymptomatic. Signs may last from a few hours up to 1 week. High mortality rate in young pigeons (1–3 months of age).
**Birds of prey**: Non-specific clinical symptoms, including weakness, anorexia, diarrhea, mild to severe depression, neurologic abnormalities. Clinical course of

disease is 24–72 hours in duration in most species; may range from 4–6 days in kestrels and 7–10 days in owls. Up to 100% mortality despite mild nature of clinical signs.

### CAUSES
**Pigeons**: Horizontal transmission via direct contact with infected birds. Free-ranging pigeons commonly infect domestic flocks. No vertical transmission reported. Carriers may infect offspring by feeding crop milk. However, squabs from uninfected parents can still become infected. In infected pigeon flocks, mature birds are typically asymptomatic carriers and intermittently shed the virus.
**Birds of prey**: Horizontal transmission via direct contact with infected birds. Consumption of infected prey species is the most likely source of infection in hawks, eagles, and owls. Scavengers may also be infected by ingesting meat of infected birds. Other free ranging non-birds of prey can also be infected with CoHV-1, usually via direct contact with infected birds.

### RISK FACTORS
**Pigeons**: Exposure to free-ranging infected pigeons or other infected species. Some breeds of pigeons may be predisposed due to inbreeding.
**Birds of prey**: Ingestion of infected pigeons or other infected prey species. Exposure to infected birds.

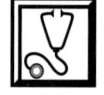

## DIAGNOSIS

### DIFFERENTIAL DIAGNOSIS
Depends on the clinical signs and signalment, but other bacterial, viral, fungal, or parasitic infections, toxin exposures, and nutritional deficiencies might cause similar broad/non-specific signs in a group of birds.

### CBC/BIOCHEMISTRY/URINALYSIS
Elevation in liver enzymes and bile acids may be seen.

### OTHER LABORATORY TESTS
The virus can be successfully isolated from necrotic foci using chicken embryos. PCR and immunofluorescence assays are available. PCR of oral swabs from live birds are an effective method of screening pigeon flocks for carriers. Loop-mediated isothermal amplification has been used for diagnosing infections in pigeons.

### IMAGING
N/A

### DIAGNOSTIC PROCEDURES
Endoscopic hepatic biopsies may be performed in more chronic presentations.

### PATHOLOGIC FINDINGS
Typically diagnosed postmortem. Multifocal, stellate, punctate, or spherical, tan lesions throughout the parenchyma of the liver, spleen, pancreas, bone marrow, kidneys, and intestinal wall. Lesions tend to congregate around reticuloendothelial tissues and hepatocytes, and eosinophilic intranuclear inclusion bodies are found in cells adjacent to necrotic regions, particularly in the liver. Upper respiratory tract and upper GI tract inflammation or ulceration (pharyngitis, esophagitis) may also be seen.

## TREATMENT

### APPROPRIATE HEALTH CARE
Treatment for this condition is primarily supportive care (particularly fluid and nutritional support).

### NURSING CARE
Affected birds often are unwilling to eat or drink, so treatment with fluid support (either IV/IO or SQ, depending on the patient's symptoms) and supportive feedings with a liquid diet may be necessary.

### ACTIVITY
N/A

### DIET
Supportive feedings with a liquid critical care diet may be necessary.

### CLIENT EDUCATION
Follow good biosecurity practices. Avoid mixing wild pigeons with domestic pigeons. Avoid feeding wild pigeons to birds of prey.

### SURGICAL CONSIDERATIONS
N/A

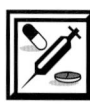

## MEDICATIONS

### DRUG(S) OF CHOICE
Acyclovir 80 mg/kg PO q8h for 10 days may reduce mortality during outbreaks (pigeons and raptors). Acyclovir 330 mg/kg PO q12h for 7–14 days has also been suggested as a treatment for raptors and owls affected by CoHV-1. There are no case reports detailing effectiveness of these treatments against CoHV-1 in either raptors or pigeons.

### CONTRAINDICATIONS
Injectable administration of acyclovir is not recommended. IM injections may cause severe muscle necrosis. IV injections may cause phlebitis and neurologic signs. Acyclovir is potentially contraindicated in dehydrated animals, animals with renal dysfunction, and

animals with neurologic deficits. However, the risk of administering treatment must be weighed with the risk of withholding treatment, as herpesvirus infection may cause all of the above symptoms.

## PRECAUTIONS
GI disturbances can occur with either injectable or oral administration. Vomiting is a known potential adverse effect at the 330 mg/kg PO q12h dosage of acyclovir.

## POSSIBLE INTERACTIONS
Unknown.

## ALTERNATIVE DRUGS
Treatment for secondary bacterial infections with broad-spectrum antibiotics may be useful. Treatment with non-steroidal anti-inflammatory pain medications to reduce inflammation and decrease discomfort associated with the viral infection may be indicated.

 FOLLOW-UP

## PATIENT MONITORING
Monitor for return to normal behavior and resolution of clinical symptoms.

## PREVENTION/AVOIDANCE
Minimize the contact of disease-free pigeons from wild birds. Avoid feeding pigeons (particularly wild pigeons) to birds of prey. Consider screening new birds with PCR prior to introducing them to breeding stock (especially if maintaining a closed flock). There are currently no commercially available CoHV-1 vaccines in the USA; however, vaccination against this disease shows promise at controlling outbreaks and preventing disease. Vaccine trials against CoHV-1 in pigeons was effective at reducing clinical signs, but not effective at preventing viral shed. Vaccine trials against CoHV-1 in kestrels and gyrfalcon hybrids was effective at preventing clinical signs and shedding of the virus.

## POSSIBLE COMPLICATIONS
N/A

## EXPECTED COURSE AND PROGNOSIS
Patients who recover will be chronic carriers for the rest of their life and may intermittently shed viral particles.

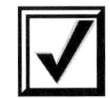 MISCELLANEOUS

## ASSOCIATED CONDITIONS
N/A

## AGE-RELATED FACTORS
N/A

## ZOONOTIC POTENTIAL
None.

## FERTILITY/BREEDING
Unknown.

## SYNONYMS
In pigeons, this disease is also known as pigeon herpesvirus or PiHV, Smadel's disease, ingluvitis of pigeons, inclusion disease, inclusion body disease, inclusion body hepatitis. In birds of prey, this disease is also known as herpesvirus hepatitis or inclusion body disease. Before sequencing studies on the virus, it was also known as falconid herpesvirus, strigid herpesvirus, and accipitrid herpesvirus.

## SEE ALSO
Adenoviruses
Herpesvirus (Duck Viral Enteritis)
Herpesvirus (Passerine Birds)
Herpesvirus (Psittacid Herpesviruses)
Liver Disease
Marek's Disease
Respiratory Infections in Backyard Chickens

## ABBREVIATIONS
CoHV-1—columbid herpesvirus-1
GI—gastrointestinal
PCR—polymerase chain reaction

## INTERNET RESOURCES
N/A

*Suggested Reading*
Gailbreath, K.L., Oaks, J.L. (2008). Herpesviral inclusion body disease in owls and falcons is caused by the pigeon herpesvirus (columbid herpesvirus 1). *Journal of Wildlife Diseases*, 44:427–433.
Phalen, D.N., Alvarado, C., Grillo, V., et al. (2017). Prevalence of columbid herpesvirus infection in feral pigeons from New South Wales and Victoria, Australia, with spillover into a wild powerful owl (*Ninox struena*). *Journal of Wildlife Diseases*, 53:543–551.
Pinkerton, M.E., Wellehan, J.F. Jr., Johnson, A.J., et al. (2008). Columbid herpesvirus-1 in two Cooper's hawks (*Accipiter cooperii*) with fatal inclusion body disease. *Journal of Wildlife Diseases*, 44:622–628.
Raghav, R., Samour, J. (2019). Inclusion body herpesvirus hepatitis in captive falcons in the Middle East: A review of clinical and pathologic findings. *Journal of Avian Medicine and Surgery*, 33:1–6.
Santos, H.M., Tsai, C.Y., Catulin, G.E.M., et al. (2020). Common bacterial, viral, and parasitic diseases in pigeons (*Columba livia*): A review of diagnostic and treatment strategies. *Veterinary Microbiology*, 247:108779.
Wernery, U., Joseph, S., Kinne, J. (2001). An attenuated herpes vaccine may protect Gyr hybrids from fatal inclusion body hepatitis: A preliminary report. *Journal of Veterinary Medicine, Series B*, 48:727–732.
Wernery, U., Wernery, R., Kinne, J. (1999). Production of a falcon herpesvirus vaccine. *Berliner und Munchener Tierarztliche Wochenschrift*, 112:339–344.
**Author**: Alicia McLaughlin, DVM, CertAqVet

H

# HERPESVIRUS (DUCK VIRAL ENTERITIS)

 **BASICS**

## DEFINITION

Duck enteritis virus (DEV) is caused by Anatid herpesvirus-1. It is a is an acute, sometimes chronic, highly contagious disease of ducks, geese, swans, and other Anseriformes of all ages, and causes considerable mortality. This disease has global distribution, as migratory waterfowl play a role in disease transmission within and between continents. The disease is characterized by vascular damage with subsequent hemorrhage and necrosis of internal organs, lesions in lymphoid organs, digestive mucosal eruptions, severe diarrhea, sudden death, and high flock morbidity and mortality (5–100%), particularly in older ducks. Adult ducks may die in good flesh. Infected ducklings frequently show dehydration, weight loss, blue beaks, and blood-stained vents. Mortality usually starts at 1–5 days after onset of clinical signs. Infection may also exhibit chronicity or latency. After primary infection has been established, DEV exhibits latent infection in trigeminal ganglia, and reactivation of the virus can occur that results in disease outburst. Recovered birds usually become disease resistant, but persist as carriers that excrete the virus in feces over a period of several months. Death rarely occurs in chronically infected flocks. Due to high mortality, condemnation, decreased egg production and hatchability, significant economic losses are associated with DEV. The Northern pintail (*Anas acuta*) and the mallard (*Anas platyrhynchos*) have been proposed as reservoir species for the virus.

## PATHOPHYSIOLOGY

DEV is a pantropic virus with rapid replication in many cell types and tissues, thereby leading to pathological lesions in many different organs. It has an incubation period of disease from 3–7 days. DEV replicates primarily in the mucosa of the digestive tract, then spreads to the bursa of Fabricius, thymus, spleen, and liver. The lining epithelial cells and lymphocytes of these organs are the principal sites for viral replication. Intranuclear viral inclusion bodies of DEV in various tissues are a hallmark finding in herpesvirus infections. Additionally, intracytoplasmic inclusion bodies in esophageal and cloacal epithelium can be seen with DEV. In adult birds, pathology is predominately noted in the digestive tract and other internal organs. In young birds, lymphoid organs, such as bursa of Fabricius and thymus, are targeted by the virus, inducing epithelial cell apoptosis and necrosis, causing depletion of

lymphocytes, and ultimately leading to immunosuppression. The resulting immune system suppression from DEV infection leads to secondary bacterial infections, such as *Pasteurella multocida*, *Riemerella anatipestifer*, and *Escherichia coli*. Transmission of DEV to susceptible birds is through direct contact with an infected duck, indirect transmission of virus from the environment, especially via a water source, or shed from latently infected or carrier birds.

## SYSTEMS AFFECTED

**GI**: Anorexia, weight loss, severe enteritis, watery or hemorrhagic diarrhea, soiled or bloodstained vent. Subsequent dehydration and increased thirst are suspected to be secondary to increased fluid loss. Multifocal ulcerations/necrosis of the mucosa and submucosa of the gastrointestinal tract, free blood in body cavities, and petechial and ecchymotic "paint brush" hemorrhages can be seen over the GI tract, pancreas, liver, and mesentery. Liver surface may have pale copper color with pinpoint hemorrhages and white foci, giving a speckled appearance. Eosinophilic intranuclear inclusions may be seen in epithelial cells of the GI tract, including the esophagus, cloaca, and liver. Occasional intracytoplasmic inclusions may be seen in epithelial cells of the esophagus and cloaca.
**Neurologic**: Depression, weakness, tremors of head and neck, prostration.
**Reproductive**: Drop in egg production (approximately 25–40% decrease) in laying hens. Adult domestic breeders tend to experience higher mortalities and persistent flock mortality.
**Cardiovascular**: Petechial and ecchymotic "paintbrush" hemorrhages on the heart, vascular damage throughout body, DIC.
**Respiratory**: Commonly have nasal discharge, may have a hoarse chirp, blue discoloration of beak reported in infected ducklings at 2–7 weeks of age.
**Ophthalmic**: Some birds may show watery ocular discharge, lacrimation, photophobia, conjunctivitis, diphtheroid plaques around the eyelids. Subsequently, some birds may refuse to drink, exacerbating dehydration. Eosinophilic intranuclear inclusions may be seen in epithelial cells of the conjunctiva and harderian gland. Occasional intracytoplasmic inclusions may be seen in epithelial cells of the conjunctiva.
**Integument**: Ruffled, unkempt appearance.
**Lymphatic/immune**: Cloacal bursa may be severely congested or hemorrhagic. Multifocal ulcerations/necrosis of the lymphoid tissues can be seen. Eosinophilic intranuclear inclusions may be seen in epithelial cells of the thymus, bursa, and spleen. Occasional intracytoplasmic inclusions may be seen in epithelial cells of the bursa.

## GENETICS
N/A

## INCIDENCE/PREVALENCE
The prevalence of latent infection is generally low in most Anseriformes except Northern pintails.

## GEOGRAPHIC DISTRIBUTION
Distribution of the virus includes North and South America, Europe and Asia. The majority of outbreaks in North America occur along the Atlantic flyway.

## SIGNALMENT
DEV is an acute, highly contagious disease of ducks, geese, swans, and other waterfowl of all ages and either sex. It is characterized by hemorrhage and necrosis in internal organs, sudden death, and high mortality, particularly in older ducks. Adult ducks may die in good flesh. Ducklings that are infected frequently show dehydration, weight loss, blue discoloration of beaks, and bloodstained vents.

## SIGNS

### Historical Findings
Poor feed efficiency, ill thrift, decreased growth rates, cachexia. Acute high and persistent mortality in waterfowl flocks, especially adult ducks in good flesh.

### Physical Examination Findings
May include inability to stand, weakness, depression, light sensitivity, inappetence, extreme thirst, ataxia, nasal discharge, soiled vent, watery or hemorrhagic diarrhea, blue beaks, bloodstained vent, acute drop in egg production of hens. An ulcerative "cold sore" lesion may be seen under the tongue.

## CAUSES
Anatid herpesvirus 1. Direct contact from infected to susceptible birds. Indirect contact with a contaminated environment.

## RISK FACTORS
Water seems to be a natural route of viral transmission. Outbreaks frequent in duck flocks with access to bodies of water cohabitated with free-living waterfowl. Carrier condition suspected in wild ducks, especially Northern pintails. Recovered birds may become latently infected carriers and may shed the virus periodically.

 **DIAGNOSIS**

## DIFFERENTIAL DIAGNOSIS

### Differentiating Similar Signs
DEV can be presumptively diagnosed based on clinical history and lesions. Lesions include multifocal ulcerations/necrosis of the mucosa and submucosa of the GI tract and lymphoid tissues, free blood in body cavities,

petechial and ecchymotic "paintbrush" hemorrhages on the heart, liver, pancreas, mesentery, and other organs. The cloacal bursa may be severely congested or hemorrhagic. Eosinophilic intranuclear inclusions may be seen in epithelial cells of the GI tract, thymus, bursa, spleen, esophagus, cloaca, liver, conjunctiva, and harderian gland. Occasional intracytoplasmic inclusions are also seen in the epithelial cells of the conjunctiva, esophagus, bursa, and cloaca. Definitive diagnosis is via viral isolation, viral detection molecular techniques, and PCR. Serologic tests are not useful for diagnosis in acute infections.

### Differentiating Causes
Diagnostic testing when indicated (e.g. viral PCR, biopsy sampling, serology, bacterial culture and sensitivity, mycobacterial and fungal cultures, Gram stain, and necropsy). Differential diagnoses may include duck viral hepatitis, pasteurellosis, other bacterial infection (mycoplasmosis, staphyloccosis, colibacillosis), necrotic and hemorrhagic enteritis, trauma, toxicosis, other viral infection (Newcastle disease, avian influenza, fowlpox), nutritional deficiencies (calcium–phosphorus imbalance, rickets). Differential diagnoses for mass mortality in waterfowls include avian cholera (*Pasteurella multocida*), botulism, Newcastle disease, and avian influenza. With DEV, typically only Anseriformes are affected and other species are spared, which is not the case with other causes of mass mortality.

### CBC/BIOCHEMISTRY/URINALYSIS
Leukocytosis may occur with secondary or concurrent systemic infection. Anemia seen with severe GI ulceration and bleeding. Hypoglycemia seen with prolonged anorexia and sepsis.

### OTHER LABORATORY TESTS
**Cytology**: Eosinophilic intranuclear inclusions may be seen in the epithelial cells of the GI tract, thymus, bursa, spleen esophagus, cloaca, liver, conjunctiva, and harderian gland, and occasional intracytoplasmic inclusion scattered in epithelial cells of the conjunctiva, esophagus, bursa, and cloaca. Occasional intracytoplasmic inclusions may be seen in epithelial cells of the conjunctiva.
**Other**: Viral isolation from liver, spleen, or kidney tissues. Conventional or quantitative real-time PCR. Serology has little diagnostic value.

### IMAGING
Survey radiographs may be normal, but may have changes should there be secondary infections affecting the GI tract, or disease affecting the liver, spleen, or other organs. Contrast radiography may be used to distinguish dilated intestinal loops from intestinal thickening seen in mycobacteriosis. Coelomic ultrasound may reveal free blood in the coelomic cavity or within organ structures. The GI tract and coelom may be evaluated endoscopically. Ulcerations and necrosis of the mucosa, submucosa, petechial or ecchymotic "paintbrush" lesions may be seen over the thoracic and coelomic organs. The cloacal bursa may be severely congested or hemorrhagic.

### DIAGNOSTIC PROCEDURES
N/A

### PATHOLOGIC FINDINGS
Hepatic necrosis and necrosis in multiple other organs with the presence of intranuclear inclusion bodies. Little or no inflammatory response is typically seen with acute and peracute disease.

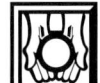 TREATMENT

### APPROPRIATE HEALTH CARE
The degree of nursing care needed is dependent on severity of disease. The disease is typically peracute and birds die before treatment can be initiated.

### NURSING CARE
Non-debilitated patients with mild lesions or symptoms may be treated on an outpatient basis if hydrated and eating well on their own, but should be kept isolated. Supportive care may be needed for anorexic, dehydrated, and/or debilitated patients, including fluids (SQ, IV, or IO), easily digestible nutrition, including gavage feeding in cases of inappetence, gastroprotectant medications in cases of GI ulceration and hemorrhage, antimicrobial and/or antimycotic medications as indicated to treat any concurrent secondary infections, and heat support for birds experiencing weight loss or negative energy balance.

### ACTIVITY
Most birds with this condition may be allowed to determine their own level of activity.

### DIET
Patients may be offered their normal diet. In cases of anorexia, weight loss, or negative energy balance, gavage feedings of easily digestible nutrition are recommended.

### CLIENT EDUCATION
Clients should be educated on disinfection protocols of contaminated areas and appropriate biosecurity practices. Avoid contact with wild, free-flying birds and water sources that are shared with wild waterfowl populations. Any underlying husbandry or diet deficiencies should be addressed.

### SURGICAL CONSIDERATIONS
N/A

 MEDICATIONS

### DRUG(S) OF CHOICE
May use analgesia when inappetence or dysphagia is present, including meloxicam (1 mg/kg PO q12h). May use gastroprotectant medications when GI ulceration is present, including famotidine (0.5 mg/kg PO q12–24h), omeprazole (0.5–1 mg/kg PO q12–24h), sucralfate (30 mg/kg PO q8–12h), and/or barium (20 ml/kg PO q24h). Bacterial—appropriate antibiotic therapy based on culture and sensitivity. Mycotic—appropriate antimycotic therapy based on culture and sensitivity. Parasite—appropriate antiparasitic therapy based on parasite identification. Antiviral against herpesviruses (e.g. aciclovir) may be tried in individual waterfowl patients.

### CONTRAINDICATIONS
Caution with use of non-steroidal anti-inflammatory medications with GI ulceration.

### PRECAUTIONS
Nystatin should not be given in cases of suspected GI ulceration, as this may result in absorption-dependent toxicity. A fecal cytology or fecal occult blood test may help to identify this condition, particularly in patients with anemia.

### POSSIBLE INTERACTIONS
N/A

### ALTERNATIVE DRUGS
N/A

 FOLLOW-UP

### PATIENT MONITORING
If inappetence, anorexia, dehydration, anemia, or significant weight loss occurs, hospitalize patient for supportive care and treatment, and obtain appropriate diagnostics. In cases of severe debilitation, severe morbidity, and latently infected individuals that may still spread disease, humane euthanasia should be considered. A closed flock policy should be enforced.

### PREVENTION/AVOIDANCE
Vaccination may be available and has been used in outbreaks in the past and in commercial duck production.

### POSSIBLE COMPLICATIONS
See Pathophysiology and Systems Affected sections.

## EXPECTED COURSE AND PROGNOSIS

Duck enteritis virus has no treatment and has a mortality rate of 5–100%. Recovered birds can become latently infected carriers and may shed the virus periodically. Immunization of breeders and ducklings with live attenuated vaccines can be performed in available countries, but chance of infection is still possible and it may not be effective in all species of ducks and water fowl.

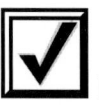

## MISCELLANEOUS

### ASSOCIATED CONDITIONS

Latently infected or carrier birds can intermittently continue to shed the virus. Secondary bacterial, mycotic, and parasitic infections may be found, due to suppression of the immune system.

### AGE-RELATED FACTORS

See Signalment section.

## ZOONOTIC POTENTIAL

DEV is not considered infectious to humans. However, it is possible for secondary bacterial, mycotic, parasitic, or other viral infections to be contracted with zoonotic potential.

## FERTILITY/BREEDING

Egg production in affected laying hens can acutely decrease. Eggs may be infected with DEV.

## SYNONYMS

Duck viral enteritis, Anatid herpesvirus-1, duck plague.

## SEE ALSO

Avian Influenza
Botulism
Bursa of Fabricius Diseases
Herpesvirus (Columbic Herpesvirus 1 in Pigeons and Raptors)
Herpesvirus (Passerine Birds)
Herpesvirus (Psittacid Herpesviruses)
Orthoavulaviruses
Pasteurellosis
Regurgitation and Vomiting

Respiratory Distress
Rhinitis and Sinusitis

## ABBREVIATIONS

DEV—duck enteritis virus
DIC—disseminated intravascular coagulopathy
GI—gastrointestinal
PCR—polymerase chain reaction

## INTERNET RESOURCES

Michigan Department of Natural Resources. Duck virus enteritis: https://www.michigan.gov/dnr/managing-resources/wildlife/wildlife-disease/wdm/duck-virus-enteritis

*Suggested Reading*
Dhama, K., Kumar, N., Saminathan, M., et al. (2017). Duck virus enteritis (duck plague): A comprehensive update. *Veterinary Quarterly*, 37:57–80.
Pendl, H., Tizard, I. (2015). Immunology. In: *Current Therapy In Avian Medicine and Surgery*, (ed. B.L. Speer), 400–432. St. Louis, MO: Elsevier.
**Authors**: Hannah Attarian, DVM, and Anthony A Pilny, DVM, DABVP (Avian)

# BASICS

## DEFINITION
A range of passerine birds have been diagnosed with herpesviruses, including finches, weavers, starlings, canaries, and cardinals. Most of these viruses have not been officially classified. The name Passerid herpesvirus-1 (PHV-1) has been suggested for a virus associated with high morbidity/mortality outbreaks in finches and has been grouped with alphaherpesviruses based on DNA analysis.

## PATHOPHYSIOLOGY
Necrosis of the trachea, syrinx, and primary bronchus; conjunctivitis with intraepithelial focal necrosis and desquamation.

## SYSTEMS AFFECTED
Respiratory, ophthalmic (conjunctiva), GI.

## GENETICS
Unknown, but there may be a species prevalence.

## INCIDENCE/PREVALENCE
There have been several outbreaks of this virus in captive flocks in Europe and North America.

## GEOGRAPHIC DISTRIBUTION
Europe and North America.

## SIGNALMENT
All ages and sexes of birds may be infected. Many different finch species are susceptible to PHV-1, but Gouldian finches appear particularly susceptible to infection and have a higher mortality rate compared with other birds (> 99% in one reported outbreak). Society finches may be more resistant to clinical disease.

## SIGNS
Conjunctivitis—unilateral or bilateral with eyelids adhered shut. Dyspnea, with clicking noises on auscultation. Weight loss, lethargy, depression, difficulty eating/drinking, hepatomegaly, regurgitation, diarrhea, biliverdinuria, sudden death. Incubation period ranges from 10–14 days. Death typically occurs within 14 days of symptom onset; can also occur in asymptomatic birds. Mortality rates range from 25–100% depending on the species involved and outbreak reported.

## CAUSES
Horizontal transmission from exposure to infected birds. Outbreaks can occur from introduction of new birds into flocks with or without sufficient quarantine, and through fomite spread (one outbreak was spread by banding young birds after the aviculturalist handled birds in the quarantine facility).

## RISK FACTORS
Any disease that causes immunosuppression could predispose birds to infection; however, most birds that have died from PHV-1 did not have evidence of other clinical disease. Gouldian finches appear to have the highest mortality rate associated with this virus. Poor biosecurity practices can spread the virus throughout breeding facilities.

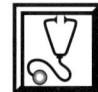

# DIAGNOSIS

## DIFFERENTIAL DIAGNOSIS
Bacterial infections (*Staphylococcus aureus*, *Chlamydia psittaci*, others); other viral infections (poxvirus, polyomavirus, eastern equine encephalitis virus); parasitic infections (*Sternostoma tracheacolum*, coccidiosis).

## CBC/BIOCHEMISTRY/URINALYSIS
Owing to the small size of passerine birds, blood diagnostic tests are seldom performed. An inflammatory leukogram or lymphocytosis may be seen on the CBC and enzymes elevation may be observed on the biochemistry.

## OTHER LABORATORY TESTS
Secondary bacterial infections with *Staph. aureus* may be seen in the conjunctiva. Electron microscopy can show aggregation of virus particles. PCR amplification and sequencing can confirm the diagnosis. Virus isolation has been attempted unsuccessfully.

## IMAGING
N/A

## DIAGNOSTIC PROCEDURES
Primarily diagnosed on postmortem examination.

## PATHOLOGIC FINDINGS
Emaciation, severe conjunctivitis, caseous yellow/white exudate in the trachea, bronchi, lungs, and/or sinuses, and splenomegaly/hepatomegaly with pinpoint depressed white foci on these organs. Histopathology findings include karyomegaly and cytomegaly with large, intensely basophilic intranuclear inclusion bodies throughout the respiratory tract, conjunctiva, proventricular glands, and lacrimal glands; hyperplasia of the bronchial epithelium; and hepatic and splenic necrosis.

# TREATMENT

## APPROPRIATE HEALTH CARE
Currently no effective treatments have been described for this pathogen.

## NURSING CARE
Affected birds often are unwilling to eat or drink, so treatment with fluid support (either IV/IO or SQ, depending on the patient's symptoms) and supportive feedings with a liquid diet may be necessary.

## ACTIVITY
N/A

## DIET
Supportive feedings with a liquid critical care diet may be necessary.

## CLIENT EDUCATION
Biosecurity and quarantine periods for finch flocks are very important. Ideally, do not mix Gouldian finches with other finch species, particularly society finches. Prognosis is poor to grave for affected birds.

## SURGICAL CONSIDERATIONS
N/A

# MEDICATIONS

## DRUG(S) OF CHOICE
No effective treatments have been described. Based on treatment of herpesvirus in other species, treatment with aciclovir 80 mg/kg PO q8h x 10 days may be helpful during outbreaks.

## CONTRAINDICATIONS
Injectable administration of aciclovir is not recommended. IM injections may cause severe muscle necrosis. IV injections may cause phlebitis and neurologic signs. Aciclovir is potentially contraindicated in dehydrated animals, animals with renal dysfunction, and animals with neurologic deficits. However, the risk of administering treatment must be weighed with the risk of withholding treatment.

## PRECAUTIONS
Gastrointestinal disturbances can occur with either injectable or oral administration of aciclovir.

## POSSIBLE INTERACTIONS
Unknown.

## ALTERNATIVE DRUGS
Treatment for secondary bacterial infections with broad-spectrum antibiotics may be useful. Treatment with non-steroidal anti-inflammatory pain medications to reduce inflammation and decrease discomfort associated with the viral infection may be indicated.

H

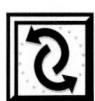 FOLLOW-UP

### PATIENT MONITORING
Monitor for return to normal behavior and resolution of clinical symptoms. Patients who recover will be chronic carriers for the rest of their life and may intermittently shed viral particles.

### PREVENTION/AVOIDANCE
Maintain closed flocks of passerines. Avoid exposure to free-ranging passerines. Quarantine new birds for at least 4 weeks before introducing them to flocks. Avoid housing Gouldian finches with other finch species, particularly society finches. No vaccine is currently available.

### POSSIBLE COMPLICATIONS
N/A

### EXPECTED COURSE AND PROGNOSIS
Mortality rate may be high with herpesviral infections in passerine birds.

 MISCELLANEOUS

### ASSOCIATED CONDITIONS
N/A

### AGE-RELATED FACTORS
N/A

### ZOONOTIC POTENTIAL
None.

### FERTILITY/BREEDING
Unknown.

### SYNONYMS
Finch cytomegalovirus (may be obsolete term).

### SEE ALSO
Herpesvirus (Columbid Herpesvirus 1)
Herpesvirus (Duck Viral Enteritis)
Herpesvirus (Psittacid Herpesviruses)
Marek's Disease
Ocular Lesions
Respiratory Distress

### ABBREVIATIONS
GI—gastrointestinal
PCR—polymerase chain reaction
PHV-1—Passerid herpesvirus 1

### INTERNET RESOURCES
N/A

*Suggested Reading*
Greenacre, C.B. (2005). Viral diseases of companion birds. *Veterinary Clinics of North America: Exotic Animal Practice*, 8:85–105.
Lee, L.F., Armstrong, R.L., Nazerian, K. (1972). Comparative studies of six avian herpesviruses. *Avian Diseases*, 16:799–805.
Paulman, A., Lichtensteiger, C.A., Kohrt, L.J. (2006). Outbreak of herpesviral conjunctivitis and respiratory disease in gouldian finches. *Veterinary Pathology*, 43:963–970.
Wellehan, J.F., Gagea, M., Smith, D.A., et al. (2003). Characterization of a herpesvirus associated with tracheitis in Gouldian finches (*Erythrura* [*Chloebia*] *gouldiae*). *Journal of Clinical Microbiology*, 41:4054–4057.
**Author**: Alicia McLaughlin, DVM, CertAqVet

# HERPESVIRUS (PSITTACID HERPESVIRUSES)

## BASICS

### DEFINITION
Herpesviruses are responsible for a variety of diseases in birds. Individuals that recover from their first infection will usually develop latent infections for prolonged periods of time. The most clinically important psittacid herpesvirus is the psittacid-alphaherpesvirus (PsAHV) type 1, which causes Pacheco's disease (upon first exposure) and internal papillomatosis (after chronic latent infection). A possible mutation of the gallid alphaherpesvirus 1 (GaAHV-1), the etiologic agent for infectious laryngotracheitis, has been involved in Amazon tracheitis disease (ATD). Other psittacid herpesviruses include PsAHV-2, which induces papillomas in African grey parrots, cacatuid-alphaherpesvirus 1 and 2 (unknown clinical significance, found in wild cockatoos), and PsAHV-3 and -5, whose genetic sequences are very similar, and both induce respiratory disease in Bourke's parrots, Eclectus, Indian ring-necked and Alexandrine parakeets. See also Appendix IV: Viral Diseases of Concern.

### PATHOPHYSIOLOGY
Pacheco's disease is an acute viremia that causes necrotizing lesions in multiple organs, including the liver, the GI tract, and the spleen. Peracute death is common, with a high mortality rate in naïve flocks, but this can vary with the species affected and the virus genotypes and strains. Birds that have survived an outbreak of Pacheco's disease can develop papillomas in their GI tract many years later, possibly following various stress factors. Depending on their size and location, papillomas can interfere with food ingestion, normal GI transit and absorption, and reproduction. Pancreatic, bile duct, and GI tract carcinomas have also been reported with PsAHV-1 latent infections. Amazon tracheitis causes an accumulation of necrotic debris in the trachea, which can result in dyspnea, occlusion, and possibly asphyxiation. PsAHV-3 and -5 cause acute dyspnea and death.

### SYSTEMS AFFECTED
Pacheco's disease and internal papillomatosis—GI, hepatobiliary, reproductive. Amazon tracheitis and PsAHV-3 and -5—respiratory.

### GENETICS
Unknown.

### INCIDENCE/PREVALENCE
Pacheco's disease outbreaks were frequent in the 1970s and 1980s until importation of wild-caught birds started to be more closely regulated. Birds imported 20–30 years ago are now more commonly seen with internal papillomatosis. Amazon tracheitis and respiratory infection by PsAHV-3 and -5 remain rare in psittacines.

### GEOGRAPHIC DISTRIBUTION
Pacheco's disease was first described in Brazil and is most commonly associated with South American parrot species. PsAHV-3 and -5 have mostly been reported in South-Eastern Asian and Australian species.

### SIGNALMENT
**Species predilections**: Varies with the genotypes and strains of the PsAHV-1. In general, macaws, Amazon parrots, cockatoos, and African grey parrots are highly susceptible. Conures are healthy carriers of some strains, but can be susceptible to others. Old World psittacines appear to be more resistant. Amazon parrots and Bourke's parakeets are susceptible to a virus related to the GHV-1. Bourke's parrots, Eclectus, Indian ring-necked and Alexandrine parakeets have shown clinical signs caused by PsAHV-3 and -5.
**Mean age and range**: Birds of all ages can be affected. However, internal papillomatosis generally occurs in older birds.
**Predominant sex**: Unknown.

### SIGNS

#### Historical Findings
Pacheco's disease—sudden death, lethargy, anorexia, regurgitation, green to yellow diarrhea, neurologic signs. Internal papillomatosis—chronic weight loss, regurgitation, infertility, papilloma in the oral cavity or in the cloaca; these can wax and wane in size. Tenesmus, blood in the droppings, passing whole seeds, dysphagia, wheezing. Amazon tracheitis—coughing, gasping, rales, anorexia, lethargy, nasal discharge, ocular discharge.

#### Physical Examination Findings
Pacheco's disease—severe depression; green staining of the cloacal feathers. Internal papillomatosis—poor body condition. Some papillomas can be observed directly or visualized by cloacoscopy. ILT/Amazon tracheitis—severe dyspnea. Mouth and beak can be bloodstained. Weight loss. Conjunctivitis. PsAHV-3 and -5—acute dyspnea.

### CAUSES
**Pacheco's disease**: Direct or indirect contact with infected birds that are shedding PsAHV-1 in their feces, their growing feather quills, and/or their pharyngeal secretions. Can occur in a closed collection after the virus is reactivated by stress in a latent carrier.
**Internal papillomatosis**: Reactivation of PsAHV-1 months or years after the primary infection. Stress and other causes of immunosuppression are suspected to play a role in this condition.
**Amazon tracheitis**: Direct contact with the respiratory secretions of infected birds (sick or latent carriers). Indirect infection also occurs (contaminated crates, litter spread in pastures, humans, etc.).
**PsAHV-3 and -5**: Unknown transmission but most likely through direct or indirect contact with infected birds.

### RISK FACTORS
**Pacheco's disease**: Mixing of birds of different origins, especially wild-caught specimens and/or from South America. Large quarantine facilities. Contact with a latent carrier of PsAHV-1. Indoor collections. High stocking density.
**Internal papillomatosis**: Previous non-lethal exposure to the PsAHV-1. Stress.
Amazon tracheitis: Recent introduction of new birds. Inadequate biosecurity.
**PsAHV-3 and -5**: Unknown.

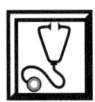

## DIAGNOSIS

### DIFFERENTIAL DIAGNOSIS

#### Pacheco's Disease
Causes of sudden death potentially associated with outbreaks: Bacterial infections causing potentially fatal hepatitis and systemic disease/septicemia—chlamydiosis, salmonellosis. Viral infections causing mortality: polyomavirus and circovirus (if young parrots are affected), adenovirus, paramyxovirus, bornavirus. Acute renal failure (gout)—high mortality, if failure in the water system. Toxicity. Causes of sudden death in one individual (not associated with outbreaks)—acute hepatic failure, heart failure, atherosclerosis, stroke, or aneurysm rupture. Trauma. Obstructive foreign body. GI perforation. Salpinx rupture/coelomitis.

#### Internal Papillomatosis
For the presence of papilloma(s): Poxvirus, papillomavirus (African grey parrots), cloacal prolapse (breeding behavior, enteritis, cloacitis), dystocia, fungal, parasitic (*Trichomonas*) or bacterial granuloma, abscess, neoplasia. For the chronic weight loss: Viral infections—bornavirus, circovirus. Mycobacterial infections. Bacterial infections: *Chlamydia psittaci*. Parasitic and fungal enteritis (*Macrorhabdus, Candida*). Chronic hepatitis ± pancreatitis. Nonobstructive foreign body. Neoplasia. Chronic renal insufficiency. Hepatic insufficiency. Atherosclerosis. Inappropriate diet quality and quantity/competition for food.

H

*Amazon Tracheitis and PsAHV-3 and 5*
Aspergillosis (*Aspergillus* spp.). Chronic respiratory disease (*Mycoplasma gallinarum* and *Escherichia coli*). Infectious coryza (*Hemophilus paragallinarum*). Infectious bronchitis (coronavirus). Avian influenza (orthomyxovirus). Newcastle disease (paramyxovirus). Swollen head syndrome (pneumovirus). Avian adenovirus. Chlamydiosis. Fowlpox (diphtheritic form). Parasitic tracheitis (*Syngamus trachea*). Tracheal foreign body. Trichomoniasis. Hypovitaminosis A.

## CBC/BIOCHEMISTRY/URINALYSIS
**Pacheco's disease**: It is rare that a bird with Pacheco's disease survives long enough to have blood collected. In experimental infections, birds develop leukopenia and a markedly increased AST.
**Internal papillomatosis**: No specific findings known. Birds with concurrent bile duct carcinomas can show elevated GGT.
**Amazon tracheitis and PsAHV-3 and -5**: Rarely performed.

## OTHER LABORATORY TESTS
PsAHV-1: Dead birds: swab of liver or spleen for PCR ± culture. Live birds: cloacal/oral swabs and blood for PCR. Amazon tracheitis: Tracheal and conjunctival swabs for PCR ± culture.

## IMAGING
**Pacheco's disease**: It is rare that a bird with Pacheco's disease survives long enough to have radiographs or ultrasound taken.
**Internal papillomatosis**: Depending on the papilloma location, radiographs could show proventricular and/or ventricular dilation and gas in the intestines (enteritis). Ultrasonography may show some abnormal findings in the liver in the case of a bile duct carcinoma.
**Amazon tracheitis**: Imaging is rarely useful for the diagnosis. Contrast tracheal radiographs could be used to differentiate ILT from a tracheal foreign body. Whole-body radiographs could be used to differentiate ILT from other diseases.

## DIAGNOSTIC PROCEDURES
"Vinegar test"—papillomatous tissue will turn white when acetic acid (5%) is directly applied. Biopsy of the papilloma. Biopsies for pancreatic and bile duct carcinoma.

## PATHOLOGIC FINDINGS
**Pacheco's disease**: May or may not have gross lesions. Generally in good body condition with ingesta in the GI tract. Enlarged, congested liver, with areas of hemorrhage and abnormal coloration (from green to brown). Enlarged discolored spleen. Multifocal congestion and hemorrhages within the kidneys, intestines, and brain. Necrotizing lesions in the liver, spleen, and

GI tract, but also many other organs, including the respiratory tract. Minimal inflammatory response. Intranuclear eosinophilic inclusion bodies (Cowdry type A).
**Internal papillomatosis**: Mucosal papillomas are typically raised, pink, and have a cauliflower-like surface. Papillomas can be unique or multiple in the GI tract. They may ulcerate and bleed. Microscopically, papillomas are formed of multiple fimbriae, each composed of a vascular core surrounded by a pseudostratified or stratified, cuboidal to columnar, epithelium. Bile duct carcinomas are multifocal and coalescing. They often replace the majority of the liver before the bird dies. They generally do not metastasize. Pancreatic duct carcinomas are grey, nodular, and coalescing.
**Amazon tracheitis**: Presence of blood, mucus, yellow caseous exudates, or a hollow caseous cast in the trachea. Microscopically, a desquamative, necrotizing tracheitis is characteristic of acute disease.
**PsAHV-3 and -5**: Pulmonary congestion and edema. Large syncytia and intranuclear inclusions in the bronchi and parabronchi (pneumonia), ± trachea, air sacs, infraorbital sinuses (less common).

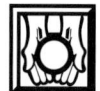

# TREATMENT
## APPROPRIATE HEALTH CARE
Birds presented alive with Pacheco's disease or Amazon tracheitis may require emergency inpatient intensive care. Birds with papillomatosis are generally outpatients.

## NURSING CARE
Birds presented alive with Pacheco's disease or Amazon tracheitis might be in shock and/or dyspnea and will require aggressive supportive care, including IO/IV fluid therapy and placement in an incubator with oxygen, if needed.

## ACTIVITY
N/A

## DIET
Assisted feeding might be required in some patients. Highly digestible pellets and formulas might be used in birds with internal papillomatosis.

## CLIENT EDUCATION
No treatment can cure a herpesvirus infection. The bird will remain a carrier if it survives the initial infection.

## SURGICAL CONSIDERATIONS
If they cause a significant problem to the bird, papillomas can be removed by surgery, cryosurgery, or staged cauterization with silver nitrate sticks (rinse with copious

amounts of fluids during the procedure). However, no technique prevents recurrence.

# MEDICATIONS
## DRUG(S) OF CHOICE
**Pacheco's disease**: Aciclovir: 80–100 mg/kg PO q8h for 10–14 days. 40 mg/kg IV/SQ/IM q8h, if cannot be given orally. 1 mg/ml in drinking water + 240 mg of medication/kg of food for 7 days (use after a single IM injection). Use of aciclovir might help reduce the morbidity/mortality, but will not cure the infection.
**Amazon tracheitis**: ILT vaccines may help reduce mortality in Amazon parrots, but more studies are needed.
**PsAHV-3 and -5**: Unknown.

## CONTRAINDICATIONS
For Pacheco's disease, any drug with potential hepatoxicity should be avoided.

## PRECAUTIONS
Aciclovir should be used with caution in patients with pre-existing renal conditions. IM injections are very irritating. Potential adverse effects include GI signs, leukopenia, anemia, and renal failure.

## POSSIBLE INTERACTIONS
Aciclovir use is contraindicated with nephrotoxic drugs and with zidovudine (antiretroviral drug).

## ALTERNATIVE DRUGS
Though other antiherpesviral drugs could potentially be used, none of them have been studied in birds.

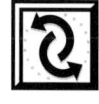

# FOLLOW-UP
## PATIENT MONITORING
Physical examinations as needed.

## PREVENTION/AVOIDANCE
For infection with PsAHV-1, avoid mixing birds from unknown sources, especially conures and other New World psittacines. PCR testing of all birds (but latent carriers can be missed). Strict hygiene and sanitation in quarantine. Vaccine is no longer available. Infection with GHV-1 and related viruses— strict hygiene. Quarantine all new birds.

## POSSIBLE COMPLICATIONS
Potentially life-threatening. Cloacal strictures following the surgical removal of papillomas.

## EXPECTED COURSE AND PROGNOSIS
Pacheco's disease is associated with a very high mortality. Papillomas vary from being insignificant to causing death after chronic

wasting disease. Amazon tracheitis are associated with mild to high mortality depending on the viral strains and other risk factors. Survivors of all these infections become latent carriers and pose a risk to other birds.

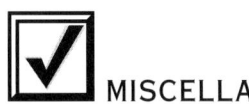 MISCELLANEOUS

### ASSOCIATED CONDITIONS
Bile duct, pancreatic, and GI tract carcinomas have been linked to the PsAHV-1.

### AGE-RELATED FACTORS
None.

### ZOONOTIC POTENTIAL
None.

### FERTILITY/BREEDING
Cloacal papillomas can interfere with breeding.

### SYNONYMS
N/A

### SEE ALSO
Adenoviruses
Anemia
Aspergillosis
Atherosclerosis
Avian Influenza
Beak Malocclusion (Lateral Beak Deformity)
Beak Malocclusion (Mandibular Prognathism)
Circovirus (Psittacines)
Circoviruses (Non-Psittacine Birds)
Cloacal Diseases
Coagulopathies and Coagulation
Foreign Bodies (Gastrointestinal)
Hemorrhage
Hepatic Lipidosis
Infertility
Iron Storage Disease
Liver Disease
Neoplasia (Gastrointestinal and Hepatic)
Nutritional Imbalances
Orthoavulaviruses
Papillomatosis, Cutaneous
Polyomavirus
Poxvirus
Renal Diseases
Respiratory Distress
Toe and Nail Diseases
Toxicity (Heavy Metals)
Trichomoniasis
Undigested Food in Droppings
Urate and Fecal Discoloration
Appendix 4: Viral Diseases of Concern

### ABBREVIATIONS
AST—aspartate aminotransferase
GGT—gamma-glutamyl transferase
GHV-1—gallid herpesvirus type 1
GI—gastrointestinal
ILT—infectious laryngotracheitis
PCR—polymerase chain reaction
PsAHV—psittacine alphaherpesvirus

### INTERNET RESOURCES
N/A

*Suggested Reading*
Henderson, E.E., Streitenberger, N., Asin, J., et al. (2022). Psittacid alphaherpesvirus 5 infection in Indian ringneck parakeets in southern California. *Journal of Veterinary Diagnostic Investigation*, 35:67–71.
Kaleta, E.F, Docherty, D.E. (2007). Avian herpesviruses. In: *Infectious Diseases of Wild Birds* (ed. N.J. Thomas, D.B. Hunter, C.T. Atkinson), 63–86. Oxford, UK: Blackwell.
Wildlife Health Australia. (2023). *Psittacid Herpesviruses in Birds in Australia: Fact Sheet.* Sydney: Wildlife Health Australia.
Tomaszewski, E.K., Wigle, W., Phalen, D. (2006). Tissue distribution of psittacid herpesviruses in latently infected parrots, repeated sampling of latently infected parrots and prevalence of latency in parrots submitted for necropsy. *Journal of Veterinary Diagnostic Investigation*, 18:536–544.
**Author**: Marion Desmarchelier, DMV, MSc, DACZM, DECZM (Zoo Health Management), DACVB
**Acknowledgements**: Shannon Ferrell, DVM, DABVP (Avian), DACZM

H

# HISTOMONIASIS

## BASICS

### DEFINITION
Avian histomoniasis is a protozoal infection caused by *Histomonas meleagridis*. It primarily affects poultry, especially chickens and turkeys, but also pheasants, chukars, grouse, peafowl, guinea fowl, and bobwhite quail.

### PATHOPHYSIOLOGY
*H. meleagridis* exists in ameboid and flagellate trophozoite forms. It reproduces by binary fission. Trophozoites shed in feces have a short survival time outside the avian host. Histomoniasis primarily targets the cecum and liver and uses a nematode (*Heterakis gallinarum*) or an earthworm as a carrier. The infection starts with ingestion of *Heterakis* eggs or earthworms containing juvenile heterakids. The parasites infest the caecal lumen, where the histomonads are released. From there, they invade the cecal mucosa, causing inflammation and subsequent damage to the liver, where they continue to reproduce. Foci of hepatic necrosis are visible about 10 days, appearing as white spots. Direct transmission within flocks through cloacal drinking is a well-known occurence in turkeys and chickens. Role of caecal microbiota has been demonstrated as essential for development of lesions.

### SYSTEMS AFFECTED
Gastrointestinal—chicken and turkeys.
Hepatobiliary (abscess)—chicken and turkeys.

### GENETICS
Certain genetic lines of poultry seem to have a different susceptibility to infection. A genetic line in turkey shows similar susceptibility to infection, but wild Canadian turkeys had a higher mortality rate and lower liver lesion rate.

### INCIDENCE/PREVALENCE
Varies geographically and among poultry populations. Prevalence may range from 1% to 30%. Outbreaks are reported frequently worldwide.

### GEOGRAPHIC DISTRIBUTION
Global, with higher prevalence in some warmer regions. Reports in wild birds have been made mainly in North America.

### SIGNALMENT
Poultry, especially chickens and turkeys, are most commonly affected, but all poultry can be affected. Chickens are often considered a reservoir for the parasite. Histomoniasis affects Galliformes almost exclusively, although rare cases in ostriches have been reported.

## SIGNS

### Historical Findings
Recent introduction of new birds or contact with infected birds. Previous exposure to turkeys or turkeys kept previously on the same field. Contact between turkeys and chickens. Clinical signs appear 1–3 weeks after infection. Mortality can reach up to 100% of the flock. Chickens are more resistant to histomoniasis than turkeys.

### Physical Examination Findings
Paleness or yellow discoloration of the comb. Affected birds are depressed, ruffled feathers, anorectic. Diarrhea with faecal material sulfur colored or containing flecks of blood and mucus.

### CAUSES
Infection with *H. meleagridis*.

### RISK FACTORS
Interactions with infected birds. Previous or current housing of turkeys in the same facility. Contact between turkeys and chickens. Presence of earthworms, which can act as intermediate hosts.

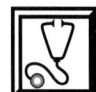

## DIAGNOSIS

### DIFFERENTIAL DIAGNOSIS
Coccidiosis, bacterial enteritis such as colibacillosis, necrotic enteritis, neoplasia.

### CBC/BIOCHEMISTRY/URINALYSIS
Elevated heterophils and monocytes. Leucocytosis. Anemia. Decreased uric acid. Transient rise in glycemia. Increased liver enzymes (AST, LDH). Decreased albumin and elevated globulin concentration.

### OTHER LABORATORY TESTS
*H. meleagridis* can be cultivated from cecal samples in infected carcasses.

### IMAGING
Not usually applicable. Liver or digestive abscess can be identified via ultrasound or CT.

### DIAGNOSTIC PROCEDURES
Necropsy and histopathological examination of affected tissues. Histopathology or cytology of cecal and liver tissues for identifying the parasite using PAS or silver stains. In vitro cultivation of cecal contents.

### PATHOLOGIC FINDINGS
Characteristic lesions in cecal and liver tissues, including necrosis and inflammation. The lumen of the ceca fills with a mixture of cecal contents, serous and hemorragic exudates, inflammatory cells, and necrotic debris. The concentric layer of this admixture forms a caseous central core. Foci in the liver appear as white spots progressing to gray

depressed area surrounded by a narrow rim of hemorrhage.

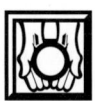

## TREATMENT

### APPROPRIATE HEALTH CARE
No treatments are currently approved to be used in poultry.

### NURSING CARE
N/A

### ACTIVITY
N/A

### DIET
N/A

### CLIENT EDUCATION
Avoid contact between chickens and turkeys.

### SURGICAL CONSIDERATIONS
N/A

## MEDICATIONS

### DRUG(S) OF CHOICE
There are no vaccinations or treatments available, since the use of imidazoles has been banned in all food-producing animals. Nitroimidazoles were generally effective for both prevention and treatment. Anthelminthic can also be used to decrease *Heterakis gallinarum* infection.

### CONTRAINDICATIONS
N/A

### PRECAUTIONS
N/A

### POSSIBLE INTERACTIONS
N/A

### ALTERNATIVE DRUGS
N/A

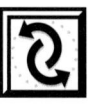

## FOLLOW-UP

### PATIENT MONITORING
N/A

### PREVENTION/AVOIDANCE
The best prevention is not to place turkeys on ranges inhabited previously by chickens or other game birds and to control earthworms. Range rotation is not practical as histomonads have tremendous survivability in *Heterakid* eggs (4 years or more). Flocks can be housed in deep stone or wire floored pens that reduce ingestion of eggs and earthworm. Anthelmintics can be used to remove *Het. gallinarum*.

## POSSIBLE COMPLICATIONS
Birds that survive several weeks become emaciated.

## EXPECTED COURSE AND PROGNOSIS
Mortality in turkey flocks can reach 80–100%.

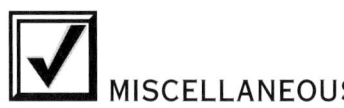 MISCELLANEOUS

### ASSOCIATED CONDITIONS
Co-infection with *Het. gallinarum*.

## AGE-RELATED FACTORS
N/A

## ZOONOTIC POTENTIAL
N/A

## FERTILITY/BREEDING
Egg drop is common.

## SYNONYMS
Blackhead disease.

## SEE ALSO
Enteritis and Gastritis
Helminthiasis (Gastrointestinal)
Liver Disease

## ABBREVIATIONS
AST—aspartate aminotransferase
CT—computed tomography
LDH—lactate dehydrogenase
PAS—periodic acid-Schiff

## INTERNET RESOURCES
N/A

*Suggested Reading*
Beer, L.C., Petrone-Garcia, V.M., Graham, B.D., (2022). Histomonosis in poultry: A comprehensive review. *Frontiers in Veterinary Science*, 9:880738.
**Author**: Minh Huynh, DVM, MRCVS, DECZM (Avian), DACZM

H

# HORNER SYNDROME

## BASICS

### DEFINITION
Horner syndrome, or oculosympathetic paresis, is characterized by miosis, enophthalmos, and protrusion of the third eyelid, which is caused by a loss of sympathetic innervation to the eye.

### PATHOPHYSIOLOGY
Horner syndrome results from damage to the oculosympathetic tract that runs from the brain to the eye and adjacent structures (e.g. resulting from trauma, infection, or neoplasia). Lesions either involve the upper motor neurons or the pre- or postganglionic sympathetic lower motor neurons that supply the eye. Reduced sympathetic stimulation of the iris dilator muscle leads to miosis of the pupil. Reduced activity of the sympathetically innervated smooth muscles in the orbital rim result in enophthalmos and associated (passive) protrusion of the third eyelid. Lack of tonic contraction of the tarsalis muscle results in ptosis or drooping of the upper eyelid. Damage is usually unilateral.

### SYSTEMS AFFECTED
**Ophthalmic**: Unilateral miosis, enophthalmos, protrusion of the nictating membrane, and ptosis.
**Nervous**: Loss of adrenergic innervation of the smooth muscle of the eyelids and feathers.
**Integument**: Erection of facial feathers.

### GENETICS
N/A

### INCIDENCE/PREVALENCE
A rare condition. A study on prevalence of among birds admitted to a wildlife hospital in Australia revealed 25 of 30,777 admitted birds (0.08%) to be diagnosed with Horner syndrome. A study evaluating presence of Horner syndrome in raptors admitted to a bird of prey clinic in the USA revealed a prevalence of 0.43% (22/5128 birds).

### GEOGRAPHIC DISTRIBUTION
N/A

### SIGNALMENT
**Species**: Horner syndrome is more commonly diagnosed in wild birds. Affected species include rainbow lorikeet (*Trichoglossus haematodus*), scaly breasted lorikeet (*Trichoglossus chlorolepidotus*), yellow-tailed black cockatoo (*Calyptorhynchus funereus*), red-bellied parrot (*Poicephalus rufiventris*), lilac-crowned parrot (*Amazona finschi*), tawny frogmouth (*Podargus strigoides*), southern boobook (*Ninox novaeseelandiae*), laughing kookaburra (*Dacelo novaeguineae*), crested tern (*Thalasseus bergii*), crested pigeon (*Ocyphaps lophotes*), Torresian crow (*Corvus orru*), grey butcherbird (*Cracticus torquatus*), eastern screech owl (*Megascops asio*), African spotted eagle owl (*Bubo africanus*), great horned owl (*Bubo virginianus*), snowy owl (*Bubo scandiacus*), boreal owl (*Aegolius funereus*), northern saw-whet owl (*Aegolius acadicus*), northern hawk-owl (*Surnia ulula*), merlin (*Falco columbarius*), Cooper's hawk (*Accipiter cooperii*), Northern goshawk (*Accipiter gentilis*), osprey (*Pandion haliaetus*), red-shouldered hawk (*Buteo lineatus*), red-tailed hawk (*Buteo jamaicensis*), and bald eagle (*Haliaeetus leucocephalus*).
**Mean age and range**: Birds with Horner syndrome appear more likely to be adult than subadult or juvenile.
**Predominant sex**: No sex predilection exists.

### SIGNS
Classic Horner syndrome is a clinical entity characterized by miosis of the pupil, enophthalmos with (passive) protrusion of the nictating membrane, ptosis or drooping of the eyelid, facial asymmetry (which is caused by unilateral ptosis and ipsilateral erection of facial feathers). Miosis may or may not always be present, and is therefore considered an unreliable marker of Horner syndrome in birds. Localization of the lesion responsible for Horner syndrome is based on history, clinical findings (including neurologic and ophthalmic examination), and pharmacologic testing. In most cases related to upper motor neuron involvement, other clinical signs (e.g. limb paresis) are present. Lesions at the postganglionic lower motor neuron level can involve peripheral branches of cranial nerves thereby resulting in cranial nerve deficits.

### CAUSES
In birds, Horner syndrome has mostly been associated with trauma (e.g. window strike, car accident). It has been diagnosed in birds in association with avulsion of the brachial plexus and pulmonary carcinoma. Other reported causes in dogs and cats include otitis media and neoplasia, although in half of cases no obvious cause is identified.

### RISK FACTORS
N/A

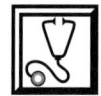

## DIAGNOSIS

### DIFFERENTIAL DIAGNOSIS
Mild anisocoria may be a normal finding in birds, and can therefore be difficult to interpret as a sole sign of Horner syndrome.

### CBC/BIOCHEMISTRY/URINALYSIS
N/A

### OTHER LABORATORY TESTS
N/A

### IMAGING
Radiographs are commonly obtained for affected birds to diagnose concurrent trauma. CT and MRI are recommended to identify anatomic lesions, such as neoplasia.

### DIAGNOSTIC PROCEDURES
Eye drops containing phenylephrine, a sympathomimetic drug, should alleviate signs of oculosympathetic palsy when denervation hypersensitivity has developed. Apraclonidine may be another accessible alternative that could be used. Damage to first or second order (but not to third order) neurons can be ameliorated by the topical application of cocaine, as this stimulates the release of sympathetic transmitters at the motor end plates of the intact third order neuron. As the iris in birds contains skeletal muscle fibers, response to phenylephrine can be diminished or suppressed in response to phenylephrine. Resolution of ptosis with phenylephrine is expected to be a more reliable indicator of Horner syndrome in birds, as composition and innervation of tarsal muscles in birds are similar to the mammalian eye.

### PATHOLOGIC FINDINGS
N/A

## TREATMENT

### APPROPRIATE HEALTH CARE
Supportive. Treatment of concurrent injuries. As trauma is a common cause of Horner syndrome, many patients will benefit from the use of NSAIDs (e.g. meloxicam) or other analgesic.

### NURSING CARE
Supportive care (assisted feeding, fluid therapy, heat supplementation) as needed for treatment of concurrent hypothermia, dehydration, or weakness.

### ACTIVITY
Birds with Horner syndrome often suffer from additional injuries that may warrant hospitalization and limited flight until injuries have resolved.

### DIET
N/A

### CLIENT EDUCATION
Horner syndrome implies significant neurologic trauma, and may be associated with a poor prognosis.

### SURGICAL CONSIDERATIONS
N/A

(CONTINUED)

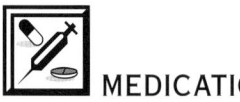

## MEDICATIONS

**DRUG(S) OF CHOICE**
N/A

**CONTRAINDICATIONS**
N/A

**PRECAUTIONS**
N/A

**POSSIBLE INTERACTIONS**
N/A

**ALTERNATIVE DRUGS**
N/A

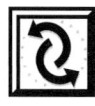

## FOLLOW-UP

**PATIENT MONITORING**
Repeated neurologic and ophthalmic evaluations may be required to monitor progress.

**PREVENTION/AVOIDANCE**
N/A

**POSSIBLE COMPLICATIONS**
N/A

**EXPECTED COURSE AND PROGNOSIS**
Horner syndrome in wild birds generally confers a poor prognosis for recovery and should be considered a significant finding during the neurologic exam. A study in birds of prey recorded complete resolution in 5/22 birds (23%). Signs resolved on average after 19.4 days (range 5–36 days) post admission. Overall prognosis for birds of prey with Horner syndrome appeared poorer than for

the reference population, possibly due to these birds having sustained more severe trauma, which would significantly decrease their chances for survival and release into the wild.

## MISCELLANEOUS

**ASSOCIATED CONDITIONS**
Concurrent traumatic injuries are reported in a large number of patients, and may include orthopedic trauma (fractures, luxations), other neurologic deficits (e.g. altered demeanor, wing paresis/paralysis, pelvic limb paresis, ataxia, vestibular syndrome), ocular trauma, wounds or hematomas, and signs of shock (dehydration, weakness, hypothermia).

**AGE-RELATED FACTORS**
N/A

**ZOONOTIC POTENTIAL**
N/A

**FERTILITY/BREEDING**
N/A

**SYNONYMS**
Oculosympathetic paresis, oculosympathetic palsy.

**SEE ALSO**
Neoplasia (Neurological)
Neurologic (Non-Traumatic Diseases)
Neurologic (Trauma)
Ocular Lesions
Trauma

**ABBREVIATIONS**
CT—computed tomography
MRI—magnetic resonance imaging
NSAIDs—non-steroidal anti-inflammatory drugs

**INTERNET RESOURCES**
N/A

*Suggested Reading*
Gancz, A.Y., Lee, S., Higginson, G., et al. (2006). Horner's syndrome in an eastern screech owl (Megascops asio). *Veterinary Record*, 159(10), 320.
Gancz, A.Y., Malka, S., Sandmeyer, L., et al. (2005). Horner's syndrome in a red-bellied parrot (*Poicephalus rufiventris*). *Journal of Avian Medicine and Surgery*, 19:30–34.
Hill, A.G. (2018). A retrospective study of Horner syndrome in Australian wild birds, 2010–2016. *Journal of Avian Medicine and Surgery*, 32:115–121.
LaChance, M.K., Fitzgerald, G., Lair, S., Desmarchelier, M.R. (2019). Horner syndrome in birds of prey. *Journal of Avian Medicine and Surgery*, 33:381–387.
Latas, P.J., Durham, B., Mansfield, S., Miller, R.L. (2021). A case study of complicated Horner's syndrome in a fledgling wild naturalized lilac-crowned parrot. *Journal of Wildlife Rehabilitation*, 41:18–22.
McLelland, J.M., McLelland, D.J., Massy-Westropp, N., et al. (2020). Horner syndrome with ipsilateral wing paresis in a wild, juvenile yellow-tailed black cockatoo (*Calyptorhynchus funereus*). *Journal of Avian Medicine and Surgery*, 34:186–191.
Williams, D.L., Cooper, J.E. (1994). Horner's syndrome in an African spotted eagle owl (*Bubo africanus*). *Veterinary Record*, 134:64–64.
**Authors**: Yvonne R. A. van Zeeland, DVM, MVR, PhD, DECZM (Avian, Small Mammal), and Nico Schoemaker, DVM, PhD, DECZM (Small Mammal, Avian)

H

# HYPERURICEMIA

 **BASICS**

## DEFINITION

Birds are uricotelic. End products of nitrogen metabolism excreted in bird urine include urates, ammonia, urea, creatinine, amino acids, and others. Uric acid (UA) is the main end product of nitrogen metabolism, representing 80% or more of the nitrogen excreted. Hyperuricemia is defined as any plasma UA concentration higher than the upper reference limit for the species. In birds, the theoretical limit of solubility of sodium urate is estimated to be 600 µmol/l (10 mg/dl). In chickens, the UA renal tubule transport system does not appear to become saturated until plasma UA levels exceed 60 mg/dl.

## PATHOPHYSIOLOGY

As the final breakdown product of dietary or endogenous purines, UA is generated by xanthine dehydrogenase (xanthine oxidase). The liver is the primary source of UA. UA is also synthesized in the kidneys, intestines, and pancreas. UA is eliminated by active tubular secretion by the cortical or reptilian nephrons. It is produced in supersaturated concentration in urine and excreted as mucopolysaccharides microspheres. Kidneys regulate UA by reabsorption, secretion, and postsecretory absorption in the proximal convoluted tubules. UA excretion is largely independent of glomerular filtration, water resorption, and urine flow rate. Levels may elevate when glomerular filtration decreases by more than 70–80% (severe dehydration) or when large numbers of renal tubules have been compromised. Birds cannot oxidize UA into the more soluble compound allantoin due to the absence of the enzyme uricase.

## SYSTEMS AFFECTED

Musculoskeletal (articular gout), renal.

## GENETICS

N/A

## INCIDENCE/PREVALENCE

N/A

## GEOGRAPHIC DISTRIBUTION

N/A

## SIGNALMENT

**Species**: UA levels can show great variability between species. Carnivorous and piscivorous birds, such as raptors and penguins, show a marked postprandial hyperuricemia in the first hours after ingestion of prey.
**Mean age and range**: A significant decreasing trend was noted with increasing age in UA. The higher levels found in nestlings were theorized to be the result of increased protein synthesis. In the orange-winged Amazon parrot (*Amazona amazonica*), UA and urea nitrogen were significantly higher in juvenile birds.
**Predominant sex**: In the collared scops owls (*Otus lettia*), UA levels were significantly higher among males than females.

## SIGNS

### General Comments

Affected birds are often asymptomatic until gout occurs, or renal function is sufficiently decreased.

### Historical Findings

Is the bird molting? Uric acid levels tend to be lower when there is higher physiologic demand for protein such as the time of molting in waterfowl. Prolonged starvation.

### Physical Examination Findings

Evidence of dehydration. Signs of articular gout include pain and swelling in the synovial joints; nodules may appear white because of tophi formation.

## CAUSES

The causes of hyperuricemia can be multifactorial but fall into two main categories: (1) Reduced renal tubular secretion of UA: Prolonged dehydration, volume depletion causes slight elevations in UA. Hypothermia. Renal disease. Damage of the proximal convoluted tubules, nephrosis. Any potential cause of nephritis such as nephrotrophic strains of infectious bronchitis virus, influenza virus, avian nephritis virus, chicken astrovirus, cryptosporidium, bacteria. Nephrotoxin exposure causing renal tubular damage: NSAIDs (e.g. diclofenac, ketoprofen), mycotoxins (e.g. oosporein, ochratoxin A), heavy metals (e.g. lead and zinc toxicity), allopurinol, organophosphate poisoning. There are a number of nutritional imbalances that can damage the kidneys, including chronic hypovitaminosis A, hypervitaminosis A, D, excess dietary calcium, high dietary fat, dietary sodium and potassium imbalances, dietary magnesium and phosphorus deficiency, as well as excess of trace elements (e.g. zinc and sodium bicarbonate supplementation). Obstructive post-renal disease. (2) Excessive production of UA: Physiologic hyperuricemia: UA levels will vary directly with dietary protein level, total food intake, and bodily requirements for amino acids. Carnivorous birds show a normal, marked postprandial hyperuricemia within the first hours after ingestion of prey. Raptors demonstrate a decline of plasma UA concentration between 8 and 23 hours after feeding. This change has also been demonstrated in broiler chickens and penguins. Flight is associated with protein catabolism and an increase in UA. Premigratory preparation in migratory birds is also associated with a rise in UA levels due increased intake of dietary protein and subsequent deamination of dietary protein for storage as fat as well as the catabolism of body protein during fasting. Prolonged starvation may also lead to increased protein catabolism (phase 3 starvation) and increased uric acid levels. Pathologic hyperuricemia can be seen with long-term, excessive high dietary protein levels. Starvation. High-protein or high-purine diet.

## RISK FACTORS

Medical conditions: Renal disease, duration of hyperuricemia—prolonged elevations increase the risk of gout developing, glomerular filtration rate, conditions that reduce include blood loss, severe dehydration, water deprivation, shock. Mycotoxicosis. Renal tubular disease. Starvation. Medications: Nephrotoxins—NSAIDs, intravenous contrast media. Environmental factors: Nutritional imbalances—excessive dietary protein, excessive dietary purines, high dietary protein + high dietary calcium, vitamin A deficiency, exposure to insecticides.

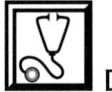 **DIAGNOSIS**

## DIFFERENTIAL DIAGNOSIS

Lipemia can cause an artifactual elevation in UA measured by the photometric uricase method. Blood samples taken via nail trim of a foot soiled with droppings can also reveal falsely elevated UA levels.

## CBC/BIOCHEMISTRY/URINALYSIS

**CBC**: Look for signs of infection or inflammation.
**Biochemistry panel**: UA is an insensitive renal function test. Normal values do not mean that kidney function is normal. Slight or mild elevations are observed in dehydrated birds because of an increase in solute concentration: As most UA is secreted from the proximal tubules and not filtered, UA levels are not affected by moderate changes in the glomerular filtration rate. In a study of dehydrated chickens, UA levels increased after 24–48 hours of water restriction but only in birds allowed free access to food. Interference with uric acid analysis on the Vetscan® (Zoetis, Parsippany, NJ) on pigmented plasma from species with canthaxanthines (e.g. flamingos) may limit to use of this analyzer in these species. Moderate to severe elevations can be caused by renal disease or a physiologic postprandial increase in carnivorous birds. UA levels do not increase significantly until there is extensive renal tubular damage and glomerular filtration decreases by more than 70–80%. UA increases and peaks approximately 2 hours after ingesting a natural meal. Levels remain elevated for at least 12 hours after feeding.

Raptors demonstrate a decline of plasma UA concentration between 8 and 23 hours after feeding. Isoflurane anesthesia resulted in decreased UA values when compared with controls in American kestrels (*Falco sparverius*). Confirm persistent hyperuricemia by obtaining a fasting UA after the patient has been clinically stabilized and rehydrated. Elevations in BUN can be seen with dehydration in birds, or after high-protein meals in carnivorous birds. GI bleeding has not been found to increase plasma uric acid in birds. In vulture species studied, the urea to UA ratio has been described as a useful tool for evaluating both prerenal azotemia and renal damage. Increases in creatinine have been linked to dehydration in pigeons. Electrolytes: In birds with gout induced by sodium bicarbonate intoxication, hypernatremia, hyperuricemia, hypokalemia, and hypochloremia were common findings among exposed birds. Moderate metabolic acidosis can be associated with hyperuricemia and can be exacerbated by damage to the proximal convoluted tubules. While UA is a weak acid and does not in itself cause acidemia, hyperuricemia is associated with decreased renal function and impaired excretion of other organic acids such as phosphoric acid. Use only appropriate reference intervals. Reported values should ideally be laboratory specific using the same analytical methods as in practice. Also evaluate previously measured values from the same individual or other health individuals of the same species.

**Urinalysis**: Indicated in birds with persistent hyperuricemia. The presence of renal casts can indicate renal pathology. Persistent hematuria has been associated with renal neoplasia, avian polyomavirus, bacterial and viral nephritis, and some forms of toxic nephropathy. Myoglobinuria can cause false positive hematuria. Porphyrinuria, as seen in lead-poisoned Amazon parrots, can result in urine that mimics hemoglobinuria, hematuria. Although proteinuria is the hallmark sign of glomerulonephritis in mammals, voided urine samples are "normally" positive for protein due to fecal contamination in the cloaca.

### OTHER LABORATORY TESTS
Confirmatory tests for gouts are (1) Murexide test: (i) Aspirate a suspect articular gout lesion, and place the sample on a microscope slide. (ii) Mix with nitric acid and allow to dry over flame. (iii) Add a drop of ammonia. (iv) Mauve color indicates UA crystals are present. (2) Polarized light on microscopy: Uric acid crystals are birefringent and will be highlighted by polarized light in cytology slides.

### IMAGING
Increased opacity may occur as a result of dehydration or renal gout. The kidneys can be evaluated by radiographs or CT.

### DIAGNOSTIC PROCEDURES
Laparoscopic examination of the kidneys and renal biopsies are often recommended in cases in which there is persistent hyperuricemia.

### PATHOLOGIC FINDINGS
There may be no pathologic changes however profound, pathologic hyperuricemia can lead to swollen kidneys with prominent lobules due to marked accumulation of urates in the tubules, urate nephrosis. Milky white kidneys. White crystalline deposits on the serosal surfaces of the pericardium, or on serosal surfaces of viscera like the liver and spleen, and skeletal muscles (visceral gout). White crystals within synovial joints (articular gout).

 ## TREATMENT

### APPROPRIATE HEALTH CARE
Treat the underlying cause of renal disease whenever possible. Patients suffering from a hyperuricemic crisis should be managed as inpatients.

### NURSING CARE
Fluid therapy. If not treated promptly and aggressively, dehydration can rapidly exacerbate renal disease and gout. Fluids can be given PO, SQ, IV, or IO routes depending on clinical circumstances. Provide nutritional support as needed.

### ACTIVITY
N/A

### DIET
Offer a balanced diet appropriate for your species of interest.

### CLIENT EDUCATION
Monitor appetite, body weight, droppings. Stress the importance of keeping the patient hydrated.

### SURGICAL CONSIDERATIONS
N/A

 ## MEDICATIONS

### DRUG(S) OF CHOICE
Reduce UA levels: There are many anecdotal reports on the use of allopurinol. It appears to be relatively safe in Galliformes, Psittaciformes, Columbiformes. Use with caution in carnivorous birds, has been shown to increase hyperuricemia and cause visceral gout.

Colchicine 0.01–0.2 mg/kg PO q12–24h; may potentiate gout formation. Urate oxidase 100–200 IU/kg IM considered a safer and more effective alternative to allopurinol, based on studies in pigeons and red-tailed hawks. Parenteral vitamin A for oliguric and anuric renal patients with hyperuricemia.

### CONTRAINDICATIONS
Stop or avoid all nephrotoxic drugs that could cause or aggravate renal disease such as aminoglycosides or sulfonamides.

### PRECAUTIONS
N/A

### POSSIBLE INTERACTIONS
Dehydration and renal disease may result in adverse responses to NSAIDs, especially cyclooxygenase inhibitors like meloxicam.

### ALTERNATIVE DRUGS
Analgesia (e.g. opioids) to alleviate the pain of articular gout. The perennial herb chicory (*Cichorium intybus* L.) has been shown to reduce serum UA levels through the inhibition of liver xanthine dehydrogenase and xanthine oxidase in quail. Another herb, the betel plant (*Piper betle* L.) has been shown to be an effective treatment for gout in broiler chickens as an alternative to allopurinol.

 ## FOLLOW-UP

### PATIENT MONITORING
Appetite, water intake. Droppings. Hydration status. CBC/chemistry panel and urinalysis.

### PREVENTION/AVOIDANCE
Ensure adequate water intake.

### POSSIBLE COMPLICATIONS
Moderate to severe hyperuricemia can result in articular or visceral gout; however, the formation of UA crystals is a complex process. It is not clear why under normal circumstances urate deposits do not occur in carnivorous birds that show postprandial hyperuricemia after ingesting a natural meal.

### EXPECTED COURSE AND PROGNOSIS
Prolonged hyperuricemia increases the risk for development of gout.

 ## MISCELLANEOUS

### ASSOCIATED CONDITIONS
Articular gout: UA crystals accumulate within synovial capsules and the tendon sheaths of joints. Visceral gout. Renal failure. Urolithiasis.

H

# HYPERURICEMIA

## AGE-RELATED FACTORS
A significant decreasing trend was noted with increasing age in UA. The higher levels found in nestlings were theorized to be the result of increased protein synthesis.

## ZOONOTIC POTENTIAL
N/A

## FERTILITY/BREEDING
N/A

## SYNONYMS
Uricacidemia

## SEE ALSO
Anorexia
Avian Influenza
Coccidiosis
Cryptosporidiosis
Dehydration
Diabetes Insipidus
Diabetes Mellitus and Hyperglycemia
Diarrhea
Emaciation
Lameness

Mycotoxicosis
Nutritional Imbalances
Orthoavulaviruses
Polydipsia
Polyuria
Renal Diseases
Sick-Bird Syndrome
Toxicosis (Heavy Metals)
Urate and Fecal Discoloration
Vitamin D Toxicosis
Appendix 8, Algorithm 14: Hyperuricemia.

## ABBREVIATIONS
BUN—blood urea nitrogen
GI—gastrointestinal
NSAIDs—non-steroidal anti-inflammatory drugs
UA—uric acid

## INTERNET RESOURCES
N/A

### Suggested Reading
Cojean, O., Larrat, S., Vergneau-Grosset, C. (2020). Clinical management of avian renal disease. *Veterinary Clinics of North America: Exotic Animal Practice*, 23:75–101.
Gumus, A., Lee, S., Ahsan, S.S., et al. (2015). Lab-on-a-bird: biophysical monitoring of flying birds. *PLoS One*, 10(4):e0123947.
Gutiérrez, J.S., Sabat, P., Castañeda, L.E., et al. (2019). Oxidative status and metabolic profile in a long-lived bird preparing for extreme endurance migration. *Scientific Reports*, 9(1):17616.
Saito, Y., Tanaka, A., Node, K., Kobayashi, Y. (2021). Uric acid and cardiovascular disease: A clinical review. *Journal of Cardiology*, 78:51–57.
Zhu, C.S., Zhang, B., Lin, Z.J., et al. (2015). Relationship between high-performance liquid chromatography fingerprints and uric acid-lowering activities of *Cichorium intybus* L. *Molecules*, 20:9455–9467.
**Author**: Christal Pollock, DVM, DABVP (Avian Practice)

## BASICS

### DEFINITION
Low blood Ca levels are responsible for a variety of clinical presentations including skeletal malformations in developing birds, a well-described neurologic/seizure disorder in grey parrots (*Psittacus erithacus*), and reproductive issues in laying hens. Low blood Mg levels are rare, but when present cause severe concurrent hypocalcemia.

### PATHOPHYSIOLOGY
Ca homeostasis is a complex, well-regulated process in birds, which involves multiple target organs, hormones, and receptors. Overall, the main cause of hypocalcemia in birds is nutritional secondary hyperparathyroidism. Bone contains 99% of Ca as hydroxyapatite. Extracellular Ca is known as total Ca and is a combination of ionized Ca and Ca bound to protein (primarily albumin) and anions. Ionized Ca is the physiologically active form and levels are very tightly regulated through hormonal mechanisms. Total Ca levels fluctuate widely with changes in protein levels and acid/base balance. The parathyroid gland secretes PTH in response to low circulating Ca levels, leading to decreased renal loss of Ca, increased Ca resorption from bones, and increased calcitriol production leading to increased intestinal absorption of dietary Ca. PTH works in concert with vitamin D. Provitamin $D_3$ is present in the skin and uropygial gland secretions. This is converted into vitamin $D_3$ (25-hydroxycholecalciferol, referred to as cholecalciferol) secondary to exposure to ultraviolet B wavelengths (290–315 nm). Cholecalciferol is primarily converted into calcitriol (1,25-dihydroxycholecalciferol) in the kidneys in response to low Ca levels. Calcitriol is the most active vitamin $D_3$ metabolite acting on the intestine to increase Ca absorption, and on osteoclasts to promote bone resorption and release of Ca and phosphorous into the bloodstream. Calcitriol also stimulates bone formation and inhibits PTH production during periods of eucalcemia. Ultimobranchial glands produce calcitonin in response to high blood levels of Ca. Calcitonin appears to inhibit osteoclast activity in bones and increase urinary Ca excretion. Egg-laying birds acquire 30–40% of required Ca from medullary bone, which is released through calcitriol and estrogen activity; 10% of Ca reserves may be required for egg production within a 24-hour period. Vitamin $D_3$ is able to be absorbed through the GI tract with 60–70% efficiency, making oral supplementation important (especially for birds not exposed to ultraviolet light). Hypocalcemia leads to enlargement of the parathyroid glands and elevated PTH. Bones become weak from Ca resorption to maintain adequate Ca levels. In adults, low Ca levels can lead to neurologic signs and seizures. In chronic egg layers, osteomalacia may lead to spontaneous fractures and decreased muscle function may lead to egg binding. Excessive dietary vitamin A and E may impact absorption of vitamin D, but this is uncommon. Mg is an essential dietary element. Mg is an intracellular cation and is integral as an activator or catalyst in over 300 enzymatic processes, most importantly in those associated with ATP. Hypomagnesemia has been induced in chickens fed on a deficient diet. Signs include hyperexcitablity, twitching, weakness, lethargy, tremors, and death. Hypomagnesemic birds are concurrently hypocalcemic, even if fed normal amounts of Ca. Their bone density (and Ca content) is increased, circulating PTH levels are high, and calcitriol levels are not elevated. The exact mechanism of how Mg inhibits circulating Ca levels is not known (although it may be associated with inhibition of calcitriol production, osteocytic dysfunction or resistance to PTH at its organs of action). Mg is present in adequate levels in seeds, nuts, and formulated diets, making deficiency rare. However, seeds and legumes contain higher levels of phytates, which can bind to Mg (and Ca). Hypomagnesemia has been reported in one neurologic hypocalcemic grey parrot that did not respond to either Ca or vitamin $D_3$ supplementation alone, but did recover after a single dose of parenteral Mg.

### SYSTEMS AFFECTED
**Endocrine/metabolic**: Main site of the disease process, leading to effects in other systems.
**Musculoskeletal**: Affected in juveniles and severe chronic hypocalcemia seen in egg laying females.
**Nervous**: Most affected in adult birds with hypocalcemia.
**Reproductive**: Affected in egg laying females.

### GENETICS
There is no genetic predisposition.

### INCIDENCE/PREVALENCE
Common in birds fed low quality diets that consist primarily of seeds.

### GEOGRAPHIC DISTRIBUTION
May affect birds anywhere.

### SIGNALMENT
**Species**: Any avian species can be susceptible, but grey parrots appear to be highly susceptible; the cause is not clear, but is postulated to be related to feeding seed diets (low in Ca and vitamin $D_3$, high in phytates) and/or a higher need for UVB exposure.
Breed Predilections: N/A
**Mean Age and Range**: Young birds are susceptible to osteodystrophy relating to transient hypocalcemia in the hen. The hypocalcemic induced seizures in grey parrots have been reported in birds 2-15 years old. However, any adult bird on an inadequate diet (and little to no UVB exposure) may develop hypocalcemia and demonstrate the classic signs of weakness, ataxia, and seizures. Any laying hen on an inadequate diet (and little to no UVB exposure) may develop osteomalacia and egg binding.
**Predominant sex**: The juvenile osteodystrophy and adult neurologic signs may occur in any sex.

### SIGNS

#### Historical Findings
Juvenile birds may come out of the nest box unable to perch or stand normally due to folding fractures. Adult birds may show (and be presented for) general sick-bird signs before the neurologic signs manifest (weakness, decreased appetite, decreased vocalization, exercise intolerance, and sitting fluffed on the bottom of the cage). Neurologic signs that owners may notice include ataxia, tremors, falling off the perch, and seizures. In addition to exhibiting the above signs, affected hens may present for straining to lay, dyspnea (due to coelomic distention), cloacal prolapse, decreased stool production, bloody eliminations, and lameness.

#### Physical Examination Findings
Juveniles—folding fractures of the long bones or curvature of the spine. Adults: Weakness, ataxia, tremors, seizures. Females: Weakness, egg present on coelomic palpation, cloacal prolapse, metabolic fractures.

### CAUSES
Low dietary Ca. Low dietary vitamin $D_3$ (or decreased vitamin D absorption due to oversupplementation of vitamins A and E). High dietary phosphorous. Chronic egg laying. Little to no UVB radiation (from specialized lights or direct sunlight). Gastrointestinal disease that leads to maldigestion or malabsorption.

### RISK FACTORS
N/A

## DIAGNOSIS

### DIFFERENTIAL DIAGNOSIS
Hypocalcemia is generally straightforward to rule in with total and ionized Ca levels in symptomatic birds. Juveniles—trauma (differentiate with history, physical examination, and radiographs). Adults: Metabolic (hypoglycemia, hepatic encephalopathy, renal failure), differentiate with chemistry panel. Toxicosis (lead, mercury, organophospahates/carbamates), differentiate

**H**

with history of exposure, chemistry panel and ionized Ca, and heavy metal testing. Infection (meningitis, meningoencephalitis); bacterial (including *Chlamydia psittaci*); parasitic; viral, including bornavirus (PDD); fungal, differentiate with history, physical examination, CBC, chemistry panel, radiographs, barium study, and specialized testing for specific etiologies. Sepsis may lead to ionized hypocalcemia, typically together with hypoglycemia. Neoplasia, differentiate through physical examination (which may demonstrate persistent neurologic deficits) and through the exclusion of all other etiologies and possibly through advanced imaging (CT). Idiopathic epilepsy, differentiate through exclusion of all other etiologies. Trauma, differentiate with history and physical examination (use alcohol to moisten feathers on head and over spine to visualize any bruising).

## CBC/BIOCHEMISTRY/URINALYSIS
Low plasma total Ca may or may not be present.

## OTHER LABORATORY TESTS
Ionized Ca is the most important value to determine true hypocalcemia. It should ideally be analyzed immediately in a blood gas/electrolyte analyzer (e.g. radiometer) or a point of care blood analyzer such as the i-Stat® (Abbott Laboratories, Abbott Park, IL). However, if the sample is frozen immediately after being spun down and sent to the laboratory on ice, useful results can be obtained (contact your lab for special instructions). The normal range in captive grey parrots is 0.96–1.22 mmol/l. Vitamin $D_3$ levels (25-hydroxycholecalciferol and 1,25 dihydroxycholecacliferol) are becoming more commonly measured, but require very specialized handling (drawn into heparin and frozen until test performed). They are considered to be useful but levels vary widely based on dietary vitamin D and UVB exposure. Reference intervals for poultry are: 25-hydroxycholecalciferol 14.5–20.0 nmol/l, 1,25 dihydroxycholecacliferol 100.0–332.8 nmol/l. PTH levels are not currently clinically feasible to obtain but may be useful in the future. Plasma Mg levels are available through most large labs. Reference intervals have been determined in several psittacine species and falcons: Grey parrot (non-reproductive) 0.82–1.07 mmol/l, Hispanolian Amazon parrot (non-reproductive) 0.82–1.07 mmol/l, hyacinth macaw 1.2 ± 0.5 mmol/l, blue and yellow macaw 1.0 mmol/l ± 0.2 mmol/l, green-winged macaw 1.3 ± 0.5 mmol/l, falcons (multiple species) 0.49–0.78 mmol/l.

## IMAGING
Whole-body radiographs and/or CT should be performed to evaluate bone malformation in young birds. Look for possible alternative diagnoses in neurologic birds. Evaluate bone density (decreased or increased due to reproductive related hyperostosis), and look for presence of eggs in reproductive females. In birds deemed unstable, a single unpositioned radiograph can reveal the presence of an egg or obvious fractures/bone density changes while minimizing stress and fracture risk (can be achieved by taking a radiograph of the bird in a radiolucent box).

## DIAGNOSTIC PROCEDURES
N/A

## PATHOLOGIC FINDINGS
Parathyroids: Classic appearance of nutritional secondary hyperparathyroidism—enlarged parathyroids with enlarged chief cells that become foamy to clear in severe disease. The chromatin becomes less condensed and the nucleus enlarges. A trabecular pattern may also be seen. Bony changes in patients with osteodystrophy: Classic appearance of rickets—elongated, disorganized zone of proliferation and wide seams of unmineralized osteoid at the trabecular periphery. Large numbers of osteoblasts are present along the trabecular periphery. Fibrous tissue proliferation is present in diseased bone.

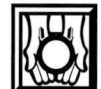

# TREATMENT

## APPROPRIATE HEALTH CARE
Juvenile birds are generally treated on an outpatient basis. Most birds are clinically normal and require diet counseling and cage modification advice. Severely affected cases may require surgery to restore better function to pelvic limbs. Adults with hypocalcemic seizures require inpatient care until the seizures resolve and the bird is able to eat and maintain hydration on its own. Follow-up with dietary counseling and supplement recommendations on an outpatient basis. Hens with egg binding – see Treatment section in Dystocia and Egg Binding chapter.

## NURSING CARE
Base supportive care on physical examination and the clinical picture. Patients may need fluid therapy based on hydration status and severity of hypovolemia – SQ for mild cases, IV/IO for severely affected birds (having vascular access also allows for more rapid administration of anticonvulsants). Supplemental gavage feedings may be required in birds who are unable to eat on their own.

## ACTIVITY
Strict cage rest until the seizures resolve and weakness improves. Making cage modifications may help prevent further injury (wrapping the perches for better grip, padding the bottom of the cage to minimize trauma if the patient falls).

## DIET
Focus on encouraging a balanced diet based on formulated pellets and a wide variety of vegetables, fruits, nuts, and grains. Ca should be around 0.5% of the diet (higher in laying hens). The Ca to phosphorous ratio should ideally be 1.5 : 1. Calcium recommendations range from 0.3–1% in laying psittacines, 1.88–3.25% in laying chickens (high end for those that lay daily). Recommended dietary Mg levels should be > 0.06%. Theoretically, this should be very easy to achieve in any diet. Sunflower seeds contain over 0.3% Mg, millet contains over 0.11% Mg, and peanuts contain over 0.16% Mg. However, phytates in seeds and legumes can bind Mg and Ca. Sprouting seeds will lower phytate levels. Mg levels in pellets range from 0.12% to 0.15%.

## CLIENT EDUCATION
Diet modification should be the primary focus. Encouraging the addition of direct sunlight exposure to the daily routine provides the bird with the best source of UVB. Alternatively, adding a UVB lamp is beneficial when direct sunlight exposure is not feasible (make sure all shielding is removed from the fixture). Discuss proximity of the lamp to birds; the bulb should be no closer than 6 inches (15 cm) and no greater than 18 inches (46 cm). Long fluorescent tube bulbs are the most consistent, and should be changed every 6 months. Other bulbs are likely to be effective, but may not be as safe (high levels may cause irritation to the cornea and/or skin around the eyes). For birds with clinical hypocalcemia with weakness and intermittent seizure activities, caging may need to be modified to provide padding in case of falls, more secure gripping surfaces for perches, and easier access to food and water. For birds that have survived a transient hypocalcemia that led to fractures, cage modifications should focus on allowing the best mobility, such as wrapping perches and placing platforms in the cage. Additionally, it is important to monitor the plantar surfaces regularly for development of pododermatitis if the bird does not ambulate normally.

## SURGICAL CONSIDERATIONS
Ca levels should be restored before significant anesthetic procedures. Very short periods of anesthesia should be used with caution if necessary for sample collection. Consider injectable or intranasal sedation instead of an inhalant.

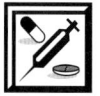

# MEDICATIONS

## DRUG(S) OF CHOICE
Ca gluconate: Dilute 10% solution 1:1 with saline or sterile water (dilute 23% solution

3:1) for IV (slow), SQ, IM injection; 50–100 mg/kg SQ, IM, slow IV; anecdotally given orally in place of Ca glubionate in its absence (50 mg/kg PO q12–24h). Vitamin $D_3$ injection, typically given in combination with vitamins A and E (vital E + A and D) 3300–6600 IU/kg IM once. Ca glubionate 150 mg/kg PO q12h or 750 mg/l drinking water, change daily (formulation not currently available). Mg sulfate injection 20 mg/kg IM once; should be considered if the plasma Mg levels are low, or if Ca and Vitamin $D_3$ supplementation do not resolve clinical signs or cause an appropriate increase in Ca. For acute seizure control, benzodiazepines are useful. Midazolam 0.1–2 mg/kg IM or IV; better IM absorption than diazepam. Diazepam 0.05–0.5 mg/kg IV.

## CONTRAINDICATIONS
N/A

## PRECAUTIONS
N/A

## POSSIBLE INTERACTIONS
Calcium may alter absorption of some medications, including doxycycline and enrofloxacin.

## ALTERNATIVE DRUGS
If cost is an issue, work towards oral supplementation as soon as possible. There is not an alternative to injectable Ca for treatment of hypocalcemic seizures.

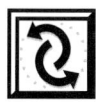 FOLLOW-UP

## PATIENT MONITORING
Seizures and neurologic signs should resolve very quickly (within hours to days) after starting treatment. Total Ca and/or ionized Ca levels should be monitored often initially to make sure the levels are rising (potentially every 1–3 days). Once the levels are noted to be rising, check every 1–2 weeks until levels are normal then monitor yearly. If vitamin D levels are measured and noted to be low, values should be monitored every 1–2 months to evaluate return to normal levels. Mg may be measured if the patient did not respond to the Ca and vitamin $D_3$ therapy as expected. If Mg level is low, it should be checked within 1 week. Low Mg levels are very uncommon so if they are

noted in a bird, the values should be evaluated yearly (together with routine blood testing).

## PREVENTION/AVOIDANCE
Providing a formulated diet with a Ca to P ration of 1.5 : 1 and magnesium level of greater than 0.6% (or higher, if this is determined for non poultry species in the future). Do not oversupplement with Ca or P, which may compete with Mg, leading to hypomagnesemia. Do not oversupplement with vitamins A or E, which may affect absorption of vitamin D.

## POSSIBLE COMPLICATIONS
Seizure activity that is persistent/ uncontrollable may lead to death. Development of a seizure focus leading to reoccurring seizures and the need for anticonvulsant therapy. Bony changes in juvenile birds may cause them to ambulate on different parts of their feet, leading to possible development of wounds or sores (pododermatitis) or arthritis.

## EXPECTED COURSE AND PROGNOSIS
If Ca levels return to normal and clinical signs resolve, the prognosis is good. If nerologic signs persisted for a prolonged period, they may continue even after resolution of Ca deficiency.

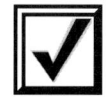 MISCELLANEOUS

## ASSOCIATED CONDITIONS
N/A

## AGE-RELATED FACTORS
Juveniles with bony changes do not often have continued hypocalcemia (it was likely related to transient hypocalcemia in the hen).

## ZOONOTIC POTENTIAL
None.

## FERTILITY/BREEDING
Hypocalcemia directly affects a hen's ability to produce and lay eggs. It must be controlled to allow for normal reproductive function.

## SYNONYMS
Calcium tetany, osteoporosis, cage layer fatigue (poultry).

## SEE ALSO
Chronic Egg Laying
Cloacal Disease
Dystocia and Egg Binding
Egg Yolk and Reproductive Coelomitis
Metabolic Bone Disease

## ABBREVIATIONS
ATP—adenosine triphosphate
Ca—calcium
CT—computed tomography
GI—gastrointestinal
Mg—magnesium
P—phosphorus
PDD—proventricular dilatation disease
PTH—parathyroid hormone
UVB—ultraviolet B

## INTERNET RESOURCES
USDA National Nutrient Database for Standard Reference (Legacy Release): https:// agdatacommons.nal.usda.gov/articles/dataset/ USDA_National_Nutrient_Database_for_ Standard_Reference_Legacy_Release/24661818

*Suggested Reading*
de Carvalho, F.M., Gaunt, S.D., Kearney, M.T., et al. (2009). Reference intervals of plasma calcium, phosphorus, and magnesium for African grey parrots (*Psittacus erithacus*) and Hispaniolan parrots (*Amazona ventralis*). *Journal of Zoo and Wildlife Medicine*, 40:675–679.
de Matos, R. (2008). Calcium metabolism in birds. *Veterinary Clinics of North America: Exotic Animal Practice*, 11:59–82.
Kirchgessner, M.S., Tully, T.N., Nevarez, J., et al. (2012). Magnesium therapy in a hypocalcemic African grey parrot (*Psittacus erithacus*). *Journal of Avian Medicine and Surgery*, 26:17–21.
Stanford, M. (2007). Clinical pathology of hypocalcaemia in adult grey parrots (*Psittacus e erithacus*). *Veterinary Record*, 161:456–457.
Stanford, M. (2006). Calcium metabolism, In: *Clinical Avian Medicine*, (ed. G.J. Harrison, L.R. Harrison), 141–151. Palm Beach, CA: Spix Publishing.
Weaver, V.M., Welsh, J. (1993). 1,25-Dihydroxycholecalciferol supplementation prevents hypocalcemia in magnesium-deficient chicks. *Journal of Nutrition*, 123:764–771.

**Author:** Anneliese Strunk, DVM, Dipl. ABVP (Avian Practice)

H

# HYPOTENSION AND HYPOVOLEMIA

## BASICS

### DEFINITION
Hypovolemia occurs when there is decreased intravascular circulating fluid volume relative to total vascular space. Hypotension is a decrease in systemic blood pressure below accepted low values. In birds, there is no accepted standard hypotensive value, and values for normotension vary among different orders of birds.

### PATHOPHYSIOLOGY
Hypovolemia can be caused by absolute fluid volume deficiency (hemorrhagic or non-hemorrhagic), relative fluid volume deficiency, or a combination of the two. Hypovolemia leads to decreased cardiac output, which results in inadequate tissue perfusion and decreased tissue oxygen delivery. This decreased perfusion (hypoperfusion) and oxygen delivery results in impaired cellular function defined as shock. When there is inadequate oxygen delivery to the cells, they switch from aerobic to anaerobic metabolism, resulting in lactic acidosis. Blood is diverted from other organs to preserve the heart and brain leading to tissue ischemia and worsening lactic acidosis leading to a further reduction in cardiac output, multiorgan failure, and death.

### SYSTEMS AFFECTED
Cardiovascular, renal/urologic, nervous.

### GENETICS
N/A

### INCIDENCE/PREVALENCE
N/A

### GEOGRAPHIC DISTRIBUTION
N/A

### SIGNALMENT
N/A

### SIGNS

#### Historical Findings
Trauma, including burns or bite wounds. Profuse regurgitation or vomiting. Abnormal droppings—diarrhea, hematochezia, melena, polyuria. Exposure to ingested or inhaled toxins (e.g. rodenticide or prescription medications). Exposure to insect bites. Any history of infection that could lead to sepsis. Recent surgery.

#### Physical Examination Findings
Altered mentation. Cyanotic, pale, or muddy mucous membranes; can be hyperemic with sepsis. Poorly palpable pulses, delayed ulnar/basilic vein refill time (> 1–2 seconds), or decreased jugular vein size and refill. Tachycardia. Decreased core body temperature; limbs can palpate warm with sepsis. Prolonged eyelid tent ± sunken eyes. Visible hemorrhage or trauma (e.g. fractures, bruising, epistaxis, purpura). Regurgitated material on face/rhampthotheca if vomiting/regurgitation. Melena, polyuria, hematochezia, hematuria if blood or volume loss is occurring from the kidneys/GI tract. Coelomic distention if there is coelomic bleeding or gastrointestinal obstruction. Burns wounds or extensive skin lesions.

### CAUSES
Hypovolemic shock. (1) Absolute fluid volume deficiency. Hemorrhagic—traumatic injury, blood loss into GI or urogenital tracts, surgery; non-hemorrhagic—vomiting/regurgitation, diarrhea, polyuria without polydipsia (e.g. renal failure, diuretic administration, osmotic diuresis from hyperglycemia), skin losses (e.g. burns, extensive skin lesions), internal fluid loss or third-space sequestration (e.g. coelom, GI). (2) Distributive shock—relative fluid volume deficiency due to expansion of the vascular space without a change in the blood volume such as use of vasodilatory drugs, anaphylaxis, SIRS, sepsis, pancreatitis, neoplasia, severe tissue trauma, neurogenic shock.

### RISK FACTORS
N/A

## DIAGNOSIS

### DIFFERENTIAL DIAGNOSIS
Hypovolemic shock: Cardiogenic shock leading to decreased cardiac output—hypertrophic or dilated cardiomyopathy, valvular disease, severe arrhythmia. Obstructive shock—pericardial tamponade, restrictive pericarditis, pulmonary thromboembolism. Undifferentiated shock—cause of shock is unknown; could be a combination of all types of shock.

### CBC/BIOCHEMISTRY/URINALYSIS

#### Complete Blood Count
Anemia due to haemorrhage. Increased PCV due to hemoconcentration. Leukopenia and heteropenia with toxic changes in cases of sepsis. Leukocytosis, heterophilia, ± monocytosis with pre-existing infection. Thrombocytopenia if this is the cause of the haemorrhage.

#### Biochemistry
Hypoproteinemia due to blood loss or hyperproteinemia and due to hemoconcentration. Hyperglycemia due to increased sympathetic tone or as a cause of osmotic diuresis. Elevated CK if there is trauma or decreased perfusion to skeletal muscles. Hyperuricemia due to hemoconcentration or renal hypoperfusion. Hypernatremia due to hemoconcentration. Hypochloremia due to profuse vomiting. Elevated bile acids and/or AST if there is hepatic hypoperfusion.

### OTHER LABORATORY TESTS
Lactate: Elevated L-lactate levels due to hypoperfusion leading to anaerobic metabolism. In mammals, lactate > 2 mmol/l is cause for concern. In birds, the value can range from 2 to 17 mmol/l, so following trends may be more helpful than absolute values, as lactate levels should decrease with improved tissue perfusion. Blood gas and acid–base evaluation: Hypoperfusion can lead to metabolic acidosis; prolonged vomiting and third spacing into the GI tract can lead to metabolic alkalosis. An increased plasma osmolarity can be caused by hemoconcentration. PT can be prolonged with clotting disorders causing hemorrhage or because of hypoperfusion; PT is reported as the most useful coagulation test in birds; reference values are available for some species.

### IMAGING
Whole-body radiographs and/or CT to evaluate the extent of trauma or to look for underlying disease. Coelomic ultrasound to evaluate for coelomic hemorrhage, coelomic effusion, gastrointestinal obstruction, and/or neoplasia.

### DIAGNOSTIC PROCEDURES
ECG for any patient with arrhythmia; this is particularly important if treatment with dobutamine is needed. Aerobic and/or anaerobic C/S collected from any obvious sources of bacterial infection. Cytologic evaluation and fluid analysis of any coelomic effusion—caution *must* be taken to ensure proper clotting before coelomoentesis is performed. Blood pressure monitoring. Direct arterial pressure monitoring is the gold standard for measuring blood pressure; arterial catheters can be placed in the superficial ulnar artery, deep radial artery, cranial tibial artery, and carotid artery. This usually requires general anesthesia, heavy sedation, or an obtunded patient. Once placed, the patient requires constant monitoring to ensure the arterial catheter is not removed. Indirect blood pressure can be measured with a sphygmomanometer, blood pressure cuff, and Doppler probe, but the results are imprecise and are better used to follow trends rather than obtain a true reading. Blood pressures can be obtained from the wing or the leg. In Amazon parrots, the cuff width should be 30–40% of the limb circumference. In red-tailed hawks, the cuff width should be 40–50% of the limb circumference. Oscillometric indirect blood pressure measurements are inaccurate and should not be used in birds.

## PATHOLOGIC FINDINGS

Depends on underlying cause of hypovolemia, hypoperfusion, or shock. Birds are more resistant to hypovolemic shock than mammals. This is due the reflex lowering of mean capillary pressure level and larger capillary surface area in skeletal muscle in birds, which allows them to mobilize fluid from the skeletal muscle and into the intravascular space. In ducks with 70% blood loss, the fluid was replaced into their intravascular space within 20 minutes. When clinical signs of shock are present in birds, they have lost 60% of their intravascular volume (vs. 25% in mammals).

 TREATMENT

### APPROPRIATE HEALTH CARE

Emergency inpatient intensive care management. Goals of treatment of hypovolemic shock are to replace circulating volume deficit, ensure return of adequate intravascular volume, and avoid tissue damage. During resuscitation, the patient should be evaluated frequently to assess response to treatment. Heart rate, respiratory rate, pulse quality, ulnar/basilic vein refill time, mucous membrane color, core body temperature, overall mentation, and urine production should improve if treatment is successful.
**Treatment of hemorrhagic hypovolemic shock**: Identify and control the source of bleeding. Fluid resuscitation with crystalloids, ± colloids, ± blood transfusion.
**Treatment of non-hemorrhagic hypovolemic shock**: Identify and treat the etiology of fluid loss. Fluid resuscitation with crystalloids, ± colloids. In human medicine, crystalloid fluid resuscitation is preferred for non-hemorrhagic volume replacement because hyperoncotic starch can lead to increased mortality and renal failure.
**Fluid resuscitation**: IV or IO catheter placement. Place IV catheter ideally in a central vein such as the jugular. If jugular catheterization is not an option, then placement of more than one peripheral IV or IO catheters is recommended.
**Fluid choices**: Isotonic crystalloids: Birds are more hypertonic than mammals and may have metabolic acidosis when in shock, so Plasmalyte-A® (Baxter Healthcare, Deerfield, IL) pH 7.4 is the best choice. Shock dose divided into 2–4 aliquots and administered over 15–20 minutes, reassessing after each dose. Colloids used to increase intravascular volume; particularly important when fluid loss is due to increased microvascular permeability (e.g. SIRS or sepsis). Do not use more than 20 ml/kg/day as this can lead to coagulopathy due to dilution of coagulation

factors and a decrease in circulating VIII and von Willebrand factor concentrations. Dose 5-ml/kg boluses over 15 minutes. Hypertonic saline increases osmotic gradient and pulls fluid from the interstitial and intracellular spaces into the intravascular space. May be particularly important in cases of head trauma; dose: 2–5 ml/kg.
**Whole blood transfusion**: Decision to transfuse is not based on PCV alone; administer in patients with tachycardia, hypoxemia, active bleeding, and/or hyperlactatemia. Blood donors must be from the same species of bird. Dose: volume depends on the extent of bleeding and the volume obtained from blood donor; administer the entire volume over 1–4 hours using a filter.
**Vasopressors**: Used *only* after the intravascular volume has been replaced or tissue perfusion will worsen. Dopamine CRI 5–10 µg/kg/minute (7 and 10 µg/kg/minute had the greatest increase in arterial blood pressure in Hispaniolan Amazon parrots with isoflurane induced hypotension). Dobutamine CRI 1–15 µg/kg/minute (15 µg/kg/minute had the greatest increase in arterial blood pressure in Hispaniolan Amazon parrots with isoflurane induced hypotension). Vasopressin CRI 0.5–5 µg/kg/minute may be helpful to restore blood pressure due to its vasoconstrictor effects, but there are no studies of its use in birds, and it may not be effective because the avian hormone is arginine vasotocin. Other vasopressors such as epinephrine (0.1–0.3 µg/kg/minute), phenylephrine (1–3 µg/kg/minute), and norepinephrine 0.1–10 µg/kg/minute can be used *temporarily* to increase blood pressure, but they cause vasoconstriction which decreases tissue and organ perfusion.

### NURSING CARE

Once stabilized, the patient will still require intensive nursing care to ensure they do not remove their IV/IO catheter, arterial catheter, or any bandages/external coaptation that have been placed. IV or IO fluid therapy is required until the patient can eat/drink on their own. If the patient is hypoglycemic, 2.5% dextrose should be added. Eye lubrication should be applied if the patient is obtunded and not blinking properly to prevent ocular ulceration. Oxygen therapy should be administered as needed. The patient's body temperature and cage temperature should be monitored to ensure that normal body temperature is maintained. Monitoring heart rate, respiratory rate, mucous membrane color, and ulnar/basilic vein refill is necessary to ensure that patient does not go into hypovolemic shock again. Monitor ins and outs, and weigh frequently to prevent fluid overloading.

### ACTIVITY

Once stabilized, the bird should be confined to a small cage with heat support, no cage bars that can be climbed, and no perches.

### DIET

Patients with hypovolemic shock should not be fed per os until they are stabilized. Once stabilized, oral intake should start with a liquid diet that is highly digestible and solid foods should only be introduced after confirmation that there is no regurgitation/vomiting, GI obstruction, or ileus.

### CLIENT EDUCATION

Loss of total circulating blood volume due to both and/or fluids loss causes hypovolemic shock. If the lost volume is not replaced quickly, this will lead to a lack of oxygen delivery to the cells and organs in the body, which might lead to multiorgan failure and death.

### SURGICAL CONSIDERATIONS

Birds with fractures associated with trauma may require surgical fixation once they are stabilized. If there is ongoing coelomic hemorrhage, emergency surgical exploratory may be necessary to find and stop the source of hemorrhage. These patients will be at a high anesthetic risk and all efforts should be made to stabilize them before surgical intervention.

 MEDICATIONS

### DRUG(S) OF CHOICE

Patients with sepsis should be treated with parenteral broad-spectrum antibiotics (see Sepsis chapter). Patients with trauma should be treated with appropriate analgesia (see Trauma chapter).

### CONTRAINDICATIONS

Owing to concerns about hypoperfusion to the kidneys, potentially nephrotoxic drugs such as NSAIDs and aminoglycosides should not be administered.

### PRECAUTIONS

Opioids should be used with caution in an obtunded patient as administration can cause respiratory depression. Dobutamine can lead to seizures (reported in dogs), which can be treated by stopping the dobutamine and administering IV diazepam. Dobutamine can cause AV block in Amazon parrots which ceases after stopping the dobutamine. Colloid use > 20 ml/kg/day can lead to coagulopathy.

### POSSIBLE INTERACTIONS

N/A

### ALTERNATIVE DRUGS

N/A

H

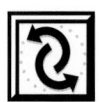

## FOLLOW-UP

### PATIENT MONITORING
If the patient survives hypovolemic shock, it will need to be closely monitored for signs or organ dysfunction with serial blood chemistry evaluation. Birds with trauma leading to fractures will need follow-up radiographs to ensure proper healing.

### PREVENTION/AVOIDANCE
N/A

### POSSIBLE COMPLICATIONS
Permanent alteration in functions such as blindness, deafness, ataxia, lameness, inability to fly. Traumatic brain injury can lead to post-traumatic seizures (see Seizures chapter). Circulatory failure leading to multiorgan function and death. Circulatory overload, transfusion reactions if whole blood is needed.

### EXPECTED COURSE AND PROGNOSIS
The prognosis depends on the etiology, the severity of the hypovolemic shock, and the patient's response to treatment. Hemorrhagic hypovolemic shock has an improved outcome when the source of bleeding can be stopped quickly and there is immediate volume resuscitation. The prognosis is worse if hypovolemic shock has progressed to multiorgan failure, if there is ongoing hypoperfusion, if there is a persistently high blood lactate concentration, or a continued requirement for vasoactive support despite intravascular volume resuscitation. Older patients with underlying comorbidities have a worse outcome.

## MISCELLANEOUS

### ASSOCIATED CONDITIONS
N/A

### AGE-RELATED FACTORS
N/A

### ZOONOTIC POTENTIAL
N/A

### FERTILITY/BREEDING
N/A

### SYNONYMS
N/A

### SEE ALSO
Hemorrhage
Seizures
Sepsis
Trauma

### ABBREVIATIONS
AST—aspartate aminotransferase
AV—atrioventricular
C/S—culture and sensitivity
CK—creatine kinase
CRI—constant rate infusion
CT—computed tomography
ECG—electrocardiogram
GFR—glomerular filtration rate
GI—gastrointestinal
MAP—mean arterial pressure
NSAIDs—non-steroidal anti-inflammatory drugs
PCV—packed cell volume
PT—prothrombin time
SIRS—systemic inflammatory response syndrome

### INTERNET RESOURCES
N/A

*Suggested Reading*
Acierno, M.J., Da Cunha, A., Smith, J., et al. (2008). Agreement between direct and indirect blood pressure measurements obtained from anesthetized Hispaniolan Amazon parrots. *Journal of the American Veterinary Medical Association*, 233:1587–1590.
Graham, J.E., Doss, G.A., Beaufrère, H. (eds.). (2021). *Exotic Animal Emergency and Critical Care Medicine.* Ames, IA: Wiley.
Pachtinger, G.E., Drobatz, K. (2008). Assessment and treatment of hypovolemic states. *Veterinary Clinics of North America: Small Animal Practice*, 38:629–643.
Schnellbacher, R.W., Da Cunha, A.F., Beaufrère, H., et al. (2012). Effects of dopamine and dobutamine on isoflurane-induced hypotension in Hispaniolan Amazon parrots (*Amazona ventralis*). *American Journal of Veterinary Research*, 73:952–958.
Taghavi, S., Nassar, A.K., Askari, R. (2023). *Hypovolemic Shock.* Treasure Island, FL: StatPearls.
**Author**: Nicole R. Wyre, DVM, DABVP (Avian and Exotic Companion Mammal), CVA, CTPEP

# BASICS

## DEFINITION
Hypothermia is subnormal core body temperature. The body temperature of birds is challenging to measure, as standard measurements taken per cloaca may not correlate well with core body temperature. In clinical practice and in experimental studies, core body temperature is measured with a long, flexible, esophageal thermometer, which is not useful in conscious birds. The core body temperature of birds is generally higher than in mammals with a higher variability than mammals. It is generally around 99–108°F (34–44°C) in most birds, depending on species and physiological status.

## PATHOPHYSIOLOGY
Hypothermia can be caused by external effects (exposure to low ambient temperatures, prolonged anesthesia, especially with ineffective warming techniques, loss of feather insulation), or can be a part of general illness, often together with hypovolemia.

## SYSTEMS AFFECTED
As in any homeothermic animal, hypothermia is detrimental and can affect all body systems. Moderate hypothermia causes shunting of blood from the extremities to preserve core body warming. Severe hypothermia leads to peripheral ischemia and necrosis, and eventually death.

## GENETICS
Some bird species are remarkably adapted to cold environmental temperatures. Nevertheless, hypothermia is possible in any bird, especially those that are ill or unprotected from extremely low ambient temperatures.

## INCIDENCE/PREVALENCE
Hypothermia is a common consequence of any illness, and drops in body temperature occur with general anesthesia.

## GEOGRAPHIC DISTRIBUTION
Colder climates pose increased risk of hypothermia for birds kept outdoors (e.g. poultry) and for birds who accidentally escape the home.

## SIGNALMENT
All birds are at risk for hypothermia when ill, undergoing sedation or general anesthesia, or in extremely cold environments. Newly hatched and older chicks without adult plumage are increasingly susceptible to hypothermia, even in moderate environmental temperatures. Birds kept outdoors or accidentally escaping are at risk of hypothermia in colder climates.

## SIGNS
### Historical Findings
Birds that are cold typically are still with a fluffed, ruffled feather appearance, which is similar to the appearance of a generally ill bird. Some birds may appear to shiver. Owners may report birds have been exposed to extreme cold.

### Physical Examination Findings
The hypothermic bird is quiet, with a fluffed, ruffled feather appearance. The extremities may be cold to the touch. Measuring body temperature in the conscious bird is difficult, so in many cases hypothermia is assumed. However, it should be measured in comatose birds, birds in shock, oiled birds, and birds under general anesthesia. Birds may respond rapidly to external warming, such as placement in a warmed incubator. As hypothermia is often associated with underlying illness, there may be physical exam findings supportive of other disease processes.

## CAUSES
Hypothermia can be a part of any disease process in birds. It is also easily produced during sedation or anesthesia, especially if heat support is inadequate. Hypothermia is also produced by overly cold ambient temperatures, even in birds thought to be adapted to cold temperatures.

## RISK FACTORS
Birds that are very young without adult plumage, older, sick, or exposed to cold temperatures for prolonged periods are at risk of hypothermia. Tropical birds may be more prone to hypothermia in low environmental temperature. Loss of feather insulation due to feather damaging behavior or plumage oil contamination may also predispose to hypothermia.

# DIAGNOSIS

## DIFFERENTIAL DIAGNOSIS
The appearance of the hypothermic bird mimics that of the generally unwell bird (lethargy, ruffled feather appearance). Some avian species, such as hummingbirds, naturally transition into a low-energy state called "torpor" overnight or when exposed to cold temperatures. This is a natural protective mechanism and should not be confused with pathologic hypothermia.

## CBC/BIOCHEMISTRY/URINALYSIS
In cases of hypothermia leading to frostbite, the biochemistry panel may reveal elevation in AST and CK. As hypothermia may arise from any underlying disease process, the CBC or biochemistry panel may reflect other underlying illness.

## OTHER LABORATORY TESTS
Other diagnostic testing should be considered as indicated to diagnose possible contributing underlying disease processes that may have facilitated hypothermia.

## IMAGING
Imaging is not typically useful for assessment of hypothermia itself, but may be useful to diagnose possible contributing underlying disease processes that may have facilitated hypothermia.

## DIAGNOSTIC PROCEDURES
Identification of suspected underlying disease processes may direct additional diagnostic testing.

## PATHOLOGIC FINDINGS
Hypothermia is difficult to diagnose on histopathology. Histopathology may reveal evidence of damage and necrosis in the heart, brain, and kidneys.

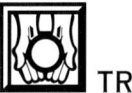

# TREATMENT

## APPROPRIATE HEALTH CARE
Hypothermia requires urgent medical intervention. Typically, if a patient can be restored to normal body temperature and normal mentation, and is able to maintain their core temperature without external heat support, they may be discharged thereafter. Other underlying disease processes may require other specific care.

## NURSING CARE
The primary treatment factor for hypothermic patients is heat support. Heat must be applied carefully, and the body must be rewarmed gradually to prevent rewarming shock and iatrogenic hyperthermia in unstable patients. Typically, a patient is placed into a heated incubator, and warmed fluid bags or heating pads are placed around the patient. Warm fluid therapy administered via direct vascular access or subcutaneously if not practical can also be helpful. Frostbite wounds should be cleaned and bandaged, but not addressed surgically without ensuring appropriate time for tissue declaration. Other nursing care will depend on any other underlying disease processes present.

## ACTIVITY
There are no specific activity restrictions for this condition; most hypothermic patients will elect to decrease movement. Patients must be protected from cold environments.

## DIET
Food should be withheld from any hypothermic patient until core body temperature improves, in order to prevent maldigestion and gastrointestinal stasis.

H

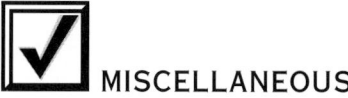

Food can be reintroduced upon restoration of normothermia, but should be restarted slowly as the body eases back to normal functions.

## CLIENT EDUCATION

Once normothermia is achieved and maintained, supportive care can focus on other underlying disease processes and/or any tissue trauma associated with frostbite lesions. Clients may need to maintain clean bandaging on frostbitten digits. Clients may need to provide additional heat support in the home environment to birds predisposed to hypothermia.

## SURGICAL CONSIDERATIONS

Surgical debridement or amputation can be considered in cases of frostbite necrosis. Amputation must be considered carefully, and is not appropriate in some situations (e.g. limb amputation in poultry or other non-flighted birds). Other surgical indications will be dependent upon any other underlying disease processes.

## MEDICATIONS

### DRUG(S) OF CHOICE

Pentoxifylline may be used in cases of frostbite, anecdotally at 15 mg/kg PO q8–12h for 2 to 6 weeks.

### CONTRAINDICATIONS

Caution should be used when using compounds known for evaporative cooling effects (e.g. isopropyl alcohol with phlebotomy, chlorhexidine for antisepsis). These products can easily contribute to or worsen hypothermia, particularly in small patients. Plucking for veterinary procedures should also be kept to a minimum.

### PRECAUTIONS

None.

## POSSIBLE INTERACTIONS

None.

## ALTERNATIVE DRUGS

Heat-supportive devices can be constructed from many on-hand materials, even when traditional heat support elements are unavailable. These include tools such as hot-water-filled exam gloves tied at the wrist, dry rice in an old sock heated in a microwave, standard fluid bags that have been maintained on a warming device.

## FOLLOW-UP

### PATIENT MONITORING

Any frostbitten wounds should be monitored daily while the tissue declares itself. General progress in terms of underlying or concurrent abnormalities should be monitored.

### PREVENTION/AVOIDANCE

Owners must be aware of temperature requirements for newly-hatched and younger birds, and risks to outdoor birds. Diligent care should be taken to prevent the escape of indoor birds.

### POSSIBLE COMPLICATIONS

Severe hypothermia leads to death. Peripheral necrosis (frostbite) can result in loss of digits, or other unprotected parts of the body, such as the combs of chickens.

### EXPECTED COURSE AND PROGNOSIS

Prognosis is highly variable and depends on the severity and duration of the hypothermia and on the inciting cause of the hypothermia (e.g. severe underlying disease vs. secondary to prolonged anesthesia). Mild, iatrogenic cases bear a good prognosis; severe cases can be fatal.

## MISCELLANEOUS

### ASSOCIATED CONDITIONS

Any underlying disease process can induce hypothermia.

### AGE-RELATED FACTORS

Newly hatched and young chicks are particularly susceptible to hypothermia due to the absence of adult plumage.

### ZOONOTIC POTENTIAL

N/A

### FERTILITY/BREEDING

N/A

### SYNONYMS

Cold shock, cold stress.

### SEE ALSO

Cere and Skin Color Changes
Hypotension and Hypovolemia
Oil Exposure
Sick-Bird Syndrome

### ABBREVIATIONS

AST—aspartate aminotransferase
CK—creatine kinase

### INTERNET RESOURCES

N/A

*Suggested Reading*
Duerr, R.S., Gage, L.J. (eds.). (2020). *Hand-Rearing Birds*, 2nd edn. Ames, IA: Wiley-Blackwell.
Scanes, C.G., Dridi, S., Sturkie, P.D. (eds.). (2022). *Sturkie's Avian Physiology*, 7th edn. St. Louis, MO: Academic Press.
Wellehan, J. (2003). Frostbite in birds: Pathophysiology and treatment. *Compendium*, 25:776–781.
**Authors:** Angela M. Lennox, DVM, DABVP (Avian and Exotic Companion Animal), DECZM (Small Mammal), and Crystal Matt, DVM

# ILEUS (FUNCTIONAL GASTROINTESTINAL, CROP STASIS)

## BASICS

### DEFINITION
Ingluvial hypomotility or crop stasis is defined as delayed emptying of material from the crop into the proventriculus. The normal crop emptying time varies depends on species, diet, time of day, feeding schedule (ad libitum vs. scheduled feeding), and age of the patient.

### PATHOPHYSIOLOGY
Ingluvial hypomotility can be caused by primary disease of the ingluvies, secondary to delayed emptying of the proventriculus and ventriculus, or secondary to systemic disease. The pathophysiology of ingluvial stasis is complicated as the majority of clinical presentations are due to disease outside of the ingluvies. Stasis can be associated with both primary infectious and non-infectious pathology. Primary ingluvial pathology is more common in juvenile and neonatal birds and less common in adults. Primary peristalsis controls the movement of food from the esophagus to the proventriculus and the filling of the crop is closely dependent on the volume of food in the proventricular and ventriculus. In fasted birds, the esophagoingluvial fissura is closed which prevents food entering the crop. Lacking a true sphincter, crop motility is commonly affected by aborad pathology. The destination of food is controlled by the contractile state of the ventriculus, mediated by the extrinsic nervous system, and the rate of passage is correlated with particle size. Any disease process that affects these systems will result in secondary ingluvial stasis.

### SYSTEMS AFFECTED
GI, nervous, respiratory.

### GENETICS
Inherited genetics is the most important factor determining the incidence of pendulous crop in turkeys.

### INCIDENCE/PREVALENCE
Hand-fed birds are more likely to develop ingluvial trauma, atonic ingluvies, and/or fistulas. Birds of prey commonly develop ingluvial bacterial dysbiosis. Chickens develop commonly develop crop stasis with a variety of conditions.

### GEOGRAPHIC DISTRIBUTION
N/A

### SIGNALMENT
All species and orders of birds could present with ingluvial stasis and hypomotility. Neonatal and juvenile birds more affected.

### SIGNS

#### General Comments
The clinical presentation of ingluvial stasis is most often secondary to a primary etiology, so clinical signs will vary. Care should be taken when examining the patient as any degree of compression of the distended crop can lead to crop material entering the oral cavity, causing choking and aspiration. If available, suction should be set up before handling the bird, as immediate removal of the crop contents or suctioning of the mouth may be necessary. Crop size and location varies among different species.

#### Historical Findings
Weight loss, crop distension, decreased fecal volume, and altered appetite (severely decreased, voracious, or picking up food and not actually ingesting it). Hand-fed (gavage) neonates may show a scab or discolored swelling on the neck or leaking food from fistula in cases of cervical esophageal perforation or crop burn. Regurgitation. Sudden death (secondary to aspiration, sepsis). Dyspnea, tachypnea, or tail bobbing in cases with suspect aspiration.

#### Physical Examination Findings
Mildly to severely distended crop, ± palpable ingluvial foreign material. Regurgitation – active or dried regurgitant on the face. Decreased fecal component of the droppings. Distended coelom if the lower GI tract is also affected. Adequate (acute) to severely decreased (chronic) muscle mass. Dyspnea, tachypnea, abnormal auscultation in cases of aspiration. Swollen, thickened, edematous skin overlying the crop, ± a visible fistula or scab in cases of crop burn or trauma. Weak/moribund especially in juveniles.

### CAUSES
**Degenerative**: Pancreatic atrophy causes secondary ingluvial hypomotility due to generalized GI dysfunction.
**Anatomic**: Esophageal strictures, atonic ingluvies secondary to overstretching, and pendulous crop in turkeys (an abnormality of the ingluvies characterized by a temporary or permanent distention with stagnant liquid or semi-liquid contents).
**Metabolic**: Any systemic disease causing generalized GI dysfunction can cause secondary ingluvial hypomotility, including severe renal failure leading to soft tissue mineralization, inadequate maintenance of body temperature in neonatal birds fed cold food, and starvation/generalized weakness. Reproductively active hens with hyperlipidemic syndrome can have delayed crop emptying/regurgitation if they have decreased perfusion to the GI tract.
**Neoplastic**: Primary GI neoplasia, including papillomatous disease, squamous cell carcinoma, basal cell carcinoma, adenocarcinoma, leiomyosarcoma, and fibrosarcoma have been described in birds; masses in the tissues of the thoracic inlet resulting in a variable obstruction of the crop include goiter (and other dysplastic lesions of the thyroid), thyroid carcinomas, and thymoma.
**Nutritional**: Hypovitaminosis A leading to squamous metaplasia of the esophagus; hypocalcemia causing generalized weakness.
**Infectious**: Bacterial—*Mycobacteria* spp. cause primary GI infection, which can cause secondary ingluvial hypomotility; many types of bacteria can cause opportunist secondary crop infections. Viral—circovirus and polyomavirus cause GI stasis, most readily identified by stasis of the crop; avian bornavirus-associated ganglioneuritis can affect any part of the GI tract including the crop; Meyer's parrot adenovirus-1 affecting the proventriculus and intestinal mucosa was reported in a juvenile Meyer's parrot presenting for ingluvial hypomotility and acute depression. Fungal—*Candida albicans* will result in a variable thickening of the mucosa and ingluvial hypomotility with dilation; *Macrorhabdus ornithogaster* affecting the isthmus can cause secondary ingluvial hypomotility and regurgitation.
**Iatrogenic**: Foreign material and food material (weeds, ingluvioliths, grit, seeds, nuts, non-toxic metal, fabric, feathers, toys, etc.) can get impacted in the crop, leading to dilation and hypomotility; feeding liquid formula to granivorous birds will lead to transient crop dilation; administration of midazolam alone or in combination with butorphanol affects GI transit time in cockatiels.
**Trauma**: Crop burns, bite wounds, and feeding tube trauma can cause tissue edema and cellulitis leading to ingluvial hypomotility.
**Toxin**: Organophosphates and lead have direct effects on nerve function that can affect motility of the GI tract; chlorophacinone toxicity causes plexus venosus subcutaneous collaris in pigeons with extensive subcutaneous hematomas near the crop and neck; omeprazole administration in juvenile chickens causes delayed crop emptying due to inhibition of acid secretion.
**Parasitic**: Primary ingluvial hypomotility can be caused by *Trichomonas gallinae*, *Capillaria* spp, *Echinura uncinata*, *Gongylonema ingluvicola*, *Dispharynx nasuata*, and *Onciola canis* infections, although *Trichomonas* is the most commonly reported parasite in psittacine birds; small intestinal cryptosporidiosis causes secondary ingluvial hypomotility due to generalized GI dysfunction.

### RISK FACTORS
All birds being tube fed are at potential risk of ingluvial trauma. Poultry that are allowed access to lush grass, sprouted grains, dried oatmeal, and soybeans.

I

# DIAGNOSIS

## DIFFERENTIAL DIAGNOSIS

Cervical airsac rupture/trauma is differentiated via palpation and passage of a feeding tube to help define the esophagus and ingluvies. Cervical hematoma presents as discoloration of the cervical skin, typically following phlebotomy of the jugular vein. Peri-ingluvial fat/soft tissue mass at the thoracic inlet can be differentiated via palpation and diagnostic imaging. Thyroid or thymus gland hypertrophy/neoplasia can be differentiated via palpation and diagnostic imaging. Aerophagia can be differentiated with radiographs.

## CBC/BIOCHEMISTRY/URINALYSIS

In cases of secondary ingluvial hypomotility, results depend on the primary disease. Primary ingluvial hypomotility rarely causes changes in the blood work that will be diagnostic. AST and/or CK may be elevated due to muscle damage associated with trauma. Leukocytosis may be seen with crop burns or severe infections. Anemia can be seen in birds with trauma or as a non-specific finding with chronic disease.

## OTHER LABORATORY TESTS

Crop cytology, Gram stain, direct microscopic examination, and C/S to identify potential primary or secondary pathogens. Microscopic examination of the feces or PCR if *M. ornithogaster* is suspected. Blood lead levels.

## IMAGING

### Radiographic Findings

Increased ingluvial size with ingesta, fluid, or gas present. Ingluvial or lower GI foreign material/metal may be visible, but radiolucent material may not be easily identified without further imaging. Mineralized neoplastic lesions may be visible. Contrast imaging is helpful to define the presence and location of radiolucent foreign material or neoplasia. With any suspicious of GI perforation, iohexol should be used in place of barium as a contrast media.

### Ultrasonography

Fluid and some intramural or intraluminal soft tissue masses may be visible within the crop.

### Advanced Imaging

CT and MRI. Fluoroscopy is helpful to confirm ingluvial hypomotility (delayed crop emptying time, esophageal bolus frequency, and crop contractions), determine whether it is segmental or affecting the entire crop, and to determine whether the motility of the remainder of the GI tract is affected. Filling defects from foreign material or neoplasia can also be delineated. Anatomical anomalies such as esophageal strictures are also easier to

see with fluoroscopy than with standard contrast radiographs. In one study of GI transit time of barium in grey parrots, one bird had a completely empty crop after 120 minutes and three birds still had material in their crop at 360 minutes. One study in blue-fronted Amazon parrots showed that the crop was completely empty in all birds after 180 minutes. Esophageal bolus frequency in cockatiels administered iohexol should be 9.2–11.1/minute. Crop contractions in Hispaniolan Amazon parrots administered barium should be 0–4.3/ minute. Crop volume, emptying time, and GI transit times vary by species.

## DIAGNOSTIC PROCEDURES

Ingluvial flush to obtain diagnostic samples for cytology, C/S, direct microscopic examination, and to remove ingluvial foreign material. Ingluviotomy and biopsy to remove foreign material and obtain diagnostic samples for histopathology, microbiology, and parasitology examination. If avian bornavirus associated ganglioneuritis is suspected, a minimum of three biopsies should be taken in vascular regions. Viral testing as recommended.

## PATHOLOGIC FINDINGS

Bacterial: Colonization of mucosa with varying inflammation. Virus: Identification of viral inclusions; many involved viruses may not have identifiable lesions in the ingluvies if it is secondarily involved in the process. Avian bornavirus-associated ganglioneuritis: Lymphoplasmacytic infiltration of the central and peripheral nervous systems. Foreign bodies and trauma: Typically, coagulative necrosis of the crop wall. Hypovitaminosis A: Squamous metaplasia of crop mucosa.

# TREATMENT

## APPROPRIATE HEALTH CARE

Patients that are self-sustaining and ambulatory can be treated as outpatients, but hospitalization and inpatient management is often appropriate when the patient is not stable.

## NURSING CARE

Supportive care may include fluid therapy (SQ, IV, or IO depending on the degree of dehydration), supplemental heat, supplemental oxygen (if any respiratory signs), analgesia, and nutritional support (gavage feeding less than the normal 3–5% of the bird's normal body weight until the crop is emptying properly). A crop support pressure bandage may be placed in birds with atonic ingluvies, pendulous crop, or after crop surgery.

## ACTIVITY

Activity should be restricted if there is any increase in respiratory effort or risk of mechanically induced regurgitation due to pressure on a distended crop.

## DIET

Diet may need to be modified to a liquid, complex carbohydrate, medium fiber content to allow easier digestion while ingluvial stasis is being resolved. Carnivores and piscivores may require food to be deboned and cleaned or temporary use of a liquid carnivore diet.

## CLIENT EDUCATION

It is important to review with the clients that ingluvial hypomotility is most commonly secondary to other problems, and typically the clinical sign of ingluvial hypomotility returns if additional pathology is present and has not been identified. Regardless, secondary factors that are identified still must be addressed in the process of management of clinical cases. Ingestion of foreign bodies is often repeated, unless future patient access to foreign material is controlled.

## SURGICAL CONSIDERATIONS

Ingluviotomy/endoscopy to remove foreign material or obtain a mucosal biopsy. Ingluvial repair should be performed to resolve crop burn/fistula only after the extent of the necrotic tissue has been defined. Esophagostomy or ingluviostomy tube placement may facilitate more regular feeding in some patients.

# MEDICATIONS

## DRUG(S) OF CHOICE

Medications will vary depending on the underlying disease. In general, parenteral medications (antibiotics for systemic infection, analgesia, Ca EDTA for lead toxicity, etc.) are preferred over oral medications as ingluvial hypomotility may lead to inadequate GI absorption. Antibiotics should be based on C/S or Gram stain results while awaiting the culture. Analgesia should be multimodal, including opioids and NSAIDs. Primary crop infections can be treated with antibiotics, antifungal, and anti-parasitic medications administered PO or via gavage directly into the crop. These drugs do not need to be systemically absorbed, and can be considered regional therapy; for example, regional therapy for ingluvial candidiasis includes nystatin 200,000–333,000 iu/kg PO q8–12h. Anti-emetics—dopamine D2-receptor antagonist used as antiemetic and gastroprokinetic metoclopramide 0.5 mg/kg SQ, IM, IV q8–12h until ingluvial hypomotility resolves, then can transition to PO. Synthetic neurokinin-1 receptor antagonist and substance P inhibitor maropitant 1.0–2.0 mg/kg SQ q12–24h based on pharmacokinetic studies in Rhode Island red chickens.

## CONTRAINDICATIONS
NSAIDs should not be used if GI ulceration is known or suspected.

## PRECAUTIONS
Midazolam 6 mg/kg IM and midazolam-butorphanol 3 mg/kg IM each have been shown to have significant effects on GI transit time and motility in birds. Metoclopramide-induced improvement in prokinetic function has not been shown to be consistent in studied avian species, and abnormal CNS signs have been observed in multiple species treated with metoclopramide. If this drug is being used and CNS signs are noted, it should be discontinued.

## POSSIBLE INTERACTIONS
None.

## ALTERNATIVE DRUGS
None.

## FOLLOW-UP

### PATIENT MONITORING
Repeat physical examination should be performed to confirm that the crop emptying is improved. If the crop does not improve, additional diagnostics and therapies are advised.

### PREVENTION/AVOIDANCE
Recommendations to prevent further events will be based on the identified or hypothesized primary etiology.

### POSSIBLE COMPLICATIONS
Atonic ingluvies may not return to normal function or may require considerable time and nursing care. Repeated clinical events are strongly suggestive that delayed ingluvial

emptying is secondary to an underlying primary condition.

## EXPECTED COURSE AND PROGNOSIS
Most presentations of primary delayed ingluvial emptying will resolve after diagnosing and appropriately treating inciting cause.

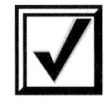

## MISCELLANEOUS

### ASSOCIATED CONDITIONS
Many conditions are associated with secondary ingluvial hypomotility.

### AGE-RELATED FACTORS
N/A

### ZOONOTIC POTENTIAL
None.

### FERTILITY/BREEDING
N/A

### SYNONYMS
Sour crop.

### SEE ALSO
Air Sac Rupture
Anorexia
Aspiration Pneumonia
Bornaviral Disease (Psittaciformes)
Coelomic Distension
Emaciation
Enteritis and Gastritis
Foreign Bodies (Gastrointestinal)
*Macrorhabdus ornithogaster*
Obesity
Regurgitation and Vomiting
Sick-Bird Syndrome
Thyroid Diseases
Toxicosis (Heavy Metal)

### ABBREVIATIONS
AST—aspartate aminotransferase
C/S—culture and sensitivity

Ca—calcium
CK—creatine kinase
CNS—central nervous system
EDTA—ethylenediaminetetraacetic acid
GI—gastrointestinal
NSAIDs—non-steroidal anti-inflammatory drugs
PCR—polymerase chain reaction

### INTERNET RESOURCES
N/A

*Suggested Reading*
Aguilar, R.F., Yoshicedo, J.N., Parish, C.N. (2012). Ingluviotomy tube placement for lead-induced crop stasis in the California condor (*Gymnogyps californianus*). *Journal of Avian Medicine and Surgery*, 26:176–181.
Kierończyk, B., Rawski, M., Długosz, J., et al. (2016). Avian crop function: A review. *Annals of Animal Science*, 16:653–678.
Martel, A., Mans, C., Doss, G.A., Williams, J.M. (2018). Effects of midazolam and midazolam-butorphanol on gastrointestinal transit time and motility in cockatiels (*Nymphicus hollandicus*). *Journal of Avian Medicine and Surgery*, 32:286–293.
Mones, A.B., Petritz, O.A., Knych, H.K., et al. (2022). Pharmacokinetics of maropitant citrate in Rhode Island red chickens (*Gallus gallus domesticus*) following subcutaneous administration. *Journal of Veterinary Pharmacology and Therapeutics*, 45(5), 495–500.
Reavill, D. (2007). The differential diagnosis. In: *Proceedings of the Annual Conference of the Association of Avian Veterinarians*: 167–173.

**Author:** Nicole R. Wyre, DVM, DABVP (Avian and Exotic Companion Mammal), CVA, CTPEP
**Acknowledgements:** Geoffrey P. Olsen, DVM, DABVP (Avian), author of first edition chapter.

I

# INFERTILITY

## BASICS

### DEFINITION
Infertility in birds can be defined as the failure to produce fertile eggs. In a wider perspective, the term infertility is erroneously used to define avian pairs that do not produce eggs, or do not seem to have interest for breeding. Finally, the widest definition may include birds that do produce fertile eggs, but there is a high percentage of embryonic deaths.

### PATHOPHYSIOLOGY
Multifactorial. All disorders that involve courtship, mating, copulation, and directly egg laying can lead to infertility.

### SYSTEMS AFFECTED
Reproductive, musculoskeletal, gastrointestinal, endocrine/metabolic, nutritional. Behavioral. Management (owner/curator).

### GENETICS
Possible, but unlikely. Eventually limited to overbred species with possible inbreeding problems (canaries, budgerigars, chicken).

### INCIDENCE/PREVALENCE
Important in breeding flocks and rare species, especially when involved in recovery, or conservation programs. Not relevant in pet birds.

### GEOGRAPHIC DISTRIBUTION
Worldwide.

### SIGNALMENT
All avian species. Canary, budgerigar, all psittacine birds, cranes, vultures. Less frequently diurnal birds of prey.

### SIGNS

#### General Comments
No eggs are laid. All (or most of the) eggs that are laid are infertile. Alternatively, there is no mating, or birds seem willing to copulate, but do not complete the act. By extension, high (or total) per cent of embryonic deaths.

#### Historical Findings
Inadequate husbandry for the species. Inadequate nest. Inappropriate diet (type and food rotation).

#### Physical Examination Findings
Often no abnormalities are noticed on physical examination. If some findings are present, they are usually related to the musculoskeletal system, the cloaca, or the eyes. Sometimes, behavioral abnormalities are noticed or reported, and signs of abnormal behavior may be evident (feather plucking, aggressivity, neophobia, continuous calling, etc).

### CAUSES
**Reproductive apparatus**: Orchitis, oophoritis, oviductitis, cystic ovary in budgerigars (*Melopsittacus undulatus*), cockatiels (*Nymphicus hollandicus*), and pheasants (*Phasianus colchicus*), hermaphroditism (true hermaphroditism is extremely rare, but wrong development of deferens is not). Lesion of the phallus (limited to ratites and waterfowl).
**Musculoskeletal apparatus**: Arthritis, arthrosis, limb deviation, bumblefoot, missing limbs, kyphosis, scoliosis.
**Gastrointestinal system**: Cloacitis, cloacal paralysis (e.g. neoplasia), cloacal papillomas. Expulsion of the semen by the female, low sperm production of the male, biochemical rejection of sperm.
**Endocrine/metabolic causes**: Low calcium blood level, pituitary gland deficiency. Lesion of the mediobasal hypothalamus in the Japanese Quail caused inhibition of the photoperiodic response and gonadal growth, hypothyroidism, autoimmune thyroiditis.
**Behavioral causes**: Wrong rearing (alone, no social contacts), wrong imprinting (especially birds of prey, waterfowls).
**Husbandry (owner/curator)**: Wrong cage/aviary, wrong nest (site, size and shape), inadequate neighbors, wrong lighting in indoor facilities, wrong facilities according to geographical location (too cold/warm; too wet/dry).
**Nutritional causes**: Ca/P unbalance, low dietary Ca, low protein in diet. Excess or deficiency in manganese, selenium, iodine, fluoride, sodium, zinc, copper, vitamin A, vitamin E, vitamin $B_{12}$, protein and linoleic acid.
**Toxic**: Aflatoxins and other mycotoxins, some drugs, may be anecdotal (metronidazole, tetracyclines, ivermectin).
**Generalized/chronic diseases**: Chlamydiosis (may cause orchitis), hepatitis (limited production of yolk proteins), many chronic diseases (for example aspergillosis), may limit egg production/laying as well as inhibiting mating behavior. Viruses, such as adenovirus, avian influenza, infection bronchitis, and avian hepatitis, may lead to egg drop, infertility, or even stopping of egg laying in poultry and waterfowl.

### RISK FACTORS
Nutritional deficiencies. Bad pair bonding. Wrong husbandry. Species-specific needs are not fulfilled.

## DIAGNOSIS

### DIFFERENTIAL DIAGNOSIS
The first important step is to determine whether there is a disease, physical impairment to breeding or fertile egg production, or a problem related to husbandry. This may also require a differentiation between eggs that do not hatch when incubated artificially, but do develop normally when incubated by the parents. Once this has been clarified, a differential diagnostic list and plan can be designed.

#### Normal Eggs Laid
**All infertile**: Viruses: Any virus able to alter the shape, pH and flora of the cloaca (herpesvirus/papillomatosis) may impede sperm vitality and fertilization of the egg. Orchitis: Bacteria, *Chlamydia psittaci*, neoplasm (especially cloaca and preen gland). No pair bonding: Healthy birds, but without copulation. Musculoskeletal problems: Arthritis, impaired limbs, inhibition to copulation due to pain and/or mechanical problems. Homosexual couple: Two males or two females housed together. DNA sexing can fail in some species, especially if poor collection technique. Abnormal development of gonads in the male bird; testicles and deferens may be altered in function and anatomy. Often seen at endoscopy.
**High number of infertile eggs**: Inadequate husbandry: Wrong perches, overly long pericloacal feathers (limited to some breeds/mutations), and any other factor related to management, that may impede a normal copulation. Competitions/disturbances of neighboring pairs, this also may disturb birds during copulation. Musculoskeletal problems: Minor forms of arthritis/arthrosis, bumblefoot, limb deviation, and lipomas may render copulation difficult, but not impossible. Viruses: Sperm vitality and fertilization of the egg may be lowered, but not completely stopped.

#### Abnormal/Misshapen Eggs Laid
By definition, metritis is an inflammatory process of the uterine portion of the oviduct (egg shell chamber). Can be bacterial, fungal, mycoplasmal, or viral. Metritis can cause abnormal shell formation. Low dietary calcium/low blood calcium; quality of the eggshell is directly related to bioavailability of calcium. Parathyroid problems, also involving the calcium metabolism.

#### Embryonic Deaths
Viruses: Species related, but adenovirus, reticuloendotheliosis virus, orthomyxovirus, paramyxovirus, polyomavirus, circovirus and herpesvirus have all been suspected or proven to cause embryonic death at different embryonic development stages. Bacteria can cause cloacitis, oviductitis, and can infect the egg content. Sometimes, bacteria can enter the eggshell directly from the environment, but in this case, a crack, or a minor fissure in the shell should be suspected. Mycoplasmas can cause metritis and embryonic death. Fungi can occasionally be cultured from dead embryos; in this case, suspect that the eggshell is not intact. Wrong incubation parameters, limited to artificial incubation and egg storing before incubation starts. Too low or too high temperature and relative humidity can lead to embryonic death.

### No Eggs Laid
Oophoritis can be infectious (viral, bacterial, or fungal), or neoplastic in origin. Whatever the cause, usually egg formation is inhibited and no eggs will be laid. Salpingitis is an inflammatory process of the proximal portion of the oviduct. Being localized in a narrow tube, like the salpinx, it usually results in the sealing of the oviduct lumen. Chronic egg binding is uncommon, but if an egg is located in the proximal coelom, not causing problems with passing feces and urine, a female bird may become egg bound for months or years. This will stop the subsequent formation and/or passage of new eggs. Homosexual pair—two males will not produce any egg. Juvenile gonads may be wrongly interpreted at endoscopy by nonexperienced avian endoscopists. Cystic ovary, supposedly due to endocrine unbalances. Outcome similar to oophoritis.

### Psittacosis
Most often the male gonads are affected, but chlamydial oophoritis has also been described. Thyroid problems cause obesity and sexual inactivity (rare). Pituitary gland diseases may affect the hypothalamic–hypophyseal–ovarian axis and cause the ovary to stop its activity. No pair bonding: When two birds have been arbitrarily selected as "a pair", mating may not occur. Very poor diet: Nutrients adequate for survival but insufficient to form and lay eggs. Wrong husbandry: Birds may be missing most/all the environmental and social stimuli that would lead to breeding. Competition/disturbances of neighboring pairs: Birds (especially males) may be so deeply involved in the competition with birds in other aviaries that they ignore their cage mate.

### CBC/BIOCHEMISTRY/URINALYSIS
CBC may be altered in case of infectious diseases affecting several organs. Rarely it will be altered in the case of poor husbandry. Biochemistry will be altered only when a specific system/organ is affected. Apart from Ca, ionized Ca and cholesterol, very little diagnostic value in avian infertility.

### OTHER LABORATORY TESTS
N/A

### IMAGING
Radiology is useful in cases of musculoskeletal problems, or when previous chronic egg binding is suspected. Endoscopy to evaluate possible homosexual pairs, or pathologies of the gonads. Ultrasound for cystic ovaries, salpingitis, retained eggs, soft-shelled eggs, and coelomitis.

### DIAGNOSTIC PROCEDURES
#### Normal Eggs Laid
**All infertile**: Egg necropsy to verify whether the eggs are infertile, or there is a very early stage embryonic death. Virology with samples collected from egg and/or parents. Bacteriology with samples collected from egg

and/or parents. Testicular biopsy to rule out orchitis or testicular tumor. Collection and evaluation of semen via electro-ejaculation, and/or manual massage. Analysis of behavior, eventually using a video recording system. Radiology to diagnose musculoskeletal problems, Endoscopy to rule out homosexual pairs or when an alteration of the male gonads is suspected.
**High number of infertile eggs**: Careful inspection of the aviary and facilities to evaluate all the risk factors that may limit a normal copulation. Analysis of behavior for competitions/disturbances of neighboring pairs. Radiology of birds to diagnose musculoskeletal problems. Viral screening.

#### Abnormal/Misshapen Eggs
Bacteriology to rule out metritis. Additional testing including fungal, mycoplasmal, or viral screening as warranted. CBC to rule out infections. Blood chemistry for evaluation of Ca and ionized Ca levels.

#### Embryonic Deaths
Viral screening of egg/embryo or parents. Microbiology, including *C. psittaci* and mycoplasma. Histopathology. In case of artificial incubation, evaluate whether the incubators are working well and monitor incubation parameters.

#### No Eggs Laid
CBC/protein electrophoresis and microbiology when oophoritis and salpingitis are suspected. Radiology to rule out ovostasis. Ultrasound to rule out cystic ovary and/or coelomitis (in the latter, aspiration of the coelomic fluid is an option). Endoscopy to rule out homosexual pair, cystic ovary, or other pathology. Psittacosis testing. Thyroid function testing. Analysis of behavior, eventually using a video recording system.

### PATHOLOGIC FINDINGS
Gross and histopathology findings will differ depending upon the main cause.

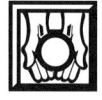 TREATMENT
### APPROPRIATE HEALTH CARE
Hospitalization and nursing of avian patients with infertility is unlikely, unless the primary cause is a generalized, or severe disease (e.g. chlamydiosis, tumor of the gonads, chronic egg binding).

### NURSING CARE
N/A

### ACTIVITY
N/A

### DIET
Diet is a significant consideration when infertility has to be addressed in a bird breeding flock. Diet will be

adjusted/modified/monitored according to species, season, and geographic location.

### CLIENT EDUCATION
If the main cause of the problem is inadequate husbandry, the client must be instructed about the best way to manage the breeding flock. This may vary dramatically with different avian species. When viral, bacterial and fungal diseases are considered the major cause of the problem, a careful education plan must be set up for the client.

### SURGICAL CONSIDERATIONS
Refer to specific publications on surgery. There is no specific procedure for avian infertility; however, the main surgical procedures that might be considered are: removal of granulomas over the ovary, coelioscopy for evaluation of gonadal abnormalities and biopsies. Hysterectomy to treat chronic egg binding. Surgery for cloacal papillomas.

 MEDICATIONS
### DRUG(S) OF CHOICE
Antibiotic therapy, ideally based on culture and sensitivity results if bacterial disease. Antifungal therapy therapy warranted if fungal disease diagnosed. Analgesics may be warranted if painful condition prohibits normal mating behavior. Other therapies based on etiology, varies based on cause.

### CONTRAINDICATIONS
NSAIDs should not be used if gastrointestinal ulceration is known or suspected to be present.

### PRECAUTIONS
NSAIDs should not be administered if renal disease is known or suspected to be present or discontinued immediately if clinical signs suggestive of renal dysfunction (such as polyuria/polydipsia) are observed.

### POSSIBLE INTERACTIONS
N/A

### ALTERNATIVE DRUGS
N/A

 FOLLOW-UP
### PATIENT MONITORING
If behavioral or management related, monitor the courtship and subsequent mating. If disease dependent, run a standard follow-up for the specific disease.

### PREVENTION/AVOIDANCE
Avoid acquiring or using old birds as breeders, unless specifically requested by the recovery program director, or in case of specific genetic needs.

## POSSIBLE COMPLICATIONS
N/A

## EXPECTED COURSE AND PROGNOSIS
Cause dependent.

## MISCELLANEOUS

### ASSOCIATED CONDITIONS
Many conditions are associated with secondary infertility. All disorders that involve courtship, mating, copulation, and egg laying can be associated with infertility.

### AGE-RELATED FACTORS
Mostly young birds (inexperience) and old birds (generalized aging) are affected.

### ZOONOTIC POTENTIAL
Only chlamydiosis is a serious threat.

### FERTILITY/BREEDING
As listed.

### SYNONYMS
N/A

### SEE ALSO
Arthritis
Ascites
Chlamydiosis
Chronic Egg Laying
Circovirus (Psittacines)
Circoviruses (Non-Psittacine Birds)
Cloacal Diseases
Coelomic Distention
Colibacillosis
Cystic Ovaries
Dystocia and Egg Binding

Egg Yolk and Reproductive Coelomitis
Herpesvirus (Columbid Herpesvirus 1 in Pigeons and Raptors)
Herpesvirus (Duck Viral Enteritis)
Herpesvirus (Passerine Birds)
Herpesvirus (Psittacid Herpesviruses)
Hypocalcemia and Hypomagnesemia
Lameness
Metabolic Bone Disease
Mycoplasmosis
Nutritional Imbalances
Obesity
Oviductal Diseases
Phallus Prolapse and Diseases
Pododermatitis
Polyomavirus
Poxvirus
Thyroid Diseases
Vitamin D Toxicosis
Xanthoma/Xanthogranulomatosis

### ABBREVIATIONS
Ca—calcium
NSAIDs—non-steroidal anti-inflammatory drugs
P—phosphorus

### INTERNET RESOURCES
N/A

*Suggested Reading*
Assersohn, K., Brekke, P., Hemmings, N. (2021). Physiological factors influencing female fertility in birds. *Royal Society Open Science*, 8:202274.
Clubb, S., Phillips, A. (1992). Psittacine embryonic mortality. In: *Psittacine Aviculture, Perspectives, Techniques and Research* (ed. R.M. Schubot, K.J. Clubb, K.J., S.L. Clubb), 318–325. Loxahatchee, FL: Aviculture Breeding and Research Center.
Crosta, L., Gerlach, H, Bürkle., M., Timossi, L. (2003). Physiology, diagnosis and diseases of the avian reproductive tract. *Veterinary Clinics of North America: Exotic Animal Practice*, 6:57–83.
Crosta, L., Petrini, D., Sawmy, S. (2021). Reproduction management of herds/flocks of exotic animals: investigating breeding failures in birds, reptiles, and small mammals. *Veterinary Clinics of North America: Exotic Animal Practice*, 24:661–695.
Fischer, D., Neumann, D., Schneider, H., Giersher, K. (2013). Assisted reproduction in two rare psittacine species: The Spix's Macaw and the St. Vincent amazon. *Proceedings of the International Conference on Avian, Herpetological and Exotic Mammal Medicine* (ICARE 2013), Wiesbaden, Germany, April 20–26:295–296.
Reuleaux, A., Siregar, B.A., Collar, N.J., et al. (2022). Productivity constraints on Citron-crested Cockatoos in a rich community of large hole-nesting birds. *Avian Research*, 13:100015.
Scanes, G.C., Dridi, S. (eds.) (2021). *Sturkie's Avian Physiology*, 7th edn. St. Louis, MO: Elsevier.
Stelzer, G., Crosta, L., Bürkle, M., Krautwald-Junghanns, M.E. (2005). Attempted semen collection using the massage technique and semen analysis in various psittacine species. *Journal of Avian Medicine and Surgery*, 19:7–13.

**Authors**: Lorenzo Crosta, DVM, PhD, DECZM, ACEPM, GP Cert (ExAp), FNOVI (Zoo-Avian) and Petra Schnitzer, DVM, MANZCVS, Med Vet, ACEPM

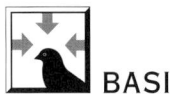

# BASICS

## DEFINITION
Iron storage disease (ISD) is used to describe the spectrum of physiologic and pathologic changes that occur with excessive iron accumulation.

## PATHOPHYSIOLOGY
Body iron content is balanced by control of dietary iron at the level of the enterocyte; there are no effective physiological methods for the removal of excess iron. Excess iron absorbed from the diet is typically stored within the hepatocytes, but can also be found in phagocytic cells in the liver and spleen, as well as the cardiomyocytes. Increased iron accumulation without evidence of associated disease is called hemosiderosis. As iron levels increase, oxidative damage to membranes and proteins can occur within the cells, resulting in cellular death and replacement by fibrosis. Disease occurs and clinical signs develop when accumulated iron affects organ function (liver, heart, spleen, pancreas). In veterinary medicine, the term hemochromatosis may be used to describe iron overload with accompanying disease. In human medicine, however, hemochromatosis refers specifically to a group of hereditary primary iron storage disease. Clinical disease is often related to liver dysfunction and failure. ISD is also suspected to promote other disease processes in birds such as diabetes mellitus (documented in toucans and parrots, iron induces oxidative stress to the B cells), and heart failure (mynahs). Other conditions reported in humans may also be relevant in birds such as neoplasia (lymphoproliferative disorders and hepatocellular carcinoma) and myopathies.

## SYSTEMS AFFECTED
Liver, endocrine, cardiac.

## GENETICS
N/A

## INCIDENCE/PREVALENCE
Unknown but seen commonly in susceptible species.

## GEOGRAPHIC DISTRIBUTION
N/A

## SIGNALMENT
Unknown but seen commonly in susceptible species.

## SIGNS
### Historical Findings
Usually non-specific.

### Physical Examination Findings
Clinical signs are generally secondary to hepatic, pancreatic, and cardiac dysfunction, and include dyspnea, abdominal distension, ascites, emaciation, depression, sudden death without premonitory signs (most frequently in toucans), reduced hemostasis. Hepatomegaly (liver enlargement) may be seen transcutaneously, directly or with the use of abdominal transillumination.

## CAUSES
Diets containing high levels of available iron compared with the natural levels of iron intake for the species. Presumptive lack of ability of ISD-susceptible species to adequately downregulate the absorption of dietary iron. Most frugivorous, nectarivorous, and palynivorous species have evolved eating a diet low in available iron. This may result from low absolute iron levels, or the presence of natural iron chelating compounds. Iron accumulation can also occur in association with systemic conditions that affect iron uptake and sequestration mechanisms (e.g. infectious diseases and some neoplasias).

## RISK FACTORS
Frugivorous birds and, to a lesser extent, insectivorous birds: Passeriformes (in particular Sturnidae, Paradisaeidae, Thraupidae, Pipridae), Trogoniformes, Psittaciformes (in particular Loriidae and South American parrots), Coraciiformes (in particular Coraciidae, Momotidae), and Bucerotiformes (in particular Bucerotidae). Diets high in iron. Diets containing heme-based sources of iron (meat) provided to non-carnivorous species as heme iron is highly bioavailable. Diets containing high levels of vitamin C (e.g. citrus fruits), which promote intestinal iron absorption. Diets containing high levels of fructose or sucrose.

# DIAGNOSIS

## DIFFERENTIAL DIAGNOSIS
**Hepatic disease**: Hepatic lipidosis, hepatic fibrosis of other causes, hepatic neoplasia, hepatic congestion (congestive heart failure), and amyloidosis, chronic hepatitis and hepatic necrosis.
**Ascites**: Reproductive disease, coelomic neoplasia, congestive heart failure, and infectious coelomitis including viral diseases.
**Diabetes mellitus**: Idiopathic destruction of B cells, corticosteroid use, and pancreatitis.

## CBC/BIOCHEMISTRY/URINALYSIS
Hematologic and biochemical changes are not consistent and may only be present in advanced disease. Anemia of chronic disease. Hypoproteinemia/hypoalbuminemia (protein electrophoresis is the only reliable measure of avian albumin). Hypoglycemia (liver failure) or hyperglycemia (diabetes mellitus). Decreased uric acid in terminal stages of liver failure. Elevated bile acids. Elevated liver enzymes (AST, GGT, GLDH, LDH). Elevated muscle enzymes (CK, AST, LDH). Increased coagulation parameters (in cases of hepatic failure).

## OTHER LABORATORY TESTS
Serum ferritin is considered the best non-invasive measurement of body iron status in mammals; however, an avian specific ferritin assay has not been developed or assessed for use in birds. Other plasma or serum analytes used in mammals, including total iron binding capacity, iron saturation, transferrin, and plasma iron have been used to limited degrees in birds to monitor treatment effectiveness but they appear to be of low value in initial diagnosis. Hepcidin assays have not been developed for birds and their usefulness is unknown.

## IMAGING
**Radiography**: Hepatomegaly, coelomic fluid, decreased air sac space, enlarged cardiac silhouette.
**Coelomic ultrasound**: Enlarged and hyperechoic liver, coelomic fluid.
**Echocardiography**: Enlarged cardiac chambers, systolic dysfunction, pericardial effusion.
**CT**: Liver attenuation tends to be increased because of the hepatic iron accumulation, however CT is not a sensitive diagnostic test for iron storage disease.
**MRI**: Has been used to estimate hepatic iron concentration in hornbills and then monitor the effects of treatment. Of limited usefulness in general clinical practice.

## DIAGNOSTIC PROCEDURES
Biopsy samples of liver are collected directly via coeliotomy (particularly if the liver is enlarged) or through coelioscopy using a rigid endoscope. The liver can be approached using the standard left lateral, right lateral, or midline approaches. The midline approach through the ventral hepatoperitoneal cavities provides the best view of both liver lobes (after incising the ventral mesenteric membrane). The liver may appear enlarged with rounded borders and may have yellowish or greenish patches that can be associated with iron accumulation. Evaluation by atomic absorption spectrophotometry, inductively coupled plasma mass spectrometry, or another analytic technique is the gold standard for assessing hepatic iron levels.

## PATHOLOGIC FINDINGS
Histopathology can be used to visually estimate the amount of iron present in hepatocytes and Kuppfer cells. Staining with Perls' Prussian blue increases the sensitivity of detection. Digital image analysis and morphologic grading scales have been used to categorize the amount of iron present. Histopathology allows the

## IRON STORAGE DISEASE

identification of hepatic pathology associated with iron overload; including necrosis, inflammation, fibrosis, and neoplasia.

# TREATMENT

## APPROPRIATE HEALTH CARE
To reduce systemic iron levels and reduce subsequent accumulation: Reduce dietary iron (see below). Phlebotomy (1% of body weight weekly). PCV should be monitored to ensure iatrogenic anemia is not induced, although lowering of the PCV is rarely encountered in these birds. Regular phlebotomy of highly susceptible species not yet suffering from ISD has been suggested for prevention. Iron chelation (see below). Treatment of concurrent disease processes (e.g. liver or cardiac failure and diabetes mellitus). Abdominocentesis may be needed to relieve dyspnea in cases with air sac compression by ascitic fluid.

## NURSING CARE
N/A

## ACTIVITY
N/A

## DIET
Diets low in available iron (30–65 mg/kg dry matter). Most avian food companies offer a low-iron pelletized diet. These diets may not consistently prevent the disease in highly susceptible species, such as toucans and mynahs. Avoid heme-based sources of iron for non-carnivorous species. Limit the amount of vitamin C in the diet (recommended dose is 50–150 mg/kg dry matter), and ideally try and give the vitamin C source separate from the iron source (vitamin C only enhances iron absorption when given at the same time). Addition of tannins to the diet can help but this should be done with caution as they can also chelate other essential trace minerals and may change palatability. The addition of decaffeinated Ceylon black tea leaves to the diet has been shown to limit iron absorption in starlings. As some bags of food may have a higher iron content than advertised, it may be advisable to measure the iron level in every new batch of food for highly susceptible species.

## CLIENT EDUCATION
Inform the client about species susceptibility and dietary causes.

## SURGICAL CONSIDERATIONS
N/A

# MEDICATIONS

## DRUG(S) OF CHOICE
Iron chelators: Deferiprone 75 mg/kg PO q24h for 90 days (studied in hornbills,

chickens, and pigeons); deferoxamine 100 mg/kg SQ q24h for 16 weeks (studied in the European starling). These treatments should always be associated with diet modifications. Urine may have a rusty color during treatment. Liver support medications such as antioxidants may be beneficial. Treatment for diabetes mellitus with insulin therapy, dietary recommendations, or glipizide may be indicated. Requirement for drugs may decrease as iron overload improves.

## CONTRAINDICATIONS
N/A

## PRECAUTIONS
N/A

## POSSIBLE INTERACTIONS
N/A

## ALTERNATIVE DRUGS
N/A

# FOLLOW-UP

## PATIENT MONITORING
Serial liver biopsies (for iron level measurement or histopathology) may be performed once or twice a year. Further developments in the use of MRI to assess hepatic iron levels may provide a non-invasive way of monitoring birds with ISD.

## PREVENTION/AVOIDANCE
See Diet section.

## POSSIBLE COMPLICATIONS
Liver failure. Cardiac failure. Diabetes mellitus. Possible decrease in fertility in Rhamphastidae. ISD has been associated with higher risk of liver neoplasia in humans and in bats, but this association has not yet been identified in birds.

## EXPECTED COURSE AND PROGNOSIS
If treated early, the prognosis is very good. If damage to the liver/heart has already occurred, the prognosis is poor. Sudden death without premonitory clinical signs has been reported in Ramphastidae. Possible association with increased risks of infection.

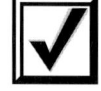

# MISCELLANEOUS

## ASSOCIATED CONDITIONS
Liver disease, diabetes mellitus, cardiac disease.

## AGE-RELATED FACTORS
N/A

## ZOONOTIC POTENTIAL
N/A

## FERTILITY/BREEDING
N/A

## SYNONYMS
N/A

## SEE ALSO
Anemia
Amyloidosis
Ascites
Coelomic Distention
Congestive Heart Failure
Diabetes Mellitus and Hyperglycemia
Hepatic Lipidosis
Liver Disease
Myocardial Diseases
Neoplasia (Gastrointestinal and Liver)
Polydipsia
Polyuria
Sick-Bird Syndrome

## ABBREVIATIONS
AST—aspartate aminotransferase
CK—creatine kinase
CT—computed tomography
GGT—gamma-glutamyl transferase
GLDH—glutamate dehydrogenase
ISD—iron storage disease
LDH—lactate dehydrogenase
MRI—magnetic resonance imaging
PCV—packed cell volume

## INTERNET RESOURCES
N/A

*Suggested Reading*
Lowenstine, L.J., Stasiak, I.M. (2015). Update on iron overload in zoologic species. In: *Fowler's Zoo and Wild Animal Medicine* (ed. R.E. Miller and M.E. Fowler), 674–681. St. Louis, MO: Elsevier.
Cork, S.C. (2000). Iron storage diseases in birds. *Avian Pathology*, 29:7–12.
Mete, A., Hendriks, H.G., Klaren, P.H.M., et al. (2003). Iron metabolism in mynah birds (*Gracula religiosa*) resembles human hereditary haemochromatosis. *Avian Pathology*, 32:625–632.
Olsen, G.P., Russell, K.E., Dierenfeld, E., Phalen, D.N. (2006). Comparison of four regimens for treatment of iron storage disease using the European starling (*Sturnus vulgaris*) as a model. *Journal of Avian Medicine and Surgery*, 20:74–79.
Seibels, B., Lamberski, N., Gregory, C.R., et al. (2003). Effective use of tea to limit dietary iron available to starlings (*Sturnus vulgaris*). *Journal of Zoo and Wildlife Medicine*, 34:314–316.
Sheppard, C., Dierenfeld, E. (2002). Iron storage disease in birds: Speculation on etiology and implications for captive husbandry. *Journal of Avian Medicine and Surgery*, 16:192–197.

**Authors:** Delphine Laniesse, DVM, DVSc, DECZM (Avian), and Hugues Beaufrère, DVM, PhD, DACZM, DABVP (Avian), DECZM (Avian)

I

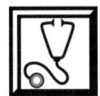 BASICS

## DEFINITION
Avian joint disease refers to conditions affecting the joints in birds, leading to pain, dysfunction, and impaired mobility. Joints involve the interface between two or more bones that interact to produce a movement. Most noticeably in avian species, the shoulder joint is formed by the meeting of three bones—the humerus, the scapula, and the coracoid. The elbow joint is formed by the humerus articulating on the radius and ulna. The carpometacarpal joint is formed by the first metacarpal bone (allula), the second and third metacarpal bone with radius and ulna. The intertarsal joint is the articulation between the tibiotarsus and the tarsometatarsus.

## PATHOPHYSIOLOGY
Inflammation of joint tissues can be due to infection, trauma, or degenerative process. Bacterial or viral agents may directly infect the joint, causing synovitis and cartilage damage. Arthritis can be localized or affecting several joint (so-called polyarthritis). Uric acid deposit can induce gout and arthritis.

## SYSTEMS AFFECTED
Musculoskeletal system.

## GENETICS
No known genetic predisposition.

## INCIDENCE/PREVALENCE
Joint disease is common in both wild and captive individuals; 3–9.8% of free-ranging hawks and pigeons had osteoarthritis in one survey. Prevalence of *Mycoplasma* and avian reovirus can be high in some poultry flocks (> 90%).

## GEOGRAPHIC DISTRIBUTION
N/A

## SIGNALMENT
Septic arthritis is specifically described in pigeons, where it can be caused by *Salmonella typhimurium* var Copenhagen. Other infectious causes include infection by *Mycoplasma* spp. including *Mycoplasma gallisepticum* and synoviae in poultry, and potentially *Mycoplasma corgypsi* in black vultures. Overweight bird in captivity. Geriatric birds. Perosis in young poultry and anatids.

## SIGNS

### Historical Findings
Lameness. Reluctance to move or fly. Altered posture. Signs of pain in general (eyes half closed, polypnea, ruffled feathers). Lethargy.

### Physical Examination Findings
Swelling and warmth around one or several joints. Pain during manipulation. Lack of mobility.

## CAUSES
Bacterial: Salmonellosis in pigeons. *Salmonella typhymurium* var Copenhagen can cause joint infections in pigeons. Infection typically occurs through ingestion of contaminated food or water. *M. gallisepticum* and *Mycoplasma synoviae* are common poultry pathogens causing synovitis and arthritis. Infection is transmitted horizontally between birds and can lead to chronic joint inflammation. Co-infection with avian reovirus are common. *M. corogypsi* in black vultures has been reported with polyarthritis. *Mycobacterium* spp. such as *M. avium* subspecies *avium* (MAA), *Mycoplasma genavense* and *M. avium* subspecies *hominisuis* can infect joints. Viral: Avian reovirus is commonly involved with mycoplasma infection and arthritis. Turkey arthritis reovirus has been established as a cause of lameness in turkeys. Fungal: Aspergillosis, caused by the fungus *Aspergillus* spp., can lead to joint involvement in turkeys. Degenerative joint disease. Trauma—luxation, fracture. Degenerative osteoarthritis can be caused by excessive tension on the joint due to inadequate substrate and/or obesity. Articular gout is caused by precipitation of uric acid tophi in the joint. Nutritional/developmental—perosis.

## RISK FACTORS
History of trauma, recent introductions of new birds, or exposure to potentially infected environments. Husbandry-related issue (substrate) and overcrowding. High-fat diet. Deficient diet (especially in manganese, choline, nicotic acid, pyridoxine, biotin, or folic acid). History of high amount of protein intake (dog and cat food, meat), erratic vitamin D supplementation, nephrotoxic drug administration (gentamicin, amphotericin B).

 DIAGNOSIS

## DIFFERENTIAL DIAGNOSIS
Some species may have physiological reversible intertarsal joint, such as the African harrier hawk (*Polyboroides typus*).

## CBC/BIOCHEMISTRY/URINALYSIS
Leukocytosis may be present. Elevated acute-phase proteins in cases of inflammation. Elevated uric acid in case of articular gout.

## OTHER LABORATORY TESTS
Joint fluid analysis for cytology and culture. Heterophils and blood may be seen in the synovial fluid. Identification of *Mycoplasma* or avian reovirus by rt-PCR on joint fluid analysis.

## IMAGING
Radiographs or other imaging modalities to assess joint structure and identify abnormalities. CT may allow better definition of bony structures. MRI may allow better definition for ligamentous structures.

## DIAGNOSTIC PROCEDURES
N/A

## PATHOLOGIC FINDINGS
Histopathology of joint tissues may reveal inflammatory infiltrates, cartilage damage, and infectious agents. In case of avian reoviral infection, arthritic lesions of tibiotarsal joints may reveal intense, diffuse lymphohistiocytic inflammation with heterophil accumulations, primarily affecting the synovial capsule and digital flexor tendon.

 TREATMENT

## APPROPRIATE HEALTH CARE
Physiotherapy, hot packs, massage can be applied if tolerated by the patient.

## NURSING CARE
Adapt the installation (accessible food and water, limiting jumping).

## ACTIVITY
Cage rest and limiting the activity may be recommended in most cases.

## DIET
Diet should be reviewed and potential source of deficiency (home-made diet) should be addressed.

## CLIENT EDUCATION
Make sure the bird is comfortable and has easy access to food and water. Client should regularly assess the bird's quality of life.

## SURGICAL CONSIDERATIONS
Severe cases of osteoarthritis may benefit from articular lavage and potentially arthrodesis. Regional limb perfusion may be used for intertarsal or tarsometatarsophalangeal joint infection. Use of antibiotic-impregnated calcium sulfate beads has been reported. Joint luxation should be stabilised surgically.

MEDICATIONS

## DRUG(S) OF CHOICE
Antibiotics for infectious arthritis (specifically targeted for *Salmonella* and *Mycoplasma* infection)—doxycycline, azithromycin, or enrofloxacin. Anti-inflammatory medications—meloxicam, grapiprant, mavacoxib, celecoxib. Analgesics—tramadol, hydromorphone, butorphanol, liposomal butorphanol, buprenorphine, gabapentin,

# JOINT DISEASES      (CONTINUED)

cannabidiol. Antifungal therapy for aspergillosis—itraconazole, voriconazole, terbinafine. Gout therapy, including allopurinol.

## CONTRAINDICATIONS
N/A

## PRECAUTIONS
Long-term anti-inflammatory drugs should be used with caution in dehydrated animals, renal-compromised birds, or species with no pharmacokinetic data.

## POSSIBLE INTERACTIONS
N/A

## ALTERNATIVE DRUGS
N/A

# FOLLOW-UP

## PATIENT MONITORING
Evaluating perching station, mobility, general demeanour.

## PREVENTION/AVOIDANCE
Correct husbandry measure (diet/substrate). Lower the density.

## POSSIBLE COMPLICATIONS
Extension of septic arthritis may lead to amputation of the affected limbs or endocarditis/discospondylitis.

## EXPECTED COURSE AND PROGNOSIS
Joint diseases are often difficult to treat in birds. Chronic lameness is expected in most cases.

# MISCELLANEOUS

## ASSOCIATED CONDITIONS
Chronic inflammation may lead to systemic amyloidosis.

## AGE-RELATED FACTORS
Geriatric birds may be more prone to degenerative osteoarthritis or articular gout.

## ZOONOTIC POTENTIAL
*Salmonella* and *Mycobacterium* can have zoonotic potential.

## FERTILITY/BREEDING
N/A

## SYNONYMS
Arthritis, osteoarthritis, septic arthritis, erosive/non-erosive arthritis.

## SEE ALSO
Hyperuricemia
Luxations
Mycoplasmosis
Perosis/Slipped Tendon
Renal Disease and Hyperuricemia
Reovirus
Tendinitis and Tenosynovitis

## ABBREVIATIONS
CT—computed tomography
MRI—magnetic resonance imaging
rt-PCR—reverse transcriptase polymerase chain reaction

## INTERNET RESOURCES
N/A

*Suggested Reading*
Azmanis, P.N., Wernick, M.B., Hatt, J.M. (2014). Avian luxations: Occurrence, diagnosis and treatment. *Veterinary Quarterly*, 34:11–21.
Leclerc, A., Goddard, N., Graillot, O., et al. (2023). Retrospective study of intertarsal joint inflammation in avian species from a zoological institution. *Journal of Avian Medicine and Surgery*, 37:235–242.
**Author**: Minh Huynh DVM, DECZM (Avian), DACZM

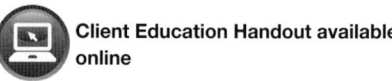

Client Education Handout available online

# BASICS

## DEFINITION
Impaired ability in ambulation, typically in response to pain, physical defect, or dysfunction of the musculoskeletal or nervous system.

## PATHOPHYSIOLOGY
Traumatic injuries to the musculoskeletal system from predators, cage mate aggression, and flight injuries are commonly seen in clinical practice. The thin cortical bone and large medullary canal combined with their high calcium content make avian bones prone to shattering upon impact. Severe and acute injuries of the pelvic limbs present as non-weight bearing of the affected limb. Mild pain may be more difficult to discern, but the bird may put less weight on the injured leg, have a weaker grip, or may be reluctant to walk. The paucity of soft-tissue surrounding the appendicular skeleton makes it prone to vascular compromise and peripheral neuropathies after traumatic injuries. Inflammation, demyelination, or compression of the nerves to the pelvis can also result in paraesthesia of the limb and changes in locomotion. Pain from pathologic fractures (osteopenia), lytic bony lesions (osteomyelitis, neoplasms of the bone), dermatologic lesions (pododermatitis), and articular gout also lead to clinical signs of lameness. Focal seizures and neurologic conditions can present as disuse or weakness of a limb or gait abnormalities. Atherosclerosis can result in intermittent lameness due to claudication, which is pain in the legs due to decrease blood flow to the limbs. Constriction injuries around the toes can lead to severe swelling and eventually necrosis of the toes and/or foot due to restricted blood flow. These types of injuries can be caused by either an annular band of fibrous tissue, string, thread, or hair wrapped around the digits or foot.

## SYSTEMS AFFECTED
**Musculoskeletal**: Fractures; osteopenia from nutritional secondary hyperparathyroidism; soft-tissue swelling or disuse atrophy of the muscle can develop.
**Skin**: Erythema; bruising; abrasions; lacerations, ulceration, constriction injuries.
**Nervous system**: Proprioceptive deficits; paresis; paralysis, focal seizures.

## GENETICS
Congenital deformities that lead to abnormal bone development have been reported.

## INCIDENCE/PREVALENCE
Impaired use of the pelvic limbs is a common presentation in clinical practice.

## GEOGRAPHIC DISTRIBUTION
N/A

## SIGNALMENT
**Species predilections**: Renal neoplasms—budgerigars. Articular gout—cockatiels, budgerigars. Ovarian neoplasia—cockatiels, chickens. Testicular neoplasia—budgerigar, cockatiel. Foot necrosis syndrome—Amazon parrots. Pododermatitis—Amazon parrots, waterfowl, poultry, raptors. Atherosclerosis—African gray parrots, Amazon parrots. Tibial dyschondroplasia—chickens, ducks, and turkeys.
**Mean age and range**: Rickets (vitamin D deficiency), splay leg, constricted toe syndrome, and dyschondroplasia tend to affect neonatal and juvenile birds. Arthritis, degenerative joint disease, osteoporosis, atherosclerosis, and neoplasms more commonly affect geriatric birds.
**Predominate sex**: Testicular tumors (males); ovarian tumors (females). Additionally, hens can develop osteopenia from chronic egg laying, making them more susceptible to pathologic bone fractures.

## SIGNS
### General Comments
Clinical signs will vary depending on the cause and location of the lameness.

### Historical Findings
Clarify with owner the onset, duration, and progression of the lameness; also determine which limb(s) may be affected. Check for a history of recent trauma. Difficulty balancing and perching may be noted as falling off the perch or spending more time on the bottom of the cage. Other findings may include a decreased appetite and activity. Feather picking or self-mutilating the affected limb may be noted.

### Physical Examination Findings
Varying degrees of non-weight bearing or ability to stand; abnormal gait or posture; may have a weak foot grip. Crepitus or laxity may be noted on palpation of the bones and joints. Bruising, swelling, bleeding, missing feathers, and open wounds may be noted on the affected limb. Paresis or paralysis of the limb. Extremities may be cold to the touch. Decreased range of motion or contracture of the limb may be noted in chronic cases. Pressure sores may be noted on the contralateral leg as a result of increased usage of the limb. Full coelomic cavity may be noted on palpation if a mass effect (renal, ovarian, testicular neoplasm) is the underlying cause of the patient's lameness; ascites may or may not be present. Color change of the cere in hormone-secreting reproductive neoplasms (budgerigars).

## CAUSES
**Musculoskeletal**: Traumatic injuries are common and can range from fractures, sprains/strain, joint luxations, and nerve plexus avulsions. Degenerative causes include arthritis, degenerative joint disease, osteomalacia, and osteoporosis. Splay leg can be due to laxities in the ligaments of the leg and/or angular deformities of bones of the pelvic limb. Tibial dyschondroplasia is a disease of fast-growing juvenile chickens, ducks, and turkeys that results in deformed bones. Articular gout. Bacterial or fungal osteomyelitis.
**Integument**: Pododermatitis (bumblefoot). Constriction injuries. Amazon foot necrosis.
**Cardiovascular**: Claudication secondary to atherosclerosis results in a shifting leg lameness and cerebrovascular ischemia. Thromboembolic disease.
**Nutritional**: Rickets (hypovitaminosis D, calcium–phosphorus imbalance). Nutritional secondary hyperparathyroidism (hypocalcemia). Selenium—vitamin E deficiency. Perosis (manganese deficiency).
**Neoplasia**: Primary or metastatic bone neoplasia. Ovarian and oviductal neoplasia. Testicular neoplasia. Renal neoplasia. Spinal neoplasia.
**Neurologic**: Toxic—heavy metal (lead, zinc); avian vacuolar myelinopathy (cyanobacteria). Focal seizures. Compression of lumbosacral plexus/ischiatic nerves by a renal or reproductive mass.
**Infectious**: Bornavius (proventricular dilatation disease); WNV; paramyxovirus; Marek's disease virus. Mycobacteria.

## RISK FACTORS
Pododermatitis—obesity in heavy-bodied birds (e.g. Amazon parrots, chickens, waterfowl); birds kept on concrete perches or hard surfaces; malnutrition. Osteopenia—chronic egg laying, nutritional secondary hyperparathyroidism (calcium deficiency). Splay leg—nutritional deficiencies (calcium, vitamin D), slick flooring with inadequate substrate. Heavy metal toxicity—pet birds allowed unsupervised free-roam at home; wildlife exposed to lead shot/sinkers. Potential sources of lead include leaded paint in homes built before 1978, caulk, linoleum, solder, and crystal rhinestones in costume jewelry or clothing. Potential sources of zinc include US pennies minted after 1982, galvanized wire and hardware (nuts, bolts). Atherosclerosis—obesity and hypercholesterolemia due to high-calorie diets and inactivity; increased estrogen levels in reproductively active hens affect lipid, calcium, and protein metabolism.

L

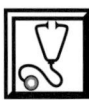

## DIAGNOSIS

### DIFFERENTIAL DIAGNOSIS
Generalized weakness from systemic disease leading to sternal recumbency could be confused with lameness. Some birds will normally hold one foot up while at rest.

### CBC/BIOCHEMISTRY/URINALYSIS
Elevated CK and AST are often noted, especially in cases of traumatic injury. Inflammatory leukograms are usually present with traumatic events; certain infectious diseases (i.e. mycobacteria) may result in severe monocytosis and heterophilia with toxic changes. Total blood calcium levels can sometimes still be in the normal range even with clear evidence of calcium deficiency and osteopenia due to the parathyroid response to hypocalcemia. Hyperuricemia can be seen in cases of articular gout.

### OTHER LABORATORY TESTS
Blood lead and zinc levels should be assessed if exposure is suspected or if metal densities are noted on radiographic films. PCR tests are available for bornavirus, WNV, and mycobacteria.

### IMAGING

#### Radiographic Findings
Evaluate for fractures, dislocations, osteomyelitis, and other bony lesions. In acute injuries, soft tissue swelling may be noted around the affected limb; in subacute or chronic disease, disuse muscle atrophy may be noted. Osteopenia may be noted in birds with nutritional secondary parathyroidism or those hens that have been chronically laying eggs. Metal densities in the GI tract are suggestive of lead and zinc toxicity; however, other metals can have the same appearance; likewise, the absence of metal densities does not rule out heavy metal toxicity. Increased tortuosity and focal and linear mineralization of the great vessels (aorta, brachiocephalic trunks) are suggestive of atherosclerosis that can lead to thromboembolic disease and claudication. Cardiomegaly and an enlarged hepatic silhouette can be seen in cases of advanced heart disease. Soft-tissue densities may be noted in the gonadorenal region if renal, ovarian, or testicular neoplasia is present; a GI barium contrast series or CT may help differentiate the soft tissue densities.

#### Ultrasonography
If soft-tissue densities are noted in the coelomic cavity, ultrasonographic examination or CT may help differentiate between different disease processes, such as renal neoplasms and reproductive disease. Echocardiography should be performed if cardiomyopathy is suspected.

#### Advanced Imaging
Infrared thermography may also help locate the source of the lameness.

### DIAGNOSTIC PROCEDURES
Fine-needle aspirate or biopsy of any bony lesions for cytologic or histopathologic examination; samples should also be collected for aerobic bacterial C/S and anaerobic bacterial and fungal culture. Electromyography and nerve conduction studies to measure muscle and nerve function. Laparoscopy allows for visualization and biopsy of any intracoelomic masses (i.e., renal, ovarian, testicular) that may be compressing the ischiatic nerve.

### PATHOLOGIC FINDINGS
Traumatic injuries: Severe tissue swelling; fractured bones; lacerations, abrasions, and avulsions of the skin. Feather destructive behavior and self-mutilation of painful areas on the limb or synsacrum. Organomegaly or neoplastic masses of the kidney, ovary, or testicles may be present. Neoplastic effusions may also be noted.

## TREATMENT

### APPROPRIATE HEALTH CARE
Assess the bird for shock and take appropriate measures as necessary. Identify and provide pain medications as needed. If osteoporosis is present, calcium supplementation may be beneficial. For splayed limbs in juveniles, hobble the pelvic limbs with non-adhesive material to bring them into appropriate alignment; must be performed early and changed frequently as bone is growing.

### Fractures/Traumatic injuries
Sedation or general anesthesia may be required if a patient is especially fractious to prevent further damage to the injured limb and/or manage pain during manipulation. External coaptation, internal fixation, external fixation, or a combination of these methods are used to stabilize fractures. All should have restricted activity/cage rest, but this alone may be appropriate for certain types of fracture (i.e. pelvic fracture). Modified Schroeder–Thomas splints or tape splints (in smaller birds) can be applied for the stabilization of tibiotarsal or metatarsal fractures. Surgical fixation with intramedullary pins, external fixators, and/or plates can be utilized in larger birds. May need distractors (tape tabs) or Elizabethan collars to prevent the bird from chewing the bandage off.

### Pododermatitis
Cover perches with bandage material or artificial turf; move the bird off hard surfaces (i.e. concrete). If the bird is obese, gradually reduce body weight and correct dietary deficiencies. Ball or other types of bandages are used to prevent and treat pododermatitis.

### NURSING CARE
Parental fluid supplementation (SC, IV, IO) if blood loss is noted in conjunction with fractures and open wounds. Aggressive fluid diuresis is recommended for patients with articular gout to prevent further progression of hyperuricemia. Low-level laser therapy (cold laser) may help alleviate pain and decrease inflammation.

### ACTIVITY
Strict cage rest is recommended for 6–8 weeks to allow fractures to heal. Cage modifications such as lowering or removal of perches is recommended for patients with perching and gait difficulties to prevent them from falling. For those patients that insist on climbing the cage bars, owners can use a large smooth-sided container lined with paper towels or newspaper as a temporary "recovery cage." Chicks with splayed limbs should be kept on surfaces that are not slick and have appropriate substrate so that they have more grip/support as they develop.

### DIET
If modifications have been made to the cage (i.e. removal of perches) bowls should be placed so food and water are easily accessible. Some birds do not eat well when bandaged or placed in an Elizabethan or bubble collar. Clipping food items or elevating the food bowls can make it easier for the bird to reach its food. Owners should weigh the bird daily to monitor food intake. Calcium and vitamin D supplementation is important, especially in egg-laying hens, to prevent osteoporosis and increased risk of fractures. Omega-3 fatty acid supplementation increases bone formation and decreases bone resorption, thus providing protection from osteoporosis.

### CLIENT EDUCATION
Bandages and splints must be kept dry and clean and should be assessed regularly to minimize complications. If the bird has difficulty balancing, enclosures will need to be modified to keep the bird comfortable and prevent it from falling; all perches should be lowered or removed. Some birds may need to be kept in a smooth-sided enclosure where they are not able to climb up the side to decrease movement and facilitate healing. Patients with permanent grip deficits benefit from enclosures that have platforms in lieu of perches. Converting to one-level caging may be appropriate for some patients.

### SURGICAL CONSIDERATIONS
Patient should be stabilized before attempting surgical fixation under anesthesia. Osteopenia may complicate the placement of surgical

hardware and delay fracture healing. Vascular compromise and peripheral neuropathy are possible surgical complications.

## MEDICATIONS

### DRUG(S) OF CHOICE
**Treatment for pain and arthritis**: Meloxicam 1–1.6 mg/kg PO, IM q12–24h; nonsteroidal anti-inflammatory medication; butorphanol tartrate 2–5 mg/kg q2–3h prn IM, IV; opioid agonist–antagonist for pain management (psittacine birds); gabapentin 10–30 mg/kg PO q8–12h; neuropathic pain medication; tramadol 5–30 mg/kg PO q6–12h; synthetic opioid; lower dose effective in raptors, psittacine birds required higher doses.
**Treatment for osteomyelitis**: Antibiotic based on culture and sensitivity.
**Treatment for lead toxicity**: Calcium EDTA 30–35 mg/kg IM, SC q12h; parental chelator for lead toxicity, maintain hydration; DMSA 40 mg/kg PO q12h; oral chelator for lead toxicosis; can be used alone or in conjunction with Ca EDTA.
**Treatment for atherosclerosis**: Isoxsuprine 10 mg/kg PO q12–24h, vasodilator; enalapril 1.25–5 mg/kg PO q8–12h, vasodilator; pentoxifylline 15 mg/kg PO q8–12h to improve peripheral perfusion.
**Treatment for articular gout**: Colchicine 0.01–0.2 mg/kg PO q12–24h, anti-inflammatory.
Treatment for hypocalcemia: Calcium glubionate 25–150 mg/kg PO q12–24h, calcium supplementation; calcium gluconate—dilute 1:1 with saline or sterile water for IV, SQ, IM injection; 5–10 mg/kg slow IV for tetany; 10–100 mg/kg SC, IM, slow IV.
**Treatment for testicular or ovarian neoplasms**: Leuprolide acetate 1500–3500 µg/kg IM q2–4w; deslorelin 4.7 mg implant SC q2–5m (synthetic GnRH agonists), long-term implant.

### CONTRAINDICATIONS
Deslorin implant in birds is considered off-label use and as an FDA-indexed drug is prohibited in the USA for the use in poultry.

### PRECAUTIONS
Polysulfated glycosaminoglycan (Adequan®, American Regent Animal Health, Shirley, NY) has been used, but fatal hemorrhage has been reported.

### POSSIBLE INTERACTIONS
N/A

### ALTERNATIVE DRUGS
Oral glucosamine, chondroitin, and omega-3 fatty acids have been used anecdotally for the treatment of osteoarthritis. Acupuncture may be useful for birds with chronic pain.

## FOLLOW-UP

### PATIENT MONITORING
Weekly assessment of bandages and splints is recommended to ensure that the lesions are healing appropriately and for any necessary adjustments. Open or infected wounds often require more frequent bandaging. Repeat radiographs can be performed in 3–6 weeks to evaluate fracture healing. Endosteal callus bone formation may be difficult to visualize radiographically.

### PREVENTION/AVOIDANCE
For birds that sustained an injury from a predator or cage mate, measures should be taken to prevent further exposure to the perpetrator. Birds at risk of osteoporosis and hypocalcemia from chronic egg-laying should be discouraged from further egg laying through behavior modification and hormonal therapies.

### POSSIBLE COMPLICATIONS
Malunion or non-union can occur with inadequate immobilization of the fracture. External coaptation may lead to joint stiffness, muscle atrophy, tendon or skin contracture, and fracture misalignment. Open fractures are at higher risk for bacterial contamination and osteomyelitis. Neurologic or vascular derangements can occur secondary to traumatic injuries. Necrosis and auto-amputation of digits may occur. Development of pressure sores on the contralateral leg, especially in heavy-bodied birds such as large chickens, waterfowl, and raptors.

### EXPECTED COURSE AND PROGNOSIS
Well-aligned, stable fractures have sufficient endosteal callus to stabilize the fracture as early as three weeks; most heal over 4–6 weeks. Lameness with renal gout and neoplasia is usually progressive over several weeks to months. Treatment of heavy metal toxicity depends on the level of toxicity and may require several courses of chelation therapy. Most patients with atherosclerosis will require lifelong heart medication. Some ovarian and testicular neoplasms may temporarily respond to repeated hormonal therapies.

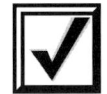

## MISCELLANEOUS

### ASSOCIATED CONDITIONS
N/A

### AGE-RELATED FACTORS
Splay leg and dyschondroplasia affect neonatal and juvenile birds. Arthritis and neoplasm more commonly affect geriatric birds.

### ZOONOTIC POTENTIAL
Mycobacteria can cause tubercular lesions of the bone marrow, resulting in unilateral or shifting leg lameness. *Mycobacterium genavense* is responsible for a majority of cases in pet birds, though *Mycobacterium avium* complex is still responsible for some infections.

### FERTILITY/BREEDING
Inability to use pelvic limbs normally to perch and balance can interfere with the bird's ability to mate. Hypocalcemic hens are at risk for egg binding and dystocia.

### SYNONYMS
Limping.

### SEE ALSO
Arthritis
Atherosclerosis
Bornaviral Disease
Dystocia and Egg Binding
Fractures
Hyperuricemia
Hypocalcemia and Hypomagnesemia
Luxations
Marek's Disease
Mycobacteriosis
Neoplasia (Integument)
Neoplasia (Neurological)
Neurologic (Non-Traumatic Diseases)
Neurologic (Trauma)
Perosis/Slipped Tendon
Pododermatitis
Toxicosis (Heavy Metals)
Trauma
West Nile Virus
Appendix 8, Algorithm 13: Lameness

### ABBREVIATIONS
AST—aspartate aminotransferase
C/S—culture and sensitivity
CK—creatine kinase
CT—computed tomography
DMSA—meso-2,3-dimercaptosuccinic acid
EDTA—ethylenediaminetetraacetic acid
GI—gastrointestinal
GnRH—gonadotropin-releasing hormone
PCR—polymerase chain reaction
PDD—proventricular dilatation disease
WNV—West Nile virus

### INTERNET RESOURCES
N/A

*Suggested Reading*
Beaufrère, H., Holder, K.A., Bauer, R., et al. (2011). Intermittent claudication-like syndrome secondary to atherosclerosis in a yellow-naped Amazon parrot

L

(*Amazona ochrocephala auropalliata*). *Journal of Avian Medicine and Surgery*, 25:266–276.

Fitzgerald, B. (2018). Diseases of pet chickens: bumblefoot. *Proceedings of the Chicagoland Veterinary Conference*. Chicago.

Guzman, D.S., Hawkins, M.G. (2023). Treatment of pain in birds. *Veterinary*

*Clinics of North America: Exotic Animal Practice*, 26:83–120.

Guzman, D.S. (2020). Avian orthopedics: put it all together. *Proceedings of the Western Veterinary Conference 2020*, Las Vegas.

Harcourt-Brown, NH (2002). Orthopedic conditions that affect the avian pelvic limb. *Veterinary Clinics of North America: Exotic Animal Practice*, 5:49–81.

Ponder, J.B., Redig, P. (2016). Orthopedics. In: *Current Therapy in Avian Medicine and Surgery* (ed. B.L. Speer), 657–667. St. Louis, MO: Elsevier.

Scagnelli, A.M., Tully, T.N. Jr. (2017). Reproductive disorders in parrots. *Veterinary Clinics of North America: Exotic Animal Practice*, 20:485–507.

**Author:** Sue Chen, DVM, DABVP (Avian)

L

# BASICS

## DEFINITION
Leukocytosis is an abnormal increase in the number of white blood cells (leukocytes) circulating in the blood.

## PATHOPHYSIOLOGY
There are several causes of leukocytosis including the following. Inflammation and antigenic stimulation, which may occur secondary to infectious and non-infectious causes. Infectious causes include bacterial, viral, parasitic, and fungal infections. Non-infectious causes of inflammation include trauma, injections, neoplasia, immune-mediated disease, and inflammation of organs such as pancreatitis and reproductive disorders (e.g. egg-yolk coelomitis). Neoplasia, including hemic neoplasia, resulting in an increased number of neoplastic leukocytes (or unidentifiable nucleated cells) in circulation, or a secondary, paraneoplastic increase in leukocytes through secretion of a substance that stimulates bone marrow release of leukocytes. Hormone-mediated, including corticosteroid leukocytosis, is most often secondary to stress or illness, and possibly catecholamine release due to excitement. Laboratory error can also occur, due to misidentification of thrombocytes or immature erythrocytes as leukocytes.

## SYSTEMS AFFECTED
Given the wide variety of causes for leukocytosis, any organ system can be affected. However, it is important to note that leukocytosis is usually an indicator or result of an underlying problem (e.g. infection, neoplasm, trauma, stress) as opposed to the primary cause of the clinical signs. The exception may be with hemic neoplasia, as the abnormal function of neoplastic leukocytes or their extreme numbers can lead to abnormal function of the bone marrow leading to cytopenias (heteropenia, thrombocytopenia, anemia), or can block blood vessels leading to necrosis in the extremities and various organs.

## GENETICS
Leukocytosis in birds is primarily a reactive response to external factors such as infections, inflammation, or stress. As such, there is no commonly encountered genetic disorder associated with this condition.

## INCIDENCE/PREVALENCE
Leukocytosis is one of the most common abnormalities observed on CBC, with most cases being due to inflammation or a stress leukogram.

## GEOGRAPHIC DISTRIBUTION
Leukocytosis can be observed on CBC of birds anywhere. The main factor that is affected by geography is the prevalence of certain infectious diseases, but they are too numerous to list.

## SIGNALMENT
**Species**: All bird species are susceptible to leukocytosis. With this said, reference intervals for the total leukocyte count and absolute values of each leukocyte should be used, as there can be significant variations in the leukocyte counts depending on the species. For example, macaws, chickens, great horned owls, and vultures tend to have higher leukocyte counts in health, as well as with stress and inflammation, than other bird species.

**Mean age and predominant sex**: Leukocytosis may occur in birds of any age and sex, although some of the underlying diseases causing these changes vary by age and sex.

## SIGNS
Leukocytosis in birds is a diagnostic sign rather than a primary clinical condition. Therefore, typical signs associated with leukocytosis itself are not readily observable. Instead, the focus lies in recognizing signs indicative of the underlying cause leading to elevated white blood cell counts. Historical findings may include reports of recent exposure to infectious agents, changes in the bird's environment, or instances of stress.

### Physical Examination Findings
**Inflammation**: Swelling, redness, or heat in specific body regions.
**Trauma**: Presence of fractures, wounds, hematomas, etc.
**Masses**: The presence of masses may indicate the presence of granulomas or tumors.
**Respiratory distress**: Labored breathing or abnormal respiratory sounds.
**Abdominal discomfort**: Palpable pain or distension in the abdominal area.
**Behavioral changes**: Altered behavior, such as lethargy, or possibly reproductive behavior if related to salpingitis or egg-yolk coelomitis.

## CAUSES
Causes of leukocytosis in birds are diverse, often reflecting underlying diseases or stressors. Grouped by pathophysiologic mechanisms: Infectious—bacterial, viral, fungal, or parasitic infections; inflammatory—tissue damage, injury, or inflammation; stress-related—environmental stressors, nutritional imbalances, or handling-related stress.

## RISK FACTORS
Dependent on underlying cause.

# DIAGNOSIS

## DIFFERENTIAL DIAGNOSIS
The differential diagnoses for leukocytosis depend in part on the type of leukocytes that are increased.
**Heterophilia**: The the most common type. Stress and excitement can cause mild mature heterophilia up to approximately twice the high end of the reference interval (mild). Severe heterophilia (70,000 cells/µl, and often higher) is most often associated with certain chronic infectious organisms, including *Aspergillus*, *Mycobacterium*, and *Chlamydia* spp. Morphological evaluation of the heterophils on the blood smear to look for evidence of a left shift or toxicity is important, and while these changes are not specific to infectious diseases, marked left shifting or severe toxicity is most often seen with bacterial infections. Mild to moderate heterophilias can be seen with a number of infectious organisms, particularly bacterial and fungal infections, trauma, neoplasia, injection of irritating substances (including some drugs or vaccines), or other non-infectious causes of inflammation such as pancreatitis, egg-yolk coelomitis. Note that bacterial infections are not always associated with a heterophilia if the infection is localized (e.g. pododermatitis) or if the rate of consumption of the heterophils is equal or higher than the rate of production by the bone marrow. Chronic myeloid/granulocytic leukemias are rare, and all other causes of heterophilia should be ruled out prior to making this diagnosis.
**Monocytosis**: Monocytosis is not typically seen with stress or excitement and mild monocytosis often accompanies heterophilia regardless of the cause. Moderate to marked monocytosis usually accompanies marked heterophilia seen with chronic infection such as *Aspergillus*, *Mycobacterium*, *Chlamydia*, or *Clostridium* spp.
**Eosinophilia**: While eosinophilia in mammals is usually associated with parasitic infections, hypersensitivity-type reactions or a paraneoplastic process, eosinophilia in birds appears to be less specific to these conditions and is often seen as part of a mixed inflammatory process or in wild birds, such as raptors, with multiple types of infectious organisms with or without non-infectious causes of inflammation. Eosinophilia is often not seen, despite parasitic infections.
**Lymphocytosis**: Can indicate antigenic stimulation, which can be present with all types of inflammation; however, it is rarely

L

## LEUKOCYTOSIS     (CONTINUED)

the predominant leukocyte type that is increased with inflammation, except perhaps with certain viral diseases or following vaccination. Anecdotally, lymphocyte counts may occasionally reach 20,000 or 30,000 cells/µl. With certain viral infections, such as highly pathogenic avian influenza, however, counts greater than this typically indicate either a lymphocytic leukemia or miscounting of thrombocytes, immature erythrocytes and/or monocytes as lymphocytes. Lymphocytic leukemias can occur spontaneously in many species, although gallinaceous birds most often have leukemia induced by viruses, including MDV, a herpesvirus, and a number of retroviruses, of which avian leukosis virus is the most common. MDV most often induces lymphoma but can also induce lymphocytic leukemias. With the retroviruses, the neoplastic lymphocytes can be small or large, and, although less common, erythrocytic or myeloid leukemias can also occur secondary to these viruses. Note that morphologically, large neoplastic lymphocytes in circulation may not be distinguishable from leukemias composed of undifferentiated cells or early precursors of other hemic cell lines.

### CBC/BIOCHEMISTRY/URINALYSIS

It is important to note that a leukocytosis is diagnosed based on the total white blood cell count (cells/µl), and further characterized by evaluation of which leukocytes are increased. Neutrophilia, monocytosis, lymphocytosis, eosinophilia, and basophilia are diagnosed by comparing the absolute values for each leukocyte type compared with species-specific reference intervals, not by the leukocyte percentages. Evaluation of leukocyte morphology on a blood smear is an important step in determining the cause of the leukocytosis. Morphological evaluation includes the following.
**Heterophils**: Determine whether there are toxic changes and a left shift, both of which often occur concurrently. Heterophils are segmented in birds, and typically have two thick sections of nuclei connected by a thin strand, which may be visible or obscured by granules. Immature heterophils have nuclei which look horseshoe shaped, bean shaped or round. Immature heterophils often have fewer pink granules, which can be round, and can have a few dark purple granules, depending on the stage of maturation. Toxic changes consist of hypogranulation, cytoplasmic basophilia, and occasionally cytoplasmic vacuolation.
**Lymphocytes**: Evaluate whether the lymphocytes appear normal (small, mature) or are atypical (too large, immature, or abnormal). If they appear normal, the top

differentials include a response to antigenic stimulation or chronic lymphocytic leukemia; if large and atypical, top differentials include an acute leukemia or blood stage (stage V) of lymphoma.
**Cell identification**: Correct identification of cell types can be a challenge in birds. Thrombocytes may be misinterpreted as small lymphocytes, particularly if the lymphocyte count is very low (which can make it difficult to know what lymphocytes should look like in that species). Identifying thrombocyte clumps, which are present on most smears, can help to establish what a thrombocyte looks like in that particular species. Heterophils and eosinophils can be challenging to differentiate. Generally, heterophils have oval granules, while eosinophils have rounds ones. Heterophils have consistently pink granules but, while eosinophils typically have pink granules, they have pale blue to even occasionally pale gray to non-staining granules in some species (mostly Psittacines). Eosinophils are also often slightly larger than heterophils, and cytoplasm, when visible, is usually more basophilic. Monocytes are typically identified by their size (since they are typically the largest leukocyte), their abundant cytoplasm, and the frequent presence of a few vacuoles. Blood smears should be evaluated for the presence of erythrocyte precursors, including polychromatophils and earlier precursors (rubricytes), which can have a similar appearance to large lymphocytes. If large numbers of polychromatophils are present, rubricytes are also likely to be present and should not be miscounted as leukocytes.

### OTHER LABORATORY TESTS
N/A

### IMAGING
Imaging, including radiographs, ultrasound, computed tomography, endoscopy, or even possibly thermal imaging can all be used to detect a number of issues including granulomas (e.g. due to aspergillosis or *Mycobacterium*), other masses (e.g. tumors), organomegaly (e.g. splenomegaly in *Chlamydia*), or effusions (e.g. egg-yolk coelomitis).

### DIAGNOSTIC PROCEDURES
Different types of diagnostic test exist to detect infectious agents, including PCR for viruses and certain other targeted organisms such as bacteria (*Mycobacterium*, for speciation), fungi and parasites, and bacterial and fungal culture and sensitivity.

### PATHOLOGIC FINDINGS
Fluid analysis, cytology, and histopathology may be able to identify various types of inflammatory lesions, infectious agents, and tumours.

## TREATMENT

### APPROPRIATE HEALTH CARE
Appropriate treatment depends on the identified cause of the leukocytosis.

### NURSING CARE
Appropriate supportive care depends on the identified cause of the leukocytosis.

### ACTIVITY
Dependent on underlying cause.

### DIET
N/A

### CLIENT EDUCATION
N/A

### SURGICAL CONSIDERATIONS
N/A

## MEDICATIONS

### DRUG(S) OF CHOICE
Appropriate medication, if needed, depends on the identified cause of the leukocytosis.

### CONTRAINDICATIONS
N/A

### PRECAUTIONS
N/A

### POSSIBLE INTERACTIONS
N/A

### ALTERNATIVE DRUGS
N/A

## FOLLOW-UP

### PATIENT MONITORING
Repeat physical examination, complete blood count and blood smear evaluation, imaging etc. can be repeated as needed for monitoring, depending on the idenfied cause of the leukocytosis.

### PREVENTION/AVOIDANCE
Dependent on underlying cause.

### POSSIBLE COMPLICATIONS
N/A

### EXPECTED COURSE AND PROGNOSIS
Dependent on underlying cause.

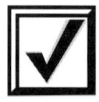

## MISCELLANEOUS

### ASSOCIATED CONDITIONS
N/A

**AGE-RELATED FACTORS**
N/A

**ZOONOTIC POTENTIAL**
N/A

**FERTILITY/BREEDING**
N/A

**SYNONYMS**
High white blood cell count, neutrophilia, monocytosis, eosinophilia, lymphocytosis, leukosis

**SEE ALSO**
Anemia
Aspergillosis

Chlamydiosis
Egg Yolk and Reproductive Coelomitis
Mycobacteriosis
Neoplasia (Lymphoproliferative)
Wounds (Including Bite Wounds, Predator Attacks)

**ABBREVIATIONS**
MDV—Marek's disease virus
PCR—polymerase chain reaction

**INTERNET RESOURCES**
Cornell University College of Veterinary Medicine. eClinPath: https://eclinpath.com

*Suggested Reading*
Brooks, M.B., Harr, K.E., Seelig, D.M., et al. (2022). *Schalm's Veterinary Hematology*. Hoboken, NJ: Wiley.
Campbell, T., Grant, K. (2022). *Exotic Animal Hematology and Cytology*, 5th edn. Hoboken, NJ: Wiley.
Pendl H., Samour, J. (2016). Hematology analyses. In: *Avian Medicine*, 3rd edn., 77–99. St. Louis, MO: Elsevier.
**Author**: Melanie Ammersbach, DVM, DACVP (Clin Path)

L

# LIVER DISEASE

## BASICS

### DEFINITION
The liver is involved with numerous systems in the body and as such is part of a wide variety of disease processes. A large number of diseases have been reported in the avian liver, and most systemic diseases will have hepatic components. Liver disease is very common in birds, both specifically and as part of systemic disease. Although generally thought of as a digestive organ, the liver plays a part in many organ systems, resulting in very wide and divergent clinical effects of liver disease. There are many types of liver diseases in birds but most can be placed into five categories: Infectious, metabolic, toxic, neoplastic, and degenerative. Many liver diseases can be caught in early subclinical stages by routine clinical evaluation. In these cases, the prognosis is much better than when treating overt clinical disease.

### PATHOPHYSIOLOGY
Because of the numerous liver diseases, the pathophysiology is widely variable. Exposure of the liver to infectious agents may occur from sepsis, by an ascending infection from the GI tract, or through the portal system. Toxins may affect the liver. Metabolic processes may cause accumulation of substances within the hepatic cells, resulting in damage to the cells. Hepatic fibrosis can occur secondary to any chronic liver condition.

### SYSTEMS AFFECTED
The liver has numerous functions and the signs can give apparent changes in many systems. Behavioral changes such as lethargy or dullness are common. GI problems such as diarrhea, steatorrhea, or anorexia are often noted in liver disease. Hemic/lymphatic/immune changes include hypoproteinemia, which may result in ascites or edema. Musculoskeletal changes often include a loss of muscle mass. Nervous problems are theoretically possible with hepatic encephalopathy. This appears to be rare in birds. Renal/urologic problems include biliverdinuria. This is one of the more specific signs of liver disease. Respiratory effort can be increased in cases where the liver is enlarged or there is ascites. Skin/exocrine changes such as poor feather quality and beak overgrowth or degradation are common.

### GENETICS
Genetically related liver diseases are not commonly reported.

### INCIDENCE/PREVALENCE
Liver disease is extremely common in birds.

### GEOGRAPHIC DISTRIBUTION
There appears to be no geographic distribution of liver disease overall, although specific diseases have higher prevalence in some areas compared to others.

### SIGNALMENT
**Species:** All birds are susceptible, although some etiologies are more common in specific bird species.
**Mean age and range:** Varies with disease.
**Predominant sex:** Most have no sex predilection.

### SIGNS

#### General Comments
Depending on the severity of the disease, physical findings may be subtle or severe.

#### Historical Findings
General malaise, often referred to as "sick-bird syndrome" is common with liver disease. Because of the digestive function of the liver, diarrhea, steatorrhea, and weight loss can occur with liver disorders. Biliverdinuria is one of the most specific of the clinical signs. When the liver fails to conjugate and excrete the biliverdin in the bile, it accumulates and is excreted in the urine.

#### Physical Examination Findings
Many birds with liver disease have a "pot-bellied" appearance due to either ascites or severe enlargement of the liver. If there has been weight loss, this appearance will be accentuated. Coagulopathies are rare but can occur with liver disease. Overgrowth and dystrophy of the beak keratin is commonly seen in chronic, low grade liver diseases, although the reason is unclear.

### CAUSES
**Infections:** Account for a large proportion of the liver disease found in birds.
Viruses: Pacheco's disease is caused by a herpesvirus and results in death without premonitory clinical signs. Polyomavirus is a systemic disease, but can affect the liver. Adenovirus, reovirus and many other viruses have been implicated in hepatitides of birds. Bacteria: Chlamydiosis caused by *Chlamydia psittaci* is a systemic infection, but hepatic signs are often prominent in the presentation. Mycobacteriosis resulting from organisms in *Mycobacterium avium intracellulare* complex also is a systemic disease with significant hepatic involvement. Opportunistic infections with a variety of bacterial species can occur by direct extension from the intestine via the biliary tree, hematogenously during sepsis, or through the portal system.

In many cases, the organism is not recovered, but the inflammatory changes within the liver suggest a previous infection. Parasites: Systemic isosporosis (formerly atoxoplasmosis) is a common and severe disease of some passerine birds. It is a systemic disease, but the liver is often involved and is one of the better sites to identify the parasites.
**Metabolic conditions:** Hepatic lipidosis is extremely common in pet birds. It often results in very chronic and low-grade disease. Excessive calorie consumption, inactivity, and nutritional imbalances appear to be responsible. Hemochromatosis is the most common disease process in many species, including mynahs, birds of paradise, and many toucan species. It can affect many organs, but often the liver is the most severely affected. Although uncommon in psittacidae, it can occur. Lories are the most commonly affected Psittacidae.
**Toxins:** Aflatoxicosis is one of the most common naturally occurring hepatotoxins. It can cause centrilobular necrosis of the liver. Iatrogenic hepatotoxins such as itraconazole will often cause acute anorexia and elevation of hepatic enzymes.
**Neoplasia:** Biliary adenocarcinoma is a common hepatic neoplasm. It has a strong association with the herpesvirus responsible for cloacal papillomas. Lymphoma is another common neoplasm of the liver. It often is multisystemic.
**Degenerative:** Chronic hepatic fibrosis is commonly found. It is a common sequela of any chronic disease state of the liver and generally remains after the primary disease has resolved.

### RISK FACTORS
Exposure to the infectious agents is the most important factor for many hepatitides. Unbalanced, high calorie diets combined with inactivity predispose birds to hepatic lipidosis. High iron diets, lack of dietary tannins, and species predilection predispose to hemochromatosis. Moldy foods predispose to aflatoxicosis. Herpesvirus infections predispose to biliary adenocarcinoma.

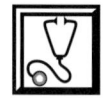

## DIAGNOSIS

### DIFFERENTIAL DIAGNOSIS
There are two phases of diagnosis. First, it must be determined if liver disease is present, then it must be determined what is causing the liver disease. The cause of liver disease may sometimes be found with tests for specific pathogens, or can be presumptive and based on risk factors such as species

(hemochromatosis) or obesity (lipidosis). There are many clinical signs of liver disease and each has its own set of differentials. Differentials for diarrhea, weight loss, and malaise include systemic disease, GI disease, or pancreatic disease. Biliverdinuria may occur with hemolysis. Enlarged coelom can occur with heart disease, reproductive disease and others. Overgrown beak may be due to knemidokoptic mange, fungal infections, or lack of wear.

## CBC/BIOCHEMISTRY/URINALYSIS
The presence and severity of liver disease can often be determined by evaluating biochemistries such as enzymes (AST, GGT, etc.), bile acids, protein, and glucose: AST elevation (hepatocellular damage). Sensitive but not specific. GGT elevation (biliary cell damage). Induced expression during cholestasis. GLDH elevation (hepatocellular necrosis). Specific but not sensitive. Bile acid elevation (functional impairment). Specific and sensitive. Hypoproteinemia (functional impairment). Hypoglycemia (functional impairment). Hematology may support an inflammatory or infectious etiology although it will not be specific.

## OTHER LABORATORY TESTS
Screening for infectious diseases may be helpful in identifying the etiology of hepatic diseases. *C. psittaci* can be detected via serology or PCR. {Mycobacterium} spp. may be detected with acid fast stains or with PCR. Herpesvirus may also be identified using PCR.

## IMAGING
Radiographs may show alterations in size of the liver. Ultrasound will give more information regarding the internal texture of the liver. CT is less commonly used, but can give a great deal of anatomical information about the liver and other internal structures. The size of the liver may be either increased or decreased in liver disease. Hepatomegaly much more common. Even some chronic fibrotic livers are quite enlarged.

## DIAGNOSTIC PROCEDURES
Liver biopsy is frequently required to definitively identify the cause of liver disease. Fine-needle aspiration can give some information, but a definitive diagnosis often requires histopathology. Endoscopic sampling of the liver is most common in birds, but open surgical biopsy or ultrasound-guided sampling are also possible.

## PATHOLOGIC FINDINGS
Gross changes range from enlargement to atrophy. There can be a variety of color changes in the liver, depending on the condition. Histopathology also varies with the specific disease process. Vacuolar changes occur with hepatic lipidosis. Inflammatory infiltrates occur with various infectious processes. Hemosiderin accumulates in the macrophages with hemochromatosis. Centrilobular necrosis occurs with aflatoxicosis.

## TREATMENT

### APPROPRIATE HEALTH CARE
The treatment of liver disease depends on treatment of the underlying etiology of the disease, as well as symptomatic management of the patient. Early cases may require very little, beyond some husbandry alterations. Others may require hospitalization and intensive care.

### NURSING CARE
Fluid therapy to achieve appropriate hydration and perfusion is appropriate. Many patients with hepatic disease will be anorectic and nutritional support is critical. Most often alimentation in the form of gavage feeding is used. Small frequent feedings may be needed to avoid regurgitation in some cases. Despite the need for nutritional improvement, the time when a patient is acutely ill may not be the appropriate opportunity to do this.

### ACTIVITY
Unless fluid lines or other supportive care prevents it, normal activity can be maintained for most birds. If the liver is extremely large, the bird should be carefully protected from falls. The liver can fracture easily, resulting in fatal hemorrhage in these cases. If there is ascites, the fluid could rupture into the air sacs and drown the bird. Increased activity is recommended for obese birds provided the previous situations are not present.

### DIET
The diet should be gradually converted to a balanced, calorically appropriate, and toxin-free diet. Diet conversion may take several weeks and close monitoring is warranted. Certain nutritional supplements may be appropriate for specific conditions of the liver. L-carnitine can improve fat metabolism in cases of hepatic lipidosis. The addition of tannins to the diet may reduce iron absorption in cases of hemochromatosis.

### CLIENT EDUCATION
A few of the liver diseases are zoonotic and this should be conveyed to the owner. There is a great deal of education involved in the dietary conversion.

### SURGICAL CONSIDERATIONS
Liver biopsy is often required for diagnosis, but is not generally used for treatment of liver disease. The only exception may be if there is an isolated tumor in an accessible part of the liver.

## MEDICATIONS

### DRUG(S) OF CHOICE
Chlamydia: Doxycycline; dosing schedules vary with preparation and species. Mycobacteria: Combined therapy with ethambutol, rifabutin, clarithromycin, or others. Long-term therapy is recommended but likely does not eliminate disease; therefore, treatment is controversial. Gram-negative bacteria: Enrofloxacin or others based on culture and sensitivity. Antioxidants such as silymarin (milk thistle) may help reduce oxidative damage and further degeneration of the hepatocytes. S-adenosyl methionine is often recommended for liver disease, but the mechanism is unclear. L-carnitine can improve fat metabolism in cases of hepatic lipidosis. Ursodiol can improve bile flow. Lactulose is often recommended, but its effect is questionable. It is generally thought to reduce GI production of ammonia, which does not appear to be a concern for most pet birds.

### CONTRAINDICATIONS
None.

### PRECAUTIONS
Hepatotoxic drugs such as itraconazole should be used cautiously in birds with hepatic disease.

### POSSIBLE INTERACTIONS
Hepatotoxic drugs such as itraconazole should be used cautiously in birds with hepatic disease.

### ALTERNATIVE DRUGS
N/A

## FOLLOW-UP

### PATIENT MONITORING
The patient's general appearance, appetite, and weight should be monitored until stable. The hepatic enzymes and bile acids should be followed to determine if therapy is effective. Frequency depends on the severity and chronicity of the condition. Acute or severe changes should be monitored more frequently (e.g. weekly) while milder or chronic disease can be monitored over a longer time frame (e.g. monthly or quarterly).

### PREVENTION/AVOIDANCE
Many liver diseases can be prevented with sound nutrition and avoidance of toxins and infectious agents.

L

## POSSIBLE COMPLICATIONS
The most common complications are failure to respond to treatment, and secondary fibrosis of the liver.

## EXPECTED COURSE AND PROGNOSIS
Subclinical liver disease often has a good prognosis. Acute hepatic diseases caused by readily treatable conditions, such as chlamydiosis, have a fair to good prognosis. However, overt signs of liver disease occur when a large proportion of the liver is damaged or nonfunctional. Because of this chronic liver disease has a guarded to poor prognosis when the patient has started to show clinical signs.

## MISCELLANEOUS

## ASSOCIATED CONDITIONS
The liver is involved in many systemic and GI disorders, primarily infectious diseases.

## AGE-RELATED FACTORS
Older patients are more likely to have chronic disorders of the liver.

## ZOONOTIC POTENTIAL
*C. psittaci* and *Mycobacterium* spp. are zoonotic.

## FERTILITY/BREEDING
No specific effects.

## SYNONYMS
Hepatic disease, hepatopathy.

## SEE ALSO
Adenoviruses
Ascites
Beak Malocclusion
Chlamydiosis
Coagulopathies
Coccidiosis (Intestinal)
Coccidiosis (Systemic)
Coelomic Distention
Hepatic Lipidosis
Herpesviruses
Iron Storage Disease
Mycobacteriosis
Neoplasia (Gastrointestinal and Hepatic)
Neoplasia (Lymphoproliferative)
Nutritional Imbalances
Obesity
Polyomavirus
Regurgitation and Vomiting
Sick-Bird Syndrome
Toe and Nail Diseases
Toxicosis (Anticoagulant Rodenticides)
Urate and Fecal Discoloration
Appendix 8 Algorithm 15: Hepatopathy

## ABBREVIATIONS
AST—aspartate aminotransferase
CT—computed tomography
GI—gastrointestinal
GGT—gamma-glutamyl transferase
GLDH—glutamate dehydrogenase
PCR—polymerase chain reaction

## INTERNET RESOURCES
N/A

*Suggested Reading*
Davies, R.R. (2000). Avian liver disease: Etiology and pathogenesis. *Seminars in Avian and Exotic Pet Medicine*, 9:115–125.
Grunkemeyer, V.L. (2010). Advanced diagnostic approaches and current management of avian hepatic disorders. *Veterinary Clinics of North America. Exotic Animal Practice*, 13:413–427.
Hung, C.S.Y., Sladakovic, I., Divers, S.J. (2020). Diagnostic value of plasma biochemistry, haematology, radiography and endoscopic visualisation for hepatic disease in psittacine birds. *Veterinary Record*, 186:563.
Nordberg, C., O'Brien, R.T., Paul-Murphy, J., et al. (2000). Ultrasound examination and guided fine-needle aspiration of the liver in Amazon parrots (*Amazona* species). *Journal of Avian Medicine and Surgery*, 14:180–184.
**Author:** Kenneth R. Welle, DVM, DABVP (Avian)

**Client Education Handout available online**

# BASICS

## DEFINITION
Lung disease is a general term that describes any infectious or non-infectious condition affecting the intrapulmonary primary bronchi, secondary bronchi, parabronchi, and parenchyma. This chapter emphasizes inflammatory lung diseases, which are disorders characterized by chronic inflammation and progressive fibrosis of the lung tissue.

## PATHOPHYSIOLOGY
Repeated insults and resulting inflammatory responses of the lung tissue can lead to chronic inflammatory disorders such as pneumoconiosis, chronic pulmonary interstitial fibrosis (CPIF), and chronic obstructive pulmonary disease (COPD). All disorders can lead to an increased thickness of the blood–air barrier and decreased gas exchange ability. Pneumoconiosis is the general term for a class of interstitial lung disease associated with inhalation of dust. The two most common types in birds are silicosis (silica dust) and anthracosis (coal dust). Compensatory polycythemia can occur in response to chronic hypoxygenation. Because the respiratory system of bird is much more efficient than it is in mammals, avian patients have a higher respiratory reserve. As a consequence, clinical signs appear later in the course of the disease and early diagnosis is difficult.

## SYSTEMS AFFECTED
Respiratory. Cardiovascular—CPIF and COPD can be associated with pulmonary arterial hypertension and secondary right heart disease. Hemic/lymphatic/immune—polycythemia can develop as a consequence of chronic hypoxygenation.

## GENETICS
N/A

## INCIDENCE/PREVALENCE
In a 19-year postmortem retrospective study, lung diseases were identified in 12.8% of captive psittacine birds and represented the primary cause of death in 51.3% of those cases. There were no mention of COPD, CPIF or pneumoconiosis. Among Amazon parrots, prevalence of CPIF is evaluated at 2–4% of birds.

## GEOGRAPHIC DISTRIBUTION
CPIF has been more frequently described in Europe.

## SIGNALMENT
CPIF—older Amazon species (average 20 years of age) may be predisposed. COPD—blue-and-gold macaw (*Ara ararauna*) are considered particularly sensitive, although other macaw species can be affected. Cockatoos may be predisposed to interstitial pneumonia associated with avian polyomavirus.

## SIGNS

### General Comments
Signs depends on severity of the disease. They often wax and wane.

### Historical Findings
Exercise intolerance. Dry and non productive "cough." Increased respiratory rate. Respiratory difficulty.

### Physical Examination Findings
Physical examination can be normal. Abnormal breathing sounds (expiratory wheeze). Open-mouth breathing. Tail bobbing. Orthopnea. Cyanosis of the beak, nail beds and facial skins in parrots with unpigmented beak, nails and unfeathered facial skin. Exertional expiratory and inspiratory respiratory distress. Signs of right heart failure including coelomic distension, heart murmur, gallop, or persistent arrhythmia.

## CAUSES
Chronic exposure and inhalation of environmental allergens, dust, irritating gas, and toxins, as well as chronic cardiac disorders and preceding microbial infections (viral, bacterial, and fungal) have been suggested to play a causative role.

## RISK FACTORS
Inadequate ventilation. Poor sanitation. Moldy food (e.g. seed mixes). Exposure to birds producing feather dust (e.g. African grey parrots, cockatoos). Exposure to airborne toxins and irritants (smoke, disinfectant, dust, aerosol). Immunosuppression from concurrent diseases, poor husbandry, or chronic stress will increase the risk of secondary bacterial and fungal infections.

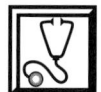

# DIAGNOSIS

## DIFFERENTIAL DIAGNOSIS
Large airway diseases (e.g. foreign body, granuloma). Coelomic space diseases (e.g. space-occupying lesion, coelomic effusion). Other pulmonary diseases (e.g. neoplasia, fungal or bacterial pneumonia). Reduced oxygen-carrying capacity of the blood (e.g. anemia, carbon monoxide toxicosis). Cardiovascular disorders (e.g. congestive left heart failure, atherosclerosis).

## CBC/BIOCHEMISTRY/URINALYSIS
CBC: Polycythemia (mean packed cell volume up to more than 70%) can be observed in case of COPD and CPIF. It is usually secondary to increased numbers of erythrocytes (erythrocytosis) or normal number of larger erythrocytes (mean corpuscular volume 0.2 fl) that contain a higher amount of haemoglobin per cell (hemoglobin content up to more than 20 g/l). RBC cytomorphology appears to be rounded in the blood film as a result of prominent expansion of the cytoplasm.

## OTHER LABORATORY TESTS
Presumptive diagnosis is based on signalment, history, and clinical findings, combined with exclusion of common diseases affecting the respiratory tract. Serology is indicated to exclude infections by *Chlamydia psittaci* and *Aspergillus* sp. Real-time PCR test performed on a swab of the conjunctiva, oropharynx, choanal and cloaca is indicated to exclude infections by *C. psittaci*. Venous blood gas measurement can reveal hypoxia ($pO_2$ as low as 34 mmHg) and hypercapnia ($pCO_2$ as high as 80 mmHg) in birds with CPIF. Culture of lung biopsies or tracheal wash can reveal bacterial or fungal secondary infections. Histopathologic examination of a lung biopsy performed under endoscopy is necessary for a definitive diagnosis of CPIF, COPD, and pneumoconiosis. It is best preceded by CT to determine an appropriate site for biopsy.

## IMAGING

### Radiographic Findings
General increase of honeycombed pattern. Dilatation of the large bronchi and rounding of the caudal edge of the lungs are non-specific radiographic signs associated with chronic lung diseases. Hyperinflation of the air sacs in cases of increased respiratory efforts. Pulmonary artery enlargement in cases of secondary pulmonary artery hypertension. Right-heart enlargement in cases of secondary right-heart cardiomyopathy. Hepatomegaly and loss of coelomic contrast associated with ascites in cases of secondary congestive right-heart failure.

### Ultrasonography
Usually unremarkable. May reveal hepatic congestion and ascites in cases of secondary congestive right heart failure.

### Advanced Imaging
In cases of lung fibrosis, generalized lung alterations, including bronchiectasis and variable thickened walls of the bronchi, may be visible on CT. Echocardiogram can document primary or secondary cardiomyopathy, pulmonary hypertension, and congestive heart failure.

## DIAGNOSTIC PROCEDURES
Air sac endoscopy may reveal moderate hypertrophy of costoseptal muscles in birds with COPD and hepatomegaly or ascites associated with venous distension in cases of

L

secondary right-sided congestive heart failure. Endoscopic lung biopsies are required for definitive diagnosis. Lower respiratory lavage may be performed to reveal secondary bacterial or fungal infections. Arrythmias can occur with severe hypoxia; low-voltage ECG has been described in cases of CPIF.

## PATHOLOGIC FINDINGS
**Pneumoconiosis**: Macroscopic miliary black foci in the lungs. Histologically, focal accumulation of dust-laden macrophages in the interatrial septa of the tertiary bronchi are characteristics. There may be infiltrates of lymphocytes and plasma cells associated with the nodule.
**COPD**: Lungs are grossly firm, with a rubbery texture, and are moderately congested. Histologically, there is extensive thickening of the interstitium with eosinophilic material and fibrous tissue with a mixed cellular infiltrate. The most common lesions are atrial smooth muscle hypertrophy and some atrial loss due to fusion and epithelial bridging. Proliferation of parabronchial lymphoid tissue and lymphoid nodule formation can occur, although less commonly.
**CPIF**: Histologic lesions are characterized by the loss of air and blood capillaries combined with interstitial fibrosis in the remaining septa. In the functional lung tissue, there will be variable amounts of smooth muscle, hypertrophy of the tertiary bronchi, edema, and congestion. In cases of pneumonia, there will be an increased number of inflammatory cells and background debris.
**Secondary pathologic findings**: Can include congestive right heart failure (hyperemia, ascites, congestion of vessels and liver) and bacterial or fungal infections.

# TREATMENT

## APPROPRIATE HEALTH CARE
Treatment is primarily symptomatic. The therapeutic goals are to resolve respiratory distress, halt progression of pulmonary fibrosis and control secondary infections. Birds with evidence of respiratory distress require emergency management and should be treated as inpatient with intensive care. 12–24 hours of stabilization may be required before performing complementary examination. Stable patients may be treated as outpatients.

## NURSING CARE
Oxygen therapy in an incubator with oxygen flow at 5 L/minute, delivering oxygen concentrations at 78–85% is indicated for birds with respiratory distress.

Humidification of air. Warmth. Fluid therapy as indicated.

## ACTIVITY
Restrict exercise level according to the degree of respiratory dysfunction.

## DIET
Assisted feeding as needed. Vitamin A and E supplementation may help reduce oxidative damage to the lungs that can result during exacerbations. A balanced omega 3:6 ratio is indicated to control excessive inflammatory response.

## CLIENT EDUCATION
The primary cause for the lung damage often remains undetected. Fibrotic changes are irreversible but clinical signs can be decreased with proper control of air quality. Long-term management is palliative and requires a strict separation of the birds from suspected sources of inhaled antigens. Good air circulation and environmental hygiene is needed. A good air filter (e.g. HEPA filter) and air humidifier located near the cage can be recommended. Never feed moldy food to birds. Minimize exposure to house dust, vapors, chemical fumes, and tobacco smoke. Birds producing feather dust can be showered more frequently and housed in a separate room. Housing outdoors when climate allows it may be indicated.

## SURGICAL CONSIDERATIONS
N/A

# MEDICATIONS

## DRUG(S) OF CHOICE
**Antianxiety/analgesic**: Recommended in cases of respiratory distress. Midazolam (0.5–3 mg/kg IM, IV, IN q8h) and/or butorphanol (0.05–6 mg/kg IM, IV q1–4h) can be given before placing the patient in the oxygen-enriched incubator.
**Anti-inflammatory drugs**: Used to decrease the inflammation responsible for the fibrosis. NSAIDs are preferred in cases of chronic obstructive pulmonary disease (e.g. meloxicam 0.1–2 mg/kg PO, IM, IV). Leukotriene antagonists (e.g. montelukast sodium 1 mg/kg PO q24h) have been anecdotally used. Steroidal anti-inflammatory drugs (e.g. dexamethasone 0.2–8 mg/kg SQ, IM, IV) are not recommended and their use should be limited to acute cases refractory to other treatments.
**Bronchodilators**: Used to relieve bronchoconstriction and decrease airway resistance. Although there may be smooth muscle contraction in macaws with COPD, the main histological lesion is hypertrophy which is unlikely to be corrected with a beta-agonist. Short-acting β2-adrenergic

agonists are considered the most effective bronchodilators. They are least toxic when given as an aerosol that is inhaled. Terbutaline can be administered parenterally 0.01–0.1 mg/kg PO, IM q6–8h initially and then continued by nebulization 0.01 mg/kg with 9 ml saline. Other drugs may include albuterol (salbutamol) 2.5 mg in 3 cc saline q4–6h for nebulization.
**Diuretics**: Recommended when heart failure is suspected. Furosemide 0.1–10 mg/kg PO, SQ, IM or IV is the preferred drug in cases of congestive heart failure.
**Antimicrobial therapy**: Recommended in birds with confirmed or suspected secondary bacterial or fungal pneumonia. Should be prescribed based on the results of C/S. For empirical treatment, broad-spectrum antibiotics are indicated in cases of bacterial infection (e.g. amoxicillin/clavulanic acid 125 mg/kg PO q12h) and azoles are indicated in cases of fungal infection (e.g. itraconazole 2.5–10 mg/kg PO q24h). Treatment should be administered for a minimum of 4 weeks.

## CONTRAINDICATIONS
Long-term corticosteroids (more than 5 days) are contraindicated because they can rapidly cause severe immunosuppression in the avian patient and predispose or exacerbate secondary infections.

## PRECAUTIONS
Birds administered antibiotics particularly long-term should also be administered an antifungal drug to reduce the incidence of secondary fungal infections. Birds receiving NSAIDs for a protracted period of time may benefit from gastroprotectant (e.g. sucralfate 25 mg/kg PO q8h) and anti-acids drugs (e.g. cimetidine 3–10 mg/kg PO, IM, IV q8–12h) to prevent gastrointestinal ulceration. African grey parrots are known to potentially be sensitive to itraconazole. Itraconazole should be used with extreme caution in patients with liver impairment.

## POSSIBLE INTERACTIONS
N/A

## ALTERNATIVE DRUGS
N/A

# FOLLOW-UP

## PATIENT MONITORING
Owners should observe clinical response to therapy and monitor respiratory rate and effort daily. Repeat physical examination, lung imaging (radiographs or preferentially CT), CBC (especially PCV) and venous blood gas analysis as indicated.

## PREVENTION/AVOIDANCE
Avoid housing susceptible birds in proximity to birds producing great amount of feather dust or other sources of dust. Bathe the birds regularly to reduce feather dust. Maintain good sanitation to reduce dust on surfaces and low levels of airborne toxins. Ensure proper ventilation and add HEPA filters throughout the house. Provide adequate nutrition and a stress-free environment.

## POSSIBLE COMPLICATIONS
Secondary pulmonary infections are possible. Pulmonary hypertension and secondary right-heart failure can develop in cases of COPD and CPIF. Endogenous lipid pneumonia can be associated with anthracosis.

## EXPECTED COURSE AND PROGNOSIS
Permanent lung damage is usually present in cases of CPOD and CPIF. Exercice intolerance often persists and crises may reoccur. Medical therapy and environmental changes can result in mild improvements of clinical signs and reduce the likelihood of severe relapse. Most birds with confirmed COPD or CPIF should be expected to have a shorter lifespan. The prognosis is guarded.

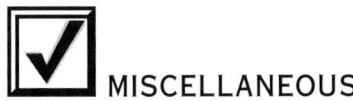

# MISCELLANEOUS
## ASSOCIATED CONDITIONS
N/A

## AGE-RELATED FACTORS
CPIF is most commonly seen in older psittacine (average 20 years of age). Severity may increase with age.

## ZOONOTIC POTENTIAL
Diseases with a zoonotic potential can be responsible for lung insults (e.g. mycobacteriosis, chlamydiosis and Newcastle disease).

## FERTILITY/BREEDING
N/A

## SYNONYMS
**Pulmonary disease**: Pulmonary disorders, small airway and parenchymal diseases.
**COPD**: Macaw pulmonary hypersensitivity, hypersensitivity syndrome, hypersensitivity pneumonitis, macaw asthma.

## SEE ALSO
Air Sac Mites
Anemia
Ascites
Aspergillosis
Aspiration Pneumonia
Avian Influenza
Congestive Heart Failure
Chlamydiosis
Herpesvirus (Columbid Herpesvirus 1 in Pigeons and Raptors)
Herpesvirus (Duck Viral Enteritis)
Herpesvirus (Passerine Birds)
Herpesvirus (Psittacid Herpesviruses)
Mycoplasmosis
Neoplasia (Respiratory)
Orthoavulaviruses
Pasteurellosis
Pneumonia
Polyomavirus
Poxvirus
Respiratory Distress
Sarcocystosis
Toxicosis (Airborne)
Toxoplasmosis

## ABBREVIATIONS
C/S—culture and sensitivity
CBC—complete blood count
COPD—chronic obstructive pulmonary disease
CPIF—chronic pulmonary interstitial fibrosis
CT—computed tomography
ECG—electrocardiogram
HEPA—high-efficiency particulate air
NSAIDs—non-steroidal anti-inflammatory drugs
$p$CO$_2$—partial pressure of carbon dioxide
PCR—polymerase chain reaction
PCV—packed cell volume
$p$O$_2$—partial pressure of oxygen
RBC—red blood cell

## INTERNET RESOURCES
N/A

*Suggested Reading*
Zandvliet, M.M.J., Dorrestein, G.M., Van Der Hage, M. (2001). Chronic pulmonary interstitial fibrosis in Amazon parrots. *Avian Pathology*, 30:517–524.
Rae, M.A., Duimstra, J.R., Snyder, S.P. (1991). Pulmonary silicosis in a blue and gold macaw. *Proceedings of the Association of Avian Veterinarians Annual Conference*, Chicago, IL: 260–262.
Taylor, M., Hunter, B. (1991). In my experience: A chronic obstructive puhnonary disease of blue and gold macaws. *Journal of the Association of Avian Veterinarians*, 5:71.
Gibson, D.J., Nemeth, M., Beaufrère, H., et al. (2019). Captive psittacine birds in Ontario, Canada: a 19-year retrospective study of the causes of morbidity and mortality. *Journal of Comparative Pathology*, 171:38–52.
**Author**: Graham Zoller, DVM, IPSAV, DECZM (Avian)

L

# LUXATIONS

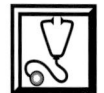

## BASICS

### DEFINITION
Luxation is complete displacement of the bony elements comprising a joint. Partial displacement is termed a subluxation. Can be described based on the two bone elements (e.g. scapulohumeral, femorotibial) and the direction (e.g. medial, lateral, craniodorsal).

### PATHOPHYSIOLOGY
Most luxations in birds, particularly free-living birds, are of traumatic etiology. Tearing or stretching of ligaments and damage to surrounding muscle results in instability of a joint. Congenital, developmental, or degenerative abnormalities can contribute to joint instability but are not well described in birds.

### SYSTEMS AFFECTED
Musculoskeletal. Skin, if the luxation is open. Neuromuscular injury to nerve, ligaments, tendons can infrequently accompany luxation.

### GENETICS
None.

### INCIDENCE/PREVALENCE
Commonly affected the elbow and shoulder of the wing and the stifle, intertarsal joint of the leg: 30% shoulder luxation; 2–12% elbow luxation. No prevalence studies for other joints.

### GEOGRAPHIC DISTRIBUTION
N/A

### SIGNALMENT
Any species. Commonly Falconiformes, Psittaciformes, Apodiformes and Anseriformes. Intensive farmed poultry present high prevalence due to rapid, abnormal weight gain. Coxofemoral luxations presented in species over 1 kg. No mean age or range, no predominant sex.

### SIGNS

#### General Comments
Clinical signs resemble an intra-articular fracture. Differentiation upon meticulous neurologic examination following an orthopedic examination by palpation under sedation. Definite diagnosis with properly positioned orthogonal view radiographs. Evaluation of underlying conditions and overall status of the bird must be addressed alongside luxation.

#### Historical Findings
Free-living birds are often found in or on the side of a road due to having collided with a motor vehicle. Captive or pet birds may have a witnessed event of flying into an object, such as a window, becoming entangled, being stepped on, or being attacked by another animal. Falconry raptors are found with extended leg on the perch.

#### Physical Examination Findings
Wing droop or lameness. Crepitation. Instability, laxity, positive withdrawal sign. Inability to fly, stand or gain height. Swelling. Bruising. Abnormal motion, rotation, or hyperextension of the affected extremity. Laceration of skin if luxation is open.

### CAUSES
Collision. Blunt trauma. Gunshot injury. Entanglement. Improper handling/capture. Viscous materials (glue, mud). Spontaneous orthopedic disease. Developmental abnormality (rupture of tibial cartilage, avulsion of flexor hallucis tendon).

### RISK FACTORS
In pet birds, allowing unsupervised and unrestricted access to the home environment increases the chances of accidental traumatic injury. Juvenile birds have inexperience in landing and flight. Improper falconry leash equipment/environment.

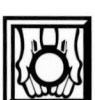

## DIAGNOSIS

### DIFFERENTIAL DIAGNOSIS
Soft-tissue injury, ligament rupture or hyperextension, articular fracture.

### CBC/BIOCHEMISTRY/URINALYSIS
CBC is advised to evaluate shock, hydration status and possible infection.

### OTHER LABORATORY TESTS
Biochemistry profile as indicator of cardiorespiratory stability to withstand general anesthesia.

### IMAGING
Orthogonal radiographs are generally sufficient for diagnosing luxation. Luxation may appear as displacement of bones from their normal articular positions or as increased joint space, depending on the degree of dislocation of the involved bones. Soft-tissue swelling is often present. It is advised to obtain whole-body radiographs in birds that have suffered trauma, rather than focusing on the area of injury, to rule out concurrent injuries. General anesthesia or sedation is usually necessary. In some complicated cases and subluxations (palatine, spinal, coracoid, coxofemoral, shoulder etc) CT is needed. MRI could be infrequently applied for meniscal/ligamental damage.

### DIAGNOSTIC PROCEDURES
Arthrocentesis and cytology/culture might be indicated in suspicion of infectious etiology or unknown joint swelling. In larger species and joints, endoscopy might be applicable to evaluate the meniscus, cruciate ligaments, and overall joint condition.

### PATHOLOGIC FINDINGS
Fibrosis, meniscal tear/rupture, intra-articular/cruciate ligament rupture, collateral ligament rupture.

## TREATMENT

### APPROPRIATE HEALTH CARE
Inpatient medical management is the appropriate therapy for concurrent traumatic injuries; temporary stabilization. Surgical management once patient is stable—necessary for best prognosis for specific luxation types. Outpatient medical management once luxation is stabilized either surgically or through external coaptation.

### NURSING CARE
Fluid therapy is indicated in patients suffering from generalized trauma. Temporary bandaging of the affected joint is indicated to prevent further soft-tissue trauma, to prevent closed luxations from becoming open, and to increase patient comfort level. Injuries of the wing distal to the elbow can be immobilized with a figure-of-eight bandage. Injuries proximal to the elbow or involving the elements of the pectoral girdle (coracoid, clavicle, and scapula) can be immobilized with a figure-of-eight bandage along with a body wrap. Injuries of the leg distal to the hock can be immobilized by taping the tarsometatarsus to the tibiotarsus with the hock in flexion. Injuries proximal to the hock can be immobilized via this type of bandage with the leg also wrapped against the body. Some luxations can be successfully managed and carry a good prognosis for full return to function when treated with bandaging alone. In birds weighing < 50 g, such as passerines, bandaging and/or cage rest may be the only realistic treatment options in some cases due to the small size of the patient. Wound care is indicated for open luxations.

### ACTIVITY
Patient activity should be restricted throughout the duration of treatment and gradually increased after surgical fixation or external coaptation is removed.

### DIET
N/A

### CLIENT EDUCATION
Guarded to poor prognosis in most cases. Surgical intervention for possible return to function is needed for specific luxation types. For return to function, early surgical intervention and postoperative physiotherapy are imperative Owner should be ready to allocate time for postoperative guided physiotherapy. Return to function might be accompanied by up to 50% ROM loss.

L

If return to full function is not an option, salvage arthrodesis should be opted. Regardless of luxation type and treatment method, degenerative joint disease may develop, requiring palliative management. Owner should be counselled regarding modification of housing to accommodate the bird's needs, if unable to fly. Falconry raptors may have reduced aerodynamic maneuverability.

## SURGICAL CONSIDERATIONS

Successful management of luxations in birds requires knowledge of avian anatomy and of the avian patient. Surgical intervention aiming to return to full function should be performed not later than three days, otherwise fibrosis occurs, inhibiting reduction. There are two major therapeutic aims: Permanent stabilization (arthrodesis) and stabilization with return to function. External coaptation may be enough for the coracoid sternum, shoulder, elbow (mild to moderate in severity), carpal, and metatarsophalangeal joints. Open surgical intervention is recommended for the elbow (severe or chronic luxation), coxofemoral, stifle, tarsal joints. Arthroplasty, femoral head osteotomy, internal and external fixations have been applied. Goniometry of the normal limb should be performed; so far, normal measurements in pigeon, cockatiels, Amazon parrots, and barred owls. HLESF allow early physiotherapy while stabilized for elbow and femorotibial joints. Metacarpophalangeal luxations have a good prognosis with type I ESF. Carpal luxations can be managed with figure-of-eight bandage or with type I ESF for 2 weeks. Elbow luxation can be managed with transarticular ESF, HLESF, type I ESF for 1 week, then removal of the ESF and figure-of-eight bandage for 7–10 days. Shoulder luxation can carry good prognosis with 2 weeks figure-of-eight and body wrap bandage. Hip luxation can be closed reduced with modified Ehmer sling bandage, if laxity persists with transfixation pin, Meij-Hazenwinkel suture stabilization or toggle pin; extra care should be taken not to damage the renal parenchyma when inserting pins. Chronic luxation could be resolved with excision arthroplasty or femoral head osteotomy. Stifle luxation in larger birds may have concomitant ligament damage; a surgical ligament repair might be attempted. Excapsular joint techniques, combination of extracapsular technique and transarticular type I HLESF have been used successfully. For permanent ankylosis triangular and linear transarticular types I and II ESF with conjoined pins can be used. Intertarsal joint luxation may be treated with transarticular type I HLESF or transarticular figure-of-eight suture with or without button system.

## MEDICATIONS

### DRUG(S) OF CHOICE

Analgesics—pain management is of the utmost importance in emergent patients and throughout the course of treatment. Opioids (buprenorphine, butorphanol, fentanyl, hydromorphone, tramadol) can be used in initial stages of treatment as well as peri- and postoperatively. NSAIDs can be used postoperatively and during the course of management (meloxicam, carprofen, ketoprofen, flunixin). Opioids or tramadol can be combined with NSAIDs for multimodal analgesia. Antibiotics are indicated perioperatively, and generally for the duration of time an ESF IM pin tie-in is in place. Culture and sensitivity should guide antibiotic selection. Antifungals should be considered prophylactically for species at higher risk of respiratory aspergillosis secondary to antibiotic therapy and for species of free-living birds at higher risk due to the stress of being held in captivity for treatment and rehabilitation.

### CONTRAINDICATIONS

Consult Food Animal Residue Avoidance Databank (FARAD.org) for antibiotic choices when managing backyard flocks.

### PRECAUTIONS

NSAIDs—avoid or use with caution in hypovolemic patients and in patients with hepatic or renal impairment.

### POSSIBLE INTERACTIONS

N/A

### ALTERNATIVE DRUGS

Gabapentin might have an effect against neuropathic pain. Intra-articular application of hyaluronic acid might help stabilization and ameliorate osteoarthritis.

## FOLLOW-UP

### PATIENT MONITORING

For luxations managed with external coaptation, bandage changes should be performed every week. ROM should be monitored with a goniometer during physiotherapy. Birds must be flight tested, observed for normal flight or locomotion/perching ability, and flight conditioned in an appropriate size aviary for the species.

For raptors, falconry techniques (creance, lure training) and hunting is recommended to assess and regain their flying ability.

### PREVENTION/AVOIDANCE

Modification of the home environment may be necessary for pet birds that incurred an injury via an accident in the home.

### POSSIBLE COMPLICATIONS

Decreased range of motion in joints secondary to bandaging—reversible in most cases following removal of bandage. In birds with leg luxation, the contralateral foot may develop bumblefoot if weight bearing is not restored to the injured leg during or following treatment. Degenerative joint disease and loss of range of motion. Osteoarthritis or soft tissue infection.

### EXPECTED COURSE AND PROGNOSIS

Highly variable and dependent on injury, selected course of treatment, and need for full function. If return to full function is not required, prognosis is for healing and acceptable outcome is good. For free-living birds requiring full function, prognosis for full return to function is poor as often they are older than 3 days and fibrosis inhibits early reduction or surgical intervention.

L

## MISCELLANEOUS

### ASSOCIATED CONDITIONS

Ligament damage, degenerative joint disease, osteoarthritis/xanthomatosis.

### AGE-RELATED FACTORS

Degenerative joint disease with fibrosis and osteophyte accumulation might progress with age.

### ZOONOTIC POTENTIAL

N/A

### FERTILITY/BREEDING

N/A

### SYNONYMS

N/A

### SEE ALSO

Arthritis
Lameness
Pododermatitis
Trauma

### ABBREVIATIONS

CBC—complete blood count
CT—computed tomography
ESF—external skeletal fixators
HLESF—hinged linear external skeletal fixation

MRI—magnetic resonance imaging
NSAIDs—non-steroidal anti-inflammatory drugs
ROM—range of movement

## INTERNET RESOURCES
N/A

*Suggested Reading*
Darrow, B., Bennett, R.A. (2021). Avian orthopedics. In: *Surgery of Exotic Animals* (ed. R.A. Bennett, G.W. Pye, eds.), 112–153. Ames, IA: Wiley.

Rasidi, E.K. (2021). Successful treatment of acute craniodorsal coxofemoral luxation in a scarlet ibis (*Eudocimus ruber*) using closed reduction and a modified Ehmer sling. *Journal of Avian Medicine and Surgery*, 35:350–360.
González, M.S. (2019). Avian articular orthopedics. *Veterinary Clinics of North America: Exotic Animal Practice*, 22:239–251.
Gjeltema, J.L., Degernes, L.A., Buckanoff, H.D., Marcellin-Little, D.J. (2018).

Evaluation of goniometry and electrogoniometry of carpus and elbow joints in the barred owl (*Strix varia*). *Journal of Avian Medicine and Surgery*, 32:267–278.
Azmanis, P.N., Wernick, M.B., Hatt, J.M. (2014). Avian luxations: occurrence, diagnosis and treatment. *Veterinary Quarterly*, 34:11–21.

**Author**: Panagiotis Azmanis DVM, PhD, DECZM (Avian)

L

# BASICS

## DEFINITION
*Macrorhabdus ornithogaster* is an anamorphic ascomycetous yeast that causes proventricular infection and associated GI disease called macrorhabdosis. A wide range of birds can be infected, often subclinically. Disease outbreaks described worldwide, commonly stress-associated in captive small psittacines and passerines, but also in wild cockatoos and finches from Australia, wild finches from Europe and rarely from North American passerine species.

## PATHOPHYSIOLOGY
*M. ornithogaster* is a large anamorphic ascomycetous yeast, a long thin rod with rounded ends that is 2–4 μm × 20–80 μm in size. Branching is rarely seen. Fecal–oral transmission. Organism colonizes the isthmus between the proventriculus and ventriculus, causing increased mucus secretion, decreased hydrochloric acid production, softening of the koilin layer and finally ulceration. Genetic variation of ribosomal DNA seems to be unsuitable for molecular epidemiology.

## SYSTEMS AFFECTED
Gastrointestinal.

## GENETICS
N/A

## INCIDENCE/PREVALENCE
Colonization in budgerigar, parrotlet, canary, and finch aviaries often is high up to 100% with a low morbidity and mortality.

## GEOGRAPHIC DISTRIBUTION
Worldwide distribution.

## SIGNALMENT
**Species**: Wide species distribution, but most often reported in budgerigars, parrotlets, lovebirds, cockatiels, grass parrots, canaries, and finches. It is sporadically reported in larger parrots, chickens, turkeys, geese, ducks, ostriches, and ibis.
**Mean age and range**: Clinical signs are usually seen in middle-aged birds, but colonisation appears to occur much earlier in life.
**Predominant sex**: None.

## SIGNS
### Historical Findings
Regurgitation. Undigested seeds in the feces. Weight loss despite apparent good appetite. Lethargy and depression. Melena as an end-stage finding. Acute anorexia, regurgitation, and death are uncommon, but reported especially in budgerigars and parrotlets. Most often without clinical signs.

### Physical Examination Findings
Emaciation. Regurgitated material and saliva on the dorsal head and face. Undigested seed in the feces. Dehydration. Depression. Melena.

## CAUSES
Infectious. Stress-related.

## RISK FACTORS
Stressors are important for pathogenesis of macrorhabdiosis, such as crowding, hygiene, diet, as well as concurrent diseases.

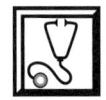

# DIAGNOSIS

## DIFFERENTIAL DIAGNOSIS
Ingluvitis, such as trichomonosis, candidosis, bacterial ingluvitis. Proventriculitis, such as cryptosporidiosis, proventricular nematodiasis, candidosis. Proventricular dilatation disease. Gastric neoplasia. Foreign body ingestion, including tricho- and phytobezoars. Heavy metal toxicosis. Renal insufficiency. Hepatic insufficiency.

## CBC/BIOCHEMISTRY/URINALYSIS
Nonspecific changes. Depending on the stage of the disease, especially with dehydration, increased total protein and hematocrit, or with proventricular ulcer, anemia characterized by decreased hematocrit.

## OTHER LABORATORY TESTS
Repeated fresh fecal wet mount, most effective in diseased birds, as they are likely to be shedding larger numbers of the organism. Examine the sample at 100× and 400× with the stage diaphragm reduced. Concentration of the yeast by preparing a macro suspension is recommended. Using a 1.5-ml microcentrifuge tube, 0.3 ml of 0.9% sodium chloride has to be placed with 0.5 g of feces, shaking the tube manually for 20 seconds and remove a drop from the meniscus of the slurry, after the solid mass has settled, for microscopical examination. Mini-Flotac technique. Fecal PCR.

## IMAGING
Plain radiography generally of limited use, aside from ruling out other causes of regurgitation, abnormal feces, and weight loss. Dilation of proventriculus and thickening of the proventriculus wall may be seen.

## DIAGNOSTIC PROCEDURES
Necropsy, for underlying diseases in individual and flock diagnosis.

## PATHOLOGIC FINDINGS
Dilation of the proventriculus with thick layer of white mucous. Ulceration junction between proventriculus and ventriculus (isthmus). Soft koilin layer with ulcerations. Emaciation. Histologically, *Macrorhabdus* is found on the surface of the isthmus glands and koilin layer, and may be located deeper within the glands and koilin layer in severe infections. Disruption of the koilin layer can occur. Inflammatory cells may be minimal. The organism will be eosinophilic when stained with hematoxylin and eosin stain. Morphologic and statistical data support a positive correlation between macrorhabdiosis and proventricular adenocarcinoma in budgerigars.

# TREATMENT

## APPROPRIATE HEALTH CARE
Inpatient medical management may be required; fluid and nutritional support are indicated if the patient is debilitated, and treatment is ideally administered via gavage. Stable birds may be managed on an outpatient basis with a water-based treatment.

## NURSING CARE
Fluid support (SQ, IV, IO) may be indicated if the bird is debilitated. Nutritional support via gavage may be indicated if anorexic or passing undigested feed.

## ACTIVITY
No restrictions indicated.

## DIET
If the patient is passing undigested seed, force feeding via gavage of a recovery formulary is required.

## CLIENT EDUCATION
If multiple birds are present, colonization with *M. ornithogaster* in other birds are very likely. If a flock disease is suspected, examinations for underlying diseases should be carried out.

## SURGICAL CONSIDERATIONS
N/A

# MEDICATIONS

## DRUG(S) OF CHOICE
Amphotericin B 100 mg/kg q12h for 30 days by oral administration. A shorter course of 14 days by direct oral administration followed by drinking water treatment (0.9 mg/ml) is possible in birds with mild clinical signs or in birds with rapid clinical improvement. Treatment did not clear, but significantly decreased the burden of *M. ornithogaster*.

**M**

# MACRORHABDUS ORNITHOGASTER

## CONTRAINDICATIONS
Medications that may be associated with gastrointestinal ulceration (e.g. NSAIDs) should be used with caution.

## PRECAUTIONS
Sodium benzoate (5 ml/L drinking water) has a very bitter taste and must be introduced gradually. Birds must be monitored closely during treatment to ensure adequate water intake. Overdosage may cause neurologic signs and death. Breeding birds may drink more water than normal, and doses should be reduced by one-quarter to one-half. Shedding and clinical signs do not consistently resolve with this treatment.

## POSSIBLE INTERACTIONS
None reported.

## ALTERNATIVE DRUGS
Altering gastric acidity has been proposed as a method for treating *Macrorhabdus*, by way of adding various vinegars or other organic acids to the water supply. However, this has not been shown to be efficacious. Nystatin reported to be effective in goldfinches (5,000 iu/bird PO q12h for 10 days). Resistance may occur. *Macrorhabdus* has responded poorly to other systemic antifungals. While fluconazole has shown promise in chickens, even low doses have resulted in toxicosis in budgerigars.

## FOLLOW-UP

## PATIENT MONITORING
Serial fecal samples should be monitored for the presence of the organism. However, as *Macrorhabdus* may be intermittently shed, eradication is difficult to achieve.

## PREVENTION/AVOIDANCE
Eggs may be pulled from the parent birds, cleaned, and hand raised to avoid transmission of *Macrorhabdus* from parent to

chick. Flock treatment via drinking water with amphotericin B can help to reduce shedding, but not eradication.

## POSSIBLE COMPLICATIONS
There has been an association with *Macrorhabdus* infection and gastric adenocarcinoma.

## EXPECTED COURSE AND PROGNOSIS
Birds that are treated earlier in the course of disease tend to have a better prognosis. More debilitated birds, or those with acute onset of signs especially melena, may continue to deteriorate and die.

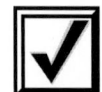

## MISCELLANEOUS

## ASSOCIATED CONDITIONS
Underlying viral, bacterial or parasitic diseases in weakened birds.

## AGE-RELATED FACTORS
N/A

## ZOONOTIC POTENTIAL
N/A

## FERTILITY/BREEDING
Infected parents may pass the organism to their offspring. Removing and cleaning eggs, followed by hand raising the chicks, prevents transmission to the chicks.

## SYNONYMS
Avian gastric yeast, megabacteriosis, virgamycosis.

## SEE ALSO
Bornaviral Disease
Candidiasis
Chlamydiosis
Coccidiosis (Intestinal)
Diarrhea
Enteritis and Gastritis

Flagellate Enteritis
Foreign Bodies (Gastrointestinal)
Helminthiasis (Gastrointestinal)
Ileus (Gastrointestinal, Crop Stasis)
Polyomavirus
Toxicosis (Ingested, Gastrointestinal)
Trichomoniasis

## ABBREVIATIONS
GI—gastrointestinal
NSAIDs—non-steroidal anti-inflammatory drugs
PCR—polymerase chain reaction

## INTERNET RESOURCES
N/A

*Suggested Reading*
Baron, H.R., Leung, K.C.L., Stevenson, B.C., et al. (2019). Evidence of amphotericin B resistance in *Macrorhabdus ornithogaster* in Australian cage-birds. *Medical Mycology*, 57:421–428.
Baron, H.R., Stevenson, B.C., Phalen, D.N. (2021). Comparison of in-clinic diagnostic testing methods for *Macrorhabdus ornithogaster*. *Journal of Avian Medicine and Surgery*, 35:37–44.
Poleschinski, J.M., Straub, J.U., Schmidt, V. (2019). Comparison of two treatment modalities and PCR to assess treatment effectiveness in macrorhabdosis. *Journal of Avian Medicine and Surgery*; 33:245–250.
Powers, L.V., Mitchell, M.A., Garner, M.M. (2019). *Macrorhabdus ornithogaster* infection and spontaneous proventricular adenocarcinoma in budgerigars (*Melopsittacus undulatus*). *Veterinary Pathology*, 56:486–493.
**Author**: Volker Schmidt, PD Dr Med Vet, DECZM (Avian and Herp)

 **Client Education Handout available online**

# BASICS

## DEFINITION
Marek's disease is caused by Marek's disease virus (MDV or Gallid alphaherpesvirus 2, previously known as MDV serotype 1) and is very common in chicken flocks. MDV is an oncogenic alphaherpesvirus belonging to the genus Mardivirus. It can be difficult to distinguish between lymphoid leukosis and reticuloendotheliosis as all are caused by viruses and have similar clinical signs.

## PATHOPHYSIOLOGY
MDV initially affects B lymphocytes but later predominantly involves T lymphocytes. It is horizontally transmitted by the respiratory route from the inhalation of infected dust or skin/feather dander. Numerous strains exist and their virulence varies (from mild to very virulent plus pathotypes), with recent emergence of more virulent strains. Gallid alphaherpesvirus 3 (serotype 2) and Meleagrid alphaherpesvirus 1 (serotype 3) are also members of the genus Mardivirus and previously grouped under the MDV group. Incubation period from time of infection to time of clinical signs can range from a few weeks to several months.

## SYSTEMS AFFECTED
Any or all of the following systems can be affected. Cardiovascular—atherosclerosis. Gastrointestinal—crop stasis due to loss of innervation of nerves supplying the crop; diarrhea, hepatomegaly. Hemic/lymphatic/immune—immunosuppression due to thymic and bursal atrophy. Musculoskeletal—stunted growth. Neuromuscular—can include paralysis due to T cell infiltration and demyelination of peripheral nerves, typically the sciatic nerves and less often the nerves of the wings or neck. Less commonly causes a transient paralysis of 1–2 days due to encephalitis. Ophthalmic—iris abnormalities due to lymphocyte infiltration (gray discoloration, unequal PLRs, misshapen iris); blindness. Renal/urologic—glomerulopathy due to immune complex deposition. Reproductive—decreased egg production and quality, reproductive tract tumors. Skin/endocrine—enlarged/swollen feather follicles visible in skin.

## GENETICS
Genetic resistance is present in some lines of birds.

## INCIDENCE/PREVALENCE
Ubiquitous in chicken flocks.

## GEOGRAPHIC DISTRIBUTION
Worldwide.

## SIGNALMENT
**Species**: Mainly chickens, to a lesser extent: turkeys, pheasants, quail, geese.
**Mean age and range**: ≥ 4 weeks of age, most commonly at 10–24 weeks.
**Predominant sex**: Females are more likely to develop tumors than males.

## SIGNS

### General Comments
Clinical signs generally seen between 10–20 weeks of age but have been reported as young as 4 weeks.

### Historical Findings
Lameness, weakness, sternal recumbency, regurgitation, head tilt, blindness, labored respirations, lethargy, diarrhea, inappetence, emaciation, dehydration, depressed egg laying, stunted growth.

### Physical Examination Findings
Unilateral leg paresis or paralysis due to lymphocyte infiltration into peripheral nerves (sciatic nerve plexus, ischiadic nerve, brachial plexus), sometimes called "fowl paralysis" or "range paralysis". May have one leg forward and one back. Iris abnormalities due to lymphocyte infiltration (gray discoloration, unequal PLRs, misshapen iris, "gray eye"). Crop stasis due to lymphocyte infiltration into vagus nerve. Enlarged/swollen feather follicles visible in skin. Abdominal distention.

## CAUSES
Inhalation of skin/feather dander from infected birds; horizontal transmission from infected birds; fomites. Virus shedding is indefinite in infectious birds. Highly contagious.

## RISK FACTORS
Concurrent infection with other immunosuppressive viruses will usually exacerbate disease (infectious bursal disease virus, chicken infectious anemia virus, reticuloendotheliosis virus). High-protein diets or selection for fast growth rate may increase susceptibility.

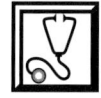

# DIAGNOSIS

## DIFFERENTIAL DIAGNOSIS
Lymphoid leukosis virus, reticuloendotheliosis, other neoplastic or visceral diseases such as ovarian or uterine adenocarcinoma.

## CBC/BIOCHEMISTRY/URINALYSIS
Leukemia may be rarely seen.

## OTHER LABORATORY TESTS
Antibody titer measurement (ELISA or virus neutralization) on serum. Virus isolation or PCR on fresh tissue, blood, serum or buffy coat.

## IMAGING
N/A

## DIAGNOSTIC PROCEDURES
Antemortem diagnostic tests are unlikely to be informative as to a specific etiologic diagnosis as many non-clinical birds are positive, but is supportive of disease in clinical cases.

## PATHOLOGIC FINDINGS
Various gross findings can be seen, depending on the phase of disease. Unilateral enlargement and loss of cross striations of the sciatic plexus/ischiadic nerves, less frequent in adult birds than in young birds. Lymphoid tumors of gonads, heart, liver, spleen, lungs, kidneys, intestines, muscles, skin. Hepatomegaly. Splenomegaly or splenic atrophy. Bursal enlargement or atrophy, less commonly involved than other organs. Vessel thickening (atherosclerosis). Kidney involvement. Ovarian involvement. Proventricular involvement. Heart involvement. Muscle involvement. Feather follicle involvement. Iris involvement with mononuclear infiltrates. Leukemia, although uncommon (lymphocytic). Various microscopic findings can be seen in cytologic or histopathologic examination, depending on the phase of disease: Perivascular infiltrations of pleomorphic lymphocytes, sometimes blastic; brain edema; glomerulopathy due to immune complexes; immunoproliferative lesions in feather pulp.

# TREATMENT

## APPROPRIATE HEALTH CARE
Treatment has been unsuccessful for birds clinically affected by any of these viruses; symptomatic infections become fatal.

## NURSING CARE
N/A

## ACTIVITY
N/A

## DIET
N/A

## CLIENT EDUCATION
When obtaining new chickens, clients should choose those that were vaccinated against MDV as day-old chicks.

## SURGICAL CONSIDERATIONS
N/A

M

# MAREK'S DISEASE　(CONTINUED)

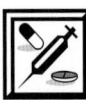

## MEDICATIONS

### DRUG(S) OF CHOICE
Treatment has been unsuccessful for birds clinically affected; symptomatic infections become fatal. However, in one study, chickens fed a diet containing the cortisol-reducing drug metyrapone showed regression or lack of Marek's disease tumors compared with a control group. Non-steroidal anti-inflammatory drugs may temporarily improve the quality of life of affected birds.

### CONTRAINDICATIONS
N/A

### PRECAUTIONS
N/A

### POSSIBLE INTERACTIONS
N/A

### ALTERNATIVE DRUGS
N/A

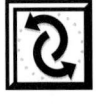

## FOLLOW-UP

### PATIENT MONITORING
N/A

### PREVENTION/AVOIDANCE
Vaccination is 90% effective, either in ovo (day 18 of incubation) or on the day of hatch, using a product containing turkey herpesvirus as well as another MDV (often CV1988/Rispens strain). Vaccination can prevent some lymphoma formation and clinical disease but does not prevent superinfection by especially virulent MDV strains. Vaccine-induced immunity takes 2 weeks to develop, so vaccinated chicks should be kept away from infection sources the first 2 weeks of life. Revaccination of an adult bird does not cause harm, but may be unnecessary, since nearly all birds will have become naturally exposed by this time. Vaccination does not prevent infection or shedding but does prevent development of disease. Genetic resistance to Marek's disease is present in some lines of birds and can be a useful component of prevention. One in vitro study suggests that treatment with meloxicam for 21 days post-infection may prevent disease by downregulating COX-2 and $PGE_2$ pathways and allowing improved T-cell function. However, it is not usually possible to identify the day of exposure in unvaccinated chicks. Hygiene, including removal of used litter and disinfection.

MDV is long-lived outside a host, retaining infectivity for 4–8 months at room temperature or for at least 10 years at 39°F (4°C). The most effective types of disinfectants are chlorine-releasing agents and iodophors; quaternary ammonium compounds are less effective and chlorhexidine is ineffective. MDV requires an extreme pH (< 3 or > 11) or temperature (> 140°F/60°C) for inactivation. Biosecurity, preventing introduction of new viral strains to a bird enclosure.

### POSSIBLE COMPLICATIONS
N/A

### EXPECTED COURSE AND PROGNOSIS
Symptomatic infections with any of these three viruses invariably become fatal.

## MISCELLANEOUS

### ASSOCIATED CONDITIONS
Atherosclerosis.

### AGE-RELATED FACTORS
N/A

### ZOONOTIC POTENTIAL
Although seropositivity has been seen in humans, there is no direct evidence of disease potential in humans.

### FERTILITY/BREEDING
Poor egg production, egg size, fertility, hatchability, and chick growth rate.

### SYNONYMS
Fowl paralysis, range paralysis, polyneuritis, neurolymphomatosis gallinarum, acute leukosis, early mortality syndrome, Alabama redleg, gray eye.

### SEE ALSO
Atherosclerosis
Dermatitis
Herpesvirus
Lameness
Neoplasia (Lymphoproliferative)
Neurologic (Non-Traumatic Diseases)
Neurologic (Trauma)
Ocular Lesions
Regurgitation and Vomiting
Respiratory Distress
West Nile Virus

### ABBREVIATIONS
COX—cyclooxygenase
ELISA—enzyme-linked immunosorbent assay
MDV—Marek's disease virus
PCR—polymerase chain reaction
$PGE_2$—prostaglandin $E_2$
PLR—pupillary light reflex

### INTERNET RESOURCES
Dinev, I. (2007). Virus-induced neoplastic diseases: Marek's disease. *Diseases of Poultry*: http://www.thepoultrysite.com/publications/6/diseases-of-poultry/201/virusinduced-neoplastic-diseases-mareks-disease
Dunn, J. (2022). Marek's disease in poultry. *Merck Veterinary Manual*: https://www.merckvetmanual.com/poultry/neoplasms/marek-s-disease-in-poultry
Wallner-Pendleton, E. Marek's disease in chickens. *PennState Extension*: https://extension.psu.edu/mareks-disease-in-chickens

*Suggested Reading*
Dunn, J.R., Gimeno, I.M. (2013). Current status of Marek's disease in the United States and worldwide based on a questionnaire survey. *Avian Diseases*, 57:483–490.
Greenacre, C. (2021). Musculoskeletal diseases. In: *Backyard Poultry Medicine and Surgery*, 2nd edn. (ed. C.B. Greenacre T.Y. Morishita), 246–249. Hoboken, NJ: Wiley.
Kamble, N., Garung, A., Kauffer, B.B., et al. (2021). Marek's disease virus modulates T-cell proliferation via activation of cyclooxygenase 2-dependent prostaglandin E2. *Frontiers in Immunology*, 12: https://doi.org/10.3389/fimmu.2021.801781.
Nair, V., Jones, R.C., Gough, R.E. (2013). Herpesviridae. In: *Diseases of Poultry*, 13th edn. (ed. D.E. Swayne, J.R. Glisson, L.R. McDougald, et al.), 258–267. Hoboken, NJ: Wiley.
Pendl, H., Tizard, I. Immunology (2016). In: *Current Therapy in Avian Medicine and Surgery* (ed. B. Speer), 406–410. St. Louis, MO: Elsevier.
Ritchie, B,W. (1995). *Avian Viruses: Function and Control*. Lake Worth, FL: Wingers Publishing.
Wakenell P. Management and Medicine of Backyard Poultry (2016). In: *Current Therapy in Avian Medicine and Surgery* (ed. B. Speer), 559–560. St. Louis, MO: Elsevier.

**Author**: Natalie Antinoff DVM, DABVP (Avian)
**Acknowledgements**: Lisa Harrenstein, DVM, DACZM, author of first edition chapter.

M

# BASICS

## DEFINITION
Metabolic bone disease (MBD) is a pathology affecting the skeleton due to a diet deficient in vitamin D, calcium, or phosphorous, or due to an incorrect calcium to phosphorous ratio. This condition may be exacerbated by limited exposure to sunlight (or another source of UV light in the range of 290–315 nm), which is required for synthesis of vitamin D. During growth, there is high bone turnover and demands for calcium, vitamin D, and phosphorous are much greater than needs for adult maintenance; therefore, this is a particularly sensitive period.

## PATHOPHYSIOLOGY
Nutritional deficiency in vitamin D, calcium, or phosphorus could manifest as various skeletal abnormalities including thin bone cortices, abnormal bone curvature causing limb deformity, stunted growth, or increased risk of bone fractures. The active form of vitamin D is important for absorption of calcium and phosphorus from the GI tract and for reabsorption of calcium in the kidneys. Circulating calcium is then used by osteoblasts and concentrates in the bone to provide physical stability, while the level of calcium in the circulation is maintained in homeostasis by interaction of several hormones, including estrogen and PTH (with calcitonin likely having a minor role). Phosphorus is maintained at homeostasis by the action of PTH and active vitamin D; both increase phosphorus absorption from the GI tract. PTH also releases phosphorus from the bone and acts to decrease its reabsorption from the urinary filtrate. A balance between dietary calcium and phosphorus is imperative to maintain the appropriate metabolism of these minerals as dietary increase in one may decrease the net absorption of the other. With a deficiency in one or more of the aforementioned nutrients, hormonal balance affecting bone turnover is altered, thereby causing abnormal bone mineralization and balance between osteoclast and osteoblast activity. This can potentially lead to decreased bone strength and to bone deformity.

## SYSTEMS AFFECTED
**Musculoskeletal**: Bone deformity. Decreased mineral density. Multiple fractures. May cause troubles in ambulation, general weakness, tremors. Beaks may be soft and bent.
**Neuromuscular**: Neuromuscular changes may accompany angular limb deformity. Hypocalcaemia may cause muscle tetanus in juvenile birds.

**Skin/exocrine**: Poor feather quality. Abnormal molting.

## GENETICS
N/A

## INCIDENCE/PREVALENCE
Incidence of this condition is lower than it was in the past, thanks to increased awareness for the need to provide appropriate nutrition. However, it is still a common condition in avian practice.

## GEOGRAPHIC DISTRIBUTION
N/A

## SIGNALMENT
All avian species may be affected. Much more common in juvenile and subadult birds.

## SIGNS
### Historical Findings
Failure to thrive, difficulty in ambulation, deformed limbs.

### Physical Examination Findings
Angular limb deformity, poor body condition, generalized weakness, poor plumage, hypocalcemic tetany.

## CAUSES
Nutritional causes for metabolic bone disease include calcium, vitamin D, and phosphorus dietary intake deficiency. Most commonly, this is iatrogenic due to inadequate nutritional intake of these nutrients. The form of vitamin D also plays an important role as vitamin $D_2$ is much less bioavailable than vitamin $D_3$. Unbalanced diets composed mostly of seeds have been found to be deficient in calcium, vitamin D, and phosphorus. In addition, the calcium to phosphorus ratio is low, thereby limiting calcium absorption. Similarly, reared carnivorous birds fed a non-supplemented all-meat diet are at risk for calcium deficiency. Vitamin D deficiency may be made worse by lack of UV light exposure. Inorganic water soluble calcium and phosphorus compounds are generally more easily absorbed than organic forms although this may also depend on the species.

## RISK FACTORS
High-fat diets are considered as an increased risk for metabolic bone disease. All-seed diets or unbalanced home-prepared diets should be considered as risk factors. An all-meat diet in a carnivorous bird or an all-seed diet in other orders without mineral supplementation are risk factors for developing this condition.

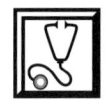

# DIAGNOSIS

## DIFFERENTIAL DIAGNOSIS
Trauma, developmental skeletal deformities.

## CBC/BIOCHEMISTRY/URINALYSIS
Decreased ionized calcium—ionized calcium provides an assessment of body calcium status whereas total calcium may be affected by other physiological factors such as plasma proteins. Hyperphosphatemia—phosphorous may be increased as a result of increased PTH, which is secondary to calcium depletion or in cases of a diet with highly skewed calcium to phosphorous ratio. Hypophosphatemia may be seen as a result of body phosphorus depletion.

## OTHER LABORATORY TESTS
Measurements of parathyroid hormone levels and 25-hydroxycholecalciferol have been used to varying levels of success in different avian species. Owing to the intricacy of these tests and the possibility of false positive results, they should not be used as screening tools, rather interpreted as part of the full clinical picture and the combination of clinical findings.

## IMAGING
Radiography is the most useful imaging modality to evaluate bone mineralization, bone deformity, and fractures. CT may also be used, particularly in larger birds, and may be a useful modality to evaluate changes in bones of the skull and the spine.

## DIAGNOSTIC PROCEDURES
N/A

## PATHOLOGIC FINDINGS
Bones may be deformed or fractured. Osteomalacia may cause soft, undermineralized long bones. The cortices may be diminished with large numbers of osteoclasts. The metaphyses may have unmineralized osteoid especially in the periphery, and the trabeculae may be lined with osteoblasts and abnormally large amounts of fibrous tissue and retained cartilage.

# TREATMENT

## APPROPRIATE HEALTH CARE
Animals with severe bone deformity may have a very guarded prognosis. External coaptation may be used to support limbs and to help correct deformities. Fractures need to be stabilized either with external cooptation, bandaging, or surgery; however, poor bone quality may decrease chances of success of a surgical procedure. Analgesia may be indicated especially if fractures are present.

## NURSING CARE
Bandaging and analgesia may be indicated to treat fractures due to metabolic bone disease. In severe cases, poor bone quality warrants limiting the bird's activity and cage padding to

M

avoid additional trauma. Weak or debilitated birds may not consume sufficient food and water voluntarily. Therefore, assisted gavage feeding and fluid support may be needed.

## ACTIVITY
Limited activity in a padded cage is indicated if a young bird has severe bone lesions or fractures. Once the bird is in a better nutritional plane and bone quality appears radiographically improved, moderate activity and gentle physiotherapy may be beneficial in establishing bone and muscle strength.

## DIET
A complete dietary assessment will provide an indication of this condition and could help in devising a plan for appropriate therapy and nutritional modifications. Diets for carnivorous birds based on meat alone are unlikely to provide sufficient calcium, whereas a diet for companion pet birds comprising seeds alone is likely to be deficient in calcium, vitamin D, and phosphorous, among other deficiencies. Formulated diets of high quality are expected to provide sufficient nutrients. Diets formulated to support the requirements of growing birds are nutrient dense and could be a good choice for a bird with apparent deficiencies. These provide a good alternative to all-seed diets or for unbalanced diets based on home-prepared foods. The nutrient requirements of carnivorous birds can be met by consumption of whole vertebrate prey. Mature prey is generally preferred to ensure calcium content and appropriate intake of fat. The recommended calcium to phosphorous ratio is generally between 1.4:1 and 2:1, with 4:1 still well tolerated. Egg-laying hens require calcium supplementation.

## CLIENT EDUCATION
Client education is highly important to manage this condition, as it is usually the result of lack of client awareness of the importance of proper nutrition. The significance of a complete diet needs to be explained to the owner as most cases of nutritional diseases, including metabolic bone disease are not only treated by proper nutrition, but are also completely preventable.

## SURGICAL CONSIDERATIONS
Some fractures that result from metabolic bone disease may need to be managed surgically. However, very poor bone quality may have a negative impact on surgical success and may affect treatment choice.

 **MEDICATIONS**

## DRUG(S) OF CHOICE
Treatment of nutritional deficiencies should be done primarily through improvement of

the diet. Additional supplementation may be considered to better address specific deficiencies for the short term; however, it should not replace improved nutrition, and care must be taken to avoid over supplementation. Calcium glubionate 25–150 mg/kg PO up to twice daily. Calcium gluconate (10%) 25–100 mg SQ or IM (diluted), injection may be painful. Vitamin D$_3$ 3300 IU/kg IM every 7 days as needed; beware of excessive use leading to hypervitaminosis D. Sunlight exposure 11–30 minutes of sunlight per day; a safer alternative to vitamin D injections. Keep the bird in appropriate temperature and avoid overheating.

## CONTRAINDICATIONS
N/A

## PRECAUTIONS
N/A

## POSSIBLE INTERACTIONS
N/A

## ALTERNATIVE DRUGS
N/A

 **FOLLOW-UP**

## PATIENT MONITORING
Monitoring of dietary changes is important to ensure owner compliance. Follow-up radiographs may be indicated every 2 weeks to monitor improvement in bone quality, or even at higher frequency if there are fractures present. Monitoring should also include ionized calcium (if decreased), body weight and condition, plumage quality, and ambulation.

## PREVENTION/AVOIDANCE
Feeding an appropriate commercially prepared balanced diet to pet birds as the main portion of the daily intake appears to be the safest way to prevent nutritional deficiencies. Wildlife rehabilitators should provide wild birds with proper nutrition according to the species. Carnivorous birds should not be fed an all-meat diet without appropriate supplementation.

## POSSIBLE COMPLICATIONS
Bone deformities may be permanent and may have severe consequences on birds including possible decrease in ambulation, risk of concurrent diseases such as pododermatitis, and risks of dystocia. Complications may vary according to the body part affected.

## EXPECTED COURSE AND PROGNOSIS
Prognosis is highly correlated with severity of the disease. Mild cases of decreased bone density but without bone deformity or

fractures have a good prognosis and will usually respond well to dietary improvement. Moderate cases with one or more fractures, poor bone mineralization or bone deformities may need extensive supportive care but have good chances of recovery albeit that bone deformities may be permanent. Severe cases with severe bone deformity or multiple fractures or complicated fractures may have a guarded prognosis, requiring much longer treatment. Euthanasia may be considered in severe cases where decreased ambulation has a significant impact on quality of life.

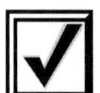 **MISCELLANEOUS**

## ASSOCIATED CONDITIONS
In many cases, the bird may be affected by multiple nutritional deficiencies, while some deficiencies may not be clinically apparent. For this reason, it is important to improve the bird's overall diet rather than supplement a single nutrient in the diet.

## AGE-RELATED FACTORS
Juvenile birds are most susceptible to this condition since bone metabolism and calcium, phosphorous, and vitamin D requirements are highest during growth. Milder clinical signs may also be seen in adult birds following a long duration of nutrient depletion.

## ZOONOTIC POTENTIAL
N/A

## FERTILITY/BREEDING
Calcium is vital for shell mineralization and smooth muscle contractions during egg laying. Since the bone is the predominant calcium store in the body, poor bone mineralization may predispose reproductive females to decreased reproductive success or even dystocia. For this reason it is important to correct the calcium, phosphorous, or vitamin D status of the bird before breeding.

## SYNONYMS
Nutritional secondary hyperparathyroidism, osteomalacia, fibrous osteodystrophy, rickets, juvenile osteoporosis, bone atrophy.

## SEE ALSO
Angel Wing
Angular Limb Deformity (Splay Leg)
Beak Malocclusion
Chronic Egg Laying
Fractures
Lameness
Luxations
Neurologic (Non-Traumatic Diseases)
Nutritional Imbalances
Polyostotic Hyperostosis/Osteomyelosclerosis
Trauma

## ABBREVIATIONS
CT—computed tomography
GI—gastrointestinal
MBD—metabolic bone disease
UV—ultraviolet

## INTERNET RESOURCES
Stanford, M. (2013). Calcium metabolism.
*Avian Medicine*, 141–151: https://
avianmedicine.net/wp/?s=calcium

*Suggested Reading*
Adkesson, M.J., Langan, J.N. (2007).
  Metabolic bone disease in juvenile
  Humboldt penguins (Spheniscus
  humboldti): investigation of ionized
  calcium, parathyroid hormone, and
  vitamin D3 as diagnostic parameters.
  *Journal of Zoo and Wildlife Medicine*,
  38:85–92.

de Matos, R. (2008). Calcium metabolism in
  birds. *Veterinary Clinics of North America:
  Exotic Animal Practice*, 11:59–82.
Koutsos, E.A., Matson, K.D, Klasing, K.C.
  (2001). Nutrition of birds in the order
  Psittaciformes: A review. *Journal of Avian
  Medicine and Surgery*, 15:257–275.
**Author**: Jonathan Stockman, DVM,
DACVIM (Nutrition)

M

# MICROSPORIDIOSIS/ENCEPHALITOZOON

 BASICS

## DEFINITION
Microsporidia are a group of obligate, intracellular, fungus-like parasitic organisms with a unique polar filament organelle used to infect a wide range of vertebrate and invertebrate hosts. While a number of microsporidian species (*Enterocytozoon bieneusi*, *Encephalitozoon cuniculi*, *Encephalitozoon intestinalis*, *Encephalitozoon hellem*) have been detected in birds (raptors, waterfowl, psittacines, passerines, and particularly pigeons), birds are *E. hellem*'s natural host. Signs of illness are uncommonly seen in infected healthy birds. No signs or non-specific general malaise may precede death in immunocompromised individuals, which are often afflicted with concurrent infections (viral, bacterial, etc.). Affected organs may include the liver, kidneys, intestines, and eyes.

## PATHOPHYSIOLOGY
The pathophysiology of most *Encephalitozoon* spp., including *E. hellem*, is believed to be similar to *E. cuniculi*: Three-phase, 3–5 weeks, direct life cycle, producing environmentally resistant spores. After ingestion, spores use their unique polar tube to penetrate intestinal cells and from there move to vascular target organs where replication occurs. After maturation, spores rupture, move through the body, and are shed through the stool and urine. *E. cuniculi* shedding starts 1 month after infection, peaks at 2 months, and declines by 3 months, thereafter becoming intermittent. Spores in avian species are not always associated with inflammation and clinical signs are often related to co-infections or illnesses especially in immune compromised individuals. Asymptomatic individuals may serve as reservoirs.

## SYSTEMS AFFECTED
Clinical signs are typically related to secondary and concurrent illnesses and immune suppression.
**Behavioral**: General malaise (quiet, fluffed, hypo/anorexia).
**Endocrine/metabolic**: Enlarged adrenal glands (likely stress induced).
**Gastrointestinal**: Diarrhea, thickening of the small intestines, glossitis.
**Hemic/lymphatic/immune**: Stress, underlying immunosuppression (often secondary to concurrent illness), bone marrow inflammation.
**Hepatobiliary**: Hepatitis, biliary hyperplasia.
**Musculoskeletal**: Weight loss from fat and muscle atrophy, weakness.
**Ophthalmic**: Conjunctivitis, keratoconjunctivitis, blepharospasm, ocular discharge, corneal neovascularization, corneal edema, conjunctival–corneal fibrinous adhesions.
**Renal/urologic**: Renal tubular disease, nephritis, urate stasis.
**Respiratory**: Dyspnea, airsacculitis.
**Skin/exocrine**: Concurrent PBFD.

## GENETICS
None.

## INCIDENCE/PREVALENCE
Unknown with companion birds being overrepresented in the literature; 29–31% of pigeon stools tested positive for microsporidial species in Spain and Brazil.

## GEOGRAPHIC DISTRIBUTION
Worldwide.

## SIGNALMENT
**Species**: Apodiformes, Anseriformes, Ciconiiformes, Columbiformes, Falconiformes, Galliformes, Gruiformes, Passeriformes, Podicipediformes, Psittaciformes, Struthioniformes, and Suliformes.
**Breed predilections**: None.
**Mean age and range**: Mass outbreaks causing mortality have been reported in nestling budgerigars, Gouldian finches, and hummingbirds.
**Predominant sex**: None.

## SIGNS

### Historical Findings
Signs reported by the owner. General malaise—quiet, fluffed, weak, weight loss, dyspnea, acute death. Asymptomatic carrier states exist.

### Physical Examination Findings
Abnormalities noted on physical examination. Clinical signs are often related to non-specific generalized wasting and concurrent illnesses. Weight loss/underconditioning. Diarrhea. Weakness. Ocular and periocular illness. Dyspnea.

## CAUSES
While multiple species of *Enterocytozoon* spp. Infect birds, *E. hellem* is the most commonly described and reported. Signs associated with infection depend on the immune status and concurrent morbidities/illness present.

## RISK FACTORS
Immune Suppression. Stress. Concurrent Illness.

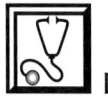 DIAGNOSIS

## DIFFERENTIAL DIAGNOSIS
N/A

## CBC/BIOCHEMISTRY/URINALYSIS
While a minimum database workup with CBC/biochemistry and fecal testing is recommended, abnormalities often correlate with concurrent morbidities and/or immune suppression.

## OTHER LABORATORY TESTS
Spores may be demonstrated via cytology with modified trichrome, periodic acid–Schiff, Ziehl–Neelsen acid–fast, Gram stain (stain Gram-positive), or immunofluorescent staining on fecal, intestines (especially jejunum, ilium), kidneys, body fluids, air sacs/lungs, and corneal impression samples. Microsporidia appear as oval to elliptical organisms with clear cytoplasm and eccentric nucleus in the apical cytoplasm of some enterocytes. PCR of fecal and tissue samples with nucleotide sequencing is more sensitive than histopathology and tissue electron microscopy. Fecal shedding is intermittent and repeated testing may be needed. Evaluations for common concurrent infections: viral testing: circovirus (PBFD), chlamydia, poxvirus, adenovirus; bacterial: *Mycobacterium*; *Macrorhabdus ornithogaster* (avian gastric yeast).

## IMAGING
Baseline radiographs are recommended as part of the minimum database and abnormalities seen are often related to concurrent morbidities (hepatitis, airsaculitis, etc.)

## DIAGNOSTIC PROCEDURES
Based on baseline blood work, radiographs, stool, and other testing the consideration of hepatic, renal, air sac, GI biopsies for histopathology and additional testing may be done (endoscopically or surgically).

## PATHOLOGIC FINDINGS
On necropsy, the most commonly affected organs include the kidneys, liver, GI tract, and eyes; however, spores have also been reported less commonly in the spleen, lungs, and air sacs. Affected organs may be related to concurrent illnesses and immune suppression. Microsporidian spores not associated with inflammation can be found in several tissues of affected birds, including the intestinal mucosa, renal tubular, bile duct, and corneal epithelium. Kidneys—lymphocytic nephritis, renal tubular distension and necrosis. Liver—multifocal necrotizing hepatitis, biliary hyperplasia. GI tract—thickening of duodenum, cloacal dilation granulomatous inflammation of serosal surfaces, enteritis with hypertrophy and necrosis of intestinal villi, severe atrophy and fusion of intestinal villi; glossitis with plaque formation (secondary to poxvirus infection). Musculoskeletal—fat and muscle atrophy. Eyes—conjunctivitis,

keratoconjunctivitis, blepharospasm, chronic epiphora, corneal neovascularization, corneal edema, conjunctival-corneal fibrinous adhesions. Air sacs—granulomatous inflammation of perirenal air sacs and connective tissue. Adrenal glands enlargement.

 TREATMENT

### APPROPRIATE HEALTH CARE
Generalized supportive care measures may be provided based on assessment (e.g. heat, fluids, assist feedings, and as needed board spectrum antibiotics) and concurrent morbidities.

### NURSING CARE
Supportive care.

### ACTIVITY
N/A

### DIET
N/A

### CLIENT EDUCATION
N/A

### SURGICAL CONSIDERATIONS
N/A

 MEDICATIONS

### DRUG(S) OF CHOICE
Albendazole 25–50 mg/kg PO q24 for 90 days. Netobimin (available in Europe) administered through drinking water at 4 g powder/400 ml water for 5 days has been used successfully in a nestling Gouldian finch mass mortality outbreak.

### CONTRAINDICATIONS
N/A

### PRECAUTIONS
No adverse reaction to albendazole were seen in two cockatoo patients; however, benzimidazoles are toxic to some avian

species (especially Columbiformes) causing medullary aplasia, GI signs, and death.

### POSSIBLE INTERACTIONS
N/A

### ALTERNATIVE DRUGS
Adjunct treatments for concurrent disease should also be considered.

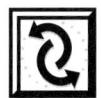 FOLLOW-UP

### PATIENT MONITORING
Patients with microsporidiosis infections should be evaluated at regular intervals. Physical examination of affected flocks and individuals, as well as repeated fecal examinations, especially due to intermittent shedding patterns, should be performed as needed.

### PREVENTION/AVOIDANCE
Maintenance of environmental hygiene: thorough cage cleaning to remove organic debris, disinfecting with quaternary ammonium compounds or 10% bleach, keeping aviaries dry to reduce the number of infectious spores; prevent overcrowding (low stocking density), elevate food and water dishes, use floor grates. Isolate and quarantine all new birds as well as any infected birds. If identified consider removing carrier birds.

### POSSIBLE COMPLICATIONS
Reinfection (or lack of clearance) is possible even with recommended prolonged treatment. Treatment and prognosis is closely tied to the degree of secondary immune suppression and/or concurrent illness(es) which cause the bulk of morbidity and mortality over the microsporidia infection itself.

### EXPECTED COURSE AND PROGNOSIS
High mortality rates accompany nestilng infections. Asymptomatic carriers may act as a reservoir of infection. Reports of treatment

are limited and more commonly affected species (pigeons) are more sensitive to benzimidazole therapy.

 MISCELLANEOUS

### ASSOCIATED CONDITIONS
Circovirus (PBFD), psittacosis, poxvirus, adenovirus, *Mycobacterium*, *M. ornithogaster*.

### AGE-RELATED FACTORS
Nestling birds suffer higher mortalities likely due to underdeveloped immune system.

### ZOONOTIC POTENTIAL
Possible zoonosis but no confirmed zoonotic cases have been reported.

### FERTILITY/BREEDING
N/A

### SYNONYMS
N/A

### SEE ALSO
N/A

### ABBREVIATIONS
GI—gastrointestinal
PBFD—psittacine beak and feather disease
PCR—polymerase chain reaction

### INTERNET RESOURCES
N/A

*Suggested Reading*
Rosell, J., Máinez, M., Didier, E.S., et al. (2016). Encephalitozoon hellem infection in aviary passerine and psittacine birds in Spain. *Veterinary Parasitology*, 219:57–60.
Snowden, K. (2004). Encephalitozoon infection in birds. *Seminars in Avian and Exotic Pet Medicine* 13:94–99.
Vergneau-Grosset, C., Larrat, S. (2015). Microsporidiosis in vertebrate companion exotic animals. *Journal of Fungi (Basel, Switzerland)*, 2(1):3.
**Author**: Julia Shakeri, DVM, DABVP (Avian), ACEPM

M

# MYCOBACTERIOSIS

## BASICS

### DEFINITION
Mycobacteriosis is infection with one or more organisms belonging to the genus *Mycobacterium*. The great majority of infections in birds are atypical, or non-tuberculous species, such as *Mycobacterium genavense* and *Mycobacterium avium*.

### PATHOPHYSIOLOGY
Source of infection is most likely environmental contamination, as atypical mycobacterial organisms are present in soil and water. In humans and other species, immunosuppression appears to be a prerequisite for infection; this has not been established in birds. Bird to bird transmission is unlikely. Rare cases of *Mycobacterium tuberculosis* were thought to have been obtained via contact with infected humans.

### SYSTEMS AFFECTED
Hepatobiliary—hepatomegaly, liver dysfunction. Lymphopoietic—splenomegaly. GI—weight loss, abnormal stools. Respiratory—air sacculitis. Skin—cutaneous nodules. Ocular—conjunctival swelling or masses.

### GENETICS
N/A

### INCIDENCE/PREVALENCE
Incidence is unknown, as many infections may be subclinical.

### GEOGRAPHIC DISTRIBUTION
Worldwide.

### SIGNALMENT
**Species**: Most birds are susceptible including passerine, psittacine, poultry, waterfowl, and many wild and zoo species.
**Species predilections**: A 2013 retrospective study of 123 cases indicate the most commonly affected psittacines were Amazon parrots (*Amazona* sp.) and grey-cheeked parakeets (*Brotogeris pyrropterus*).
**Mean age and range**: All ages are susceptible, but this tends to be a disease of older birds, as the organism is slow-growing and disease is chronic.
**Predominant sex**: Both sexes are susceptible.

### SIGNS

#### Historical Findings
Owners may note non-specific chronic signs including weight loss and lethargy.

#### Physical Examination Findings
Signs are often nonspecific and relate to the affected body system, but in all advanced cases signs include weight loss and lethargy. Birds with primary GI disease may present with weight loss, abnormal stool, and other

symptoms referred to the GI tract. Birds with respiratory infections may present with abnormal respirations (rate/effort), audible respiratory sounds (wheeze/click). The ocular or dermal forms may present as conjunctival or skin masses. Birds with hepatic form present for vague illness culminating in signs attributable to hepatic enlargement (enlarged coelom, respiratory distress, coelomic fluid). As disease is generally chronic, owners may report long-term vague symptoms. Physical examination findings are again dependent on body system affected, and can include reduced pectoral muscle mass (weight loss), dyspnea (increased respiratory rate and effort), enlarged coelomic space, and evidence of a coelomic mass or fluid. Masses may appear on the conjunctiva or any portion of the skin. Several anecdotal cases reported masses at the site of tattoo placement used to permanently identify gender after surgical sexing (ventral patagium).

### CAUSES
*M. genavense* is the most common cause of mycobacteriosis in pet birds (psittacines and passerines) while *M. avium* tends to predominate in wild and zoo birds. A variety of other mycobacterial species have also been isolated from cases of avian mycobacteriosis. In most cases, source of atypical mycobacterial organisms is unknown, but can be presumed to be water, food, and soil. Multiple infections within groups of birds are rarely reported. The sources of confirmed *M. tuberculosis* cases are apparently infected human owners (reverse zoonosis).

### RISK FACTORS
Risk factors for birds have not been determined, but may be exposure to soil. However, surveys of tap water have also been positive for atypical mycobacterial organisms. Infections of immunocompetent humans are extremely rare, and most infections are a consequence of severe immunocompromise. The role of immunosuppression in atypical mycobacterial infections in birds is uncertain. Zoo birds with prolonged exposure with positive birds have been shown to be at an increased risk of getting infected.

## DIAGNOSIS

### DIFFERENTIAL DIAGNOSIS
Owing to the wide range of body systems affected and chronic nature of the disease, the differential diagnosis list is extensive in most cases and includes numerous other infectious, neoplastic, or metabolic diseases. In cases of dermal or conjunctival masses, differential diagnoses include inflammation, infection, cysts, and neoplasia.

### CBC/BIOCHEMISTRY/URINALYSIS
A commonly reported finding in birds with systemic mycobacterial infections is marked elevation of the leukocytes, with monocytosis. However, birds with local lesions, and some birds with systemic disease, may not present with CBC abnormalities. Biochemistry alterations reflect disease of the body system affected and general debilitation, for example, elevated AST and bile acids in advanced hepatic forms, and hypoalbuminemia in chronic GI cases. All chronic inflammatory and infectious processes tend to produce anemia in birds, and in many cases, non-regenerative in nature.

### OTHER LABORATORY TESTS
Protein electrophoresis may support chronic inflammatory/infectious disease. In birds with GI infections, non-staining bacterial rods may appear in fresh fecal cytologic preparations. Suspect samples can be submitted for acid-fast staining. C/S of mycobacterial organisms is possible, but challenging, as most organisms are difficult to grow. Acid-fast staining or PCR for *M. avium* or *M. genavense* from tissue biopsies, especially the spleen and liver, are considered the most sensitive method for diagnosis. Another commercially available test for *Mycobacterium* diagnosis is next-generation DNA sequencing. This tool is able to identify low numbers of *Mycobacterium* organisms without requiring active growth via culture.

### IMAGING
Plain radiography may reflect abnormalities of the affected system, for example, hepatic silhouette enlargement, enlarged bowel loops, and pulmonary nodules. Contrast radiography is extremely useful to distinguish between proventricular and hepatic disease in cases of a widened proventricular and hepatic silhouette, and to give more information on GI transit time. Ultrasound may help to confirm hepatomegaly.

### DIAGNOSTIC PROCEDURES
Acid-fast staining on tissue biopsies and PCR testing on tissue remains the most useful diagnostic test both for confirmation of infection. Speciation can be performed based on PCR for selected *Mycobacterium* spp. or culture and molecular techniques for other *Mycobacterium* spp. Speciation may be warranted in atypical mycobacteriosis cases or to rule out the presence of tuberculous mycobacteria, especially if the bird is in contact with immunocompromised people. Samples may include feces (but not specific as environmental *Mycobacterium* may normally be present in feces), masses, and organ specimens (spleen, liver, lung, bowel).

## PATHOLOGIC FINDINGS

Histopathologic changes consistent with mycobacteriosis include granulomatous inflammation with foamy macrophages containing acid-fast microorganisms.

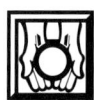

# TREATMENT

### APPROPRIATE HEALTH CARE

Prior to considering treatment, the organisms should be positively identified by species to rule out rare cases of *M. tuberculosis* or other tuberculous *Mycobacterium* sp., which are of severe zoonotic risk to humans. Most experts agree birds with *M. tuberculosis* should be euthanized. It should be kept in mind that treatment protocols require daily administration of medications for a year or more. It is likely that even birds treated with long-term therapy may never clear disease; as such, prolonged therapy with multidrug regimens has the potential to result in multidrug-resistant mycobacterial organisms. It may be warranted to consult with a human physician prior to initiating treatment on a pet bird. The zoonotic potential of NTM is unclear and human infection from birds have not yet been reported.

### NURSING CARE

Birds with chronic disease are often debilitated and require advanced supportive care. In severe cases, this may require hospitalization to correct fluid deficits and provide nutritional support.

### ACTIVITY

For very ill birds, activity should be limited until the bird is well enough to avoid injury from falls.

### DIET

All ill birds benefit from an appropriate diet based on current research. For most psittacine birds, this consists of a formulated diet with limited produce and other table foods. Anorexic or hyporexic birds benefit from tube feeding with a highly digestible, liquid diet designed for ill or recovering birds.

### CLIENT EDUCATION

Clients must be aware of the zoonotic potential of this disease and discuss this with their physician (see Treatment and Zoonoses sections). Owners should also be aware that treatment is long term, as long as 1 year or more, and is unlikely to be curative.

### SURGICAL CONSIDERATIONS

Local skin or conjunctival masses may be removed entirely. Removal of individual coelomic masses may be of benefit; however, disease is often systemic.

# MEDICATIONS

### DRUG(S) OF CHOICE

Reviews of outcomes of large numbers of pet birds treated for mycobacteriosis with specific drug combinations at specific dosages are unavailable. A 2014 study in ring-necked doves showed poor organism clearance in birds treated for 180 days with a 3-drug combination. A 2020 case report showed failure of a multiagent protocol to clear *M. avium* from a pigeon flock. Treatment is based upon drug combinations used in humans and other animals for similar microbacterial species. Without benefit of C/S (which is available but difficult and expensive), the practitioner is advised to research medications currently used for similar organisms in human patients. Drugs reported used for mycobacteriosis in birds include enrofloxacin, rifampin, rifabutin, ethambutol, clarithromycin, isoniazid, and others. Drug dosages are entirely extrapolated from other species. It should be noted that some countries restrict the use of human antituberculous drugs in other species because of the growing risk of antibiotic resistance.

### CONTRAINDICATIONS

There is too little information on the use of antituberculous drugs in birds to determine contraindications.

### PRECAUTIONS

Owner's physician should be consulted prior to instituting any treatment. Euthanasia should be strongly considered in cases of definitive diagnosis of mycobacteriosis on a bird with contact with immunocompromised people.

### POSSIBLE INTERACTIONS
N/A

### ALTERNATIVE DRUGS
None.

# FOLLOW-UP

### PATIENT MONITORING

Treatment efficacy is sometimes difficult to judge, due to the widespread nature of some forms of the disease. Clinical abnormalities may appear to resolve. Birds that exhibit changes in CBC, such as marked heterophilia and anemia, may show marked improvement with treatment. Birds with GI forms of the disease may be screened for the presence of acid-fast bacteria; however, it should be kept in mind that shedding of mycobacterial

organisms is sporadic. Birds with hepatic form diagnosed via biopsy and histopathology may benefit from repeat biopsy. Regardless, it is difficult to prove "cure" even after long-term therapy. Current literature suggests elimination of disease is unlikely.

### PREVENTION/AVOIDANCE

As the source of atypical mycobacteriosis is often unknown, prevention of reinfection is difficult. Organisms have been commonly found in soil, food, and water.

### POSSIBLE COMPLICATIONS

Outcome likely depends on the chronicity of the disease and degree of body system damage. Birds with severe hepatic mycobacteriosis, for example, may succumb to liver failure despite elimination of the organisms. Poor treatment compliance in humans and other species is linked to risk of organism resistance and ultimately treatment failure. Therefore, treatment must be administered regularly and for the recommended course (often more than 1 year). This may prove difficult for some owners. Recent data suggest that even prolonged therapy in avian species is unlikely to clear disease.

### EXPECTED COURSE AND PROGNOSIS

Long-term retrospective outcome studies are unavailable in birds. There are numerous single reports (both documented and anecdotal) of apparent treatment successes. However, other reports indicate the disease may be difficult to completely eradicate and may reappear after many years. Excision of single dermal or conjunctival masses may be curative. The prognosis for birds with systemic disease is uncertain.

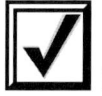

# MISCELLANEOUS

### ASSOCIATED CONDITIONS
N/A

### AGE-RELATED FACTORS

As it is a chronic condition, diagnosis is rarely obtained in young birds (under 2 years of age).

### ZOONOTIC POTENTIAL

As mentioned above, *M. tuberculosis* and other tuberculous *Mycobacterium* sp. are of severe zoonotic risk to humans. Most experts agree birds with *M. tuberculosis* should be euthanized. Treatment of birds with atypical mycobacterial infections should consider the stage of infection and potential contact with immunocompromised people.

M

## MYCOBACTERIOSIS

### FERTILITY/BREEDING

Birds with GI forms of mycobacteriosis should not raise chicks.

### SYNONYMS

Tuberculosis, TB, non-tuberculous mycobacteria.

### SEE ALSO

Anemia
Anorexia
Ascites
Coelomic Distention
Diarrhea
Enteritis and Gastritis
Infertility
Lameness
Liver Disease
Sick-Bird Syndrome

### ABBREVIATIONS

AST—aspartate aminotransferase
C/S—culture and sensitivity
CBC—complete blood count
GI—gastrointestinal
NTM—non-tuberculous mycobacteria
PCR—polymerase chain reaction

### INTERNET RESOURCES

Most state department of agriculture websites have specific information on mycobacteriosis. In some states, mycobacteriosis is a reportable disease.

*Suggested Reading*

Lennox, A.M. (2007). Mycobacteriosis in companion psittacine birds: A review. *Journal of Avian Medicine and Surgery*, 21:181–187.

Palmieri, C., Roy, P., Dhillion, A.S., Shivaprasad, H.L. (2013). Avian mycobacteriosis in psittacines: A retrospective study of 123 cases. *Journal of Comparative Pathology*, 148:126–138.

Saggese, M.D., Tizard, I., Gray, P., Phalen, D.N. (2014). Evaluation of multidrug therapy with azithromycin, rifampin, and ethambutol for the treatment of *Mycobacterium avium* subsp avium in ring-necked doves (*Streptopelia risoria*): an uncontrolled clinical study. *Journal of Avian Medicine and Surgery*, 28:280–289.

VanDerHeygen, N. (1997). Clinical manifestations of mycobacteriosis in pet birds. *Seminars in Avian and Exotic Pet Medicine*, 6:18–24.

Ledwon, A., Miasko, M., Napiokowska, A., et al. (2020) Case study and attempt of treatment of mycobacteriosis cause by *Mycobacterium avium* in a parental flock of meat-breed pigeons. *Avian Diseases*. 64:335–342.

Riggs, G. (2012). Avian mycobacterial disease. In *Fowler's Zoo and Wild Animal Medicine Current Therapy* (ed. R.E. Miller M.E. Fowler), 266–274. St. Louis, MO: Saunders.

Washko, R.M., Hoefer, H., Kiehn, T.E., et al. (1998). *Mycobacterium tuberculosis* infection in a green-winged macaw (*Ara chloroptera*): report with public health implications. *Journal of Clinical Microbiology*, 36:1101–1102.

**Authors:** Angela M. Lennox, DVM, DABVP (Avian and Exotic Companion Animal), DECZM (Small Mammal), and Crystal Matt, DVM

**M**

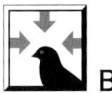

# BASICS

## DEFINITION
The term mycoplasmosis means an infectious and clinically apparent disease caused by any *Mycoplasma* spp. The clinical importance in birds is usually within the respiratory, the locomotory, or the urogenital tract. *Mycoplasma* spp. are widely distributed bacterias in all animal taxa and plants. Their importance ranges from commensals, secondary pathogenic to highly pathogenic contagious pathogens. They usually occur at epithelial or mucous membranes, but some species are able to live intracellularly. *Mycoplasma* spp. lack a cell wall and are surrounded by a thin membrane. They therefore have an amorphic appearance, are motile and are naturally resistant against any antibiotics that affects the cell wall. They are not very stable outside the host and deteriorate quickly in ultraviolet light. Due to their very small genome (some species < 600 kbp) they have limited metabolic pathways and require special media to be cultured in a laboratory. As laboratory methods to detect mycoplasmas, such as culture, are very difficult and PCR protocols focus on various species, mycoplasmas might not be detected, even if they are clinically suspected.

## PATHOPHYSIOLOGY
*Mycoplasma* spp. usually focus on epithelial cells in the respiratory tract, joint tissue, and urogenital tract. They produce an inflammatory response, often characterized by lymphocytes and monocytes. They do not usually induce purulent inflammation. If such is present, secondary pathogenic bacteria have complicated the infection. Morbidity associated with infections in a collection is usually very high, but mortality is low to medium and, often, more chronic diseases are described. Acute mycoplasma infection can be caused by *M. gallisepticum*, with a high mortality, especially in chicks and young birds. High mortalities described in free-ranging finches are more often due to loss of vision from a severe eye infection and not from *Mycoplasma* as a direct cause. Chronic *Mycoplasma* infections are usually fatal if untreated.

## SYSTEMS AFFECTED
**Musculoskeletal**: *Mycoplasma synoviae*, *Mycoplasma gallisepticum* and *Mycoplasma meleagridis* especially cause joint swelling, limb deformities, abnormal gait.
**Ophthalmic**: *M. gallisepticum*, *M. synoviae* (and other *Mycoplasma* spp.) cause conjunctivitis and ocular discharge.

**Respiratory**: *M. gallisepticum* and sometimes also *M. synoviae* causes, sinusitis, aerosacculitis and pneumonia.
**Reproductive**: *M. synoviae* causes egg apex abnormalities, *M. synoviae*, *M. gallisepticum* and *M. meleagridis*, *Mycoplasma iowae* uterus infections and veneral diseases, and low hatching rate of eggs. Other *Mycoplasma* species are found in semen and eggs but do not seem to cause problems.

## GENETICS
N/A

## INCIDENCE/PREVALENCE
Both *M. gallisepticum* and *M. synoviae* have a worldwide distribution and appear regularly in poultry. The poultry industry therefore has a no-tolerance policy for *Mycoplasma* in parent flocks. *M. synoviae* is regularly detected in egg-laying hybrid chickens, but its detection does not automatically mean that it is causing a severe problem. Detection of *M. gallisepticum* is usually clinically relevant. Introduction of mycoplasmas into a poultry flock is usually through other poultry as carriers or inanimate vectors. The role of wild birds for poultry seems to be not as important as previously thought. The prevalence of *Mycoplasma* spp. is highly varied between the different avian groups, so interpretation of their detection in a clinical environment is difficult. Prevalence varies in non-poultry birds. Raptors and storks have a very high prevalence of Mycoplasma spp. in their respiratory tract and seem to carry them as commensals. Here, the occurrence of the bacteria in a sick bird might not lead to a diagnosis and species identification is necessary to differentiate the typical *Mycoplasma* sp. for those birds from potentially pathogenic *Mycoplasma* sp. Nightingales, tits, and psittacines do not carry mycoplasmas at all and detecting the bacteria in these birds may be a relevant finding. In some avian species like crows, prevalence is intermediate and *Mycoplasma* spp. are more often detected in clinically affected birds rather than healthy ones, making interpretation even more difficult. In a flock, treatment usually does not lead to a *Mycoplasma*-free status and carrier birds might remain.

## GEOGRAPHIC DISTRIBUTION
Worldwide, as carried by Passerines, Galliformes, raptors, Anseriformes.

## SIGNALMENT
**Species**: All birds seem to be susceptible with varying prevalence and specific mycoplasma species. Galliformes, house finches, American goldfinches, Columbiformes, psittacines, raptors, Anseriformes are known to be clinically affected. Some songbirds seem to be

*Mycoplasma* free, whereas raptors and storks usually have *Mycoplasma* in their microflora.
**Mean age and range**: All ages are susceptible.
**Predominant sex**: Both sexes are susceptible.

## SIGNS
### Historical Findings
In flocks, respiratory signs and conjunctivitis are regularly reported. Sometimes joint swellings, increased mortality in chickens or a low hatching rate of brooding eggs are mentioned.

### Physical Examination Findings
*M. gallisepticum*, *M. synoviae* (other *Mycoplasma* spp.?): Respiratory signs— conjunctivitis, ocular and nasal discharge often dried. Impaired breathing. Later, tracheitis, sinusitis and pneumonia, especially if infection is complicated by other bacteria. Reduced egg production, egg apex abnormalities, increased embryonic death, dwarfing and toe curling in embryos. Weight loss. Reduced growth rate. Swollen joints, lameness. Abnormal gait. *M. meleagridis*: Skeletal disease including slipped tendons in turkeys. *M. sturni*: May have some pathogenic potential (conjunctivitis and respiratory) in crows and some songbirds, but reported also as commensal.

## CAUSES
So far, 26 avian *Mycoplasma* spp. have been described, but many more undescribed species are present. It was thought that *Mycoplasma* spp. have a high host specificity, but it seems not as strict as previously assumed. *Mycoplasma* spp. are described across many avian families, and even mammalian mycoplasmas have been detected in birds. Whereas in poultry some *Mycoplasma* spp. are well described as pathogenic and causing high economic losses (*M. gallisepticum*, *M. meleagridis*, *M. synoviae*, and *M. iowae*) the role of other *Mycoplasma* spp. in birds is not well understood. In poultry, several more *Mycoplasma* spp. are known but their role in respiratory diseases seem to be minor. It can be assumed that some species like *M. gallisepticum* and *M. synoviae* are clinically suspicious in any bird species where they are detected. *M. gallisepticum* is also responsible for massive clinical outbreaks in free-ranging finches.

## RISK FACTORS
Transmission seem to be easy and morbidity is high. It appears via aerosols, food and water, and through vertical transmission. Development of clinical disease depends on the *Mycoplasma* sp., the strain and the immune status of the host. Chicks and young birds are thus usually more susceptible for clinical disease.

M

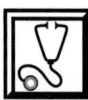

## DIAGNOSIS

### DIFFERENTIAL DIAGNOSIS
Avian influenza, chlamydiosis, Newcastle disease. Infectious bronchitis. Infectious laryngotracheitis. Poxvirus. Vitamin A deficiency. *Bordetella avium*. Reovirus (viral arthritis). *Staphylococcus/Streprococcus*. *Pasteurella*. *Ornithobacterium rhinotracheale*. *Avibacterium paragallinarum*. Gout. Marek's disease.

### CBC/BIOCHEMISTRY/URINALYSIS
The white blood cell count may show a heterophilia and in chronic disease, monocytosis may also be present. Chronic cases may also show a nonregenerative anemia. Biochemistry is usually normal.

### OTHER LABORATORY TESTS
*Mycoplasma* spp. are difficult to culture and takes several days. Therefore, direct detection of the pathogen using PCR protocols are preferable. In species where *Mycoplasma* spp. are common (poultry, raptor, storks) and a clinical disease caused by this pathogen is suspected, a specific PCR focusing on *M. gallisepticum* and *M. synoviae* is preferable. In other avian species or if other *Mycoplasma* spp. are suspected, a *Mycoplasma* genus-specific PCR is preferable. If this test is positive, the species can be identified by sequencing the PCR product or by using additional species-specific PCRs. In cases where species identification is not possible by PCR, *Mycoplasma* culture can be an option. It should be noted that swabs taken for culture must be transported in special media. If the birds have already received antibiotic treatment, *Mycoplasma* culture usually fails. In chronic cases, or when evaluating flocks, serological tests to detect species species-specific antibodies can be used— usually ELISA or serum agglutination tests, which are commercially available for *M. gallisepticum*, *M. synoviae*, and *M. meleagridis*.

### IMAGING
Whole-body radiographs may exhibit signs of air sacculitis, including air sac lines on both lateral and ventrodorsal projections. The appearance of the lungs on radiographs may show increased radio-opacity of the lung fields. Soft-tissue swelling of joints may also be present. Skull radiographs may not have enough resolution to show sinusitis. Skull CT or MRI can show evidence of sinusitis. An endoscopic examination of the air sacs and lungs is preferable and may be best to detect early evidence of cloudy air sacs or pus, mucus, or fluids covering the air sacs can be seen. Air sac biopsies might be used for histopathologic examination to reveal

lymphoplasmocytic infiltrations associated with *Mycoplasma* infections.

### DIAGNOSTIC PROCEDURES
*Mycoplasma* can be usually found in the trachea. Tracheal swabs are best for culture and PCR. If joints are affected, synovial aspirates can be used. In case of low hatchability of brooding eggs, esophagus of the embryo and/or the yolk-sac membrane are the best samples. Serum is best for serology.

### PATHOLOGIC FINDINGS
Histologically, inflammation including lymphoplasmocytic infiltration and necrosis will be present in tissues infected with *Mycoplasma*.

## TREATMENT

### APPROPRIATE HEALTH CARE
Affected flocks or individuals should be treated with an antibiotic. Keep in mind that in flock treatment, carrier birds remain and clinical disease will reappear, especially if younger birds are introduced. Individual patients might need supportive care, especially when the respiratory system is affected. Oxygen supply, nasal and sinus flushing, or even air sac catheters might be necessary. Nebulization therapy is usually advantageous. In poultry breeding flocks, the culling of the entire flock should be considered. Antibiotic treatment or egg treatment reduces vertical transmission but does not prevent it.

### NURSING CARE
Fluid and nutritional support may be necessary in birds that are anorexic and dehydrated due to this disease. Young birds especially require heat support.

### ACTIVITY
If there are skeletal and joint signs, activity should be restricted until the patient improves.

### DIET
N/A

### CLIENT EDUCATION
N/A

### SURGICAL CONSIDERATIONS
N/A

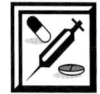

## MEDICATIONS

### DRUG(S) OF CHOICE
Any antibiotic focusing on the bacterial cell wall is inefficient. Macrolides like tylosin, azithromycin, erythromycin, or tetracyclines,

and as a reserve antibiotic quinolones (enrofloxacin) can be used. Sensitivity tests for *Mycoplasma* require culture and minimum inhibitory concentration values and are only done in a very few laboratories. Antibiotic use is not therefore usually based on a sensitivity test.

### CONTRAINDICATIONS
If antibiotics are used, restrictions for their use in food animals must be considered. Backyard chickens are usually also food-producing animals by law. Gentamicin is sometime recommended for use against *Mycoplasma*, but should not be used systemically in birds as it can be nephrotoxic.

### PRECAUTIONS
N/A

### POSSIBLE INTERACTIONS
N/A

### ALTERNATIVE DRUGS
Eradication, not treatment, is recommended for flocks.

## FOLLOW-UP

### PATIENT MONITORING
Patients with a severe dyspnea should be closely monitored. If *Mycoplasma* sp. is the primary pathogen, treatment results in a quick improvement. Regularly infections are complicated by other bacteria or even viruses and those cases do not respond well to treatment. Longer supportive care is then necessary.

### PREVENTION/AVOIDANCE
Contact between the flock and free-ranging birds should be limited. Birds introduced in the flock should be examined by PCR for the presence of *Mycoplasma* spp. In species where the bacteria are usually present in their microflora, PCR should focus on *M. gallisepticum* and *M. synoviae* which should not be present. In poultry, serological tests for *M. gallisepticum* and *M. synoviae* can be of advantage to detect carrier birds, as they usually have specific antibodies. Hatching eggs should only be taken from *Mycoplasma*-free flocks. For *M. gallisepticum* and *M. synoviae*, live and inactivated vaccines are available. These vaccines are registered for poultry; experience in other birds is rare, especially as their use is off-label and may be prohibited. In poultry, vaccines usually work very well in preventing clinical signs. It should be noted that, despite vaccination, field infections are still possible. In vaccinated birds, serological tests are of limited value as they cannot distinguish between antibodies directed against the vaccine and field infections. Parent poultry flocks

(producing hatching eggs) are therefore not vaccinated. Backyard poultry with repeated problems with *Mycoplasma* should be vaccinated, which also means that vaccination must continue in future generations so as not to risk reccurrence of the disease. Live vaccine can be detected by PCR for several weeks, so PCR testing for *Mycoplasma* cannot be done at least 6–8 weeks after using a live vaccine, or a positive result requires differentiation of vaccine strain from field strain.

## POSSIBLE COMPLICATIONS
Decreased egg production. Decreased meat production. Long-term respiratory and skeletal disease. Poor developing chronically diseased chicks.

## EXPECTED COURSE AND PROGNOSIS
Treated birds are considered lifelong carriers. Clinical prognosis is usually good after specific antibiotic treatment.

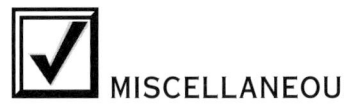

## MISCELLANEOUS

### ASSOCIATED CONDITIONS
N/A

### AGE-RELATED FACTORS
N/A

### ZOONOTIC POTENTIAL
The zoonotic potential of avian *Mycoplasma* spp. seems to be very limited and has been documented only for *Mycoplasma lipofasciens*, with very light respiratory signs for a few days. However, *Mycoplasma* do survive in the nose and hair of humans for some days. Therefore, humans are considered a vector for transmission between flocks. Caution should be taken when going to different flocks when *Mycoplasma* is suspected.

### FERTILITY/BREEDING
Poultry testing positive for *M. gallisepticum* and *M. synoviae* should not be used for breeding. *Mycoplasma* infections lead to a low hatchability, embryo dwarfing and curled toes. In turkeys, a venereal disease with a reduced fertility is described. In falcons, *Mycoplasma* spp. were detected in semen samples but semen quality was comparable to *Mycoplasma*-negative samples. Egg quality is reduced after *M. synoviae* infections. In sum, reproductivity of a flock is decreased after *M. gallisepticum*, *M. synoviae*, *M. meleagridis*, and *M. iowae* infection, but might also be with other *Mycoplasma* sp.

### SYNONYMS
*M. synoviae*—infectious synovitis, avian mycoplasmosis, infectious sinusitis and mycoplasma arthritis. *M. gallisepticum*—chronic respiratory disease of chickens.

### SEE ALSO
Angular Limb Deformity (Splay Leg)
Infertility
Joint Diseases
Lameness
Pneumonia
Rhinitis and Sinusitis
Respiratory Infections of Backyard Chickens
Respiratory Distress

### ABBREVIATIONS
CT—computed tomography
ELISA—enzyme-linked immunosorbent assay
MRI—magnetic resonance imaging
PCR—polymerase chain reaction

## INTERNET RESOURCES
Most state/country departments of agriculture websites have specific information on *Mycoplasma*. In some states/countries, *Mycoplasma* infection is a reportable disease.

*Suggested Reading*
Ferguson-Noel, N., Armour, N.K., Amir, H., et al. (2020). Mycoplasmosis. In: *Diseases of Poultry*, 14th edn. (ed. D.E. Swayne, M. Boulianne, C.M. Logue, et al.), Volume II, 907–965. Ames, IA: Wiley-Blackwell.
Lierz, M. (2010). Importance of Mycoplasmas in non-poultry birds. *Proceedings of the Association of Avian Veterinarians Annual Conference*.
Lierz, M., Hagen, N., Hafez, H.M. (2008). Occurence of mycoplasmas in free-ranging birds of prey in Germany. *Journal of Wildlife Diseases*, 44:845–850.
Möller Palau-Ribes, F., Enderlein, D., Hagen, N. et al. (2016). Description and prevalence of *Mycoplasma ciconiae* sp. nov. isolated from white stork nestlings (*Ciconia ciconia*). *International Journal of Systemic Evolutionary Microbiology*, 66:3477–3484.
Ziegler, L., Möller Palau-Ribes, F., Schmidt L., Lierz, M. (2017). Occurrence and relevance of *Mycoplasma sturni* in free-ranging corvids in Germany. *Journal of Wildlife Diseases*, 53:228–234.
Fischer, L., Möller Palau-Ribes, F., Kipper, S. et al. (2022). Absence of *Mycoplasma* spp. in nightingales (*Luscinia megarhynchos*) and blue (*Cyanistes caeruleus*) and great tits (*Parus major*) in Germany and its potential implication for evolutionary studies in birds. *European Journal of Wildlife Research*, 68:1–4.
**Authors**: Michael Lierz, DZooMed, DECZM (Wildlife Population Health) DECPVS, Prof Dr Med Vet

M

# MYCOTOXICOSIS

 BASICS

## DEFINITION
Mycotoxins are secondary metabolites produced by a wide range of fungi, most commonly molds. When present in feeds, feedstuffs, and litter, mycotoxins can produce a variety of pathologic changes, referred to as mycotoxicoses, in birds and other animals. Although hundreds of mycotoxins affect birds, only a small subset are considered a major concern in avian species, with some causing significant economic losses in the poultry industry. Mycotoxins that have a significant impact on avian health include the following.
**Aflatoxins**: Includes more than a dozen related furanocoumarin metabolites produced by *Aspergillus flavus*, *Aspergillus parasiticus*, and *Aspergillus nomius*. Aflatoxin B1 is the most common, toxic, and carcinogenic member of the group.
**Ochratoxin and citrinin**: Structurally related metabolites produced by *Aspergillus* and *Penicillium* spp. that cause indistinguishable clinical syndromes. *Aspergillus ochraceus* and *Penicillium verrucosum* are most often associated with mycotoxicoses. Ochratoxin A is the most prevalent and toxic.
**Fusariotoxins**: Produced by *Fusarium* spp. and several other genera, these toxins include fumonisins, moniliformin, zearalenone, and trichothecenes (multiple toxins with deoxynivalenol, diacetoxyscirpenol, satratoxin, and T-2 toxin considered the most concerning in birds). Deoxynivalenol (vomitoxin) is the most encountered but least acutely toxic trichocethene mycotoxin in poultry. T-2 toxin, on the other hand, is one of the most acutely toxic trichothecenes. Zearalenone has limited toxicity to birds. Moniliformin is the cause of "spiking mortality syndrome," which leads to acute death of young chicks.
**Oosporein**: Nephrotoxins produced by *Oospora colorans*, *Chaetomium trilaterale*, *Chaetomium aureum*, and numerous other filamentous fungi.
**Ergotism**: Alkaloid toxins produced by *Claviceps* spp.

## PATHOPHYSIOLOGY
The toxicopathology of most mycotoxins is centered around inhibition of protein synthesis, which makes tissues with high levels of protein synthesis and turnover more susceptible. The mechanism of action and target organ(s) varies between the different mycotoxins, with the liver, kidneys, GI tract, and immune system most affected. Recent studies suggest that there may be physiological (especially GI) and immunological effects of mycotoxins at lower, more common levels of contamination (below regulatory levels set by legislative authorities).

## SYSTEMS AFFECTED
**Behavioral**: Refusal to feed, lethargy.
**Hepatobiliary**: Primary site of action with severe changes to the liver (necrosis, fatty infiltration, hemorrhage, fibrosis) and biliary system.
**Renal/urologic**: Primary site of action with severe changes to the kidneys (renomegaly, necrosis), gout.
**Hemic/lymphatic/immune**: Bursal atrophy, thymic atrophy, impaired immunity, anemia, clotting deficiency, haemorrhage.
**GI**: Enteritis, ulceration, oral mucosal lesions.
**Nervous**: Seizures, opisthotonos, ataxia.
**Reproductive**: Affects egg production, hatchability, fertility, and sexual maturity.
**Skin/Exocrine**: Ulcerations, comb and digit gangrege (especially ergotism), feather and pigmentation changes.
**Endocrine/metabolic**: Pancreatitis.
**Cardiovascular**: Vasoconstriction, cardiomegaly and pericardial edema.
**Musculoskeletal**: Cachexia, rickets and tibial dyschondroplasia.
**Respiratory**: Dyspnea rarely reported.

## GENETICS
Genetics may play a role in the susceptibility to some mycotoxins.

## INCIDENCE/PREVALENCE
Mycotoxins are prevalent in most feed ingredients. A worldwide survey revealed that 81% of grain and feed samples tested positive for at least one mycotoxin. However, contamination of feedstuffs at toxic levels is typically low.

## GEOGRAPHIC DISTRIBUTION
Worldwide distribution. Mycotoxin contamination is typically more problematic in climates with high temperatures and humidity.

## SIGNALMENT
**Species**: All avian species can be affected. Mycotoxicoses have been reported in poultry, wild birds, and companion avian species. Poisoning is much less common in companion birds, such as psittacines, compared with poultry, due to differences in housing and feeding. Within poultry, generalized species susceptibility in descending order is ducks, turkeys, geese, pheasants, chickens. However, species sensitivity varies greatly by toxin. Chickens are highly sensitive to oosporein but relatively resistant to aflatoxins and fumonisins. Ducks are highly sensitive to fumonisins and trichothecenes. Turkeys are sensitive to aflatoxins and more resistant to fumonisins.
**Breed predilections**: Broiler breeds are highly susceptible to ochratoxin/citrinin.
**Mean age and range**: Any age can be affected, but younger birds are more susceptible to the pathologic effects.
**Predominant sex**: None.

## SIGNS
### General Comments
Acute toxicity events caused by ingestion of high levels of mycotoxins can cause overt clinical signs including mortality; however, chronic low-level toxicity is more common and can lead to more insidious symptoms such as reduced productivity and secondary infections due to immunosuppression. Mycotoxin-induced immunosuppression has been associated with disease outbreaks, vaccination failures, and poor antibody levels, likely due to lymphoid depletion and inhibition of development of the bursa of Fabricius. Symptoms vary based on the type of toxin, co-contamination with other mycotoxins, dose ingested, duration of exposure, species, age, and nutritional and physiologic status of the animal.

### Historical Findings
Impaired production efficiency of poultry in the absence of any obvious infectious diseases, environmental or management factors, or nutritional deficiencies may be caused by mycotoxicoses. Historical exposure to wet, spoiled, or moldy feed increases the index of suspicion.

### Physical Examination Findings
**General**: Inappetence/decreased feed intake, reduced growth, lethargy, weakness, depression.
**Aflatoxins, ochratoxin, citrinin, fusariotoxins**: Hepatic, immunologic, GI, renal, and hematopoietic dysfunction characterized by bruising, secondary infections, undigested food in stool, diarrhea, polyuria, polydipsia, and dehydration. Neurologic symptoms include ataxia, inability to fly, convulsions, opisthotonos, flaccid paralysis of wings/neck, seizures, and coma. Reduced egg production and weight, delayed sexual maturity, decreased hatchability, decreased semen volume and fertility, and reduced eggshell quality may occur. Poor feathering and pigmentation alterations, abnormal vocalizations, huddling, and hypothermia reported. Carcinogenic effects of aflatoxins are not a concern in poultry but may be in pet psittacine birds with long-term exposure. Fusariotoxins cause epithelial lesions with ulceration, crusting, and necrosis on the oral mucosa, feet, and legs; comb cyanosis; and constrictive lesions on the digits (dry gangrene). Dyspnea and cyanosis reported with moniliformin toxicosis.
**Oosporein**: Articular gout, dehydration, polydipsia, diarrhea, decreased egg production, listlessness, ataxia.
**Ergotism**: Necrosis/gangrene of the beak/toes/adnexa (comb, wattles), altered feather development, enteritis.

## CAUSES
All feedstuffs have the potential to be contaminated with mycotoxins pre- or post-harvest (during storage, transport,

processing, or feeding). Commonly contaminated feedstuffs include peanuts, corn, barley, rye, wheat, oats, buckwheat, rice, and sorghum. T-2 toxin and satratoxins are also found in contaminated litter. Wild birds may be intoxicated by consuming grains from damaged, fungus infested standing crops. Backyard poultry and wild birds may be exposed through access to compost heaps, fertilizers, potting soil, and decaying fruits and vegetables. Whole kernel peanuts, Brazil nuts, moldy grains, corn, and moldy cheese are sources of mycotoxins for companion avian species.

### RISK FACTORS
Season, location of grain cultivation, temperatures, water availability, and time of harvest can cause plant stress, making plants more vulnerable to fungal infection and subsequent mycotoxin production. Improper storage of feedstuffs and feed at high temperatures and humidity and insect damage can also predispose to mycotoxin contamination. Mycotoxins have an additive effect with other toxins (including other mycotoxins), infectious agents, or nutritional deficiencies.

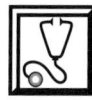

## DIAGNOSIS
### DIFFERENTIAL DIAGNOSIS
Owing to the wide variety of clinical signs and organ systems affected, many infectious and non-infectious differential diagnoses exist, including infectious diseases (aspergillosis, mycobacteriosis, avian cholera, duck viral enteritis, *Sarcocystis*, coccidiosis, toxoplasmosis, chlamydiosis, campylobacteriosis, salmonellosis), neoplasia, amyloidosis, hepatic lipidosis, water deprivation/salt toxicity, and other toxins (pesticides, heavy metal, plants, botulism). Differentials for reproductive changes include heat stress, excess sulphonamides or nicarbazin, DDT insecticide, avian influenza, infectious bronchitis, infectious bursal disease, and Newcastle disease virus. Ruleouts for oral mucosal and skin lesions include avian pox virus, candidiasis, trichomoniasis, gout, copper sulfate toxicosis, quaternary ammonium disinfectants, and nutritional deficiencies (vitamin A, panthothenic acid, biotin).

### CBC/BIOCHEMISTRY/URINALYSIS
Bloodwork changes are non-specific and vary based on the toxin. The most common changes include decreased total protein, albumin, and globulins; elevated liver enzymes, hyperbilirubinemia, hypocholesterolemia; elevated uric acid; anemia, thrombocytopenia, prolonged whole-blood clotting time and prothrombin time, and leukopenia.

### OTHER LABORATORY TESTS
Although mycotoxicoses may be suspected based on feeding history, clinical signs, and pathologic lesions, definitive diagnosis requires identification and quantification of the specific mycotoxin in patient samples or the feed. The most sensitive, selective, and accurate mycotoxin analytical method is liquid chromatography coupled to (tandem) mass spectrometry. This method can detect hundreds of mycotoxins in a single sample, including mycotoxins not routinely screened for or regulated in feedstuffs.

### IMAGING
May confirm organomegaly or help rule out other differential diagnoses.

### DIAGNOSTIC PROCEDURES
N/A

### PATHOLOGIC FINDINGS
The most prominent changes include:
**Aflatoxin, ochratoxin, citrinin**: Hepatomegaly or cirrhosis (chronic), gall bladder distension, renomegaly, visceral and articular gout (ochratoxin/citrinin), splenomegaly, pacreatomegaly, petechiation, visceral hemorrhages, lymphoid atrophy (spleen, thymus, bursa of Fabricius). Histopathologic analysis shows fatty infiltration of hepatocytes, hepatocyte degeneration, focal hemorrhages, extensive hepatic fibrosis, nodular lymphoid infiltration, biliary hyperplasia, interstitial nephritis, and enteritis.
**Fusariotoxins**: GI lesions (hyperemic mucosa, catarrhal enteritis. ulceration, necrosis, hemorrhage, enlarged proventriculus/ventriculus), visceral hemorrhages, ascites, cardiomegaly, pericardial edema, rickets, tibial dyschondroplasia, hepatomegaly, biliary hyperplasia, renomegaly, pancreatomegaly, lymphoid atrophy. Several toxins cause ulcerations and necrosis of the rictus, hard palate, choana, and tongue. Irritation of the respiratory tract occurs with satratoxin.
**Oosporein**: Large pale kidneys with extensive visceral and articular gout and multifocal proximal tubular necrosis on histopathology.
**Ergotism**: Vascular changes and associated lesions in the intestines, liver, kidney, heart, and brain. Dermal necrosis, vesicles, and ulcers noted from contact.

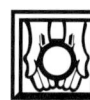

## TREATMENT
### APPROPRIATE HEALTH CARE
Flock management for poultry, inpatient medical management for individual cases in companion birds.

### NURSING CARE
Treatment is centered around supportive care as no antidotes exist for mycotoxicoses. Address any concurrent disease processes to

help alleviate disease interactions. Intoxicated animals can be treated with probiotics, vitamin and trace mineral supplementation (such as vitamin E, vitamin C, selenium), and fluid therapy. Vitamin K and silymarin supplementation are recommended in cases with liver dysfunction. During acute ingestion of the individual patient, crop lavage can be performed followed by administration of activated charcoal. Intravenous fluid administration is recommended in affected psittacines to maintain hydration.

### ACTIVITY
N/A

### DIET
The most important therapeutic step is immediate removal of the suspected contaminated feed and replacement with unadulterated feed. Increased dietary protein levels may aid recovery.

### CLIENT EDUCATION
Discuss proper diet, feed storage, disinfection, and quality control measures with owners/poultry raisers.

### SURGICAL CONSIDERATIONS
N/A

## MEDICATIONS
### DRUG(S) OF CHOICE
There are no specific antidotes for any mycotoxins. Tremors and seizures should be controlled with antiepileptic medications such as diazepam, midazolam, or phenobarbital with mannitol in cases of refractory seizures where cerebral edema is suspected. Broad-spectrum antibiotics are indicated in cases with secondary infections due to immunosuppression (often oxytetracycline in livestock).

### CONTRAINDICATIONS
Mycotoxins target the liver and kidneys; dysfunction in these organs may affect drug choices.

### PRECAUTIONS
N/A

### POSSIBLE INTERACTIONS
N/A

### ALTERNATIVE DRUGS
N/A

## FOLLOW-UP
### PATIENT MONITORING
Clinical assessment of mentation, hydration, nutritional status, neurologic signs, and fecal output/consistency is recommended with

repeated CBC/biochemistries to assess organ damage.

### PREVENTION/AVOIDANCE

Mycotoxin concentration feed limits have been set by legislative authorities (eg: FDA, European Union); however, forage and animal bedding is not regulated for the presence of mycotoxins. Management practices that prevent mold growth and mycotoxin formation during manufacture, transport, and storage are essential for prevention. Preharvest control: Agronomic practices to minimize plant stress, fungal invasion, and toxin accumulation (e.g. proper irrigation, insect control, pesticide application, proper fertilization, timely planting and harvesting). Post-harvest control: Proper storage and handling of feedstuffs to prevent fungal growth (controlled temperature and moisture, insect/rodent prevention). Monitoring with feed assays is recommended. Counteracting strategies: The use of nutritionally inert adsorbents (aka mycotoxin binders) to bind mycotoxins in the animal's GI tract and reduce bioavailability is the most common detoxification approach but does not work for all mycotoxins. Enzymatic or microbial detoxification (i.e. biotransformation or biodetoxification) and bioprotection are additional, newer strategies.

### POSSIBLE COMPLICATIONS

Permanent organ damage and dysfunction (e.g. liver, kidney, immune) is possible in survivors, depending on the toxin and avian species affected.

### EXPECTED COURSE AND PROGNOSIS

Recovery can be prolonged for many mycotoxicoses but is possible. Prognosis is guarded if patients are leukopenic.

 MISCELLANEOUS

### ASSOCIATED CONDITIONS

None.

### AGE-RELATED FACTORS

Younger avian patients are more susceptible to some mycotoxicoses, possibly due to increased intestinal absorption.

### ZOONOTIC POTENTIAL

There is a danger of passage of mycotoxins within the food chain via meat, viscera, and eggs. Levels of mycotoxin residues in food for human consumption are regulated by government organizations.

### FERTILITY/BREEDING

Several mycotoxins reduce egg production, reduce hatchability, reduce semen production, and increase embryo death.

### SYNONYMS

Chaetomidin (oosporein), vomitoxin (deoxynivalenol), X disease of turkeys (aflatoxicosis).

### SEE ALSO

Anemia
Anorexia
Cardiac Disease
Coagulopathies and Coagulation
Dehydration
Diarrhea
Enteritis and Gastritis
Hemorrhage
Hepatic Lipidosis
Hyperuricemia
Infertility
Liver Disease
Neoplasia
Neurologic (Non-Traumatic Diseases)
Neurologic (Trauma)
Oral Plaques
Pancreatic Diseases
Polyuria
Renal Diseases
Seizures

### ABBREVIATIONS

DAS—diacetoxyscirpenol
DDT—dichlorodiphenyltrichloroethane
GI—gastrointestinal

### INTERNET RESOURCES

Cornell University Cornell University College of Veterinary Medicine (2012). Mycotoxins: https://partnersah.vet.cornell.edu/content/mycotoxins
Hines, E., Lorenzoni, G. (2023). Mycotoxins and their effect on poultry and swine production: https://extension.psu.edu/mycotoxins-and-their-effect-on-poultry-and-swine-production
Poultry DVM. Mycotoxicosis: http://www.poultrydvm.com/condition/mycotoxicosis
Sandu, D. (2023). Mycotoxicoses in poultry. *MSD Veterinary Manual*: https://www.merckvetmanual.com/poultry/mycotoxicoses-in-poultry/mycotoxicoses-in-poultry

*Suggested Reading*
Hoerr, F.J. (2013). Mycotoxicoses. In: *Diseases of Poultry*, 14th edn. (ed. D.E. Swayne, M. Boulianne, C.M. Logue, et al.), 1330–1348. Ames, IA: Wiley.
Murugesan, G.R., Ledoux, D.R., Naehrer, K, et al. (2015). Prevalence and effects of mycotoxins on poultry health and performance, and recent development in mycotoxin counteracting strategies. *Poultry Science*, 94:1298–1315.
Sobhakumari, A, Poppenga, R.H., Tawde, S. (2018). Avian toxicology. In: *Veterinary Toxicology: Basic and Clinical Principles*, 3rd edn. (ed. R.C. Gupta), 711–731. St. Louis, MO: Elsevier.

**Author**: Brynn McCleery, DVM, DABVP (Avian Practice)

M

# BASICS

## DEFINITION
Myiasis is infestation of the live animal body with larval forms of flies.

## PATHOPHYSIOLOGY
As in mammals, flies are attracted to injured or necrotic tissue or accumulated waste. A few fly species may damage normal, intact skin, such as *Cochliomyia hominivorax* (screwworm), but this is rare in the USA, and is only sporadically reported in infected imported livestock. Screwworm infestation is a reportable disease. Myiasis from common species (such as *Lucilia sericata*, the common greenbottle fly) is more common.

## SYSTEMS AFFECTED
The skin and underlying tissues are most commonly affected. The eye, oral cavity, ear, and vent may be affected, especially if these structures are diseased. In cases of severe primary trauma, secondary myiasis can affect medullary bone and intracoelomic organs.

## GENETICS
There is no genetic predisposition to myiasis.

## INCIDENCE/PREVALENCE
Myiasis is more commonly seen in wild birds and birds housed outdoors, such as poultry. Outdoor-housed pet birds may be affected, and potentially indoor-housed birds in situations where conditions favor fly infestation. This is a rare problem in healthy birds. Most affected birds are debilitated to some degree.

## GEOGRAPHIC DISTRIBUTION
Myiasis is seen in warmer environments or in warmer seasons with habitat suitable for flies.

## SIGNALMENT
Any debilitated exposed bird can be susceptible to myiasis.

## SIGNS
### General Comments
Most birds with myiasis are debilitated or injured and live in an environment suitable for flies.

### Historical Findings
Owners are often unaware of the presence of fly larvae, as they are hidden under feathers. They may report a foul odor and general unwell behavior, including decreased activity and appetite. An injury, or accumulation of feces on the ventrum or near the cloaca may be present and obvious. In most cases, birds are housed outdoors or have exposure to the outdoors. However, some owners are unaware of the presence of a significant fly infestation, or may even notice live maggots in the enclosure and present the bird for treatment suspecting endoparasites.

### Physical Examination Findings
The presence of fly larvae confirms the diagnosis. In most cases, these are associated with an injury or area of diseased skin and often necrosis. Maggots may be found in feces adhered to the bird's feathers, often near the vent. In some cases, they may be found in the conjunctiva, oral cavity, ears, or vent.

## CAUSES
With a few unusual exceptions, most flies are not attracted to normal birds and do not proliferate with proper husbandry. Waste accumulation, skin injury, and general debilitation contribute to myiasis under suitable conditions.

## RISK FACTORS
Being geriatric, injured, or debilitated increases risk of myiasis. Additionally, conditions of poor husbandry, especially improper disposal of waste, is another predisposing factor.

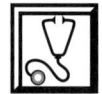
# DIAGNOSIS

## DIFFERENTIAL DIAGNOSIS
No other conditions mimic myiasis when larval flies are confirmed. The incidental presence of non-parasitic insects (e.g. mealworms attracted to food waste) could suggest myiasis.

## CBC/BIOCHEMISTRY/URINALYSIS
CBC and biochemistry changes reflect underlying injury or illness, and include alterations in the leukogram and possible elevations of AST and CK due to soft tissue damage.

## OTHER LABORATORY TESTS
Myiasis may predispose to secondary bacterial infection. C/S help to direct optimal antimicrobial therapy.

## IMAGING
Imaging is useful to help determine the extent of tissue damage, especially in cases of trauma (e.g. presence of fractures). Imaging may also reveal a cause of general disease (e.g. organ enlargement, presence of ventricular foreign bodies).

## DIAGNOSTIC PROCEDURES
Identification of suspected underlying or secondary conditions may direct additional diagnostic testing.

## PATHOLOGIC FINDINGS
Live maggots are usually associated with damaged or abnormal tissue. Histopathology reveals generalized necrosis, and may give information on tissue conditions predisposing to myiasis.

# TREATMENT

## APPROPRIATE HEALTH CARE
The areas affected by myiasis must be treated as appropriate; this may include surgical excision or debridement with healing by second intention. Secondary or underlying conditions are addressed, and general supportive care is initiated.

## NURSING CARE
Fluid deficits plus maintenance are calculated and delivered parenterally, or orally when practical. Wound care is variable, and depends on the type and extent of the wound. Some wounds may be disrupted by birds, and should be protected by bandaging, or if necessary, Elizabethan or other style collars.

## ACTIVITY
Birds with open wounds or tissue predisposed to myiasis must be protected from flies. In most cases, this is best done by housing indoors. Construction of flyproof outdoor enclosures can be done, but is challenging.

## DIET
Sick birds must be provided with ample high-quality nutrition and have waste or soiled food removed promptly.

## CLIENT EDUCATION
Complete written instructions for client aftercare should be provided, together with the warning that healing wounds are susceptible to repeated myiasis and must be carefully protected.

## SURGICAL CONSIDERATIONS
Infected wounds should be addressed as indicated; treatment may include surgical excision for primary healing, or debridement and healing by second intention. Severe necrosis of limbs may necessitate amputation. Amputation must be considered carefully, and is not appropriate in some situations (e.g. limb amputation in poultry or other non-flighted birds).

# MEDICATIONS

## DRUG(S) OF CHOICE
Antiparasitics are used to kill live larvae. Choices include nitenpyram, which is used anecdotally in birds per cloaca, orally, or suspended in water directly over the larvae.

M

There are not established dosages, but anecdotally one tablet per average sized hen or larger bird of prey has been used with apparent success. Afoxolaner has been described for myiasis in dogs and fluralaner for cats. Afoxolaner has been used for treatment of ectoparasites in a variety of zoo birds at 2.5 mg/kg topically, and fluralaner has been used for treatment of ectoparasites in poultry at 1.5 g/100 L water. Both could be considered for myiasis. Directly spraying wounds with antiparasitics/repellents for other species may be harmful to the wound and potentially toxic to birds. Antimicrobials are selected ideally from C/S of infected wounds; however, empirical antimicrobials appropriate for the species can be selected. Myiasis is often associated with a painful injury, and analgesics are appropriate.

### CONTRAINDICATIONS
None.

### PRECAUTIONS
Some medications are prohibited in poultry, even if the individual bird is a pet and not intended for food. Practitioners must be aware of prohibited classes of drugs (e.g. fluoroquinolones) and avoid them.

### POSSIBLE INTERACTIONS
N/A

### ALTERNATIVE DRUGS
Live maggots and ova can be individually removed by hand. This may not be difficult for smaller wounds.

 FOLLOW-UP

### PATIENT MONITORING
General progress in terms of underlying or concurrent abnormalities are monitored. Wounds are monitored for proper healing.

### PREVENTION/AVOIDANCE
Ideal nutrition and husbandry, especially removal of uneaten food and waste, are important for all patients. For outdoor birds, strategies to reduce fly populations (baits, traps, removal of waste and other attractions) are important.

### POSSIBLE COMPLICATIONS
Myiasis can lead to death when severe or untreated. This is usually the result of local infection, sepsis, or general debilitation.

### EXPECTED COURSE AND PROGNOSIS
When underlying causes and wounds or abnormal tissues are treated, prognosis is very good.

 MISCELLANEOUS

### ASSOCIATED CONDITIONS
N/A

### AGE-RELATED FACTORS
Very young or older, debilitated birds may be more prone to myiasis.

### ZOONOTIC POTENTIAL
Myiasis may signal an environmental health hazard for humans (e.g. presence of excessive waste).

### FERTILITY/BREEDING
N/A

### SYNONYMS
Fly strike, maggot infestation.

### SEE ALSO
Dermatitis
Trauma

### ABBREVIATIONS
AST—aspartate aminotransferase
C/S—culture and sensitivity
CBC—complete blood count
CK—creatine kinase

### INTERNET RESOURCES
Williams, R.E. (2010). Control of poultry pests. Purdue University, Poultry Extension E-3-W, Livestock and Poultry: https://extension.entm.purdue.edu/publications/E-3.pdf

*Suggested Reading*
Herdt, P.D., Boutreus, A., Hoye, K.V., et al. (2019). Effect of a drinking water conditioner of stability and efficacy of fluralaner in laying hens infested with poultry red mites. *Avian Diseases*, 3:97–101.
Jaramillo, E.Y., Nunez, C.R., Zavala, M. de los Á Álvarez, et al. (2020). Use of afoxolaner for the treatment of lice in different genera (*Chrysolophus* spp, *Lophura* spp, *Phasianus* spp, and *Syrmaticus* spp) and species of pheasants and west Mexican chachalacas (*Ortalis poliocephala*). *Veterinary Parasitology*, 280:106065.
Morishita, T.Y., Greenacre, C.B. (eds.). (2021). *Backyard Poultry Medicine and Surgery: A guide for veterinary practitioners.* Ames, IA: Wiley.

**Authors:** Angela M. Lennox, DVM, DABVP (Avian and Exotic Companion Mammal), DECZM (Small Mammal); Crystal Matt, DVM

M

# BASICS

## DEFINITION
Cardiovascular disease as a whole is common in companion birds and is becoming increasingly better recognized. Myocardial diseases encompass a wide range of conditions whose ultimate consequence is frequently heart failure. Disorders of the myocardium can have a degenerative, infectious, inflammatory, metabolic, nutritional, or toxic basis or are classified as idiopathic. The diagnosis and treatment of myocardial disease is complicated by technical limitations brought on by the small size and unique anatomy of birds, the potential variability of clinical manifestations, limited sensitivity or practicality of available investigative methods, extrapolation of therapeutics from small animal and human medicine, and limited treatment options depending on the primary etiology.

## PATHOPHYSIOLOGY
Myocardial diseases include dilated cardiomyopathy (DCM), hypertrophic cardiomyopathy, ischemic injury and chronic degenerative changes, myocarditis, epicarditis, or endocarditis of bacterial, fungal, viral, parasitic, or non-infectious origin, damage due to nutritional deficiencies or imbalances, iron storage disease, trauma, or toxin exposure, and neoplasia. Many of these diseases have the potential endpoint of myocardial failure involving either the left or right ventricle or both, resulting in systolic and/or diastolic failure and low-output or congestive heart failure (CHF) clinical scenarios.

## SYSTEMS AFFECTED
Owing to the central and fundamental role of the heart in the health and function of all other body systems, nearly all organs can be affected by myocardial disease to some degree. Multiple organ systems may be affected by the underlying disease process responsible for the myocardial disease.
**Cardiovascular and endocrine/metabolic**: Via systolic and/or diastolic dysfunction, stroke volume and cardiac output may become inadequate to maintain arterial blood pressure and tissue perfusion, resulting in lethargy, weakness, and multi-organ dysfunction. Failure to empty the venous reservoirs is manifested by vascular congestion and transudation of fluid within tissues and body cavities (CHF). Disease progression is a consequence of chronic compensatory neuroendocrine activation involving, in part, increased sympathetic tone and the renin–angiotensin–aldosterone system, which cause increases in heart rate and contractility, vasoconstriction, retention

of water and sodium to increase circulatory volume, and increased venous pressure. Congestive signs may be characterized by peripheral venous and organ congestion, ascites, pericardial effusion, pulmonary and peripheral edema, or a combination of these factors.
**Respiratory**: Myocardial failure results in respiratory embarrassment due to intracoelomic air sac compression (caused by ascites and organomegaly), pulmonary congestion and edema, cardiac tamponade, or a combination of these symptoms.
**Hepatobiliary/renal**: Hepatomegaly (sometimes together with ascites in the hepatoperitoneal cavities) and renomegaly can develop in cases of CHF due to passive venous congestion. This, together with reduced arterial blood pressure and tissue perfusion, can negatively impact the function of both organs.
**Hemic/lymphatic/immune**: Splenomegaly may result from congestion or from an immune response to the underlying disease process, which might also produce hematologic changes such as a leukocytosis. Polycythemia frequently develops as a consequence of chronic hypoxia.
**Nervous/neuromuscular/musculoskeletal**: Reduced arterial blood pressure and tissue perfusion, together with neurologic damage can produce altered mentation or other neurologic deficits, syncope, and seizures. Cachexia and generalized weakness often accompany cardiac disease and failure.
**Gastrointestinal**: Gastrointestinal function and motility can decrease with myocardial disease and failure due to congestion and reduced arterial blood pressure and tissue perfusion.
**Behavioral**: Changes are often subtle, but include lethargy, reduced appetite, and reduced activity level, stamina, and interest in normal activities.

## GENETICS
Understanding of the genetic factors underlying myocardial disease and congenital cardiac defects in birds is limited. Genetic, as well as other factors, have been proposed to play a role in the etiology of spontaneous DCM and ascites syndrome in poultry species. The genetic basis for cardiovascular disease in birds is an area of ongoing research.

## INCIDENCE/PREVALENCE
Cardiac diseases have been recognized predominately in poultry and companion psittacine birds. The most commonly reported disease entities in some taxonomic groups are CHF in psittacines; cardiomyopathies, infectious disease, and ascites syndrome in chickens and turkeys; and viral myocarditis in birds of prey. The relatively few published studies examining the prevalence of cardiac disease in psittacines

have shown a prevalence between 5.2% and 36%. In one postmortem study, 58% of birds with cardiac disease had died of CHF and the remaining 42% had cardiac lesions that were considered incidental and secondary to systemic infectious diseases including pulmonary aspergillosis, bacterial septicemia, avian polyomavirus infection, and avian bornavirus infection. Another postmortem study in psittacines identified a similar spectrum of infectious disease states as the prior study, but also found that atherosclerotic disease and CHF accounted for the majority of non-infectious cardiovascular diseases. These findings are consistent with the author's experience, in which cardiac disease most consistently takes the form of CHF subsequent to advanced atherosclerotic disease, and as such, age and species groups represented mirror those with higher prevalence of atherosclerosis. Cases of infectious disease are encountered less frequently and those of DCM, neoplasia, toxin exposure, and other causes only sporadically.

## GEOGRAPHIC DISTRIBUTION
There is no specific geographic distribution.

## SIGNALMENT
**Species**: Any species of bird can develop myocardial disease, but it is most often recognized in companion psittacine birds, poultry species, birds of prey, pigeons, and waterfowl (e.g. ducks, geese, and swans). Species predisposed to atherosclerotic disease, to include several psittacine species, pigeons, raptors, turkeys, and chickens, may have a higher predilection for ischemic cardiomyopathy.
**Mean age and range**: Any age may be affected, but chronic degenerative disease and underlying atherosclerotic disease are more likely to develop with advancing age, including in psittacines over 20 years of age.
**Predominant sex**: Overall, there is no specific sex predilection for myocardial disease, except where atherosclerotic disease is an underlying factor; female psittacines are at higher risk than males and the opposite is true in turkeys and chickens.

## SIGNS

### General Comments
Myocardial disease most often manifests clinically when heart failure develops; other clinical manifestations depend on the underlying etiology. Clinical signs may be absent earlier in the course of disease.

### Historical Findings
Signs are often non-specific, including sudden death, lethargy, depression, weakness, reduced activity level, reduced appetite, and exercise intolerance. Other reported signs may include respiratory distress, coelomic distention, falling or collapse, syncope, and seizures.

M

# MYOCARDIAL DISEASES     (CONTINUED)

M

### Physical Examination Findings
Tachycardia, arrythmia, murmur, poor pulse quality or deficits, exercise intolerance, tachypnea, dyspnea, harsh lung sounds, cyanosis, pallor, coelomic distention, extension of the liver lobes caudal the sternal margin, peripheral venous congestion, peripheral edema, failure to absorb subcutaneous fluids. Altered mentation, paresis, ataxia, syncope, seizure, blindness, anisocoria, vestibular signs, other neurologic deficits.

## CAUSES

### Degenerative
**Hypertrophic cardiomyopathy**: Usually the product of pressure and volume overload states (cardiomyopathy of overload) and are discussed in more detail in the CHF chapter.
**Ischemic injury**: Ischemic cardiomyopathy and infarction have been reported in birds of prey and in pigeon and quail models of atherosclerosis. Myocardial changes consistent with ischemic injury, including myocardial necrosis, inflammation, degeneration, and fibrosis, have been associated with atherosclerosis of the coronary arteries in psittacines. Myocardial necrosis likely reflects recent injury, while degenerative and fibrotic changes reflect chronic, ongoing injury. These changes have the potential to produce arrhythmias. Arrhythmias could result in sudden death while systolic and diastolic myocardial dysfunction may ultimately culminate in congestive heart failure. Acute myocardial infarction is thought to be rare in psittacines.

### Infectious Myocarditis, Endocarditis, Epicarditis
Bacterial and fungal infections can occur by hematogenous spread or by extension from infected adjacent tissues.
**Bacterial**: Including but not limited to *Chlamydia psittaci*, *Mycobacterium* spp., *Escherichia coli*, *Salmonella* spp., *Listeria monocytogenes*, *Pasteurella multocida*, *Riemerella anatipestifer* (turkeys, ducks), *Mycoplasma* spp., *Erysipelothrix rhusiopathiae*, *Enterococcus* spp., *Streptococcus* spp., *Staphylococcus* spp., *Enterobacter cloacae*, *Pseudomonas aeruginosa*, *Lactobacillus jensenii*.
**Fungal**: *Aspergillus* spp., *Candida* spp., Zygomycetes. *Aspergillus* spp. infection can spread to the heart from the adjacent lungs and air sacs and disseminated infection with *Aspergillus* spp., *Candida* spp., and Zygomycetes can have cardiac involvement by angioinvasion and hematogenous spread.
**Viral**: Avian bornavirus (causing avian ganglioneuritis): Inflammatory infiltrates are frequently found in the epicardium and myocardium, as well as myocardial necrosis and fibrosis, potentially resulting in myocardial dysfunction, arrhythmias, and sudden death.

**Avian polyomavirus**: Polyomavirus infection produces myocarditis with necrosis and hemorrhage in psittacines and finches. West Nile virus—myocarditis and necrosis has been documented in several psittacine species and is a common feature of the disease in North American birds of prey. Avian influenza virus, Eastern equine encephalitis virus, avian leukosis virus, parvovirus (geese, Muscovy ducks), avian encephalomyelitis virus, reovirus, avian paramyxovirus I, psittacine poxvirus.
**Parasitic**: *Sarcocystis* spp. and *Toxoplasma gondii* (both reported to cause myocarditis and necrosis associated with protozoal cysts within cardiomyocytes), filarioid nematodes (found in wild-caught cockatoos), *Trichomonas gallinae* (pigeons), *Atoxoplasma serini* (passerines), *Leucocytozoon* spp.

### Inflammatory (Non-Infectious)
Visceral gout (inflammatory reaction can accompany urate deposition in the myocardium and epicardium).

### Idiopathic
DCM is myocardial disease resulting in ventricular dilation, thinning of the myocardium, and systolic and diastolic dysfunction. By definition, the condition cannot be fully explained by the effects of abnormal loading, so should not be confused with the chamber dilatation that develops as an endpoint of pressure or volume overload states. Well-known disorder of turkey poults; cause is unknown but is associated with rapid growth and production. Histopathologic lesions include degeneration of myofibers with vacuolation, secondary endocardiosis, focal infiltration of lymphocytes, and secondary changes in the liver. There are scant reports of DCM in other species of birds, but they include a whooper swan (*Cygnus cygnus*) and a captive red-tailed hawk (*Buteo jamaicensis*). In both cases, the myocardium was histologically normal and no specific cause could be identified. Scarcely reported in psittacines and is generally considered idiopathic. Myocardial degeneration and fibrosis may develop for undetermined reasons.

### Metabolic/Nutritional
Fatty infiltration into the myocardium associated with obesity, iron storage disease, vitamin E/selenium deficiency (associated with myocardial degeneration), calcium/phosphorous imbalance, and vitamin D$_3$ toxicity (can cause cardiac and vascular mineralization), excessive dietary sodium or potassium.

### Neoplastic
Cardiac neoplasms include hemangioma and hemangiosarcoma, rhabdomyoma and rhabdomyosarcoma, fibrosarcoma, melanosarcoma, and lymphosarcoma.

### Toxic
Furazolidone (nitrofuran antibiotic that induces DCM in chicks, ducklings, and turkey poults when fed at a concentration of ≥ 300 ppm), lead toxicosis (lesions can include myocardial degeneration and necrosis, fibrinoid necrosis of myocardial arterioles, and subsequent thrombosis and infarction), zinc toxicosis, avocado (persin), various toxic plants (Cassia, rapeseed), mycotoxins, some rodenticides, ionophores, doxorubicin.

## RISK FACTORS
There are many potential risk factors for myocardial disease considering the wide variety of causes. These include husbandry and dietary factors, housing (outdoor vs. indoor) and lifestyle (including lack of exercise), infectious disease exposure, toxin exposure, and concurrent or predisposing conditions.

# DIAGNOSIS

## DIFFERENTIAL DIAGNOSIS
Differential diagnoses will include other cardiovascular diseases, neurologic diseases, respiratory diseases, or intracoelomic pathology producing similar clinical signs and physical examination findings. As these may be vague and non-specific, a comprehensive diagnostic workup will be required to identify and characterize cardiovascular disease and rule out other causes. Definitive premortem diagnosis of specific myocardial disease is challenged by limitations in diagnostic sample types (e.g. histologic samples) that can be collected antemortem, particularly in an unstable patient. However, careful history collection together with systematic, stepwise diagnostic investigation, can allow cardiac disease differentials to be progressively narrowed down.

## CBC/BIOCHEMISTRY/URINALYSIS
Hematology may show polycythemia if there has been chronic hypoxia. Hematocrit values of 60% or greater should be suspicious for chronic heart or respiratory diseases when obvious dehydration is not present. Other hematologic changes may be seen with infectious processes, usually reflecting stress, inflammation, or infection. Biochemical changes may occur due to concurrent changes in the liver (elevated AST or bile acids) or kidneys (elevated uric acid). Cardiac troponin T and I can be measured but limited information is available in birds on validated assays. Plasma lipoproteins may be measured in relation to atherosclerosis dyslipidemic risk factors.

## OTHER LABORATORY TESTS
If an infectious disease etiology is suspected, pathogen-specific serologic assays may be useful in achieving a definitive diagnosis.

## IMAGING
Radiographic findings may include cardiomegaly, pulmonary congestion or edema, coelomic effusion, hepatomegaly, or splenomegaly. Echocardiography may demonstrate pericardial effusion, thinning of cardiac muscle with dilated cardiomyopathy, or thickened cardiac muscle with hypertrophic cardiomyopathy. Contractility can be subjectively assessed. Using a standard transcoelomic approach, only two views are available in most birds, a four-chamber view, and an aortic outflow view. Cross-sectional views are not possible with this approach and cardiac measurements cannot be accurately made.

## DIAGNOSTIC PROCEDURES
Electrocardiography may be helpful in identification of arrhythmia or other electrical activity of the heart.

## PATHOLOGIC FINDINGS
See Systems Affected, Signs, and Causes sections. Gross pathologic findings in heart disease may include pericardial effusion, hypertrophy or dilation of the ventricles, or valvular endocarditis. Histopathology may include inflammation of the myocardium, fibrosis, or atherosclerotic plaques.

## TREATMENT

### APPROPRIATE HEALTH CARE
Treatment of cardiac diseases involves treatment of the underlying cause, if known, and treatment of the CHF that often results from these diseases.

### NURSING CARE
Stress should be minimized in avian heart patients. Social arrangements should be adjusted to avoid conspecific aggression, and other sources of stress should be removed.

### ACTIVITY
Limitations should be individually applied and focused on ensuring easy access to food and water, and protection from injury.

### DIET
Diet modifications are not advised in birds with unmanaged cardiovascular disease. Adjustments in diet if needed can be considered once the patient's underlying disease process is managed.

### CLIENT EDUCATION
General treatment and prognosis information should be discussed. Clients should be taught to watch for signs of decompensation such as tachypnea, dyspnea, lethargy, and/or dysrexia, as these are indications for a repeat examination and adjustments in therapy.

## SURGICAL CONSIDERATIONS
Pericardiocentesis may be used if there is significant pericardial effusion. Endoscopic creation of a pericardial window may be useful for chronic pericarditis. Otherwise, surgical treatment is not practical for the treatment of heart disease in birds.

## MEDICATIONS

### DRUG(S) OF CHOICE
Therapeutics must be evaluated and applied based on the primary etiology present. Since the myocardium can be affected by a wide range of primary disease processes successful, management must be based on a definitive diagnosis. Considerations for primary myocardial disease include ACE inhibitors (enalapril), beta-blockers (carvedilol), and/or primary ionotropes (pimobendan). Depending on the state in which the patient presents, additional therapy to reduce volume overload or manage CHF could include but is not limited to diuretics (furosemide) and/or additonal vasodilators (isoxsuprine).

### CONTRAINDICATIONS
Identification of the primary etiology is pivotal to clinical improvement. Lack of diagnosis in cases of myocardial disease can lead to repeated poor outcomes.

### PRECAUTIONS
N/A

### POSSIBLE INTERACTIONS
None.

### ALTERNATIVE DRUGS
None.

## FOLLOW-UP

### PATIENT MONITORING
Patient follow up is dependent on the primary etiology. Therapy and patient status should be evaluated q3–4w to facilitate adjustments in dosing or therapeutic plan. Continued follow-up is reasonable on a q3–6m basis or as needed based on recrudescence of clinical signs.

### PREVENTION/AVOIDANCE
This is dependent on the primary disease process resulting in myocardial pathology. See atherosclerosis for prevention guidance specific to this etiology.

### POSSIBLE COMPLICATIONS
N/A

## EXPECTED COURSE AND PROGNOSIS
Survival times vary based on the severity of disease at the time of presentation and underlying reason for disease. Early detection and treatment may result in more prolonged survival.

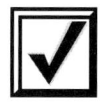

## MISCELLANEOUS

### ASSOCIATED CONDITIONS
Atherosclerosis, CHF.

### AGE-RELATED FACTORS
Although cardiovascular disease may increase in frequency with age, there are no adjustments to the diagnosis and treatment associated with age.

### ZOONOTIC POTENTIAL
Some infectious etiologies (e.g. *Chlamydia psittaci*) for myocardial disease are zoonotic.

### FERTILITY/BREEDING
Patients with cardiovascular disease should not be used for breeding, nor should reproduction be encouraged.

### SYNONYMS
N/A

### SEE ALSO
Atherosclerosis
Bornaviral Disease (Aquatic Birds)
Bornaviral Disease (Psittaciformes)
Chlamydiosis
Congestive Heart Disease
Obesity
Respiratory Distress
Toxicosis (Ingested, Gastrointestinal)

### ABBREVIATIONS
ACE—angiotensin-converting enzyme
AST—aspartate aminotransferase
CHF—congestive heart failure
DCM—dilated cardiomyopathy
HCM—hypertrophic cardiomyopathy

### INTERNET RESOURCES
N/A

*Suggested Reading*
Fitzgerald, B.C. (2022). Cardiovascular diseases in pet birds: Therapeutic options and challenges. *Veterinary Clinics of North America: Exotic Animal Practice*, 25:469–501.
Fitzgerald, B.C., Beaufrère, H. (2015). Cardiology. In: *Current Therapy in Avian Medicine and Surgery* (ed. B.L. Speer), 252–328. St. Louis, MO: Elsevier.
**Authors**: Brenna Fitzgerald, DVM, DABVP (Avian), and Bianca Murphy, DVM, DABVP (Avian)

M

# NEOPLASIA (GASTROINTESTINAL AND HEPATIC)

 BASICS

## DEFINITION
GI neoplasia refers to a tumor of the tissues related to the GI tract, which include the oral cavity, esophagus, crop, proventriculus, ventriculus, small and large intestines. Hepatic neoplasia refers to a tumor of the liver or a tumor relating to the liver. Neoplasms of the GI tract and the liver can be primary or secondary (metastasis), benign, or malignant.

## PATHOPHYSIOLOGY
Various neoplasms of the GI tract and hepatobiliary system have been reported in Psittacines. Secondary metastasis of other tumor types is uncommon to these internal organs. Documented tumor types in avian species include: GI—leiomyosarcoma, papillomatosis, squamous cell carcinoma, adenocarcinoma, lymphoma; hepatobiliary—papillomatosis, cholangiocarcinoma, carcinoma, adenoma.

## SYSTEMS AFFECTED
GI—oral cavity, esophagus, crop, proventriculus, ventriculus, small intestines, large intestines. Liver—hepatic tissue, biliary tract. Secondary systems can be affected if metastasis occurs.

## GENETICS
N/A

## INCIDENCE/PREVALENCE
Uncommon.

## GEOGRAPHIC DISTRIBUTION
N/A

## SIGNALMENT
Leiomyosarcoma of the GI tract has been reported in budgerigars and lovebirds. Papillomatosis primarily affects New World psittacines, especially macaws, Amazon parrots, and hawk-headed parrots. Cholangiocarcinomas are most frequently described in Amazon parrots.

## SIGNS

### Historical Findings
Typical presenting complaints include hemorrhage from the vent, coelomic distension, lethargy and inability to perch, weight loss, cloacal prolapse, agitation, non-specific debilitation, regurgitation, dark red-brown stools, yellow-orange stools with undigested whole seeds, beak overgrowth or irregularities, and polyuria. Oral tumors can result in dyspnea, recurrent infections, dysphagia, and nasal discharge. Bile duct

neoplasia can result in cloacal prolapse, weight loss, anorexia, seizures and trembling, and coma.

### Physical Examination Findings
On physical examination, a large, coelomic mass may be palpated (leiomyosarcoma), mass(es) may be noted on cloacal eversion (papilloma, carcinoma), chronic stomatitis with necrosis (squamous cell carcinoma of the oral cavity), and thickening of the crop or esophageal wall with plaque-like masses (squamous cell carcinoma). Antemortem diagnosis of many of these neoplasm types is challenging.

## CAUSES
Papillomas in parrots have been linked to a herpesviral etiology. Additionally, a weak but potential link between papillomatosis and bile duct carcinomas has been theorized. A link between vitamin A deficiency and squamous cell carcinoma has been suggested as a progression from the metaplasia created by the deficiency. Intestinal adenocarcinoma in chickens has been linked to avian leucosis virus subgroup J. Lymphoid neoplasia of the GI tract and liver has been linked to Marek's disease (herpesvirus), lymphoid leukosis, or reticuloendotheliosis.

## RISK FACTORS
Papillomas primarily affect New World psittacines, especially macaws, Amazon parrots, and hawk headed parrots.

 DIAGNOSIS

## DIFFERENTIAL DIAGNOSIS
Non-neoplastic: *Macrorhabdus ornithogaster*, avian bornavirus (proventricular dilation disease), mycobacteriosis, heavy metal toxicity, parasitic causes, foreign body.

## CBC/BIOCHEMISTRY/URINALYSIS
Bloodwork should be performed to evaluate the overall health of the patient, and to determine whether there are any abnormal blood counts that could be related to the neoplastic process. Cytopenias, anemia, and leukocytosis may all be reported with varying types of neoplasia. Anemia is a frequent finding as a result of hemorrhage from the GI tract. Additionally, biochemistry profiles may demonstrate organ involvement associated with the tumor, or organ dysfunction related to the age of the patient or the presence of other disease processes. Hypercalcemia of malignancy has been previously documented in avian patients.

## OTHER LABORATORY TESTS
Fine-needle aspirate and cytology (with or without ultrasound guidance). Biopsy and histopathology of the lesion (punch biopsy, core needle [Tru Cut™, Merit Medical Systems, South Jordan, UT], laparoscopic for internal organs).

## IMAGING
Radiographs, ultrasound and CT can all have utility in the assessment of avian neoplasia. They help to demonstrate the extent of the lesion, invasiveness of the disease, and also to stage the animal (evaluate for metastasis). Many malignant tumors will spread to other organs, with the most common location of metastasis being the lungs, but other locations such as coelomic organs and bone may be involved, depending on the tumor type. Although radiographs provide some utility in assessment, contrast-enhanced CT provides a much better overall picture of the coelomic organs, as well as a more global evaluation of the primary lesion and potential for metastatic lesions. Contrast radiography can be helpful in GI neoplasia to help distinguish irregular distention, thickening of the proventriculus and ventriculus, or irregular or incomplete filling of the GI tract.

## DIAGNOSTIC PROCEDURES
Following acquisition of a biopsy, immunohistochemical testing may be required to obtain a definitive diagnosis when cell morphology alone does not provide enough information; however, the canine and feline antibodies that are used may not cross-react with avian tissues and therefore, must be a consideration when additional testing is undertaken. In addition to these challenges, there are also no established positive controls in avian patients, which creates difficulties when interpreting the results.

## PATHOLOGIC FINDINGS
Pathology findings will depend on the type of tumor that is present in the avian patient.

 TREATMENT

## APPROPRIATE HEALTH CARE
Treatment of the tumor will depend on the type of tumor, invasiveness, and presence or absence of metastasis. Many of the GI and hepatic neoplasms are diagnosed postmortem and extensive metastasis is noted. In the case of cloacal papillomas, surgical removal can be attempted, but recurrence is common. There is a single case of an antemortem diagnosis of cholangio carcinoma in a yellow-naped

N

Amazon parrot that was treated with carboplatin. SCC: Treatment for SCC is typically a combination of surgical excision and radiation therapy. Additionally, intralesional chemotherapy with carboplatin and cisplatin have been attempted with limited success.

## NURSING CARE
Avian patients that are diagnosed with GI and hepatic neoplasia should be provided with supportive care to ensure that they maintain a good quality of life that is pain and as stress free as possible. Depending on the needs of the patient, analgesia, antibiotics, or oxygen therapy may be useful to maintain the comfort of the avian patient.

## ACTIVITY
Avian patients that have been diagnosed with gastrointestinal and hepatic neoplasia should be allowed to choose their own level of activity.

## DIET
No specific dietary recommendations.

## CLIENT EDUCATION
Avian owners are more aware of treatment options for GI and hepatic neoplasia in domestic animal species and humans. As a result, there is an increasing demand for advanced diagnostic and therapeutic options for companion avian species. In any sick avian patient, it is always important to discuss the risks of handling, diagnostics, and treatment, including death. Prognosis and consideration for euthanasia may also be necessary discussions with the owner. At this time, there is no established standard of care for avian neoplasia and most of the dosages are extrapolated with an unknown array of adverse effects.

## SURGICAL CONSIDERATIONS
Surgical excision with adequate margins is an ideal treatment option for many neoplastic processes. This should only be undertaken after a patient has a definitive diagnosis, has been fully staged, and evidence of metastasis has been ruled out. Additionally, the risks of surgery and anesthesia in the avian patient must be fully disclosed to the owner, with a risk versus benefit approach investigated prior to surgery. In cases where inadequate margins

are obtained after surgery, additional treatment options should be explored depending on the tumor type, including additional surgery, radiation therapy, systemic or local chemotherapy. Complete surgical excision in the case of GI and hepatic neoplasia is unlikely to be possible.

## MEDICATIONS
### DRUG(S) OF CHOICE
Chemotherapy may be a therapeutic option, targeted towards the tumor type. Supportive care including analgesics (opioids, NSAIDs), antibiotics, or antifungals may also be considered.

### CONTRAINDICATIONS
N/A

### PRECAUTIONS
Chemotherapy doses are typically extrapolated from what is known in canine and feline patients, and these may not be the correct dose for avian species. Although in dogs and cats, body surface area is used to calculate chemotherapy dosages, it is unknown if this is appropriate for avian patients. Adverse effects of certain chemotherapeutics have been reported in avian species.

### POSSIBLE INTERACTIONS
N/A

### ALTERNATIVE DRUGS
N/A

## FOLLOW-UP
### PATIENT MONITORING
The most important factor to monitor in patients with neoplasia is quality of life. Each patient should be routinely evaluated for changes in respiration, appetite, and ability to perform normal behaviors.

### PREVENTION/AVOIDANCE
N/A

### POSSIBLE COMPLICATIONS
N/A

## EXPECTED COURSE AND PROGNOSIS
In general, the prognosis for many of the avian GI and hepatic neoplasms is guarded to poor, with many of the tumors being diagnosed postmortem.

## MISCELLANEOUS
### ASSOCIATED CONDITIONS
Herpesvirus.

### AGE-RELATED FACTORS
N/A

### ZOONOTIC POTENTIAL
N/A

### FERTILITY/BREEDING
N/A

### SYNONYMS
N/A

### SEE ALSO
N/A

### ABBREVIATIONS
CT—computed tomography
GI—gastrointestinal
NSAIDs—non-steroidal anti-inflammatory drugs
SCC—squamous cell carcinoma

### INTERNET RESOURCES
N/A

*Suggested Reading*
Styles, D.K., Tomaszewski, E.K., Jaeger, L.A., Phalen, D.N. (2004). Psittacid herpesviruses associated with mucosal papillomas in neotropical parrots. *Virology*, 325:24–35.
Sundberg, J.P., Junge, R.E., O'Banion, M.K., et al. (1986). Cloacal papillomas in psittacines. *American Journal of Veterinary Research*, 47:928–932.
Zehnder, A., Hawkins, M., Koski, M., et al. (2010). Therapeutic considerations for squamous cell carcinoma: An avian case series. Paper presented at: 31st Annual Proceedings of the Association of Avian Veterinarians, San Diego, August 2–5.
**Author**: Sara Gardhouse, DVM, DABVP (Exotic Companion Mammal), DACZM

N

# NEOPLASIA (INTEGUMENT)

## BASICS

### DEFINITION
Integumentary neoplasia refers to a tumor related to the integument or skin, which includes the epidermis, dermis, hypodermis, associated glands, feathers, beak, and nails. Integumentary neoplasms can be primary or secondary (metastasis), benign, or malignant.

### PATHOPHYSIOLOGY
Both benign and malignant neoplasia of the integument has been reported in avian species. Squamous cell carcinoma (SCC): malignant neoplasia of the epithelial cells—feathered skin, beak, uropygial gland. Lipoma: Benign neoplasia of the adipose tissue—most commonly found in the subcutaneous tissues, but can arise anywhere on the body. Xanthoma: Non-neoplastic dermal mass composed of cholesterol and lipid-laden macrophages—most commonly found in the skin and subcutaneous tissues of psittacines and gallinaceous birds, locations—dorsum, wings, upper legs. Cutaneous lymphoma: Head, periocular, neck.

### SYSTEMS AFFECTED
Integument: Epidermis, dermis, hypodermis, associated glands (uropygial gland), feathers/follicles, nails, beak. Secondary systems can be affected if metastasis occurs.

### GENETICS
N/A

### INCIDENCE/PREVALENCE
Unknown.

### GEOGRAPHIC DISTRIBUTION
N/A

### SIGNALMENT
SCC commonly affects cockatiels, Amazon parrots, and conures. Lipoma: obese birds, especially budgerigars, Quaker parrots, Amazon parrots, macaws. Xanthoma: obese birds with hyperlipidemia, concurrent trauma to the affected area.

### SIGNS
#### Historical Findings
Typical presenting complaints include detection of a mass on the body of the bird. Additionally, weakness, lethargy, and weight loss may be detected depending on the progression and advanced stage of the disease.

#### Physical Examination Findings
There is no known age or sex predisposition reported with integumentary neoplasia in avian species. Certain avian species have been documented to more commonly have specific types of integumentary neoplasia. SCC comprises ill-defined, often ulcerated, pink, raised, proliferative, and infiltrative masses.

Lipoma is well circumscribed, typically non-infiltrative but can be infiltrative, usually within the subcutaneous tissues. The most common location for lipomas has been documented to be the pericloacal region. Xanthoma is a friable, well-vascularized yellow to orange mass. Lymphoma is diffuse swelling or multifocal nodules of the head, periocular area, and/or neck (most commonly).

### CAUSES
N/A

### RISK FACTORS
In certain integumentary neoplasms, obesity and diet are thought to play a role in the underlying etiology.

## DIAGNOSIS

### DIFFERENTIAL DIAGNOSIS
Feather cysts. Infectious: Bacterial—staphylococci, streptococci, *Bacillus* species; fungal—dermatophytosis, *Cryptococcus*, *Malassezia*; parasitic—*Knemidocoptes mutans* (scaly face or leg mite), feather mites; viral—psittacine beak and feather disease. Inappropriate nutrition.

### CBC/BIOCHEMISTRY/URINALYSIS
SCC: often no changes on bloodwork. Lipoma: often no changes on bloodwork. Xanthoma: hyperlipidemia may be present. Lymphoma: often no changes on bloodwork, but the presence of a lymphocytosis (often severe) should raise concern. Additionally, paraneoplastic hypercalcemia and monoclonal hyperglobulinemia have both been documented in cases of lymphoma in avian species.

### OTHER LABORATORY TESTS
Fine-needle aspirate and cytology: Certain tumors exfoliate well with aspirate or impression smear and cytology, while others do not. SCCs exfoliate well. Lipomas often result in a fatty layer on the slide that dissolves when staining is attempted, or a layer of well-differentiated adipocytes in some cases may be seen. Lysis of the cells associated with sampling is, however, common. In cases of liposarcoma, the adipocytes are often immature and less well circumscribed. Xanthomas will appear as cholesterol clefts and multinucleated giant cells on cytologic evaluation. Lymphoma can often be diagnosed fine-needle aspiration and cytology. Biopsy and histopathology are gold standard for definitive diagnosis.

### IMAGING
Radiographs, ultrasound and CT can all have utility in the assessment of avian neoplasia. They help to demonstrate the extent of the

lesion, invasiveness of the disease, and also to stage the animal (evaluate for metastasis). Many malignant tumors will spread to other organs, with the most common location of metastasis being the lungs, but other locations such as coelomic organs and bone may be involved, depending on the tumor type. Although radiographs provide some utility in assessment, contrast-enhanced CT provides a much better overall picture of the coelomic organs, as well as a more global evaluation of the primary lesion and potential for metastatic lesions.

### DIAGNOSTIC PROCEDURES
Following acquisition of a biopsy, immunohistochemical testing may be required to obtain further characterization of the diagnosis when cell morphology alone does not provide enough information; however, the canine and feline antibodies that are used may not cross-react with avian tissues and therefore, must be a consideration when additional testing is undertaken. In addition to these challenges, there are also no established positive controls in avian patients which creates difficulties when interpreting the results. In the case of lymphoma, the T cell marker, CD3 has been demonstrated to cross-react well among species, with less consistent cross-reaction demonstrated with the B cell markers CD79a and BLA36.

### PATHOLOGIC FINDINGS
Pathology findings will depend on the type of tumor that is present in the avian patient.

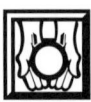

## TREATMENT

### APPROPRIATE HEALTH CARE
Treatment of the tumor will depend on the type of tumor, invasiveness, and presence or absence of metastasis.
**SCC**: Best treated surgically with the ultimate goal of complete excision with complete margins. However, in situations where this cannot be achieved, local radiation therapy may provide benefit, either strontium for superficial lesions or orthovoltage radiation therapy for deeper or larger lesions, although typically these tumors are thought to be more radiation resistant in other species. Intralesional chemotherapy and cryotherapy may also be alternative options.
**Lipoma**: Surgical excision is appropriate in cases where the tumor is large, growing rapidly, or becomes ulcerated.
**Xanthoma**: Xanthomas are not true neoplasms, so unless the mass is causing functional problems or is constantly being traumatized, no treatment is necessary.
**Lymphoma**: Treatment of lymphoma will depend whether the disease is systemic or

AVIAN 285

(CONTINUED) NEOPLASIA (INTEGUMENT)

local (based on staging). In cases of systemic disease, chemotherapy is the recommended treatment, compared with cases of local disease, where radiation therapy may be recommended.

## NURSING CARE
Avian patients that are diagnosed with integumentary neoplasia should be provided supportive care to ensure that they maintain a good quality of life that is pain and as stress free as possible. Depending on the needs of the patient, anti-inflammatories or opioids may be indicated to maintain the comfort of the avian patient. Additionally, treatment with antibiotics or antifungals may be indicated in cases of secondary infection.

## ACTIVITY
Avian patients that have been diagnosed with integumentary neoplasia should be allowed to choose their own level of activity.

## DIET
Dietary changes to reduce body weight are recommended in obese patients with lymphoma. Additionally, pilot studies may demonstrate utility of L-carnitine to reduce body weight and the size of subcutaneous lipomas in budgerigars. Dietary changes to reduce body weight are recommended in obese patients with xanthomas. Additionally, a diet supplemented with vitamin A or precursors may help to reduce the size of these masses.

## CLIENT EDUCATION
Avian owners are more aware of treatment options for integumentary neoplasia in domestic animal species and humans. As a result, there is an increasing demand for advanced diagnostic and therapeutic options for companion avian species. In any sick avian patient, it is always important to discuss the risks of handling, diagnostics, and treatment, including death, especially in birds that are in respiratory distress. Prognosis and consideration for euthanasia may also be necessary discussions with the owner. At this time, there is no established standard of care for avian neoplasia and most of the dosages are extrapolated with an unknown array of adverse effects.

## SURGICAL CONSIDERATIONS
Surgical excision with adequate margins is an ideal treatment option for many neoplastic processes. This should only be undertaken after a patient has a definitive diagnosis, has been fully staged, and evidence of metastasis has been ruled out. Additionally, the risks of surgery and anesthesia in the avian patient must be fully disclosed to the owner, with a risk versus benefit approach investigated prior to surgery. In cases where inadequate margins are obtained after surgery, additional treatment options should be explored depending on the tumor type, including additional surgery, radiation therapy, systemic or local chemotherapy.

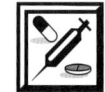

## MEDICATIONS

### DRUG(S) OF CHOICE
Chemotherapy may be a therapeutic option, targeted towards the tumor type. Supportive care including analgesics (opioids, NSAIDs), antibiotics, or antifungals may also be considered.

### CONTRAINDICATIONS
N/A

### PRECAUTIONS
Chemotherapy doses are typically extrapolated from what is known in canine and feline patients, and these may not be the correct dose for avian species. Although in dogs and cats, body surface area is used to calculate chemotherapy dosages, it is unknown whether this is appropriate for avian patients. Adverse effects of certain chemotherapeutics have been reported in avian species.

### POSSIBLE INTERACTIONS
N/A

### ALTERNATIVE DRUGS
N/A

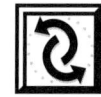

## FOLLOW-UP

### PATIENT MONITORING
The most important factor to monitor in patients with neoplasia is quality of life. Each patient should be routinely evaluated for changes in respiration, appetite, and ability to perform normal behaviors.

### PREVENTION/AVOIDANCE
N/A

### POSSIBLE COMPLICATIONS
N/A

### EXPECTED COURSE AND PROGNOSIS
The prognosis for avian integumentary neoplasia will vary on the tumor type. However, for many of the local tumors, complete treatment and cure may be possible.

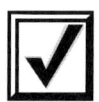

## MISCELLANEOUS

### ASSOCIATED CONDITIONS
N/A

### AGE-RELATED FACTORS
N/A

### ZOONOTIC POTENTIAL
N/A

### FERTILITY/BREEDING
N/A

### SYNONYMS
N/A

### SEE ALSO
N/A

### ABBREVIATIONS
NSAIDs—non-steroidal anti-inflammatory drugs
SCC—squamous cell carcinoma

### INTERNET RESOURCES
N/A

*Suggested Reading*
De Voe, R.S., Trogdon, M., Flammer, K. (2004). Preliminary assessment of the effect of diet and L-carnitine supplementation on lipoma size and bodyweight in budgerigars (*Melopsittacus undulatus*). *J Avian Med Surg.*, 18:12–18.
Nemetz, B. (2004). Strontium-90 therapy for uropygial neoplasia. In: *Proceedings of the Annual Conference of the Association of Avian Veterinarians, 25th Annual Conference*, January.
Zehnder, A., Swift, L., Sundaram, A. (2014). Multi-institutional survey of squamous cell carcinoma in birds. In: *35th Annual Conference Association of Avian Veterinarians*.

**Author**: Sara Gardhouse, DVM, DABVP (Exotic Companion Mammal), DACZM

N

# NEOPLASIA (LYMPHOPROLIFERATIVE)

 BASICS

## DEFINITION
Lymphoid neoplasia is a type of malignant cancer that initiates from the reticuloendothelial and lymphatic systems. Recent research has found that the distinction between lymphoma and leukemia may not be as obvious as previously thought. As a generalization, most pathologists term lymphoma as predominantly affecting organs or creating solid masses. Lymphoma may also include involvement of the blood and bone marrow. Lymphoma can be characterized as T cell or B cell immunophenotype. Leukemia tends to involve the blood and/or the bone marrow primarily.

## PATHOPHYSIOLOGY
Lymphoid neoplasias typically arise from lymphocytes and lymphoid tissues, but it is also possible for them to originate from any other tissue located within the body, or they can originate from the bone marrow.

## SYSTEMS AFFECTED
**Hematology**: Predominantly the lymphocytes (small cells, typically chronic; large cells, typically acute); bone marrow.
**Alimentary**: The spleen and liver are predominantly affected in avian species; however, the GI tract, including the proventriculus and intestines, can be involved.
**Cutaneous**: There have been reported cutaneous T cell lymphoma cases in birds.
**Other organ systems**: Included typically as a result of metastases and can include the CNS (brain and spinal cord), urogenital (kidneys), respiratory (lungs), cardiac (heart).

## GENETICS
There is no reported genetic predisposition to lymphoma or leukemia.

## INCIDENCE/PREVALENCE
The true prevalence is unknown but preliminary research through the Exotic Species Cancer Research Alliance (ESCRA) has found that lymphoma or leukemia is approximately 8% of all avian cancers and is the most commonly reported and submitted type of avian cancer (Harrison unpublished data).

## GEOGRAPHIC DISTRIBUTION
A geographic distribution has not been reported for lymphoma or leukemia in birds.

## SIGNALMENT
**Species**: Species that have had cases of lymphoma reported in are the African grey parrot, African penguin, Amazon parrot, bald eagle, black swan, blue-and-yellow macaw, blue fronted Amazon parrot, budgerigar, canary, cockatiel, cockatoo, crested wood partritge, European starling, great horned owl, great Indian hill mynah, green winged macaw, helmented guineafowl, Humboldt penguin, jackdaw, java sparrow, junglefowl, macaroni penguin, merlin, orange-winged Amazon parrot, ostrich, peafowl, peregrine falcon, pink-backed pelican, red-crowned crane, ruff, salmon-crested cockatoo, scarlet macaw, sulphur-crested cockatoo, sun conure, tragopan, umbrella cockatoo, wild Okinawa rail, yellow-naped Amazon parrot, yellow-headed Amazon parrot.
**Species predilection**: Canaries are the most common to develop cutaneous lymphoma, and in this situation, males have been reported to have more cases than females.
**Predominant sex**: There are no published data that indicate that one sex is more prone to developing this condition. Preliminary unpublished data from ESCRA do not indicate that there is difference in the sex of the bird developing lymphoma or leukemia.

## SIGNS
### General Comments
Lymphoid neoplasia can affect all tissues in the body, with some that occur more often than others. Clinical signs and physical examination findings can vary depending on where the bird is affected.

### Historical Findings
Owner reported clinical signs can consist of anorexia, weight loss, depression, paresis, coelomic distension, paralysis, paresis, diarrhea, regurgitation, melena, hematochezia, dyschezia, and apparent blindness.

### Physical Examination Findings
The most common presentation of lymphoid neoplasia in birds tends to be multicentric, or throughout the body ± blood and bone marrow. Clinical signs related to this are non-specific, such as depression, anorexia, weight loss, and muscle wasting.
**Hematology**: Pale mucous membranes, petechia, ecchymotic hemorrhages, epistaxsis.
**Alimentary**: Coelomic masses, splenic mass, ascites, biliverdinuria, regurgitation, diarrhea, hematochezia, melena, straining to defecate.
**Cutaneous**: Nodules, plaques, ulcerations, non-healing wounds, nodules, which can be around the head and neck or diffusely throughout the body.

## CAUSES
There are viral causes of lymphoma in poultry, such as lymphoid leukosis, an Alpharetrovirus within the family of Retroviridae which can cause a B cell lymphoma. An additional viral disease, Marek's disease, is an alphaherpesvirus that can produce T cell lymphomas primarily in poultry. Reticuloendotheliosis virus can produce B cell lymphomas in the bursa and non-bursal T cell lymphomas have been reported experimentally but not clinically. Infections with reticuloendotheliosis have been found in poultry, turkeys (including wild turkeys), ducks, geese, quail, and likely many other avian species.

## RISK FACTORS
N/A

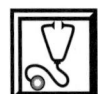 DIAGNOSIS

## DIFFERENTIAL DIAGNOSIS
Sepsis (bacterial or fungal), other bacterial infection that can cause hepatic or splenic enlargement (*Mycobacteria* spp. or *Chlamydia psittaci*) viral infection, localized granuloma (*Mycobacteria* spp. or fungal) other neoplasia (benign or malignant).

## CBC/BIOCHEMISTRY/URINALYSIS
### Complete Blood Count
Anemia and leukopenia have been reported in an Amazon parrot. Leukemia is defined as a hematopoietic neoplasm arising in the bone marrow or is present in the blood of neoplastic cells of hematopoietic origin. Acute leukemia has immature cells of myeloid or lymphoid origin, which may include blast cells. By the World Health Organization definition, an acute leukemia must have > 20% blast cells. Chronic leukemia has mature cells and can be of lymphoid or myeloid origin. For those with leukemia, a marked leukocytosis and mature lymphocytosis has been reported. Non-specific findings such as non-regenerative anemia secondary to chronic inflammation or disease, are common. Pancytopenia with non-regenerative anemia, heteropenia, and thrombocytopenia was reported in a Pekin duck that had lymphocytic leukemia.

### Biochemistry
Hypercalcemia and hyperglobulinemia has been reported an Amazon parrot. Other abonormalities could be attributed to the organs affected with metastases, such as liver involvement (elevation of serum AST, GGT, and bile acids). Renal involvement would cause elevations of uric acid. Other generalized serum chemistry findings could be elevations in AST or CPK, particularly if the bird is recumbent, or has muscle wasting.

## OTHER LABORATORY TESTS
Confirmatory testing for evaluating leukemia can involve a bone marrow biopsy. Additional testing, such as PCR testing for MDV, avian leukosis virus or reticuloendotheliosis virus can be peformed on tissues samples collected via biopsy or at necropsy. Poultry with MDV typically have high viremia titers and are PCR positive.

## IMAGING
Metastases checks should always be performed, with ultrasound, radiographs, and CT. MRI can be used to evaluate for CNS lesions, although depending on the size of the bird, CT and MRI may be less valuable in differentiating lesions in smaller-sized organs. CT with contrast can help to identify masses within the body, however, and this must be done with the use of an IV catheter.

## DIAGNOSTIC PROCEDURES
Bone marrow aspiration from the tibiotarsus can be performed to confirm lymphoma diagnosis if there is lymphocytosis present.

## PATHOLOGIC FINDINGS
### Gross Pathololgic Findings
Grossly, the most commonly reported body systems are hepatic and GI. There are typically metastases present and are considered to be multicentric. Metastasis can occur to any organ/organ system. Affected organs may also appear paler than normal. Organomegaly may also be observed in the spleen, liver, and kdneys. Coelomic effusion may be diagnosed when there is metastatic disease and there is serosal involvement. Cutaneous lesions tend to involve the dermis. Grossly, cutaneous lesions could range from plaques to ulcerations to raised nodules, with the head and neck most commonly affected. Gross lesions within other organ systems can appear as white to tan nodules of varying sizes. Secondary lesions such as decreased muscle mass, absence of fat, bacterial or fungal infections may be diagnosed.

### Histopathologic Findings
Grading of lymphoma in humans is done according to how the cells look and behave in comparison with normal cells. These subtypes consist of indolent (low grade, slow growing), or aggressive (high grade, fast growing). Overall, the tumors were found to have sheets of round cells with round to oval nuclei, with a majority of cases having infiltrative growth patterns. The majority of cases had homogenous populations of round cells. Mitotic count varied in cases depending on severity. Immunohistochemistry should be used to confirm B-cell or T-cell lymphoma, although non-B, non-T cell lymphoma cases have been reported. All B cell lymphoma cases were diagnosed as multicentric, all involved the GI system, and the majority of them involved the intestines. B cell lymphomas had varied histological features and mitotic counts, but the most common size of the neoplastic cells was large. B cell lymphomas tended to be in the GI and urogenital systems. T cell lymphomas had no pattern for anatomic location or cellular characteristics, although they did tend to affect the respiratory system. All non-B, non-T cell lymphomas have been diagnosed in cockatiels.

## TREATMENT
### APPROPRIATE HEALTH CARE
In typical treatments of cancer, the goal of complete surgical removal and radiation is aiming for a cure. Unfortunately, in the case of lymphoma or leukemia, surgical removal is not possible. Complete, whole body radiation has been attempted, but was not successful in a black swan. Chemotherapy is typically used to achieve remission, which is the control of the animal's cancer for greater than a 6-month time frame.

### Radiation therapy
Radiation treatments overall tend to have varying treatment responses in avian patients. Additionally, birds have been found to have a very high radiation threshold. Radiation has been used in other species as either a whole body treatment, or as a treatment for cutaneous lymphoma. Of the birds treated, the following treatments were used: Orthovoltage teletherapy 40 Gy treated for10 fractions of 4 Gy/fraction in an African grey parrot with malignant lymphoreticular neoplasia in the right periorbital region. Outcome: Feather loss where radiated; additionally, ocular changes of the right eye was noted as well as right-sided nasal discharge. The swelling decreased significantly initially but grew back to 50% of its original size within 2 months. Megavoltage teletherapy 32 Gy treated for 4 fractions of 8 Gy/fraction in a female Congo African grey parrot with bursal lymphoma. Outcome: No response to treatment. External beam radiation therapy 2.0 Gy total dose divided into 10 fractions of 20 cGy, each treatment every 2–3 days over 31 days in whole-body black swan T cell lymphocytic leukemia. Outcome: No adverse effects or clinical disease; remission never achieved, no change in coelomic size or number of masses, died 433 days post treatment.

### NURSING CARE
Care is dependent on the clinical signs the patient presents with. Typically, birds present as anorexic or depressed, and supportive care such as fluid therapy and nutritional support should be initiated. This can include IV or IO catherization and fluids. If the respiratory tract is compromised with metastases or the animal is overly depressed, oxygen therapy and heat support are warranted. If ascites is present, coelomocentesis can be performed to relieve pressure and to help the bird short term, but this is typically a poor prognostic indicator. Chemotherapy medications can decrease the overall WBC count, which can predispose to secondary bacterial infections or potentially secondary fungal infections. If this

occurs, treat with the appropriate medication based on C/S for bacterial infections and appropriate antifungal treatment based on the medication that is best for the avian patient.

### ACTIVITY
The activity of the patient at the time of diagnosis and treatment chosen will determine the activity level the bird should be allowed. If surgical removal was performed, activity should be restricted for 2 weeks or until the site is healed and sutures removed. If the bird is treated with chemotherapy, dependent on the chemotherapy, the bird should be limited to one area (cage) as there are human safety concerns over exposure to the drug, which is eliminated in the feces or urine. If radiation treatment has been used, the bird's activity should be limited at least on the day of treatment to allow for adequate recovery from anesthesia.

### DIET
Weight loss is a common sequelae of cancer and cancer treatments. Proper nutrition should be encouraged during this period. Feed may be needed to be supplemented with an oral feeding formula via gavage to maintain appropriate caloric input for the avian patient.

### CLIENT EDUCATION
It is important to discuss potential treatment options ranging from palliative care to chemotherapy and/or radiation. It is also important to discuss that although there are some reported survival times, these are not definitive, as research is still being undertaken to gain a better understanding of survival time. The treatment protocols in this chapter are individually published case treatments that may or may not work on different birds with different stages of diagnoses, additional research is currently in progress to evaluate these therapies. Additionally, owners should be aware of any potential risks such as secondary bacterial or fungal infection, anesthetic death during diagnostics or treatments, and continued progression of disease.

### SURGICAL CONSIDERATIONS
Surgical removal of a solitary mass tends to contribute to a positive outcome in other species; however, lymphoma tends to be multicentric, which makes surgical removal not possible.

## MEDICATIONS
### DRUG(S) OF CHOICE
Oral chemotherapy treatments are typically the easiest to administer, particularly chemotherapeutics that can cause necrosis if they are administered extravascularly. Various IV medications have been used, including

N

## NEOPLASIA (LYMPHOPROLIFERATIVE) (CONTINUED)

vincristine; IM cyclophosphamide; SQ L-asparaginase; and PO prednisone/ prednisolone, chlorambucin, and cyclophosphamide. Specific treatments and outcomes used in a variety of patients are listed below.

**Black swan with chronic T-cell lymphocytic leukemia:** Treated with 2 mg chlorambucil PO every 48 hours; no response after 2 months, discontinued. Treatment with L-asparaginase 400 iu/kg SQ and lomustine 60 mg/m² orally q3 w was then initiated. Prednisolone 0.5 mg/kg PO s.i.d. was started (itraconazole was also initiated); 2 months later there was no response to treatment. Palliative radiation was initiated at this time. The bird died 450 days post diagnosis.

**Juvenile blue-and-gold macaw with cutaneous pseudolymphoma:** Treated with chlorambucil (20 mg/m² PO q14 d for 3 treatments). Elevations in AST and ALT were noted during treatment. Nodules resolved but splenomegaly persisted 5 months post-treatment but was normal sized 2.5 years later. Chemistry abnormalities were also resolved 2.5 years later and the bird was apparently normal at that time.

**Cockatiel with chronic lymphocytic leukemia:** Chlorambucil 2 mg/kg orally q3.5 d dependent on owner compliance. Treatment stabilized but did not cause any regression of disease. The bird was euthanized 8 months after treatment started (15 months after initial diagnosis).

**Double yellow-headed Amazon parrot with T cell lymphocytic leukemia:** Treated with chlorambucil 2 mg/kg orally twice a week. Antibiotics were also administered. There was no response to treatment after 40 days and the bird was euthanized.

**Green-winged macaw with T cell lymphocytic leukemia:** Prednisone 1 mg/kg orally s.i.d., chlorambucin 1 mg/kg orally twice weekly (discontinued after 6 weeks due to thrombocytopenia); cyclophsophamide 5 mg/kg orally 4 days/week with daily prednisone for 32 weeks.

**Lineolated parakeet with chronic lymphocytic leukemia:** Prednisone 1 mg/kg orally once a day and a single treatment of cyclophosphamide 50 mg/kg IM), chlorambucil 1.5 mg/kg orally q3–4 d planned. Patient became anorexic and lethargic after cyclophosphamide injection and PCV and WBC decreased significantly 5 days after injection and owner elected euthanasia.

**Moluccan cockatoo with lymphoma and leukemic profile:** Treated with cyclophosphamide and L-asparaginase but developed toxic GI symptoms. The animal was then treated with vincristine sulfate (0.5–0.75 mg/m² q4 w), prednisone (0.45 mg/kg PO q12h) and chlorambucil

(1 mg PO twice weekly). The animal had resolution of the solid tumors and the leukemia was stable.

**Pekin duck with lymphocytic leukemia and malignant lymphoma:** Vincristine (0.1 mg/kg IV once weekly/biweekly) and chlorambucil (2 mg/kg PO twice weekly) for 17 weeks. Initially there was a response to treatment but then quality of life decreased at 17 weeks and was euthanized.

**Umbrella cockatoo with non-epitheliotropic cutaneous B cell lymphoma with leukemic profile:** Treated with vincristine 0.1 mg/kg IV q1–3 w, and chlorambicil 2 mg/kg PO twice weekly. Chlorambucil was received for 17 weeks and vincristine was given on weeks 1, 4, 5, 7, 8, 11, 12, and 14. At week 17, this bird became fluffed, depressed, anorexic, and was anemic, so chemotherapy was discontinued. Lymphocytosis was present still at this time. At 29 weeks, the bird was determined to be in complete remission, which lasted 8+ years.

### CONTRAINDICATIONS
N/A

### PRECAUTIONS
N/A

### POSSIBLE INTERACTIONS
N/A

### ALTERNATIVE DRUGS
There have been reports of potential adverse effects of prednisone/prednisolone in birds, causing immunosuppression, diabetes mellitus, hyperadrenocorticism, and hepatic damage; however, advantageous effects of treatment may exceed the risks, and multiple birds have been treated with long-term prednisone/prednisolone treatments and have not developed adverse effects from this medication. Other potential treatment options could include other NSAIDs, such as meloxicam for palliative care at 1 mg/kg s.i.d. or b.i.d. Herbal therapies and acupuncture may also help with pain relief and nausea.

### FOLLOW-UP

### PATIENT MONITORING
N/A

### PREVENTION/AVOIDANCE
N/A

### POSSIBLE COMPLICATIONS
Recurrence of lymphoma/leukemia is likely at some point. Adverse effects of chemotherapy or anesthetic medications can occur and can range from depression, anorexia, sloughing of tissue, respiratory depression, cardiac depression, and death. As there are no pharmacokinetic or pharmacodynamic

studies in all bird species, many medication doses for chemotherapy are based on canine or feline doses and frequency, which may not be adequate to treat a bird or may be toxic.

### EXPECTED COURSE AND PROGNOSIS
Prognosis is dependent on stage of lymphoma or leukemia at diagnosis. The average ESCRA reported survival time in months for avians with lymphoma is 34 months and the average avian leukemia survival time is 6.2 months. Additional cases are being diagnosed and treated earlier, which could extend survival times.

### MISCELLANEOUS

### ASSOCIATED CONDITIONS
Secondary bacterial infections are most commonly associated with treatment or severe lymphoid neoplastic infections. In some instances, treatment with antibiotics concurrently with chemotherapies may be warranted. Secondary fungal infections could occur, but are typically more common with wildlife patients, which could also be related more to the immunosuppressive effects of stress in addition to lymphoid neoplasia.

### AGE-RELATED FACTORS
Prevalence increases with age, but if disease occurs in younger animals it tends to be more aggressive.

### ZOONOTIC POTENTIAL
N/A

### FERTILITY/BREEDING
If the reproductive tract is affected by metastatic lymphoma, reproductive potential will likely be reduced or completely diminished.

### SYNONYMS
Lymphoma, malignant lymphoma, lymphosarcoma, lymphoproliferative neoplasia, leukemia, acute myeloid leukemia, chronic lymphocytic leukemia.

### SEE ALSO
Anemia
Ascites
Cere and Skin Color Changes
Coelomic Distention
Infertility
Liver Disease
Marek's Disease
Neurologic (Non-Traumatic Diseases)
Neurologic (Trauma)
Retroviruses in Galliformes
Sick-Bird Syndrome

### ABBREVIATIONS
AST—aspartate aminotransferase
C/S—culture and sensitivity

CNS—central nervous system
CT—computed tomography
ESCRA—Exotic Species Cancer Research Alliance
GGT—gamma-glutamyl transferase
GI—gastrointestinal
MDV—Marek's disease virus
MRI—magnetic resonance imaging
PCR—polymerase chain reaction
WBC—white blood cell

### INTERNET RESOURCES

Cornell University School of Veterinary Medicine. eClinpath: https://eclinpath.com
Exotic Species Cancer Research Alliance: https://escra.cvm.ncsu.edu
Merck Veterinary Manual: https://www.merckvetmanual.com/bird-owners/disorders-and-diseases-of-birds/cancers-and-tumors-of-pet-birds?query=avian%20cancers

*Suggested Reading*
Gibson, D.J., Nemeth, N.M., Beaufrère, H., et al. (2021). Lymphoma in psittacine birds: A histological and immunohistochemical assessment. *Veterinary Pathology*, 58:663–673.
Gosbell, M., Luk, K., Macwhirter, P. (2021). Chronic lymphocytic leukemia in a cockatiel (*Nymphicus hollandicus*). *Journal of Avian Medicine and Surgery*, 35:341–349.
Hammond, E.E., Sanchez-Migallon Guzman, D., Garner, M.M., et al. (2010). Long-term treatment of chronic lymphocytic leukemia in a green-winged macaw (*Ara chloroptera*). *Journal of Avian Medicine and Surgery*, 24:330–338.
Kollias, G.V., Homer, B., Thompson, J.P. (1992). Cutaneous pseudolymphoma in a juvenile blue and gold macaw (*Ara Ararauna*). *Journal of Zoo and Wildlife Medicine*, 23:235–40.
Osofsky, A., Hawkins, M.G., Foreman, O., et al. (2011). T-Cell chronic lymphocytic leukemia in a double yellow-headed Amazon parrot (*Amazona ochrocephala oratrix*). *Journal of Avian Medicine and Surgery*, 25:286–294.
Rivera, S., McClearen, J.R., Reavill, D.R. (2009). Treatment of nonepitheliotropic cutaneous B-cell lymphoma in an umbrella cockatoo (*Cacatua alba*). *Journal of Avian Medicine and Surgery*. 23:294–302.
Sinclair, K.M., Hawkins, M.G., Wright, L., et al. (2015). Chronic T-cell lymphocytic leukemia in a black swan (*Cygnus atratus*): Diagnosis, treatment, and pathology. *Journal of Avian Medicine and Surgery*, 29:326–335.

**Author:** Tara M. Harrison, DVM, MPVM, DCZM, DACVPM, DECZM (Zoo Health Management), CVA

N

# NEOPLASIA (NEUROLOGIC)

## BASICS

### DEFINITION
Primary tumors within the CNS are divided into those arising from neuroepithelial tissues, meninges, germ cell tumors, and the pituitary. Non-neuroepithelial neoplasms (craniopharyngioma) and cysts (epidermoid and dermoid cysts), as well as primary lymphomas of the CNS, are also recognized; however, these tumors are not covered in this chapter. Brain metastasis from other tumors are also seen in birds. The following are those neurologic tumors described in birds.

**Tumors of neuroepithelial tissue:** Gliomas—astrocytic tumors, derived from astrocytes. The high grade astrocytoma is a glioblastoma (glioblastoma multiforme); oligodendroglial tumor derived from oligodendrocytes; other gliomas—mixed such as oligoastrocytoma, which contains glial cells of different types; ependymal tumors arise from ependymal tissue; ependymoma. Choroid plexus tumors—choroid plexus papilloma; pineal tumor; pineocytoma (benign); pineoblastoma (malignant). Embryonal tumors—medulloblastoma; primitive neuroectodermal tumors, a small-cell tumor arising from a progenitor cell population capable of divergent differentiation along neuronal, ependymal, glial, and possibly mesenchymal cell lines; neuroblastoma, an embryonal neoplasm with limited neuronal differentiation.
**Tumors of the meninges:** Meningioma.
**Germ cell tumors:** Teratoma.
**Pituitary tumors:** Adenomas, adenocarcinomas.

### PATHOPHYSIOLOGY
Predisposing factors have not been described with most avian CNS tumors. However, FGV, which belongs to avian leukosis virus subgroup A, induces "fowl glioma" in domestic chickens (*Gallus gallus domesticus*). This disease is characterized by multiple nodular gliomatous growths of astrocytes.

### SYSTEMS AFFECTED
All tumors of the CNS, benign and malignant, can result in significant neurologic dysfunction simply as a mass effect within the skull. Some may also be functional tumors (pituitary and pineal tumors). CNS—changes in appetite, seizures, ataxia, paresis. Endocrine—polydipsia and polyuria. Ophthalmic—blindness, exophthalmia. Reproductive—ovarian inactivity (functional pineal gland tumor). Respiratory—invasive growth into respiratory sinus. Skin —feather color changes, altered molt.

### GENETICS
No significant genetic predisposition has been identified. Some tumors are congenital such as teratomas.

### INCIDENCE/PREVALENCE
Tumors of the CNS are rare, based on avian submissions to one pathology service retrospective study at < 1% (6/557) of all tumors diagnosed (all avian species including domestic fowl). In an Australian survey of neoplasms in avian species excluding domestic fowl, 0.7% (3/383) were primary CNS tumors. A review of pet bird tumors, both from the literature as well as submissions to a teaching hospital, found CNS tumors at 0.9% (15/1539), 10 of which were pituitary tumors.

### GEOGRAPHIC DISTRIBUTION
N/A

### SIGNALMENT
No specific age or sex predilection with one exception. Pituitary tumors are more common in young to middle-aged budgerigars.

### SIGNS
**Gliomas:** Astrocytoma—transitory torticollis, retropulsion (walking backwards), and ataxia. Glioblastoma—progressive weakness, weight loss, exophthalmos, ataxia, seizures, and a resting tremor. Oligodendroglioma—not reported. Oligoastrocytoma—unexpected death. Ependymoma—head tilt, ataxia.
**Choroid plexus tumors:** Choroid plexus papilloma—not reported.
**Pineal tumor:** Pineocytoma—ovarian inactivity. Pineoblastoma—intermittent diarrhea, weight loss, polydipsia, head tilt, weakness.
**Embryonal tumors:** Medulloblastoma—ataxia, intention tremors. Primitive neuroectodermal tumors. Neuroblastoma—mass in the left orbit of the eye.
**Tumors of the meninges:** Meningioma—not reported.
**Germ cell tumors:** Teratoma—head tilt, circling, and facial nerve paralysis.
**Pituitary tumors:** Exophthalmia, ocular chemosis, blindness, localized pruritus, abnormal feather molt, polyuria, polydipsia, weight loss, ataxia, and depression.

### CAUSES
Underlying causes or genetic alterations are unknown for most avian CNS tumors. FGV induces "fowl glioma" in domestic chickens.

### RISK FACTORS
Risk factors are unknown.

## DIAGNOSIS

### DIFFERENTIAL DIAGNOSIS
Any disease process that involves the CNS.

#### Infectious
**Virus:** Bornavirus—cachexia, ingluvial stasis, gastric and intestinal dilatation, regurgitation, ataxia, ataxia, paresis, proprioceptive deficits, head tremors, and death. Eastern equine encephalitis—high mortality, depression, anorexia, hemorrhagic gastroenteritis regurgitating food, sternal recumbency. Western equine encephalitis—anorexia, weight loss, weakness, depression, drowsiness, stupor, ataxia, and incoordination. Avian orthoavulavirus 1 (paramyxovirus 1)—polydipsia, ataxia, poor balance, torticollis, head tremors, inability to fly, and diarrhea. West Nile virus—ataxia, tremors, weakness, seizures, and abnormal head postures and movement prior to death.
**Bacteria:** *Listeria monocytogenes*, *Enterococcus* species, and *Salmonella* species.
**Fungus:** *Aspergillus* species, *Dactylaria gallopava*.
**Protozoa:** *Tetratrichomona gallinarum*—ataxia, blindness, intermittent seizures. Sarcocystosis—severe weakness, dyspnea, fresh blood in oral cavity, head twitching and torticollis. Atoxoplasmosis (systemic isosporosis)—respiratory distress, emaciation, dyspnea, tail-bobbing, and hypothermia. Amebic meningoencephalitis—anorexia, dyspnea, depression, head shaking, nasal discharge. *Toxoplasma gondii*—anorexia, prostration, weight loss, diarrhea, and dyspnea.
**Metazoa:** Schistosomiasis encephalitis—circling, flapping wings, head tilt. *Baylisascaris procyonis*—seizures, torticollis, opisthotonus, head-tilt, circling, ataxia, paralysis, and visual deficits.

#### Non-infectious
**Nutritional:** Encephalomalacia (hypovitaminosis E)—tremor, incoordination, and recumbency.
**Toxin:** Lead toxicity—dehydration, depression, polyuria, passive regurgitation, neurologic deficits (flipping backwards), ataxia, paralysis of wings or legs, seizures, head tilt, lime-green feces. Sodium toxicity—lethargic, stiff and posteriorly extended legs, dyspnea, anorexia.
**Miscellaneous:** Lafora bodies in a cockatiel. Cerebellar degeneration and/or hypoplasia. Ischemic stroke.

### CBC/BIOCHEMISTRY/URINALYSIS
These tests would be used to identify other disease conditions and/or to monitor the effects of attempted therapy (chemotherapy or radiation).

### OTHER LABORATORY TESTS
Bacterial and/or fungal cultures from the respiratory or digestive tracts to monitor for secondary disease conditions.

## IMAGING
Although antemortem confirmed diagnosis of a CNS tumor is not reported, both CT and MRI, with or without contrast are potential diagnostic imaging techniques. Contrast-enhancing masses can be seen using CT and MRI as shown in multiple case reports. Resolution may be limited, however, considering the small size of most birds. Standard radiographic study of the skull may provide identification of any associated skeletal abnormalities.

## DIAGNOSTIC PROCEDURES
Neurologic examination should localize the lesions: brain, spinal cord, or neuromuscular system.

## PATHOLOGIC FINDINGS
### Gliomas
**Astrocytoma**: Astrocytomas are usually fairly uniform with hyperchromatic nuclei and abundant cytoplasm. Cell process can be seen with silver stains. Few mitotic figures are present.
**Glioblastoma**: It is cellular and has a pleomorphic histologic appearance. Some cells resemble differentiated astrocytes and others are elongated and fusiform with numerous mitotic figures. Multiple giant cells or multinucleated cells may be present. Glioblastoma typically occur in the cerebrum and occasionally the cerebellum.
**Oligodendroglioma**: The characteristic features of oligodendrogliomas include sheets of uniform cells with the "honeycomb" cell pattern which is described as a feature of delayed fixation of the tumor tissues. Microvascular proliferation is another characteristic feature of this tumor. Multifocal microcystic areas and accumulation of mucinous-like material are also frequent findings in oligodendrogliomas. Mitoses are infrequent. Immunohistochemistry is frequently used to further characterize these tumors. In poultry, this is more common in adult birds and originates in the periventricular areas of the third ventricle.
**Oligoastrocytoma**: Oligoastrocytomas are mixed gliomas with neoplastic oligodendrocytes and astrocytes that are either intermingled or separated into distinct clusters.
**Ependymoma**: A mass arising from the lateral ventricle in a domestic fowl, having some characteristics of an ependymoma. The growth was expansive, non-invasive and subdivided into major and minor lobules composed of neuroglial cells.

### Choroid plexus tumors
**Choroid plexus papilloma**: These tumors present as well-defined papillary structures within ventricles. They are gray-white to red. Histologically, the tumors have a vascular connective tissue stroma covered by epithelial cells that are cuboidal or columnar and resemble normal choroid plexus.

### Pineal tumor
**Pineocytoma**: Pineocytoma is a circumscribed encapsulated cellular mass generally embedded between folia of the rostral cerebellar vermis. These benign tumors present as lobulated nodular growths of the gland. The lobules are composed of columnar epithelium and surrounding parafollicular cells. Pineocytomas are rarely seen and best described in poultry.
**Pineoblastoma**: A friable suprathalamic grey mass located on midline that compresses adjacent structures. Composed of sheets and cords of cells having a round to oval nuclei and small to moderate amounts of vacuolated basophilic cytoplasm. Occasional rosettes.

### Embryonal tumors
**Medulloblastoma**: Medulloblastoma is considered an embryonic neoplasm that grossly is well defined and histologically is composed of anaplastic cells that may form rosettes.

### Primitive neuroectodermal tumors
**Neuroblastoma**: Grayish-white soft nodular mass found in the rostral part of the left cerebrum.

### Tumors of the meninges
**Meningioma**: These tumors are usually solitary within the meninges and are of variable shape. They are firm and gray-white to yellow. Microscopically, tumor cells usually have abundant cytoplasm and are fusiform. Whorls and bundles of neoplastic cells are the most common pattern.

### Germ cell tumors
**Teratoma**: A teratoma may be defined as a tumor composed of multiple cell types and tissues arising from the germ cells of two (diadermic) or three (tridermic) embryonic layers (ectoderm, endoderm and mesoderm). Extragonadal sites of development include the pineal gland, cerebellum, and spinal cord.

### Pituitary tumors
These tumors are usually red-brown and may extend outside of the sella tursica if large. Histologically, adenomas comprise large epithelial cells that are usually devoid of granules. These cells form nests and lobules with minimal stroma. Cells making up carcinomas are more anaplastic and there may be mitotic figures seen. Tumor lobules and cords are infiltrative into surrounding tissue. For many of the tumors in budgerigars, immunohistochemistry is commonly positive for growth hormone, consistent with somatotroph tumors. Distant metastasis (liver, midbrain and air sacs) have been recorded for the budgerigar somatotroph pituitary tumors.

 TREATMENT

### APPROPRIATE HEALTH CARE
General supportive care measures warranted based on degree of signs.

### NURSING CARE
Fluid therapy, nutritional support, seizure management.

### ACTIVITY
Cage rest in the case of severe neurologic impairment.

### DIET
Supportive feeding may be needed if bird is not eating enough to maintain weight.

### CLIENT EDUCATION
Humane euthanasia may be indicated if quality of life is severely impaired. Adapting cage environment may be helpful (low perches, incubator set up, food and water bowls in easy reach).

### SURGICAL CONSIDERATIONS
Surgical treatment has not been reported.

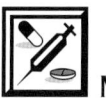 MEDICATIONS

### DRUG(S) OF CHOICE
N/A

### CONTRAINDICATIONS
N/A

### PRECAUTIONS
N/A

### POSSIBLE INTERACTIONS
N/A

### ALTERNATIVE DRUGS

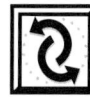 FOLLOW-UP

### PATIENT MONITORING
N/A

### PREVENTION/AVOIDANCE
N/A

### POSSIBLE COMPLICATIONS
N/A

### EXPECTED COURSE AND PROGNOSIS
All the CNS tumors warrant a guarded to terminal prognosis. Distant metastasis (liver, midbrain and air sacs) have been recorded for the budgerigar somatotroph pituitary tumors.

N

## NEOPLASIA (NEUROLOGIC)

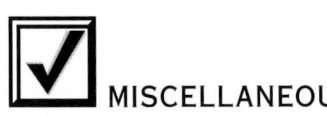

## MISCELLANEOUS

**ASSOCIATED CONDITIONS**
N/A

**AGE-RELATED FACTORS**
Pituitary tumors are more common in young to middle-aged budgerigars.

**ZOONOTIC POTENTIAL**
None.

**FERTILITY/BREEDING**
N/A

**SYNONYMS**
N/A

**SEE ALSO**
Bornaviral Disease (Psittaciformes)
Diarrhea
Emaciation
Neoplasia (Lymphoproliferative)
Neurologic (Non-Traumatic Diseases)

Neurologic (Trauma)
Ocular Lesions
Polydipsia
Polyuria
Sarcocystosis
Seizures
Sick-Bird Syndrome
Toxicosis (Environmental/Pesticides)
Toxicosis (Heavy Metals)
Toxicosis (Iatrogenic)
West Nile Virus

**ABBREVIATIONS**
CNS—central nervous system
CT—computed tomography
FGV—fowl glioma-inducing virus
MRI—magnetic resonance imaging

**INTERNET RESOURCES**
N/A

*Suggested Reading*
Langohr, I.M., Garner, M.M., Kiupel, M. (2012). Somatotroph pituitary tumors in budgerigars (*Melopsittocus undulatus*). *Veterinary Pathology* 49:503–507.
Leach, M.W. (1992). A survey of neoplasia in pet birds. *Seminars in Avian and Exotic Pet Medicine* 1:52–64.
Schmidt, R.E., Reavill, D.R., Phalen, D. (2015). *Pathology of Pet and Aviary Birds*. 2nd edn. Hoboken, NJ: Wiley Blackwell.
Suchy, A., Weissenböck, H., Schmidt, P. (1999). Intracranial tumours in budgerigars. *Avian Pathology*, 28:125–130.
Zehnder, A., Graham, J., Reavill, D., McLaughlin, A. (2016). Neoplastic diseases in avian species. In: *Current Therapy in Avian Medicine and Surgery* (ed. B. Speer B), 107–141. St. Louis, MO: Elsevier.

**Authors:** Drury R. Reavill, DVM, DABVP (Avian/Reptile & Amphibian), DACVP (deceased), Hugues Beaufrère, DVM, PhD, DACZM, DABVP (Avian), DECZM (Avian)

N

## BASICS

### DEFINITION
Renal neoplasia refers to a tumor of the tissues related to the kidneys.

### PATHOPHYSIOLOGY
Renal neoplasia has been reported in many avian species, but has most commonly been documented in the budgerigar. The most commonly reported tumor type in non-domestic free-ranging and captive birds is renal carcinoma, although adenoma, nephroblastoma, cystadenoma, fibrosarcoma, lymphosarcoma, and other neoplastic diseases have also been reported. Myeloproliferative disease, histiocytosis, and malignant melanoma have also been reported to affect the avian kidney. In chickens, infectious type C retrovirus, including avian leukosis virus (ALV) and sarcoma virus (SV), have been commonly documented to cause carcinomas of the urogenital tract. Similar associations in psittacines such as budgerigars, have not been documented.

### SYSTEMS AFFECTED
Renal; secondary systems can be affected if metastasis occurs.

### GENETICS
N/A

### INCIDENCE/PREVALENCE
Unknown, but most commonly reported in budgerigars.

### GEOGRAPHIC DISTRIBUTION
N/A

### SIGNALMENT
Certain tumor types are seen in certain species more commonly: Budgerigars—renal carcinoma and adenocarcinoma; chickens, small passerines—embryonal nephroma (nephroblastoma). More commonly reported in male than female birds and more commonly in psittacines than passerines. In one study investigating 74 budgerigars, 47/74 birds (63.5%) had renal tumors and were diagnosed most commonly within 5 years of age.

### SIGNS

#### Historical Findings
The most common presenting complaint is a unilateral or bilateral lameness or paresis/paralysis that results from compression of the lumbar and sacral nerve plexi, passing through (lumbar), or dorsal to (sacral) the kidney. These clinical signs may also result from the expansion of the tumor into the synsacrum.

#### Physical Examination Findings
Unilateral or bilateral lameness or paresis. Skeletal muscle atrophy and osteopenia of the affected side. Coelomic distension/enlargement.

Diarrhea. Dyspnea. Weight loss. Clinical findings of systemic disease may be noted in cases of lymphoma or metastasis of the primary tumor.

### CAUSES
N/A

### RISK FACTORS
N/A

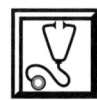

## DIAGNOSIS

### DIFFERENTIAL DIAGNOSIS
Trauma (in cases of lameness), granulomatous disease, abscess, infectious disease (bacterial, parasitic (renal *Coccidia*, sarcocystis, *Microsporidia*, *Cryptosporidia*, flukes), viral, fungal), nutritional (hypercalcinosis, hypovitaminosis A), gout.

### CBC/BIOCHEMISTRY/URINALYSIS
Bloodwork should be performed to evaluate the overall health of the patient, and to determine whether there are any abnormal blood counts that could be related to the neoplastic process. Cytopenias, anemia, and leukocytosis may all be reported with varying types of neoplasia. Biochemistry profiles may demonstrate organ involvement associated with the tumor, or organ dysfunction related to the age of the patient or the presence of other disease processes. Hypercalcemia of malignancy has been previously documented in avian patients. Unlike in mammals, BUN only occurs in small amounts in avian plasma and is also secreted solely by glomerular filtration, making it a poor indicator of renal function; however, it has been documented that BUN can provide a reasonable assessment of a bird's hydration status and the presence (or absence) prerenal dehydration. Uric acid is the major breakdown product of protein in avian species. Uric acid is produced and secreted in the liver, kidney, and pancreas, and is subsequently eliminated by tubular secretion, independent of glomerular filtration, water resorption, and urine flow rate. The uric acid is not thought to be significantly affected by the hydration status of the patient, and therefore, should provide a reasonable understanding of the renal status of the avian patient; however, commonly, hyperuricemia is not detected until late in the disease process. Some studies have indicated that bilateral renal involvement is more likely to result in an elevation in uric acid. Urinalysis is not commonly performed in avian species because of the anatomical and physiological adaptions that occur. Urine is expelled into the cloaca and is often mixed with feces at the time of excretion from the body. Additionally, urine can reflux into the lower GI tract,

where water and electrolyte reabsorption may occur.

### OTHER LABORATORY TESTS
Fine-needle aspiration and cytology of the lesion (with or without ultrasound guidance). Biopsy and histopathology of the lesion (punch biopsy, core needle [Tru Cut™, Merit Medical Systems, South Jordan, UT], laparoscopy).

### IMAGING
Radiographs, ultrasound and CT can all have utility in the assessment of avian neoplasia. They help to demonstrate the extent of the lesion, invasiveness of the disease, and also to stage the animal (evaluate for metastasis). Many malignant tumors will spread to other organs, with the most common location of metastasis being the lungs, but other locations such as coelomic organs and bone may be involved, depending on the tumor type. Although radiographs provide some utility in assessment, contrast-enhanced CT provides a much better overall picture of the coelomic organs, as well as a more global evaluation of the primary lesion and potential for metastatic lesions.

#### Radiographic Findings
The lateral radiograph provides the greatest utility in assessing the size and shape of the avian kidney. When the kidney is enlarged, there will be evidence of loss of the dorsal diverticulum of the abdominal air sac dorsal to the kidney. Additionally, when kidneys are of normal size and shape, the ventral border should not extend past a horizontal line drawn parallel to the spine passing through the ventral border of the acetabulum. Addition of GI contrast can also provide additional information about the origin of a coelomic mass.

#### Ultrasonography
Ultrasound of the avian urogenital tract is challenging but may aid in differentiating renal neoplasia from oviductal disease or a liver mass; however, this is often done in the hands of a skilled ultrasonographer. The size of the avian patient may also limit the utility of this imaging modality. Typically, renal neoplasia results in compression of the abdominal air sacs and intestinal displacement, and therefore, the renal mass can often be identified as a round, non-homogeneous structure.

### DIAGNOSTIC PROCEDURES
Following acquisition of a biopsy, immunohistochemical testing may be required to obtain a definitive diagnosis when cell morphology alone does not provide enough information; however, the canine and feline antibodies that are used may not cross-react with avian tissues and so must be a consideration when additional testing is

**N**

undertaken. In addition to these challenges, there are also no established positive controls in avian patients, which creates difficulties when interpreting the results.

### PATHOLOGIC FINDINGS
Pathology findings will depend on the type of tumor that is present in the avian patient.

## TREATMENT

### APPROPRIATE HEALTH CARE
Treatment of the tumor will depend on the type of tumor, invasiveness, and presence or absence of metastasis.

### NURSING CARE
Avian patients that are diagnosed with respiratory neoplasia should be provided supportive care to ensure that they maintain a good quality of life that is pain and as stress free as possible. Depending on the needs of the patient, anti-inflammatories, opioids, or fluid support may be indicated to maintain the comfort of the avian patient. Fluid therapy may aid avian patients with an elevated uric acid.

### ACTIVITY
Avian patients that have been diagnosed with respiratory neoplasia should be allowed to choose their own level of activity. Additionally, if lameness or paresis is noted, modifications to the home environment may be necessary to ensure that the bird is able to access food, water, and the basic necessities.

### DIET
No specific dietary recommendations.

### CLIENT EDUCATION
Avian owners are more aware of treatment options for renal neoplasia in domestic animal species and humans. As a result, there is an increasing demand for advanced diagnostic and therapeutic options for companion avian species. In any sick avian patient, it is always important to discuss the risks of handling, diagnostics, and treatment, including death. Prognosis and consideration for euthanasia may also be necessary discussions with the owner. At this time, there is no established standard of care for avian neoplasia and most of the dosages are extrapolated with an unknown array of adverse effects.

### SURGICAL CONSIDERATIONS
Surgical excision with adequate margins is an ideal treatment option for many neoplastic processes. This should only be undertaken

after a patient has a definitive diagnosis, has been fully staged, and evidence of metastasis has been ruled out. Additionally, the risks of surgery and anesthesia in the avian patient must be fully disclosed to the owner, with a risk versus benefit approach investigated prior to surgery. In cases where inadequate margins are obtained after surgery, additional treatment options should be explored depending on the tumor type, including additional surgery, radiation therapy, systemic or local chemotherapy. In the case of renal neoplasia, surgery would be extraordinarily challenging and likely associated with high rates of mortality. The access to the respective renal arteries is typically restricted by the tumor making ligation and hemostasis virtually impossible.

## MEDICATIONS

### DRUG(S) OF CHOICE
Chemotherapy may be a therapeutic option, targeted towards the tumor type. A renal adenocarcinoma in a male budgerigar temporarily responded to carboplatin. Supportive care including analgesics (opioids, NSAIDs), antibiotics, or antifungals may also be considered.

### CONTRAINDICATIONS
N/A

### PRECAUTIONS
Chemotherapy doses are typically extrapolated from what is known in canine and feline patients, and these may not be the correct dose for avian species. Although in dogs and cats, body surface area is used to calculate chemotherapy dosages, it is unknown whether this is appropriate for avian patients. Adverse effects of certain chemotherapeutics have been reported in avian species.

### POSSIBLE INTERACTIONS
N/A

### ALTERNATIVE DRUGS
N/A

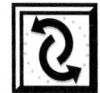

## FOLLOW-UP

### PATIENT MONITORING
The most important factor to monitor in patients with neoplasia is quality of life. Each patient should be routinely evaluated for

changes in respiration, appetite, and ability to perform normal behaviors.

### PREVENTION/AVOIDANCE
N/A

### POSSIBLE COMPLICATIONS
N/A

### EXPECTED COURSE AND PROGNOSIS
In general, the prognosis for avian renal neoplasia is poor. In reported cases of renal neoplasia, most birds lived < 3 months after initial diagnosis.

## MISCELLANEOUS

### ASSOCIATED CONDITIONS
N/A

### AGE-RELATED FACTORS
N/A

### ZOONOTIC POTENTIAL
N/A

### FERTILITY/BREEDING
N/A

### SYNONYMS
N/A

### SEE ALSO
N/A

### ABBREVIATIONS
BUN—blood urea nitrogen
CT—computed tomography
GI—gastrointestinal
NSAIDs—non-steroidal anti-inflammatory drugs

### INTERNET RESOURCES
N/A

*Suggested Reading*
Neumann, U., Kummerfeld, N. (1983). Neoplasms in budgerigars (*Melopsittacus undulatus*): clinical, pathomorphological and serological findings wiht special consideration of kidney tumours. *Avian Pathology*, 12:353–362.
Schmidt, R., Reavill, D., Phalen, D. (2003). *Pathology of Pet and Aviary Birds* (ed. R. Schmidt, D. Reavill, D. Phalen). Ames, IA: Iowa State Press.
Simova-Curd, S., Nltzl, D., Mayer, J., Hatt, J.M. (2006). Clinical approach to renal neoplasia in budgerigars (*Melopsittacus undulatus*). *Journal of Small Animal Practice*, 47:504–511.
**Author:** Sara Gardhouse, DVM, DABVP (Exotic Companion Mammal), DACZM

N

# NEOPLASIA (REPRODUCTIVE)

## BASICS

### DEFINITION
Reproductive neoplasia are abnormal new growths of tissue, which develop faster than adjacent normal tissues of the reproductive tract and in an uncoordinated, persistent manner.

### PATHOPHYSIOLOGY
Neoplasia development is a multistep process involving an accumulation of changes and/or errors in cellular DNA. It occurs with disruption of the genes that control cell growth and differentiation.

### SYSTEMS AFFECTED
Reproductive:
**Ovary**: Adenocarcinoma*/adenoma, carcinomatosis*, granulosa cell tumor*, carcinoma, cystadenocarcinoma, ovarian hemangiosarcoma—metastasis to the pericardium and epicardium, leiomyosarcomas/leiomyoma, teratoma, dysgerminoma, fibrosarcoma, lipoma, lymphomatosis, arrhenoma, ovarian Sertoli cell tumor, myxoma—poultry.
Oviduct: Adenocarcinoma*/adenoma—adenocarcinomas may originate in the ovary or in the upper portion of the magnum of the oviduct, less frequently in the infundibulum or uterus (shell gland). Adenocarcinomas of the magnum are extremely malignant, with metastasis to the lungs and other viscera via hematogenous emboli. A distinction between an oviduct and ovarian origin cannot be made in advanced cases most of the time. Leiomyoma* of the mesosalpinx—usually located centrally in the ventral ligament of the oviduct; common tumor in chickens. Carcinoma. Carcinomatosis.
**Testis**: Seminoma*—most diagnosed testicular tumor in birds. Usually benign; reports of malignant tumors with metastasis to the kidney, spleen, liver, pancreas, lung, heart, peritoneum. Usually unilateral. Occurs in Galliformes, Anseriformes, Psittaciformes, Passeriformes, Bucerotiformes. Sertoli cell tumor*. Interstitial cell tumor*. Lymphosarcoma. Teratoma/teratocarcinoma. Leydig cell tumor. Tubular adenoma. Carcinomatoid embryoma. Anaplastic tumor. Sarcoma. Spindle cell sarcoma.
**Epididymis and ductus deferens**:
Leiomyosarcoma. Carcinoma.
(* Most common reproductive neoplasms in avian species.)

### GENETICS
Like humans, chickens with ovarian adenocarcinoma expressed increased p53 mutations on their genes, which correlated with the number of lifetime ovulations; increased expression of HER-2/neu, which was associated with more advanced disease; upregulation of COX-1 compared with COX-2.

### INCIDENCE/PREVALENCE
Ovarian neoplasia occurs more commonly than oviductal tumors in avian species. Reproductive neoplasia represents up to 22% of all neoplasm in ornamental and pet birds and is the second most frequent location of neoplasms after the tegument. Prevalence of Sertoli cell tumors may be as high as 1.7% in male budgerigar; 45% of white leghorn hens from 2- to 7-years of age developed reproductive neoplasia over a 3-year period, of which 32% were ovarian tumors, 8% oviductal tumors, and 5% leiomyomas of the suspending ligament of the oviduct. Adenocarcinomas and carcinomatosis represent 75–80% of all the reproductive neoplasia in poultry hens. Reported incidence of reproductive neoplasia in cranes was 9.1%, with 100% metastasis.

### GEOGRAPHIC DISTRIBUTION
Worldwide.

### SIGNALMENT
**Species**: Budgerigars, cockatiels, and poultry are more prone to ovarian/oviductal adenocarcinoma. Female and male budgerigars are more prone to granulosa cell tumors and testicular neoplasia, respectively.
**Breed predilections**: None.
**Mean age and range**: The prevalence of spontaneous reproductive neoplasia increases with age: 4–20% of ovarian neoplasia in 2.5- to 3.5-year-old hen compared with 40% in 6-year-old poultry hens. Ovarian adenocarcinoma is uncommon in hens < 2 years of age.
**Predominant sex**: None.

### SIGNS
#### General Comments
Male and female birds can present with similar clinical signs.

#### Historical Findings
Fluffed feathers, lethargy, abnormal feces (odor, size).

#### Physical Examination Findings
Coelomic distension. Dyspnea. Ascites. Lethargy. Unilateral lameness; left-sided in female psittacines and poultry if compression of the lumbar or sacral nerve plexus; right- or left-sided in males. Cyanosis of the pelvic limbs if compression of the ischiatic nerve and blood vessels. Chronic weight loss. Inappetence. Poor or altered reproductive performance, cessation of egg laying in females. Change of cere color in male and female with sexual dimorphism. Behavioral changes: Reproductive behaviors in females.

Increased aggressiveness or feminization from Sertoli cell tumors.

### CAUSES
Spontaneous neoplasia of the reproductive tract can occur in all avian species. Lymphoid leukosis (retrovirus) and Marek's diseases virus (herpesvirus) can induce neoplasia of the reproductive tract in poultry.

### RISK FACTORS
Spontaneous neoplasia of the reproductive tract can occur in all avian species. Lymphoid leukosis (retrovirus) and Marek's diseases virus (herpesvirus) can induce neoplasia of the reproductive tract in poultry.

## DIAGNOSIS

### DIFFERENTIAL DIAGNOSIS
Coelomitis, egg-yolk coelomitis, cystic right oviduct (poultry), infectious bronchitis virus (poultry), oviductal impaction, oviductal rupture, renal neoplasia, cardiac diseases, and atherosclerosis.

### CBC/BIOCHEMISTRY/URINALYSIS
Standard hematological and biochemical evaluation are seldom helpful with avian neoplasia of the reproductive tract. Anemia may occur with birds with reproductive neoplasia secondary to bleeding from the tumor or metastasis to the bone marrow.

### OTHER LABORATORY TESTS
Measurement of sexual hormone levels (LH, FSH) is not available in clinical settings.

### IMAGING
#### Coelomic Radiographic Findings
Radiographs may confirm a mass effect in the dorsocaudal coelomic cavity in the projection area of the reproductive tract. The ventriculus is usually displaced caudoventrally with ovarian or testicular tumors. Diagnosis of neoplasia may be difficult to obtain, as it may be difficult to distinguish normal enlargement of the reproductive tract from neoplasia. Polyostotic hyperostosis may be present as a paraneoplastic syndrome with functional ovarian and oviductal neoplasms or testicular Sertoli cell tumors.

#### Coelemic Ultrasonography
Ultrasonography can be more sensitive than radiographs by providing more accurate information regarding the appearance of the reproductive tract. Because of the gonad location, air sac presence, and the small size of most birds, this imaging technique often requires an experienced examiner to obtain diagnostic quality images. Most of time, fine-needle aspiration of the reproductive tract for cytology cannot be safely done with avian patients.

N

# NEOPLASIA (REPRODUCTIVE)  (CONTINUED)

### Advanced Imaging
CT and MRI are the most sensitive tools to evaluate the reproductive tract in avian species.

### DIAGNOSTIC PROCEDURES
Coelioscopy is often required and is the diagnostic procedure of choice to visualize the reproductive tract, as well as providing definitive diagnosis through biopsy and histopathology of suspected lesions.

### PATHOLOGIC FINDINGS
Ovarian ADs present as small, round, white, and firm nodules on the ovarian surface that can progress into a cauliflower-like mass, whereas oviductal adenocarcinomas are individual or clustered, sessile, gray, and firm masses. In case of metastasis, numerous masses on serosal surfaces of the pancreas, oviduct, mesentery, and/or intestines are commonly observed. Granulosa cell tumors usually are yellow, round, and lobulated mass with an extremely friable consistency, which may become very large. Leiomyomas are usually small, white, nodules with a characteristic white, glistering appearance on the cut surface. Many testicular tumors are cystic.

## TREATMENT

### APPROPRIATE HEALTH CARE
Treatment for most neoplastic diseases of the avian reproductive tract is typically unrewarding, as it is common for birds to present when the tumor is large or when other secondary clinical conditions, including metastasis, are present. Intensive care treatment is recommended with birds presenting with marked coelomic distension, ascites, dyspnea, or poor general condition. As neoplasia of the reproductive may have a slow and chronic progression, some avian patients may receive a medical management as an in/outpatient, depending on their clinical signs and their owner's abilities to detect small changes in their bird. If a surgical plan is elected, patients should always be first stabilized (see Surgical Considerations section).

### NURSING CARE
Birds with dyspnea may benefit from oxygen therapy. Therapeutic coelomocenthesis is recommended in birds with ascites to improve breathing pattern or comfort, as well as punction of accessible cystic lesions. Appropriate analgesia should be provided if the condition is causing pain or discomfort.

### ACTIVITY
Activity should be restricted in case of severely ill patients. In case of limb lameness, perches should be covered with an elasticated bandage and lowered in the cage to help the bird moving around.

### DIET
Nutritional support should be provided to birds with anorexia or dysorexia.

### CLIENT EDUCATION
Risks related to biopsy of the gonads to reach a final diagnosis and expected prognosis should be discussed with the owners. Owner's behavior mimicking avian sexual behaviors should be discontinued.

### SURGICAL CONSIDERATIONS
**Female reproductive tract**:
Salpingohysterectomy can be performed in case of oviductal neoplasia, if the patient is stable. Partial or complete ovariectomy is a high-risk procedure reserved to experienced surgeons. Multiple small veins often connect the ovary directly into the common iliac vein. Venous bleeding from a lacerated common iliac vein often is the cause of life-threatening hemorrhage during ovariectomy. Attempt to medically or behaviorally downregulate the bird's reproductive activity to reduce ovary vascularity should be attempted prior to surgery.

**Male reproductive tract**: In case of early diagnosis, orchidectomy can be performed by an experienced surgeon with a good prognosis without metastasis. Several methods have been described: simple extraction (caponization), laser ablation, intracapsular suction, en-bloc surgical excision, and minimally invasive endoscopic orchiectomy. Presurgical administration of megestrol acetate (1–3 mg/kg, PO, q24 h) have been described for 7–10 days prior to surgery to reduce testicular size and limit blood supply. In the case of cystic testicular tumors, aspiration of the cyst during surgery may reduce the mass size and facilitate its removal.

## MEDICATIONS

### DRUG(S) OF CHOICE
The use of synthetic GnRH including leuprolide acetate injection or substained-release deslorelin acetate implants have been described with variable response in birds with neoplasia of the reproductive tract: Ovarian adenocarcinomas in two cockatiels were managed with periodic coelomocentesis and GnRH agonist administration for 9 and 25 months, respectively. A positive response to GnRH agonist therapy was documented in only one of the two birds. Doses as high as 1500–3500 mg/kg of leuprolide acetate were used. Deslorelin acetate implants were found to be superior to leuprolide acetate injections both for consistent control of secondary effects from ovarian carcinoma and tumor growth in 1 cockatiel. Female birds with ovarian adenocarcinoma that responded to GnRH agonists usually required ever-increasing doses, with deslorelin giving about 4–5 months of relief and leuprolide about 2 weeks; 7/8 budgerigars with suspected Sertoli cell tumors showed marked improvement of their general condition and return to normal cere color following single or repeated 4.7 mg deslorelin acetate implant administration. Mean time to recurrence of symptoms was approximately 20 weeks. Carboplatin chemotherapy has been described to treat nonresectable testicular tumors, but no conclusive data regarding its efficacy are available to date. One cockatiel with incomplete removal of a seminoma was treated with orthovoltage radiation, which resulted in complete resolution with an 18-month follow-up.

### CONTRAINDICATIONS
N/A

### PRECAUTIONS
Only one report exists of suspected anaphylactic reaction and death in two elf owls following administration of leuprolide acetate. Exacerbation of the clinic signs may be observed during the first week following deslorelin acetate implant placement or first 48–72 hours following leuprolide acetate injection in birds.

### POSSIBLE INTERACTIONS
N/A

### ALTERNATIVE DRUGS
N/A

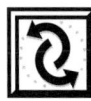

## FOLLOW-UP

### PATIENT MONITORING
Follow-up imaging is usually recommended at first every 2–4 weeks to monitor the reproductive tract size and appearance and then every 4 months with deslorelin acetate implant. Serum triglyceride levels has been used an indicator of ovarian or testicular Sertoli cell tumor activity to monitor treatment effect. Subjective evaluation of serum lipemia has been described to monitor the response of this ovarian carcinoma in cockatiel.

### PREVENTION/AVOIDANCE
Purchasing poultry vaccinated for Marek's disease and coming from lymphoid leukosis-free breeders should be recommended.

### POSSIBLE COMPLICATIONS
Sudden death or sudden worsening of the general conditions may be observed.

## EXPECTED COURSE AND PROGNOSIS

Prognosis for long-term recovery is grave with very few reports of successful treatment. Prognosis of ovarian adenocarcinoma is worse if ascites is present, as ascites and loss of body condition usually develop with extensive tumor growth or metastasis. One cockatiel with ovarian adenocarcinoma was controlled through surgical and GnRH agonists for a 5-year 10-month period.

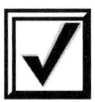 **MISCELLANEOUS**

## ASSOCIATED CONDITIONS

Egg retention, ascites, cystic ovarian disease, medullary polyostotic hyperostosis, abdominal hernias, oviductal impaction, oviductal prolapse, coelomitis.

## AGE-RELATED FACTORS

See Signalment section.

## ZOONOTIC POTENTIAL

N/A

## FERTILITY/BREEDING

Bird with reproductive neoplasia should not be bred.

## SYNONYMS

Reproductive neoplasia, neoplasm of the reproductive tract.

## SEE ALSO

Ascites
Dystocia
Egg Yolk and Reproductive Coelomitis
Marek's Disease
Retroviruses in Galliformes

## ABBREVIATIONS

COX—cyclooxygenase
CT—computed tomography
FSH—follicle-stimulating hormone
GnRH—gonadotropin-releasing hormone
LH—luteinizing hormone
MRI—magnetic resonance imaging

## INTERNET RESOURCES

N/A

*Suggested Reading*

Carrasco, D.C., González, M.S. (2017). Reproductive disorders in commonly kept fowl. *Veterinary Clinics of North America: Exotic Animal Practice*, 20:509–538.

Echols, S., Speer, B. (2022). Avian reproductive tract diseases and surgical resolutions. *Clinical Theriogenology*, 14:32–43.

Hakim, A.A., Barry, C.P., Barnes, et al. (2009). Ovarian adenocarcinomas in the laying hen and women share similar alterations in p53, ras, and HER-2/neu. *Cancer Prevention Research*, 2:114–121.

Kapsetaki, S.E., Compton, Z., Dolan, J., et al. (2023). Life history and cancer in birds: clutch size predicts cancer. *bioRxiv*, 2023-02.

Mans, C., Pilny, A. (2014). Use of GnRH-agonists for medical management of reproductive disorders in birds. *Veterinary Clinics of North America: Exotic Animal Practice*, 17:23–33.

**Author**: Noémie Summa, DMV, IPSAV (Zoological Medicine), DACZM

N

# NEOPLASIA (RESPIRATORY)

 **BASICS**

## DEFINITION
Respiratory neoplasia refers to a tumor of the tissues related to the respiratory tract, which include nasopharyngeal, sinusal, laryngeal, syringeal, tracheal, pulmonary, and air sac tissues. Respiratory neoplasms can be primary or secondary (metastasis), benign, or malignant.

## PATHOPHYSIOLOGY
Primary respiratory neoplasia in psittacines is uncommon, although documented cases exist. Secondary metastasis to the respiratory tract of birds has also been reported with numerous tumor types. Squamous cell carcinoma of the infraorbital sinus and oral cavity. Nasal adenocarcinoma. Bronchial carcinoma. Air sac cystadenocarcinoma. Pulmonary adenocarcinoma. Respiratory hamartoma. Poorly differentiated carcinomas in cockatiels. Pulmonary carcinoma.

## SYSTEMS AFFECTED
Respiratory—nasopharyngeal, sinusal, laryngeal, syringeal, tracheal, pulmonary, and air sac tissues. Secondary systems can be affected if metastasis occurs.

## GENETICS
N/A

## INCIDENCE/PREVALENCE
Uncommon.

## GEOGRAPHIC DISTRIBUTION
N/A

## SIGNALMENT
There is no known age or sex predisposition reported with respiratory neoplasia in avian species. Certain avian species have been documented to more commonly have specific types of respiratory neoplasia.

## SIGNS
### Historical Findings
Typical presenting complaints include respiratory clinical signs, in addition to weakness and lethargy.

### Physical Examination Findings
Severe respiratory signs including respiratory distress involving increased respiratory rate and effort, and open beak breathing are reported. Avian patients are typically weak, critical, and often unstable patients at the time of presentation.

## CAUSES
N/A

## RISK FACTORS
N/A

 **DIAGNOSIS**

## DIFFERENTIAL DIAGNOSIS
Infectious respiratory disease (bacterial, viral, fungal). Toxin exposure.

## CBC/BIOCHEMISTRY/URINALYSIS
Bloodwork should be performed to evaluate the overall health of the patient, and to determine whether there are any abnormal blood counts that could be related to the neoplastic process. Cytopenias, anemia, and leukocytosis may all be reported with varying types of neoplasia. Additionally, biochemistry profiles may demonstrate organ involvement associated with the tumor, or organ dysfunction related to the age of the patient or the presence of other disease processes. Hypercalcemia of malignancy has been previously documented in avian patients.

## OTHER LABORATORY TESTS
Fine-needle aspirate and cytology of the lesion (with or without ultrasound guidance). Biopsy and histopathology of the lesion (punch biopsy, core needle [Tru Cut™, Merit Medical Systems, South Jordan, UT], laparoscopic for internal organs).

## IMAGING
Radiographs, ultrasound and CT can all have utility in the assessment of avian neoplasia. They help to demonstrate the extent of the lesion, invasiveness of the disease, and also to stage the animal (evaluate for metastasis). Many malignant tumors will spread to other organs, with the most common location of metastasis being the lungs, but other locations such as coelomic organs and bone may be involved depending on the tumor type. Although radiographs provide some utility in assessment, contrast-enhanced CT provides a much better overall picture of the coelomic organs, as well as a more global evaluation of the primary lesion and potential for metastatic lesions.

## DIAGNOSTIC PROCEDURES
Following acquisition of a biopsy, immunohistochemical testing may be required to obtain a definitive diagnosis when cell morphology alone does not provide enough information; however, the canine and feline antibodies that are used may not cross-react with avian tissues and so must be a consideration when additional testing is undertaken. In addition to these challenges, there are also no established positive controls in avian patients which creates difficulties when interpreting the results.

## PATHOLOGIC FINDINGS
Pathology findings will depend on the type of tumor that is present in the avian patient.

 **TREATMENT**

## APPROPRIATE HEALTH CARE
Treatment of the tumor will depend on the type of tumor, invasiveness, and presence or absence of metastasis. In general, neoplasms of the respiratory tract in avian species tend to be locally invasive with common metastasis to the coelomic organs and bones. There are few reports of treatment given the aggressive nature of these tumors, with many birds succumbing to the tumor or euthanasia due to the severity and quality of life concerns. Treatment for squamous cell carcinoma is typically a combination of surgical excision and radiation therapy. Additionally, intralesional chemotherapy with carboplatin and cisplatin have been attempted with limited success. Surgical amputation of the wing has been described to obtain complete margins when the tumor is localized to the humerus.

## NURSING CARE
Avian patients that are diagnosed with respiratory neoplasia should be provided supportive care to ensure that they maintain a good quality of life that is pain and as stress free as possible. Depending on the needs of the patient, oxygen therapy, anti-inflammatories, or opioids may be indicated to maintain the comfort of the avian patient.

## ACTIVITY
Avian patients that have been diagnosed with respiratory neoplasia should be allowed to choose their own level of activity, as overexertion could cause episodes of weakness, collapse, and respiratory distress.

## DIET
No specific dietary recommendations.

## CLIENT EDUCATION
Avian owners are more aware of treatment options for respiratory neoplasia in domestic animal species and humans. As a result, there is an increasing demand for advanced diagnostic and therapeutic options for companion avian species. In any sick avian patient, it is always important to discuss the risks of handling, diagnostics, and treatment, including death, especially in birds that are in respiratory distress. Prognosis and consideration for euthanasia may also be necessary discussions with the owner. At this time, there is no established standard of care for avian neoplasia and most of the dosages are extrapolated with an unknown array of adverse effects.

**N**

## SURGICAL CONSIDERATIONS

Surgical excision with adequate margins is an ideal treatment option for many neoplastic processes. This should only be undertaken after a patient has a definitive diagnosis, has been fully staged, and evidence of metastasis has been ruled out. Additionally, the risks of surgery and anesthesia in the avian patient must be fully disclosed to the owner, with a risk–benefit approach investigated prior to surgery. In cases where inadequate margins are obtained after surgery, additional treatment options should be explored depending on the tumor type, including additional surgery, radiation therapy, systemic or local chemotherapy.

 MEDICATIONS

### DRUG(S) OF CHOICE

Chemotherapy may be a therapeutic option, targeted towards the tumor type. Supportive care including analgesics (opioids, NSAIDs), antibiotics, or antifungals may also be considered.

### CONTRAINDICATIONS
N/A

### PRECAUTIONS

Chemotherapy doses are typically extrapolated from what is known in canine and feline patients, and these may not be the correct dose for avian species. Although in dogs and cats, body surface area is used to calculate chemotherapy dosages, it is unknown if this is appropriate for avian

patients. Adverse effects of certain chemotherapeutics have been reported in avian species.

### POSSIBLE INTERACTIONS
N/A

### ALTERNATIVE DRUGS
N/A

 FOLLOW-UP

### PATIENT MONITORING

The most important factor to monitor in patients with neoplasia is quality of life. Each patient should be routinely evaluated for changes in respiration, appetite, and ability to perform normal behaviors.

### PREVENTION/AVOIDANCE
N/A

### POSSIBLE COMPLICATIONS
N/A

### EXPECTED COURSE AND PROGNOSIS

In general, the prognosis for avian respiratory neoplasia is guarded to poor, with many of the tumors behaving in a locally invasive manner, with metastasis.

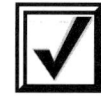 MISCELLANEOUS

### ASSOCIATED CONDITIONS
N/A

### AGE-RELATED FACTORS
N/A

### ZOONOTIC POTENTIAL
N/A

### FERTILITY/BREEDING
N/A

### SYNONYMS
N/A

### SEE ALSO
N/A

### ABBREVIATIONS
CT—computed tomography
NSAIDs—non-steroidal anti-inflammatory drugs

### INTERNET RESOURCES
N/A

*Suggested Reading*
Baumgartner, W.A., Guzman, D.S.M., Hollibush, S., et al. (2008). Bronchogenic adenocarcinoma in a hyacinth macaw (*Anodorhynchus hyacinthinus*). *Journal of Avian Medicine and Surgery*, 22:218–225.
Garner, M.M., Latimer, K.S., Mickley, K.A., et al. (2009). Histologic, immunohisto-chemical, and electron microscopic features of a unique pulmonary tumor in cockatiels (*Nymphicus Hollandicus*): Six cases. *Veterinary Pathology*, 46:1100–1108.
Raidal, S.R., Shearer, P.L., Butler, R., Monks, D. (2006). Airsac cystadenocarcinomas in cockatoos. *Australian Veterinary Journal*, 84:213–216.
**Author**: Sara Gardhouse, DVM, DABVP (Exotic Companion Mammal), DACZM

N

# NEURAL LARVA MIGRANS

## BASICS

### DEFINITION
Neural larva migrans (NLM) is cerebrospinal nematodiasis. This is produced by migration of nematode larvae through the brain and spinal cord and causing severe neurological signs and lesions that often result in death. *Baylisascaris* spp. are a well-recognized cause of cerebrospinal nematodiasis of North American mammals and birds.

### PATHOPHYSIOLOGY
Raccoons are infected by *Baylisascaris* by ingestion of eggs or larvae in tissues of paratenic hosts. The nematodes mature in their intestines and eggs are shed in their feces. Infection of birds occurs when they ingest eggs from contaminated environments. After the eggs hatch, larval nematodes will aggressively migrate through the tissues of the bird, resulting in neurologic damage. A few migrating larvae can cause fatal CNS disease.

### SYSTEMS AFFECTED
**Nervous**: CNS is primary infected.
**Ophthalmic**: Focal choroiditis and larval granuloma in ocular muscle have been reported in experimental infection.
**Digestive**: Very uncommon to see lesions of the larval migrations in birds.

### GENETICS
None.

### INCIDENCE/PREVALENCE
High disease prevalence and mortality when exposed to a contaminated environment.

### GEOGRAPHIC DISTRIBUTION
North America for *Baylisascaris* spp.

### SIGNALMENT
Species: > 90 avian species including chickens, turkeys, ostriches, emus, pigeons, doves, quails, pheasants, partridges, blue jays, robins, and psittacines (cockatoos, macaws, Patagonian conures, cockatiels, lorikeet, lovebirds).

### SIGNS
*Historical Findings*
Exposure to contaminated environment and/or and/or transport containers. Gradual onset and slow progression of neurologic symptoms over a period of several weeks or acute presentation.

*Physical Examination Findings*
Loss of equilibrium. Increasing ataxia. Circling. Torticollis. Head tilts. Visual defects. Unable to stand or walk. Nystagmus. Incoordination. Extensor rigidity.

### CAUSES
*Baylisascaris procyonis* is the most common cause of visceral, ocular larva migrans (OLM), and NLM with the raccoon as

primary host. *Baylisascaris columnaris* that cycles through skunks and *Baylisascaris melis* of badgers show less tendency to result in OLM and NLM. Report of *Toxocara cati* from lesions of NLM in North Island brown kiwi (*Apteryx mantelli*). *Chandlerella quiscali* has been associated with NLM in emus.

### RISK FACTORS
Outdoor aviary. Sharing space in areas frequented by raccoons.

## DIAGNOSIS

### DIFFERENTIAL DIAGNOSIS
Viral (Newcastle disease, avian influenza A virus, West Nile virus), bacterial, fungal or protozoal encephalitis, Heavy metal toxicosis, insecticide toxicosis, hepatic encephalopathy, otitis media and interna, and trauma.

### CBC/BIOCHEMISTRY/URINALYSIS
CBC and biochemistry are usually within normal limits. Compared with mammals, peripheral eosinophilia has not been documented in birds with NLM. Increased AST and CK levels may be seen with muscular lesions secondary to neurologic signs.

### OTHER LABORATORY TESTS
Serology may be used in antemortem diagnosis. However, these techniques require species-specific reagents that have not been standardized for birds.

### IMAGING
Advanced imaging such as computed tomography and magnetic resonance imaging may be recommended, although absence of visible lesions should not exclude NLM.

### DIAGNOSTIC PROCEDURES
Cerebrospinal fluid may be analysed, although the only reported analysis of cerebrospinal fluid from a macaw with confirmed NLM secondary to *B. procyonis* did not reveal eosinophilia as it would in mammals.

### PATHOLOGIC FINDINGS
Diagnosis of NLM is difficult because of the paucity of larvae in the avian CNS in most cases. Gross necropsy may show malacia and hemorrhage in the brains, although absent to minimal lesions are more common. Histologic lesions within the brain and/or spinal cord include leukomalacia, axonal degeneration, multifocal white matter vacuolation, non-suppurative inflammatory reaction with gliosis and/or perivascular lymphoplasmacytic cuffing. In some cases, the migration tracks of the nematodes can be identified. The third-stage larvae of *Baylisascaris* sp. cannot be differentiated,

so species determination is usually not possible on histological examination.

## TREATMENT

### APPROPRIATE HEALTH CARE
Emergency inpatient intensive care management should be provided with fluid the appropriate analgesia.

### NURSING CARE
Routine supportive and nursing care should be provided. Perching and substrates should be adapted to the neurologic condition of the affected birds.

### ACTIVITY
Activity should be restricted in case of severely ill patients. Perches should be covered with elasticated bandage and lowered in the cage to help in preventing falls and trauma. The bottom of the cage should be padded.

### DIET
Nutritional support should be provided if birds cannot eat on their own.

### CLIENT EDUCATION
Owners should be aware of the poor prognosis and high mortality rates associated with NLM in birds.

### SURGICAL CONSIDERATIONS
N/A

## MEDICATIONS

### DRUG(S) OF CHOICE
Treatment for NLM is generally unsuccessful. While anthelmintics can successfully eliminate *B. procyonis* worms from the intestines of raccoons, they are generally unsuccessful against NLM in aberrant hosts.

### CONTRAINDICATIONS
N/A

### PRECAUTIONS
Killing NLM could worsen neurological clinical signs secondary to increased inflammation related to dead nematodes.

### POSSIBLE INTERACTIONS
N/A

### ALTERNATIVE DRUGS
N/A

## FOLLOW-UP

### PATIENT MONITORING
Patients usually die before follow-up due to poor prognosis.

## PREVENTION/AVOIDANCE

Emphasis needs to be placed on preventing disease as treatment option are unsuccessful with NLM. Thorough cleaning of the environment with identifying raccoon latrines and removal of contaminated soil or contaminated bedding material. Thorough cleaning of any cages that have housed raccoons, skunks, or badgers. Control rodents, as they can carry *Baylisascaris* spp. eggs into the aviary. Avoiding the use of natural materials in exhibits, such as logs, limbs, or rocks collected from surrounding areas, unless decontaminated. Control methods of wild raccoons on zoo grounds. Bait deworming of stable local raccoon populations. Prophylactic treatment of the food with pyrantel tartrate or with ivermectin at regular intervals has been described to reduce the risks in birds in exhibits or enclosures at increased risk of exposure to *B. procyonis* ova.

## POSSIBLE COMPLICATIONS

*B. procyonis* eggs may remain infective for years and are difficult to destroy.

## EXPECTED COURSE AND PROGNOSIS

The prognosis for individuals affected with *B. procyonis* NLM is typically very poor.

 MISCELLANEOUS

## ASSOCIATED CONDITIONS

OLM or other aberrant migration uncommon.

## AGE-RELATED FACTORS

None.

## ZOONOTIC POTENTIAL

Humans are also susceptible to *Baylisascaris* infection.

## FERTILITY/BREEDING

N/A

## SYNONYMS

Cerebrospinal nematodiasis.

## SEE ALSO

Toxoplasmosis

## ABBREVIATIONS

AST—aspartate aminotransferase
CBC—complete blood count
CK—creatine kinase
CNS—central nervous system
NLM—neural larva migrans
OLM—ocular larva migrans

## INTERNET RESOURCES

N/A

*Suggested Reading*
Diab, S.S., Uzal, F.A., Giannitti, F., Shivaprasad, H.L. (2012). Cerebrospinal nematodiasis outbreak in an urban outdoor aviary of cockatiels (*Nymphicus hollandicus*) in southern California. *Journal of Veterinary Diagnostic Investigation*, 24: 994–999.
Pilny, A.A., Reavill, D. (2020). Emerging and re-emerging diseases of selected avian species. *Veterinary Clinics of North America: Exotic Animal Practice*, 23: 429–441.
Russell, D., Smith, D., Crawshaw, G., et al. (2005). Neural larva migrans due to *Baylisascaris procyonis* in captive lovebirds and lorikeets: A case series. In: *2005 Proceedings AAZV, AAWV, AZA/NAG Joint Conference.*American Association of Zoo Veterinarians: 135.

**Author**: Noémie Summa, DMV, IPSAV (Zoological medicine), DACZM

N

# NEUROLOGIC (NON-TRAUMATIC DISEASES)

## BASICS

### DEFINITION
Any condition that causes damage or deterioration to the nervous system, via trauma, toxin, infection/inflammation, or organ failure.

### PATHOPHYSIOLOGY
Toxicities: Organophosphates act as anticholinesterases, allowing excessive acetylcholine at the neuromuscular junctions resulting in tremoring, weakness or paralysis. Heavy metals such as lead or zinc will damage the nervous system. Infectious diseases damage to the nervous system, usually by causing cell death. In some cases, this is due to direct infection (e.g., *Chlamydia psittaci*, paramyxovirus-3), or indirectly by damage from the host immune system. Atherosclerosis causes hypoxic damage to the CNS and secondary seizures. Neoplasia causes space occupying lesions (e.g. Marek's disease, pituitary adenomas, cerebellar neuroectodermal tumors). Seizures may result from nutritional deficiencies in vitamins $B_1$, $B_2$, $B_6$, $B_{12}$, $D_3$, E, as well as selenium, calcium, and phosphorus. Dyslipidemia/lipid emboli secondary to hyperestrogenism of reproductively active hens, characterized by excessive lipid circulating, causing vascular sludging and lipid emboli. The resulting hypoxic cell damage can lead to neurologic signs such as head tilt. Lipid storage diseases can cause neurodegeneration from the accumulation of lipopigments within neurons.

### SYSTEMS AFFECTED
Nervous. Musculoskeletal—paresis/paralysis. Cardiovascular—vascular damage by lead, or due to atherosclerosis. GI—regurgitation, undigested seeds, weight loss.

### GENETICS
See Incidence/Prevalence section.

### INCIDENCE/PREVALENCE
Amazons and grey parrots may be more prone to atherosclerosis and secondary seizures. Muscovy ducks may be particularly sensitive to duck viral enteritis, and mallard ducks are more resistant to the disease.

### GEOGRAPHIC DISTRIBUTION
N/A

### SIGNALMENT
**Species**: All avian species can be affected.
**Species predilections**: Grey parrots, silky chickens, budgerigars, red-lored Amazons, Muscovy ducks.
**Mean age and range**: Any age can be affected, but older patients may be more

susceptible to atherosclerotic or neoplastic causes of neurologic signs.
**Predominant sex**: Reproductively active females are susceptible to dyslipidemia/lipid emboli, and will be more likely to succumb to hypocalcemia. Other causes of neurologic disease show no sex predilection.

### SIGNS

#### Historical Findings
Owners may note acute or chronic progression of neurologic signs.

#### Physical Examination Findings
Seizures. Blindness. Ataxia. Paresis/paralysis. Changes in mentation or equilibrium. Muscle tremors or fasciculation. Acute death with no clinical signs.

#### Cranial Nerve Exam
Cranial nerve (CN) exam may reveal: CN I (olfactory) deficits may result in altered appetite and eating habits. CN II (optic) damage will result in blindness, decreased or absent menace. CN III (oculomotor) dysfunction may result in ventrolateral deviation of globe, or drooping of the upper eyelid. Iris constriction may also be affected, but less so due to the presence of striated muscle within the iris. CN IV (trochlear) dysfunction will lead to dorsolateral deviation of the globe. CN V (trigeminal) has three branches with sensory and motor functions. Dysfunction of the ophthalmic branch will show loss of sensation around the face and beak. Dysfunction of the maxillary branch will lead to loss of sensation of the face, beak, and/or mouth/palate. Dysfunction of the mandibular branch will lead to decreased bite strength and closing, and inability to close eye. CN VI (abducens) deficits will result in inability to move the nictitating membrane (third eyelid). CN VII (facial) deficits will result in lack of response to facial sensation and possible facial droop or asymmetry. Taste sensation is also innervated by CN IX, and may be difficult to evaluate in birds. CN VIII (vestibulocochlear) deficits will result in hearing loss, and/or loss of equilibrium (nystagmus, head tilt or circling toward the affected side). CN IX (glossopharyngeal) and CN X (vagal) nerve anastomoses in birds and are evaluated together. Deficits will result in lack of tongue sensation, dysphagia, regurgitation, voice changes or loss. CN XI (accessory) dysfunction may result in poor neck mobility. CN XII (hypoglossal) dysfunction will result in deviation of the tongue toward the affected side, decreased mobility or tone, or change in or absence of voice. Eye movement is the result of interactions with a variety of cranial

nerves (III, IV, VI and VIII), the brainstem and the cerebellum. Problems with any of these nerves may lead to strabismus. The palpebral reflex can be evaluated to assess both CN V and CN VII. CN V, IX, X, XI, and XII control tongue movement, beak strength and swallowing.

#### Postural/Gait Examination Findings
Vestibular or cerebellar lesions may result in postural changes like head tilts, or twisting of the body, or intention tremors. Central vestibular signs may also be associated with changes in mental status, postural reaction deficits, or vertical nystagmus. Decreased or asymmetric wing retraction or grip strength. Crossed extensor reflexes are associated with upper motor neuron lesions and can be an indicator of severe spinal cord lesions. Knuckling over, or a loss of conscious proprioception, indicates that there is a lesion in the peripheral and/or central nervous system. Dysfunction of the pudendal nerves results in decreased cloacal reflex. Muscle atrophy.

### CAUSES
Organophosphates toxicities, heavy metals. Infectious/inflammatory. Viral: PDD, a bornavirus, and Marek's disease (herpesvirus in poultry). Newcastle disease (paramyxovirus), Duck viral enteritis (herpesvirus in waterfowl), West Nile virus, and duck viral hepatitis (picornavirus). Bacterial: Botulism caused by *Clostridium botulinum* enterotoxin, chlamydiosis caused by *Chlamydia psittaci*, general septicemia. Avian vacuolar myelopathy is a rare neurologic disease caused by a toxin from a novel cyanobacteria (*Stigonematales*). Fungal, such as aspergillosis. Parasitic (aberrant larval migrans with *Baylisascaris*, toxoplasmosis, sarcocystosis, etc.). Yolk emboli secondary to egg-yolk ceolomitis. Trauma. Dietary or nutritional: Hypocalcemia (especially in gray parrots). Specific vitamin, calcium, phosphorus, or selenium nutritional deficiencies in young psittacines. Metabolic causes, such as hepatic encephalopathy, although controversy exists as to whether hepatic encephalopathy can occur in birds, as nitrogenous waste products are not the end product in birds as they are in mammals. Neurologic signs can occur with severe hepatic disease. Atherosclerosis. Lafora body neuropathy—reported in cockatiels. Congenital causes such neuronal ceroid lipofuscinosis, iron storage diseases, lysosomal storage diseases.

### RISK FACTORS
Supervised or unsupervised time outside of a cage that might allow exposure to toxins or injuries. Exposure to other birds or animals.

Nutritionally inadequate diet. Reproductive activity. Certain breeds: Bald eagles (avian vacuolar myelopathy); toucans, mynahs, birds of paradise, lorikeets, starlings (iron storage disease).

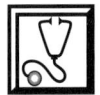

# DIAGNOSIS

## DIFFERENTIAL DIAGNOSIS
Any disease or trauma that leads to depression, ataxia or muscle weakness. Myopathy/muscular dystrophy-like syndrome (rare).

## CBC/BIOCHEMISTRY/URINALYSIS
CBC: A marked leukocytosis, often with a monocytosis, may be seen with chlamydiosis. Anemia may be seen with neuronal ceroid Lipofuscinosis. Biochemistry profile: Decreased total blood calcium levels may be seen with hypocalcemia. Hypoglycemia may be seen in very young birds. Elevations in AST and/or bile acids may be elevated in hepatic encephalopathy. Cholesterol/triglycerides may be elevated in atherosclerosis and dyslipidemia syndrome. Urinalysis: Hematuria may be seen with lead toxicosis, particularly in amazon parrots.

## OTHER LABORATORY TESTS
Ionized calcium levels may be useful in suspect cases when total calcium is normal but history or clinical signs warrant further investigation for hypocalcemia. Avian bornavirus PCR testing may be helpful in birds showing clinical signs. Chlamydiosis PCR testing for the presence of *Ch. psittaci*. Electromyography values can determine the health of the muscle cell and the integrity of the motor unit (lower motor neuron and associated muscle fibers) to differentiate peripheral nerve damage from primary muscle disease.

## IMAGING
### Radiographic Findings
Metallic densities consistent with heavy metal toxicity. Fractures of the spine or skull suggesting a traumatic cause to neurologic signs. Dilated proventriculus/ventriculus in the case of PDD. Calcified major blood vessels may be identified on radiographs, suggesting atherosclerosis.

### Advanced Imaging
CT and MRI are useful in evaluating structures within the head and spine, space occupying lesions, areas of trauma or other abnormalities. MRI is the preferred imaging modality to evaluate brain and spinal cord for lesions like hydrocephalus, but require longer anesthesia times to perform. CT is often faster and less expensive.

## DIAGNOSTIC PROCEDURES
Histopathology (crop/GI biopsy or necropsy) remains the most definitive diagnostic tool in PDD.

## PATHOLOGIC FINDINGS
**Neuronal ceroid lipofuscinosis**: Gross examination would be unremarkable. Histologic findings include neuronal intracytoplasmic eosinophilic and or golden/brown globular and granular material within the brain and spinal cord.
Duck viral enteritis: A herpesvirus. Hemorrhage and erosions under the tongue, esophagus, intestinal mucosa and cloaca. Annular rings of hemorrhage may be present in the intestines. Intranuclear inclusion bodies may be seen in liver and areas of the GI mucosa.
**Newcastle's disease**: A paramyxovirus. Hemorrhage throughout the GI tract and tracheitis. Pericardial effusion and cardiomegaly may be seen. Inflammation of the kidneys and brain is seen microscopically.

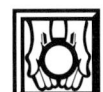

# TREATMENT

## APPROPRIATE HEALTH CARE
Identify and treat the underlying condition. Inpatient treatment is often required cases of ongoing seizure activity, anorexia, lethargy, recumbency, dysphagia, ataxia, or coma. Hypoglycemia, even after seizure activity, is rare, but normoglycemia must be maintained. Appropriate antimicrobial therapy (antibiotics, antifungals). In cases of suspected atherosclerosis, isoxsuprine or pentoxifylline may improve cerebral blood flow.

## NURSING CARE
Fluid therapy if unable to maintain hydration. This may be delivered via SC, IV or IO routes. Nutritional support via gavage or feeding tube if the patient is unable to feed itself. A padded cage may need to be provided if the bird is unable to stand, ataxic, or seizures repeatedly.

## ACTIVITY
If the patient is weakened or has difficulty climbing, then perches, food and water sources may need to be placed lower in the cage to allow the patient access.

## DIET
In cases where the patient is eating, it is advisable to offer the patient's regular diet, even if it is substandard to assure that the patient continues to eat. Mineral and vitamin deficiencies may be supplemented orally or parenterally. When the patient has recovered, transitioning to a better balanced diet may be performed. If the patient is unable to feed itself, nutritional support via gavage or feeding tube should be performed using a resuspended balanced hand feeding formula.

## CLIENT EDUCATION
Exposure to sources of infection, toxins, or trauma need to be eliminated. The importance of an appropriate diet.

## SURGICAL CONSIDERATIONS
Placement of a ventricular feeding tube via ingluviotomy may be indicated for greater ease of assisted feeding during prolonged recoveries. Removal of heavy metal foreign bodies via gastric lavage, endoscopy, or surgery.

# MEDICATIONS

## DRUG(S) OF CHOICE
**For controlling seizures**: Midazolam 0.5–1.0 mg/kg IM. May be repeated up to 3 times if necessary. May also be administered intracloacally—use double the dose. Diazepam may also be administered via continuous IV or IO infusion at 1 mg/kg/h if further seizure control is needed. Once seizures have been controlled for 12–24 hours, diazepam is tapered to zero over the next 12–24 hours. If further seizure control is needed, phenobarbital may be infused at 2–10 mg/kg/h. Once the seizures have been stopped, phenobarbital may be used for long-term seizure control at 2–7 mg/kg PO q12h. Levetiracetam 60 mg/kg IM; can use for long-term seizure control at dosing up to 100 mg/kg PO q8h.
**Cerebral edema**: Mannitol 0.5–1.0 g/kg IV over 20 minutes. This may be repeated up to 3 times in a 24-hour period.
**Chlamydiosis**: Doxycycline 75–100 mg/kg IM q5–7d for a minimum of 45 days, or 25–50 mg/kg PO q24h for 45 days.
**PDD**: Currently, treatment with NSAIDs has shown some success at reducing clinical signs. Meloxicam 0.5 mg/kg PO q12–24h. Treatment is usually lifelong.
**Lead toxicity**: See Heavy Metal Toxicosis chapter.
**Hypocalcemia**: See Hypocalcemia/Hypomagnesemia chapter.
**Dyslipidemia syndrome/lipid emboli**: See Dyslipidemia/Hyperlipidemia chapter. Dilution of the vascular sludge with crystalloid diuresis is a mainstay. Cholesterol-lowering statin drugs may be compounded and tried in birds. These include atorvastatin 3 mg/kg q24h, simvastatin 1 mg/kg q24h, lovastatin 6 mg/kg q24h.

## CONTRAINDICATIONS
Avoid steroids in birds with neurologic disease. Birds seem to be more sensitive to the immunosuppressive effects of steroids, and

N

this might worsen clinical signs, particularly if the cause is infectious. Steroid use may also lead to hyperglycemia, which is shown to have a poorer prognosis in head trauma.

### PRECAUTIONS
Phenobarbital may not reach therapeutic levels and may be ineffective to control seizures in some avian species (e.g. grey parrots). Levetiracetam may be more appropriate.

### POSSIBLE INTERACTIONS
N/A

### ALTERNATIVE DRUGS
N/A

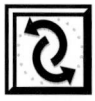 FOLLOW-UP

### PATIENT MONITORING
Successive neurologic exams essential to monitor response to treatment and prognosis. If seizures are being controlled with phenobarbital, blood levels should be checked 2–3 weeks after starting therapy. If seizures are being controlled with levetiracetam and zonisamide, blood levels can be monitored to verify therapeutic (based on humans) dosing.

### PREVENTION/AVOIDANCE
Eliminating or limiting exposure to toxins or infectious agents that cause neurologic disease. Screening birds for *Ch. psittaci* prior to introducing them into flocks can reduce the risk.

### POSSIBLE COMPLICATIONS
Some neurologic signs may be permanent, and may persist even after treatment.

### EXPECTED COURSE AND PROGNOSIS
Varies with the cause. Congenital abnormalities carry a poor prognosis. Toxicoses have a better prognosis with early treatment.

 MISCELLANEOUS

### ASSOCIATED CONDITIONS
N/A

### AGE-RELATED FACTORS
N/A

### ZOONOTIC POTENTIAL
Chlamydiosis and Newcastle disease are reportable diseases. They are also zoonotic. Chlamydiosis can cause a serious respiratory disease, and Newcastle disease can cause conjunctivitis in people.

### FERTILITY/BREEDING
N/A

### SYNONYMS
N/A

### SEE ALSO
Atherosclerosis
Avian Influenza
Bornaviral Diseases
Botulism
Dyslipidemia/Hyperlipidemia
Hypocalcemia and Hypomagnesemia
Liver Disease
Mycotoxicosis
Neoplasia (Neurologic)
Neurologic (Trauma)
Otitis
Orthoavulaviruses
Seizures
Sick-Bird Syndrome
Toxicosis (Environmental/Pesticides)
Toxicosis (Heavy Metals)
Toxicosis (Iatrogenic)
Toxicosis (Ingested, Gastrointestinal)
Trauma
West Nile Virus
Appendix 8, Algorithm 9: Neurologic Signs

### ABBREVIATIONS
AST—aspartate aminotransferase
CN—cranial nerve
CNS—central nervous system
CT—computed tomography
GI—gastrointestinal
MRI—magnetic resonance imaging
NSAIDs—nonsteroidal anti-inflammatory drugs
PCR—polymerase chain reaction
PDD—proventricular dilatation disease

### INTERNET RESOURCES
N/A

*Suggested Reading*
Evans-Reid, E.E., Jones, M.P., Crews, A.J., Newkirk, K. (2012). Neuronal ceroid lipofuscinosis in a mallard duck (*Anas platyrhynchos*). *Journal of Avian Medicine and Surgery*, 26:22–28.
Petritz O.A. (2015). Avian Neurology. *Proceedings of the Pacific Veterinary Conference*, CA.
Antinoff, N., Orosz, S.E. (2012). Don't be nervous! A Clinician's approach to the avian neurologic system. *Proceedings of the Association of Avian Veterinarians Annual Conference*, Louisville, KT.
Clippinger, T.L., Bennett, R.A., Platt, S.R. (2007). The avian neurologic examination and ancillary neurodiagnostic techniques: A review update. *Veterinary Clinics of North America. Exotic Animal Practice*, 10:803–836.
Johnson-Delaney, C.A., Reavill, D. (2009). Toxicoses in birds: Ante- and postmortem findings for practitioners. *Proceedings of the Association of Avian Veterinarians Annual Conference*, Milwaukee, WI.
Orosz, S.E., Bradshaw, G.A. (2007). Avian neuroanatomy revisited: From clinical principles to avian cognition. *Veterinary Clinics of North America. Exotic Animal Practice*, 10:775–802.

**Author:** Stephen Dyer, DVM, DABVP (Avian)

N

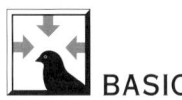

# BASICS

## DEFINITION
Any traumatic event that causes damage to the nervous system.

## PATHOPHYSIOLOGY
Trauma that results in injuries to intracranial or spinal structures. These can result in traumatic brain injury (TBI). TBI is divided into primary and secondary effects. Primary injury occurs at the time of impact and the severity of the damage is determined by the force of the impact. These injuries include cerebral lacerations from skull fractures, direct neuronal–axonal damage, cortical contusions, and intracranial hemorrhage. In most cases, these types of direct parenchymal damage to the brain are beyond the treatment of clinicians. Secondary injuries to neuronal tissues occur due to glutamate release resulting in ATP depletion and the failure of autoregulation systems that help maintain adequate blood flow to the brain. These lead to the production of reactive oxygen species and proinflammatory cytokines. Secondary injuries occur in the minutes to days following the trauma. Systemic factors include hypoxia, hypotension, electrolyte and acid-base disturbances, and systemic inflammation. Treatment is focused on recognizing and minimizing secondary injuries.

## SYSTEMS AFFECTED
Nervous. Ophthalmic. Musculoskeletal—paresis/paralysis.

## GENETICS
N/A

## INCIDENCE/PREVALENCE
TBI may be one of the more common reasons for admissions of wild birds.

## GEOGRAPHIC DISTRIBUTION
This can occur anywhere.

## SIGNALMENT
All avian species can be affected.

## SIGNS
### Historical Findings
Owners may note acute appearance of neurologic signs, trauma may or may not have been observed.

### Physical Examination Findings
Seizures. Blindness. Ataxia. Head tilt. Circling. Visible bruising under the skull. Intraocular haemorrhage. Aural haemorrhage. Paresis/paralysis. Changes in mentation or equilibrium. Muscle tremors or fasciculation. Acute death with no clinical signs.

### Cranial Nerve Examination
Menace is a reflex involving the cerebellum, CN II (optic nerve, sensory) and CN V (trigeminal nerve, motor). Pupillary light reflex involves tests the function of CN II (sensory) and CN III (oculomotor, motor). In birds, this made more challenging by the presence of striated muscle in the iris allowing for a voluntary override. This may be minimized by checking this early in the exam. Birds have a complete decussation of the optic nerve, but may still have some consentual light reflex due to the incomplete bony septum between the orbits allowing light to reach the contralateral retina. Globe position can be altered by CN III deficits (ventrolateral deviation), CN IV deficits (trochlear, dorsolateral deviation) or CN VI (abducens, medial deviation). Third-eyelid position is difficult to evaluate due to the presence of striated muscle. Palpebral reflex tests the function of sensory and motor components within the trigeminal nerve (CN V). Facial expressions may test CN VII, but this is often impractical due to the presence of feathering and limited facial musculature compared with that of mammals. Nystagmus can indicate damage to the vestibulocochlear nerve (CN VIII) or the brainstem.

### Postural/Gait Examination Findings
Vestibular or cerebellar lesions may result in postural changes like head tilts, or twisting of the body, or intention tremors. Central vestibular signs may also be associated with changes in mental status, postural reaction deficits, or vertical nystagmus. Decreased or asymmetric wing retraction or grip strength. Crossed extensor reflexes are associated with upper motor neuron lesions and can be an indicator of severe spinal cord lesions. Knuckling over, or a loss of conscious proprioception, indicates that there is a lesion in the peripheral and/or central nervous system. Dysfunction of the pudendal nerves results in decreased cloacal reflex. Muscle atrophy.

## CAUSES
Vehicular trauma, window strikes, ceiling fan injuries, closing doors, conspecific aggression (bird bites), interspecific aggression (dog or cat bites).

## RISK FACTORS
Supervised or unsupervised time outside of a cage that might allow exposure to injuries. Exposure to other birds or animals.

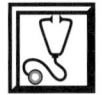

# DIAGNOSIS

## DIFFERENTIAL DIAGNOSIS
Any disease or trauma that leads to depression, ataxia or muscle weakness (heavy metal toxicity, avian ganglioneuritis/PDD, lysosomal storage disease. Myopathy/muscular dystrophy-like syndrome (rare).

## CBC/BIOCHEMISTRY/URINALYSIS
CBC: Minimum database for head trauma, and may reveal other concurrent morbitities. Biochemistry profile: Minimum database for head trauma and may reveal other concurrent morbitities.

## OTHER LABORATORY TESTS
To rule out other causes of neurologic signs. Ionized calcium levels may be useful in suspect cases when total calcium is normal but history or clinical signs warrant further investigation for hypocalcemia. Avian blood lead levels > 10 mg/dl are suggestive of lead toxicosis in the presence of clinical signs; > 20 mg/dl are considered diagnostic. Elevated serum zinc levels suggest zinc toxicosis. Avian bornavirus PCR testing may be helpful in birds showing clinical signs. Chlamydiosis PCR testing for the presence of *Chlamydia psittaci*. Electromyography values can determine the health of the muscle cell and the integrity of the motor unit (lower motor neuron and associated muscle fibers) to differentiate peripheral nerve damage from primary muscle disease.

## IMAGING
### Radiographic Findings
Fractures of the spine or skull suggesting a traumatic cause to neurologic signs. Other other causes may be suspected, such as heavy metal with the presence of metallic densities, or avian ganglioneuritis/PDD with dilation of the GI tract.

### Advanced Imaging
CT or MRI useful in evaluating structures within the head and spine, space occupying lesions, areas of trauma or other abnormalities.

## DIAGNOSTIC PROCEDURES
N/A

## PATHOLOGIC FINDINGS
Gross lesions may include hemorrhage of the skull, meninges, and brain, as well as skull fractures. Histologic lesions may also include malacia.

# TREATMENT

## APPROPRIATE HEALTH CARE
Identify and treat the underlying condition. Inpatient treatment is often required cases of ongoing seizure activity, anorexia, lethargy, recumbency, dysphagia, ataxia, or coma. Hypoglycemia, even after seizure activity, is rare, but normoglycemia must be maintained.

Hyperglycemia must also be avoided, shown to exacerbate secondary brain injury. Correction of hypovolemia is critical to maintaining cerebral perfusion. Hypotension leads to significantly worse outcomes.

### NURSING CARE
Fluid therapy to maintain hydration. Oral gavage may be used with mild dehydration and minimal clinical signs. Much more commonly, this may be delivered via SQ, IV or IO routes. Oxygen support with 40% oxygen. Unlike with other emergencies, avoid overheating; placing birds in 70–75°F (21–24°C) environments will avoid the increased cerebral metabolism and demand that occurs at higher temperatures. Nutritional support via gavage or feeding tube if the patient is unable to feed itself. A padded cage may need to be provided if the bird is unable to stand, ataxic, or seizures repeatedly.

### ACTIVITY
If the patient is weakened or has difficulty climbing, then perches, food, and water sources may need to be placed lower in the cage to allow the patient access.

### DIET
In cases where the patient is eating, it is advisable to offer the patient's regular diet, even if it is substandard to assure that the patient continues to eat. Mineral and vitamin deficiencies may be supplemented orally or parenterally. When the patient has recovered, transitioning to a better balanced diet may be performed. If the patient is unable to feed itself, nutritional support via gavage or feeding tube should be performed using a resuspended balanced hand feeding formula.

### CLIENT EDUCATION
Exposure to sources of trauma need to be eliminated. Some neurologic deficits may become permanent, even with swift intervention.

### SURGICAL CONSIDERATIONS
Placement of a ventricular feeding tube via ingluviotomy may be indicated for greater ease of assisted feeding during prolonged recoveries.

## MEDICATIONS
### DRUG(S) OF CHOICE
For controlling seizures, midazolam 0.5–1.0 mg/kg IM; may be repeated up to 3 times if necessary. May also be administered intracloacally—use double the dose. Diazepam may also be administered via continuous IV or IO infusion at 1 mg/kg/h if further seizure control is needed. Once seizures have been controlled for 12–24 hours, the diazepam is tapered to zero over the next 12–24 hours. If further seizure control is needed, phenobarbital may be infused at 2–10 mg/kg/h. Once the seizures have been stopped, phenobarbital may be used for long term seizure control at 2–7 mg/kg PO q12h. Levetiracetam 60 mg/kg IM; can be used for long-term seizure control at dosing up to 100 mg/kg PO q8h. Recent studies suggest that hypertonic saline may be superior to mannitol in reducing cerebral edema, although both have been used for this purpose. Intravascular effects of hypertonic saline in increasing intravascular volume may only last 15 minutes, but these saline induced decreases in intracranial pressure may last much longer. Hypertonic saline benefits may also include shrinkage of endothelial cells improving cerebral blood circulation, a reduction in cerebrospinal fluid production and immunomodulary effects. 7.5% NaCl is administered at 4 ml/kg IV. Mannitol 0.5–1.0 grams/kg IV over 20 minutes. This may be repeated up to 3 times in a 24-hour period.

### CONTRAINDICATIONS
Avoid steroid use in birds with neurologic disease. Birds seem to be more sensitive to the immunosuppressive effects of steroids, and this might worsen clinical signs, particularly if the cause is infectious. Steroid use may also lead to hyperglycemia, which is shown to have a poorer prognosis in head trauma.

### PRECAUTIONS
Avoid overheating. Correct hypovolemia before administering mannitol.

### POSSIBLE INTERACTIONS
N/A

### ALTERNATIVE DRUGS
N/A

## FOLLOW-UP
### PATIENT MONITORING
Successive neurologic exams are essential to monitor response to treatment and prognosis.

### PREVENTION/AVOIDANCE
Eliminating or limiting exposure to sources of trauma (e.g. ceiling fans, other animals).

### POSSIBLE COMPLICATIONS
Some neurologic signs may be permanent, and may persist even after treatment.

### EXPECTED COURSE AND PROGNOSIS
Varies with the severity of the primary trauma and the speed with which the secondary brain injury can be slowed or reversed.

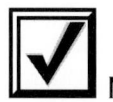

## MISCELLANEOUS
### ASSOCIATED CONDITIONS
N/A

### AGE-RELATED FACTORS
N/A

### ZOONOTIC POTENTIAL
N/A

### FERTILITY/BREEDING
N/A

### SYNONYMS
N/A

### SEE ALSO
Atherosclerosis
Avian Influenza
Bornaviral Diseases
Botulism
Dyslipidemia/Hyperlipidemia
Hypocalcemia and Hypomagnesemia
Liver Disease
Mycotoxicosis
Neoplasia (Neurologic)
Neurologic (Non-Traumatic Diseases)
Otitis
Orthoavulavirus
Seizures
Sick-Bird Syndrome
Toxicosis (Environmental/Pesticides)
Toxicosis (Heavy Metals)
Toxicosis (Iatrogenic)
Toxicosis (Ingested, Gastrointestinal)
Trauma
West Nile Virus
Appendix 8, Algorithm 9: Neurologic Signs

### ABBREVIATIONS
ATP—adenosine triphosphate
CN—cranial nerve
CT—computed tomography
GI—gastrointestinal
MRI—magnetic resonance imaging
NSAID—nonsteroidal anti-inflammatory drug
PCR—polymerase chain reaction
PDD—proventricular dilatation disease
TBI—traumatic brain injury

### INTERNET RESOURCES
N/A

AVIAN 307

(CONTINUED)                                    NEUROLOGIC (TRAUMA)

*Suggested Reading*

Powers L.V. (2018). Treatment of beak and skull injuries and psittacine birds. *AAVUC-UPAV.*

Jolly, M. (2015). Treatment of traumatic brain injury in morepork owls: a review of diagnostic and treatment options. *AAVAC-UPAV.*

Antinoff, N., Orosz, S.E. (2012). Don't be nervous! A clinician's approach to the avian neurologic system. *Proceedings of the Association of Avian Veterinarians Annual Conference*, Louisville, KT.

Clippinger, T.L., Bennett, R.A., Platt, S.R. (2007). The avian neurologic examination and ancillary neurodiagnostic techniques: A review update. *Veterinary Clinics of North America. Exotic Animal Practice*, 10:803–836.

Orosz, S.E., Bradshaw, G.A. (2007). Avian neuroanatomy revisited: From clinical principles to avian cognition. *Veterinary Clinics of North America. Exotic Animal Practice*, 10:775–802.

**Author**: Author Stephen Dyer, DVM, DABVP (Avian)

N

# NUTRITIONAL IMBALANCES

 **BASICS**

## DEFINITION

Nutritional deficiency can be defined as an insufficient intake of a bioavailable nutrient essential to support a given physiological state. There are approximately 30 essential nutrients in birds; however, the requirements likely vary greatly between species according to their natural habitat and diet. Despite these differences, analysis of crop content of free-living nestling parrots of different species and geography appears similar in its nutritional content. Theoretically, a deficiency state is possible for any essential nutrient; however, some deficiencies have only been experimentally produced, whereas others are commonly seen in practice. Deficiencies are more likely to have a clinical manifestation during times of growth, reproduction, stress, or disease; however, birds that appear healthy to the owner may have subclinical deficiencies that may increase the risk of morbidity or they may have mild signs. A classic example of a deficient diet in pet birds is a seed-only diet. This type of diet is deficient in many essential nutrients including total protein, vitamin A, vitamin D, calcium, and phosphorous.

## PATHOPHYSIOLOGY

The predominant cause of nutritional deficiencies is poor diet. Less commonly, primary malabsorption may also cause nutritional deficiencies. An all-seed diet, unbalanced home-prepared diets, and poor quality commercial feeds have all been demonstrated as causes of nutritional imbalances. As many nutrients are required for energy metabolism, a high-fat or calorically dense diet may lead to relative deficiencies. Each deficiency may cause characteristic pathology (e.g. iodine deficiency will affect thyroid function and may cause goiter, whereas vitamin A deficiency may cause squamous metaplasia affecting the epithelium and mucus membranes).

## SYSTEMS AFFECTED

Any system may be affected depending on the type of deficiency or imbalance. Common examples include behavioral—changes in vocalization patterns have been observed in cockatiels fed a vitamin A/carotenoid deficient diet; endocrine/metabolic—iodine deficiency may cause goiter in budgerigars; however, this is not usually accompanied by decreased thyroid hormones in circulation.

**Gastrointestinal**: Vitamin A deficiency may cause squamous metaplasia, which may manifest as oral plaques or a decrease in number or appearance of the choanal papillae (species dependent).

**Hemic/lymphatic/immune**: Vitamins A and E have a role as immune modulators and deficiencies in these vitamins may exacerbate other morbidities.

**Hepatobiliary**: Biotin deficiency may cause hepatic lipidosis in cockatiels.

**Musculoskeletal**: Vitamin D, calcium, and phosphorus deficiencies or imbalances may cause metabolic bone disease and developmental pathology.

**Nervous**: Thiamine deficiency may cause neurologic signs. Most commonly seen in pescivorous birds that have ingested thiaminase-containing fish. Vitamin E deficiency may cause encephalomalacia and generalized neurologic signs.

**Neuromuscular**: Calcium deficiency may cause seizures or seizure-like muscle tremors; African grey parrots appear to be particularly susceptible. Magnesium deficiency may exacerbate clinical signs associated with calcium deficiency, as it can regulate secretion of the parathyroid hormone and can affect calcium metabolism. Vitamin E deficiency may cause torticollis.

**Ophthalmic**: Vitamin A deficiency may cause pathologic keratinization of the conjunctival mucus membranes, swelling, irritation, severe pain, and in advanced cases inability to open the eyes.

**Renal/urologic**: Vitamin A deficiency may cause squamous metaplasia affecting the renal tubules and subsequently renal disease.

**Reproductive**: Vitamin D and/or calcium deficiencies may predispose females to dystocia or egg binding and abnormal shell production. Vitamin A deficiency may cause embryonic death or congenital defects. Respiratory vitamin A deficiency may cause crusting around the nares or cere. Vitamin A deficiency may predispose birds to secondary respiratory infection.

**Skin/exocrine**: Vitamin A deficiency may cause poor plumage, decreased coloring (as carotenoids play a part in synthesis of some pigments). Vitamin A deficiency may cause uropygial gland (preen gland) disorders such as inflammation and impaction. Protein deficiency may cause an abnormal and thin plumage. Specifically, methionine deficiency has been associated with streaks across the feathers known as stress bars.

## GENETICS
N/A

## INCIDENCE/PREVALENCE

The prevalence of nutritional imbalance is still considered high, despite increased awareness to the importance of incorporation of formulated pelleted diet in pet bird nutrition. Wild birds nursed by good Samaritans may also present with nutritional deficiencies.

## GEOGRAPHIC DISTRIBUTION
N/A

## SIGNALMENT

**Species**: Any species may be affected; however, deficiencies are less likely in birds that are allowed to roam freely and select food on their own (such as roaming wild birds, backyard poultry, or waterfowl).

**Mean age and range**: Any age could be affected, growing animals and reproducing animals are more vulnerable.

**Predominant sex**: Females are more likely to be affected during reproduction. Otherwise, both sexes are equally at risk.

## SIGNS

### Historical Findings

Comprehensive diet history should always be included as part of the medical history. This should include type of diet fed, amounts offered and consumed, and frequency and type of treats provided. Other pertinent information regarding previous diets, length of time fed current diet, and any information regarding bodyweight fluctuations should also be noted.

### Physical Examination Findings

Obesity. Failure to thrive. Blunted choanal papillae. Poor body condition. Poor plumage. Neurologic signs. Weakness/tremors. Limb deformity.

## CAUSES

Nutritional deficiencies are the result of an imbalanced diet, most commonly an all-seed diet or an imbalanced home-prepared diet that consists of human food items. Vitamin E and thiamine deficiencies have been described in piscivorous birds as fish may contain thiaminase that breaks down thiamine and fatty fish contain high levels of lipids, which may become oxidized and may reduce availability of vitamin E.

## RISK FACTORS

History of an imbalanced diet; all-seed diets, unbalanced home-cooked diets, and inappropriate diets for a reared wild bird are all possible risk factors. High fat may increase the risk for nutritional deficiencies if diets are not balanced.

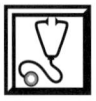 **DIAGNOSIS**

## DIFFERENTIAL DIAGNOSIS

Dermatologic pathologies resulting from vitamin A deficiency may need to be differentiated from neoplastic, traumatic, or infectious processes depending on appearance and location. Seizures and neurologic abnormalities caused by calcium deficiency or thiamine deficiency need to be differentiated from neurologic disease associated with trauma, infection, inflammation, or idiopathic processes. Skeletal pathology caused by calcium, phosphorous, or vitamin D deficiency should be differentiated from congenital abnormalities, infectious diseases causing abnormal growth, protein/energy malnutrition, or trauma.

## CBC/BIOCHEMISTRY/URINALYSIS
CBC: Deficiencies of folate or iron may cause nonregenerative anemia; however, these conditions are not commonly seen. Riboflavin and pyridoxine deficiencies may cause an increase in heterophil counts and a decrease in lymphocyte counts. Biochemistry: Hypocalcemia may be seen in birds on a calcium deficient diet; however, normal total calcium does not rule out hypocalcemia and ionized calcium measurement may be indicated to assess the bird's calcium status. Hypomagnesemia may accompany hypocalcemia. Hyperuricemia may result from kidney disease secondary to vitamin A deficiency.

## OTHER LABORATORY TESTS
Specific tests are available to diagnose specific nutritional deficiencies (e.g. thiamine deficiency may be diagnosed by decreased serum transketolase activity). However, common deficiencies such as vitamin A deficiency cannot be easily diagnosed using blood tests alone.

## IMAGING
Skeletal pathology resulting from vitamin D, phosphorous, or calcium deficiencies may be viewed on radiographs. Coelomic ultrasound may be beneficial in evaluating parenchymatic changes associated with hepatic lipidosis due to biotin deficiency or for the diagnosis of hepatopathies associated with vitamin A, copper, or iron accumulation.

## DIAGNOSTIC PROCEDURES
Hepatic biopsies are used for quantification and diagnosis of vitamin A deficiency or toxicity. Skin biopsies may be useful in diagnosing vitamin A deficiency, which characteristically manifests as squamous metaplasia. Deficiencies in B vitamins may be detected with high-performance liquid chromatography, for instance for detection of thiamine deficiency. Thiamine deficiency may also be diagnosed with an erythrocyte transketolase assay. Low or borderline-low plasma ionized calcium may be a finding in birds with calcium or severe vitamin D deficiency. Response to therapy may also be the diagnostic method employed in some cases where the index of suspicion for a

nutritional deficiency is high (e.g. resolution of goitre in response to correction of iodine intake or improvement in ophthalmic or respiratory signs in response to an improved diet with sufficient vitamin A).

## PATHOLOGIC FINDINGS
Vitamin A deficiency may cause pathology affecting epithelial tissues throughout the body; specifically, epithelial turn over and keratinization. These non-specific changes are called squamous metaplasia. Pathology associated with calcium, phosphorous, or vitamin D deficiency includes skeletal changes. Postmortem findings in birds with severe nutritional imbalances are beyond the scope of this section and may be found elsewhere.

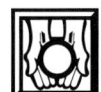

## TREATMENT

### APPROPRIATE HEALTH CARE
Most often patients diagnosed with nutritional deficiencies may be managed as outpatients with recommendations to correct the diet and additional supplementation if needed. Vitamin A deficiency causing respiratory disease, seizures due to hypocalcemia, severe respiratory distress due to goiter, and dystocia due to calcium deficiency are some examples of nutritional deficiencies that need to be addressed urgently with supportive care in parallel with dietary correction and supplementation.

### NURSING CARE
Nursing care is required in cases of birds presenting with acute clinical signs as described above. Oxygen support, medical seizure management, and fluid therapy may be needed in cases of acute respiratory distress or seizures. Calcium by injection may help with seizure control in birds presenting with acute hypocalcemia and may also assist in dystocia with a possible nutritional background. Budgerigars with goiter due to iodine deficiency presenting with acute respiratory distress may need oxygen support. Injectable glucocorticoids may be used as emergency treatment to relieve goiter associated dyspnea.

### ACTIVITY
There is no need for activity alteration in most cases. Birds suffering from nutritional deficiencies affecting their bone health may need to be restricted in activity until bone quality improves.

### DIET
Unbalanced diet should be addressed to resolve most nutritional deficiencies.

Current recommendations for psittacine diets are that 50–75% of the daily caloric intake to be provided by commercial pelleted diets and the rest from a selection of fruits, vegetables, and small amounts of seeds, grains and nuts. The nutritional content of common food items may be found on nutrient databases online, such as FoodData Central.

### CLIENT EDUCATION
Client education is key for the management of poor nutrition. The importance of balanced nutrition should be discussed as part of a wellness examination or a new-bird examination. For pet psittacines, directions should be provided to allow the owner to select from good-quality commercial formulated pelleted diets. Providing the bird several diets as options may be a good way to find a preferred diet and make dietary transition an easier process. An appropriate treat/produce allowance should also be included.

### SURGICAL CONSIDERATIONS
N/A

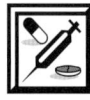

## MEDICATIONS
### DRUG(S) OF CHOICE
Vitamin and mineral supplementation may be included in the management of nutritional deficiencies, especially in acute cases or short term while the patient is transitioned to an appropriate diet. Calcium gluconate (10%) 5–100 mg/kg IM/slow IV may be given to psittacines or raptors in acute hypocalcemia. May cause arrhythmias, so monitor heart rate while administering. Magnesium sulphate 20 mg/kg IM single treatment (or as needed) for hypomagnesemia. Iodine (sodium iodide 20%) 2 mg (0.01 ml)/bird IM as needed. Vitamin A 20,000–30,000 iu/kg IM. Thiamine 1–3 mg/kg IM every 7 days. Vitamin $D_3$ 3300 iu/kg IM every 7 days as needed. Beware of excessive use leading to hypervitaminosis D. Moderate sunlight exposure (11–30 minutes/day, avoiding overheating) may be used in conjunction or as replacement.

### CONTRAINDICATIONS
None.

### PRECAUTIONS
None.

### POSSIBLE INTERACTIONS
N/A

### ALTERNATIVE DRUGS
N/A

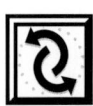

## FOLLOW-UP

### PATIENT MONITORING
Monitoring of response to treatment and dietary modification is important to assess accuracy of diagnosis and owner compliance. Diet transition may be challenging in many cases and owners can find the process exasperating without proper guidance.

### PREVENTION/AVOIDANCE
Providing a balanced diet and avoiding all-seed or home-prepared unbalanced diets.

### POSSIBLE COMPLICATIONS
Changes to the respiratory and oral epithelium may cause ulcerations and secondary infections.

### EXPECTED COURSE AND PROGNOSIS
Most clinical signs described above are expected to resolve with appropriate nutrition. Some anatomic changes associated with chronic deficiencies may be permanent.

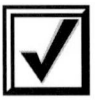

## MISCELLANEOUS

### ASSOCIATED CONDITIONS
N/A

### AGE-RELATED FACTORS
Growing animals and reproducing females are generally more susceptible to clinical manifestation. It is also hypothesized that geriatric animals in general have altered nutritional requirements and may be more prone to clinical deficiencies.

### ZOONOTIC POTENTIAL
None.

### FERTILITY/BREEDING
Reproducing females have higher energy and nutrient demands. Calcium metabolism is paramount for eggshell deposition, embryonic tissues, and contractions during egg laying; therefore, deficiencies in either calcium or vitamin D may predispose a bird to egg binding or dystocia. Vitamin A is associated with successful breeding; therefore, it is necessary to ensure that the reproductive female is fed an appropriate diet even prior to breeding.

### SYNONYMS
Nutritional deficiencies, nutritional insufficiency, dietary imbalance.

### SEE ALSO
Beak Malocclusion (Lateral Beak Deformity)
Chronic Egg Laying
Dystocia and Egg Binding
Hypocalcemia and Hypomagnesemia
Infertility
Lameness
Iron Storage Disease
Metabolic Bone Disease
Obesity
Oral Plaques
Pododermatitis
Rhinitis and Sinusitis
Seizures
Thyroid Diseases
Toe and Nail Diseases
Trauma
Vitamin D Toxicosis

### ABBREVIATIONS
N/A

### INTERNET RESOURCES
US Department of Agriculture. FoodData Central: https://fdc.nal.usda.gov
Nutrition Advisory Group to the Association of Zoos and Aquariums: http://nagonline.net.

*Suggested Reading*
Brightsmith, D.J. (2012). Nutritional levels of diets fed to captive Amazon parrots: does mixing seed, produce, and pellets provide a healthy diet? *Journal of Avian Medicine and Surgery*, 26:149–160.
Cornejo, J., Dierenfeld, E.S., Renton, K., et al. (2022). Nutrition of free-living neotropical psittacine nestlings and implications for hand-feeding formulas. *Journal of Animal Physiology and Animal Nutrition*, 106:1174–1188.
Fidgett, A.L., Gardner, L. (2014). Advancing avian nutrition through best feeding practice. *International Zoo Yearbook*, 48:116–127.
Hess, L., Mauldin, G., Rosenthal, K. (2002). Estimated nutrient content of diets commonly fed to pet birds. *Veterinary Record*, 150:399–404.
Koutsos, E.A., Matson, K.D., Klasing, K.C. (2001). Nutrition of birds in the order Psittaciformes: A review. *Journal of Avian Medicine and Surgery*, 15:257–275.
Schmidt, R.E., Reavill, D.R., Phalen, D.N. (2003). *Pathology of Pet and Aviary Birds*, 2nd edn. Ames, IA: Wiley-Blackwell.
**Author:** Jonathan Stockman, DVM, DACVIM (Nutrition)

**Client Education Handout available online**

# BASICS

## DEFINITION
Obesity is one of the most common nutritional diseases of pet birds and is defined as those whose body weight exceeds optimal by > 20%.

## PATHOPHYSIOLOGY
Obesity occurs when energy intake chronically exceeds energy expenditure due to: (1) lower metabolic requirement (some species); (2) increased efficiency of energy absorption; (3) decreased energy expenditure; or (4) increased intake (e.g. high-calorie diets, poor nutritional content, or poor biofeedback of satiation).

## SYSTEMS AFFECTED
**Dermatological**: Lipomas, xanthomatosis, pododermatitis.
**Reproductive**: Infertility, dystocia.
**Cardiovascular**: Atherosclerosis, heart failure.
**Hepatic**: Hepatic lipidosis.
**Respiratory**: Air sac impingement by visceral fat.
**Gastrointestinal**: Lipomas and fatty deposits may cause crop impingement leading to regurgitation.
**Endocrine**: Hypothyroidism.

## GENETICS
There may be a genetic basis for obesity.

## INCIDENCE/PREVALENCE
Common in captive species with high caloric intake.

## GEOGRAPHIC DISTRIBUTION
Worldwide among captive avian species.

## SIGNALMENT
**Species**: Common in many companion birds. Amazons, budgerigars, quaker parrots, rose-breasted and sulfur-crested cockatoos, pigeons, and waterfowl are particularly susceptible.
**Mean age and range**: Risk may increase with age and subsequent decrease in metabolic rate.
**Predominant sex**: Both sexes equally susceptible.

## SIGNS
### Historical Findings
Exercise intolerance. Seed-based diet (especially sunflower, safflower, hemp, rape, nyjer, spray millet). Other high fat diet ("table food" nuts, especially peanuts/peanut butter, cheese, eggs, etc). Limited exercise/sedentary lifestyle.

### Physical Examination Findings
Pectoral soft tissue may bulge bilaterally to keel. Excessive fat in coelom, axillae/flank, and subcutis. Excessive caudal coelomic fat can cause Coelomic distention. Skin may

have yellowish tint from underlying fat or xanthomatosis. Lipomas may be present, particularly over cranial sternum and crop area. Skin over lipomas may be xanthomatous, ulcerated, or focal necrosis may occur. Keel bone may be difficult to palpate. Plumage may appear to have bald patches due to dilation of aptera from subcutaneous fat. A wide-based stance may be present. Dyspnea due to compression of abdominal and caudal thoracic air sacs by visceral fat (especially Amazon parrots, budgerigars, cockatiels, Pionus parrots).

## CAUSES
Excess consumption of foods high in simple starches or fats. Excess consumption of deficient diets to satisfy nutritional demands. Behavioral polyphagia secondary to boredom. Lower energy requirements in some species (budgerigars, quakers, and rose-breasted cockatoos are suspected examples). Lack of sufficient exercise either through behavioral tendencies (Amazon parrots) or husbandry deficiency. Hypothyroidism is sometimes speculated but is difficult to confirm using laboratory testing and may be overdiagnosed.

## RISK FACTORS
See Signalment section.

# DIAGNOSIS

## DIFFERENTIAL DIAGNOSIS
**Differentiating similar signs**: Sick birds may appear bulked due to fluffed plumage. Palpation of the keel and pectoral muscles will distinguish the obese bird from the sick bird, which is often underweight. Caudal coelomic distention can also be caused by organomegaly, masses, or ascites.
**Differentiating causes**: An exhaustive history of diet both offered and consumed should be taken, including all treats, as well as frequency and amounts fed, to elucidate if and how excess calories are provided. A thorough history of opportunities for activity should be taken, including cage size, time and activities outside cage, and access to swings and ladders.

## CBC/BIOCHEMISTRY/URINALYSIS
Complete blood count is typically normal. Biochemistry panel may be normal or may show elevations in liver enzymes or hypercholesterolemia. Lipemia may be present and may indicate hepatic lipidosis, with or without liver enzymes elevations.

## OTHER LABORATORY TESTS
Separate addition of cholesterol may need to some biochemical panels. Persistently elevated cholesterol may warrant a lipoprotein electrophoresis. Serum thyroxine

levels and TSH stimulation testing are needed to confirm suspected hypothyroidism.

## IMAGING
Obesity may complicate radiography due to loss of caudal coelomic detail and increased soft-tissue density overlying the air sacs. The liver silhouette is frequently enlarged with loss of the cardiohepatic "waist."

## DIAGNOSTIC PROCEDURES
N/A

## PATHOLOGIC FINDINGS
N/A

# TREATMENT

## APPROPRIATE HEALTH CARE
In patients of adequate health based on physical examination, radiography, and CBC/biochemistry panel evaluations, decreasing dietary caloric content and increasing activity is usually the most effective treatment for obesity. Concurrent illnesses (hepatic, renal, other metabolic, infectious, etc.) should be addressed prior to initiating changes in diet or activity.

## NURSING CARE
Weight loss should be monitored closely so as not to exceed 3% of body weight/week. Weight loss in excess of 3% body weight/week in obese birds may result in hepatic lipidosis.

## ACTIVITY
Activity may be increased through opportunities to increase flight or walking locomotion and other environmental enrichment activities including the encouragement of foraging behaviors. Cage furniture such as swings and ladders can encourage physical activity. Increasing cage size may benefit some birds. Time outside the cage can be increased to encourage flying, climbing, and play. Many birds (particularly Amazons, budgerigars, cockatiels, and cockatoos) enjoy a variety of music, and can be encouraged to bob and "dance" with their owners to music the bird likes. This may be of most use for very overweight and sedentary birds to begin increasing activity without overstressing extremely unfit individuals. Increased frequency of bathing can add flapping, feather shaking, and active grooming. Increased diversity of activities in addition to providing foraging activities may help decrease polyphagia secondary to boredom.

## DIET
Foraging toys and techniques can help slow the rate of calorie intake, known to be more rapid in captivity. Although dietary improvements may be needed, changes should

O

# OBESITY                                              (CONTINUED)

be gradual to prevent anorexia due to aversion or non-recognition of the novel food item. Reductions in food volume, fat content, and changes in overall dietary composition may be needed. An ideal diet is 80% commercial pellet to 20% fruit and vegetables on a dry weight, except macaws, which require a greater amount of fat in their diet, and cockatiels consuming greater than 50% pellets, which may be at risk for renal dysfunction. Transitioning to a pelleted diet can take many months, particularly if it is a novel food to the bird. Many repeated offerings of novel foods are required before it will be tasted and eventually accepted, similar to mammalian species: 10–13 months of consistently offering a food may be required in very novelty-phobic individuals. During the transition phase, birds will often fling their pellets with a sharp head flick. Although this resembles a human expression of disgust, it may simply signify the end of that particular tasting experience and should in no way discourage the owner from continuing to present the desired new diet. Pellets can be offered near a preferred perch or in a preferred food dish or foraging toy to increase appeal. Small birds are more likely to pick at pellets spread on a flat surface on plain white paper or on a mirrored surface. For highly bonded birds, the owner may pretend to eat the food to generate interest. For birds that already eat one non-seed food item, only that food and pellets may be offered in the morning, when appetite is highest. Seeds may be withheld and presented later in the day. (Note: it is very important that this technique only be attempted in birds that have been assessed as healthy enough to endure a brief fast if they refuse this meal, preferably via a thorough physical examination and minimal database of radiographs, CBC, and biochemistry chemistry panel.)

## CLIENT EDUCATION
See Diet and Prevention/Avoidance sections.

## SURGICAL CONSIDERATIONS
Lipomas may require surgical resection if correction of diet and activity do not cause reduction, particularly in cases of significant crop impingement or necrosis. Some lipomas are very vascular, and hemostatic techniques may be needed.

# MEDICATIONS

## DRUG(S) OF CHOICE
L-carnitine (1000 mg/kg of feed) for lipomas. L-thyroxine (0.1 mg/4 oz drinking water for

1–4 months) to be used for documented hypothyroidism only.

## CONTRAINDICATIONS
The use of thyroid hormone treatment is not recommended in obesity of non-thyroid origin, as dangerous cardiovascular complications can ensue.

## PRECAUTIONS
See Appropriate Health Care and Nursing Care sections.

## POSSIBLE INTERACTIONS
N/A

## ALTERNATIVE DRUGS
N/A

# FOLLOW-UP

## PATIENT MONITORING
See Appropriate Health Care and Nursing Care sections.

## PREVENTION/AVOIDANCE
Birds should be fed a species-appropriate high-quality, nutritionally sound diet. Ample opportunity for exercise must be provided, as well as encouragement for sedentary individuals.

## POSSIBLE COMPLICATIONS
Associated hepatic lipidosis can affect drug metabolism, particularly of anesthetics. Hypercholesterolemia, atherosclerosis, and heart failure have all been associated with chronic obesity. Visceral fat deposits can cause air sac impingement, compromising respiratory effort. Fatty or lipomatous deposits over the crop can cause regurgitation. Incidence of dystocia may be increased. Pododermatitis and arthritis may be exacerbated.

## EXPECTED COURSE AND PROGNOSIS
Dietary improvements and increased activity can be difficult to achieve, as they usually require changes in both owner and patient behavior. Owing to the high metabolic rate of birds, husbandry corrections often reverse obesity and prevent complications.

# MISCELLANEOUS

## ASSOCIATED CONDITIONS
See Possible Complications section.

## AGE-RELATED FACTORS
See Signalment section.

## ZOONOTIC POTENTIAL
N/A

## FERTILITY/BREEDING
Both male and female fertility may be impaired, although the mechanism of this is not completely understood.

## SYNONYMS
N/A

## SEE ALSO
Atherosclerosis
Coelomic Distention
Hepatic Lipidosis
Dyslipidemia/Hyperlipidemia
Infertility
Nutritional Imbalances
Pododermatitis
Regurgitation and Vomiting
Thyroid Diseases
Xanthoma/Xanthogranulomatosis

## ABBREVIATIONS
TSH—thyroid-stimulating hormone

## INTERNET RESOURCES
N/A

*Suggested Reading*
Koutsos, E., Gelis, S., Echols, M.S. (2016). Advancements in nutrition and nutritional therapy. In: *Current Therapy in Avian Medicine and Surgery* (ed. B.L. Speer), 142–150. St. Louis, MO: Elsevier.
Macwhirter, P. (1994). Malnutrition. In: *Avian Medicine: Principles and Application* (ed. B.W. Ritchie, G.J. Harrison, L.R. Harrison), 842–861. Lake Worth, FL: Wingers Publishing.
McDonald, D. (2006). Nutritional considerations: Section I. In: *Clinical Avian Medicine* (ed. G.J. Harrison, T.L. Lightfoot), Vol. I, 86–107. Palm Beach, FL: Spix Publishing.
Reid R.B., Perlberg W. (1998). Emerging trends in pet bird diets. *Journal of the American Veterinary Medical Association*, 212:1236–1237.
Rupley, A.E. (1997). Nutritional diseases. In: *Manual of Avian Practice*, 298–301. Philadelphia, PA: Saunders.
Smith, J.M, Roudybush, T.E. (1997). Nutritional disorders. In: *Avian Medicine and Surgery* (ed. R.B. Altman, S.L. Clubb, G.M. Dorrestein, K. Quesenberry), 501–516. Philadelphia, PA: Saunders.
**Author**: Julia Shakeri, DVM, DABVP (Avian Practice)
**Acknowledgements**: Elisabeth Simone-Freilicher, DVM, DABVP (Avian Practice), author of first edition chapter.

# BASICS

## DEFINITION
Any abnormality of the eye or associated structures. The most common ophthalmologic lesions including cataracts, conjunctivitis, periocular swelling, uveitis and retinal detachment are addressed.

## PATHOPHYSIOLOGY
**Cataracts**: A cataract is opacity of any part of the lens or its capsule. Cataracts may be associated with malformation, genetic disorders, nutritional deficiency, trauma, senescence, toxicity, or other ocular disorders.
**Conjunctivitis**: Conjunctivitis is inflammation of the conjunctiva and is one of the most common ocular lesions in pet birds. Common causes of conjunctivitis include vitamin A deficiency, infection, and toxins. Inflammation can be secondary to trauma, such as that experienced during handling, shipping, self-induced, or from a conspecific.
**Periocular swelling**: Periocular swelling involves focal or diffuse disorders of the eyelids, infraorbital sinus, or nasal gland. Common causes of periocular swelling include trauma, infections, neoplasia, and nutritional deficiency.
**Uveitis**: Uveitis is the term for inflammation of the uvea and can be divided into categories based on location—anterior, intermediate, posterior, and panuveitic. Causes of uveitis can include trauma, infection, immune-mediated, and neoplasia.
**Retinal disease**: Retinal detachment can be either retinal separation or a tear. Retinal separation occurs between the retinal pigment epithelium and neural retinal, resulting in subretinal fluid, exudate, etc. A retinal tear is most often due to trauma in raptors.

## SYSTEMS AFFECTED
**Ophthalmic**: This is the primary system affected.
**Behavioral**: Birds may present for anorexia or behavior changes if vision is compromised.
**Gastrointestinal**: Birds may present for anorexia or non-specific signs of illness.
**Hemic/lymphatic/immune**: In immune-mediated conditions.
**Reproductive**: Reproduction may be affected if vision is compromised.
**Respiratory**: Birds may have abnormal respiration if disease extends into the sinuses or upper airway.
**Skin/exocrine**: Birds may present for visible swellings or skin discoloration.

## GENETICS
Hereditary cataract has been reported in Norwich and Yorkshire canaries. Cataract and optic nerve hypoplasia has been reported in turkeys.

## INCIDENCE/PREVALENCE
Conjunctivitis is one of the most common ocular lesions in pet birds. *Mycoplasma gallisepticum* has caused outbreaks of conjunctivitis in wild house finches. Hyphema was the most frequent ocular finding in a retrospective survey of ocular examinations in raptors. 15.4% of 24 psittacines in quarantine that died were found to have cataracts.

## GEOGRAPHIC DISTRIBUTION
Worldwide distribution.

## SIGNALMENT
**Species**: All avian species are susceptible to these conditions. Pet psittacine birds and passerines (conjunctivitis), raptors secondary to trauma (uveitis), canaries (cataracts).
**Mean age and range**: Aged birds are more likely to have cataracts. All age ranges can be affected by these conditions.
**Predominant sex**: None.

## SIGNS

### General Comments
Signs can be non-specific or birds may present with visible lesions.

### Historical Findings
Owners may report gradual or sudden changes in behavior or appearance based on the condition. Squinting indicates that the affected eye is painful.

### Physical Examination Findings
**Periocular swelling**: Eyelids and/or periocular areas may appear uniformly or focally swollen, erythematous, and/or scaly; palpebral fissure width may be reduced; nictitans may be prolapsed; eyelid and periocular feather loss; discharge to the point of eyelids matted together; conjunctival hyperemia or swelling and/or facial swelling; facial rubbing.
**Corneal pathology**: Ulceration detected with application of fluorescein stain. Cornea scars are opaque, but fluorescein negative. Psittacines and aged falcons often develop crystalline corneal deposits.
**Conjunctivitis**: Hyperemia, blepharospasm, variable photophobia, chemosis, serous to mucopurulent discharge; nictitans mobility may be impaired; eyelid margins may be sealed together; periocular feather loss and self-trauma may occur.
**Cataracts**: Lens opacities identified by direct or retroillumination may be focal to diffuse, dyscoria and posterior synechiae in cases with previous or current uveitis, lens luxation or subluxation in chronic cataracts, vision loss depending on extent of disease, globe size reduced in cases of congenital microphthalmos or acquired phthisis.
**Uveitis**: Photophobia, blepharospasm, corneal edema, aqueous flare, hypopyon, vitreous opacity, hypotony or secondary

glaucoma, miosis, dyscoria, iris thickening or discoloration, rubeosis irides, and or posterior synechiae are signs of uveitis. Aqueous flare may be detected with a bright light source focused to the smallest diameter possible, in a darkened room, with the examiner looking perpendicular to the direction of the light beam. Focal to diffuse retinal edema, hemorrhage, retinal detachment, and vitreal opacity may be present in cases of active posterior uveitis. Diffuse corneal edema, posterior synechiae, anterior synechiae, secondary glaucoma, cataract, retinal atrophy, chronic detachment, and blindness can be sequelae of chronic uveitis.
**Retinal detachment**: Retinal detachment may be serous, with fluid accumulation between the retina and retinal pigmented epithelium. Detachment may also be the result of a tear in the retina, often visible on ophthalmoscopy. Retinal tears occur most often as the result of trauma, especially in raptors.

## CAUSES
**Cataracts**: Hereditary cataract in canaries, in association with crooked toe in Brahma chickens, maternal vitamin E deficiency in turkeys can cause cataract in offspring, blunt or perforating trauma, aging change, dinitrophenol fed to chicks, avian encephalomyelitis, and chronic uveitis and retinal degeneration.
**Conjunctivitis**: Trauma, vitamin A deficiency, infectious causes (bacteria, mollicutes including *Mycoplasma*, *Ureaplasma*, *Acholeplasma*, viruses, nematodes, and trematodes). Bacterial causes can include *Pseudomonas*, *Staphylococcus*, *Pasteurella*, *Citrobacter*, *Escherichia coli*, *Actinobacter*, *Actinobacillus*, *Erysipelothrix*, *Clostridium botulinum*, *Mycobacteria* sp., *Bordetella avium*, *Chlamydia psittaci*, *Haemophilus*, *Salmonella* sp., *Aeromonas*. Fungal causes can include *Candida* and *Aspergillus* sp. Viral causes include poxviruses, herpesviruses, avian influenza virus, paramyxovirus, adenovirus, cytomegalovirus, and others. Parasitic causes can include *Ceratospira*, *Oxyspirura*, *Philophthalmus*, *Thelazia*, *Serratia*, and cryptosporidium. Photosensitization from certain plants, chemical/ammonia burn, foreign bodies and neoplasia have also been associated with conjunctivitis.
**Periocular swelling**: Many of the same causes of conjunctivitis listed above including trauma, infections (bacterial, parasitic, viral), nutritional deficiency, and neoplasia. In addition to the above differentials, *Knemidokoptes pilae*, infraorbital sinusitis, and nasal or salt gland inflammation can result in periocular swelling.
**Uveitis**: Blunt or perforating trauma (often involving hemorrhage), corneal ulceration,

O

viral (including herpesvirus-induced lymphomatosis and West Nile virus), bacterial (*Pasteurella*, salmonellosis, *Mycoplasma*, others), mycotic (*Aspergillus*), protozoal infection (toxoplasmosis), and neoplasia can also cause uveitis.

**Retinal detachment**: Common sequela of trauma, especially in raptors.

### RISK FACTORS
Birds on inadequate diets may be predisposed to ocular lesions related to hypovitaminosis A. Birds housed in unsanitary conditions may be predisposed to ammonia or other irritant-induced conjunctivitis. Inappropriate housing may predispose to traumatic injury. Vitamin E deficiency in turkey hens results in cataracts of offspring. Brahma chickens with crooked toes have been reported to develop spontaneous cataracts.

## DIAGNOSIS

### DIFFERENTIAL DIAGNOSIS
Subcutaneous emphysema from air sac trauma or leakage can give the appearance of pathology around the neck and face. Ink from newsprint or toys and even owner lipstick can cause discoloration around the eyes. Upper respiratory disease or regurgitation can cause matting of the feathers around the face and eyes that could be mistaken for ocular disease. Ocular disease in poultry is often a manifestation of systemic disease.

### CBC/BIOCHEMISTRY/URINALYSIS
Blood work may or may not be helpful depending on etiology of disease. CBC changes may be present with infectious or chronic disease. A minimum diagnostic database is helpful to rule out underlying disease.

### OTHER LABORATORY TESTS
*Chlamydia, Mycoplasma*, viral, fungal, and parasitic screening tests are indicated if signs warrant. Bacterial or fungal cultures may be indicated. Paranasal flush or aspirates can be submitted for cytologic examination and/or culture.

### IMAGING
Radiographs of the head and whole body may be indicated as part of a complete workup and to rule out underlying respiratory disease. CT may be more helpful for evaluating sinuses than plain radiography. Contrast radiography has been reported. Ultrasound can be helpful to assess the globe and surrounding tissues.

### DIAGNOSTIC PROCEDURES
Complete ophthalmologic examination is crucial for any ocular or orbital problem. This includes fluorescein stain and tonometry. An otoscope without a cone provides magnification for examination of the anterior chamber. The direct ophthalmoscope set on the slit beam in a darkened room may be used to detect aqueous flare. Posterior segment examination may be performed with either a direct ophthalmoscope, or with a Finoff transilluminator and lens (40–60 diopters). Consider consultation with a board-certified ophthalmologist when feasible. Topical mydriatics used for mammals are not useful in birds due to the presence of skeletal muscle in the iris. Additional diagnostic procedures that may be warranted include exfoliative conjunctival or corneal cytologic examination (including Gram, acid-fast, Giminez, periodic acid–Schiff stains if warranted), biopsy, (rarely, aqueous or vitreous paracentesis), and other procedures as indicated. Skin scraping or tape preps can help rule out parasitic causes such as *Knemidokoptes*.

### PATHOLOGIC FINDINGS
The presence of intracellular bacteria in heterophils or epithelial cells can be seen with bacterial infections. Epidermal hyperplasia with ballooning degeneration, intraepithelial vesicles, and eosinophilic intracytoplasmic inclusion are seen on histopathologic examination of skin biopsies in cases of poxvirus. Conjunctival cytologic examination of birds with chlamydia may reveal conjunctival epithelial cell hyperplasia, inflammatory cell infiltrate, intracytoplasmic chlamydial elementary bodies on Giemsa- or Gimenez-stained samples, and antigen may be demonstrated by IFA. *Mycoplasma* inclusions are small basophilic dots on the surface of epithelial cells. Neoplastic cells may be seen on cytologic or biopsy samples in cases of neoplasia.

## TREATMENT

### APPROPRIATE HEALTH CARE
Birds with ocular lesions can generally be managed on an outpatient basis unless significant pathology is present.

### NURSING CARE
Supportive care as indicated including fluid therapy and gavage feeding in anorexic patients. Warm compresses and ocular flushing may help loosen up caked debris resulting in eyelid matting. In cases of suspected infectious disease, birds should be isolated. Protective gear should be worn by caretakers if zoonotic disease is suspected. Elizabethan or protective collars may be helpful in cases of self-trauma. Supportive care and management of secondary bacterial and fungal infections may be the only treatment option for some viral diseases.

### ACTIVITY
No activity restriction is indicated unless patient is systemically ill or if vision is impaired. Confining the patient to a smaller area may help facilitate treatment.

### DIET
Birds on an inadequate diet should be converted to an appropriate diet. Assisted feeding may be indicated if vision is impaired or the bird is not eating.

### CLIENT EDUCATION
Owners should be educated on proper nutrition for their bird. If the event was caused by trauma or excessive restraint, owners should be counselled on ways to avoid future trauma and proper restraint techniques.

### SURGICAL CONSIDERATIONS
Foreign bodies, including conjunctival nematodes and trematodes, should be removed. Cataract surgery can be considered in cases of cataracts; this should be performed with a veterinary ophthalmologist. Temporary tarsorrhaphy is an option for protection of the cornea in cases of severe ulceration. Enucleation or modified evisceration may be indicated in cases of neoplasia or painful conditions refractory to therapy. Eyelid repair may be indicated in cases of eyelid laceration.

## MEDICATIONS

### DRUG(S) OF CHOICE
Systemic antibiotic, antifungal, antiparasitic, or antiviral therapies as warranted. Broad-spectrum topical ophthalmic antibiotics (e.g. bacitracin-polymyxin B-neomycin, tetracycline, chloramphenicol, gentamycin, fluoroquinolone) are indicated in some cases of infectious conjunctivitis, keratoconjunctivitis, and uveitis. Systemic NSAIDs are warranted in cases of severe inflammation or uveitis. Topical NSAIDs including flurbiprofen or diclofenac can help control local inflammation. Mydriasis cannot realistically be obtained with topical therapy in birds, so pupil preservation is best controlled by reducing inflammation. Lubricating therapies should be instituted if lagophthalmos is present or associated with eyelid swelling. Parenteral vitamin A (10,000–25,000 iu/300 g body weight) is helpful in vitamin A deficiency.

### CONTRAINDICATIONS
Topical steroids or NSAIDs should not be used in cases of corneal ulceration. Follow FARAD guidelines in food animal species, including poultry and waterfowl.

## PRECAUTIONS

Systemic or topical medication (especially corticosteroid) therapy is not without risk and potential adverse effects or complications should be discussed with owners prior to treatment. Corticosteroid therapy may exacerbate underlying viral or bacterial disease. Oil/petrolatum-based ointments can cause greasy residue on feathers; water-based formulations preferred whenever feasible.

## POSSIBLE INTERACTIONS

Topical and/or systemic steroid therapy could result in generalized immunosuppression so judicious use is recommended.

## ALTERNATIVE DRUGS

TPA (tissue plasminogen activator) has been administered intravitreally in cases of intraocular hemorrhage. Safety and efficacy of topical and oral medications to control glaucoma in mammals have not been extensively investigated in birds but can be considered in cases of glaucoma. Dorzolamide and timolol have been used to treat glaucoma in a caique. Timolol should be used with caution in small birds.

 FOLLOW-UP

## PATIENT MONITORING

Follow-up ophthalmologic examination will help determine response to therapy. More frequent visits are warranted in cases of corneal ulceration or severe disease.

## PREVENTION/AVOIDANCE

Vaccination of poultry for Marek's disease and avian encephalomyelitis may be warranted. Vaccines for other viral diseases including poxvirus and West Nile virus can be considered. Identify and treat minor corneal ulceration early to prevent progression. Treat traumatic injury and uveitides aggressively and early. Quarantine new additions to the aviary or flock and isolate affected birds early.

## POSSIBLE COMPLICATIONS

Severe corneal pathology may result in globe rupture. Blindness can result from severe or untreated disease. Corticosteroid therapy may exacerbate underlying viral or bacterial disease.

## EXPECTED COURSE AND PROGNOSIS

Course and prognosis depends on the disease condition. Minor disease can be self-resolving or responsive to therapy and associated with a good outcome. Severe disease can result in progressive pathology refractory to therapy.

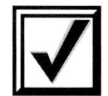 MISCELLANEOUS

## ASSOCIATED CONDITIONS

Other lesions, including fractures, may be present in cases of trauma so thorough physical examination is warranted. Any of these ocular conditions can be related to systemic disease and/or secondary complications. Most ocular disease in poultry is secondary to systemic pathology, including fowl cholera, mycoplasmosis, infectious coryza.

## AGE-RELATED FACTORS

Aged birds may have higher morbidity and mortality than younger birds. Cataracts are more common in aged birds.

## ZOONOTIC POTENTIAL

Infectious disease causes including *Chlamydia, Salmonella, Mycobacteria,* influenza, and paramyxoviruses are potentially zoonotic.

## FERTILITY/BREEDING

Birds with vision impairment or systemic disease may have reduced fertility or difficulty breeding.

## SYNONYMS

*Chlamydia*—parrot fever. *Knemidokoptes pilae*—scaly face and leg mite.

## SEE ALSO

Adenoviruses
Air Sac Rupture
Aspergillosis

Bordetellosis
Cryptosporidiosis
Mycobacteriosis
Mycoplasmosis
Neoplasia (Lymphoproliferative)
Neoplasia (Neurologic)
Nutritional Imbalances
Orthoavulaviruses
Respiratory Distress
Rhinitis and Sinusitis
Salmonellosis
Toxicosis (Airborne)
Trauma
West Nile Virus
Also individual viral diseases

## ABBREVIATIONS

CT—computed tomography
IFA—immune fluorescence assay
NSAIDs—non-steroidal anti-inflammatory drugs

## INTERNET RESOURCES

Pollock, C. Raptor ophthalmology: Ocular lesions. *LafeberVet*: http://lafeber.com/vet/raptor-ophthalmology-ocular-lesions
US Food Animal Residue Avoidance Bank: www.farad.org

*Suggested Reading*
Abrams, G., Paul-Murphy, J., Murphy, C. (2002). Conjunctivitis in birds. *Veterinary Clinics of North America: Exotic Animal Practice.* 5:287–309.
Kern, T. (1997). Disorders of the special senses. In: *Avian Medicine and Surgery* (ed. R.B. Altman, S.L. Clubb, G.M. Dorrestein, K. Quesenberry), 563–580. Philadelphia, PA: Saunders.
Montiani-Ferreira, F., Moore, B.A., Ben-Shlomo, G. (eds.). (2022). Part IV. Aves. In: *Wild and Exotic Animal Ophthalmology*, 321–627. New York, NY: Springer Nature.
Murphy, C., Kern, T., McKeever, K, et al. (1982). Ocular lesions in free-living raptors. *Journal of the American Veterinary Medical Association*, 181:1302–1304.
**Authors**: Jennifer E. Graham, DVM, DABVP (Avian/ECM), DACZM, and Ruth M. Marrion, DVM, DACVO, PhD

O

# OIL EXPOSURE

## BASICS

### DEFINITION
Oil exposure in birds is defined as a contamination of external structures and/or internal ingestion or inhalation of petroleum-based or other types of oil. This exposure can occur on an individual basis or can affect large populations of wild birds. In both cases, the type of oil will affect the outcome of exposure and can lead to both short- and long-term effects on a wide variety of body systems.

### PATHOPHYSIOLOGY
Environmental sources of oil include, but are not limited to, natural seeps, pipeline breaks, drilling platform or well accidents, tanker collisions, illegal/deliberate releases, and dumping of waste oil by the general public. In addition, the individual bird can encounter cooking or waste oil within a household setting. Birds can be exposed to oil during any of their daily activities, including feeding, loafing, flying, breeding, nesting, and raising young. External contamination leads to disruption of feather alignment and possible skin and corneal irritation/burns. Internal contamination can occur from ingestion of oil through feeding in contaminated waters or from preening of oiled feathers. Exposure to highly refined fuels, such as jet or diesel fuels, can result in inhalation of highly volatile fumes that lead to respiratory and neurological abnormalities.

### SYSTEMS AFFECTED
**Skin/exocrine:** Oil disrupts the microscopic alignment of hooks and barbules on feathers, resulting in the inability of birds to maintain waterproofing. This, in turn, can lead to loss of buoyancy in the water, exposure to environmental elements resulting in hypo- or hyperthermia and loss of flight capability. Highly volatile fuels can also cause varying degrees of skin irritation or burns through direct contact with exposed areas.
**GI:** Ingestion of oil causes direct inflammatory effects on the GI tract as well as an alteration in electrolyte and water transport across the intestinal mucosa. Inability to feed normally in the wild or in captivity during rehabilitation activities can result in malnutrition and weight loss.
**Hepatobiliary:** Liver abnormalities result from exposure to polyaromatic hydrocarbons and other toxic components of oil.
**Hemic/lymphatic/immune:** Ingestion of crude oil has been linked to development of hemolytic anemia in different avian species. Anemia of chronic disease and malnutrition is also seen. Petroleum exposure results in direct suppression of immune system

function and this is exacerbated by immunosuppression resulting from the stress of oiling and captivity during rehabilitation.
**Reproductive:** Exposure to oil can result in failed reproduction in the short-term due to loss of breeding activity, contamination of eggs or young with oil and disruption of normal reproductive hormonal levels. Long-term population effects on reproductive success have been documented following large-scale oil spills.
**Musculoskeletal:** Malnutrition often results in pectoral muscle (most prominently) atrophy seen on admission to rehabilitation. Secondary problems related to captive care include keel, hock and foot sores resulting from abnormal pressure points on the bird's body when it is held out of the water for prolonged periods of time.
**Endocrine/metabolic:** Internal exposure to oil may result in impairment of salt gland function, resulting in osmoregulatory dysfunction.
**Behavioral:** Any wild bird contaminated with oil that is subsequently captured and then brought into rehabilitation experiences a large amount of stress during the entire process. This results in behavior consistent with that of a wild animal that believes it is in constant danger until the moment of release back to the wild.
**Respiratory:** Inhalation of highly volatile fumes from refined fuels can result in direct damage to exposed areas of the respiratory tract. It is also hypothesized to increase absorption of smaller aromatic hydrocarbons and to reduce ability to dive in water for aquatic birds.
**Nervous:** Exposure to highly volatile fumes from refined fuels can result in neurological abnormalities, including ataxia and seizure activity.
**Ophthalmic:** Highly volatile fuels can cause corneal irritation or burns through direct contact or via exposure to fumes from the oil.

### GENETICS
N/A

### INCIDENCE/PREVALENCE
Birds can be exposed to oil almost anywhere in their habitat, although there is increased incidence of oiling in areas where oil is extracted, transported, or refined. Incidence may rise in winter months due to the increased possibility of storms leading to transport spills. In addition, many seabirds congregate in large numbers on the open ocean during this period, making them more vulnerable to oiling.

### GEOGRAPHIC DISTRIBUTION
Worldwide—especially in developed countries which use large quantities of petroleum products.

### SIGNALMENT
All avian species, no specific age or sex predilection, although seabirds and waterfowl are especially vulnerable.

### SIGNS
#### General Comments
Some types of refined oils will be clear in coloration and difficult to discern on feathers. In some instances, wild birds will die from problems associated with oil exposure before they reach land and are never found during search and collection efforts. More heavily oiled birds in the marine environment are often found first and brought for rehabilitation because they are more incapacitated from the oil. Ironically, trace to lightly oiled birds are often in poorer shape by the time they are weakened enough from oil exposure to be captured.

#### Historical Findings
In most areas of the USA, the National Response Center (telephone: +1 800-424-8802) will advise the responsible agencies (Coast Guard, Environmental Protection Agency, state and federal natural resource agencies) about the event. In some regions, however, state agencies take the lead for initial incident notification. An incident command system is then instituted for the spill response. If an individual oiled bird is found with possible petroleum contamination, it is recommended that the state wildlife agency be contacted as this bird may be part of a larger spill event. Trained wildlife response personnel are engaged by the spiller (the responsible party) to conduct wildlife operations. The general public should be discouraged from search and collection of wild birds during an oil spill incident. An individual oiled bird, whether wild or owned, may be brought to a veterinary practice for care after being found oiled. Outside the USA, many regions have advanced oil spill contingency planning in place; many of which that include wildlife operations. For large scale spills (i.e. tier 3 responses) or in regions where planning is not fully developed, Oil Spill Response Limited (telephone: +44 (0) 2380331551), the largest international industry-funded cooperative, is available 24 hours a day, 365 days of the year to attend spills of oil, chemicals and other hazardous substances worldwide (http://www.oilspillresponse.com/services/member-response-services).

#### Physical Examination Findings
Oil contaminated feathers and skin—in most instances, this is fairly obvious, although highly refined fuels may be colorless and vapors may have dissipated by the time the

bird is found. Feathers may be matted, wet, feel oily, and smell like the petroleum product. Oil may occlude the nares or the oropharyngeal area—the bird may be in respiratory distress. Increased respiratory effort, rate, abnormal respiratory tract sounds with inhalation of toxic fumes. Neurological signs including ataxia, seizures with exposure to toxic fumes. If the cornea or periocular area is irritated or burned, epiphora, conjunctival redness/swelling, corneal edema or ulceration will be seen. Hypo- or hyperthermia, depending on environmental factors. Thin to emaciated body condition unless found within the first 24–48 hours of oiling. Dehydration. Evidence of regurgitation and diarrhea. Anemia. If the bird has been out of the water for prolonged periods, it may show evidence of pressure sores on the keel, posterior aspects of the hocks and the feet.

## CAUSES
Cooking or motor oils. Petroleum products—crude, gasoline, intermediate distillates (diesel, jet fuels), heavy distillates (lubricants, waxes), residues (heavy fuel oils, asphalt, tar, coke).

## RISK FACTORS
Birds of the open ocean (shearwaters, petrels, fulmars, albatrosses) are likely to encounter petroleum released with drilling platform accidents, tanker accidents, or illegal discharges. These birds are especially vulnerable because they live far away from land and often drown when their waterproofing is compromised with oil exposure, so they are less apt to be collected when conducting shoreline response. Birds that inhabit coastal areas and only come to land to breed (loons, grebes, auks, gannets/boobies) are similar to open ocean birds and often live in areas with heavy tanker traffic, but they are more likely to be encountered. Birds that inhabit near shore environments (pelicans, wading birds, gulls, terns, shorebirds) are less vulnerable because they can get to land more easily and do not require a fully aquatic environment, but they often live in environments with multiple sources of potential oil release. Waterfowl (ducks, geese, swans) are, in general, more hardy than birds in the above categories.

## DIAGNOSIS

### DIFFERENTIAL DIAGNOSIS
External contamination with another substance (e.g. dispersants used during oil spill responses, but rare exposure), household solvents, glues. Internal exposure to other inhaled or ingested toxins (e.g. Teflon®, poisonous plants, heavy metals). Infectious diseases leading to multisystemic signs—polyomavirus, herpesvirus, mycobacteriosis, chlamydiosis.

## CBC/BIOCHEMISTRY/URINALYSIS
CBC may reveal evidence of anemia, increased white blood cell count due to direct effects of oil or secondary bacterial and fungal infections. PCV/TS are often sampled every 2–3 days while in care. Biochemistry panels may show low total protein levels (malnutrition, hepatic dysfunction), hypoglycemia, hepatic and renal enzyme abnormalities, electrolyte disturbances resulting from malnutrition, dehydration and the multisystemic effects of the toxic components in oil. No single analyte, however, has conclusively been found to rule in oil exposure as the cause of morbidity.

## OTHER LABORATORY TESTS
Contaminated feathers can be "fingerprinted" to identify the specific composition of the oil that is present. This is a process using gas chromatography/mass spectrometry and is only available through certain laboratories. ELISA, often used for soil testing, has been used to detect polyaromatic hydrocarbons in oil from feathers, but is not yet validated.

## IMAGING
Radiographs may be useful in discerning respiratory abnormalities (inhalant toxicity, aspergillosis infections secondary to immune suppression and captive environment), organomegaly such as an enlarged hepatic silhouette or adrenal hyperplasia, and thickened GI tract walls. Not a primary method of diagnosis for oil exposure.

## DIAGNOSTIC PROCEDURES
Can place a few feathers in a pan of water and watch for an oil sheen to appear—not considered a specific test of oil contamination, since the sheen may be from other substances. Fluorescein tests to reveal possible corneal ulceration. Endoscopy may show ingested oil within the GI tract. Laparoscopy may reveal evidence of secondary bacterial or fungal infections.

## PATHOLOGIC FINDINGS
Necropsies of oiled birds cannot be performed in large oil spill events in the USA, as the bodies are considered legal evidence, unless permission is obtained from the proper authorities. Gross necropsy lesions highly variable. Oil may be present on feathers, in oropharyngeal area, trachea, or in the GI tract. Lining of the GI tract may be inflamed or hemorrhagic. Lungs may appear hemorrhagic with exposure to volatile fumes. Salt glands and adrenal glands may be enlarged. No specific or consistent lesions in birds exposed to oil.

## TREATMENT

### APPROPRIATE HEALTH CARE
All personnel working with oiled birds during a spill response should wear appropriate personal protective equipment and should have received hazardous materials training. Search and collection of oiled birds during large-scale oil spills is only conducted by trained personnel. When birds are found during search and collection, they are initially stabilized in the field. This involves removing any oil occluding eyes, nares and glottis and impairing movement of wings and legs as well as administration of a balanced electrolyte solution via gavage if the bird is normothermic and is not neurologically impaired, otherwise IV or SQ fluid administration may be required. Birds may also need to be treated for hypo-or hyperthermia with the use of warm or cold packs appropriate for field use. Because birds affected during large-scale oil spills are considered legal evidence for use in damage assessment proceedings against the responsible party, a strict chain of custody procedure is followed during their time in captivity. The location where birds are found is documented with GPS readings, and an individual leg band is placed on the bird (or other means of identification) so that it can be tracked throughout the rehabilitation process. When a bird reaches the rehabilitation center, it is given a thorough physical examination with documentation of the extent of oiling, is photographed and a small sample of oiled feathers is taken for legal purposes. Any abnormalities noted on physical examination require appropriate medical care. Because a large number of birds are often seen during spill responses, treatment is often given on a "herd health" basis administered for the "average" bird rather than tailored to each individual. Triage is an essential part of the rehabilitation process during an oil spill response. Decisions are made based on the resources available, health status of the bird, and other general factors, for example, the historical success of rehabilitation of the species. This means that euthanasia plays a significant role in oiled wildlife response efforts.

### NURSING CARE
Scrupulous attention should be paid to disinfection and cleanliness during all procedures in oiled bird care. Because these birds are often immunocompromised, every step should be taken to decrease the incidence of secondary bacterial or fungal infections. Aspergillosis is the most common infectious disease seen in an oil spill response, and prophylactic antifungal medications (in addition to facilities maintaining 10–15 air exchanges/hour and an attention to reducing stressors) are often administered to decrease the possibility of this infection. Initial care for dehydrated oiled birds consists of fluid administration given either IV or orally via

O

gavage. Hetastarch therapy for hypoproteinemic birds may be used in individual cases at 15 ml/kg divided 3–4 times per day followed by maintenance fluids. Oil is gently removed from eyes with an ophthalmic irrigation solution, and from the nares and/or glottis using dampened gauze sponges. Body temperature abnormalities (normal 102–105°F/38.9–40.5°C) should be corrected, and facilities housing seabirds should be kept at 75–85°F (23.9–29.4°C) to assist in maintain body temperatures and to reduce preening activity. For seabirds that are not used to being out of the water, padded wraps to decrease the incidence of pressure sores over hocks and feet can be helpful. Keel wraps are sometimes placed to decrease pressure sores over this area. Protective wraps, however, must be applied by skilled rehabilitators so that they do not constrict the animal.

### Feeding
High calorie nutritional slurries [e.g. Emeraid Piscivore® (Lafeber, Cornell, IL) slurry at 10% fat], are also administered via gavage, usually alternating with oral electrolyte fluids. Birds are encouraged to self-feed by offering appropriate food items, such as whitebait or night smelt for piscivores. Obligate marine species are given additional salt in their feedings while housed on land or in fresh water.

### Housing
A decision must be made whether to house a bird individually or in a group pen. In general, birds that are gregarious in the wild (e.g. pelicans or common murres) can be housed together. Birds are housed in indoor pens until they are cleaned and then are moved to outdoor aviaries or pools appropriate to the species once cleared for prerelease conditioning.

### Washing, Rinsing, and Drying
A 1–2% dishwashing solution at 104–106°F (40–41°C) is used to bathe oiled birds. The water is placed into appropriately sized tubs and the bird is moved from tub to tub until the bath water is clean. All soap must then be rinsed off thoroughly to ensure proper waterproofing. This requires rinsing with water at 104–106°F using a high-pressure, adjustable nozzle and making sure to get every portion of the bird's feathers clean. When a bird is properly rinsed, the water will bead off the feathers and the bird's feathers will appear dry. Birds are dried off using incubators, heat lamps, or warm air pet dryers set on "low". They should be closely monitored to make sure that they are not overheating. Most birds will preen their feathers back into alignment in this time period.

### ACTIVITY
Oiled birds are housed in indoor pens that restrict their activity before cleaning. After cleaning, these birds can be moved to outdoor aviaries or pools in order to condition them prior to release.

### DIET
See above. If the bird is regurgitating, losing weight and/or has diarrhea, the veterinarian may choose to focus on rehydration methods and back off gavage feeding of nutritional slurries.

### CLIENT EDUCATION
If an owned bird becomes oiled within the household, clients should be instructed in methods to limit further access to sources of oil in the future. Appropriate education should also be given to address individual problems associated with the oiling incident, such as proper wound care or dietary considerations.

### SURGICAL CONSIDERATIONS
N/A

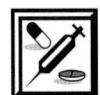 MEDICATIONS

### DRUG(S) OF CHOICE
Antibiotics: Amoxicillin/clavulinic acid 125 mg/kg PO q12h. Enrofloxacin 10–20 mg/kg PO, SC, IM q12–24h. Antifungals: Itraconazaole 20 mg/kg PO q24h. Analgesics: Meloxicam 0.5–2.0 mg/kg PO q12–24h. Ophthalmic medications: Avoid use of petroleum based ointments. Ciprofloxacin drops—one drop in affected eye(s) q4–6h. Salt 250 mg/kg PO every other day. Sucralfate 25 mg/kg PO q8h before food or other drugs. Vitamin supplementation: Vitamin $B_1$ for those birds eating thawed frozen fish (1–2 mg/kg PO q24h). Commercial vitamin for fish-eating birds (Mazuri® Auklet Supplements, Mazuri Exotic Animal Nutrition, St. Louis, MO).

### CONTRAINDICATIONS
Repeated injections of enrofloxacin are associated with severe muscle necrosis.

### PRECAUTIONS
Avoid use of antibiotics and glucocorticoids unless clinically necessary, as these medications may increase the risk of aspergillosis and other infectious diseases in immunocompromised oiled birds.

### POSSIBLE INTERACTIONS
N/A

### ALTERNATIVE DRUGS
Alternative antibiotics and antifungal medications can be used based on culture and sensitivity results.

 FOLLOW-UP

### PATIENT MONITORING
**Pre-release conditioning**: Once birds are cleaned and medical issues such as malnutrition

and anemia are resolved, they are moved into outdoor aviaries or pools for pre-release conditioning and observation of waterproofing, appetite and behavior.
**Release evaluation**: Criteria used to determine suitability for release include behavior, such as diving appropriately in pools, body weight/condition, waterproofing, normal blood values, and resolution of all other abnormalities noted during the rehabilitation process (e.g. wounds healed).
**Post-release**: Every bird should be permanently banded/ringed so that post-release reporting can be done. Monitoring via radio and satellite telemetry has been used in certain species following large-scale oil spill incidents.

### PREVENTION/AVOIDANCE
Recognize potential for oil exposure in the household and take steps to cover and safely dispose of any cooking or waste oil in this setting. The Oil Pollution Act 1990 mandates that each state in the USA should have a contingency plan for oiled wildlife response. It also requires every company that moves petroleum in the USA to have a "plan to prevent spills that may occur" and have a "detailed containment and cleanup plan" for oil spills.

### POSSIBLE COMPLICATIONS
Many oiled birds will succumb or must be euthanized due to the effects of oil or as a result of the secondary effects of captive care. These complications are discussed in the Systems Affected section.

### EXPECTED COURSE AND PROGNOSIS
The success of treatment for oil exposure varies widely depending on factors such as the type of oil spilled, the amount of oiling on the bird, the species of bird affected, preplanning for spill response, the expertise of response personnel and many others considerations.

 MISCELLANEOUS

### ASSOCIATED CONDITIONS
N/A

### AGE-RELATED FACTORS
N/A

### ZOONOTIC POTENTIAL
During an oil spill response, there is potential for a large number of captive wild birds to be housed together indoors. Some of these birds may become ill with infectious diseases such as aspergillosis or chlamydiosis, which are potentially zoonotic. In addition, stressed birds may be shedding GI pathogens such as *Campylobacter* or *Salmonella*. As stated before, it is imperative that personnel

working with oiled birds be familiar with and follow protocols designed to minimize exposure to zoonotic agents.

## FERTILITY/BREEDING
See Reproduction in the Systems Affected section.

## SYNONYMS
N/A

## SEE ALSO
Anemia
Aspiration Pneumonia
Coagulopathies
Dehydration
Diarrhea
Emaciation
Enteritis and Gastritis
Hemorrhage
Hypothermia
Infertility
Liver Disease
Neurologic (Trauma)
Ocular Lesions

Pneumonia
Regurgitation and Vomiting
Respiratory Distress
Seizures
Trauma

## ABBREVIATIONS
ELISA—enzyme-linked immunosorbent assay
GI—gastrointestinal
GPS—Global Positioning System
PCV—packed cell volume
TS—total solids

## INTERNET RESOURCES
International Bird Rescue: www.bird-rescue.org
University of California Davis School of Veterinary Medicine. Oiled Wildlife Care Network: https://owcn.vetmed.ucdavis.edu
Tristate Bird Rescue & Research: https://tristatebird.org/oil-spill-response-and-services

*Suggested Reading*
Jessup, D.A., Leighton, F.A. (1996). Oil pollution and petroleum toxicity to wildlife. In: *Noninfectious Diseases of*

*Wildlife* (ed. A. Fairbrother, L.N. Locke, G.L. Hoff), 141–156. Ames, IA: Iowa State University Press.
Leighton, F.A., Peakall, D.B., Butler, R.G. (1983). Heinz-body hemolytic anemia from the ingestion of crude oil: a primary toxic effect in marine birds. *Science* 220: 871–873.
Mazet, J.A.K., Newman, S.H., Gilardi, K.V.K., et al. (2002). Advances in oiled bird emergency medicine and management. *Journal of Avian Medicine and Surgery* 16(2):146–149.
Tseng, F.S. (1999). Considerations in care for birds affected by oil spills. *Seminars in Avian and Exotic Pet Medicine* 8:21–31.
USGS (1999). Oil. In: *Field Manual of Wildlife Diseases* (ed. M. Friend, J.C. Franson), 309–315. Information and Technology Report 1999-001. Reston, VA: Biological Resources Division, US Geological Survey.

**Authors**: Florina S. Tseng, DVM, and Mike Ziccardi, DVM, MPVM, PhD, DACZM

O

## ORAL PLAQUES

## BASICS

### DEFINITION
Oral plaques are generally yellow, creamy, or white raised lesions on the mucosa of the oropharynx. In birds, oral plaques are most commonly caused by hypovitaminosis A, or infections with avian poxvirus, herpesvirus (pigeons, doves, owls, canaries, Amazons, Bourke's parakeets), bacteria, *Candida* (most commonly *Candida albicans*), *Trichomonas* (*Trichomonas gallinae*, *Trichomonas columbae*) or *Capillaria* spp.

### PATHOPHYSIOLOGY
Hypovitaminosis A causes squamous metaplasia resulting in hyperkeratotic squamous cells which plug the mucous and salivary glands, causing swelling and nodules. The mucous itself is thicker and tenacious, and when combined with exfoliated cornified squamous cells, will appear as mucosal plaques. Candidiasis is an opportunistic disease most commonly caused by *C. albicans*, although *Candida parapsilosis* and, rarely, other species have been reported. Infection may be superficial or may invade deeply into mucosa, particularly in the crop. Suppression of normal oral or ingluvial flora by antibiotics (typically tetracyclines) can predispose patients. May also be a secondary pathogen following lesions caused by bacteria, viruses, or hypovitaminosis A. Avian poxvirus is transmitted through biting insects or conspecific aggression resulting in skin trauma. The virus stimulates epithelial cell DNA synthesis, resulting in hyperplasia. The exudative lesions often become secondarily infected, resulting in plaques, swellings, or caseous plugs throughout the mucosa of the oropharynx. Amazon parrots are considered especially susceptible to a diphtheritic form of avian poxvirus, although this is seen much less now that fewer birds remain from the imported population. Herpesvirus results in fibrinonecrotic pseudomembranes secondary to inflammatory and necrotic debris. A mutation of the herpesvirus which causes infectious laryngotracheitis virus in chickens is believed to be responsible for a severe upper respiratory disease in Amazon parrots and Bourke's parakeets, also called Amazon tracheitis virus.

### SYSTEMS AFFECTED
**GI**: Oral plaques can cause dysphagia, pharyngitis. *Candida* and *Trichomonas* commonly affect the crop, and sometimes lower GI tract. *Mycobacterium* spp. can form granulomas throughout the lower GI tract. Capillaria may be found in the oropharynx, esophagus, crop, and small intestine. Avian poxvirus lesions may be found in the crop.

**Renal**: Hypovitaminosis A-associated squamous metaplasia of renal tubular epithelium, resulting in kidney dysfunction.
**Respiratory**: Lesions associated with the glottis or proximal trachea can cause cough or dyspnea. Hypovitaminosis A-associated squamous metaplasia of upper respiratory epithelium, predisposing patient to sinusitis, rhinitis. *Trichomonas* and herpesvirus can affect the larynx and trachea. Avian poxvirus can affect the trachea, air sacs and lungs. *Trichomonas* may extend widely from original lesions.
**Skin/exocrine**: Avian poxvirus often results in skin lesions, particularly of the face and feet. Herpesvirus may result in foot lesions. *Mycobacterium* spp. may cause granulomatous swellings at any location.
**Ophthalmic**: Avian poxvirus can cause blepharitis, chemosis, conjunctivitis, ulcerative lesions of the eyelids, secondary keratitis, corneal ulcers, and corneal perforation.

### GENETICS
N/A

### INCIDENCE/PREVALENCE
Oral plaques are generally considered common in wild birds admitted to wildlife centers. Prevalence depends on the cause.

### GEOGRAPHIC DISTRIBUTION
Worldwide.

### SIGNALMENT
Generally seen in very young patients or adults with underlying disease causing immunocompromise.

### SIGNS
#### Historical Findings
Inappetance or anorexia. Dysphagia. Gaping, yawning, repeated tonguing of oral mucosa. Regurgitation or vomiting, increased upper GI transit time (especially with crop involvement). Dyspnea, cough (especially when glottis and proximal trachea affected). Halitosis (especially candidiasis).

#### Physical Examination Findings
May include dehydration, weight loss, and weakness secondary to negative energy balance. Oral plaque lesions on the oropharyngeal mucosa may be diphtheritic or caseous—(avian poxvirus, herpesvirus, *Candida*, *Trichomonas*, *Capillaria*); granulomas—(mycobacterial, other bacteria, fungal); hyperkeratotic—(hypovitaminosis A). Easily removed (hypovitaminosis A, *Trichomonas*). Difficult to remove (bacterial, avian poxvirus). Gray or brown, fibrinous, and friable ("wet" form of avian poxvirus).

### CAUSES
Nutritional deficiency (generally seed-based diet): hypovitaminosis A. Bacterial: often Gram-negative (*Escherichia coli*, *Klebsiella* spp., *Pseudomonas aeruginosa*, *Pasteurella* sp.), more

rarely Gram positive (*Staphylococcus* spp.), anaerobic, or mycobacterial. Choanal bacterial lesions are sometimes seen with sinusitis. Fungal: *Candida* spp. Parasitic: *Trichomonas*. Viral: Avian poxvirus, herpesvirus, which may occur concurrently in pigeons with trichomoniasis, causing more severe lesions.

### RISK FACTORS
See Signalment section.

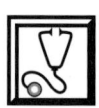

## DIAGNOSIS

### DIFFERENTIAL DIAGNOSIS
#### Differentiating Similar Signs
Dried food can accumulate in the mucosa and resemble plaques; this is often dependent on diet and eating habits. Hypovitaminosis A can cause a pustular glossitis along the lateral surfaces of the tongue and around the glottis. Although at first glance these may resemble plaques, careful inspection will reveal that these lesions are not superficial like oral plaques, but instead are composed of purulent or caseous material within the salivary pores lining the tongue. These may require debridement in addition to vitamin A supplementation to resolve. Pigeons may present with sialolithiasis, concretions in the caudal pharynx originating from the salivary glands.

#### Differentiating Causes
On physical examination, hypovitaminosis A also presents with blunting of the choanal papillae. This blunting usually appears as a very even, symmetrical scalloping, rather than the irregular erosion seen secondary to chronic sinusitis. Poxvirus usually presents with crusty or nodular lesions of the head, legs, and feet. Lesions may be swabbed for cytology, direct saline microscopy, and Gram stain. Additional diagnostic testing when indicated (e.g. acid-fast stain, mycobacterial or viral PCR, bacterial C/S, mycobacterial and fungal cultures). Lesions refractory to treatment should be biopsied to rule out underlying neoplasia, especially squamous cell carcinoma.

### CBC/BIOCHEMISTRY/URINALYSIS
In non-systemic cases, hemogram and biochemical profiles may be normal. Leukocytosis may occur with secondary or concurrent systemic infection. Anemia seen with severe GI ulceration and bleeding. Hypoglycemia seen with prolonged anorexia. Hyperuricemia seen secondary to hypovitaminosis A squamous metaplasia of renal tubule epithelium.

### OTHER LABORATORY TESTS
#### Cytology
May see squamous cells with abundant basophilic keratin granules, often together in rafts or sheets with hypovitaminosis A.

Secondary bacterial infection may or may not be present. Inflammatory cells are usually not a component. May see bacteria, or "ghost rods" with mycobacterial infections. May see oval darkly basophilic budding yeast with *Candida*. The presence of pseudohyphae (slender unbranched chains of tubular cells) is suggestive of tissue invasion. May see basophilic piriform flagellated protozoa with an undulating membrane with *Trichomonas*. A wet mount of the lesions is more sensitive to diagnose trichomoniasis. Intracytoplasmic (Bollinger) or intranuclear inclusion bodies with avian poxvirus. Intranuclear (Cowdry) bodies with herpesvirus. *Capillaria* spp. eggs.

### Microscopic Examination
For direct microscopic examination for motile *Trichomonas*, an esophageal swab may be performed with a wet cotton-tipped applicator with sterile saline. A water droplet from the swab is then expressed onto a slide. Warming may improve motility and detection of the organism.

### IMAGING
Survey radiographs are often normal, but delayed motility and gastrointestinal dilation may be noted with lower GI involvement. Contrast radiography may be used to distinguish dilated intestinal loops from intestinal thickening seen in mycobacteriosis. Skull CT may help to delineate complex lesions with extension into adjacent structures.

### DIAGNOSTIC PROCEDURES
Lesion biopsy may be indicated, depending on the cause.

### PATHOLOGIC FINDINGS
Depends on the underlying disease.

## TREATMENT
### APPROPRIATE HEALTH CARE
The degree of nursing care needed is dependent on severity of disease.

### NURSING CARE
Non-debilitated patients with mild lesions and signs may be treated on an outpatient basis if hydrated and eating well on their own. Supportive care may be needed for anorexic, dehydrated, and/or debilitated patients, including fluids (SQ, IV, or IO), easily digestible nutrition, including gavage feeding in cases of inappetence, and heat support for birds experiencing weight loss or negative energy balance.

### ACTIVITY
Most birds with this condition may be allowed to determine their own level of activity.

### DIET
Although dietary improvements may be needed, changes should be gradual and deferred until the patient has recovered.

### CLIENT EDUCATION
The overall predisposing factors that led to the disease need to be addressed. Clients should be educated on nutritional requirements for their particular species. Any underlying husbandry deficiencies should be addressed.

### SURGICAL CONSIDERATIONS
In very severe cases, debridement of the lesions under sedation may be needed.

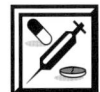

## MEDICATIONS
### DRUG(S) OF CHOICE
May use analgesia when inappetence or dysphagia is present, including meloxicam 0.5–1 mg/kg PO q12h. Hypovitaminosis A—vitamin A 5000–20,000 iu/kg IM. *Candida*—for superficial infections nystatin 300,000 iu/kg PO q12h; however, dose volume is large and requires direct contact with lesions to be effective. For severe infections, fluconazole 2–5 mg/kg PO q24h, itraconazole 10 mg/kg PO q12h for 21 days, or voriconazole 15–20 mg/kg PO q12h. *Trichomonas*—metronidazole 20–50 mg/kg PO q12h for 3–5 days, ronidazole 6–10 mg/kg PO q24h for 7–14 days, or carnidazole 20–30 mg/kg PO q12h for 3–5 days. Bacterial—appropriate antibiotic therapy based on culture and sensitivity. Pigeon herpesvirus—treat topically and systemically with acyclovir 80 mg/kg PO q8h for 7–10 days, or 40 mg/kg IV/SQ q8h. Amazon tracheitis (herpesvirus)—successful specific treatment has not been reported. Avian poxvirus—vitamin A, treatment of secondary bacterial infections if present. *Capillaria*—fenbendazole 100 mg/kg PO, or oxfendazole 10–40 mg/kg PO, repeat in 14 days.

### CONTRAINDICATIONS
Metoclopramide and cisapride have not been proven to be effective for improving crop motility.

### PRECAUTIONS
Fenbendazole can cause toxicity in a number of species, including pigeons and doves, vultures, storks, cockatiels and lories. Nystatin should not be given in cases of suspected GI ulceration, as this may result in absorption-dependent toxicity. Fecal cytology or fecal occult blood test may help identify this condition, particularly in patients with anemia.

### POSSIBLE INTERACTIONS
N/A

### ALTERNATIVE DRUGS
N/A

## FOLLOW-UP
### PATIENT MONITORING
If inappetence, anorexia, dehydration, or significant weight loss occurs, hospitalize patient for supportive care and treatment, and obtain appropriate diagnostics.

### PREVENTION/AVOIDANCE
Birds should be fed a species-appropriate high-quality, nutritionally sound diet. Owners should observe good hygiene, and housing, nest boxes, food, and water supply should be carefully kept as clean as possible. Flock biosecurity measures should be observed. Routine treatment of pigeons for trichomoniasis is recommended to reduce shedding. Pigeons should not be fed to raptors, to prevent the transmission of *Trichomonas* and herpesviruses. A vaccine for avian poxvirus is available for pigeons, doves, and canaries. The vaccine is recommended only for healthy flocks to prevent viral recombination.

### POSSIBLE COMPLICATIONS
See Pathophysiology and Systems Affected sections.

### EXPECTED COURSE AND PROGNOSIS
Following treatment, prognosis is good for bacterial and nutritional plaques or candidiasis in patients who are not seriously debilitated. Recovery from nutritional plaques is usually within 2–3 weeks. Recovery from the non-septicemic form of avian poxvirus is usually 3–4 weeks, if uncomplicated by secondary bacterial or fungal infections. Some strains in passerines and columbids can leave survivors prone to tumor formation. The diphtheritic ("wet") and septic forms are associated with high mortality. Survivor immunity may be life-long. Amazon tracheitis virus is usually lethal, and recovery may be as long as 9 months. Acyclovir may reduce mortality in pigeon herpesvirus. Psittacine birds are prone to relapses of trichomoniasis. Significant morbidity and mortality can be seen. Recovery following treatment may be as rapid as 1–2 days. Mycobacterial lesions carry a guarded prognosis and treatment is controversial due to zoonotic potential, particularly in susceptible individuals.

## MISCELLANEOUS
### ASSOCIATED CONDITIONS
Chronic and recurrent trichomoniasis in pigeons is associated with concurrent herpesvirus.

O

# ORAL PLAQUES

## AGE-RELATED FACTORS
Juveniles and subadults are considered more susceptible to various infectious agents causing oral plaques such as *Trichomonas*, *Capillaria*, and viruses.

## ZOONOTIC POTENTIAL
*Mycobacteria* spp. can be infectious to humans. The potential varies with species within this genus, and the degree to which it occurs is controversial.

## FERTILITY/BREEDING
N/A

## SYNONYMS
N/A

## SEE ALSO
Aspergillosis
Aspiration
Candidiasis
Ileus (Functional Gastrointestinal, Crop Stasis)
Flagellate Enteritis
Helminthiasis (Gastrointestinal)
Herpesvirus (Columbid Herpesvirus 1 in Pigeons and Raptors)
Herpesvirus (Duck Viral Enteritis)
Herpesvirus (Passerine Birds)
Herpesvirus (Psittacid Herpesviruses)
Marek's Disease
Mycobacteriosis
Neoplasia (Gastrointestinal and Hepatic)
Neoplasia (Respiratory)
Nutritional Imbalances
Poxvirus
Regurgitation and Vomiting
Respiratory Distress
Rhinitis/Sinusitis
Tracheal and Syringeal Diseases
Trichomoniasis
Appendix 8, Algorithm 8: Oropharyngeal Lesions
Also individual viral diseases

## ABBREVIATIONS
C/S—culture and sensitivity
CT—computed tomography
GI—gastrointestinal
PCR—polymerase chain reaction

## INTERNET RESOURCES
N/A

*Suggested Reading*
Chaves Hernandez A.J. (2014). Poultry and avian diseases. In: *Encyclopedia of Agriculture and Food Systems*, 2nd edn. (ed. N.K. Van Alfen), 504–520. St. Louis, MO: Elsevier.
Gelis, S. (2006). Evaluating and treating the gastrointestinal system. In: *Clinical Avian Medicine* (ed. G.J. Harrison, T.L. Lightfoot), Vol. I, 411–440. Palm Beach, FL: Spix Publishing.
Hoefer, H.L. (1997). Diseases of the gastrointestinal tract. In: *Avian Medicine and Surgery* (ed. R.B. Altman, S.L. Clubb, G.M. Dorrestein, K. Quesenberry), 419–453. Philadelphia, PA: Saunders.
Lumeij, J.T. (1994). Gastroenterology. In: *Avian Medicine: Principles and Application* (ed. B.W. Ritchie, G.J. Harrison, L.R. Harrison), 482–521. Lake Worth, FL: Wingers Publishing.
**Authors**: Hannah Attarian, DVM, and Anthony A Pilny, DVM, DABVP (Avian)
**Acknowledgements**: Adapted from first edition authored by Elisabeth Simone-Freilicher, DVM, DABVP (Avian)

O

**BASICS**

## DEFINITION
Avian avulaviruses (AAvV) are enveloped, single-stranded, negative-sense RNA viruses in the family *Paramyxoviridae* subfamily *Avulavirinae*, divided into 3 genera (*Metaavulavirus*, *Orthoavulavirus*, and *Paraavulavirus*) with 22 unique members (AAvV-1 to -22; previously known as avian paramyxoviruses), the most important species being avian orthoavulavirus 1 (OAvV-1), which is synonymous with Newcastle disease virus (NDV); the World Organisation for Animal Health (WOAH) still uses NDV to refer to OAvV-1 viruses. A wide variety of domestic and wild avian species are susceptible to AAvV-1 infection. Newcastle disease indicates a syndrome/disease caused in poultry species by virulent isolates of OAvV-1, also known as virulent Newcastle disease virus. Low-virulence isolates of OAvV-1 rarely cause clinical disease, almost exclusively in younger or immunosuppressed birds. OAvV-1 strains are pathotyped by the ability to cause disease in naive chickens (*Gallus gallus*). Pathotypes in increasing order of virulence are asymptomatic enteric, lentogenic, mesogenic, neurotropic velogenic, and viscerotropic velogenic. The intracerebral pathogenicity index in specific pathogen-free day-old chickens is used to standardize the virulence of OAvV-1 strains: 0.0–0.2, asymptomatic enteric; 0.2–0.5, lentogenic; 1.0–1.5,mesogenic; > 1.5 velogenic. Pathotype definitions may not be applicable to OAvV-1 infection in species other than domestic fowl, as species clinical signs may vary widely. Pigeon paramyxovirus serotype 1 (PPMV-1) denotes a variant of virulent OAvV-1 (viruses in genotype VI) that commonly circulates in Columbiformes worldwide, including domestic pigeons (*Columba livia domestica*). As PPMV-1 are virulent OAvV-1 viruses, they infect and may cause severe disease in non-Columbidae species. Avian metapneumoviruses (aMPV) includes enveloped, single-stranded, negative-sense RNA viruses in the family *Paramyxoviridae*, subfamily *Pneumovirnae*, genus *Metapneumovirus*; aMPVs are divided genetically into four subtypes (A, B, C, D). Primarily a cause of respiratory disease in turkeys (*Meleagris gallopavo*) and chickens, aMPVs have been isolated from waterfowl and gamefowl.

## PATHOPHYSIOLOGY
AAvV attaches to the host cell membrane via the hemagglutinin–neuraminidase protein, and the envelope fuses with the plasma membrane through the fusion protein in a pH-independent mechanism. Upon fusion, the viral ribonucleoprotein is released into the cytoplasm, where transcription of virus genes and full genome replication is carried out by the viral polymerase. Virions are released by budding. Virus is shed in feces and oropharyngeal secretions. Transmission is fecal–oral, aerosol, or contact with mucous membranes (especially conjunctiva). Pests (flies, mice), humans, and vehicles may act as fomites. The most important determinant of virulence for OAaV-1 is the cleavage site of the fusion protein. In virulent OAvV-1 strains, this protein is cleaved intracellularly by furin-like enzyme, leading to systemic infection. In non-virulent strains, the fusion protein is cleaved extracellularly by trypsin-like enzymes, limiting infection to the epithelium of the upper respiratory and GI tracts; in these cases, bacterial coinfection can worsen the disease. Most susceptible species to virulent OAvV-1 are Galliformes, such as chickens, turkeys, and pheasants. aMPV primarily targets respiratory epithelium, albeit it may target respiratory macrophages. aMPV attaches to the host cell and enters the cytoplasm where replication takes place. Virions are released by budding. Transmission is unpredictable, only contact confirmed to spread virus. *Escherichia coli* co-infection is believed to worsen clinical disease.

## SYSTEMS AFFECTED
AAvV—variable by host species and serotype. For virulent OAvV-1, primarily targeted are the lymphoid organs (including mucosa-associated lymphoid tissues), nervous and respiratory systems. aMPV—primarily respiratory, variable by host species.

## GENETICS
Fayoumi chickens have been reported to be partially resistant to development of clinical signs upon OAvV-1 infection, compared with inbred white leghorn chickens, although these differences are not relevant for clinical practice.

## INCIDENCE/PREVALENCE
OAvV-1: Poultry species (especially gallinaceous species) are considered the main reservoir of virulent OAvV-1 strains. Asymptomatic–enteric pathotype may be common in wild birds. A specific variant (genotype V) of virulent OAvV-1 may be endemic in Phalacrocoracidae (cormorants and shags) in North America. A specific variant (genotype VI; also known as PPMV-1) of virulent OAvV-1 is endemic in Columbiformes worldwide. OAvV-1 is distributed worldwide; Newcastle disease is common in poultry in Africa, Asia, Central America, and parts of South America; sporadic in other parts of the world. AAvV-2 to -22: Unknown, likely variable by species. aMPV: Common in poultry, variable in wild birds.

## GEOGRAPHIC DISTRIBUTION
Worldwide.

## SIGNALMENT
AAvVs infect a wide variety of avian species. Common species associations are: OAvV-1—any avian species, chickens considered most susceptible. PPMV-1 (OAvV-1 genotype V variant)—pigeons and doves, can infect other species and may cause disease (especially poultry). AAvV-2—chickens, Gouldian finch, orange-collared sparrow and house wren, ruddy turnstone, robin, canary, parrot, eagle, pheasant. AAvV-3—turkeys, chicken, ostrich, Psittaciformes and Passeriformes, parakeet. AAvV-4—ducks, mallard, serology in chickens. AAvV-5—budgerigars. AAvV-6—domestic ducks, mallard, serology in chicken. AAvV-7—hunter-killed dove, turkeys, ostriches, collard doves. AAvV-8—Canada geese, serology in wild fowl and mallards, wild ducks. AAvV-9—domestic ducks, migratory waterfowl. AAvV-10—rock hopper penguins (*Eudyptes chrysochome*), Magellanic peguins (*Spheniscus magellanicus*). AAvV-11—common snipe (*Gallinago gallinago*). AAvV-12—Eurasian wigeon (*Anas penelope*). AAvV-13—geese, white-fronted geese. AAvV-14—duck fecal sample. AAvV-15a—white-rumped sandpiper. AAvV-15b and AAvV-17—wild birds. aMPV—turkeys, chickens, numerous wild birds.

## SIGNS
### General Comments
Newcastle disease (caused by virulent OAvV-1 in susceptible species): Incubation period 2–15 days (average 5–6 days).

### Historical Findings
**Newcastle disease**: Galliformes (chickens, turkeys, pheasants); marked, peracute increase in mortality, sudden drop in egg production, misshapen eggs. Neurologic, GI, and/or respiratory signs. Viscerotropic velogenic disease carries up to 100% mortality and is associated with GI signs. Neurotropic velogenic disease carries around 50% mortality; respiratory, and neurologic

signs predominate. Other pathotypes show low to no mortality. Quail (*Coturnix japonica*): Moderate mortality (< 50%), neurologic signs. Psittacines: Species with reported infections include *Neophema* spp., budgerigars, yellow-headed Amazons (*Amazona oratrix*), yellow-naped Amazons (*Amazona auropalliata*). Malaise, respiratory signs may be reported. Raptors: Disease has been reported in falcons (*Falco* spp.). Neurologic ± GI signs are seen. Variable in other species.

**PPMV-1:** Pigeons: Variable morbidity (30–100%) and mortality (≤ 77% adults, ≤ 95% juveniles). GI and neurologic signs. Poor feather quality.

**AAvV 2–7:** Variable by serotype, host species. Generally a combination of GI, respiratory, and/or neurologic signs.

**AAvV 8–22:** Asymptomatic or unclear clinical picture.

**aMPV:** Turkeys: Severe morbidity (up to 100%), variable mortality (up to 50%), severely decreased egg production, respiratory signs. Chickens: Variable morbidity (up to 80%), low mortality, decreased egg production, swollen head, respiratory signs.

*Physical Examination Findings*
**Newcastle disease:** Vary by host species and pathotype of virus. Most often a combination of respiratory, GI, and neurologic signs. Chickens and turkeys: Viscerotropic—lethargy, facial swelling, conjunctivitis, mucoid oral discharge, dyspnea, cyanosis (especially comb), diphtheritic mucous membranes; neurotropic—hypermetria, head and muscle tremors, head tilt, unilateral paralysis; mesogenic—respiratory signs; neurologic signs—head tremors, head tilt, paralysis; lentogenic—respiratory signs (rare and mild, especially as a reaction to spray vaccination). Psittacines: Lethargy, oculonasal discharge, conjunctivitis, dyspnea; neurologic signs–falcons; neurotropic—hyperesthesia, clonic spasms, ataxia, head tremors, dysphagia, tongue paresis, ptyalism, amaurosis, third-eyelid paresis/paralysis, progressive pelvic limb paralysis, convulsions; viscerotropic—severe depression, mucoid diarrhea and hematochezia, constant vocalization.

**PPMV-1:** Pigeons: Ataxia, head tilt, limb paresis, pecking aside seeds, darrhea, poorly developed feathers if infected during molt.

**AAvV-2:** Turkeys: Respiratory signs (mild to severe), sinusitis, decreased egg production. Chickens: catarrhal tracheitis, mild enteritis, and GALT hyperplasia.

**AAvV-3:** Psittacines and passerines: Acute pancreatitis and CNS symptoms, worsening CNS signs with excitement, death, circling, head tilt, ataxia, opisthotonos, steatorrhea, weight loss, dyspnea. Red-crowned parakeets: enlarged liver and spleen, lymphocyte

infiltration in the kidneys, moderate lymphoid cell infiltration in hepatic and pulmonary tissue. Chickens and turkeys: Enlarged pancreas with focal necrosis.

**AAvV-4:** Chickens: Catarrhal tracheitis, mild enteritis, and GALT hyperplasia, mild interstitial pneumonia and lymphocytic infiltrates in the pancreas.

**AAvV-5:** Budgerigars: Death, depressed mentation, dyspnea, diarrhea, hemorrhages in the proventriculus, duodenum, jejunum, and rectum, discoloration of the liver and splenomegaly, head tilt (torticollis).

**AAvV-6:** Turkeys: Respiratory signs (mild), decreased egg production. Chickens: Catarrhal tracheitis, mild enteritis, and GALT hyperplasia, mild interstitial pneumonia and lymphocytic infiltrates in the pancreas.

**AAvV-7:** Turkeys: Rhinitis, dyspnea, enlarged pancreas and airsacculitis. Doves: Enlarged and congested livers and spleens.

**AAvV 8–10, 13–15, 17:** Asymptomatic.

**aMPV:** Turkeys: Snicking, rales, sneezing, nasal discharge, coughing, head shaking, foamy ocular discharge, swollen infraorbital sinuses, submandibular edema, uterine prolapse (secondary to cough). Chickens: Nasal discharge, foamy ocular discharge, peri/infraorbital sinus swelling, rales, head tilt, ataxia, opisthotonus.

## CAUSES
Newcastle disease: virulent form of OAvV -1. PPMV-1. AAvV 2–17, aMPV: Relevant virus.

## RISK FACTORS
OAvV-1: Exposure of poultry species to migratory birds, illegally acquired birds, unvaccinated birds, or pigeons. PPMV-1: Exposure to pigeon/dove racing or trade events. Raptors: feeding on pigeons and quail, use of pigeons in training. aMPV and many AAvV: Exposure to wild birds.

# DIAGNOSIS
## DIFFERENTIAL DIAGNOSIS
**Newcastle disease:** Poultry: Depending on clinical signs, variable list, including high-pathogenicity avian influenza, infectious bronchitis, infectious laryngotracheitis, mycoplasmosis, fowl cholera, aspergillosis, avian metapneumovirus, other bacterial infections. Other host species: Variable by clinical signs.

**PPMV-1:** Pigeons: Salmonellosis, adenovirus type 1. Other species: Variable by clinical signs.

**AAvV 2–17:** Variable by clinical signs.

**aMPV:** Low pathogenicity avian influenza, infectious laryngotracheitis, fowl cholera, mesogenic vNDV, other AAvV.

## CBC/BIOCHEMISTRY/URINALYSIS
Variable results, depending on systems affected and severity of infection.

## OTHER LABORATORY TESTS
**ND:** Contact regulatory authorities for guidance in sample acquisition from suspect cases. Viral isolation (VI): VI: Tracheal, oropharyngeal, or cloacal swabs; organ tissue samples—used to inoculate embryonated chicken eggs. May take up to seven days. HA assay: Performed on samples after virus isolation. HI assay: Performed with OAvV-1 antiserum on samples with a positive HA. OAvV-1 antiserum may cross-react with AAvV-3 and 7, rarely -2 and -4. Monoclonal antibodies may reduce cross-reactions. Molecular diagnostics: real-time rt-PCR on Matrix gene most commonly used, followed by real-time rt-PCR for putative fusion cleavage site. Genetic variation between viruses may reduce sensitivity. Once outbreak strain is determined, specific primers may be generated. Serology generally not diagnostically useful due to widespread vaccination in poultry. May be used to monitor flock immunity. HI and ELISA assays are used most to detect and quantify antibodies to OAvV-1. ELISA usually specific to host species.

**PPMV-1:** VI: Brain samples ideal (virus persists 5 weeks), cloacal swabs (virus persists 3 weeks); rtT-PCR more sensitive than VI.

**AAvV 2–17:** Combination of VI and HA.

**aMPV:** Viral DNA identification: VI: Sample oculonasal discharge, choana, sinus or intranasal scrapings. Best done as early as possible. Successful VI more difficult in severely affected birds. rt-PCR generally highly sensitive. Some kits only test for certain subtypes. Serology: ELISA: Variable sensitivity depending on subtype of virus. Virus neutralization and indirect immunofluorescence also available.

## IMAGING
Variable results depending on systems affected, severity of infection.

## DIAGNOSTIC PROCEDURES
N/A

## PATHOLOGIC FINDINGS
**AAvV:** Variable, depending on species and systems affected.

**OAvV-1:** Virulent strains: necrosis of lymphoid organs, haemorrhages throughout the visceral organs, hemorrhages in mucosa-associated lymphoid tissues in the GI tract, including the proventriculus and cecal tonsils. Non-virulent strains: mild lesions, mainly catarrhal inflammation of respiratory tract that may become more severe (fibrinous) due to secondary bacterial infection.

**aMPV**: Turkeys: Tracheal deciliation, mucoid exudate in turbinates and trachea, reproductive-associated coelomitis, misshapen eggs, airsacculitis, pericarditis, pneumonia, perihepatitis. Chickens: Yellow gelatinous to purulent edema of subcutaneous tissues of head.

# TREATMENT

## APPROPRIATE HEALTH CARE
For poultry affected by Newcastle disease, culling is usually carried out, as implemented by local veterinary authority. Proper biosecurity measures. Vaccination is carried out in poultry using live attenuated (lentogenic strains) and inactivated vaccines. AAvV and aMPV inactivated by most disinfectants, including bleach, ethanol, quaternary ammonia, iodophors. Removal of organic matter before application of disinfectants is critical. Avoid high stocking density and multi-age stock. Provide adequate ventilation and high-quality litter. Remove manure frequently.

## NURSING CARE
Symptomatic care indicated by patient, situation. Fluid therapy, oxygen therapy, hand feeding, supplemental heat may all be indicated.

## ACTIVITY
N/A

## DIET
N/A

## CLIENT EDUCATION
Proper biosecurity measures.

## SURGICAL CONSIDERATIONS
N/A

# MEDICATIONS

## DRUG(S) OF CHOICE
No antiviral drugs are known to treat AAvV or aMPV. Secondary infections common, especially respiratory. Select antimicrobials based on pathogen, sensitivity, location of infection, and patient species.

## CONTRAINDICATIONS
N/A

## PRECAUTIONS
Drug selection in food-producing animals should be made in compliance with regulatory statutes.

## POSSIBLE INTERACTIONS
N/A

## ALTERNATIVE DRUGS
N/A

# FOLLOW-UP

## PATIENT MONITORING
vND: Alert authorities—notifiable disease to WOAH. Monitor clinical status of both sick and asymptomatic exposed animals. Infected patients should be isolated for 14 days (aMPV) or 30 days (AAvV) beyond resolution of clinical signs. AAvV: Repeat testing (VI, rt-PCR) of recovered patients to determine if virus being shed.

## PREVENTION/AVOIDANCE
Proper biosecurity measures. Avoid contact with birds of unknown health status; 30-day quarantine for all new birds. Newcastle disease: Vaccines available, used in numerous species. Vaccination may substantially reduce clinical disease, cannot completely prevent virus replication/shedding. Protocols for poultry vary and are informed by husbandry and geographic location. Vaccination of falcons is recommended immediately after importation or as soon as moult is finished and training begins. Unvaccinated "sentinel" birds may be used. AAvV 2-17: Vaccines may be available against certain virus subtypes in specific species. aMPV: Vaccines available for turkeys and chickens. Protection, especially in chickens, may not be complete.

## POSSIBLE COMPLICATIONS
Secondary infections (especially respiratory).

## EXPECTED COURSE AND PROGNOSIS
Newcastle disease: Falcons—grave; death in 3–7 days. Psittacines—guarded to grave. Infected psittacines may intermittently shed virus for extended periods (> 1 year). Chickens—viscerotropic grave, up to 100% mortality; neurotropic guarded, ~50% mortality; mesogenic—good, low to no mortality. PPMV-1: Pigeons—guarded, highly variable mortality; poultry—as for Newcastle disease. AAvV-2: Good. AAvV-3: Turkeys—good; psittacines and passerines—guarded to grave, up to 100% mortality (may be species-dependent). AAvV-5: Budgerigars—grave, up to 100% mortality. AAvV-4, 8–17: Unknown, likely species dependent. aMPV: Turkeys—variable mortality (0.4–50%) depending on age, vaccination status. Uncomplicated infections resolve in 10–14 days. Chickens—good-to-variable morbidity, low mortality.

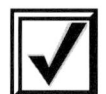

# MISCELLANEOUS

## ASSOCIATED CONDITIONS
Secondary respiratory infections.

## AGE-RELATED FACTORS
Juveniles may be more susceptible.

## ZOONOTIC POTENTIAL
OAvV-1 is rarely isolated from humans and there is no evidence of human-to-human transmission. It usually occurs in those who work closely with poultry or have lab infections. The most common symptom is a self-limiting conjunctivitis. aMPV: Clinical disease not reported, but turkey production workers have tested seropositive.

## FERTILITY/BREEDING
AAvV and aMPV may cause severe reproductive losses.

## SYNONYMS
Newcastle disease: Exotic Newcastle disease, pseudo-fowl pest, pseudo-fowl plague, avian pest, avian distemper, Tetelo disease, Ranikhet disease, Korean fowl plague. AAvV-2: Yucaipa virus. AAvV-5: Kunitachi virus. aMPV: Avian pneumovirus, turkey rhinotracheitis, swollen head syndrome, avian rhinotracheitis.

## SEE ALSO
Aspergillosis
Avian Influenza
Circoviruses
Herpesviruses
Mycoplasmosis
Neurologic (Non-Traumatic Diseases)
Pasteurellosis
Pneumonia
Respiratory Distress
Rhinitis and Sinusitis
Salmonellosis
Seizures
West Nile Virus
Also individual named viral diseases

## ABBREVIATIONS
AAvV—avian avulavirus
aMPV—avian metapneumovirus
APMV—avian paramyxovirus
CNS—central nervous system
ELISA—enzyme-linked immunosorbent assay
GALT—gastrointestinal-associated lymphoid tissue
GI—gastrointesinal
HA—hemagglutination
HI—hemagglutination inhibition
HN—hemagglutinin-neuraminidase
OAvV—avian orthoavulavirus
PPMV-1—pigeon paramyxovirus serotype-1
rt-PCR—reverse transcriptase PCR
VI—virus isolation
WOAH—World Organisation for Animal Health

## INTERNET RESOURCES
Center for Food Safety and Public Health, Iowa State University.Biosecurity website for livestock and poultry farmers: www.cfsph. iastate.edu

O

# Orthoavulaviruses

Cornell University, Cornell Wildlife Health Lab. Avian avulavirus (paramyxovirus): https://cwhl.vet.cornell.edu/disease/avian-avulavirus-paramyxovirus
US Department of Agriculture. Defend the Flock Program: http://www.aphis.usda.gov/animal_health/birdbiosecurity

*Suggested Reading*
Capua, I., Alexander, D.J. (eds) (2009). *Avian Influenza and Newcastle Disease: A Field and Laboratory Manual.* Milan, Italy: Springer-Verlag Italia.
Cattoli, G., Susta, L., Terregino, C., Brown, C. (2011). Newcastle disease: a review of field recognition and current methods of laboratory detection. *Journal of Veterinary Diagnostic Investigation*, 23:637–656.
Suarez, D., Miller, P.J., Koch, G., et al. (2020). Newcastle disease, other avian paramyxoviruses, and avian metapneumovirus infections. In: *Diseases of Poultry*, 14th edn. (ed. D.E. Swayne), 89–138. Hoboken, NJ: Wiley.

**Authors:** Sunoh Che, DVM, MSc, PhD, DACVPM, and Leonardo Susta, DVM, PhD, DACVP

# BASICS

## DEFINITION
Otitis is defined as inflammation of any of the structures of the ear. It can be further localized based on one of three locations: (1) Otitis externa includes inflammation of the structures surrounding the ear opening and any structures leading to the tympanic membrane, such as the external ear canal or external acoustic meatus. Unlike mammals, birds lack an auricle that can become inflamed. (2) Otitis media is inflammation of the tympanic membrane and structures in the tympanic cavity. Structures in the tympanic cavity include muscles, ligaments, the columella (the single auditory ossicle in birds), and the paratympanic organ (presumably serving as a barometer and altimeter). The tympanic cavity in birds pneumatize most of the bones of the neurocranium and, in most birds, the quadrate and mandibular bones. (3) Otitis interna is inflammation of tissues associated with the membranous labyrinth. This includes the cochlea, the *Macula lagenae* (presumably a magnetic field receptor), and the vestibular apparatus (utriculus, sacculus, and three semicircular canals).

## PATHOPHYSIOLOGY
Otitis is an inflammatory reaction in one of the three areas of the ear. Infection is the most common cause for the inflammatory reaction. Otitis externa may result from extension of otitis media past the tympanic membrane, or bacteria, fungi, or parasites on the skin near the ear opening entering the canal. As the tympanic cavity pneumatizes parts of the skull, infectious otitis media may extend to the medullary cavity of these bones. The close topographical relationship of CN VII to the external ear canal and middle ear cavity can lead to CN VII deficits with otitis externa and media. The spatial proximity of the middle and inner ear to the brain and the short CN VIII in birds makes ascending and descending otitis media/interna to and from the brain very likely. Neoplastic processes can invade the ear from other areas of the skull or originate in the ear canal. Topical aminoglycoside application generates free radicals within the inner ear, with subsequent permanent damage to sensory cells and neurons of the cochlea (permanent hearing loss) and/or vestibular apparatus (vertigo, ataxia, and/or nystagmus). Because birds can regenerate and replace hair cells of the inner ear, the hearing loss in birds may *not* be permanent as it is in mammals.

## SYSTEMS AFFECTED
**Nervous**: Otitis can lead to deafness, vestibular disease, CN VII deficits, and encephalitis.
**Ophthalmic**: As a continuation of an upper respiratory or infraorbital sinus infection, conjunctivitis may also be present.
**Respiratory**: If otitis interna/media is secondary to an upper respiratory infection, there may be signs of respiratory disease.
**Skin/exocrine**: If otitis externa is present, there may be discharge and feather loss near the ear opening.
**Gastrointestinal**: Severely affected birds may be anorexic.

## GENETICS
Eclectus parrots and macaws hatch with a thin membrane covering their ear canals that has tiny openings evident by day 2 in eclectus and day 23 in macaws. If this membrane remains intact, it can lead to inflammation of the outer ear canal.

## INCIDENCE/PREVALENCE
Otitis externa, otitis media, and otitis interna are uncommon to rare conditions in all orders of birds. Of the three locations for disease, otitis externa is the most common. Bacterial infection is the most common cause of otitis externa. Otitis media and interna remain rare disease diagnoses in birds.

## GEOGRAPHIC DISTRIBUTION
N/A

## SIGNALMENT
Lovebirds are prone to otitis externa; birds of prey have large middle ear cavities which could increase their susceptibility to otitis media.

## SIGNS
### Historical Findings
Otitis externa—owners may report increased scratching or rubbing of the skin and feathers near the ear opening. The owners may report feather loss near the ear opening. Crusted feathers and discharge around the ear opening may be seen. Otitis media/interna—owners may report lack of balance as evidenced by falling off the perch, an inability to perch, an inability to fly, a head tilt, nystagmus, and/or head swaying. Observant owners may notice decreased hearing or louder vocalization if the hearing has been compromised.

### Physical Examination Findings
**Otitis externa**: External examination of the ear opening may reveal loss of the ear coverts/auriculars surrounding the ear opening, active or dried discharge from the canal, growths or skin thickening near the ear opening, or periauricular swelling, pain, and erythema.

**Otitis media/interna**: Otoscopic examination (using a small cone) may reveal a ruptured, swollen, or thickened tympanic membrane. Signs of vestibular disease such as a head tilt, torticollis, proprioceptive deficits, ataxia, nystagmus, and head swaying may be present. Decreased or absent response to loud noises can be noted if the hearing has been affected.
**Associated signs**: Changes in mentation, blindness, seizures, and head pressing if the otitis is associated with encephalitis. Ocular or nasal discharge, periocular swelling, conjunctivitis, sneezing, and a change in the auscultation of the air sacs if otitis is associated with respiratory or the infraorbital sinus disease.

## CAUSES
**Anatomic**: Retained ear canal membrane in post-hatchling eclectus and macaws.
**Neoplastic**: Squamous cell carcinoma of the ceruminous gland of the ear; non-specified benign neoplasia causing hemorrhage from the ear was reported in an Amazon parrot.
**Nutritional**: Hypovitaminosis A leading to squamous metaplasia may predispose to opportunistic bacterial and/or fungal otitis.
**Infectious (bacterial)**: Otitis interna—*Salmonella enterica arizonae* was reported in turkey poults with meningoencephalitis spreading to the inner ear via CN VIII causing otitis interna; *Pseudomonas aeruginosa* was reported to cause otitis interna in a little bustard; otitis media—*P. aeruginosa* was reported to cause otitis media in an African grey parrot, turkeys, and chickens; *Proteus mirabilis* causes otitis media in poultry; *Mycoplasma gallisepticum* causes otitis media in turkeys; *Ornithobacterium rhinotracheale* was reported to cause otitis media and cranial osteomyelitis in red-legged partridges. Otitis externa—*Corynebacterium kroppenstedtii* was reported to cause otitis externa in a lovebird; *Mycobacterium* spp. have been reported to cause a mass protruding from the left ear in a pionus parrot; *P. aeruginosa*, *Klebsiella* sp., *Enterobacter* sp., *Staphylococcus aureus*, and *Kocuria kristinae* have been indicated to cause otitis externa.
**Infectious (viral)**: Paramyxovirus causes otitis interna; poxvirus can cause proliferative lesions near the opening of the external ear causing otitis externa; circovirus was reported to cause fibroepithelial hyperplasia of the external acoustic meatus in a kakariki; herpesvirus (psittacid herpesvirus 3) was reported to cause primary respiratory disease and secondary otitis media in Bourke's parrots.
**Infectious (fungal)**: *Candida* spp., *Microsporum gallinae*, *Aspergillus* sp. can cause dermatitis that can extend to the external ear.

O

**Parasitic:** *Cryptosporidium baileyi* was reported to cause otitis media in a Saker falcon); ectoparasites such as *Knemidocoptes*, harvest mites, and fleas (*Echidnophaga gallinacean*) can localize on the head and enter the external ear canal.

**Iatrogenic:** Foreign material such as food or regurgitated material can lodge in the ear canal.

**Traumatic:** Traumatic injury to the head can lead to hemorrhage, swelling, inflammation, or fracture of the skull and associated external, middle, and inner ear, which could result in transient or permanent deafness and vestibular disease.

**Toxic:** Ototoxicity of the inner ear can occur with the application of topical aminoglycoside antibiotics in a patient without an intact tympanic membrane; streptomycin and gentamicin are primarily vestibulotoxic, and amikacin, neomycin, dihydrostreptomycin, and kanamycin are primarily cochleotoxic.

## RISK FACTORS
N/A

## DIAGNOSIS

### DIFFERENTIAL DIAGNOSIS
Otitis externa: No other disease condition will result in skin and feather changes around the external ear opening. Otitis media and interna: Neurologic signs associated with this condition can also be caused by CNS disease and any disease condition that causes whole body weakness and vestibular signs.

### CBC/BIOCHEMISTRY/URINALYSIS
Possibly increased white blood cell count due to an absolute heterophilia. Chronic disease may lead to a monocytosis and non-regenerative anemia of chronic inflammation. Plasma biochemistry: Not associated with abnormalities.

### OTHER LABORATORY TESTS
Bacterial and fungal infections can be diagnosed via C/S. Cytology, Gram stain, and skin scrapings can be used to diagnose parasitic disease and decide on empirical antimicrobial therapy while awaiting culture results. Biopsy of any tumor, growth, or irregular swelling. Viral testing as necessary.

### IMAGING
Radiographs are not helpful in demonstrating the anatomic structure of most birds. Dorsoventral and lateral projections can be useful in Psittaciformes. For most species, CT scan and/or MRI are the preferred diagnostic imaging modalities.

### DIAGNOSTIC PROCEDURES
Rigid endoscopy with a 1.9-mm scope can be used to examine the external ear canal and tympanic membrane, to obtain a biopsy, to remove foreign material, or to obtain a sample for cytology and culture and sensitivity.

### PATHOLOGIC FINDINGS
Inflammation and infectious disease organisms can be seen on tissue samples from areas affected by otitis.

## TREATMENT

### APPROPRIATE HEALTH CARE
Most of these patients are stable and do not require in-hospital treatment. Most patients are treated as outpatients. In some cases, debridement of discharge in or around the external ear canal may be needed.

### NURSING CARE
Nursing care is necessary in cases where otitis media/externa is present, and the patient has severe vestibular disease and cannot perch nor stand properly. In these cases, most patients also need to be support fed as they are anorexic. Necessary care may include a padded enclosure with no perches until the patient is more stable. Assist feedings and parenteral fluids may be necessary until the patient is stable and able to drink and eat on its own.

### ACTIVITY
N/A

### DIET
N/A

### CLIENT EDUCATION
If the patient has torticollis or a head tilt as a result of otitis media/interna, these conditions may not fully resolve once the disease condition has been treated. Clients should be instructed on how to set up an enclosure for a patient with a chronic head tilt or torticollis. Hearing loss in birds may not be permanent if it is caused by loss of the hair cells in the inner ear.

### SURGICAL CONSIDERATIONS
N/A

## MEDICATIONS

### DRUG(S) OF CHOICE
Antibiotic selection is based on culture and sensitivity results. Antibiotics can be given orally. They can also be applied to the area around the opening of the ear canal and into the ear canal. Topical water-based or ophthalmic antibiotic solutions are preferable to oil-based preparations. NSAIDs to decrease pain and inflammation— meloxicam 1.0 mg/kg PO q12h. Possible saline ear canal flushes. Analgesics as necessary.

### CONTRAINDICATIONS
Aminoglycosides should be avoided as they are toxic to inner ear structures. Topical and systemic steroids are contraindicated as they may exacerbate signs associated with infection.

### PRECAUTIONS
Avoid vigorous flushing around the opening of the ear canal.

### POSSIBLE INTERACTIONS
N/A

### ALTERNATIVE DRUGS
Topical acetic and boric acid commercial solution if a bacterial infection is suspected.

## FOLLOW-UP

### PATIENT MONITORING
Follow up within 1 week of diagnosis and treatment to observe effectiveness of antimicrobials in case of bacterial or fungal disease.

### PREVENTION/AVOIDANCE
N/A

### POSSIBLE COMPLICATIONS
Long-term hearing loss. Long-term difficulty balancing and flying.

### EXPECTED COURSE AND PROGNOSIS
Uncomplicated infection that is susceptible to drug treatment should resolve in 10–14 days. More complicated disease associated with osteomyelitis may take much longer to resolve. Disease involving structures associated with balance and proprioception may not recover to a normal state.

## MISCELLANEOUS

### ASSOCIATED CONDITIONS
Upper respiratory disease.

### AGE-RELATED FACTORS
N/A

### ZOONOTIC POTENTIAL
N/A

### FERTILITY/BREEDING
N/A

### SYNONYMS
N/A

### SEE ALSO
Hypocalcemia and Hypomagnesemia
Lameness
Neural Larva Migrans
Neurologic (Non-Traumatic Diseases)
Neurologic (Trauma)

Toxicosis (Environmental and Pesticides)
Toxicosis (Heavy Metals)
Neoplasia (Neurological)
Orthoavulaviruses
Rhinitis and Sinusitis
Seizures
Trauma
West Nile Virus

## ABBREVIATIONS
C/S—culture and sensitivity
CN—cranial nerve
CNS—central nervous system
CT—computed tomography
MRI—magnetic resonance imaging
NSAIDs—non-steroidal anti-inflammatory drugs

## INTERNET RESOURCES
N/A

*Suggested Reading*
Bonsmann, A., Stoffel, M.H., Burkhart, M., Hatt, J.M. (2016). Anatomical atlas of the quail's ear (*Coturnix coturnix*). *Anatomia, Histologia, Embryologia*, 45:399–404.
Martel, A., Haesebrouck, F., Hellebuyck, T., Pasmans, F. (2009). Treatment of otitis externa associated with *Corynebacterium kroppenstedtii* in a peach-faced lovebird (*Agapornis roseicollis*) with an acetic and boric acid commercial solution. *Journal of Avian Medicine and Surgery*, 23:141–150.
Rival, F. (2005). Auricular diseases in birds. In: *Proceedings of the 8th European Association of Avian Veterinarians Conference*, Arles, France, April 24–30, 333–339.
Scala, C., Langlois, I., Lemberger, K. (2015). Bilateral granulomatous and fibrinoheterophilic otitis interna due to *Pseudomonas aeruginosa* in a captive little bustard (*Tetrax tetrax*). *Journal of Avian Medicine and Surgery*, 29:120–124.

**Author**: Nicole R. Wyre, DVM, DABVP (Avian and Exotic Companion Mammal), CVA, CTPEP

**Acknowledgements**: 1st edition author, Karen Rosenthal, DVM, MS

O

# OVARIAN DISEASES

## BASICS

### DEFINITION
The most common diseases affecting the ovary in psittacine, galliforme and anseriforme patients are cystic ovarian disease, ovarian neoplasia, and oophoritis, which is an infectious or inflammatory disease of the ovary. Cystic ovarian disease is somewhat common in a variety of pet bird species, but occurs in higher frequency in budgerigars, cockatiels, canaries, and pheasants. The exact cause is unknown, although an endocrine imbalance is suspected. The disease is characterized by a single or multiple cystic structures on the ovary. Ovarian neoplasia can occur in any species and predominantly affects mature or older avian subjects. Cockatiels, budgerigars, and chickens are more commonly affected. The ovary is usually consumed by a proliferative, firm, multinodular mass when first identified or visually examined. The physical appearance may either be a flattened mass with a grainy surface or an enlarged ovary with a multitude of varying sized follicles. Ovarian neoplasms are typically classified by tissue of origin. Oophoritis is an inflammation of the ovary. The etiology of the inflammatory process may be infectious (bacterial, fungal, viral), neoplastic or an inflammatory process spread by disease in an adjoining abdominal coelomic organ.

### PATHOPHYSIOLOGY
Cystic ovarian disease is suspected to be an endocrine related disease affecting the ovary of a variety of avian species. A secondary condition is hyperostosis of long bones, noted both on radiographic appearance and histopathology sections of bones of the extremities. The cause of ovarian neoplastic diseases is usually either of a genetic predisposition in psittacines or of a herpesvirus-induced disease, also known as Marek's disease, in gallinaceous birds. In chickens, ALV can create neoplastic disease of the ovary. Ovarian adenocarcinoma is also common in laying chickens. Oophoritis is most often caused by retrograde migration of bacteria from the cloaca up the oviduct to access the ovary and abdominal coelom. Viral diseases and, less often, systemic fungal diseases may also affect the ovary. Ovarian neoplasms may cause in inflammatory reaction of the ovarian tissue as the mass grows. Inflammatory disease processes of local organs such as the kidney, pancreas, and intestinal tract may also cause inflammation to the ovary.

## SYSTEMS AFFECTED
**Reproductive**: One or more cystic structures may be noted on the ovary. Abdominal distension is a common secondary clinical sign. Reproductive performance may be affected negatively. Infertility is common in both disease states. Oviductal neoplasms may occur concomitantly with ovarian neoplasms.

**Musculoskeletal**: Hyperostosis of the bones of the extremities is commonly noted on radiographs in both diseases. Pectoral muscle mass loss is common in advanced stages of both disease states.

**Hepatobiliary**: Metastasis of ovarian carcinomas to the liver, spleen or other internal organs may occur.

**Gastrointestinal**: Abdominal herniation with incorporated loops of bowel may occur with advanced cases of either disease. Feces may collect on the vent or even pile up due to abdominal distension and dorsal displacement of the vent by the swollen abdomen or by distension from abdominal herniation.

**Neuromuscular**: Left-leg lameness may occur if the neoplasm applies pressure to the ischiatic nerve.

**Behavioral**: Affected birds may show nesting behavior. If abdominal distension is severe, patients may show lethargy, ataxia, or respiratory distress.

## GENETICS
Suspected to be genetically inherited in budgerigars and cockatiels.

## INCIDENCE/PREVALENCE
Cystic ovarian disease and oophoritis are fairly common conditions in cockatiels and budgerigars. Can be noted in a variety of other species. Eclectus parrots seem to have a higher incidence among the larger psittacines. Ovarian neoplasia—psittacines, budgerigars, and cockatiels are overrepresented, suspected to be from a genetically inherited trait. In chickens that have not been vaccinated for Marek's disease and/or have been exposed to carrier birds or birds symptomatic of Marek's disease, the incidence is fairly high. ALV tends to occur in lower numbers in domestic poultry, but is a well-known factor causing ovarian cancer, as well as other neoplastic diseases within the abdominal coelom. Ovarian adenocarcinoma is common in laying chickens.

## GEOGRAPHIC DISTRIBUTION
N/A

## SIGNALMENT
**Species**: Can occur in any avian species.
**Breed predilections**: Budgerigar, cockatiel, eclectus parrot, poultry.

**Mean age and range**: Affected birds are sexually mature and have usually had several seasons of production or breeding.
**Predominant sex**: Female.

## SIGNS
### General Comments
Initially, the signs of ovarian cysts and oophoritis are hidden from human inspection until the patient becomes clinically affected. Large ovarian cysts and ovarian neoplastic masses often create abdominal distension from just the sheer size of the cyst/neoplasm or from ascites. Infertility may be noted in breeder birds and initiate the reason for an endoscopic view of the ovary. Radiographs often reveal bilateral hyperostosis of long bones (radius, ulna, femur and tibiotarsus). In severely affected birds, all bones may show a bright homogeneous, mineral opacity. Large cysts or neoplasms will often reveal a soft-tissue dense mass immediately cranial to the anterior renal pole on a true lateral radiographic projection. Some birds exhibit nesting behavior for long periods of time with no egg production. Generalized lethargy and weight loss occurs more often in chickens with either Marek's disease or ALV.

### Historical Findings
Many cases are presented as egg bound, due to the abdominal distension with no recent egg production. Breeders note infertility as a reason for the examination.

### Physical Examination Findings
Most cases of cystic ovarian disease, oophoritis, and ovarian neoplasia present with some degree of abdominal distension. Abdominal palpation often reveals a fluid filled abdomen with no egg present. In severe cases of abdominal distension caused by large ovarian cysts or ascites, dypsnea and exercise intolerance may be noted.

## CAUSES
Endocrine-related metabolic imbalances are assumed to be the initiating factor for cystic ovarian disease in psittacines and passerines. Ovarian neoplasia may be an end-stage disease of cystic ovarian disease. Lymphoma of the ovary secondary to Marek's disease is common in chickens. Other ovarian neoplasias may occur without a specific etiologic agent.

## RISK FACTORS
Allowing chronic hormonal stimulation in species known to be prone to excessive egg laying (budgerigars, cockatiels, and eclectus) may predispose to cystic ovarian disease. Marek's-related ovarian lymphoma is common in backyard flocks or small breeder setups where baby chicks are exposed to carrier or unvaccinated adults.

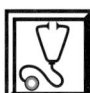

# DIAGNOSIS

## DIFFERENTIAL DIAGNOSIS

Abdominal swelling due to ascites may be secondary to peritonitis, liver disease, cardiac disease, or oophoritis. Abdominal swelling with a firm intracoelomic mass may be caused by a retained egg, ectopic egg, or a neoplastic disease of an abdominal organ. Dyspnea due to abdominal distension may be also noted with ascites, neoplasia of an abdominal organ that has displaced, or compressed abdominal air sacs. Any infectious, inflammatory, fungal, metabolic, or neoplastic disease affecting the ovary or oviduct may be implicated with respect to infertility issues.

## CBC/BIOCHEMISTRY/URINALYSIS

CBC in cases of cystic ovarian disease will vary from normal to a picture of an inflammatory hemogram where ascites is a part of the clinical picture. Some cases of oophoritis may show an elevated WBC count with basophilia and in severe cases, a left shift of the heterophilic series. Ovarian neoplastic diseases often reveal normal hemograms unless lymphoid neoplasia is involved. Lymphoma of the ovary is a common sequelae in Marek's and ALV. As with other lymphoid neoplastic diseases, circulating anaplastic or neoplastic lymphocytes may be apparent in WBC differential counts of these two viral diseases. PCV may be low if there has been metastasis to the bone marrow. Blood chemistry profiles generally show elevations of AST and CK, indicative of muscle loss and/or internal inflammatory disease.

## OTHER LABORATORY TESTS
N/A

## IMAGING

### Radiographic Findings

Whole-body survey radiographs in pure cystic ovarian diseases may show a fluid or soft tissue dense, spherical space-occupying mass or masses juxtaposed to the cranial pole of the renal silhouette on the lateral view. Cases involving ascites will produce a homogeneous fluid density encompassing the vast majority or the entire space of the abdominal coelom. Homogenous osseous density of long bones, termed hyperostosis, is a common finding in ovarian cystic disease and many cases of ovarian neoplastic disease. This infers an endocrine imbalance involving calcium mobilization. Ovarian neoplasias produce a soft-tissue dense space-occupying mass cranial to the cranial division of the kidney in a lateral view. The shape may be lobulated to spherical. Barium contrast radiography has a great benefit in relation to space occupying abdominal masses. On a lateral projection, barium-filled loops of intestines are displaced ventrally in cases of ovarian cysts and medium to large size ovarian neoplasms. Ventrodorsal radiographic projections of both ovarian cystic disease and ovarian neoplasia generally reveal displacement of barium-filled ventriculus and/or intestinal loops to the center or right side of the abdominal coelom. Rarely will cases of oophoritis be noticeable radiographically.

### Ultrasonography

Ultrasonography of the abdominal coelom is extremely valuable if performed and read by a radiologist or someone with vast experience and training in identifying anatomical abnormalities of the avian ovary. Ultrasonography of the normal ovarian ducts and ovaries is challenging, and visualization of the ovaries depends on their size and quality of the ultrasound equipment and user experience. Ovarian follicles appear as rounded, variably echogenic structures, where the echogenicity changes with maturation, increasing in echogenicity as the yolk develops. Ovarian cysts can be single or multiple. Occasionally, effusion of an undetermined source may be the only finding when ovarian cysts are present. They appear sonographically as clearly defined, rounded anechoic, thin-walled compartments with distal acoustic enhancement. Ovarian neoplasms typically appear as large masses. They are well-defined structures, usually easily detected, large, rounded masses of mixed echogenicity, seen sonographically as having a marked focal or diffuse homogenous echotexture. Again, oophoritis cases may not be identified by abdominal coelomic ultrasound.

### Advanced Imaging

Coelomic CT has the potential to be valuable in mid- and large-size Psittacines, Galliformes and Anseriformes. There are several limiting factors in reference to the ability of the scan to deliver an accurate diagnostic image. An extremely critical factor is the capability of the CT unit. Many machines used in the veterinary market are not advanced enough to provide images on small patients with small size pathological issues. Slices smaller than 2 mm are generally needed to diagnose masses or cystic structures in our avian patients. Secondly and equally important, the size of the patient and the corresponding size of the mass must be of adequate size for the specific machine being used to identify the pathological abnormality on the ovary.

## DIAGNOSTIC PROCEDURES

Abdominal coelomic endoscopy is extremely diagnostic in cases of all cases of oophoritis, cystic ovarian disease, and ovarian neoplasia where ascites is not the predominating clinical presentation. Cystic masses on the ovary may be an incidental finding in cases of infertility investigation or when radiographs indicate potential ovarian disease. Solid, nodular soft tissue masses both small and large can be visualized on endoscopy of the left abdominal coelom in cases of ovarian neoplastic diseases. C/S of the ovary is essential for directing treatment for cases of oophoritis. Suspected cases of a virus-induced neoplastic process in chickens will need blood tests, biopsy, or necropsy submission for an accurate diagnosis of ALV or Marek's disease.

## PATHOLOGIC FINDINGS

Depending on the severity of the ovarian cystic disease, surgical or gross necropsy findings reveal one of the following: One large cystic structure attached to the surface of the ovary that may be several mm to cm in diameter, depending on the species involved or numerous medium-sized ovarian cystic structures that fill up a large area in the abdominal coelom. The cysts are well encapsulated and filled with either clear fluid or yolk material. In cockatiel species, the cysts often take up 50–75% of the abdominal coelom. These cysts are easy to aspirate with a 25–26 gauge needle or winged infusion set attached to a 3- to 12-cc syringe. Care must be taken in small species not to suction the entire amount of the fluid contents, as this may create a metabolic imbalance by drawing off fluid that contains protein and electrolytes that the patient uses to create a homeostatic metabolic environment. These cystic structures are loosely attached to the ovarian parenchyma yet often have a vascular supply at the attachment site. Endoscopic visualization of a patient with oophoritis may reveal a mucoid to cheesy material on the surface of the ovary. The vasculature will generally be more prominent as it tries to help combat the inflammation. Cultures are advisable to identify a bacterial involvement in the disease etiology. With advanced training and experience, an endoscopic or open laparotomy may be essential to take a biopsy of the ovary to obtain the most diagnostic sample for this disease. Ovarian neoplastic disease may take on several shapes and sizes in avian species. These cancerous masses generally involve the entire ovarian parenchyma. Ovarian neoplasms may create dozens of medium size follicles that take up a large portion of the left and right cranial abdominal coelom. Certain types of ovarian neoplasms may produce a large solid mass that engulfs the entire ovary. The following

O

types of ovarian tumors have been reported: Lymphoma, adenocarcinoma, leiomyosarcoma, adenoma, and granulosa cell tumors. In poultry, Marek's-induced lymphoma is very common. Granulosa cell tumors are yellow-lobulated, irregular masses that are friable. They may become quite large and may fill the abdominal cavity. Ovarian carcinomas are variably sized, firm, gray-white, and multilobular. They may implant on serosal surfaces of adjacent organs, the mesentery, and body wall. They may also metastasize. Arrhenoblastomas are gray-white, lobulated masses comprising structures resembling seminiferous tubules. Carcinomatosis has been reported in poultry as a sequelae to ovarian neoplastic disease. Histopathology of ovarian cystic disease reveals cysts lined by flattened cells caused by trapped surface mesothelium. Granulosa cells line follicular cysts. In reference to histopathology of ovarian neoplastic disease, the findings will vary greatly depending on the specific cell type of ovarian neoplasm present. Granulosa cell tumors are composed of nests and trabeculae of slightly pleomorphic cells with eosinophilic cytoplasm and vesicular nuclei separated by variable amounts of stroma. Histologically, carcinomas are composed of poorly differentiated epithelial cells forming cords, acini, and papillary structures.

# TREATMENT

## APPROPRIATE HEALTH CARE
Patients exhibiting symptoms of lethargy, abdominal distension, and/or dyspnea will benefit by being hospitalized in a quiet, warm environment. Dyspneic patients should be placed in an oxygen cage. Cases presenting with a large fluid distended abdomen, will need cystocentesis to remove up to 50% of the suspected ascitic fluid to relieve some of the abdominal pressure and the air sac displacement.

## NURSING CARE
Placing the patient in a warmed hospital cage that is secluded and has dimmed lighting will help the bird's homeostasis mechanisms. Anorectic patients will need gavage feeding an avian nutrient formula for sick birds. Intravenous fluids may be required for critically depressed patients. Patients with ovarian neoplasia need supportive care of heat, fluids and nutrition while medical or surgical management is contemplated. Removal of the female from any conspecific male birds, nesting material, or hiding places, and removal of mirrors and other self-stimulating objects from the cage or home environment is advised for female birds with

cystic ovarian disease. Birds with ascites or large fluid-filled cysts should have the fluid aspirated to relieve the physical pressure of the fluid or cyst on the respiratory system.

## ACTIVITY
If the patient is totally non-symptomatic, no restriction on activity will be necessary. Weak or lethargic patients need to be hospitalized in a quiet, warm environment. Restricted activity may be beneficial in both cases to conserve the patient's strength and keep respiratory efforts at a baseline level.

## DIET
N/A

## CLIENT EDUCATION
Cystic ovarian disease is a chronic recurring condition. Lifelong changes will be necessary to help control the disease. Manipulation of the environment is essential to diminish hormonal stimulation that may lead to ovarian cyst formation. Changes to the home environment must include removal of all nest boxes, nesting materials, and mirrors. Preferably, the female should be kept in a different room from any conspecific male, and owners should refrain from stroking or petting the bird on her back, and should not let the bird hide under blankets, sheets, or towels. Owners must watch for signs of abdominal swelling, respiratory distress, or nesting-type behavior. Recurring symptoms must be attended to quickly. Avian patients with ovarian cancer are in need of frequent reassessments. Even with surgical removal or debulking, chemotherapy, or radiation therapy, neoplasms of the ovary may grow at an extraordinary rate. Abdominal swelling or pressure on surrounding renal tissue needs to be rechecked on a routine basis, the timing of which will depend on the species, size of the original mass, and overall health of the patient. A recheck examination by endoscopy, radiology, or ultrasonography is required to reassess and evaluate true changes in size of the neoplasm. Prevention is key in reference to ALV and Marek's-induced disease in chickens. Vaccinating baby chicks against Marek's disease before they are allowed to have contact with the soil or purchasing vaccinated chicks is an extremely valuable preventative measure.

## SURGICAL CONSIDERATIONS
Surgery for correction of ovarian cystic disease is risky and should only be attempted by an accomplished avian surgeon and only after abdominocentesis and medical therapy have failed. Exploratory surgery will be a challenge on these patients. Their respiratory status is challenged by the shear size of the mass. They are generally in a catabolic state and if the abdominal air sacs are incised and the cystic fluid enters this space, the patient

may drown. The patient should be placed on a surgical board with head elevated The surgical approach may either be with the patient in dorsal recumbancy for a left lateral approach or in right lateral recumbancy for a left lateral approach. Extreme care must be taken on the surgical approach. Inside the coelom, the intestinal loops are often displaced and may be in a location that will interfere with the usual entry location. Once in the abdominal coelom, the cystic structure is identified and often aspirated to collapse the structure so the ovary and surrounding structures may be identified. Once all vital structures (kidney, intestinal loops, ureter) have been identified, the surgeon may either ligate the cystic structure with Hemoclips or a surgical ligature. Radiosurgical excision with and without endoscopy has been performed. Extreme care must be taken not to ligate the anterior pole of the kidney, the renal artery, or the ureter. The larger the species, the easier it is to visualize the vital structures around the ovary. Ovarian neoplastic diseases are generally very difficult to resolve surgically. In large species (macaws, raptors, chickens, ducks), there exists the potential for a successful surgical outcome. In general, ovarian neoplasms encompass the entire ovary and are closely attached to the cranial pole of the left kidney, making surgical or radiosurgical excision difficult and risky.

# MEDICATIONS

## DRUG(S) OF CHOICE
There are several therapeutic options for treating ovarian cysts in the avian patient; hCG has been used for decades in avian patients to control excessive layers. Leuprolide acetate, a GnRH agonist, has been used for over two decades to treat excessive egg laying in psittacines. Deslorelin acetate, an implant formulation of a GnRH agonist, has recently been used anecdotally to treat a variety of ovarian diseases in avian species. Reports from several practitioners reveal some cases have shown diminishment of cyst size with the use of deslorelin acetate. Cabergoline, a potent dopamine receptor agonist, may be used to treat cystic ovary patients. It works in humans by reducing prolactin release from the pituitary gland. Dosages for the various pharmaceutical agents mentioned above are cabergoline 10–20 ug/kg s.i.d. or as needed, deslorelin acetate implant 4.7 mg, hCG 500–1000 units/kg IM on days 1, 3, 7 q3–6w, leuprolide acetate 200–800 µg/kg q14d for 3 treatments (average dosage recommendation is

500 μg/kg); ovarian neoplastic masses have shown size reduction with the use of deslorelin acetate. Chemotherapy may be beneficial in certain cases that are diagnosed by laparoscopic or open laparotomy biopsy. If the etiology for a case of oophoritis is bacterial in nature and a culture of the ovary is obtained, an appropriate antibiotic therapy will be necessary. The use of meloxicam, a non-steroidal anti-inflammatory drug, is also advisable. Viral etiologies generally are not responsive to treatment. Some fungal etiologies may respond to antifungal medications and meloxicam.

### CONTRAINDICATIONS
N/A

### PRECAUTIONS
Medroxyprogesterone acetate has been used in years past to treat excessive egg laying and ovarian cyst formation. This drug has been proven to cause fatal hepatic lipidosis in avian species. It is not recommended for use since other safer alternatives are available. The use of deslorelin acetate in non-ferret species is considered extra-label and is prohibited by Virbac. Use in chickens, a food animal as categorized by the FDA, may be illegal.

### POSSIBLE INTERACTIONS
N/A

### ALTERNATIVE DRUGS
An holistic supplement consisting of palm fruit and raspberries has been shown to diminish egg laying in psittacines and therefore may be of benefit to shrink ovarian cysts. Alternative treatments or therapies have not been documented to provide a benefit for ovarian neoplastic diseases.

 FOLLOW-UP

### PATIENT MONITORING
Weekly, monthly or quarterly recheck appointments are recommended to assess shrinkage of the cystic or neoplastic ovarian mass. Referral to a facility that has endoscopy, ultrasound or CT capability will provide more accurate assessment of changes in size of the mass.

### PREVENTION/AVOIDANCE
Hormone stimulation is the main at home avoidance therapy that will be useful to slow or prevent recurrence of cystic structures. In specific reference to chickens, vaccinating day old chicks against Marek's disease or purchasing Marek's vaccinated young chicks is the best way to prevent Marek's-associated ovarian lymphosarcoma.

### POSSIBLE COMPLICATIONS
In reference to ovarian cystic disease, recurrence is likely. Close attention needs to be paid to abdominal swelling, dyspnea, lethargy, depression, and/or anorexia. Patients with bacterial or fungal oophoritis will generally improve with the proper treatment course. Patients with ovarian neoplastic masses may show acute symptoms of depression, lethargy, anemia, and/or dyspnea at any time frame post diagnosis or initiation of therapy.

### EXPECTED COURSE AND PROGNOSIS
Both diseases have a high potential for progression of the disease. Death or elective euthanasia may be possible outcomes for both ovarian cystic disease and ovarian neoplastic diseases.

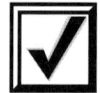 MISCELLANEOUS

### ASSOCIATED CONDITIONS
Cases of ovarian cystic disease, oophoritis, and ovarian neoplastic diseases may cause abdominal distension, dyspnea, and/or ascites.

### AGE-RELATED FACTORS
All three conditions occur in mature female birds.

### ZOONOTIC POTENTIAL
N/A

### FERTILITY/BREEDING
All three diseases often result in an infertile hen.

### SYNONYMS
Ovarian cysts
Carcinomatosis

### SEE ALSO
Ascites
Cere and Skin, Color Changes
Chronic Egg Laying

Coelomic Distention
Dystocia and Egg Binding
Egg Yolk and Reproductive Coelomitis
Infertility
Lameness
Neoplasia (Lymphoproliferative)
Neoplasia (Reproductive)
Oviductal Diseases

### ABBREVIATIONS
ALV—avian leukosis virus
AST—aspartate aminotransferase
C/S—culture and sensitivity
CK—creatine kinase
CT—computed tomography
GnRH—gonadotropin-releasing hormone
hCG—human chorionic gonadotropin
PCV—packed cell volume
WBC—white blood cell

### INTERNET RESOURCES
N/A

*Suggested Reading*
Bowles, H.L. (2002). Reproductive diseases of pet bird species. *Veterinary Clinics of North America: Exotic Animal Practice*, 5:489–506.
Hofbauer, H., Krautwald-Junghanns, M.E. (1999). Transcutaneous ultrasonography of the avian urogenital tract. *Veterinary Radiology & Ultrasound*, 40:58–64.
Keller, K.A., Beaufrère, H., Brandao, J., et al. (2013). Long-term management of ovarian neoplasia in two cockatiels (*Nymphicus hollandicus*). *Journal of Avian Medicine and Surgery*, 27:44–52.
Mans, C., Pilny, A. (2014). Use of GnRH-agonists for medical management of reproductive disorders in birds. *Veterinary Clinics of North America: Exotic Animal Practice*, 17:23–33.
Scagnelli, A.M., Tully, T.N. (2017). Reproductive diseases in parrots. *Veterinary Clinics of North America: Exotic Animal Practice*, 20:485–507.
Schmidt, R.E., Reavill, D.R., Phalen, D.N. (2003). Reproductive system. In: *Pathology of Pet and Aviary Birds*, 2nd edn., 109–120. Ames, IA: Wiley.
**Author**: Gregory Rich, DVM, BS Medical Technology

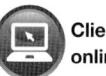 **Client Education Handout available online**

# OVIDUCTAL DISEASES

## BASICS

### DEFINITION
The oviduct is the structure that handles the ova following ovulation. Various segments of the oviduct are responsible for specific aspects of egg development. The oviductal segments from cranial to caudal are the infundibulum, magnum, isthmus, uterus, and vagina. There is a discrete sphincter between the uterus and vagina. The vagina opens into the urodeum of the cloaca. Most birds only have a left ovary and oviduct. Various disease processes can affect the oviduct and can result in salpingitis and/or impaction of the oviduct, dystocia, etc. Neoplasia is also occasionally found to affect the oviduct.

### PATHOPHYSIOLOGY
Any disorder that creates inflammation or other changes in anatomy in the oviduct can affect normal egg formation, leading to development of abnormal eggs and/or obstruction. Nutritional disease that results in hypocalcemia can affect normal muscle function of the oviduct, as well as impacting egg shell formation. Ascending or systemic bacterial, fungal, and viral infections can lead to salpingitis, and some pathogens have tropism for the oviduct. Neoplastic conditions of the oviduct can become secondarily infected or lead to abnormal egg development and impaction as well. Occasionally, oviductal torsion or herniation is encountered.

### SYSTEMS AFFECTED
Reproductive tract.

### GENETICS
There does not appear to be a genetic predisposition of oviductal disease in birds.

### INCIDENCE/PREVALENCE
Incidence and prevalence are unknown across all avian species. In domestic poultry, oviductal disease is a common finding, especially in older birds. Anecdotally, it is common in various non-domestic species in managed care.

### GEOGRAPHIC DISTRIBUTION
N/A

### SIGNALMENT
**Species**: Female birds of any species can be affected by oviductal disease; however, prolific, heavy-laying species seem predisposed. Domestic chickens and ducks, cockatiels, and various finch species are often diagnosed with oviductal disorders.
**Mean age and range**: Older female birds that have been reproductively productive are predisposed to oviductal disease.

**Predominant sex**: Female.

### SIGNS
#### General Comments
Clinical signs associated with oviductal disease can be subtle and non-specific. Occasionally, birds with diseased oviducts may strain or have some discharge from the vent. Often, symptoms are vague such as lethargy, anorexia/weight loss, and fluffed feathers.

#### Historical Findings
A common history for a bird with oviductal disease is an acute change in egg laying behavior and/or the observation of changes in the appearance of the eggs being passed. A classic presentation is a bird that has been laying heavily for a period of time will begin passing soft-shelled or deformed eggs, followed by complete cessation of laying. Occasionally, cases present in more chronic stages, where laying ceased many months to years prior to presentation. It is important to understand that birds that have never laid an egg can also be affected by oviductal disease.

#### Physical Examination Findings
Usually, physical examination findings are non-specific (poor body condition, dehydration, etc.). Examination findings specific to oviductal disease typically manifest as coelomic distention. Oviductal disease can result in coelomic effusion resulting in grossly apparent coelomic distention. Occasionally, the oviduct may be apparent during coelomic palpation. Changes in the oviduct near the cloaca can cause deformation and dysfunction of the vent, resulting in abnormal conformation and/or external accumulation of feces and urates. If eggs are available for examination, they may have soft shells, defects in the shells, a foul smell, and be streaked with blood and/or purulent material. Occasionally, inspissated yolk material or pus may be passed.

### CAUSES
Infectious organisms that can cause primary salpingitis in birds include bacteria (*Escherichia coli*, *Gallibacterium anatis*, *Mycoplasma* spp., *Riemerella anatipestifer*, etc.), viruses (avian influenza, herpesvirus, adenovirus, paramyxovirus, coronavirus, etc.) and fungi (*Aspergillus* sp., etc.). Malnutrition resulting in inadequate mineral stores for normal eggshell formation and poor oviductal motility can lead to impaction and secondary infection. Oviductal torsions, body-wall herniation and incarcerations, and traumatic injuries due to fracture of intraoviductal eggs are occasionally encountered. Uterine carcinoma or adenocarcinomas are the most common neoplasms associated with the avian oviduct.

### RISK FACTORS
Chronic egg laying, excessive body condition/ coelomic fat, malnutrition, trauma while gravid, and egg binding can predispose birds to developing oviductal disorders. Exposure to potential pathogens with tropism for the oviduct. Long-term exposure to estrogenic compounds has been associated with oviductal disease in domestic poultry.

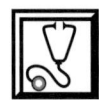

## DIAGNOSIS

### DIFFERENTIAL DIAGNOSIS
Diagnosis of oviductal disease is usually straightforward and involves a careful history, physical examination and imaging. Further support and/or characterization of the disease is possible via advanced imaging, clinical pathology, and laparoscopy. Differentials include ovarian disease, egg-yolk peritonitis/ coelomitis, dystocia.

### CBC/BIOCHEMISTRY/URINALYSIS
A leukocytosis is sometimes present, being primarily heterophilic or monocytic depending on the chronicity of the disease process. A non-regenerative anemia may also be noted secondary to chronic disease. The chemistry panel may show hypercalcemia and hyperphosphatemia as well as hyperproteinemia (particularly hyperglobulinemia) if reproductive activity is still occurring. Other chemistry changes associated with injury or dysfunction of other coelomic organs may be observed if the oviductal disease has created coelomitis.

### OTHER LABORATORY TESTS
Cytology of impression smears from oviductal tissue or discharge, if available, can provide useful information. C/S or specific molecular diagnostics of tissue or discharge can also be useful in diagnosis and direction of therapy. If biopsies are collected or salpingectomy performed, histopathology is indicated. Definitive diagnosis, as well as identification of healthy margins, will help to direct further therapy. If coelomic fluid or oviductal fluid is present, it can be aspirated and cytology and C/S performed on it.

### IMAGING
Plain radiography with often show a mass effect in the coelomic region if the oviduct is enlarged. Fluid accumulation within the coelom can also be appreciated with plain radiographs. Further imaging is usually required to definitively identify disease of the oviduct however. CT, preferable with contrast, can be effective in identifying the oviduct and characterizing disease of the organ. If there is significant expansion of the

coelomic visceral mass or coelomic effusion, an adequate acoustic window may exist for meaningful ultrasonographic examination of the coelom.

## DIAGNOSTIC PROCEDURES
Laparoscopic examination is often used to diagnose oviductal disease definitively. Laparoscopy can be challenging if air sac space is limited for manipulation of the scope. Care should be taken when coelomic effusion is present, as perforation of the coelomic membrane can result in fluid entering the air sacs/lungs, and effectively can drown the patient. If the oviduct is accessible, it is possible to collect biopsies from the serosal surface. However, perforation of the oviduct can result in introduction of material from the lumen into the coelom, so caution is recommended. Intraluminal examination of the oviduct via endoscopy is also possible. Accessing the oviduct through the cloaca may be challenging, depending on how disease has affected the anatomy.

## PATHOLOGIC FINDINGS
The pathologic findings affecting the oviduct can range from acute salpingitis of varying severity with or without a suppurative component to a more chronic granulomatous inflammatory condition. The presence of material within the oviduct is variable, but often there is intraluminal inspissated yolk material or purulent material present. Adenocarcinoma is occasionally noted to affect the avian oviduct and can be difficult to impossible to differentiate from an inflammatory condition grossly. Benign neoplastic change of the oviduct is possible but not commonly encountered.

## TREATMENT

### APPROPRIATE HEALTH CARE
Cessation of further reproductive activity is typically indicated in cases of oviductal disease. Treatment with GnRH agonist medications, such as leuprolide and deslorelin, has proven effective in curtailing ovarian activity and subsequent egg laying in avian species (at least transiently). Other hormones have been used in avian patients with variable results. In cases of infectious salpingitis (bacterial or fungal), antimicrobial therapy is indicated based on cytology, C/S. NSAIDs are also typically indicated. Other non-specific treatments such as fluid therapy and nutritional support should be employed as needed. Attempts can be made to treat cases of oviductal disease conservatively and preserve the reproductive capabilities of the bird. In cases in which there is inspissated material within the lumen of the oviduct,

administration of prostaglandin E2 to relax the Urodeovaginal spincter and prostaglandin F2α to stimulate oviductal contraction may be effective in clearing the oviduct of unwanted material. Alternatively, salpingotomy followed by flushing of the oviduct can be attempted. Conservative therapy is not often successful, with salpingohysterectomy often necessary for definitive treatment of oviductal disease.

### NURSING CARE
Many cases of oviductal disease are chronic and patients are relatively stable. However, the occasional bird will present in the terminal stages of disease or suffering from dehydration, malnutrition, and possibly sepsis and/or organ failure, and will require intensive nursing care for effective therapy. Fluid and nutritional therapy can be critical in addition to more specific therapies to address the oviductal disease.

### ACTIVITY
No activity restrictions accompany the treatment of avian oviductal disease.

### DIET
Disease of the avian oviduct can sometimes be secondary to malnutrition. Diets deficient in vitamin A, vitamin D, calcium and other minerals can lead to malformed eggs and potential dystocia. When treating cases of oviductal disease, in addition to providing adequate caloric intake, complete diets should be offered to support normal oviductal function.

### CLIENT EDUCATION
Clients working with high risk species should be well-versed regarding nutritional requirements and management tools to help limit excessive egg laying. Recognition of the signs of oviductal disease is also important.

### SURGICAL CONSIDERATIONS
Salpingohysterectomy is often necessary to definitively treat oviductal disease in birds. A left flank approach is usually employed to facilitate removal of the oviduct. Often transection of the last left rib is necessary to achieve proper exposure. Salpingohysterectomy is typically a fairly straightforward procedure, even with a diseased oviduct. Ligation of the oviduct's blood supply in the mesosalpinx is made much easier and safer with the use of hemostatic clips and cautery. The oviduct should be ligated and removed as close to the cloaca as possible. When disease is limited to the oviduct, salpingohysterectomy can be curative. Surgical cure is possible even in cases of neoplasia if disease-free margins are attainable and metastasis has not occurred. Often, removal of the oviduct causes suppression of ovulation in avian patients. However some birds will ovulate

following salpingohysterectomy and develop yolk coelomitis. Ovariectomy is difficult and the risk of haemorrhage is high, due to the anatomy of the ovary and ovarian artery and often diminutive size of avian patients. Iatrogenic damage to the left adrenal and cranial pole of the kidney is also a concern.

## MEDICATIONS

### DRUG(S) OF CHOICE
NSAIDs, antibiotic and antifungal medications, and hormone agonists/analogues are frequently indicated in treatment of oviductal disease in birds. Addition of other medications is usually based on the unique needs of individual cases. Empirically chosen antibiotics should reflect the common occurrence of *E. coli* and other Gram-negative isolates and *Mycoplasma* sp. as causative agents of salpingitis. The GnRH agonists leuprolide acetate and deslorelin are frequently used to discontinue reproductive activity in avian patients. It should be understood that long-acting GnRH agonists will initially stimulate reproductive activities prior to downregulation. The use of depot leuprolide is well described in the available literature and a number of different protocols are described. A dose of 250–750 µg/kg IM q2–6w is recommended. Recommendations for deslorelin use vary according to species with a 4.7-mg implant resulting in suppression in most birds, although time of effect can be variable. If prostaglandin therapy is attempted, prostaglandin E2 is dosed at 0.02–0.1 mg/kg applied topically to the uterovaginal sphincter. Prostaglandin F2α is dosed at 0.02–0.1 mg/kg IM or intracloacal once.

### CONTRAINDICATIONS
N/A

### PRECAUTIONS
N/A

### POSSIBLE INTERACTIONS
N/A

### ALTERNATIVE DRUGS
N/A

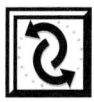

## FOLLOW-UP

### PATIENT MONITORING
Physical examination to determine resolution of disease or recurrence pattern. Follow-up imaging of the coelom via ultrasound or CT may be indicated to monitor ovarian development and possible ovulation and

development of yolk coelomitis. Coelomocentesis may be required if effusion is present.

### PREVENTION/AVOIDANCE

Proper diet (including maintenance of normal body condition) and avoidance of management systems that encourage overproduction of eggs can help avoid oviductal disease. Allowing birds to incubate eggs or use of dummy eggs can help limit egg production, as can manipulation of light cycles and caloric intake in some species. Proper hygiene of substrate and nesting material may help to avoid ascending infections.

### POSSIBLE COMPLICATIONS

If medical treatment is pursued, irreversible scarring of the oviduct may occur rendering it permanently non-functional. Therefore, the next time the bird ovulates the ova may not be handled appropriately and disease may recur. If salpingohysterectomy is performed and ovarian activity continues, internal ovulation may occur resulting in egg-yolk peritonitis/coelomitis. GnRH agonists can be administered prophylactically in an attempt to avoid this complication.

### EXPECTED COURSE AND PROGNOSIS

Recurrence of disease is common in birds that are treated medically. Birds that have salpingectomies usually have no further problems, but should be monitored for future ovarian function.

 MISCELLANEOUS

### ASSOCIATED CONDITIONS

Misovulated ova ("internal laying"), egg-yolk peritonitis.

### AGE-RELATED FACTORS

Older female birds that have been reproductively productive are predisposed to oviductal disease.

### ZOONOTIC POTENTIAL

N/A

### FERTILITY/BREEDING

Birds suffering from oviductal disease are often rendered infertile. Cases of mild salpingitis or dystocia that are treated medically have the best chance of retaining their reproductive capabilities.

### SYNONYMS

N/A

### SEE ALSO

Adenoviruses
Ascites
Aspergillosis
Avian Influenza
Chronic Egg Laying
Cloacal Diseases
Coelomic Distention
Colibacillosis
Dystocia and Egg Binding
Egg Yolk and Reproductive Coelomitis
Hypocalcemia and Hypomagnesemia

Infertility
Mycoplasmosis
Neoplasia (Reproductive)
Nutritional Imbalances
Orthoavulaviruses

### ABBREVIATIONS

C/S—culture and sensitivity
CT—computed tomography
GnRH—gonadotropin-releasing hormone
NSAIDs—non-steroidal anti-inflammatory drugs

### INTERNET RESOURCES

N/A

*Suggested Reading*
Divers, S.J. (2010). Avian endosurgery. *Veterinary Clinics of North America: Exotic Animal Practice*, 13:203–216.
Guzman, D.S.M. (2016). Avian soft tissue surgery. *Veterinary Clinics of North America: Exotic Animal Practice*, 19:133–157.
Lierz, M., Petriz, O.A., Samour, J. (2016). Reproduction. In: *Current Therapy in Avian Medicine and Surgery* (ed. B.L. Speer), 433–460. St. Louis, MO: Elsevier.
Mehler, S.J., Bennett, R.A. (2022). Avian reproductive procedures. In: *Surgery of Exotic Animals* (ed. R.A. Bennett, G.W. Pye), 163–174. Hoboken, NJ: Wiley-Blackwell.
Rubin, J.A., Runge, J.J., Mison, M., et al. (2016). Surgery. In: *Current Therapy in Avian Medicine and Surgery* (ed. B.L. Speer), 631–667. St. Louis, MO: Elsevier.
**Author**: Ryan DeVoe, DVM, DACZM

# BASICS

## DEFINITION
Pain is defined by IASP as "an unpleasant sensory and emotional experience associated with, or resembling that associated with, actual or potential tissue damage". In animals, the following definition is common: "An aversive sensory and emotional experience representing awareness by the animal of damage or threat to the integrity of its tissues; it changes the animal's physiology and behaviour to reduce or avoid damage, to reduce the likelihood of recurrence, and to promote recovery" (Molony and Kent 1997). The term nociception is used when evaluating measurable responses to specific noxious stimulus like the ones used in animal models.

## PATHOPHYSIOLOGY
The classical ascending pathways for pain involve activation of receptors or channels (nociceptors). This is responsible for the creation of action potentials (i.e. transduction of noxious stimuli into electrical impulses). There are three types of nociceptors: (1) mechanical receptors, for sharp or pricking stimuli; (2) thermal receptors, for burning or freezing stimuli; (3) polymodal receptors for slow burning stimuli. Transmission by the afferent or sensory fibers of peripheral nerves to the dorsal horn of the spinal cord (C and Aδ fibers). Modulation at the spinal cord and brain. Perception of the unpleasant experience in the brain. The descending pathways are less define but also thought to play a role in the physiology of pain. There are different types of pain, depending on the classification: Nociceptive, inflammatory, and neuropathic pain. Nociceptive pain occurs in the absence of tissue damage and serves a protective function. Inflammatory occurs when inflammatory mediators are involved. Neuropathic pain occurs when primary damage with damage or alterations in the physiology or anatomy of the sensory nervous system. Acute, chronic. Central, peripheral. Somatic, visceral. Mild, moderate, severe.

## SYSTEMS AFFECTED
Behavioral, cardiovascular, endocrine/metabolic, gastrointestinal, hemic/lymphatic/immune, hepatobiliary, musculoskeletal, nervous, neuromuscular, ophthalmic, renal/urologic, reproductive, respiratory, skin/exocrine.

## GENETICS
N/A

## INCIDENCE/PREVALENCE
N/A

## GEOGRAPHIC DISTRIBUTION
N/A

## SIGNALMENT
N/A

## SIGNS

### General Comments
Even if animals cannot verbally express their emotions, it is very likely that they all can still experience pain or a pain-like status that causes discomfort and/or stress. Pain may be difficult to see in prey species as they will try to hide it.

### Historical Findings
Non-specific signs like anorexia, decreased activity behaviors, lack of vocalization, lack of preening, feather-damaging behavior or self-mutilation, and abnormal body posture or flight might be observed. Socially, birds might withdraw from the rest of the flock or change temperament.

### Physical Examination Findings
Increased heart rate, increased respiratory rate in acute pain. During manipulation, agitation and vocalization could be present and the bird could attempt to withdraw.

## CAUSES
Similar to mammals; trauma (fractures, wounds), non-traumatic wounds, surgical wounds, neoplasia, other inflammatory processes, neuropathic pain.

## RISK FACTORS
N/A

# DIAGNOSIS

## DIFFERENTIAL DIAGNOSIS
Stress (e.g. not used to being handled), sedation, abnormal behavior, weakness.

## CBC/BIOCHEMISTRY/URINALYSIS
Leukocytes, proteins, and globulines may be increased with inflammatory pain but very low specificity.

## OTHER LABORATORY TESTS
Plasma corticosterone may be increased with stress but very low specificity.

## IMAGING
N/A

## DIAGNOSTIC PROCEDURES
Below are behavioral and postural parameters that can be used to evaluate pain in birds (Mikoni et al., 2023). Parameters should be evaluated in the context of appropriateness for the avian species being evaluated, and are summarized based on historic studies performed on birds in pain, but have not been validated. For each category, expected normal behavior is listed first, with the changes being progressive with increased levels of pain.
**Mentation**: Alert and attentive, quiet, depressed.
**Environmental interaction**: Engaged and interactive with environment (toys, conspecifics, food/water dishes, observers/caregivers). Reserved and interacts with less with environment than expected. Largely inactive/resting and not engaging with surroundings.
**Perching**: Easily maneuvers onto perch and is able to traverse along it without difficulty. Able to initially maneuver onto perch, but then remains largely within the same spot once perched. Unable to or does not perch and remains on floor of enclosure.
**Maintenance behaviors**: Performs maintenance behaviors (preening, shaking plumage, scratching, stretching, wiping beak, etc.) readily. Performs maintenance behaviors at a decreased frequency than expected. Does not perform any noticeable maintenance behaviors when observed.
**Locomotion**: Moving frequently and easily around enclosure, either horizontally or, where appropriate, vertically. Will occasionally move self to different locations within cage, but slowly. Largely immobile during the observation period.
**Focal preening of singular area**: Minimal to no increase in attention to one spot repeatedly (grooms all body parts similarly when preening body). Occasional pecking/biting at one spot repeatedly. Significant overgrooming/biting at one spot repeatedly.
**Body posture**: Body and neck held erect and engaged. Body erect, but with neck and head lowered and held closer to chest. Body held low or against vertical surface (wall, enclosure side, and so forth), or body lying fully on the floor.
**Appetite**: Visits feeder/food dish readily while awake. Visits feeder at a reduced frequency compared with patient's normal. Does not visit feeder at all during observed period while awake. See suggested readings for other scales used in experimental designs.
**Other diagnostic tools**: Measurement of blood pressure (direct more reliable than indirect) (usually increased with pain), use of ECG and/or Doppler during anesthesia (increased heart rate), use of capnography during anesthesia (increased respiratory rate). Response to treatment can be used also the discern from sedation in some cases.

## PATHOLOGIC FINDINGS
N/A

P

# TREATMENT

## APPROPRIATE HEALTH CARE
Immobilisation of the painful area (bandages), ice packs, protection of painful wounds (bandages), avoid pressure on/contact with the painful area. Laser therapy, acupuncture, massage.

## NURSING CARE
General supportive care.

## ACTIVITY
Immobilization of the painful area, if unstable, is generally recommended.

## DIET
N/A

## CLIENT EDUCATION
Pain scales used to monitor patient progression of pain by owners have not been validated in birds, but recognition of normal and abnormal behaviors, together with simple descriptive pain intensity scales (e.g. absent, mild, moderate, severe), numeric (e.g. 1–10), or visual analog scales can be used.

## SURGICAL CONSIDERATIONS
Any surgery may cause pain, so pain management should be part of the anesthesia protocol. The pain protocol should be adjusted to the known severity of pain caused by the procedure in other species. Vagal response with decreased of heart rate and respiratory rate can happen during manipulation of painful lesions (e.g. during fracture repair).

# MEDICATIONS

## DRUG(S) OF CHOICE
The drugs and doses below are generalizations in psittacines and raptors based on a limited number of species studies. Caution is recommended when extrapolating dosages between species due to high interspecies pharmacokinetic variability and other physiological differences in their response to these drugs. For more accurate dosing recommendations and a detailed list of specific species studied, as well as information in other species or drugs not mentioned, please see the references provided below. The authors recommend reviewing other texts for the exact mechanism of action of the drugs described.

### Opioids
**Butorphanol**: Psittacines—short lived and for moderate pain, 5 mg/kg IM/SQ q2–3h, 1 mg/kg/h IV CRI after a loading dose of 2–3 mg/kg. Raptors—seems ineffective based on studies in American kestrels, which resulted in hyperalgesia in males at the higher doses.

**Buprenorphine**: Psittacines—seems to have little efficacy or to be ineffective based on studies in grey parrots, cockatiels and orange-winged Amazon parrots. Raptors—for moderate pain, 0.1–0.6 mg/kg IM q 6–12h based on studies in American kestrels; 0.3–1.8 mg/kg IM q24h or q42–72h based on studies on red-tailed hawks.

**Hydromorphone**: Raptors—for moderate to severe pain, 0.1–0.6 mg/kg IM q3–6h based on studies in American kestrels and great horned owls. Psittacines—for moderate to severe pain, 1 mg/kg IM q6h based on studies in orange-winged Amazon parrots, but caused agitation so lower doses between 0.5 and 1 mg/kg recommended clinically. No effect in cockatiels with doses up to 0.6 mg/kg IM and higher doses might be needed.

**Fentanyl**: Raptors—for severe pain, 10–30 mcg/kg/h IV CRI, based on studies on red-tailed hawks. Psittacines—not recommended due to the high rates required and depressive effect on heart rate and blood pressure at these rates based on studies in Hispaniolan Amazon parrots.

**Tramadol**: Psittacines—for mild to moderate pain, 30 mg/kg PO q6–8h, 5 mg/kg IV q4h based on studies on Hispaniolan Amazon parrots. Caution when administering parenteral doses due to increase bioavailability when compared with oral administration. Raptors—for mild to moderate pain, 5 mg/kg PO q6–8h in American kestrels and q12h in bald eagles, 10–15 mg/kg IV/IM based on studies on hawks.

### Non-Steroidal Anti-Inflammatory Drugs
**Meloxicam**: Raptors 0.5–1.6 mg/kg IM, PO q12h, based on the studies on American kestrels, great horned owls, and red-tailed hawks. Psittacines 0.5–1.6 mg/kg IM, PO q12–24h. Significant differences between species in dose and frequency, use species-specific dose when information is available. Hispaniolan Amazon parrots 1.6 mg/kg PO q12h. Grey parrot 1 mg/kg q24h PO. Poor oral absorption and very short half-life in cockatiels suggest higher and/or more frequent dosing.

**Gabapentinoids**: Psittacines 15–30 mg/kg PO q8–12h based on studies in Hispaniolan Amazon parrots. Raptors: 11 mg/kg q8h based on studies in great horned owl.

### Other
**Local anesthetics**: Benzocaine for topical use. Lidocaine 2–4 mg/kg perineurally or locally. Bupivacaine 2 mg/kg max perineurally or locally.

**Canabinoids**: Psittacines 30/32.5 mg/kg of CBD/CBDA-rich hemp extract q12h PO based on studies on orange-winged Amazon parrots. CBD alone needs higher doses and more frequent administration based on other studies in Hispaniolan Amazon parrots.

## CONTRAINDICATIONS
The authors recommend also reviewing general adverse effects and contraindications in other texts. Morphine may cause hyperalgesia in some birds. Hydromorphone may cause agitation and nausea-like behaviors in some birds. Naloxone, naltrexone (opioid antagonists) may cause hyperalgesia. Diclofenac is toxic in Gyps vultures, Steppe eagles, and possibly other avian species; not recommended for use. Ibuprofen and ketoprofen can also cause toxicity in Gyps vultures.

## PRECAUTIONS
N/A

## POSSIBLE INTERACTIONS
N/A

## ALTERNATIVE DRUGS
N/A

# FOLLOW-UP

## PATIENT MONITORING
Pain scales can be used to monitor progression of the pain/effectiveness of the analgesia given. They can be repeated 2–3 times daily. Return to normal behavior and appetite can also indicate improvement. Response to treatment should be used to review and adjust pain management protocol as needed.

## PREVENTION/AVOIDANCE
Adequate pain management protocol in cases in which pain is known to occur (e.g. surgeries, small painful procedures).

## POSSIBLE COMPLICATIONS
Feather-damaging behavior, self-mutilation, other abnormal behavior (e.g. stereotypies, pica).

## EXPECTED COURSE AND PROGNOSIS
Depends on the cause and the severity of the pain and presence or not of complications.

# MISCELLANEOUS

## ASSOCIATED CONDITIONS
N/A

## AGE-RELATED FACTORS
N/A

## ZOONOTIC POTENTIAL
N/A

## FERTILITY/BREEDING
N/A

## SYNONYMS
Nociception.

## SEE ALSO
Trauma

## ABBREVIATIONS
CBC—cannabidiol
CBDA—cannabidiolic acid
CRI—constant rate infusion
IASP—International Association for the Study of Pain
PD—pharmacodynamic
PK—pharmacokinetic

## INTERNET RESOURCES
International Association for the Study of Pain: www.iasp-pain.org

*Suggested Reading*
Beausoleil, N.J., Holdsworth, S.E., Lehmann, H. (2021). Avian nociception and pain. *Sturkie's Avian Physiology*, 7th edn. (ed. C.G. Scanes, S. Dridi), 223–231. St. Louis, MO: Elsevier.
Desmarchelier, M., Troncy, E., Beauchamp, G., et al. (2012). Evaluation of a fracture pain model in domestic pigeons (*Columba livia*), *American Journal of Veterinary Research*, 73:353–360.
Guzman, D.S., Hawkins, M.G. (2023). Treatment of pain in birds. *Veterinary Clinics of North America: Exotic Animal Practice*, 26:83–120.
Mazor-Thomas, J.E., Mann, P.E., Karas, A.Z., Tseng, F. (2014). Pain-suppressed behaviors in the red-tailed hawk (*Buteo jamaicensis*). *Applied Animal Behaviour Science*, 152:83–91.
Mikoni, N.A., Guzman, D.S., Paul-Murphy, J. (2023). Pain recognition and assessment in birds. *Veterinary Clinics of North America: Exotic Animal Practice*, 26:65–81.
Molony, V., Kent, J.E. (1997). Assessment of acute pain in farm animals using behavioral and physiological measurements. *Journal of Animal Science*, 75:266–272.
Paul-Murphy, J.R., Sladky, K.K., Krugner-Higby, L.A., et al. (2009). Analgesic effects of carprofen and liposome-encapsulated butorphanol tartrate in Hispaniolan parrots (*Amazona ventralis*) with experimentally induced arthritis. *American Journal of Veterinary Research*, 70:1201–1210.

**Authors**: Delphine Laniesse, DVM, DVSc, DECZM (Avian), and David Sanchez-Migallon Guzman, LV, MS, DECZM (Avian, Small Mammal), DACZM

P

# PANCREATIC DISEASES

## BASICS

### DEFINITION
Any disease process that directly affects the structure and/or function of a bird's pancreas. These include pancreatitis, exocrine pancreatic insufficiency (EPI), diabetes mellitus, neoplasia, pancreatic atrophy, pancreatic necrosis, cystic pancreas amyloidosis.

### PATHOPHYSIOLOGY
Pancreatitis is an inflammatory condition of the pancreas. Damage to the acinar cell walls results in the leakage of digestive enzymes (primarily protease, trypsin, and phospholipase) within the pancreatic parenchyma, resulting in autodigestion. EPI is associated with insufficient synthesis and/or secretion of pancreatic enzymes from the tubuloacinar glands. This can be associated with inadequate enzyme production by the pancreatic acinar cells or by obstruction of the pancreatic ducts. Primary neoplasia of the pancreas includes adenoma, adenocarcinoma, lymphoma, pancreatic duct carcinoma, and islet cell carcinoma. Metastatic neoplasia can also invade the avian pancreas. Pancreatic atrophy occurs secondary to the loss of functional pancreatic tissues, often with subsequent pancreatic fibrosis. Pancreatic necrosis is typically an acute disease process where the pancreatic tissue rapidly degenerates. Cystic pancreas and amyloidosis are rarely reported and are typically considered incidental findings on necropsy.

### SYSTEMS AFFECTED
**Behavioral**: Bird may exhibit signs of pain, depression, or feather destructive behaviors (particularly over the ventral coelom).
**Endocrine**: Diabetes mellitus.
**GI**: Altered GI motility secondary to local chemical coelomitis. Enhanced vascular permeability may also lead to focal or generalized coelomitis.
**Hemic/lymphatic/immune**: Leukocytosis.
**Hepatobiliary**: Hepatic lesions may result from fatty infiltrates, cholestasis, leukocytic infiltrates, or focal damage by pancreatic enzyme release.
**Respiratory**: Inflammation, organomegaly, and coelomic effusion may compromise air sac volume.
**Skin**: Feather loss if bird is exhibiting feather destructive behaviors.

### GENETICS
Quaker parrots have a high instance of acute pancreatic necrosis, which may be associated with hyperlipidemia. *Neophema* spp. are more likely to suffer from chronic pancreatitis secondary to paramyxovirus.

### INCIDENCE/PREVALENCE
Unknown. Due to difficult antemortem diagnosis, most pancreatic diseases are identified postmortem. The postmortem prevalence of acute pancreatic necrosis has been estimated at 12.9% in quaker parrots.

### GEOGRAPHIC DISTRIBUTION
N/A

### SIGNALMENT
**Species**: Pancreatitis has been documented in a multitude of avian species. EPI has been reported in a sulfur-crested cockatoo, yellow-naped Amazon parrot, cockatiel, macaw, chickens, pigeons, quail, and an Indian hill mynah. Primary pancreatic neoplasia has been documented in ducks, guinea fowl, chickens, cockatiels, Amazon parrots, eclectus parrot, and macaws. Metastatic pancreatic neoplasia has been reported in ducks, a great tit, a golden eagle, an Adelie penguin, a domestic pigeon, and a long-legged buzzard. Pancreatic atrophy has been reported in chickens, ostriches, budgerigars, a blue and gold macaw, and a peregrine falcon. Pancreatic necrosis occurs most commonly in quaker parakeets, but has also been documented in chickens, turkeys, magpies, cockatoos, an Amazon parrot, a kiwi, and a red-tailed hawk. Pancreatic cysts have been documented in chickens. Pancreatic amyloidosis has been reported in Pekin ducks, swans, Japanese quail, and an Australian diamond firetail finch.
**Mean age and range**: Not documented.
**Predominant sex**: None.

### SIGNS

#### General Comments
Pancreatic diseases are often undiagnosed antemortem because symptoms can be vague and non-specific.

#### Historical Findings
Lethargy, weakness. Anorexia, poor appetite, although an increased appetite can be seen with EPI and diabetes. Depression, recumbency. Vomiting, regurgitation. Diarrhea, voluminous foul-smelling droppings. Undigested food in the feces, oily feces. Polyuria, polydipsia. Weight loss, failure to thrive. Feather-damaging behaviors, aggression. Labored breathing.

#### Physical Examination Findings
Poor body condition, emaciation. Dehydration. Coelomic distension (fluid or masses), with subsequent decreased or absent abdominal air sac sounds. Coelomic pain. Feather loss, particularly over the ventral coelom. Pasted vent. Dried vomitus on head feathers.

### CAUSES
Pancreatitis can be idiopathic, or associated with infection of the pancreas with bacteria (including *Mycobacterium* spp. and *Chlamydia*), viruses (West Nile virus, paramyxovirus, reovirus, adenovirus, herpesvirus, coronavirus, avian influenza, polyomavirus, poxvirus, duck hepatitis virus, avian encephalomyelitis virus, infectious bronchitis virus, and gyrovirus-3), fungi (*Aspergillus*), or parasites (nematodes, trematodes, coccidia, cryptosporidia). It can also be caused by obesity, toxins (primarily zinc, mycotoxins, and selenium), neoplasia, trauma, or secondary to egg-yolk coelomitis or medroxyprogesterone therapy. EPI can be idiopathic, congenital, or secondary to any disease process that causes damage to the pancreatic acinar cells or obstruction of the pancreatic ducts (pancreatitis, pancreatic atrophy, pancreatic necrosis, or neoplasia). Pancreatic neoplasia is often idiopathic, but infection with herpesvirus in psittacines, retrovirus (avian osteoperosis virus strain Pts-56) in guinea fowl, and reticuloendotheliosis virus in domestic geese have been linked to pancreatic neoplasia. Pancreatic atrophy can be caused by pancreatitis, pancreatic necrosis, prolonged caloric deficiency, zinc toxicosis, pancreatic duct obstruction, atherosclerosis of the pancreatic vasculature, or selenium deficiency. Chicken parvovirus has been shown to cause pancreatic atrophy in broilers. Pancreatic necrosis is often idiopathic, but other potential causes include acute pancreatitis, high-fat diets, zinc or levamisole toxicity, and infection (adenovirus, avian influenza, herpesvirus, polyomavirus, poxvirus, West Nile virus, pigeon paramyxovirus, and *Chlamydia*). Pancreatic amyloidosis usually associated with systemic amyloidosis.

### RISK FACTORS
Obesity. High-fat diets.

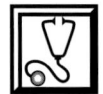

## DIAGNOSIS

### DIFFERENTIAL DIAGNOSIS
Primary GI disease (ingluvitis, gastroenteritis, GI ulceration, foreign body, obstruction, PDD). Hepatobiliary disease (cholangiohepatitis, biliary outflow obstruction, toxic injury). Secondary causes of weight loss and chronic diarrhea (hepatic failure, kidney failure, PDD). Secondary causes of coelomic effusion (heart disease, liver disease, neoplasia, egg yolk coelomitis). Secondary causes of coelomic organomegaly (liver disease, reproductive tract disease, neoplasia). Secondary causes of polyuria/polydipsia (primary renal disease, reproductive tract disease, endocrinopathy, diabetes insipidus).

**(CONTINUED)**

## CBC/BIOCHEMISTRY/URINALYSIS

Lipemia. Elevated triglycerides and cholesterol. Elevated amylase (> 1100 iu/dl) and/or lipase. Elevated AST, ALT, ALP, CK. Hyperglycemia (typically > 1000 mg/dl with diabetes). Leukocytosis. Glucosuria, ketonuria.

## OTHER LABORATORY TESTS

Lower increases of amylase and lipase may be associated with extrapancreatic causes, such as renal disease, GI disease, or glucocorticoid or medroxyprogesterone administration. Fecal amylase and trypsin levels may be reduced, whereas fecal starch and fat levels may be elevated. Trypsin-like immunoreactivity is species specific and has not been studied in birds. Cobalamin and folate levels have also not been assessed in birds. Blood triglyceride levels can be assessed after administration of corn oil alone or mixed with pancreatic enzymes. Assessing blood insulin, glucagon, or fructosamine levels may be beneficial in the diagnosis of diabetes. Blood zinc levels may be indicated if zinc intoxication is suspected. PCR or antibody testing for suspected viral, bacterial, chlamydial, or fungal infection. Protein electrophoresis may show decreased protein levels if EPI is present, or increased globulins if inflammation is present.

## IMAGING

Coelomic ultrasound may demonstrate coelomic effusion or masses. The pancreas can be partially visualized between the descending and ascending duodenum, but unless there is profound enlargement or a mass present, it may be difficult to image. Although the pancreas is not visible radiographically, coelomic visceral enlargement, ascites, hepatomegaly, or other systemic problems that may be correlated with pancreatic disease may be noted. MRI and CT may show pancreatic enlargement or masses in the area of the pancreas.

## DIAGNOSTIC PROCEDURES

Biopsy of the pancreas via coelioscopy or coeliotomy can be diagnostic, but focal lesions may be missed.

## PATHOLOGIC FINDINGS

**Pancreatitis**: The pancreas may be grossly firm, irregular, or hemorrhagic, and may contain mycobacterial or fungal granulomas, or suppurative lesions. A purulent exudate or coelomic effusion may be present. Infiltration of the pancreas with lymphocytes, heterophils, or histiocytes may occur, and fibrin deposition may be noted. Bacteria, parasites, or viral inclusion bodies may be evident. Fibrosis can be seen with chronic pancreatitis.
**EPI**: May be caused by pancreatitis or pancreatic atrophy, so pathologic changes

associated with these diseases may be present. Occlusion of the pancreatic ducts may also be present, due to hyperplasia, neoplasia, inflammatory exudates, or the presence of nematodes or trematodes.
**Diabetes mellitus**: Degenerative changes may be seen in the pancreatic islets, including hypoplasia, atrophy, and/or vacuolation of islet cells.
**Neoplasia**: Masses and coelomic effusion may be grossly present. Primary or metastatic neoplastic cells are noted within the pancreatic parenchyma.
**Pancreatic atrophy**: The pancreas is small and possibly irregular, with shrinkage of acinar cells and loss of zymogen granules. Acini are irregular, and the cells usually contain clear cytoplasm. Fibrosis may be present.
**Pancreatic necrosis**: The pancreas is firm and pale, with variable hemorrhage and adjacent fat necrosis. Histological abnormalities include coagulative necrosis of pancreatic acini, hemorrhage within the pancreatic lobules, and multifocal necrosis of adjacent mesenteric fat. Coelomic effusion may be present.
**Zinc toxicity**: Parenchymal mottling may be noted. The primary histological lesion is degranulation and vacuolation of the acinar cells. Cellular necrosis, mononuclear inflammatory infiltrates, and interstitial fibrosis may also be present.

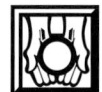

## TREATMENT

### APPROPRIATE HEALTH CARE

Aggressive inpatient treatment is indicated with pancreatitis (especially acute pancreatitis), pancreatic necrosis, and unregulated diabetes. Uncomplicated EPI and pancreatic atrophy may be treatable on an outpatient basis.

### NURSING CARE

Aggressive fluid therapy is indicated to correct hypovolemia and dehydration, and to maintain adequate pancreatic microcirculation. Fluids can be administered IV, IO, SQ, or PO. A balanced electrolyte solution, such as lactated Ringer's solution, is typically the first choice. Addition of colloids may be indicated if the bird is in shock or is profoundly hypovolemic. Pain management is typically indicated. Both narcotic analgesics and NSAIDs may be used. Antibiotics are indicated if a bacterial etiology is suspected. Antiemetic medications may be warranted if the bird is actively vomiting or regurgitating, or if GI ileus is present. The use of pancreatic enzymes may benefit pancreatitis patients, as well as birds with EPI. In critical cases, a plasma transfusion might be indicated, in

order to replace protease inhibitors and decreasing further pancreatic damage.

### ACTIVITY

Limited activity may be beneficial with active disease and during recovery.

### DIET

Continue to feed normally unless intractable vomiting or regurgitation is present. Birds should ideally not be fasted due to their high metabolic rate. Syringe, gavage, and enteral feeding via an esophagostomy or duodenostomy tube may be indicated in anorectic animals. Low-fat diets are indicated. A formulated diet would be optimal. Seed-based diets should be avoided due to high fat content and lower digestibility. The addition of pancreatic enzymes to the diet is indicated with EPI.

### CLIENT EDUCATION

Discuss the need for aggressive treatment in critically ill patients. Discuss the difficulty of obtaining a diagnosis antemortem, and the possible need for more invasive diagnostics. Discuss the need for lifelong medical therapy for animals with EPI or diabetes. Make sure that the client is aware birds with pancreatic diseases often come with a guarded to poor prognosis.

### SURGICAL CONSIDERATIONS

Pancreatic biopsy obtained either endoscopically or via coeleotomy is often necessary to confirm the diagnosis. The placement of an esophagostomy or duodenostomy feeding tube may be indicated. Extrahepatic biliary obstruction secondary to pancreatic disease may require surgical correction. In the case of pancreatic neoplasia, surgery may be indicated to obtain biopsies, and/or remove or debulk the tumor(s). The presence of coelomic effusion, organomegaly, or coelomic masses may compromise the air sacs, increasing the risk for anesthetic complications.

## MEDICATIONS

### DRUG(S) OF CHOICE

Antiemetic drugs and GI motility stimulants may be indicated if vomiting, regurgitation, or ileus is present; metoclopramide 0.3–0.5 mg/kg IV, IM, PO q8–12h, cisapride 0.5–1.5 mg/kg PO q8h, maropitant 1–2 mg/kg SQ, PO (questionable efficacy in birds). Antibiotics if evidence of bacterial or chlamydial infection is present. Therapy should be based on bacterial C/S results, if possible. Pain management is indicated with pancreatitis, pancreatic necrosis, and neoplasia; butorphanol 0.5–4 mg/kg IM, IV q1–4h, tramadol 11–30 mg/kg q6–12h (questionable efficacy in some species), meloxicam 0.5–1 mg/kg

# PANCREATIC DISEASES

IM, IV, PO q12–24h, carprofen 2–10 mg/kg IM, IV, PO q12–24h. Powdered pancreatic enzymes are indicated in cases of EPI, and may also benefit some patients with pancreatitis. The use of omega 6 and 3 fatty acids may help to reduce hyperlipidemia and pancreatic inflammation. The use of insulin and/or oral hypoglycemic medications may be indicated if diabetes is present. Chelation therapy is indicated if zinc toxicity is present. Chemotherapy protocols may be indicated in cases of primary or metastatic pancreatic neoplasia.

## CONTRAINDICATIONS
Anticholinergics. Corticosteroids (unless part of a chemotherapy protocol). Diuretics.

## PRECAUTIONS
Tetracyclines may increase fibrosis in cases of chronic pancreatitis.

## POSSIBLE INTERACTIONS
N/A

## ALTERNATIVE DRUGS
Plant-based organic enzyme supplements have been marketed for birds. The efficacy of these products in cases of EPI is questionable.

 FOLLOW-UP

## PATIENT MONITORING
Amylase and lipase levels should be rechecked 1–2 weeks after the patient is discharged. Patients that survive pancreatitis or pancreatic necrosis should be monitored closely for the development of EPI and diabetes.

## PREVENTION/AVOIDANCE
Reduce weight if obese. Avoid high-fat diets, and attempt to convert birds from a seed-based diet to a formulated diet.

## POSSIBLE COMPLICATIONS
Failed response to medical therapy. Other life-threatening disease may be linked to these diseases.

## EXPECTED COURSE AND PROGNOSIS
The prognosis is good for patients with mild pancreatitis, EPI, and diabetes mellitus. The prognosis is poor to grave for patients with necrotizing pancreatitis, pancreatic necrosis, or malignant neoplasia.

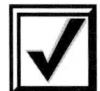 MISCELLANEOUS

## ASSOCIATED CONDITIONS
**Life-threatening**: Coelomitis. Coelomic effusion. Hepatobiliary damage from cholestasis or due to leakage of pancreatic enzymes. Metastasis of malignant pancreatic neoplasia. **Non-life-threatening**: Diabetes mellitus. EPI.

## AGE-RELATED FACTORS
N/A

## ZOONOTIC POTENTIAL
Some causative agents of pancreatitis are potentially zoonotic (e.g. *Chlamydia*, *Mycobacterium*, avian influenza virus).

## FERTILITY/BREEDING
Birds with congenital pancreatic abnormalities should not be bred.

## SYNONYMS
N/A

## SEE ALSO
Chlamydiosis
Coelomic Distention
Diabetes Mellitus
Egg Yolk Coelomitis
Toxicosis (Heavy Metals)
Ileus (Functional Gastrointestinal, Crop Stasis)
Mycobacteriosis
Orthoavulaviruses

Regurgitation and Vomiting
Undigested Food in Droppings

## ABBREVIATIONS
ALP—alkaline phosphatase
ALT—alanine aminotransferase
AST—aspartate aminotransferase
C/S—culture and sensitivity
CK—creatine kinase
CT—computed tomography
EPI—exocrine pancreatic insufficiency
GI—gastrointestinal
MRI—magnetic resonance imaging
NSAIDs—non-steroidal anti-inflammatory drugs
PCR—polymerase chain reaction
PDD–proventricular dilation disease

## INTERNET RESOURCES
Veterinary Information Network: http://www.vin.com/VIN.plx

*Suggested Reading*
de Matos, R., Monks, D. (2016). Diseases of the endocrine system: Protein hormones. In: *Current Therapy in Avian Medicine and Surgery* (ed. B.L. Speer), 385–399. St. Louis, MO: Elsevier.
Doneley, R. (2010). Disorders of the avian pancreas. In: *Avian Medicine and Surgery in Practice: Companion and Aviary Birds*, 182–184. London, UK: Manson Publishing.
Doneley, R. (2001). Acute pancreatitis in parrots. *Australian Veterinary Journal*, 79:409–411.
Pilny, A.A. (2008). The avian pancreas in health and disease. *Veterinary Clinics of North America: Exotic Animal Practice*, 11:25–34.
Schmidt, R.E., Reavill, D.R. (2014). Lesions of the avian pancreas. *Veterinary Clinics of North America: Exotic Animal Practice*, 17:1–11.
**Author**: David E. Hannon, DVM, DABVP (Avian)

# PAPILLOMATOSIS (CUTANEOUS)

# BASICS

## DEFINITION
Cutaneous papillomas are considered benign neoplasms, characterized by hyperplasia of the epithelium. Papillomas are colloquially referred to as cutaneous or skin warts and are typically of either viral (papillomaviruses or herpesviruses) or unknown origin. Psittacid alphaherpesvirus is associated with cloacal papillomatosis in psittacine species and is discussed in the Herpesvirus (Psittacid Herpesviruses) chapter.

## PATHOPHYSIOLOGY
Papillomaviruses are generally considered host specific, although recent evidence may challenge this hypothesis. These viruses typically affect the featherless skin, most commonly associated with the skin of the eyelids, at the junction of the beak and face, and on the feet and legs. Transmission is thought to be by direct contact with infected birds, or a contaminated environment through traumatic wounds, but this has not been proven. Infection with papillomaviruses of the epidermal basal cells can result in wart-like lesions of the skin or a persistent asymptomatic infection.

## SYSTEMS AFFECTED
Skin (dermis, epithelium).

## GENETICS
There is no known genetic basis for cutaneous papillomas in birds.

## INCIDENCE/PREVALENCE
Incidence and prevalence of cutaneous papillomatosis is unknown. One study from the early 1970s of wild chaffinches (*Fringilla coelebs*) demonstrated a prevalence of 1.8%. Cutaneous papillomatosis in psittacine species is considered rare. In a recent publication in which papillomavirus genomic sequencing was evaluated in several wild bird species without clinical signs, prevalence varied from 0% to 29.4%, depending on species sampled.

## GEOGRAPHIC DISTRIBUTION
Cutaneous papillomatosis is can potentially affect birds anywhere in the world, with no clear seasonal pattern. However, in a recent study of wild birds without clinical signs, using genomic sequencing, PCR-positive birds were more common in spring compared with fall months in Canada.

## SIGNALMENT
**Species**: All avian species are considered susceptible. Currently, eight avian papillomavirus types have been described in nine bird species from six avian orders.

Papillomavirus DNA has been detected in skin lesions of chaffinch (*Fringilla coelebs*), greenfinch (*Carduelis chloris*), canary (*Serinus canaria*), brambling (*Fringilla montifringilla*), northern fulmar (*Fulmarus glacialis*), African grey parrot (*Psittacus erithacus erithacus*), yellow-necked francolin (*Francolinus leucoscepus*), mallard duck (*Anas platyrhynchos*), Adélie penguin (*Pygoscelis adeliae*), and a red-billed gull (*Chroicocephalus novaehollandiae scopulinus*). Papilloma-like viral particles have been observed using electron microscopy in skin lesions from a gannet (*Morus bassanus*), canaries, and a brambling. In addition to the papillomavirus types that were associated with disease in birds, papillomaviruses were identified in clinically normal Adélie penguins, yellow-necked francolins, canaries, mallard ducks, Atlantic puffin (*Fratercula arctica*), American herring gulls (*Larus smithsoniasnus*), and black-legged kittiwakes (*Rissa tridactyla*).
**Mean age and range**: All ages appear to be susceptible. In a recent study in Canada, genetic sequencing across four wild bird species demonstrated a higher prevalence in adults compared with juveniles.
**Predominant sex**: Both equally susceptible.

## SIGNS
Skin lesions include papules, nodules, or discrete masses on the feet, legs, or around the eyes and commissures of the beak. In a Yorkshire canary, tongue lesions were positive for papillomavirus. Masses may be focal to multifocal and are hyperplastic with a cauliflower-like or wart-like appearance (e.g. papilliferous).

## CAUSES
Papillomaviruses (DNA viruses) are suspected as the cause of most cutaneous papillomas, but not all cutaneous papillomas contain viral particles. A novel herpesvirus (psittacid herpesvirus 2) was found to be associated with a cutaneous papilloma and a cloacal papilloma in an African grey parrot.

## RISK FACTORS
A traumatic disruption in the epidermis can allow papillomaviruses to invade the basal cells. It is thought that debilitation and immunosuppression may predispose some individuals to papillomavirus infection. An additional potential risk factor is exposure to any avian species with cutaneous papillomas.

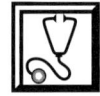

# DIAGNOSIS

## DIFFERENTIAL DIAGNOSIS
Soft tissue sarcoma or other epithelial tumors, poxvirus, bacterial or fungal cutaneous abscesses, *Knemidokoptes* mites.

## CBC/BIOCHEMISTRY/URINALYSIS
No specific blood parameter changes are associated with avian cutaneous papillomatosis.

## OTHER LABORATORY TESTS
N/A

## IMAGING
N/A

## DIAGNOSTIC PROCEDURES
The diagnosis of skin disease has traditionally relied on biopsy and histopathologic examination of skin lesions. Electron microscopy of tissue preparations from cutaneous papillomas was used to confirm the presence of papilloma viral particles in several species. More recently, molecular tools, such as PCR and/or immunohistochemistry, are increasingly used to analyze tissue samples. Oropharyngeal/cloacal swabs have recently been used for genome-sequencing for identifying papillomaviruses in wild birds.

## PATHOLOGIC FINDINGS
**Gross lesions**: White to gray, fleshy, or cauliflower-like growths, most typically on a short stalk.
**Histopathologic lesions**: Papillary mass with pedunculated fibrovascular connective tissue stalk, stratified squamous epithelium covered with a hyperkeratotic layer, with or without the presence of basophilic intranuclear inclusion bodies at junction of keratinized and non-keratinized epithelium. In the dermis, lymphocytes and heterophils are occasionally present.

# TREATMENT

## APPROPRIATE HEALTH CARE
Outpatient supportive care.

## NURSING CARE
Supportive care may include wound care, fluid support, NSAIDs (e.g. meloxicam), and appropriate antimicrobials.

## ACTIVITY
N/A

## DIET
N/A

## CLIENT EDUCATION
If a pet bird is affected, warn client that little is known about transmission, but contact transmission may be important, so other birds in the household may be susceptible.

## SURGICAL CONSIDERATIONS
Surgical excision of papillomatous lesions may be an option, especially if function (e.g. flight, vision, ability to eat) is affected. The lesions can be surgically excised using scalpel blade, cautery, laser, or cryosurgery, but the papillomas may recur.

P

## MEDICATIONS

### DRUG(S) OF CHOICE
No antiviral drugs are known to be effective. Administering anti-inflammatory drugs and appropriate antibiotics for any secondary bacterial infections, based on bacterial culture and antibiotic sensitivities, may be prudent.

### CONTRAINDICATIONS
N/A

### PRECAUTIONS
N/A

### POSSIBLE INTERACTIONS
N/A

### ALTERNATIVE DRUGS
N/A

## FOLLOW-UP

### PATIENT MONITORING
Monitor areas of excised papillomas for recurrence or conversion to neoplastic masses.

### PREVENTION/AVOIDANCE
In captive facilities, such as zoos, aquaria, or wildlife rehabilitation centers, do not mix uninfected birds with known papillomavirus infected birds. Prevent chronic foot and leg trauma with appropriate substrate.

### POSSIBLE COMPLICATIONS
Recurrence of the papilloma after excision or secondary microbial (e.g. bacterial, fungal) infection at the surgical site.

### EXPECTED COURSE AND PROGNOSIS
Cutaneous papillomas may spontaneously regress or may never resolve on their own and continue to proliferate. If functional capacity, such as vision or ability to eat, is affected, the prognosis may be guarded to poor. Benign papillomas may evolve into neoplastic epithelial lesions.

Papillomaviruses have the potential to cause neoplasia in birds as is the case in mammals. Firm masses under a wing and on a digit of the foot on a mallard duck were diagnosed as having mesenchymal dermal neoplasms (spindle-cell sarcomas) with basophilic intranuclear inclusion bodies for which next-generation sequencing determined these inclusions to be a novel papillomavirus. In a red-billed gull (*Chroicocephalus novaehollandiae scopulinus*) with clinical signs and histopathology results consistent with papillomas, one of the papilloma lesions also demonstrated histopathologic evidence of that it had progressed to an in-situ carcinoma.

## MISCELLANEOUS

### ASSOCIATED CONDITIONS
In free-ranging finches in the UK from multiple species—39 chaffinches, 4 bullfinches (*Pyrrhula pyrrhula*), 1 greenfinch, and 1 goldfinch (*Carduelis carduelis*)—hyperplastic lesions of the hind limbs commonly contained both papillomavirus DNA and leg mites, suggesting that dual infection may be important for lesion development in some passerine species.

### AGE-RELATED FACTORS
N/A

### ZOONOTIC POTENTIAL
N/A

### FERTILITY/BREEDING
N/A

### SYNONYMS
N/A

### SEE ALSO
Herpesvirus (Passerine Birds)
Herpesvirus (Psittacid Herpesviruses)

### ABBREVIATIONS
NSAIDs—non-steroidal anti-inflammatory drugs
PCR—polymerase chain reaction

### INTERNET RESOURCES
N/A

*Suggested Reading*
Canuti, M., Munro, H.J., Robertson, G.J., et al. (2019). New insight into avian papillomavirus ecology and evolution from characterization of novel wild bird papillomaviruses. *Frontiers in Microbiology*, 10:701.
Lawson, B., Robinson, R.A., Fernandez, J.R., et al. (2018). Spatio-temporal dynamics and aetiology of proliferative leg skin lesions in wild British finches. *Scientific Reports*, 8:14670.
Phalen, D. (1997). Viruses. In: *Avian Medicine and Surgery* (ed. R.B. Altman S.L. Clubb, G.M. Dorrestein, K. Quesenberry), 281–322. St. Louis, MO: Saunders.
Styles, D.K., Tomaszewski, E.K., Phalen, D.N. (2005). A novel psittacid herpesvirus found in African grey parrots (*Psittacus erithacus erithacus*). *Avian Pathology*, 34:150–154.
Truchado, D.A., Williams, R.A.J., Benitez, L. (2018). Natural history of avian papillomaviruses. *Virus Research*, 252:58–67.
Truchado, D.A., Moens, M.A.J., Callejas, S., et al. (2018). Genomic characterization of the first oral avian papillomavirus in a colony of breeding canaries (*Serinus canaria*). *Veterinary Research Communications*, 42:111–120.
**Author**: Kurt K. Sladky, MS, DVM, DACZM, DECZM (Zoo Health Management & Herpetology)

P

# BASICS

## DEFINITION
Pasteurellosis or avian cholera is a bacterial infection of free-ranging birds caused by *Pasteurella multocida*, a Gram-negative, aerobic/facultative anaerobic species of bacteria. *P. multocida* causes disease in a wide variety of mammalian and avian species and has been reported in more than 100 species of bird. At least 16 serotypes of *P. multocida* exist that cause disease in wild bird populations, which are differentiated from those causing disease in domestic fowl. Serotype 1 is most frequently identified in waterfowl outbreaks along the North American migratory flyways, with the exception of the Atlantic flyway. Pasteurellosis is primarily a disease of wild waterfowl, with outbreaks occurring on wintering and breeding grounds where birds are in close proximity and in high concentrations. Frequency and incidence of outbreaks have increased since the disease was first described in the mid-1940s, due in large part to the loss of wetland habitat, forcing more and more birds to congregate in smaller areas. Avian cholera has been called the most significant infectious disease of North American waterfowl.

## PATHOPHYSIOLOGY
Acute pasteurellosis is an extremely rapidly progressing disease, resulting in death within 6–48 hours following exposure. Exposure to *P. multocida* can occur via mucous membranes of the upper respiratory and GI tracts. Infection can occur through ingestion of contaminated food or water, direct contact between infected and non-infected birds, aerosolization of organisms from the surface of contaminated water (bathing, landing on/taking off from water), or through wounds in the skin. Deceased birds may shed very large numbers of the organism into the environment. *P. multocida* can persist in water for weeks to months, prolonging outbreaks if proper site management is not implemented. Once the organism enters the body, the disease process progresses rapidly to septicemia, endotoxemia, and death. Severity of signs and rapidity of progression are related to the specific strain the virulence of that strain, species affected, sex, age, immune status due to previous exposure, concurrent injury/illness, route of exposure, and exposure dose. While a chronic carrier state has been defined for *P. multocida* infections in poultry, this has not been established as a potential source of infection in wild birds.

## SYSTEMS AFFECTED
**Cardiovascular**: Death from *P. multocida* usually occurs as a result of circulatory collapse due to hypovolemic shock ± consumptive coagulopathy.

**Respiratory**: Infected birds may have severe upper respiratory discharge and respiratory distress.

**Neuromuscular**: Infected birds may display a variety of neurologic signs ranging from lethargy to erratic flight, sometimes attempting to land on water significantly above the water's surface.

## GENETICS
N/A

## INCIDENCE/PREVALENCE
Pasteurellosis has been called a "disease for all seasons." However, outbreaks are most commonly associated with circumstances where large numbers of birds have congregated in a small area and when birds are under increased stress, such as migration or nesting/breeding.

## GEOGRAPHIC DISTRIBUTION
Major outbreaks among waterfowl have occurred during both spring and summer migration along all four North American migratory flyways. Pasteurellosis gained more recognition as a significant disease of free-ranging waterfowl in North America in the 1970s. Locations that experience the most frequent and significant pasteurella outbreaks are located along major migratory flyways and include California's Central Valley, Klamath Basin at the California/Oregon border, the Texas Panhandle, and the Platte River Basin in Nebraska. Pasteurella outbreaks in wild waterfowl are related to loss of habitat by increasing concentrations of birds.

## SIGNALMENT
Waterfowl, such as ducks and geese, and coots are most frequently affected in large outbreaks of *P. multocida*. Scavenger species, such as gulls, raptors, and corvids, are also commonly affected when attracted to large numbers of carcasses at an outbreak site, becoming infected by consuming infected tissues.

## SIGNS
Often, affected birds are found dead without clinical signs. However, when clinical signs are present, they can include lethargy; birds do not try to evade capture and may die within a matter of minutes after capture. Convulsions. Swimming in circles. Opisthotonos. Erratic flight; attempting to land before water's surface. Mucous discharge from mouth. Bloody nasal discharge. Soiled vent. Pasty, yellow droppings/bloody droppings.

## CAUSES
Multiple serotypes of *P. multocida* cause pasteurellosis in free-ranging birds. Serotypes that cause disease in wild birds are different from those that cause disease in captive poultry. There is also a differentiation of serotypes on the Atlantic flyway of the USA compared with the rest of the country. The sources of outbreaks remain unknown, in both wild and domestic populations of affected birds, nor where the bacteria reside when not causing disease. The circumstances that lead to outbreaks are also largely unknown.

## RISK FACTORS
High concentrations of birds in close proximity in wintering and breeding grounds. Continued destruction of wetlands has led to increased population densities on the remaining sites, increasing the likelihood of outbreaks.

# DIAGNOSIS

## DIFFERENTIAL DIAGNOSIS
Botulism. Heavy-metal toxicosis. Organophosphate/carbamate toxicity. Duck viral enteritis. Highly pathogenic avian influenza.

## CBC/BIOCHEMISTRY/URINALYSIS
Due to acute progression of the disease, finding for these diagnostics are usually unremarkable.

## OTHER LABORATORY TESTS
Culture of heart blood, liver, bone marrow. Can persist for weeks in bone marrow, so scavenged portions can be used for diagnostics. Coccobacilli on smear of heart blood.

## IMAGING
Imaging is generally not feasible because of the acute progression of the disease.

## DIAGNOSTIC PROCEDURES
Pasteurella serotyping. Culture of liver, bone marrow, or heart blood of recently deceased individuals. Identification of large numbers Gram-negative coccobacilli on heart blood smear is highly suggestive.

## PATHOLOGIC FINDINGS
Histopathology findings nonspecific in acute deaths. Affected birds typically in good body condition. Food in upper GI tract, indicating acute death. Hemorrhages on the surface of the heart muscle and along the coronary band. Small white-yellow foci within the hepatic parenchyma. May also see darkening, copper tone, swelling, and fracture of the liver upon handling. Hemorrhages on the surface of the ventriculus. Ropey nasal discharge. Intestines contain thick, yellowish fluid or clear mucous. Intestinal contents and nasal discharge contain very large numbers of *P. multocida* organisms.

# TREATMENT

## APPROPRIATE HEALTH CARE
The degree of health care provided is based on the severity of the clinical signs. Due to the peracute nature of this disease in wild

P

birds, as well as the difficulty in treating large population of potentially affected birds, antibacterial treatment and nursing care are usually not feasible. In a captive bird setting, treatment should be based on clinical signs, organ systems affected, and the results of C/S of appropriate samples.

## NURSING CARE
Nutritional and fluid support should be provided to patients too debilitated to eat and drink on their own. Thermal support should also be provided as needed. Basic cleanliness should be maintained in patients who are recumbent and unable to preen. Large waterfowl, such as geese, who are sternally recumbent, should be housed on heavily padded substrate or on a cushion that elevates the keel above the substrate to avoid development of decubital ulcers along the keel. Birds unaccustomed to spending prolonged time out of water may also develop abrasions/ulcerations on the plantar surfaces of their feet/hocks as well, so appropriate substrate and protective wraps are indicated. Many species of waterfowl are susceptible to secondary fungal infections caused by *Aspergillus* spp., and prophylactic treatment with antifungal agents may be indicated.

## ACTIVITY
N/A

## DIET
N/A

## CLIENT EDUCATION
N/A

## SURGICAL CONSIDERATIONS
N/A

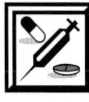

## MEDICATIONS
### DRUG(S) OF CHOICE
Antibiotic therapy should be based on C/S in individual birds but is impractical for treatment of flocks of wild birds. Canada geese have been treated successfully with intramuscular injections of oxytetracycline, followed by a 30-day treatment course of tetracycline-infused feed.

### CONTRAINDICATIONS
N/A

### PRECAUTIONS
N/A

### POSSIBLE INTERACTIONS
N/A

### ALTERNATIVE DRUGS
*P. multocida* tends to be susceptible to a variety of antibiotics commonly used in veterinary medicine (e.g. enrofloxacin, amoxicillin-clavulanate, tetracyclines, sulfonamides).

## FOLLOW-UP
### PATIENT MONITORING
N/A

### PREVENTION/AVOIDANCE
Surveillance of sites where waterfowl congregate is the most important defence against large outbreaks for *P. multocida*. At sites where an outbreak has occurred, or suspected outbreak is occurring, collection of carcasses will mitigate further contamination of the environment. Removal of carcasses, which can act as decoys, will also decrease attraction of other birds to a contaminated area and prevent scavenging of infected carcasses. Scavenger species, such as gulls and corvids, do not succumb to *P. multocida* infection as rapidly as do waterfowl, and may therefore spread the organism far from the original outbreak site. Habitat management is another facet of the prevention/management of *P. multocida* outbreaks. Contaminated areas may be drained and water diverted to another, uncontaminated location, or flooded to decrease the overall concentration of the organism in the environment. Hazing practices may also be employed to prevent congregation of birds at a contaminated site. A killed vaccine has been developed which has been shown to be effective in preventing disease in Canada geese. However, immunity is short-lived, only lasting for approximately 12 months, making its application for *P. multocida* management in migratory waterfowl limited. Canada geese have also been treated successfully post-exposure with oxytetracycline injections, followed by administration of tetracycline in feed, but again, application to large numbers of free-ranging birds would be difficult.

### POSSIBLE COMPLICATIONS
N/A

### EXPECTED COURSE AND PROGNOSIS
*P. multocida* infection in wild birds is typically a peracute to acute disease process, usually resulting in death within a matter of hours. Due to the rapid progression of this septicemic disease, prognosis for survival and recovery is poor.

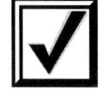

## MISCELLANEOUS
### ASSOCIATED CONDITIONS
N/A

### AGE-RELATED FACTORS
Chickens more susceptible as they reach maturity. Ducks > 4 weeks. Turkeys, young to mature.

### ZOONOTIC POTENTIAL
Infection with *P. multocida* is not considered a high human health risk because of differences in species susceptibilities to different strains. Most pasteurella infections in humans are the result of domestic animal bites; however, individuals working at outbreak sites or performing necropsies on suspected *P. multocida* infected birds should take appropriate precautions and wear appropriate personal protective equipment to prevent passage of disease.

### FERTILITY/BREEDING
N/A

### SYNONYMS
Fowl cholera, avian cholera, avian hemorrhagic septicemia.

### SEE ALSO
Avian Influenza
Botulism
Herpesvirus (Columbid Herpesvirus 1 in Pigeons and Raptors)
Herpesvirus (Duck Viral Enteritis)
Herpesvirus (Passerine Birds)
Toxicosis (Environmental/Pesticides)
Toxicosis (Heavy Metals)
Salmonellosis
Sepsis
Wounds (Including Bite Wounds, Predator Attacks)

### ABBREVIATIONS
C/S—culture and sensitivity
GI—gastrointestinal

### INTERNET RESOURCES
N/A

*Suggested Reading*
Franson, J.C., Friend, M., Gibbs, S.E.J., Wild, M.A. (1999). Avian cholera. In: *USGS Field Manual of Wildlife Diseases: General Field Procedures and Diseases of Birds*, 75–92. Madison, WI: US Geological Survey.
Samuel, M.D., Boltzer, R.G., Wobeser, G.A. (2007). Avian cholera. In: *Infectious Diseases of Wild Birds* (ed. N.J. Thomas, B. Hunter, C.T. Atkinson), 239–269. Ames, IA: Blackwell Publishing.
Wobeser, G.A. (1997). Avian cholera. In: *Diseases of Wild Waterfowl*, 2nd edn., 57–69. New York: Plenum Press.
**Author:** Shannon M. Riggs, DVM, DABVP (Avian)

# BASICS

## DEFINITION
Avian patagium disease refers to a condition affecting the patagium, the thin membranous structure of skin and connective tissue that supports the wings and legs of birds. It may involve inflammation, infection, trauma, or neoplasia within the patagium.

## PATHOPHYSIOLOGY
Patagial disease can result from various factors, including trauma, infectious agents, or underlying systemic diseases, leading to inflammation, edema, and impaired wing function. Superficial chronic ulcerative dermatitis (SCUD) is an inflammatory condition worsened by bacterial infection (often *Staphylococcus* spp.), which may evolve into chronic condition. Patagial trauma is frequent in wild bird affected by barbwire trauma or kite trapping. Patagial retraction is frequent in birds with wing injury and prolonged wing bandage or cage rest.

## SYSTEMS AFFECTED
Integumentary system (patagium and skin).

## GENETICS
N/A

## INCIDENCE/PREVALENCE
Varies among bird species and populations. SCUD may have an epizootic appearance, with several birds affected among the same flock.

## GEOGRAPHIC DISTRIBUTION
N/A

## SIGNALMENT
Gray parrot, lovebird, and cockatiels are known to present with SCUD, but many other parrot species can be affected.

## SIGNS

### Historical Findings
Unable to fly. Feather-damaging behavior. Bleeding from the wing. Lethargy.

### Physical Examination Findings
Swelling or thickening of the patagium. Decreased wing mobility. Feather loss. Redness or discoloration of the patagium. Ulceration and bleeding. Crusting and fibrotic lesions.

## CAUSES
Trauma: Injuries to the wings or patagium, including bites or collisions. Retraction: Previous history of trauma, prolonged inability to fly, bandages. Infectious agents: Bacterial or fungal infections affecting the patagium (*Staphylococcus* spp.). Underlying systemic conditions, such as nutritional deficiencies or metabolic disorders, impacting the health of the patagium. Neoplasia. Squamous cell carcinoma.

## RISK FACTORS
Traumatic events. Poor nutrition. Human proximity and manipulation may influence the normal flora of the bird skin and predispose to SCUD.

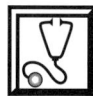

# DIAGNOSIS

## DIFFERENTIAL DIAGNOSIS
Wing injuries. Dermatitis. Systemic diseases affecting wing function.

## CBC/BIOCHEMISTRY/URINALYSIS
May show leukocytosis in cases of infectious or inflammatory patagium disease. Elevated acute phase proteins in cases of inflammation.

## OTHER LABORATORY TESTS
Cytology and microbial cultures of affected patagium tissues.

## IMAGING
Radiographs or other imaging modalities to assess wing structure and identify abnormalities such as bone lysis, fracture, or infection.

## DIAGNOSTIC PROCEDURES
Biopsy of the patagium for histopathological examination.

## PATHOLOGIC FINDINGS
Histopathology may reveal inflammation, infection, or structural abnormalities in the patagium tissues.

# TREATMENT

## APPROPRIATE HEALTH CARE
Use of a Elizabethan collar may be required to prevent self inflicted trauma.

## NURSING CARE
Supportive care.

## ACTIVITY
Minimal extension of the wing is required until the cutaneous tissue is healed. After this period, the wing must be extended gradually to regain full elasticity of the patagium.

## DIET
Optimal diet is important for wound healing. Omega-3 supplementation may be beneficial to reduce inflammation.

## CLIENT EDUCATION
Basic hygiene and use of glove to touch the wound.

## SURGICAL CONSIDERATIONS
Patagial laceration may be repaired surgically. The tendon of the propatagium must also be repaired if lacerated. Patagial dermatitis related to SCUD may require wound debridement until a healthy granulation bed is formed.

# MEDICATIONS

## DRUG(S) OF CHOICE
Antibiotics (amoxiccilin clavulanate, doxycycline, azithromycin) or antifungal medications (itraconazole) for infectious patagium disease. Anti-inflammatory drugs—meloxicam. Topical ointment—poloxamer gel with antibiotics, silver sulfadiazine, intrasite gel.

## CONTRAINDICATIONS
N/A

## PRECAUTIONS
N/A

## POSSIBLE INTERACTIONS
N/A

## ALTERNATIVE DRUGS
N/A

# FOLLOW-UP

## PATIENT MONITORING
Frequent wound checks are recommended over a course of 2–3 months.

## PREVENTION/AVOIDANCE
N/A

## POSSIBLE COMPLICATIONS
Chronic ulceration may lead to osteomyelitis, elbow arthritis, and endocarditis.

## EXPECTED COURSE AND PROGNOSIS
In case of SCUD, the wound healing process is long (2 months) and recurrence is frequent. In case of patagial tear, the functional prognosis is fair to poor, depending on the severity of the trauma.

# MISCELLANEOUS

## ASSOCIATED CONDITIONS
N/A

P

## PATAGIUM DISEASES

### AGE-RELATED FACTORS
N/A

### ZOONOTIC POTENTIAL
Methicillin-resistant *Staphylococcus aureus* has been described.

### FERTILITY/BREEDING
N/A

### SYNONYMS
None.

### SEE ALSO
Dermatitis
Fractures
Joint Diseases
Luxations

### ABBREVIATIONS
SCUD—superficial chronic ulcerative dermatitis

### INTERNET RESOURCES
N/A

*Suggested Reading*
Abou-Zahr, T., Carrasco, D.C., Dvm, N.S., et al. (2018). Superficial chronic ulcerative dermatitis (SCUD) in psittacine birds: review of 11 cases (2008–2016). *Journal of Avian Medicine and Surgery*, 32:25–33.
**Author**: Minh Huynh, DVM, DECZM (Avian), DACZM

P

# BASICS

## DEFINITION
Perosis or avian slipped tendon is a condition where the gastrocnemius tendon displaces laterally or medially from the caudal/plantar aspect of the intertarsal joint.

## PATHOPHYSIOLOGY
The pathophysiology in non-poultry avian species is not well researched. Perosis in broiler chicken develops mainly due to manganese, zinc, choline, or biotin deficiency, and rapid growth. Other trace elements and amino acids might also play a role. The condition appears In broiler chickens around 14–35 days. There is disruption in ligament and bone formation around the tarsal joint. This disruption affects the position of the Achilles tendon, which emerges from the trochlear groove, and the joint appears dislocated.

## SYSTEMS AFFECTED
Musculoskeletal—affecting the tibiotarsus, tarsal joint, tarsometatarsus, and/or the gastrocnemius tendon.

## GENETICS
Suspected in poultry to have some genetic relationships but not definitively proven.

## INCIDENCE/PREVALENCE
Rare in adults. Uncommon in chicks with proper diet. Common in chicks with improper diet or growth/weight monitoring.

## GEOGRAPHIC DISTRIBUTION
N/A

## SIGNALMENT
**Species**: All avian species. Seen in poultry, waterfowl, ratites, falcons and parrot species.
**Mean age and range**: Neonates, fledglings.
**Predominant sex**: None.

## SIGNS
### Historical Findings
Inability to stand and swelling of the hock joint reported by the owner.

### Physical Examination Findings
Acute lameness and inability to stand and/or walk. Upon palpation, the "slipped" tendon may be visibly deviated laterally or more commonly medially. In the acute phase, the tendon may be manually positioned caudally upon extension of the tarsal joint but deviates when the joint is flexed. Edema is present in the acute phase, leading to progressive joint inflammation and tendonitis. Angular limb deformity may be present.

## CAUSES
Deficiency in biotin, choline, methionine, manganese/zinc. Valgus/varus malposition. Trauma.

## RISK FACTORS
Chicks and fledglings with rapid growth. Heavy-bodied species with relatively shorter legs (i.e. waterfowl). Species with long legs in relation to body size. Inadequate diet. Lack of exercise or water for swimming; overcrowding.

# DIAGNOSIS

## DIFFERENTIAL DIAGNOSIS
Intertarsal joint luxation, angular limb deformity, infectious arthritis (mycoplasmosis), collateral ligament rupture, intertarsal meniscal damage, intra-articular fracture, degenerative joint disease.

## CBC/BIOCHEMISTRY/URINALYSIS
Often within normal limits unless secondary inflammation or infection has developed to a point where the white blood cell count begins to increase.

## OTHER LABORATORY TESTS
N/A

## IMAGING
Radiographs should be performed to rule out any underlying pathology to the joint or bones. CT is helpful to define the anatomical structures in chronic severe cases.

## DIAGNOSTIC PROCEDURES
If fistula present, sterile swab for C/S test for antibiotic choice.

## PATHOLOGIC FINDINGS
Inflammation of the tissues around the tarsal joint and calcaneal tendon. Purulent fistula.

# TREATMENT

## APPROPRIATE HEALTH CARE
Initial joint stabilisation until further diagnostics. Outpatient management in mild cases. Inpatient management in severe cases with surgical management for 48 hours to ensure stability and prevent complications.

## NURSING CARE
Care should include proper drug administration, weight reduction, surgical site monitoring, adequate diet and force feeding in case of anorexia, movement restriction, clean environment; water avoidance for waterfowl and wading birds.

## ACTIVITY
Slick surfaces in the brooder or nest box should be avoided with the proper use of substrates, such as shaving, carpet, and so on.

Waterfowl should be encouraged to exercise through swimming.

## DIET
A well-balanced diet should be provided, avoiding excessive protein and calorie intake. Since excessive caloric intake is a risk factor, monitoring daily weight gain is vital in prevention and therapeutics. The daily weight gain should be appropriate for the species but on average is around 10% daily. Leg and tendon issues may be exacerbated with excessive calcium supplementation, leading to decreased manganese absorption.

## CLIENT EDUCATION
Due to the varying levels of prognosis, client education about expectations of outcome is very important.

## SURGICAL CONSIDERATIONS
If no inflammation, early reposition and splint for 1–3 weeks may hold the tendon in place. Tenorrhaphy: The soft tissues are dissected, and the tendon sheath is sutured to the periosteum along the trochlear ridge. In addition, deepening the trochlear groove has been used in conjunction with this technique or as a single technique, with variable success. Another technique describes the placement of staples or K-wire into each distal tibiotarsal condyle with sterile cable meshed between and over the tendon to hold it in place. A less invasive approach with variable success is the external use of sutures to hold the tendon over the caudal position. If angular limb deformity coexists, it should be adequately corrected with wedge/diamond osteotomy and ESF. In case of failure of the above surgical techniques, arthrodesis with transarticular ESF is recommended.

P

# MEDICATIONS

## DRUG(S) OF CHOICE
NSAIDs may be used in management of the pain and inflammation associated with the stresses on the joints/bones.

## CONTRAINDICATIONS
None.

## PRECAUTIONS
None.

## POSSIBLE INTERACTIONS
None.

## ALTERNATIVE DRUGS
Intra-articular application of hyaluronic acid (low molecular weight) every 10 days might help stabilization and ameliorate osteoarthritis.

## FOLLOW-UP

### PATIENT MONITORING
Patients should be monitored daily for progress of therapy and complications; weight management to avoid overweight, fast growth and imbalanced caloric load; goniometry to ensure proper return to range of movement.

### PREVENTION/AVOIDANCE
Most nutritional deficiencies can be prevented by placing chicks on a balanced and appropriate diet for the species. Daily monitoring of weight (same time of day before feeding) is extremely important to adjust the caloric input to regulate a slow steady weight gain.

### POSSIBLE COMPLICATIONS
Arthritis/osteomyelitis. Ankylosis of the intertarsal joint. Degenerative joint disease. Unilateral pododermatitis. Surgical implant failure. Angular limb deformity due to incorrect splinting position. Constrictive blood flow and edema and/or discomfort.

### EXPECTED COURSE AND PROGNOSIS
Depending on the severity presented during the initial examination. Mild cases may be managed medically with a fair prognosis but more advanced cases that require surgical correction have a guarded to poor prognosis.

## MISCELLANEOUS

### ASSOCIATED CONDITIONS
Valgus/varus deformity. Collateral ligament rupture. Intertarsal joint luxation. Curled toes.

### AGE-RELATED FACTORS
Commonly diagnosed in nestlings, fledglings.

### ZOONOTIC POTENTIAL
N/A

### FERTILITY/BREEDING
N/A

### SYNONYMS
Slipped tendon.

### SEE ALSO
Angular Limb Deformity (Splay Leg)
Joint Diseases
Toe and Nail Diseases

### ABBREVIATIONS
C/S—culture and sensitivity
CT—computed tomography
ESF—external skeletal fixation
NSAIDs—non-steroidal anti-inflammatory drugs

### INTERNET RESOURCES
N/A

*Suggested Reading*
Darrow, B., Bennett, R.A. (2021). Avian orthopedics. In: *Surgery of Exotic Animals* (ed. R.A. Bennett, G.W. Pye), 112–153. Ames, IA: Wiley.
Erdélyi, K., Tenk, M., Dan, A. (1999). Mycoplasmosis associated perosis type skeletal deformity in a saker falcon nestling in Hungary. *Journal of Wildlife Diseases*, 35:586–590.
Rath, N.C., Durairaj, V. (2022). Avian bone physiology and poultry bone disorders. In *Sturkie's Avian Physiology*, 6th edn. (erd.C.G. Scanes), 529–543. St. Louis, MO: Elsevier.
Zadravec, M., Matko, M., Azmanis, P. (2022). Slipped tendon of M. gastrocnemious in an adult breeding female Gyrfalcon (Falco rusticolus) treated using Hyaluronic Acid (Suplasyn). Proceedings of 5th International Conference for Avian Herpetological and Exotic Mammal Medicine, Budapest, 27–31 March.
**Author**: Panagiotis Azmanis DVM, PhD, DECZM (Avian), Dip ZooMed

**P**

# BASICS

## DEFINITION
Only 3% of bird species have a phallus: an intromittent (protruding) form in ratites (ostriches, emus, cassowaries, rheas, tinamous, kiwis), and Anseriformes (ducks, geese, swans); a non-intromittent form in Galliformes (chickens, turkeys, grouse, quail, pheasants, peafowl, guineafowl, partridge) and Emberizidae (towhees, juncos, buntings, New World sparrows). Only in males, the structure is derived from the internal cloacal wall, which is generally associated with sperm competition. In the Argentine lake duck (*Oxyura vittata*), the corkscrew-shaped phallus can approach 16 in. (6.2 cm) in length. This condition can cause concern for a client or "good Samaritan" because the phallus is visibly protruding from the cloaca.

## PATHOPHYSIOLOGY
The intromittent phallus normally lies on the cloacal floor and becomes erect due to lymphatic engorgement produced by the left and right lymphatic bodies. Semen then travels in a groove, the phallic sulcus. In all intromittent phallic species except the ostrich, the phallus has a blind-ended, long, hollow tube, which, with lymphatic engorgement, inverts out like a latex glove finger. The left lymphatic body is larger than the right, and this incongruity causes the erect phallus's spiral twist. With the non-intromittent phallus, two lateral folds on the ventral edge of the vent become engorged, protruding that edge, which the male quickly contacts to the female's protruding oviduct, with semen transferring down the groove and into the oviduct. Vasa parrots (*Coracopsis vasa*, *Coracopsis nigra*) have an intermediate form, with a fleshy bag-like protrusion (1½ × 2 in./4 × 5 cm in size) from the male's cloaca inserted into the female's cloaca, with copulation lasting up to 100 minutes. This protrusion can be physiologically prolapsed in the species during the breeding season, and should not automatically be considered a pathological prolapse. Except in the Vasa parrot example, if the phallus does not return fully into the cloaca, it would considered a pathological prolapse requiring veterinary assistance.

## SYSTEMS AFFECTED
**Reproductive**: May limit reproductive success, trauma to phallus and/or cloacal tissue.

**Behavioral**: Usually occurs during breeding season in seasonal species, can include self-mutilation of phallus if causing discomfort, also may be associated with chronic masturbation on inanimate objects.
**GI**: Caking may lead to inability to empty GI system in timely manner.
**Renal/urologic**: Urate caking may block outflow of ureters, leading to primary renal disease.
**Skin/exocrine**: Chronic prolapse may cause urate/fecal caking of vent region skin and feathers.
**General**: Generalized weakness may lead to prolapse.

## GENETICS
N/A

## INCIDENCE/PREVALENCE
Unknown.

## GEOGRAPHIC DISTRIBUTION
Likely worldwide.

## SIGNALMENT
**Species**: Ostriches, rheas, emus, cassowaries, tinamous, kiwis, ducks, geese, swans.
**Mean age and range**: Mature males and immature males attempting to breed.
**Predominant sex**: Male.

## SIGNS
### Historical Findings
Breeding season; usually female present, may have been competing males, possible diarrhea/polyuria of explosive nature or chronic.

### Physical Examination Findings
Phallus hanging partway or completely out of cloaca; may exteriorize during defecation or urination. Tissue may appear normal (usually a pale white or yellow) or may be necrotic and inflamed. May be fecal, with urate caking around vent on feathers. Diarrhea and/or polyuria may be noted. In some cases, the phallus may only extrude when bird becomes sexually stimulated by presence of female, male competitors, or even a human owner (other animal) to which it has "mate bonded." Bird may have generalized weakness or have systemic neurologic disease.

## CAUSES
Trauma during successful breeding or breeding fatigue are the most likely causes. GI/cloacal disease—cryptosporidiosis and histomoniasis have both been documented causes in ostrich chicks. Mycoplasmosis and neisseriosis (suspected sexually transmitted "goose gonorrhea" in geese and erysipelothricosis in a duck) should be considered secondarily, especially if more

than one bird is affected. Generalized weakness may lead to prolapse and inability to retract, likewise any severe systemic neurologic disease, such as Eastern or Western equine encephalitis viruses or West Nile virus, should be on the differential list. Frostbite may cause or exacerbate a prolapse.

## RISK FACTORS
Breeding season, poor male to female ratio, male competitors, unreceptive females, immature males around females, cold weather.

# DIAGNOSIS

## DIFFERENTIAL DIAGNOSIS
Cloacal prolapse, intestinal prolapse, oviductal prolapse, GI foreign body protruding from cloaca, foreign body adhered to feathers around vent, neoplasia.

## CBC/BIOCHEMISTRY/URINALYSIS
Possibly leukocytosis if site is infected or inflamed, possible polycythemia or hyperproteinemia.

## OTHER LABORATORY TESTS
Fecal floats, direct smears, fecal acid-fast stains, fecal cultures or microbiomes if evidence of concurrent diarrhea or if there is a flock issue, infectious agent-specific PCR diagnostics.

## IMAGING
N/A

## DIAGNOSTIC PROCEDURES
N/A

## PATHOLOGIC FINDINGS
Grossly, the phallus would be engorged, possibly necrotic or traumatized. Other lesions noted in the cloacal or phallic tissue may indicate an underlying etiology such as an infectious agent.

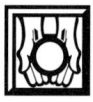

# TREATMENT

## APPROPRIATE HEALTH CARE
Surgical management once stable. If amputating, may be outpatient postoperatively. If tacking back in, consider inpatient observation postoperatively to assess need to progress to amputation or retacking.

## NURSING CARE
Keep phallus lubricated and moist, ideally with a water-soluble lubricant.

# PHALLUS PROLAPSE      (CONTINUED)

## ACTIVITY
Separate the affected individual away from females and potentially other males. Best to keep in quiet, dark area to encourage limited activity and excitement until the issue is resolved.

## DIET
Only if dietary issues causing GI disease led to prolapse.

## CLIENT EDUCATION
N/A

## SURGICAL CONSIDERATIONS
Ideally, the phallus can be replaced into the cloaca. However, in most cases, the bird strains to push it back out immediately or the phallus reprolapses with defecation or urination. In these cases, placing two simple interrupted sutures to decrease the size of the cloacal opening but still allow defecation and urination may buy some time for the tissue to detumesce and be kept within the cloaca. Suture selection should depend on the size of the bird, but often suture strength required is greater than expected. If the phallus will not stay when replaced, 4-0 mono-filament absorbable suture can be tried to gently tack the phallus to its resting position within the cloacal mucosa. If those sutures are not holding, the tissue is necrotic or inflamed, or the client does not want to attempt salvage, then a phallectomy can be performed. As the structure is only used for copulation, not urination, there is no urethra to rebuild. In some cases, the use of a lidocaine/ bupivacaine/sodium bicarbonate local ring and deeper block may suffice for analgesia, without needing to resort to general anesthesia. The block is applied proximal to where the amputation is planned. The phallus can be a vascular organ, so expect moderate site hemorrhage with a local block. Depending on the size of the phallus, hemoclips, vessel sealing devices, $CO_2$ laser, electrocautery, or transfixation or circumferential sutures may be used for ligation, depending on size of phallus, equipment available, and surgeon experience and comfort level. The author usually places the ligation just proximal to a crushing hemostat clamp, then cuts distal to that clamp, slowly removing the clamp. How far proximal on the phallus one attempts amputation may depend on access, equipment, and surgical expertise. Often small "stumps" that are left can be retained by the bird within the cloaca with no apparent long-term repercussions. Too aggressive an amputation may lead to damage of the cloaca, slippage of ligation and secondary hemorrhage during recovery, or deformation of the cloaca, leading to defecation and urination issues. In most cases, the bird's body appears to "self-amputate" the ligation site over time and sutures or hemoclips are shed out unnoticed over the next few weeks to months.

# MEDICATIONS

## DRUG(S) OF CHOICE
Application of a hypertonic sugar solution may be of assistance. If sutures are placed on the cloaca, the application of a DMSO gel or infusion of the cloaca with DMSO may help to reduce inflammation and may lead to phallus erection reduction. Antibiotics should be considered if the tissue appears necrotic or infected. If amputation is performed, consider prophylactic antibiotics because of the location (cloaca) of the surgery. Analgesia should be considered. NSAIDs and opioids may be warranted, depending on species and studies supporting analgesic effects of a particular drug and dose with that species. An underlying cause may warrant direct treatment of that disease to manage the animal holistically and also prevent recurrence.

## CONTRAINDICATIONS
If bird is considered a food animal, all applicable laws should be considered, and the use of medications severely limited.

## PRECAUTIONS
N/A

## POSSIBLE INTERACTIONS
N/A

## ALTERNATIVE DRUGS
N/A

# FOLLOW-UP

## PATIENT MONITORING
Visual reassessment of the phallus or amputation site should be performed daily to weekly until considered resolved. Experienced veterinarians may be able to manually palpate the phallus or stalk.

## PREVENTION/AVOIDANCE
Avoid breeding situations. Neutering or sterilizing birds is still extremely difficult and has high mortality risks; therefore, this should only be contemplated by an experienced surgeon or as a supplemental procedure of last resort.

## POSSIBLE COMPLICATIONS
Inability to breed, cloacal feces or urate leakage, and partial permanent mild prolapse of phallus, stalk, cloaca.

## EXPECTED COURSE AND PROGNOSIS
Medical management generally has a guarded prognosis since most cases present in an advanced state to a veterinarian. While amputation may lead to inability to sire offspring (or not), if done correctly most birds have a good prognosis, unless underlying health issues led to the problem and were uncorrectable.

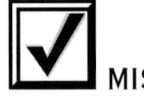

# MISCELLANEOUS

## ASSOCIATED CONDITIONS
N/A

## AGE-RELATED FACTORS
Usually only in mature males during breeding season.

## ZOONOTIC POTENTIAL
N/A

## FERTILITY/BREEDING
While some birds may still be able to successfully father offspring, phallectomy may lead to inability to naturally successfully copulate, an important consideration for valuable breeders. Ostriches seem to have been reported to have a higher risk of unsuccessful siring.

## SYNONYMS
N/A

## SEE ALSO
Cloacal Diseases
Coccidiosis
Cryptosporidiosis
Foreign Bodies (Gastrointestinal)
Helminthiasis
Infertility
Neural Larva Migrans
Trauma

## ABBREVIATIONS
DMSO—dimethyl sulfoxide
GI—gastrointestinal
NSAIDs—non-steroidal anti-inflammatory drugs
PCR—polymerase chain reaction

## INTERNET RESOURCES
N/A

*Suggested Reading*
Carnaccini, S., Ferguson-Noel, N.M., Chin, R.P., et al. (2016). A novel *Mycoplasma* sp. associated with phallus disease in goose breeders: pathological and bacteriological findings. *Avian Diseases*, 60:437–443.
Echols, S., Speer, B. (2022). Avian reproductive tract diseases and surgical resolutions. *Clinical Theriogenology*, 14: 32–43.

P

Holubová, N., Tůmová, L., Sak, B., et al. (2020). Description of *Cryptosporidium ornithophilus* n. sp. (*Apicomplexa: Cryptosporidiidae*) in farmed ostriches. *Parasites & Vectors* 13:340.

Kimura, T., Rocha, G., da Rocha Neto, H., et al. (2022). Prolapse and amputation of phallus in a greater rhea (*Rhea americana*) kept in captivity: Case report. *Research, Society and Development*, 11: e41411326015.

Silva, A. P., Cooper, G., Blakey, J., et al. (2020). Retrospective summary of *Erysipelothrix rhusiopathiae* diagnosed in avian species in California (2000–19). *Avian Diseases*, 64:499–506.
**Author**: Eric Klaphake, DVM, DACZM

P

# PNEUMONIA

 **BASICS**

## DEFINITION
Inflammation of the lung parenchyma secondary to infectious etiologies (bacterial, fungal, viral, parasitic), toxin exposure, or foreign material inhalation. Commonly associated with inflammation in the airsacs (airsacculitis).

## PATHOPHYSIOLOGY
Birds have a very specialized, efficient respiratory system with lungs that are adhered to the dorsolateral body wall. Gas exchange occurs in air capillaries, which communicate with other airways (as opposed to the blind sacs of mammalian alveoli). Birds have a system of airsacs, which have very little blood supply and minimal cilia (only in limited areas near the lungs), thus are not able to clear out items via the mucociliary apparatus. Most of them are dependent, leading to deposition of inhaled particles, which cannot exit the body, and thus create a source of inflammation as the body tries to wall them off. Pathogens may enter the respiratory tract by inhalation or hematogenous spread. Infections in the upper respiratory tract may spread into the lower tract. The avian immune system is effective in encapsulating sources of infection/inflammation over time, preventing exposure of the etiologic agents to the immune system and blood supply, making identification challenging and treatment more difficult.

## SYSTEMS AFFECTED
Respiratory.

## GENETICS
N/A

## INCIDENCE/PREVALENCE
Common in pet birds and poultry.

## GEOGRAPHIC DISTRIBUTION
Unlimited distribution.

## SIGNALMENT
All species and ages, both sexes. Hand-fed birds (especially young) are more susceptible to aspiration pneumonia. Several species of birds including arctic species, penguins, pelagic birds, waterfowl, raptors, and grey parrots, among others, may be predisposed to aspergillosis or fungal pneumonia.

## SIGNS
### General Comments
If a bird presents for respiratory distress, discuss with the owner the possible risk of acute decompensation and death from handling. Place in oxygen before and during examination and between diagnostic tests.

Birds have a very efficient respiratory system, and oxygen may not alleviate respiratory distress.

### Historical Findings
Owners may note mild to severe signs including general sick-bird signs (lethargy, depression, inappetence, weight loss, decreased activity, fluffed, sitting on the bottom of the cage), progressive exercise intolerance, voice change/loss of voice (if associated with lesions in syrinx/caudal trachea), open-beak breathing, increased respiratory effort (tail bob, exaggerated keel movement), coughing (may need to differentiate from mimicking a human coughing sound).

### Physical Examination Findings
Respiratory rate and effort should be evaluated before birds are handled. Assess for tail bob, exaggerated keel movement, open-beak breathing, extended neck. If dyspnea is noted, place patient in oxygen cage for 5–10 minutes before the examination. Take exam in stages if dyspnea worsens during handling. Carefully hold all dyspneic birds upright (especially if coelomic distention is noted). Signs of pneumonia on physical examination include increased respiratory rate and effort (tail bob); increased or rough lung sounds may be heard on auscultation of dorsal body wall; increased airsac sounds on ventral auscultation; open-beak breathing, thin body condition. Return to a prehandling respiratory rate may be prolonged in birds with pneumonia.

## CAUSES
### Infectious
**Bacterial**: May be inhaled/aspirated or spread hematogenously (sepsis); Gram-negative pathogens commonly noted although Gram-positive organisms have also been reported (*Streptococcus* spp., *Staphylococcus* spp.). Specific etiologies include *Nocardia*, *Chlamydia psittaci*, *Mycobacterium* (*Mycobacterium avium* complex, *Mycobacterium genavense*), *Mycoplasma* spp.
**Fungal**: Including *Aspergillus* spp., *Penicillium* spp., *Zygomycetes* (including *Mucor*, *Rhizopus*, *Absidia*), *Trichosporon* spp., *Candida albicans*; cryptococcal pneumonia may be associated with cryptococcal sinusitis.
**Viral**: Including polyomavirus, herpesvirus, poxvirus, paramyxovirus (including END), avian influenza.
**Parasitic**: Including *Sarcocystis* spp. (*Sarcocystis falcatula* most significant) especially in Old World Psittacines; *Sternostoma tracheolum* (airsac mites in canaries and finches); Nematodes such as

*Serratospiculum* sp., *Cyathostoma* sp., *Syngamus* sp.; Trematodes such as *Bothriogaster variolaris*, *Szidatitrema* sp.
### Non-Infectious
**Aspiration**: Especially hand-fed birds.
**Airborne toxins**: Most commonly related to exposure to pyrolysis products from overheating pans coated with PTFE; also includes exposure to aerosol sprays, paint fumes, cigarette smoke, fumes from burned food and self-cleaning ovens; most often causes acute death but birds that survive demonstrate signs of pneumonia.

## RISK FACTORS
Malnutrition. Birds on an all-seed (vitamin A deficient) diet are more prone to hypovitaminosis A, which can promote squamous metaplasia within the respiratory tract. Hand feeding. Systemic disease or immune suppression. Exposure to airborne irritants (cigarette smoke, dust, burning food, or coated pans). Poor husbandry (inadequate diet, unsanitary conditions). Stress. Use of immunosuppressive drugs such as corticosteroids.

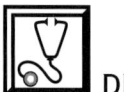 **DIAGNOSIS**

## DIFFERENTIAL DIAGNOSIS
Upper airway disease (including nasal, glottis and tracheal disease)—differentiate with imaging and physical examination. Heart failure—differentiate with physical examination (auscultation), radiographs and ultrasound. Pulmonary hypersensitivity is most common in macaws exposed to dust-producing birds; differentiate with history, radiographs, and hematocrit (the hematocrit is very high in birds with hypersensitivity). Pulmonary neoplasia—differentiate with CT, biopsy and CBC. Trauma—differentiate with history and CT. Any source of coelomic distention which compresses airsacs (fluid accumulation from coelomitis, heart or liver failure; organomegaly; neoplasia, etc.)—differentiate with physical examination, radiographs, ultrasound, CT.

## CBC/BIOCHEMISTRY/URINALYSIS
CBC: A leukocytosis may be present (if the lesions are localized to the airsacs or are well walled off in the lung parenchyma, there may be little to no elevation in the WBC count). The leukogram may vary depending on the etiologic agent. Bacterial infections are more likely to cause heterophilia with or without a left shift. Fungal, chlamydial, or mycobacterial infections may produce a monocytosis, which may only be a relative

P

monocytosis with an otherwise normal WBC count. If gas exchange is impaired for a long enough time (or in cases of pulmonary hypersensitivity), polycythemia may occur. Conversely, anemia may be present related to chronic disease. Chemistry panel: Creatine kinase may be elevated if the infection is adjacent to or invading the muscle surrounding the lungs, but otherwise the chemistry panel helps identify other concurrent disease processes which may affect the treatment plan.

### OTHER LABORATORY TESTS
Protein electrophoresis may help to confirm the presence of inflammation in the absence of a leukocytosis. Molecular diagnostics and serology may be available for specific etiologic agents. Bacterial and fungal culture and sensitivity are very important; submit tracheal wash samples or tissue from lung and airsac biopsies. NGS can also be performed on the same samples submitted for culture, and can identify and quantify the most prevalent bacterial and fungal organisms. Cytology should be performed if a tracheal wash sample is obtained. Histopathology should be performed on any biopsies taken. Fecal examination (centrifugal flotation ± sedimentation) if parasites are suspected.

### IMAGING
Whole-body radiographs are important to identify abnormalities in the lung fields and airsacs. On the lateral view, patchiness to the normal "honeycomb" appearance may suggest pulmonary infiltrates or granulomas; thickening of the airsac membranes ("airsac lines") and opacities within the airsacs may be recognized. On the ventrodorsal view, asymmetry to the lung fields and lateral airsacs may be noted. The pectoral muscles overlap the lung tissue, making interpretation of lungs on the ventrodorsal view challenging. CT with iodinated contrast is very useful to identify lesions in the lungs and airsacs and to differentiate primary respiratory disease from other coelomic disease.

### DIAGNOSTIC PROCEDURES
Transtracheal wash is a technique that allows sampling without surgery. Use 0.5 to 1.0 ml/kg saline in an anesthetized patient; submit sample for cytology as well as aerobic and fungal cultures and NGS. Celioscopy is a minimally invasive technique to visualize the airsacs and caudoventral border of the lungs. The aisacs should be completely clear and the lungs should be bright pink without any exudate or hemorrhage. Biopsies should be obtained of any lesions and lung tissue and submitted for histopathology and aerobic and fungal culture and NGS. Tissue should be saved in the freezer for possible molecular diagnostics as directed by the histopathologic findings.

### PATHOLOGIC FINDINGS
The lungs may appear hemorrhagic or have white or yellow patches on the surface when visualized. Airsacs may have increased vascularity or may contain white to yellow caseous plaques (fungal plaques may appear fluffy). Parasites may be grossly visible. Histology will demonstrate inflammation characteristic of the etiologic agent. Polyomavirus—mononuclear infiltration. Herpesvirus—edema and congestion; presence of large syncytia within bronchi and parabronchi, with large amphophilic-to-eosinophilic intranuclear inclusion bodies. Inflammation primarily within the parabronchi composed of foamy macrophages, pale basophilic mucus, homogeneously eosinophilic edema fluid, fibrin, cellular debris, and sloughed necrotic epithelial cells. Poxvirus—epithelial hyperplasia of the airways. Inhaled bacteria—intraluminal hemorrhage, a small amount of suppurative inflammation and fibrin deposition. Hematogenous bacteria—more severe effacement of parenchyma with hemorrhage, congestion, fibrinopurulent exudate, and intralesional bacteria. Nocardiosis and mycobacteriosis—parenchymal granulomatous lesions. Mycoplasma pneumonia—lymphocytic infiltrates which may develop into lymphoid nodules. Fungal infections—granulomatous lesions in the lungs and airsacs. Sarcocystis—severe pulmonary congestion, edema, or hemorrhage. Airsac mites—when present in the parabronchi cause infiltration of lymphocytes, plasma cells, and macrophages. Nematodes and trematodes—granulomatous lesions, consolidation, necrosis. Toxin exposure—edema and hemorrhage within the gas exchange tissues. Foreign body inhalation—initially characterized by hemorrhage, congestion, edema and fibrin deposition; chronic lesions are characterized by accumulations of lymphocytes, macrophages, and multinucleated giant cells. Lipid pneumonia—multifocal alveolar histiocytosis characterized by accumulation of foamy macrophages and interstitial infiltration of a small numbers of lymphocytes and heterophils, multifocal anthracosis, and intense congestion.

### TREATMENT

### APPROPRIATE HEALTH CARE
Inpatient care is required for birds that require oxygen or supportive care (fluids, feeding). Outpatient care is feasible for birds that are stable off of oxygen and are eating and maintaining hydration.

### NURSING CARE
Fluid therapy as needed based on deficits (SQ or IV/IO) to maintain hydration. Oxygen may be required (measure respiratory rate on and off of oxygen to determine if it is helping).

### ACTIVITY
Keep quiet and warm, minimize activity. Birds with respiratory compromise may not tolerate exercise well.

### DIET
Offer patient's normal diet. Gavage may be needed if decreased appetite noted.

### CLIENT EDUCATION
Respiratory disease carries a guarded prognosis and may require very long-term and aggressive therapy (granulomas are hard to penetrate with medications and some may need to be surgically debrided). Aggressive care as quickly as possible will increase the chances of recovery.

### SURGICAL CONSIDERATIONS
Birds with pneumonia will likely require ventilatory support during anesthesia. They may not respond as well to gas anesthetics if too much functional tissue is affected. Be prepared to place an airsac cannula if there is suspicion that the trachea or syrinx is involved. However, if there is severe lung parenchymal disease (affecting air exchange tissues), the airsac cannula may not help.

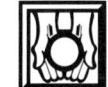

### MEDICATIONS
### DRUG(S) OF CHOICE
Base on culture/sensitivity or NGS, when possible. If testing is possible, use a broad-spectrum combination of antibiotics. Doses are for psittacines, unless otherwise noted. Treatment should persist for at least 1 month, and repeat radiographs, CBC, ± CT or endoscopy should be used to determine if treatment may be discontinued.

#### Antibiotics
Very debilitated or septic birds may require injectable antibiotics for a few days then switched to oral versions. Ceftazidime 50–100 mg/kg IM or IV q4–8h. Piperacillin/tazobactam 100 mg/kg IM or IV q6–12h. Ticarcillin/clavulanic acid 200 mg/kg IM q12h. Long-acting doxycycline injection (drug of choice for *Mycoplasma* and *Chlamydia*) 75–100 mg/kg IM q5–7d for 4–6 weeks. Enrofloxacin—wide dose range; historically 5–15 mg/kg b.i.d. was recommended and may still be efficacious; currently 15–30 mg/kg q24h accepted for SQ, IM, PO (IM dose should be used only

P

once to minimize muscle trauma, dilute SQ dose in fluids to minimize tissue trauma), no anaerobic coverage, not approved in food producing birds. Amoxicillin/clavulanic acid 125 mg/kg PO b.i.d. Trimethoprim/ sulfamethoxazole 30–100 mg/kg PO q12–24h. Doxycycline (drug of choice for *Mycoplasma* and *Chlamydia*) 25–50 mg/kg PO q12–24h. Marbofloxacin 2.5–5 mg/kg PO q24h (effective against *Mycoplasma* and *Chlamydia*). Azithromycin (used for primarily intracellular infections, like *Chlamydia psittaci*, 10–20 mg/mg PO q48h for at least 5 treatments for non-intracellular infections (macaws); 40 mg/kg PO q24h for 30 days for intracellular infections (macaws); 40 mg/kg PO q48h for 21 days for intracellular infections (cockatiels).

### Nebulized Medications
Accepted as beneficial. Twice daily treatment is recommended for at least 15-minute sessions. Create a nebulization chamber out of a large plastic storage container or a carrier wrapped in a clear plastic garbage bag. For treatment of the lung and airsacs, the nebulized particles should be < 3–5 μm in diameter (this information is available in nebulizer package inserts). Saline (0.9%) and sterile water may reduce viscosity of secretions on without any additives. Enrofloxan 10 mg/ml saline. Amikacin 5–6 mg/ml saline. Piperacillin 10 mg/ml saline. Terbutaline 0.01 mg/kg with 9 ml saline— bronchodilation. N-acetyl-L-cysteine 22 mg/ml in sterile water—mucolytic agent; tracheal irritation/reflex bronchoconstriction noted in mammals, use preceded by bronchodilators in mammals.

### Other Medication
Ivermectin is the drug of choice for tracheal mites; 0.2 mg/kg topically over the right jugular once every 2 weeks for 3 doses.

## CONTRAINDICATIONS
N/A

## PRECAUTIONS
Some birds may not tolerate medications as well as others and adverse reactions are possible despite all precautions. In general, hypovolemia and dehydration should be corrected before starting most therapeutic agents. Trimethoprim/sulfa and enrofloxacin may cause vomiting. Doxycycline may cause regurgitation and should be used at a lower dose range in macaws and cockatoos. Alterations in liver or kidney function might affect medication choices (i.e. imidazoles should be used with caution in patients with altered liver function, azithromycin should not be used in birds with liver or renal disease,

doxycycline should be used with caution in birds with liver disease). Sulfa antibiotics should not be used in birds with dehydration, liver disease or bone marrow suppression. Nebulized amikacin is unlikely to cause renal dysfunction, but should be used with caution in patients with existing renal disease.

## POSSIBLE INTERACTIONS
Do not use amoxicillin/clavulanic acid with allopurinol. Foods containing calcium, aluminum, magnesium, or iron may interfere with absorption of oral doxycycline and enrofloxacin.

## ALTERNATIVE DRUGS
Omega 3 fatty acid supplementation may help as an adjunct treatment (for its anti-inflammatory effects), but does not replace the need for antimicrobials if indicated.

 **FOLLOW-UP**

## PATIENT MONITORING
CBC should be performed regularly (weekly to start with, then monthly to every 6 months for fungal or other granulomatous disease). Radiographs or CT should be performed at least before cessation of treatment to confirm absence of disease. Long-term infections should be monitored with radiographs or CT every 3–6 months. Follow up endoscopy to visualize previously diseased lungs and airsac spaces may be necessary to determine whether imaging changes are related to active disease or scar tissue.

## PREVENTION/AVOIDANCE
Ensure good ventilation, clean housing, regular exposure to direct sunlight, nutritionally balanced diet.

## POSSIBLE COMPLICATIONS
Permanent damage may lead to residual exercise intolerance or potentially lack of response to treatment. Initial improvement then recrudescence if treatment discontinued too early.

## EXPECTED COURSE AND PROGNOSIS
Prognosis is variable depending on etiology. Simple bacterial infections may clear up in weeks, but fungal and other granulomatous infections may take months (to years) of treatment.

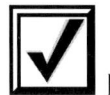 **MISCELLANEOUS**

## ASSOCIATED CONDITIONS
Upper airway disease.

## AGE-RELATED FACTORS
Young birds with aspiration pneumonia are more likely to develop infections of multiple etiologies due to immune suppression. Older birds, especially after being fed a lifetime of seeds or being exposed to long-term second-hand smoke, may be more at risk due to immune suppression.

## ZOONOTIC POTENTIAL
*Chlamydia psittaci* is zoonotic. Mycobacterial infections are potentially zoonotic and careful consideration should be taken when determining if treatment is warranted. *Paramyxovirus* that causes END may cause mild disease in humans. Avian influenza is also potentially zoonotic.

## FERTILITY/BREEDING
Note regulations for use of therapeutics in poultry. No antibiotics are approved for laying hens but withdrawal times can be determined. Fluoriquinolones, nitroimidazoles, glycopeptides, and cephalosporins are all prohibited for use in food animals. Access the Food Animal Residue Avoidance Databank for egg withdrawal times for non prohibited drugs (http://www.farad.org).

## SYNONYMS
Lower respiratory tract disease.

## SEE ALSO
Aspergillosis
Aspiration Pneumonia
Avian Influenza
Coelomic Distension
Herpesvirus (Columbid Herpesvirus 1 in Pigeons and Raptors)
Herpesvirus (Duck Viral Enteritis)
Herpesvirus (Passerine Birds)
Herpesvirus (Psittacid Herpesviruses)
Mycobacteriosis
Orthoavulaviruses
Polyomavirus
Poxvirus
Respiratory Distress
Toxicosis (Airborne)
Tracheal and Syringeal Disease

## ABBREVIATIONS
CBC—complete blood count
CT—computed tomography
END—exotic Newcastle disease
NGS—next-generation sequencing
PTFE— polytetrafluoroethylene
WBC—white blood cell

## INTERNET RESOURCES
Food Animal Residue Avoidance Databank: http://www.farad.org

### Suggested Reading
Balsamo, G., Maxted, A.M., Midla, J.W. (2017). Compendium of measures to control *Chlamydia psittaci* infection among humans (psittacosis) and pet birds (avian

chlamydiosis), 2017. *Journal of Avian Medicine and Surgery*, 31:262–282.

Crosta L. (2021). Respiratory diseases of parrots: anatomy, physiology, diagnosis and treatment. *Veterinary Clinics of North America: Exotic Animal Practice*, 24:397–418.

Hillyer, E.V., Orosz, S., Dorrestein, G.M. (1997). Respiratory system. In: *Avian Medicine and Surgery* (ed. R.B. Altman, S.L.

Clubb, G.M. Dorrestein, K. Quesenberry), 387–411. Sy. Louis, MO: Saunders.

Sanchez-Migallon Guzman, D., Beaufrère, H., Welle, K.R., et al. (2023). Birds. In: *Carpenter's Exotic Animal Formulary* (ed. J.W. Carpenter, C.A. Harms), 6th edn., 222–443. St. Louis, MO: Elsevier.

Schmidt, R.E., Reavill, D.R., Phalen, D.N. (2015). *Pathology of Pet and Aviary Birds*, 2nd edn. Ames, IA: Wiley.

Tully, T.N., Harrison G.J. (1994). Pneumonology, In: *Avian Medicine: Principles and Application* (ed. B.W. Ritchie, G.J. Harrison, L.R. Harrison), 556–581. Lake Worth, FL: Wingers Publishing.

**Author**: Anneliese Strunk, DVM, DABVP (Avian Practice)

P

# PODODERMATITIS

 **BASICS**

## DEFINITION
Avian pododermatitis, also known as bumblefoot, is a catch-all term for inflammatory, infectious, and/or degenerative conditions of the avian foot. The condition can range from smoothing of the epidermis, mild swelling and redness of the plantar surfaces of the feet and toes, to ulceration and/or hyperkeratosis and potentially cellulitis and osteomyelitis. Strictly speaking, pododermatitis is inflammation of the dermal structures of the feet; however, this term is often used interchangeably with bumblefoot in avian species. Etiology may vary according to species and specific environmental conditions, diet, and management systems.

## PATHOPHYSIOLOGY
Regardless of the inciting cause, ischemic conditions and/or vascular congestion are often important features in the development of bumblefoot. Standing for abnormally long periods of time and lack of adequate exercise can contribute to vascular congestion and pressure injury to tissues. Poor hygiene and inappropriate substrates and perching can cause bumblefoot via excessive wear/pressure or maceration of the plantar tissues of the feet, with resultant disruption of the epidermis. Extension of infectious disease to deeper tissues resulting in cellulitis, tenosynovitis, and osteomyelitis may follow. Malnutrition can also cause or exacerbate bumblefoot. Hypovitaminosis A with squamous metaplasia of the plantar epithelium can predispose birds to plantar erosions and damage to deeper tissues. Biotin deficiency has also been cited as a predisposing factor in poultry.

## SYSTEMS AFFECTED
Typically, bumblefoot begins as a disorder of the skin, but the disease can progress to affect all of the anatomic structures of the feet.

## GENETICS
No genetic predisposition is appreciated.

## INCIDENCE/PREVALENCE
Bumblefoot is primarily a disease of birds in managed care and is almost always related to deficiencies in husbandry. Incidence and prevalence are therefore variable and dependent on specific husbandry conditions.

## GEOGRAPHIC DISTRIBUTION
N/A

## SIGNALMENT
**Species**: Heavy-bodied species and species that in a natural state spend most the time flying or swimming, such as birds of prey (*Accipitridae*), parrots (*Psittacidae*), penguins (*spheniscidae*), storks (*Ciconiidae*), cranes (*Gruidae*), flamingos (*Phoenicopteridae*), waterfowl and shorebirds (*Anseriformes*), are predisposed to pododermatitis, although all species can be affected.
**Mean age and range**: All ages are susceptible.
**Predominant sex**: Both sexes are susceptible, although the larger sex of some dimorphic species are more frequently affected due to relatively increased body weight.

## SIGNS
### General Comments
Bumblefoot can assume a variety of presentations depending on the inciting cause and chronicity. A number of classification systems are described in various publications. In one simple classification scheme, three grades are described. With grade I bumblefoot, lesions are mild, localized, and characterized as either degenerative or proliferative. In degenerative conditions, the normally pebbled skin on the plantar surface of the feet becomes smooth and thin. In proliferative conditions, hyperkeratosis occurs resulting in "corns" and cracking on the plantar surfaces. With grade II bumblefoot, bacterial or fungal infections begin to play a role in the disease process. *Staphyloccocus aureus*, *Enterococcus faecalis*, *Escherichia coli*, *Pseudemonas* spp., and occasionally yeast or fungi, are often encountered. There is typically a noticeable inflammatory component to type II pododermatitis. In grade III bumblefoot, the changes are typically chronic, infected, and involve deeper soft and bony tissues of the feet. In some chronic cases, a static condition can develop in which a heavy eschar develops over an ulcer on the plantar aspect of the foot. In these cases, over time, excessive fibrous connective tissue can develop under the eschar, which may eventually cause significant discomfort and lameness.

### Historical Findings
Typically, predisposing factors can be identified in the history or physical examination. Often, there is history of an injury to the pelvic limbs resulting in direct injury to the feet and/or resulting in uneven weight bearing. Persistently wet or unhygienic substrate conditions or inappropriate perching (inappropriate size, shape, and surface) can result in acute bumblefoot. Management circumstances in which birds are standing for long periods of time and not exercising adequately can predispose to development of bumblefoot. Birds that are overweight or malnourished (hypovitaminosis A) are at increased risk. Birds that have been previously affected by bumblefoot are predisposed to recrudescence of disease.

### Physical Examination Findings
Bumblefoot can affect one or both pelvic limbs, resulting in varying degrees of lameness. With mild cases, clinical signs can be as seemingly insignificant as minor smoothing of the keratinized skin on the plantar surfaces of the toes and feet. Advanced cases may present with swelling of the toes and feet, ulcerations with eschar formation on the plantar surfaces. Joint effusion and abscessation of the soft tissues and joints may also be encountered.

## CAUSES
Causes of bumblefoot include both acute and chronic trauma, and poor hygiene. Lacerations, puncture wounds, and abrasions can become secondarily infected leading to bumblefoot. Abnormal wear on weight-bearing surfaces as may occur with sedentary birds with lack of opportunity or motivation for exercise, or those suffering from degenerative joint disease, and obesity, can also lead to bumblefoot. Malnutrition due to hypovitaminosis A or lack of appropriate biotin can increase risk for bumblefoot.

## RISK FACTORS
The risk factors for bumblefoot are conditions that result in abnormal trauma to the structures of the feet, or change the skin and other tissue's ability to withstand normal wear. Risk factors include, but are not limited to, obesity, inactivity, inappropriate substrate and/or perches, poor hygiene and/or chronically wet substrate. Traumatic injuries to the feet and limbs can create portals for ingress of infective organisms, resulting in bumblefoot. Degenerative conditions of the pelvic limbs can also lead to bumblefoot, as abnormal forces are applied to the structures of the feet. When injuries or degenerative conditions affect a pelvic limb, it is not uncommon for bumblefoot to develop in the contralateral foot.

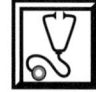 **DIAGNOSIS**

The diagnosis of bumblefoot is relatively straightforward; however, diagnostics beyond a physical examination are often required to characterize the diagnosis and direct therapy.

## DIFFERENTIAL DIAGNOSIS
Neoplasia, articular gout, poxvirus, or papillomavirus infections and acariasis affecting the structures of the feet can sometimes mimic bumblefoot.

## CBC/BIOCHEMISTRY/URINALYSIS
CBC, protein electrophoresis and acute phase protein measurement, such as amyloid A, often show signs of inflammation.

Changes in the differential may reflect the duration of the disease process. A chemistry panel is indicated to evaluate organ function; systemic amyloidosis may be encountered as a sequela to chronic cases of bumblefoot.

## OTHER LABORATORY TESTS

Fine-needle aspiration and impression smears of affected tissue for cytology, as well as culture/sensitivity and molecular diagnostics are often useful in diagnosis and direction of therapy. If joints are noted to be distended, arthrocentesis may be indicated. Biopsies and histopathology of affected tissue can provide extremely important information, especially in cases that are proliferative and/or do not respond to therapy as expected.

## IMAGING

High-detail radiographs of the feet are indicated to rule out osteomyelitis of the bony structures of the feet. Fistulograms using iodinated contrast material can also be useful. Angiography using iodinated contrast materials suitable for IV administration may be a worthwhile diagnostic to characterize the blood supply to the feet. Ultrasonography with a high-frequency transducer is an effective imaging modality in larger species, and can be especially helpful in identifying pockets of fluid and evaluating the vasculature structures of the feet. Stand-off pads can facilitate effective imaging of structures just under the skin. CT with systemic or regional administration of iodinated contrast material may also provide useful information. Thermography has been described as useful in detecting subclinical bumblefoot in poultry. This modality may be useful in evaluation of cases of lameness with no external lesions or in the monitoring of cases under treatment.

## DIAGNOSTIC PROCEDURES
N/A

## PATHOLOGIC FINDINGS

Dermatitis, cellulitis, tenosynovitis, and osteomyelitis are common findings in bumblefoot cases. Vasculitis with thrombosis and loss of blood supply to affected tissue are also frequently encountered. Lack of adequate vascular supply is a very important finding, as it will dramatically affect the bird's ability to recover and resolve bumblefoot lesions.

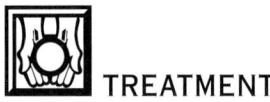

## TREATMENT

### APPROPRIATE HEALTH CARE

Patients that are self-sustaining and ambulatory are typically treated as outpatients, but brief hospitalization may be appropriate for initiation of analgesic therapy and collection of baseline diagnostic data (including screening radiographs). Debilitated patients may need extended periods of hospitalization for supportive care until stable. Correction of husbandry deficiencies and other predisposing factors is critical to addressing bumblefoot in avian patients. In very mild cases, correction of these predisposing factors may be adequate for complete resolution of the lesions. In mild cases in which the plantar skin is intact, protective bandaging and NSAIDs may be sufficient to reverse the process and allow the skin to heal and resume its normal conformation. In more severe cases where ulceration, abscessation, and necrotic tissue are present, surgical debridement is necessary. Debridement needs to be precise and delicate to preserve vital structures if possible. Bandaging is an important aspect of treating bumblefoot in avian patients. Wet-to-dry bandages can be an effective debridement technique, especially in early management of severely infected and necrotic lesions. Many different bandaging schemes are described, but all share the common goal of relieving pressure on the lesion and encourage circulation of blood to the plantar structures. Donut-shaped pads can be fashioned out of various pliable materials and incorporated into the bandage. Custom shoes configured using silicone or other similar materials may also be considered. Great care needs to be taken to avoid creating restriction of circulation and/or excessive pressure at the contact points of any pad or shoe incorporated into the bandage. Wrapping the toes with soft-cast padding or other similar materials at the contact points can help avoid the development of iatrogenic lesions. The use of VAC devices is often discussed as a possible option in treating severe bumblefoot lesions in birds, but implementation of this modality is challenging. In terrestrial birds that are not inclined to chew vacuum lines, VAC therapy can be considered as a possible option for treatment in the early stages of treatment. The benefit of VAC therapy should be considered in light of the limitations it will have on activity. Adjunctive therapy of bumblefoot with photobiomodulation may be beneficial and at least help speed healing. Multiple doses of 3–4 J/cm$^2$ over the course of a number of weeks may be required to see a positive effect.

### NURSING CARE

Management of substrate, perching, and bandage is critical in the treatment of bumblefoot. If bandage or shoe application is indicated, meticulous maintenance is necessary. Quarters for convalescing birds should be managed such that the bandages stay clean and dry until scheduled changes. If a bandage is noted to appear soiled or wet, it should be changed immediately. It is recommended that bandages should be changed every 24–72 hours, depending on lesion severity. The need for sedation or anesthesia and/or analgesia for bandage changes can be decided on a case by case basis. If the bird vigorously resists bandaging and appears overly stressed by the bandage change procedure, anesthesia is warranted.

### ACTIVITY

In most cases, activity and exercise should be encouraged and maximized. Birds with bumblefoot should be kept in lean body condition to avoid excessive pressure on the structures of the feet. Exercise will also encourage circulation of blood and lymph in the feet. Flighted birds should be given as much opportunity to fly as possible.

### DIET

Birds suffering from bumblefoot should have their vitamin A status and body condition critically evaluated with adjustments made as necessary. Vitamin A supplementation should be pursued carefully as oversupplementation can easily occur. In most cases, oral supplementation is preferred over parenteral delivery. Often, providing a balanced diet is sufficient and specific vitamin A administration is not necessary. Supplementation with biotin can also be considered. Body condition should be kept as lean as possible to minimize pressure on the bird's feet. Providing a healthy diet in appropriate proportions combined with adequate exercise will help to keep birds as lean as possible in captive situations.

### CLIENT EDUCATION

Bumblefoot is typically a disorder of animals in managed care and is directly related to deficiencies in husbandry and diet. Most cases of bumblefoot can be avoided with proper education of caretakers and implementation of a minimum standard of husbandry. Caretakers working with high-risk species, such as waterfowl and falcons, should be aware of the risk factors for development of bumblefoot and should monitor their charges closely. Some species can develop severe bumblefoot within days of the introduction of inappropriate perching and substrate. Thus, caretakers must be properly educated regarding appropriate perching and substrate management for the species they work with.

### SURGICAL CONSIDERATIONS

Surgical intervention is often indicated in cases of bumblefoot. Surgical procedures should be carefully planned as clumsy and over-aggressive debridement can result in damage to vital structures of the feet and can

P

affect the long-term outcome of the case. Magnification can be helpful. Necrotic tissue should be carefully removed with efforts to identify and preserve tendons, ligaments, joint capsules, vasculature, and nerves, if possible. Resultant surgical defects can be closed primarily or allowed to heal via second intention depending on the level of residual contamination/necrotic tissue present. In cases where joints or tendon sheaths are affected or abscessed, indwelling catheters can be placed to allow repetitive local therapy via flushing or delivery of medications. Pedicle advancement flap skin grafts or other grafting techniques may be used to close defects on the plantar surfaces of the feet. These procedures can be considered in chronic cases with persistent open plantar lesions. Following the application of advancement flaps, careful bandaging and antisepsis is necessary.

 MEDICATIONS

## DRUG(S) OF CHOICE
There are no medications that are uniformly indicated in cases of bumblefoot; selection of medication(s) should be based on the specifics of individual cases. Oral and parenteral NSAIDs are frequently indicated in cases of bumblefoot. Meloxicam, ketoprofen, and carprofen are commonly used in avian patients and are typically well tolerated and seemingly effective in avian patients. In cases likely to be experiencing moderate to severe discomfort, opiate medications such as tramadol, butorphanol, and nalbuphine can be considered, as well as strategic application of local anesthetics. Antimicrobial therapy is indicated when open lesions are present or there is obvious evidence of infection. Drug choice should ideally be based on culture results, although *Staph. aureus*, *Ent. faecalis* and *E. coli* are commonly encountered isolates. In addition to systemic antibiotics, regional perfusion of the affected limb(s) can be considered to promote generation of high concentrations of drug in the target tissues which decreasing potential risk for adverse systemic effects. Use of vascular access ports has been described in avian patients and can be considered for long-term parenteral antibiotic therapy. Since in many cases of bumblefoot, blood flow to the lesion(s) is impaired, efforts to promote perfusion are indicated. Pentoxifylline at a dose of 15 mg/kg PO q8–12h for 6–8 weeks has been used with seemingly positive effect.

### Topical Medications
Various topical medications are used in the treatment of bumblefoot. Antimicrobial creams or ointments are used when open lesions are present. Silver sulfadiazine cream is very frequently used when open lesions are present. Pluronic gel compounded to contain an appropriate antibiotic can be effective in local treatment of infectious processes. Mixtures containing dimethyl sulfoxide, various corticosteroids, NSAIDs, and antibiotics are described for use in treatment of bumblefoot and labeled with names such as "Bumble-Be-Gone." These mixtures should be used with caution, especially when containing corticosteroids, as birds tend to be quite sensitive to the adverse effects of corticosteroids. Topical application of materials such as granulated sugar, raw or medical honey, and papaya can be safe and effective as part of the therapeutic approach for open bumblefoot lesions. These materials can be incorporated into wet-to-dry bandages and aid dramatically with antisepsis, debridement, and encouragement of granulation tissue formation. There are many topical products available that may have some application in the treatment of avian bumblefoot. Various topical antimicrobial products, as well as collagen-containing products, platelet-derived growth factor, and platelet-rich plasma may all have applications, depending on the specific features of the case.

## CONTRAINDICATIONS
NSAIDs should be used with caution in birds with existing or suspected renal disease. If topical medications containing corticosteroids are used, care should be taken to monitor for signs of adverse effects. Even topical corticosteroid administration can result in systemic effects, including immunosuppression.

## PRECAUTIONS
N/A

## POSSIBLE INTERACTIONS
N/A

## ALTERNATIVE DRUGS
N/A

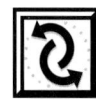 FOLLOW-UP

## PATIENT MONITORING
Therapy for bumblefoot is often necessarily protracted, requiring weeks to months depending on the severity of disease. Birds that have previously been affected by bumblefoot are predisposed to recurrence of disease in the future, even after many months to years. Cases that appear to be going well will often abruptly worsen, so close monitoring by caretakers and frequent rechecks are recommended. The follow-up schedule will, of course, depend on the individual case, but in severe cases rechecks every 1–2 weeks may be warranted until the lesions appear to be improving. Following apparent resolution of lesions, the bird should be rechecked at monthly intervals for 2–3 months and then every 6 months until the bird is determined to be stable. Serial CBCs, chemistry panels, and cultures of open lesions are often indicated to provide optimal care for birds suffering from bumblefoot. Serial imaging via radiography, CT, ultrasonography, and thermography can also be useful, especially in cases that are not responding as expected to therapy.

## PREVENTION/AVOIDANCE
Optimal nutrition, maintenance of healthy body condition, and adequate exercise are all central to prevention of bumblefoot in captive birds. Appropriate substrate and perching, including hygiene, are also important in prevention of bumblefoot. Immediate and aggressive therapy of traumatic lesions to the feet or toes is also important.

## POSSIBLE COMPLICATIONS
In cases of unilateral bumblefoot, it is not uncommon to see lesions develop in the contralateral foot due to uneven weight bearing. Chronic bumblefoot can also lead to degenerative conditions of the joints of the pelvic limbs. Systemic amyloidosis may be encountered in birds with long-standing bumblefoot lesions. The liver, spleen, kidneys, and heart are commonly affected by amyloidosis in these cases. Biopsies of affected tissues are necessary to diagnose the condition. Birds with chronically infected bumblefoot lesions are also at risk for sepsis and bacterial seeding of visceral organs. As a result, hepatic abscessation and development of endocarditis is occasionally encountered. Localized and systemic tetanus has rarely been reported in birds with lesions infected with *Clostridium tetani*.

## EXPECTED COURSE AND PROGNOSIS
Mild cases of bumblefoot hold a good to fair prognosis based on causative factors and can be expected to make fast and complete recoveries with appropriate therapy and husbandry modification. More severe or chronic cases carry a guarded prognosis. Treatment of severe cases can take many months and recrudescence of disease following apparently successful therapy is common. In very severe cases in which septic arthritis, tenosynovitis and/or osteomyelitis is present, the prognosis is poor for complete recovery and euthanasia may even be considered.

P

(CONTINUED)

 **MISCELLANEOUS**

**ASSOCIATED CONDITIONS**
Amyloidosis, sepsis, endocarditis, osteomyelitis, infectious arthritis, degenerative joint disease.

**AGE-RELATED FACTORS**
Older, chronically affected birds are likely to be affected by associated conditions as listed above.

**ZOONOTIC POTENTIAL**
N/A

**FERTILITY/BREEDING**
N/A

**SYNONYMS**
Bumblefoot.

**SEE ALSO**
Angular Limb Deformity
Arthritis
Cere and Skin Color Changes
Dermatitis
Ectoparasites (Mites)
Ectoparasites (Ticks, Lice, Dipterans)
Fractures
Lameness
Luxations
Nutritional Imbalances
Obesity
Papillomatosis (Cutaneous)
Perosis
Poxvirus
Toe and Nail Diseases
Trauma

**ABBREVIATIONS**
CBC—complete blood count
CT—computed tomography
NSAIDs—non-steroidal anti-inflammatory drugs
VAC—vacuum-assisted closure

**INTERNET RESOURCES**
Ash, L. (2020). The modern apprentice: Falconry, ecology, eduction—Perches: http://www.themodernapprentice.com/perches.htm

*Suggested Reading*
Barboza, T., Beaufrère, H., Moens, N. (2020). Effects of perching surfaces and foot bandaging on central metatarsal foot pad weight loading of the peregrine Falcon (*Falco peregrinus*). *Journal of Avian Medicine and Surgery*, 34:9–16.
Blair, J. (2013). Bumblefoot: A comparison of clinical presentation and treatment of pododermatitis in rabbits, rodents, and birds. *Veterinary Clinics of North America: Exotic Animal Practice*, 16:715–735.
Doneley, R.J.T., Smith, B.A., Gibson, J.S. (2015). Use of a vascular access port for antibiotic administration in the treatment of pododermatitis in a chicken. *Journal of Avian Medicine and Surgery*, 29: 130–135.

Erlacher-Reid, C., Dunn, J.L., Camp, T., et al. (2012). Evaluation of potential variables contributing to the development and duration of plantar lesions in a population of aquarium-maintained African penguins (*Spheniscus demersus*). *Zoo Biology*, 31:291–305.
Harcourt-Brown, N.H. (1996). Foot and leg problems. In: *BSAVA Manual of Raptors, Pigeons and Waterfowl* (ed. P.H. Benyon, N.A. Forbes, N.H. Harcourt-Brown), 163–167. Ames, IA: Iowa State University Press.
Knafo, S.E., Graham, J.E., Barton, B.A. (2019). Intravenous and intraosseous regional limb perfusion of ceftiofur sodium in an avian model. *American Journal of Veterinary Research*, 80:539–546.
Remple, J.D. (2006). A multi-faceted approach to the treatment of bumblefoot in raptors. *Journal of Exotic Pet Medicine*, 15: 49–55.
Sanders, S., Whittington J., Bennett P., et al. (2013). Advancement flap as a novel treatment for pododermatitis lesion in a red-tailed hawk (*Buteo jamaicensis*). *Journal of Avian Medicine and Surgery*, 27: 294–300.
**Author**: Ryan de Voe, DVM, DACZM

 **Client Education Handout available online**

P

# POLYDIPSIA

 **BASICS**

## DEFINITION
Abnormal or excessive water consumption (thirst), typically greater than 100 ml/kg/day. Many birds, such as carnivores and frugivores, obtain their water intake requirements through their diet, and some small xerophilic species can survive on metabolic water produced from a dry diet in the absence of water intake. However, the water consumption rate of most species follows a regular relation with body mass. Birds weighing 100 g or more drink approximately 5% of their body mass per day, but as the body mass decreases, water consumption rates rise, up to about 50% for birds weighing 10–20 g. Birds with salt glands drinking salt water may drink substantially more than those without salt glands.

## PATHOPHYSIOLOGY
Water consumption is controlled by interactions between the kidneys, pituitary gland, and hypothalamus. Polydipsia (PD) usually occurs as a compensatory response to polyuria (PU) to maintain hydration. Occasionally PD may be the primary process and PU is the compensatory response. In that case, the patient's plasma becomes relatively hypotonic because of excessive water intake, and ADH secretion is reduced, resulting in PU.

## SYSTEMS AFFECTED
**Cardiovascular:** Alterations in circulating fluid volume.
**Endocrine/metabolic:** The hypothalamus and pituitary gland play a role in compensation to PD.
**Renal/urologic:** Kidneys.

## GENETICS
Strains of Japanese quail and leghorn chickens with hereditary diabetes insipidus have been described.

## INCIDENCE/PREVALENCE
N/A

## GEOGRAPHIC DISTRIBUTION
N/A

## SIGNALMENT
Congenital causes of PD may be seen in younger animals. Most of the conditions that cause PD are more common in middle-aged to older birds. Psychogenic PD is often associated with juvenile hand-reared cockatoos.

## SIGNS
Excessive water consumption.

## CAUSES
### Primary Polydipsia
Behavioral problems, pyrexia, pain, hypotension, and any disease process that directly affects the anterior hypothalamic thirst center (psychogenic polydipsia). It has also been reported secondary to lithium administration. Mild hepatoencephalopathy and altered function of portal osmoreceptors can cause PD in mammals and may have a similar effect in birds. Hepatoencephalopathy, due to increased ammonia, has not been proven to occur in birds at this time. NSHP due to calcium use exceeding dietary intake and subsequent stimulation of the parathyroid gland, may have an effect on the thirst center in the brain, resulting in PD.

### Secondary Polydipsia
Can occur with any disease process that also causes polyuria.
**Renal disease:** Nephrogenic diabetes insipidus. Inflammatory—glomerulonephritis (chlamydia, polyoma virus, paramyxovirus, poxvirus, reovirus, adenovirus, herpesvirus, aspergillosis), hypercalcemic nephropathy, renal gout, bacterial pyelonephritis, yolk coelomitis. Degenerative—hypovitaminosis A, obstructive uropathy (urolith, cloacolith, neoplasia, egg binding), polycystic kidney disease, amyloidosis, mineralization, nephrosis. Toxic—heavy metals (lead, zinc, mercury), acetone, aflatoxin, ethylene glycol, drug-induced (allopurinol, aminoglycosides, cephalosporins, sulfonamides, tetracyclines, nonsteroidal anti-inflammatory drugs), hypervitaminosis D, caffeine, theobromine. Renal ischemia—hypoperfusion (dehydration, anesthesia, hypovolemia, atherosclerosis). Neoplasia (adenocarcinoma, nephroblastoma).
**Systemic or metabolic disease:** CDI. Liver disease. Pancreatitis. GI disease (diarrhea, hexamitiasis in pigeons). Septicemia. Localized abscess, salpingitis. Neoplasia (pituitary or pineal adenoma/adenocarcinoma).
**Metabolic:** Diabetes mellitus. Disseminated intravascular coagulopathy. Hypercalcemia. Hyperthyroidism. HAC.
**Dietary:** Breeding/feeding offspring. Excessive dietary sodium.
**Other:** Stress/excitement. Congenital/genetic.

## RISK FACTORS
Renal disease or liver disease. Administration of diuretics, corticosteroids, or anticonvulsants.

 **DIAGNOSIS**

## DIFFERENTIAL DIAGNOSIS
If associated with excessive weight loss, consider renal failure, pyelonephritis, liver failure, diabetes mellitus, neoplasia, hyperthyroidism. If associated with polyphagia, consider diabetes mellitus, hyperthyroidism. If associated with hypercalcemia, consider hypervitaminosis D, normal egg production, reproductive tract disease, neoplasia. If associated with coelomic distention, consider liver disease, reproductive disease, neoplasia, normal egg production. If associated with a behavioral or neurological disorder, consider hepatic failure, primary PD, CDI, heavy metal or salt intoxication.

## CBC/BIOCHEMISTRY/URINALYSIS
Serum sodium levels may help differentiate primary PD from primary PU. Hyponatremia or decreased serum osmolarity suggests primary PD, whereas hypernatremia or increased serum osmolarity indicates primary PU. Increased uric acid level may be indicative of renal failure, but dehydration, lipemia, high-protein diet, or muscle catabolism may also cause hyperuricemia. Persistent hyperuricemia after rehydration and fasting is indicative of renal disease. Decreased uric acid levels are indicative of liver dysfunction. Elevated levels of AST and bile acids may indicate liver disease. Persistent hyperglycemia is indicative of diabetes mellitus. Hypercalcemia may be present with normal egg production, reproductive tract disease, neoplasia, or hypervitaminosis D. Hyperphosphatemia and hyperkalemia may also occur with renal failure. Hyperkalemia with concurrent hyponatremia are suggestive of HAC in mammals, but this has yet to be determined in birds. Hypoalbuminemia (as determined by plasma EPH) supports renal or hepatic causes of PU/PD. Heterophilia suggests infectious or inflammatory disease. Alterations in urine specific gravity are not as reliable as an indicator of renal tubular disease in birds, as is seen with mammals, due to the bird's limited ability to concentrate urine. Glucosuria and ketonuria are indicative of diabetes mellitus, but urine glucose may be increased with fecal contamination. Proteinuria may indicate renal disease, but avian urine normally contains much higher protein levels than mammalian urine. Proteinuria may also be associated with fecal contamination. Avian urine is typically isosmotic because the predominant reptilian-type nephrons cannot concentrate urine beyond plasma osmolality, making assessment of urine specific gravity difficult. Hyposthenuria in a dehydrated bird may indicate an inability to concentrate urine.

## OTHER LABORATORY TESTS
Serum EPH may show hypoproteinemia secondary to a protein-losing nephropathy, or elevated globulin levels indicating an inflammatory or infectious disease process. Since urine samples are typically contaminated with GI flora, urine cultures

tend to be non-diagnostic, unless an uncontaminated urine sample can be obtained directly from the ureter. PCR testing for suspected pathogens (e.g. *Aspergillus*, polyomavirus, paramyxovirus) that can potentially cause PU/PD might be rewarding. Assessment and comparison of plasma and urine osmolality may be beneficial in determining if a bird is able to concentrate its urine. Assessment of circulating levels of AVT can be used to rule out diabetes insipidus, but normal values have not been established for most species.

### IMAGING
Plain and contrast radiography, ultrasound, CT, and MRI can all be used to image coelomic structures, such as the kidneys, liver, and reproductive tract, and may also demonstrate coelomic masses or effusion.

### DIAGNOSTIC PROCEDURES
Water deprivation testing is useful in ruling out diabetes insipidus and psychogenic PD. This test should only be considered after all other possible causes of PU/PD have been ruled out.
**Traditional water deprivation test**: The bird is weighed, and blood and urine samples are collected for assessment of PCV, total solids and osmolality of blood, and specific gravity and osmolality of urine. The bird is then placed in a cage with no food or water for the duration of the test. Blood and urine parameters are evaluated every 3–4 hours for 12–48 hours, depending on the species and physical condition of the bird (smaller birds should be evaluated more frequently). The test should be discontinued when the patient demonstrates the ability to concentrate its urine or loses 4–5% of body weight. Birds with psychogenic polydipsia should develop more concentrated urine and an increase in PCV, total solids, and plasma osmolality, consistent with dehydration. Birds with diabetes insipidus become dehydrated but maintain dilute urine.
**Gradual water deprivation test**: This test is preferred over the traditional water deprivation test because it allows the kidneys and cloaca to respond gradually to increasing plasma osmolality. The bird's average water intake is determined, and then reduced by 10% over 3–5 days. Final deprivation should be done in the hospital. At this point, the traditional water deprivation test protocol should be followed.
**Vasopressin/desmopressin response test**: This test is used to distinguish between CDI and NDI. Vasopressin and desmopressin are ADH analogues. Administration to birds with CDI should result in increased urine specific gravity and osmolality. Birds with NDI will not respond.

### PATHOLOGIC FINDINGS
N/A

 TREATMENT

### APPROPRIATE HEALTH CARE
Treat the underlying cause of PD whenever possible.

### NURSING CARE
Serious medical consequences are rare if the patient has free access to water and is willing and able to drink. Until the mechanism of PD is understood, discourage owners from limiting access to water. Treatment should be directed at the underlying cause. PD patients should be provided with free access to water unless they are vomiting. If the patient is vomiting, replacement maintenance fluids should be administered after the patient has been assessed and appropriate diagnostic samples have been obtained. Parental fluids should also be administered when other conditions limit oral intake or dehydration persists despite PD. Base fluid selection on knowledge of the underlying cause for fluid loss. In most avian patients, Normosol®-R (Hospira, Inc., Lake Forest, IL), Plasmalyte-R® (Baxter Healthcare, Deerfield, IL), Plasmalyte-A® (Baxter Healthcare, Deerfield, IL), and 0.9% NaCl are acceptable replacement fluid. Primary PD should be treated by limiting water intake to a normal daily volume. The patient should be monitored closely to avoid iatrogenic dehydration. Monitor body weight, hydration status (moistness of mucus membranes, skin turgor, eye position), perfusion parameters (mentation, mucus membranes color, CRT, pulse quality, heart rate, temperature of extremities), droppings.

### ACTIVITY
N/A

### DIET
Nutritional support. Provide adequate nutrition and calories. Gradually transition the bird to a healthy, balanced diet.

### CLIENT EDUCATION
Monitor appetite, body weight, droppings. Stress the importance of keeping the patient hydrated.

### SURGICAL CONSIDERATIONS
N/A

 MEDICATIONS

### DRUG(S) OF CHOICE
Varies with underlying cause.

### CONTRAINDICATIONS
Do not administer ADH or any of its synthetic analogs (desmopressin, vasopressin) to patients with primary PD because of the risk of inducing water intoxication.

### PRECAUTIONS
Until renal and hepatic failure have been excluded as potential causes for PU/PD, use caution in administering any drug that is eliminated via these pathways.

### POSSIBLE INTERACTIONS
N/A

### ALTERNATIVE DRUGS
N/A

 FOLLOW-UP

### PATIENT MONITORING
Hydration status by clinical assessment of hydration and serial evaluation of body weight. Fluid intake and urine output provide a useful baseline for assessing adequacy of hydration therapy.

### PREVENTION/AVOIDANCE
Complete water deprivation.

### POSSIBLE COMPLICATIONS
Dehydration.

### EXPECTED COURSE AND PROGNOSIS
Depends on the etiology of polydipsia.

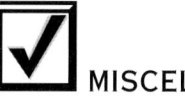 MISCELLANEOUS

### ASSOCIATED CONDITIONS
N/A

### AGE-RELATED FACTORS
N/A

### ZOONOTIC POTENTIAL
N/A

### FERTILITY/BREEDING
N/A

### SYNONYMS
N/A

### SEE ALSO
Dehydration
Diabetes Insipidus
Diabetes Mellitus and Hyperglycemia
Liver Disease
Neoplasia (Neurologic)
Polyuria
Renal Diseases
Thyroid Diseases
Toxicosis (Vitamin D)
Appendix 8, Algorithm 10: Polydipsia

P

# POLYDIPSIA

## ABBREVIATIONS
ADH—antidiuretic hormone
AST—aspartate aminotransferase
AVT—arginine vasotocin
CDI—central diabetes insipidus
CRT—capillary refill time
CT—computerized tomography
EPH—electrophoresis
GI—gastrointestinal
HAC—hyperadrenocorticism
MRI—magnetic resonance imaging
NDI—nephrogenic diabetes insipidus
NSHP—nutritional secondary
hyperparathyroidism
PCR—polymerase chain reaction

PD—polydipsia
PU—polyuria

## INTERNET RESOURCES
N/A

*Suggested Reading*
Echols, M.S. (2006). Evaluating and treating the kidneys. In: *Clinical Avian Medicine* (ed. G.J. Harrison, T.L. Lightfoot), Vol. I, 451–492. Palm Beach, FL: Spix Publishing.
Hudelson, K.S., Hudelson, P.M. (2006). Endocrine considerations. In: *Clinical Avian Medicine* (ed. G.J. Harrison, T.L. Lightfoot), Vol. I, 541–557. Palm Beach, FL: Spix Publishing.
Lennox, A.M., Doneley, R. (2004). Working up polyuria and polydipsia in a parrot. *Proceedings of the Association of Avian Veterinarians Annual Conference*, 59–66.
Oglesbee, B. (2003). Approach to the polydipsic/polyuric bird. *Proceedings of the Western Veterinary Conference Annual Conference*.
Polzin, D.J. (2021). Polyuria and polydipsia. In: *The 5-Minute Veterinary Consult: Canine and Feline*, 7th edn. (ed. L.P. Tilley, F.W.K. Smith Jr., M.M. Sleeper, B.M. Brainard), 1113–1114. Chichester, UK: Wiley.
**Author**: David E. Hannon, DVM, DABVP (Avian)

P

# BASICS

## DEFINITION
Avian polyomavirus (APV) infection is a non-enveloped virus in the family Polyomaviridae, which has been documented to affect avian psittacine neonates as well as adults. Clinical signs range from feather dystrophy and depression to slow crop emptying and death in budgerigar species. Non-budgerigar psittacines may show slow crop emptying, diarrhea, subcutaneous hemorrhages, and/or acute death in neonates to subclinical infections in adult parrots. Canaries and finches have been shown to be clinically susceptible to APV.

## PATHOPHYSIOLOGY
Infection with APV generally takes place 7–14 days after direct exposure to an infected or carrier bird. Dander or body fluids from an infected or carrier bird may also transmit viral particles to a naïve bird by human hands, articles of clothing, or feeding utensils. On a cellular level, APV causes massive internal hemorrhages, hepatic necrosis, myocardial cell necrosis and/or atrophy of lymphoid tissue in all species infected. In budgerigars, APV can be detected in skin and feather follicles.

## SYSTEMS AFFECTED
### Budgerigar Species
**Feather**: Follicle cellular lysis and necrosis causing lack of down feather formation and generalized feather dystrophy.
**Skin**: Hemorrhages can be detected on the skin in a variety of locations.
**Hepatobiliary**: Hepatocellular swelling and necrosis.
**Spleen**: Splenomegaly, cellular swelling and necrosis.
**Cardiovascular**: Pericardial effusion, karyomegaly and myocardial cell necrosis.
**Renal**: Karyomegaly and cellular necrosis.

### Non-Budgerigar Psittacines
**Hepatobiliary**: Hepatocellular necrosis, generally severe.
**Spleen**: Karyomegaly and cellular necrosis.
**Renal**: Karyomegaly and cellular necrosis.
**Skin**: Subcutaneous hemorrhages.
**Cardiac**: Karyomegaly and pericardial effusion.
**Hemic/lymphatic**: Karyomegaly of vessel walls, atrophy of lymphoid tissue in the spleen and bursa.

## GENETICS
N/A

## INCIDENCE/PREVALENCE
Higher incidence is noted in the spring and summer. This increase coincides with hatching season. Prevalence is higher in aviaries that do not practice proper a "closed aviary" concept.

## GEOGRAPHIC DISTRIBUTION
APV can be found in all geographic regions where budgerigar and non-budgerigar psittacine parrots are being raised in an avicultural environment.

## SIGNALMENT
**Species**: Budgerigar, non-budgerigar psittacines and passerines. Eclectus parrots, caiques and hawkhead parrots are more susceptible to fatal polyomavirus infections.
**Mean age and range**: All neonatal and juvenile psittacines are susceptible. Sudden death in birds < 3 weeks of age post exposure to carrier or clinically infected birds. Adult budgerigars and non-budgerigar species may become subclinical carriers.

## SIGNS
Sudden to peracute death in birds < 3 weeks of age is common. Subcutaneous hemorrhages, delayed crop emptying, regurgitation, and diarrhea are common in non-budgerigar psittacines. Feather dystrophy is common in budgerigars that survive the initial infection.

### Historical Findings
Owners usually report poor crop emptying, regurgitation, diarrhea or acute death in neonatal psittacines. Breeders/owners of budgerigars usually notice feather abnormalities or acute death in neonates and fledglings.

### Physical Examination Findings
On physical examination of budgerigar babies, subcutaneous hemorrhages and/or feather abnormalities may be noted prior to death or in older survivors. Non-budgerigar species often show lethargy, slow crop emptying, diarrhea, and subcutaneous hemorrhages.

## CAUSES
Exposure to carrier birds or birds clinically infected with polyomavirus is the most common cause of infection. The virus may also be carried on the owner's hands from one bird to the next. Contaminated feeding utensils, water and food bowls and caging material may also serve as fomites. Housing multiple species of non-vaccinated baby psittacines together increases the risk of infection.

## RISK FACTORS
Stress of travel, inadequate environmental temperature, and/or overcrowding may lower an individual's ability to fight off infection.

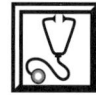

# DIAGNOSIS

## DIFFERENTIAL DIAGNOSIS
Any cause of acute death in psittacine neonates should be considered until testing or histopathology accurately identifies the causative agent. Viral diseases such as Pacheco's, PBFD, and adenovirus must be on a rule-out list. Systemic infections such as bacterial sepsis or chlamydiosis may create similar internal organ pathology.

## CBC/BIOCHEMISTRY/URINALYSIS
Patients that are infected but not near death may show elevated white blood cell counts, low PCV and generally have extremely elevated AST and CK enzymes.

## OTHER LABORATORY TESTS
Specific antemortem diagnostic tests involve oral, cloacal or fecal DNA probe testing for viral particles. Paired serum samples to show increases in antibody titers are useful in survivors.

## IMAGING
N/A

## DIAGNOSTIC PROCEDURES
N/A

## PATHOLOGIC FINDINGS
Gross necropsy findings in fatal APV infections are fairly classic and generally involve noting subcutaneous hemorrhages on the crop, abdominal skin, patagium, and/or torso. Most cases have a pale oral cavity. A variety of feather abnormalities may be noted, specifically in young budgerigar cases. Internal gross lesions often reveal serosal hemorrhages on many organs, hydropericardium, hepatomegaly, splenomegaly, ascites, and myocardial hemorrhages. Histopathological lesions in both groups often reveal hepatic, splenic, and myocardial necrosis. Intranuclear inclusions may be noted in heart, liver, splenic, and renal tissues. Inclusions in feather follicles may also be seen in budgerigar species.

# TREATMENT

## APPROPRIATE HEALTH CARE
Supportive care with nutritional support, IV or IO fluids and warmth are helpful but may not slow the progression of signs. Interferon and other immune stimulation may provide help in isolated cases.

## NURSING CARE
Patients suspected of having a PMV infection should be under strict quarantine in either the veterinary clinic or hospital, or at the owner's home or aviary. All humans coming in contact with infected and clinical birds should wear protective clothing that can be discarded after handling known positive cases. These birds should be treated or fed last.

## ACTIVITY
N/A

## DIET
N/A

P

## POLYOMAVIRUS (CONTINUED)

### CLIENT EDUCATION

Clients with diseased or infected carrier birds should be advised to stay away from pet stores, bird fairs, or other breeder's facilities until their home or aviary has been properly disinfected. They need to be advised that bird dander from infected birds can transmit to naive birds without direct contact. Environmental testing for APV is highly recommended. Feeding utensils, nest boxes, cages, counter tops, floors, and walls of the home or aviary should all have DNA probe testing to identify APV-positive zones that need disinfection. Prevention is the key to APV. APV vaccination has been approved for all psittacines > 5 weeks of age and repeated 2–4 weeks later. Vaccinated APV-negative birds are resistant to infection, and hence eliminate spread to other birds.

### SURGICAL CONSIDERATIONS

N/A

## MEDICATIONS

### DRUG(S) OF CHOICE

No antiviral medications are effective. Interferon has been used with mixed results.

### CONTRAINDICATIONS

N/A

### PRECAUTIONS

N/A

### POSSIBLE INTERACTIONS

N/A

### ALTERNATIVE DRUGS

N/A

## FOLLOW-UP

### PATIENT MONITORING

Serologic testing of the affected bird(s) to determine their seroconversion is helpful to determine if they are still infected. Environmental disinfection and DNA probe testing is critical to make sure the locale where the infected bird(s) originated from is critical to protect other birds and prevent the spread of the virus to other locations.

### PREVENTION/AVOIDANCE

Vaccination of psittacine birds can help protect naive birds and eliminate spread to other birds/facilities. Neonates and adult psittacines can be vaccinated, especially those that will be exposed to non-vaccinated birds from other breeders or homes. A large percentage of infected budgerigar and non-budgerigar psittacine neonatal patients often expire within 2 weeks of exposure. Vaccination will not be effective in neonates that have recently been infected with the virus. Surviving budgerigar and non-budgerigar patients may take 1–2 weeks to begin acting normally. Feather growth abnormalities are common in surviving budgerigar species. APV is very stable in the environment for long periods of time. Environmental disinfection with 10% sodium hypochlorite, 70% ethanol and Avinol-3™ (Veterinary Products Laboratories, Phoenix, AZ) have all been shown to effectively inactivate the virus.

### POSSIBLE COMPLICATIONS

Increased susceptibility to other infectious diseases.

### EXPECTED COURSE AND PROGNOSIS

Most neonate and juvenile birds with clinical disease will die within 2 weeks of exposure. Surviving budgerigar and non-budgerigar patients may take 1–2 weeks to begin acting normally. Feather growth abnormalities are common in surviving budgerigar species.

## MISCELLANEOUS

### ASSOCIATED CONDITIONS

See above.

### AGE-RELATED FACTORS

Sudden death in birds <3 weeks of age post exposure to carrier or clinically infected birds. Adult budgerigars and non-budgerigar species may become subclinical carriers.

### ZOONOTIC POTENTIAL

N/A

### FERTILITY/BREEDING

Decreased egg hatchability and early embryonic deaths may occur in budgerigar species.

### SYNONYMS

Papovavirus (previous classification), budgerigar fledgling disease.

### SEE ALSO

Anemia
Coagulopathies
Feather Disorders
Hemorrhage
Infertility
Liver Disease
Sick-Bird Syndrome
Toxicosis (Heavy Metals)

### ABBREVIATIONS

APV—avian polyomavirus
AST—aspartate aminotransferase
CK—creatine kinase
PBFD—psittacine beak and feather disease
PCV—packed cell volume

### INTERNET RESOURCES

N/A

*Suggested Reading*
Garcia, A.P., Latimer, K.S., Niagro, F.D., et al. (1994). Diagnosis of polyomavirus-induced hepatic necrosis in psittacine birds using DNA probes. *Journal of Veterinary Diagnostic Investigation*, 6:308–314.
Ritchie, B.W. (1995). Papovaviridae. In: *Avian Viruses: Function and Control*, 127–170. Lake Worth, FL: Wingers Publishing.
Ritchie, B.W., Latimer, K.S., Leonard, J., et al. (1999). Safety, immunogenicity and efficacy of an inactivated avian polyomavirus vaccine. *American Journal of Veterinary Research*, 59:143–148.
Ritchie, B.W., Niagro, F.D., Latimer, K.S., et al. (1993). Efficacy of an inactivated polyomavirus vaccine. *Journal of the Association of Avian Veterinarians*, 7:187–192.
Ritchie, B.W., Niagro, F.D., Latimer, K.S., et al. (1991). Polyomavirus infections in adult psittacine birds. *Journal of the Association of Avian Veterinarians*, 5:202–206.
**Author:** Gregory Rich, DVM, BS Medical Technology

**Client Education Handout available online**

# POLYOSTOTIC HYPEROSTOSIS

## BASICS

### DEFINITION
Polyostotic hyperostosis describes the radiographic appearance of the avian skeleton as it relates to female reproductive hormonal state. It is characterized by generalized increased medullary opacity to some or all bones that is typically seen starting 10–14 days before egg formation.

### PATHOPHYSIOLOGY
Polyostotic hyperostosis is a commonly observed finding on radiographs of the female avian patient. The pathogenesis remains unknown, as the condition is seen in birds with reproductive-associated activity and birds suffering from reproductive disorders. Bone marrow ossification occurs secondary to rising estrogen levels and is a physiologic change related to normal egg laying. Bone marrow ossification may also relate to a pathologic change such as neoplasia and bone marrow disease and in males under paraneoplastic estrogen production. The increased opacity relates to calcium mobilization and storage for use in eggshell formation.

### SYSTEMS AFFECTED
**Musculoskeletal**: Increased bone opacity from calcium storage in the avian skeleton.
**Reproductive**: A finding in reproductively active female birds.

### GENETICS
No genetic predisposition, as it most often occurs as a normal physiologic change.

### INCIDENCE/PREVALENCE
The finding is common in reproductively active hens but is not generally considered a pathologic condition in itself.

### GEOGRAPHIC DISTRIBUTION
N/A

### SIGNALMENT
**Species**: No species predilection, as it is seen in all species of birds but is most commonly seen as associated with reproductive disorders in budgerigars and cockatiels.
**Mean age and range**: Sexually mature hens (sexual and hormonal maturity varies widely among species).
**Predominant sex**: Females of egg-laying age. Although rare, this condition can occasionally occur in male birds in association with gonadal tumors or disease.

### SIGNS
#### General Comments
The skeleton may increase in weight by up to 25% by the replacement of hematopoietic tissue with medullary bone.

#### Historical Findings
Behavioral changes secondary to hormonal changes. Aggressive behaviors such as cage or nest protection. Broodiness and nesting behaviors, hiding, paper shredding. Egg laying, which may be chronic and uncontrolled. Fecal retention secondary to normal nesting behavior. Lethargy, weakness, or decreased appetite may be observed in birds with chronic egg laying.

#### Physical Examination Findings
No directly attributable physical exam findings. Body weight may increase in relation to reproductive state. An egg may be palpable in the coelomic cavity.

### CAUSES
Reproductive activity and hormonal changes, estrogen production. Egg laying. Calcium mobilization for egg shell formation.

### RISK FACTORS
A poor diet without appropriate vitamins and calcium supplementation may lead to pathology.

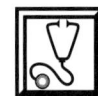

## DIAGNOSIS

### DIFFERENTIAL DIAGNOSIS
Osteomyelosclerosis—disease occurs in non-laying hens and cocks as a result of specific pathology. Osteopetrosis—induced by avian leukosis virus in chickens. Neoplasia, including metastatic disease—uncommon, but may represent alterations secondary to reproductive tract neoplasia. Metabolic bone disease—a decreased overall opacity to bones that can result in weakness, lethargy, and pathologic fractures. Coelomic distension—may indicate a reproductively active hen with reproductive tract enlargement. Various bone marrow diseases may lead to increased medullary opacification, but typically does not lead to mineral opacities. These may include Mycobacteriosis, West Nile virus, leukemia, and severe leukocytosis.

### CBC/BIOCHEMISTRY/URINALYSIS
A mild anemia and leukocytosis may be seen in reproductive females. Hypercalcemia is commonly seen as a normal physiologic response to egg laying. Hypercholesterolemia and hypertriglyceridemia may be seen as a physiologic response to egg laying in the ovulating hen. Hyperuricemia occurs during egg laying from compression of renal parenchyma.

### OTHER LABORATORY TESTS
EPH—hyperglobulinemia may be seen in egg-laying birds.

### IMAGING
Standard radiography is the primary method of identification. Generalized increased medullary opacity of some or all bones (primarily long bones) is observed. Radiography is also useful for evaluation of concurrent or associated medical conditions.

### DIAGNOSTIC PROCEDURES
N/A

### PATHOLOGIC FINDINGS
Polyostotic hyperostosis is not considered a pathologic finding on its own. It can be seen in birds that have gonadal tumors.

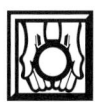

## TREATMENT

### APPROPRIATE HEALTH CARE
Treatment is only required for polyototic hyperostosis associated with an abnormal medical condition.

### NURSING CARE
As appropriate for other medical conditions that may be diagnosed; no direct care.

### ACTIVITY
No restriction of activity level is required in a healthy egg-laying hen.

### DIET
Hens should be on appropriate calcium supplementation such as eggshell powder, mineral blocks, calcium powder, calcium suspension, and cuttlebone.

### CLIENT EDUCATION
May indicate future egg laying. May indicate reasons for behavior changes. Clients should be educated about chronic egg laying, egg binding, yolk coelomitis, and other reproductive diseases of pet birds. Leuprolide acetate can be administered if the hen starts to exhibit reproductive behaviors.

### SURGICAL CONSIDERATIONS
Surgery is only indicated with concurrent reproductive disease and may include salpingohysterectomy.

## MEDICATIONS

### DRUG(S) OF CHOICE
No direct treatment for the radiographic finding. Leuprolide acetate, a long-acting GnRH analog used to prevent ovulation and egg production. Doses vary: 700–800 µg/kg IM for birds < 300 grams, 500 µg/kg IM for birds > 300 grams q21–30d. Deslorelin acetate implants can also be used for management of reproductive conditions in birds.

### CONTRAINDICATIONS
N/A

### PRECAUTIONS
N/A

P

## POSSIBLE INTERACTIONS
N/A

## ALTERNATIVE DRUGS
N/A

## FOLLOW-UP

### PATIENT MONITORING
Routine radiography is useful to determine the presence of increased ossification and to determine reproductive status.

### PREVENTION/AVOIDANCE
Discourage excessive egg laying by reducing the photoperiod to no more than 10 hours/day by covering the cage at night, keep the hen separate from any mate or perceived mates, reduce foods high in fat and overall quantity of food, and remove nests and nesting material. Leuprolide acetate can be administered monthly or seasonally or when the hen is exhibiting reproductive behavior to prevent ovulation and egg laying. A deslorelin acetate implant can also be placed and may prevent egg laying for several months.

### POSSIBLE COMPLICATIONS
N/A

### EXPECTED COURSE
### AND PROGNOSIS
N/A

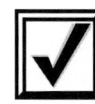

## MISCELLANEOUS

### ASSOCIATED CONDITIONS
Reproductive activity. Egg laying. Hormonal behaviors.

### AGE-RELATED FACTORS
N/A

### ZOONOTIC POTENTIAL
N/A

### FERTILITY/BREEDING
Since elected sterilization is not routine, any female bird can lay eggs. Breeding of pet birds should be discouraged.

### SYNONYMS
Egg-laying bones, osteomyelosclerosis.

### SEE ALSO
Cere and Skin Color Changes
Chronic Egg Laying
Dystocia and Egg Binding
Neoplasia (Lymphoproliferative)
Neoplasia (Reproductive)
Ovarian Diseases
Oviductal Diseases
Toxicosis (Vitamin D)

### ABBREVIATIONS
EPH—protein electrophoresis
GnRH—gonadotropin-releasing hormone

### INTERNET RESOURCES
Pollock, C. (2012). Reproductive emergencies in birds. *Lafeber Vet*: https://lafeber.com/vet/reproductive-emergencies

*Suggested Reading*
Hadley T., (2010) Management of Common Psittacine Reproductive Disorders in Clinical Practice. *Veterinary Clinics of North America: Exotic Animal Practice*, 13:429–438.
Baumgartner, R., Hatt, J.-M., Dobeli, M., Hauser, B. (1995). Endocrinologic and pathologic findings in birds with polyostotic hyperostosis. *Journal of Avian Medicine and Surgery*, 9:251–254.
Bowles, H.L. (2006). Evaluating and treating the reproductive system. In: *Clinical Avian Medicine* (ed. G.J. Harrison, T.L. Lightfoot), Vol. 2, 519–540. Palm Beach, FL: Spix Publishing.
Pollock, C.G., Orosz, S.E. (2002). Avian reproductive anatomy, physiology, and endocrinology. *Veterinary Clinics of North America: Exotic Animal Practice*, 5:441–474.
Stauber, E., Papageorges, M., Sande, R., Ward, L. (1990). Polyostotic hyperostosis associated with oviductal tumor in a cockatiel. *Journal of the American Veterinary Medical Association*, 196:939–940.

**Author**: Anthony A. Pilny, DVM, DABVP (Avian)

P

# BASICS

## DEFINITION
Polyuria (PU) is defined as a true and persistent increase in urinary output and water intake. PU is a non-specific sign.

## PATHOPHYSIOLOGY
Normal urine output and water intake vary immensely among different bird species, age, and physiologic state. Urine output is dependent on GFR, tubular reabsorption of solutes and water, and patency of the urinary tract. The medullary or mammalian nephrons contain a loop of Henle, which concentrates urine. A countercurrent multiplier present within the medullary cone is capable of producing concentrated urine, but the degree of concentration is much less in birds compared with mammals. Urine may flow via retrograde peristalsis from the urodeum into the coprodeum and distal portion of the colon, where water and sodium are reabsorbed in the ceca (when present) and rectum. This can create considerable differences between the osmolality of ureteral urine and that of voided urine, particularly in dehydrated birds. In a study of dehydrated pigeons, voided urine was 30% more concentrated than that obtained via ureteral cannulation.

## SYSTEMS AFFECTED
Endocrine/metabolic. GI system—ceca, rectum, cloaca play a role in reabsorption of ureteral water. Behavioral—polydipsia. Urinary and osmoregulatory system.

## GENETICS
N/A

## INCIDENCE/PREVALENCE
N/A

## GEOGRAPHIC DISTRIBUTION
N/A

## SIGNALMENT
PU can be observed with a variety of conditions and in any avian species: Genus *Neophema*—PMV-3, a potential cause of PU. Chickens, guinea fowl (*Numida meleagris*), grey parrots (*Psittacus erithacus*)—adenovirus causing pancreatic disease. Finches and canaries—bacterial nephritis. Pigeons—*Salmonella*, PMV-1. Raptors—lead poisoning.

## SIGNS

### General Comments
Is PU truly present? Birds with PU may be presented for "diarrhea." Evaluate the volume and color of urine and urate components. Is the urine output normal for the species and age of the bird?

### Historical Findings
Is PU a transient or persistent finding? Is there polydipsia (PD)? Is there a history of exposure to renal disease risk factors such as heavy metals, nephrotoxic drugs, supplementation with excessive levels of vitamin D$_3$? Does the bird consume high moisture food items like fruit, gruel, water-laden vegetables, nectar? Is there a history of breeding or feeding offspring? Has a change in appetite been recognized (anorexia, polyphagia)?

### Physical Examination Findings
Measure body weight. Evaluate hydration status (moistness of mucus membranes, skin turgor, eye position). Evaluate perfusion parameters (mentation, mucus membrane color, capillary refill time, pulse quality, heart rate, temperature of the extremities). Perform a complete physical examination to evaluate body condition and identify additional clinical signs that may further characterize underlying disease. Evaluate fresh droppings to minimize any confusion between PU versus diarrhea.

## CAUSES
Prerenal disease: Increased intake of fluids—psychogenic polydipsia, fluid administration (overhydration); dietary imbalances: hypervitaminosis D, excessive dietary sodium; drugs—diuretics, glucocorticoids, endogenous (stress) or exogenous; *Escherichia coli* endotoxin; electrolyte abnormalities—hypercalcemia; hormonal conditions—diabetes insipidus, diabetes mellitus, hyperadrenocorticism, hypoadrenocorticism, hyperthyroidism, pituitary adenoma/carcinoma. Liver disease (severe hepatopathy). Pancreatitis. Salpingitis or localized abscess. Sepsis. Renal disease or gout: PU/PD is an uncommon sign of renal disease in the bird—inflammation of the kidney or structural changes can interfere with its ability to concentrate urine; important causes of infectious nephritis associated with PU include salmonellosis, adenoviral disease affecting the pancreas, psittacid herpesvirus-1, IBV, PMV-1, PMV-3, avian polyomavirus, West Nile virus, sarcocystosis, psittacosis; exposure to toxins—heavy metals (e.g. zinc, lead), nephrotoxic drugs (e.g. aminoglycosides, sulfonamides). Postrenal disease: Postobstructive diuresis (urolithiasis, cloacolith, neoplasia, egg binding). Older birds (especially cockatiels and budgerigars) on poor diets may develop PU/PD, lethargy, hyperuricemia when abruptly converted to a formulated diet. This may be due to reduced renal and hepatic function from a life-long deficiency in vitamin A and certain amino acids. PU is a common manifestation of many systemic diseases, but the mechanism

of action is unknown and resolution of PU occurs with resolution of the systemic disease.

## RISK FACTORS
**Medical conditions**: GFR, conditions that reduce blood loss, severe dehydration, shock. Inflammation (chronic). Immunocompromise. Old age. Systemic hypertension. Uncontrolled diabetes mellitus.
**Medications**: Nephrotoxins—NSAIDs, intravenous contrast media, etc.
**Environmental factors**: Poor husbandry. Adverse conditions that might lead to dehydration. High moisture conditions that promote the development of moldy feed (mycotoxicosis). Improper nutrition.

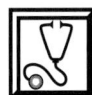

# DIAGNOSIS

## DIFFERENTIAL DIAGNOSIS
Diarrhea (increased fluid in feces). Normal droppings in nectar-eating birds like lories and lorikeets, birds with diets high in fruits, water-laden vegetables, birds on gruels, tube feeding, or hand-feeding formulas, breeding birds, or birds feeding young. Transient PU as a stress response.

## CBC/BIOCHEMISTRY/URINALYSIS
Complete blood count or at least hematocrit/total protein. Biochemistry panel including blood glucose, blood urea nitrogen, creatinine (useful indicator of prerenal dehydration); uric acid; albumin, total protein; sodium. Urinalysis is indicated in birds with persistent PU. Birds with diabetes mellitus often have urine glucose concentrations > 2000 mg/dl. Specific gravity ranges from 1.005 to 1.020 in most polyuric birds.

## OTHER LABORATORY TESTS
Increased amylase concentrations have been reported in some pancreatitis cases. Lactate. Blood lead/zinc levels. Serology as indicated. Plasma and urine osmolality may help distinguish between causes of PU, especially when diabetes insipidus or psychogenic polydipsia are suspected. Protein electrophoresis.

## IMAGING
Survey radiographs. Contrast studies of the GI tract can help isolate the location of the kidneys and the source of organomegaly. Sonographic evaluation of coelomic organs. Alternate imaging techniques include nuclear scintigraphy to evaluate renal function. MRI, CT. Do not perform intravenous excretory urography in birds with severe renal compromise.

## DIAGNOSTIC PROCEDURES
Water deprivation testing can be used to distinguish psychogenic polydipsia and

P

diabetes insipidus from other causes of PU. Laparoscopic examination of the kidneys and renal biopsy.

## PATHOLOGIC FINDINGS
Depending on the underlying site of disease, signs of inflammation, organomegaly, edema, etc. may be visible in adrenal glands, brain, GI tract, kidneys, liver, pancreas. Reproductive tract.

# TREATMENT

## APPROPRIATE HEALTH CARE
Treat the underlying cause of PU whenever possible.

## NURSING CARE
Unless PU is caused by overhydration, careful attention to fluid therapy is required to prevent significant abnormalities in hydration. Monitor body weight, hydration status (moistness of mucus membranes, skin turgor, eye position), perfusion parameters (mentation, mucus membrane color, CRT, pulse quality, heart rate, temperature of extremities), droppings.

## ACTIVITY
N/A

## DIET
Nutritional support. Provide adequate nutrition and calories. Gradually transition the bird to a healthy, balanced diet.

## CLIENT EDUCATION
Monitor appetite, body weight, droppings. Stress the importance of keeping the patient hydrated. Long-term prognosis.

## SURGICAL CONSIDERATIONS
N/A

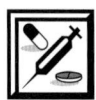

# MEDICATIONS

## DRUG(S) OF CHOICE
Although PU is an uncommon sign of renal disease, consider antibiotic therapy if nephritis is suspected, since 50% of avian nephritis cases are associated with bacterial infection.

## CONTRAINDICATIONS
Diuretics could exacerbate fluid loss and dehydration. Stop or avoid all nephrotoxic drugs that could cause or aggravate renal disease, such as aminoglycosides or sulfonamides.

## PRECAUTIONS
Drugs primarily cleared by renal tubular secretion or filtration (e.g. penicillin) may demonstrate a shorter half-life or fail to reach therapeutic plasma levels in the polyuric patient.

## POSSIBLE INTERACTIONS
Dehydration can result in adverse responses to NSAIDs, especially cyclooxygenase inhibitory drugs like meloxicam.

## ALTERNATIVE DRUGS
Medical management of diabetes mellitus can include insulin, glipizide. Analgesia (e.g. opioids) for renal tumor patients.

# FOLLOW-UP

## PATIENT MONITORING
Activity level. Appetite and water intake. Droppings. Body weight. Hydration status (moistness of mucus membranes, skin turgor, eye position). Perfusion parameters (mentation, mucus membrane color, CRT, pulse quality, heart rate, temperature of extremities).

## PREVENTION/AVOIDANCE
Water deprivation.

## POSSIBLE COMPLICATIONS
Dehydration.

## EXPECTED COURSE
## AND PROGNOSIS
N/A

# MISCELLANEOUS

## ASSOCIATED CONDITIONS
Dehydration.

## AGE-RELATED FACTORS
N/A

## ZOONOTIC POTENTIAL
N/A

## FERTILITY/BREEDING
Polyuria can be a normal finding in breeding birds or birds feeding offspring.

## SYNONYMS
N/A

## SEE ALSO
Adenoviruses
Bornaviral Diseases
Chlamydiosis
Dehydration
Diabetes Insipidus
Diabetes Mellitus and Hyperglycemia

Herpesvirus (Columbid Herpesvirus 1 in Pigeons and Raptors)
Herpesvirus (Duck Viral Enteritis)
Herpesvirus (Passerine Birds)
Herpesvirus (Psittacid Herpesviruses)
Hyperuricemia
Liver Disease
Neoplasia (Neurologic)
Orthoavulaviruses
Pancreatitis
Polydipsia
Polyomavirus
Renal Disease
Salmonellosis
Sarcocystosis
Thyroid Diseases
Toxicicosis (Heavy Metals)
Toxicosis (Ingested, Gastrointestinal)
Toxicosis (Vitamin D)
Urate and Fecal Discoloration
West Nile Virus
Appendix 8, Algorithm 11: Polyuria

## ABBREVIATIONS
CRT—capillary refill time
CT—computed tomography
GFR—glomerular filtration rate
GI—gastrointestinal
IBV—infectious bronchitis virus
MRI—magnetic resonance imaging
NSAIDs—non-steroidal anti-inflammatory drugs
PD—polydipsia
PMV—paramyxovirus
PU—polyuria

## INTERNET RESOURCES
N/A

*Suggested Reading*
DiGeronimo, P.M., Crossland, N.A., Jugan, A., et al. (2018). Diabetes mellitus with concurrent cerebellar degeneration and necrosis in a domestic goose (*Anser anser domesticus*). *Journal of Avian Medicine and Surgery*, 32:122–127.
Lightfoot, T.L. (2010). Geriatric psittacine medicine. *Veterinary Clinics of North America: Exotic Animal Practice*, 13:27–45.
Łukaszuk, E., Stenzel, T. (2020). Occurrence and role of selected RNA-viruses as potential causative agents of watery droppings in pigeons. *Pathogens*, 9:1025.
Phalen, D.N. (2020). Diseases of the avian urinary system. *Veterinary Clinics of North America: Exotic Animal Practice*, 23:21–45.
Scope, A., Schwendenwein, I. (2020). Laboratory evaluation of renal function in birds. *Veterinary Clinics of North America: Exotic Animal Practice*, 23:47–58.
**Author**: Christal Pollock, DVM, DABVP (Avian Practice)

# BASICS

## DEFINITION
Avian poxviruses are large (150–250 ×
265–350 nm) double-stranded, enveloped
DNA viruses. Poxviruses are in the
*Chordopoxvirinae* subfamily of the *Poxviridae*
family. They have been identified in 374
species from 23 orders. Disease from
infection is most commonly categorized as
cutaneous or "dry" (nodules and crusting
lesions on unfeathered skin) and diphtheroid
or "wet" (fibronecrotic membranes of the
upper gastrointestinal or respiratory systems).
Septicemic disease is also possible; animals
become acutely depressed and die. Mortality
rates are higher with diphtheroid and
septicemic disease. Poxviruses can delay
weight gain and reduce egg laying in chicken
and turkey flocks.

## PATHOPHYSIOLOGY
Poxviruses replicate in the cytoplasm of
epithelial cells and the virus induces a
hyperplastic host response. Infection may be
limited to the cells around the site of
inoculation, but in some cases viremia
develops. Viral replication in the liver and
bone marrow then leads to a secondary
viremia and replication in multiple organs.
Disease is more severe in viremic birds.
Poxviruses cannot penetrate intact epithelium
and infections depend on disruption of
epithelial integrity. Direct, indirect, ingestion,
and inhalation may be sources of
transmission. Biting insects are considered a
major vector. In domestic species, the
incubation period is typically 5–10 days and
flock outbreaks last 2–3 months; flocks may
be chronically infected. The form of disease
(cutaneous, diphtheroid, or septicemic) and
severity of infection varies with route of
inoculation, viral strain, viral load, and
immune status of the bird. Flocks may have
multiple forms in a single outbreak, and
individual birds within a flock may have
more than one form. Birds that survive
infection typically have a protective immune
response to that strain. In recovered birds, a
carrier state is possible. Strains are named for
the species in which they were first identified;
molecular evaluation is not complete for all
strains identified. There are 12 strains
identified by the International Committee on
Taxonomy of Viruses: canarypox, fowlpox,
juncopox, mynahpox, pigeonpox,
psittacinepox, quailpox, sparrowpox,
starlingpox, turkeypox, flamingopox,
penguinpox. Fowlpox from chickens (*Gallus
gallus domesticus*) is the type species. Strains
are typically specific to individual species and
disease tends to be more severe in adapted
hosts, although this is not universal.

## Cutaneous Pox
Cutaneous (dry) pox starts as papule and
vesicle formation in areas of unfeathered skin.
Vesicles rupture, leaving erosions that scab.
Secondary bacterial or fungal infection is
common. Lesions typically take about
1 month to heal in domestic species and up
to 3 months or more in wild species.
Secondary infections can complicate healing
and can lead to chronic wounds.
Occasionally, skin lesions are dark, discolored
areas without papule/vesicle formation.
Scarring, digit loss, and hypopigmentation
may be present after healing. Cutaneous pox
frequently develops in Psittaciformes,
Falconiformes, Passeriformes, Galliformes,
and waterfowl, and is the primary form
identified in free-ranging wild birds.
Mortality rates tend to be low unless lesions
are severe and limit basic behaviors
(e.g. feeding).

## Diphtheroid Pox
Diphtheroid (wet) pox occurs on mucosa.
Erosions fill with fibronecrotic material and
may develop on the tongue, hard palate,
larynx, trachea, bronchi, esophagus, or crop.
Secondary bacterial or fungal infections are
common. Diphtheroid pox often develops in
Psittaciformes, Columbiformes, and
Galliformes. It is more common in domestic
or captive wild species and is not identified
frequently in free-ranging wild birds.
Mortality rates are high. Wet pox is the form
historically associated with Amazon parrots
(*Amazona* spp.) at import stations.

## Septicemic Pox
Septicemic pox causes severe disease. Animals
become acutely depressed and dyspneic and
frequently die. Multiple organs may be
impacted. Necrosis of the heart and liver, as
well as air sacculitis, pneumonia, peritonitis,
and necrotic debris in the alimentary tract
have been described. Septicemic pox is
frequently reported in captive canaries
(*Serina* spp.).

## SYSTEMS AFFECTED
Skin, respiratory, gastrointestinal,
ophthalmic, hemic/lymphatic/immune.

## GENETICS
N/A

## INCIDENCE/PREVALENCE
The incidents rate ranges from 0–50% across
various species in captive and free-range
settings, often falling in the 5–20% range. In
captive psittacines in North America, disease
is uncommon; however, canary and chicken
flocks are often infected. Vaccination is
common in commercial chicken flocks as
part of routine management. Clinical disease
in pet canaries is uncommon.

## GEOGRAPHIC DISTRIBUTION
Worldwide, except the Arctic and Antarctic.

## SIGNALMENT
**Species**: While strains appear specific for
individual species, some strains can infect
non-adapted hosts. Disease may be more or
less severe in the aberrant host. All species
should be considered susceptible to potential
infection to a species-specific strain.
Captive-bred pet parrots, birds largely held
indoors, or held outdoors with good
protection from insect pests are less
commonly affected. In psittacines, disease
was most often associated with importation
of birds from the wild. South and Central
American Amazon and pionus (*Pionus* spp.)
parrots, macaws (e.g., *Ara* spp.), lovebirds
(*Agapornis* spp.), quaker parrots (*Myiopsitta
monachus*), and conures (e.g., *Aratinga* spp.)
were considered most susceptible. During
this period, disease in African species,
cockatoos, and cockatiels was less common.
Poxvirus is commonly reported in domestic
chickens and pigeons (*Columba livia
domestica*) and disease can be severe.
**Mean age and range**: Any age, disease may
be more common and/or severe in juvenile
birds.

## SIGNS

### Historical Findings
There may be a history of recent additions to
the flock. In outdoor-housed flocks, weather
changes that increase insect populations (e.g.
warm, moist conditions) may be reported. In
cutaneous pox, caregivers typically note lesion
development around the face or digits. Signs
may be chronic and multiple birds in a flock
may be affected. Birds with severe lesions
may have trouble eating or finding food due
to proliferations around the mouth or eyelids,
or may have reduced mobility due to severe
lesions on the digits. In diphtheroid pox,
caregivers may appreciate lethargy, anorexia,
increased breathing rate or effort, open-beak
breathing, or reduced appetite. Septicemic
pox may be reported as acute depression,
increased respiratory rate or effort, and death.

### Physical Examination Findings
Cutaneous pox typically presents as
proliferative, crusted lesions around the
palpebral margins, oral commissure, wattles,
digits, and other unfeathered regions. In
some species (e.g. penguins), lesions may be
noted on the wings and cloaca. Mobility
issues may be noted due to impingement of
digit motion or pain. Diphtheroid pox
presents with a moist, fibronecrotic
membrane in the oral cavity that is tightly
adhered to underlying tissue. Stridor,
dyspnea, and/or tachypnea may be present if
lesions are in the respiratory system.
Cutaneous and diphtheroid lesions
hemorrhage readily if disturbed. Animals may
be thin or in good body condition,
depending on duration of signs and whether

P

lesions impact eating and drinking. Animals may be dehydrated. Septicemic pox may present with severe depression and respiratory changes, animals may be in appropriate body condition but dehydration and other signs of severe disease are expected.

## CAUSES
Clinical signs are related to epithelial hyperplasia and secondary bacterial or fungal infection.

## RISK FACTORS
Conditions that increase population density (e.g. fall flocking behavior, high-density commercial farming), reduce immune function (e.g. transportation stress), and increase insect vectors (e.g. warm, moist weather) can increase disease.

# DIAGNOSIS

## DIFFERENTIAL DIAGNOSIS
Cutaneous—bacterial infection, papillomavirus, *Knemidokoptes* mite infection, *Trichophyton gallinae* infection (favus). Diphtheroid—herpesvirus (infectious laryngotracheitis virus), fungal infection (e.g. candidiasis, aspergillosis), hypovitaminosis A, trichomoniasis. Septicemic—bacterial sepsis, pneumonia, toxin, any cause of acute mortality.

## CBC/BIOCHEMISTRY/URINALYSIS
Changes consistent with secondary disease conditions (e.g. leukocytosis with secondary bacterial infection).

## OTHER LABORATORY TESTS
N/A

## IMAGING
N/A

## DIAGNOSTIC PROCEDURES
Clinical signs are suggestive. Cytology and/or histology of lesions demonstrate large intracytoplasmic vacuolar inclusions (Bollinger bodies) that push the nucleus to the margin of the cell and contain small, round, pale eosinophilic inclusions consistent with pox infection. Molecular diagnostics (e.g. TaqMan PCR with sequencing) is appropriate for research projects or other cases where definitive diagnosis is necessary. Contour feathers have been shown to be a reliable source for viral DNA, reducing risk from biopsy in living animals, particularly small species. Viral isolation from diseased tissue or blood (in septicemic cases) can also be used for definitive diagnosis. Secondary infections are common, and lesions are often inflammatory; poxvirus infection appears associated with immunosuppression in some outbreaks. Serology may support exposure to the virus.

## PATHOLOGIC FINDINGS
Gross findings include lesions as noted above. In addition, intestinal thickening and splenic, liver, and pulmonary congestion may be noted. Histopathology changes in cutaneous pox include epidermal hyperplasia and hypertrophy. Large, granular eosinophilic inclusions are noted in epithelial cells above the basal layer. While inclusions are typically intracytoplasmic, in some infections, intranuclear inclusions have also been reported. Necrosis and secondary bacterial or fungal infection near the surface of the lesion is common. In the diphtheroid form, serous membranes have severe fibrinous inflammation and liver necrosis may be present. In the septicemic form, pulmonary changes such as edema and fibrinous pneumonitis develop.

# TREATMENT

## APPROPRIATE HEALTH CARE
There is no direct treatment for poxvirus. Management is based on appropriate supportive care in individual animals and population management strategies for flocks. Cutaneous lesions are often minor and self-limiting. If severe proliferation or secondary infection is present, standard treatments should be implemented. Crusts may be removed (e.g. moistened and slowly broken down, surgically debulked). Topical antimicrobials, systemic antibiotics and antifungals, analgesics, and anti-inflammatory medication may be indicated. Ocular medications may be appropriate if palpebral integrity is compromised. Diphtheroid cases may need hospitalization for intensive supportive care. If patients are admitted, care must be taken to prevent transmission to other in-hospital patients.

## NURSING CARE
If animals are eating and ambulating normally, little supportive care is needed with cutaneous disease. If lesions are severe and animals have been unable to eat or drink, fluid and nutrition support is appropriate. In diphtheroid and septicemic forms of the disease, oxygen therapy and more aggressive fluid and nutritional support may be indicated. Nebulizing may be considered in birds with severe respiratory compromise.

## ACTIVITY
N/A, except as appropriate for managing general condition.

## DIET
N/A, unless base diet is considered inappropriate for species.

## CLIENT EDUCATION
Clients should be instructed that poxviruses are long-lasting in the environment. Appropriate cleaning and other forms of environmental management (e.g. dust control) should be implemented. Pest control methods (e.g. mosquito reduction or netting, treatment for mites) should be reviewed. Enhanced biosecurity measures should be implemented (e.g. isolation of clinically affected and exposed birds, work with clinically affected birds last, separate tools for clinically affected birds). Vaccination for certain species should be discussed (e.g. domestic chicken, turkey, quail).

## SURGICAL CONSIDERATIONS
If lesions are significant, debridement or surgical removal may be appropriate.

# MEDICATIONS

## DRUG(S) OF CHOICE
There is no treatment for poxvirus but topical antimicrobials, systemic antibiotics and antifungals, analgesics, and anti-inflammatory medication may be indicated. Ocular medications may be appropriate if palpebral integrity is compromised.

## CONTRAINDICATIONS
N/A

## PRECAUTIONS
N/A

## POSSIBLE INTERACTIONS
N/A

## ALTERNATIVE DRUGS
N/A

# FOLLOW-UP

## PATIENT MONITORING
Typically, once lesions are healing, birds will recover. Follow-up schedules should be based on severity of clinical disease. Clinicians should discuss flock management options with owners.

## PREVENTION/AVOIDANCE
Prevention is primarily through maintaining appropriate environmental conditions, biosecurity, and management of insect vectors. Unlike many enveloped viruses, virions remain viable in the environment for longs periods of time and are resistant to disinfection. Contaminated perches, nest boxes, bedding, and other housing materials should be destroyed. Virions can be inactivated with 1% potassium hydroxide, 2% NaOH, 5% phenol, and steam, or exposure to 50°C for 30 minutes or 60°C for

8 minutes. Virkon® S (Lanxess, Baytown, TX) appears to be effective. Infected and exposed birds should be isolated. Vaccines for some strains are available (e.g. fowlpox) and may be appropriate. Many commercially produced chickens are vaccinated as juveniles. Protection is generally strain specific. The vaccine may not protect fully against some wild strains. Vaccination of clinically ill birds is not recommended; at the start of an outbreak, unaffected birds can be vaccinated for flock protection.

## POSSIBLE COMPLICATIONS
Complications from poxvirus infection are primarily related to secondary infections, as noted above. Permanent scarring (e.g. digit loss, palpebral anatomy) may develop in some cutaneous cases. *Poxviridae* may have oncogenic properties; skin tumors in Columbiformes and pulmonary tumors in canaries have been reported.

## EXPECTED COURSE AND PROGNOSIS
Prognosis for cutaneous form is often good. Diphtheroid and septicemic forms are often fatal.

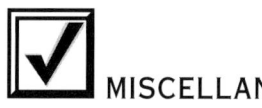 MISCELLANEOUS

## ASSOCIATED CONDITIONS
N/A

## AGE-RELATED FACTORS
N/A

## ZOONOTIC POTENTIAL
N/A

## FERTILITY/BREEDING
May reduce breeding success; disease in chicks may be more severe than in adults.

## SYNONYMS
N/A

## SEE ALSO
Aspergillosis
Candidiasis
Ectoparasites (Mites)
Ectoparasites (Ticks, Lice, Dipterans)
Herpesvirus (Columbid Herpesvirus 1 in Pigeons and Raptors)
Herpesvirus (Duck Viral Enteritis)
Herpesvirus (Passerine Birds)
Herpesvirus (Psittacid Herpesviruses)
Nutritional Imbalances
Oral Plaques
Papillomatosis
Pneumonia
Respiratory Distress
Trichomoniasis

## ABBREVIATIONS
PCR—polymerase chain reaction

## INTERNET RESOURCES
American Association of Zoo Veterinarians. Infectious Diseases Manual: https://www.aazv.org/page/754
Hyline International. (2019). *Vaccination Recommendations*. Technical Update: https://www.hyline.com/Upload/Resources/TU%20VACC%20ENG.pdf
International Committee on Taxonomy of Viruses. Subfamily *Chordopoxviridae*

*Genus: Aviooxvirus*: https://ictv.global/report/chapter/poxviridae/poxviridae/avipoxvirus

*Suggested Reading*
Baek, H.E., Bandivadekar, R.R., Pandit, P., et al. (2020). TaqMan quantitative real-time PCR for detecting Avipoxvirus DNA in various sample types from hummingbirds. *PLoS One* 15(6):e0230701.
Giotis, E.S., Skinner, M.A. (2019). Spotlight on avian pathology: Fowlpox virus. *Avian Pathology*, 48:87–90.
McInnes, C.J., Damon, I.K., Smith, G.L. et al. (2023). ICTV Virus Taxonomy Profile: Poxviridae 2023. *Journal of General Virology*, 104(5): https://doi.org/10.1099/jgv.0.001849.
Tripathy, D.N., Reed, W.M. (2020). Pox. In: *Disease of Poultry*, 14th edn., vol I. (ed. D.E. Swayne, M. Boulianne, C.M. Logue, et al.), 364–381. Hobkoken, NJ: Wiley & Sons, Inc.
van Riper C., III, Forrester, D.J. (2007). Avian pox. In: *Infectious Diseases of Wild Birds* (ed. N.J. Thomas, D.B. Hunter, C.T. Atkins), 131–176. Ames, IA: Blackwell.
Weli, S.C., Tryland, M. (2011). Avipoxiruses: Infection biology and their use as vaccine vectors. *Virology Journal*, 8:49.
Williams, R.A.J., Truchado, D.A., Benitez, L. (2021). A review on the prevalence of poxvirus disease in free-living and captive wild birds. *Microbiology Research*, 12(2):2.

**Authors**: Katharina B. Hagen, DMV, and Leigh Ann Clayton, DVM, DABVP (Avian, Reptile–Amphibian Practice), eMBA

P

# PROBLEM BEHAVIORS: AGGRESSION, BITING AND SCREAMING

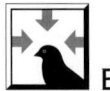 **BASICS**

## DEFINITION

There are different scientific levels of analysis relevant to understanding and solving behavior problems. Each level addresses different sources of influence and strategies for change. In this chapter, the behavioral level of analysis is presented, also known as behavior analysis. Behavior analysis is the scientific investigation of environmental influences on behavior. Applied behavior analysis (ABA) is the behavior-change technology based on this science.
The essential focus of ABA is learning (i.e. behavior change due to contact with the environment). The term "environment" includes all the stimuli, events, and conditions that the animal experiences, including the interactions between caregivers and their birds. As such, the appropriate unit of analysis in ABA is individual learner (bird), client (or other caregivers), and ever-changing environment. From the behavioral perspective, a problem behavior is defined as any activity that is the result of learning processes and occurs at a strength that is: (1) problematic to the client; (2) negatively impacts the bird's health and welfare; or (3) interferes with the bird's ability to live successfully in human care. Strength refers to any measurable characteristic of behavior (e.g. frequency, rate, duration, and intensity).

## PATHOPHYSIOLOGY

In this context, the problem behaviors of interest are neither a result nor a symptom of underlying pathophysiology. Rather, problem behaviors are the result of functionally related antecedents (events that occur before the behavior) and functionally related consequences (events that occur after the behavior). These correlates comprise the three-term contingency: antecedent–behavior–consequence (ABC). As behavior never occurs in the absence of antecedents and consequences, the three-term contingency is the smallest meaningful unit of behavior analysis. Antecedents signal the behavior–consequence contingency ahead and consequences provide the feedback about the adequacy of past behavior. Consequences are also the purpose for behaving, that is, that which we behave to gain or escape. For example, given too little to do (antecedent), many birds learn to scream (observable behavior), to gain attention (consequence). Given an imposing hand (antecedent), many birds learn to bite (observable behavior), to escape being touched or picked up (consequences). In both cases, it is reasonable

to predict that unless something changes, the birds will continue to scream and bite because doing so is purposive, neither willy-nilly nor the result of alleged character traits (e.g. vicious, neurotic). Biting and screaming persist because they control functional outcomes.

## SYSTEMS AFFECTED
Behavioral.

## GENETICS
At both the population level (evolutionary history) and individual level (personality), inherited behavioral tendencies influence and are influenced by learning outcomes. Like a Gordian knot, the co-influences of biology and the environment are inextricably intertwined. However, most reported problems with pet birds (e.g. screaming, biting, inactivity) have not been associated with genetic markers.

## INCIDENCE/PREVALENCE
No conclusive data are currently available. However, problem behaviors are commonly reported by clients and are likely the main reason that clients relinquish birds.

## GEOGRAPHIC DISTRIBUTION
Problem behaviors are ubiquitous.

## SIGNALMENT
**Species**: No conclusive data currently available.
**Mean age and range**: All.
**Predominant sex**: No conclusive data currently available.

## SIGNS

### General Comments
The behavior of interest is dependent on certain environmental conditions (i.e. predicted by specific antecedents and maintained by functional consequences). In discussions with veterinarians, clients may present behavior problems with hypothetical constructs and intangible labels such as vicious, aggressive, territorial, dominant, attention seeking, jealous, hormonal, and fearful, instead of describing what an animal does in certain conditions. Behavioral descriptions include observable responses such as screaming, biting, lunging, flying at people or other pets, chewing unapproved household items, and inactivity.

### Historical Findings
Insufficiencies in the environment account, at least partly, for most common problem behaviors. Changes in the environment can improve these problems and may ameliorate them entirely.

### Physical Examination Findings
Physical examination is often normal; comorbid medical problems are possible (e.g. poor skin and feather condition, overweight,

pododermatitis). Clinicians anecdotally report an increase in behavior problems as parrots mature from juvenile to adult.

## CAUSES
Problem behaviors are most often the result of general lack of knowledge about how behavior works, which translates to insufficient environmental arrangement and training skills. Specifically, clients inadvertently reinforce undesirable ("wrong") behaviors, create persistent undesirable behaviors with intermittent reinforcement, and insufficiently reinforce desired ("right") behaviors. Understanding the behavior ABCs is a powerful tool to reveal the ways in which functional misbehavior is shaped. By asking, "What sets the occasion for the behavior?" and, "What does the bird get or get out of (or away from) by doing the behavior?" clinicians and clients can identify antecedents that predict the behavior and consequences that maintain the behavior. For example, lunging and biting often occur when a hand approaches the bird and are maintained by escape of the aversive stimuli (e.g. the clients, the approaching hand, being touched, being picked up); screaming often occurs when there is limited social interaction and maintained by intermittent attention (good or bad, obvious or subtle), and chewing and inactivity are often the result of a lack of stimulus diversity or experience using enrichment devices.

## RISK FACTORS
Few clients have had the opportunity to learn about the ABCs of behavior or to develop skills in deliberate application of positive reinforcement for developing desired behaviors. Clinicians can review basic concepts with clients and support them in building positive reinforcement training. Behavior discussions and analysis can be integrated into annual exams. By identifying the antecedents to and consequences of the undesirable behavior, clinicians and clients can start to predict and resolve problematic behavior. Additionally, desired behavior can be identified and supported through appropriate antecedent arrangement and consequence delivery (positive reinforcement). Each case needs to be evaluated independently. However, some patterns are common. For example, lunging or biting (aggression) may be associated with a history of a client forcing or coercing the parrot to come to them or be near them. This is often associated with stepping onto a hand to control the bird's movement, bring it close to people, and/or touch the bird. If, as the hand approaches, behavior consistent with discomfort (or a "no, not now" request from the bird) is ignored and the bird is forced to

step up, biting may develop. After a bite, the hand is removed, and the bird avoids the step up or close contact with the person. To address this, the client can remove their hand at a much earlier signal from the bird (such as walking or leaning away). The client can focus on arranging the environment to avoid the need to step up (such as creating paths for the bird to use) and/or retraining step up using positive reinforcement. Deliberately training behavior involves shaping the behavior, reinforcing gradual steps toward the desired behavior.

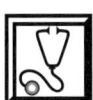

## DIAGNOSIS

### DIFFERENTIAL DIAGNOSIS
Physical and ethological correlates for problem behavior should be considered. However, many clients and veterinarians underestimate learning as the reason for undesirable behavior that has become problematic. A detailed evaluation of the antecedents and consequences of specific undesirable behaviors are generally rewarding for addressing the behavior and training more desirable behaviors.

### CBC/BIOCHEMISTRY/URINALYSIS
N/A

### OTHER LABORATORY TESTS
N/A

### IMAGING
N/A

### DIAGNOSTIC PROCEDURES
The diagnostic protocol in the ABA model is centered on identifying the ways in which antecedents set the occasion for the behavior and consequences reinforce or punish the behavior, thereby increasing or decreasing the probability of the behavior occurring again. The following key questions facilitate diagnostic ABCs: (1) What does the behavior look like? Use observable descriptions not hypothetical constructs or intangible labels. (2) What antecedent conditions predict when the behavior will occur? Consider when the behavior is most likely. (3) What is the immediate consequence of the behavior? Consider what change in the environment occurs immediately following the behavior. (4) Will the behavior likely increase (maintain) or decrease if nothing changes? Additional information may be obtained by also asking, "Under what conditions does the bird not exhibit the behavior, that is, when is the bird successful?" In all cases, it is important to remember that the undesirable (to the client) behavior has function for the bird. If there are multiple undesirable behaviors identified, the functional

assessment (and then treatment plan) is completed for each behavior. If it helps the client, it can be useful to complete a functional assessment for multiple undesirable behaviors at one time. However, it is typical for clients and clinicians to focus on treating one undesirable behavior at a time.

### PATHOLOGIC FINDINGS
N/A

## TREATMENT

### APPROPRIATE HEALTH CARE
An effective treatment protocol requires a direct link between diagnosis and treatment (Table 1). Once the ABCs are identified, treatment consists of systematically redesigning the environment to replace the problem behavior with an existing alternative and to teach new skills. For each problem behavior, answering the following questions will inform the treatment plan: (1) What acceptable alternative behavior can the bird do to get the same functional outcome? As an example, instead of biting to remove your hand from the cage, the parrot could lean back. This allows the bird an alternative behavior (leaning back) to get the same functional outcome (hand leaving cage) instead of biting. (2) What new skill do you (the client) want the bird to learn? As an example, the parrot could step onto a transport stick (instead of the client's hand/arm) to move around the home. This allows the bird to develop a behavior that can be important for its care. Essential strategies include differential selection of alternative or incompatible behavior, whereby reinforcers are contingently delivered for acceptable, desired behaviors. But a behavior cannot be reinforced until it occurs. This is problematic for new behaviors. Waiting for the complete, desired behavior to occur and capturing it with reinforcement is not reliable, and the desired behavior may not happen at all. Shaping (differential reinforcement of successive approximations) is the solution to this challenge. It is the procedure of reinforcing a graduated sequence of subtle changes toward the final behavior, starting with the closest response the bird already does. Shaping starts by reinforcing the first approximation every time it is offered, until it is performed without hesitation. Next, an even closer approximation is reinforced, at which time reinforcement for the first approximation is withheld. Once the second approximation is performed without hesitation, an even closer approximation is reinforced while withholding reinforcement

for all previous approximations. In this way, the criterion for reinforcement is gradually shifted, incrementally closer and closer to the target behavior. Finally, every instance of the target behavior is reinforced. If the bird experiences difficulty at any criterion, the trainer can back up and repeat the previous successful step, or the trainer can reinforce even smaller approximations. As an example, to shape a step up behavior, the approximations might look like the following: The bird looks at the perch; the bird leans toward the perch; the bird steps toward the perch; the bird lifts a foot and touches the perch; the bird touches the perch and lean its weight onto the foot; the bird lifts its other foot toward the perch; the bird holds the perch with both feet. At that point, longer duration, movement of perch, and additional variables could be added. Note that, the perch is held far enough away that the bird must move toward it. This creates a clear choice to engage with the client and this choice is easy for the client to see. This distance and ability to say "no" or "yes" is an important component of creating clarity in communication between client and bird. Data should be taken to ensure that the intervention is heading in the right direction and trigger revisions to the plan if it is not progressing. Training new behavior is a skill, and seeking support of a trained professional who is accomplished at positive reinforcement and working with parrots can be useful to support clients.

### NURSING CARE
N/A

### ACTIVITY
N/A

### DIET
If the bird is on an inappropriate diet for the species, dietary modification should be implemented as part of a holistic wellness program. Ensuring that diets are provided in a manner that supports natural time budgets for foraging activity is an important component to providing basic care and good welfare. Parrot species in the wild spend hours foraging for food. Reserving favored food items for positive reinforcement training can be useful in maintaining and training behavior.

### CLIENT EDUCATION
Educating clients and providing ongoing support are critical to effective intervention. As clients are responsible for implementing the plan, it must be created in collaboration with them.

### SURGICAL CONSIDERATIONS
N/A

P

## PROBLEM BEHAVIORS: AGGRESSION, BITING AND SCREAMING (CONTINUED)

**Table 1**

| Examples of how to use key questions to prompt functional evaluation of problem behavior and identify treatment options. | | |
| --- | --- | --- |
| *Question* | *Purpose of Question* | *Example* |
| What does the behavior look like? | Describe it in observable (operational) terms, without labels. | Typical label: Behavior A—the bird is aggressive. Behavior B—the bird is territorial. |
| | | Operationalized behaviors: Behavior A—the bird bites hands. Behavior B—the bird lunges and bites other bird's leg. |
| What conditions predict when the behavior will occur? | Antecedent evaluation. Identify the relevant environmental stimuli that cue or set the stage for the behavior. | Behavior A happens when the bird is in the cage, the client's hand is within 6 in. |
| | | Behavior B happens when both birds are on the play-gym and food is in one bowl. |
| What does the bird get or get away from by doing the behavior? | Consequence evaluation. Identify the relevant environmental stimuli that are reinforcing (maintaining) the behavior. | After behavior A happens, the hand is pulled away and the bird is not touched. |
| | | After behavior B happens, the other bird leaves the area and the bird has access to the food. |
| Under what conditions does the bird not exhibit the behavior? | Identify the environment when the bird is most successful. This step helps clients realize that the bird is successful under certain conditions. | Behavior A is least likely to happen when the bird is on a table or the hand is still and bird has walked toward the hand. |
| | | Behavior B is least likely to happen when food is put in multiple food bowls on the play-gym or there is no food present. |
| What do you want the bird to do instead? | Treatment. Identify another behavior the bird can do in place of the problem behavior for the same outcomes. | For behavior A, the bird can lean away to remove hand. The bird can learn with shaping to step up for valued reinforcers. |
| | | For behavior B, the birds can eat from separate bowls once two bowls are installed, or food can be omitted from the play area. |

## MEDICATIONS

### DRUG(S) OF CHOICE

If abnormal neurophysiology is suspected based on lack of response to appropriate plans, medication such as selective serotonin reuptake inhibitors (e.g. fluoxetine), tricyclic antidepressants (e.g. clomipramine) and benzodiazepines (e.g. diazepam) may be considered. It is inappropriate to expect medication to compensate for a poor environment. Reproductive cycles may exacerbate behavior problems and temporary administration of medications that reduce reproductive hormones, such as GnRH agonists (e.g. leuprolide acetate for depot suspension), may be appropriate as part of a comprehensive management strategy.

### CONTRAINDICATIONS
N/A

### PRECAUTIONS
N/A

### POSSIBLE INTERACTIONS
N/A

### ALTERNATIVE DRUGS
N/A

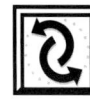

## FOLLOW-UP

### PATIENT MONITORING

Varies with the case. A single meeting is often sufficient to develop a plan that clients can implement. Routine (typically weekly) communication may help support the clients through the initial implementation phase. Behavior discussions should be part of annual wellness exams.

### PREVENTION/AVOIDANCE

It is possible to build desirable behavior repertoires deliberately and proactively in birds. Clinicians can work with clients to understand how to use ABA technology to develop basic skills in parrots, such as step up and create enriching environments. They can prepare clients with juvenile parrots for common changes that occur as the bird matures. Clients can set up the home environment to make the "right" behaviors more likely through thoughtful antecedent arrangement and thoughtful delivery of valuable outcomes. Clients can support their bird's welfare by ensuring the

P

bird's behavior has meaning through empowerment, choices, and environments rich with stimulus diversity. Most parrots are wild animals, they are not domesticated. Deliberate, thoughtful arrangement of the environment, including training skills, is important for the bird's welfare. Clinicians can incorporate behavioral questions into annual wellness exams and be part of an integrated care group if undesirable behaviors are developing. They may also have a role in supporting clients in training husbandry behaviors such as target training, moving from one area to another, stepping up onto a perch, allowing the body to be touched, nail trimming, holding wings out and up, and transportation training. Clinicians can partner with an educated behavior consultant experienced in working with companion parrots and their caregivers.

## POSSIBLE COMPLICATIONS

Fluent behavior can be suppressed but not eliminated. Thus, problem behaviors can recover because of inadvertent reinforcement or when the context cues in which the behavior was learned reappear. Care must be taken to avoid either event. The treatment plan should be faithfully implemented again if this occurs.
When force and coercion is a lifestyle, rather than a very occasional event, animals have too little control over their own outcomes. This lack of empowerment is correlated with physiologic changes consistent with lower immunity and higher inflammatory parameters and suboptimal welfare. Clients should be approached with empathy and support. Typically, client intentions are well meaning. They lack the knowledge and support to effectively implement positive reinforcement training. The full ramifications of understanding ABC can be upsetting to some clients, and the clinician can support them by focusing on opportunities and positive interactions.

## EXPECTED COURSE AND PROGNOSIS

A well-designed intervention typically produces initial responsiveness quickly, within a week. However, the longer the problem behavior has been rehearsed the longer it may take to change. Also, behavior problems can become more persistent with repeated failed interventions.

 MISCELLANEOUS

### ASSOCIATED CONDITIONS
N/A

### AGE-RELATED FACTORS
N/A

### ZOONOTIC POTENTIAL
N/A

### FERTILITY/BREEDING
N/A

### SYNONYMS
Some common labels used with pet parrots that bite or scream include viscous, aggressive, hormonal, territorial, dominant, and fearful.

### SEE ALSO
Feather-Damaging and Self-Injurious Behavior

### ABBREVIATIONS
ABA—applied behavior analysis
ABC—antecedent–behavior–consequence
GnRH—gonadotropin-releasing hormone

### INTERNET RESOURCES
Articles and examples of using applied behavior analysis with parrots and other animals: Behavior Works (Susan Friedman's site); behaviorworks.org
Support for enrichment, behavior consultation, and training behaviors with parrots: The Gabriel Foundation; thegabrielfoundation.org/behavior-consultations

Articles and examples of using applied behavior analysis with birds and other animals: Natural Encounters Inc.; naturalencounters.com
Articles and examples of positive reinforcement training with many species, find interested trainers in your area: Karen Pryor's Clicker Training; clickertraining.com
Articles and examples of positive reinforcement training, find interested trainers in your areas: International Association of Animal Behavior; https://iaabc.org

*Suggested Reading*
Clayton, L.A., Friedman, S.G., Evans, L.A. (2012). Management of specific and excessive posturing behavior in a hyacinth macaw (*Anodorhynchus hyacinthinus*) by using applied behavior analysis. *Journal of Avian Medicine and Surgery*, 26:107–110.
Friedman, S.G. (2007). A framework for solving behavior problems: Functional assessment and intervention planning. *Journal of Exotic Pet Medicine*, 16:6–10.
Friedman, S.G., Haug, L.I. (2010). From parrots to pigs to pythons: Universal principles and procedures of learning. In: *Behavior of Exotic Pets* (ed. V.V. Tynes), 190–205. Chichester, UK: Wiley.
Friedman, S.G., Edling, T.M., Cheney, C.D. (2006). Concepts in behavior: Section I. In: *Clinical Avian Medicine* (ed. G.J. Harrison, T.L. Lightfoot), Vol. I, 46–59. Palm Beach, FL: Spix Publishing.
Heidenreich, B. (2005). *The Parrot Problem Solver: Finding solutions to aggressive behavior.* Neptune City, NJ: TFH Publications.
Stelow, E. (2021). Avian behavior consultation for exotic pet practitioners. *Veterinary Clinics of North America: Exotic Animal Practice*, 24(1):103–117.
**Authors**: Leigh Ann Clayton, DVM, DABVP (Avian Practice, Reptile–Amphibian Practice), and Susan G. Friedman, PhD

 **Client Education Handout available online**

P

# REGURGITATION AND VOMITING

## BASICS

### DEFINITION
Regurgitation is the retrograde expulsion of ingesta from the esophagus, including the crop. Vomiting is the retrograde expulsion of ingesta from the proventriculus, ventriculus, or intestine. Because of the anatomic arrangement of the ventriculus, vomiting from the intestine is rare in birds. Both vomiting and regurgitation are usually active processes in birds. The rule that regurgitation occurs passively and vomiting is active is not valid in birds. The origin of the expelled ingesta can be determined based on the pH. The pH of the proventriculus should be very acidic, and the pH of the crop and esophagus should be close to neutral.

### PATHOPHYSIOLOGY
Following stimulation of the GI tract, vestibular system, or central nervous system, signals are sent to the GI tract and a coordinated contraction of the smooth and skeletal muscles propel ingesta back into and subsequently out of the mouth.

### SYSTEMS AFFECTED
GI; the respiratory system may develop aspiration pneumonia or rhinitis.

### GENETICS
There does not appear to be a genetic component.

### INCIDENCE/PREVALENCE
Regurgitation and vomiting are common clinical signs.

### GEOGRAPHIC DISTRIBUTION
N/A

### SIGNALMENT
**Species**: These signs can occur in birds of any species, age, or sex.
**Mean age and range**: None.
**Predominant sex**: Behavioral regurgitation is somewhat more common in male birds.

### SIGNS
#### General Comments
These are clinical signs rather than a disease. However some findings are common.

#### Historical Findings
Owners may witness the expulsion of material from the mouth. Undigested, mucus-coated food may be found in the enclosure.

#### Physical Examination Findings
Dried food or mucus may be matting the feathers of the head (often referred to in lay press as head sweating). Sour or fetid breath odor can occur, especially when there is infection in the crop. Distended, fluctuant, or thickened crop can be noted during examination.

## CAUSES
Regurgitation and vomiting can be behavioral conditions, usually related to misplaced courtship or sexual behavior toward objects or people. Normal casting behavior in raptors involves vomiting up the indigestible components of their prey. The casts are formed in the ventriculus. Crop or esophageal disorders: Bacterial, yeast, or *Trichomonas* infections are common in the crop. Bacterial infections often result in sour, mucous exudate in the crop. Yeast (*Candida* spp.) and *Trichomonas* infections often cause thickened crop walls. Foreign bodies in the crop are usually quite large or they will pass down to the ventriculus. They are generally readily palpable. Ingluvioliths are usually urate stones and result from coprophagia. They are readily palpable on examination. Burns or fistulae occur commonly in handfed baby birds from overheated or unevenly heated formula. These birds may have severe infections. Proventricular or ventricular diseases: Infectious—ABV, PDD, *Macrorhabdus ornithogaster*, *Candida* spp., *Cryptosporidium* spp. Other parasites. *Mycobacterium* spp. Foreign bodies, including heavy metals, usually will be trapped in the ventriculus. The outflow is particle size dependent. Heavy metals have the additional risk of inhibiting motility and eroding the mucosa. Neoplasia in the GI tract occurs most commonly at the isthmus between the proventriculus and ventriculus. Most commonly, the birds die from rupture and subsequent hemorrhage of the mass. Ulcers can occur in the stomach or intestine. *Macrorhabdus* infection is a major cause in small species. Stress, NSAIDs, and heavy metals are risk factors for any species. Koilin dysplasia is a rare condition, but can result in obstruction of the ventricular outflow. Obstructive conditions of the GI tract: Uncommon. The ventriculus strains out most foreign bodies before they reach the intestine. When they do occur, they are severe and acute. Intussusception occasionally occurs. Motion sickness occurs in many birds. Sometimes there is a significant stress component involved. The birds are generally healthy otherwise. Extreme polydipsia can result in regurgitation, especially if the bird is handled. The overfilled, distended crop readily refluxes the contents. Iatrogenic (drugs, anesthetics) regurgitation is relatively common. Macaws appear particularly prone to this condition.

## RISK FACTORS
Social and imprinting factors can affect behavioral regurgitation. Poor sanitation of environment, water, and food can result in bacterial overgrowth and infection of the upper GI tract. Immunosuppression or immunologic immaturity can allow infections to take hold more easily. Exposure to

infectious agents is necessary for primary pathogens to affect the bird. Some, such as ABV, have very long incubation periods. Access to foreign material is a risk factor for birds with a tendency to consume them.

## DIAGNOSIS

### DIFFERENTIAL DIAGNOSIS
Regurgitation and vomiting are signs. Differentials include upper GI diseases and behavioral alterations.

### CBC/BIOCHEMISTRY/URINALYSIS
There are no specific changes peculiar to this clinical sign. Any changes very much depend on the specific cause and the severity of the disease. Infectious causes of vomiting and regurgitation may show inflammatory responses on CBC. Electrolyte alterations may occasionally occur. If severe, biochemical alterations may occur due to catabolic effects.

### OTHER LABORATORY TESTS
Cytology, culture, molecular diagnostics from fecal, crop or gastric (proventricular, or ventricular) samples can help identify infections. Special stains may be needed to identify some organisms. Acid-fast stains are useful for identifying *Cryptosporidium* or *Mycobacterium* spp. Fecal flotation and direct (wet mount) examination should be used to help identify parasites. Direct examination also allows visualization of *M. ornithogaster*. *Macrorhabdus* PCR provides more sensitive screening for this gastric yeast. ABV PCR may have some utility; however, this should be interpreted carefully. Not all infected birds test positively, and many asymptomatic birds test positively. Testing for antiganglioside antibodies is controversial, but could provide additional information on PDD status.

### IMAGING
Radiography, possibly including positive contrast can help determine if there is gastric or intestinal involvement. Fluoroscopy with contrast can be useful to determine motility. CT, with or without contrast provides superior images of the gastrointestinal tract. Ultrasound may be helpful for detecting some conditions.

### DIAGNOSTIC PROCEDURES
Testing the pH of the expelled material can help to distinguish between vomiting and regurgitation. Crop biopsy with histopathology is still the most definitive diagnostic test for PDD. A full-thickness biopsy, incorporating visible vessels (and the associated but difficult to see nerves) is needed. However, this test has low sensitivity and is invasive. Endoscope-assisted gastric lavage can be used to inspect the lining of the stomach. This is often done in conjunction

with the crop biopsy, using the crop incision as an access point to the coelomic esophagus. Endoscopy of the crop, proventriculus, or ventriculus may be indicated in some cases. Coelomic endoscopy may be indicated in other cases.

### PATHOLOGIC FINDINGS
Findings are highly variable and depend on the specific cause of the vomiting or regurgitation. Lymphoplasmacytic ganglioneuritis is the key pathologic finding of PDD.

 **TREATMENT**

### APPROPRIATE HEALTH CARE
Treatment of identified cause of the problem is necessary to resolve the problem long term. Hospitalization may be required during the initial phase of treatment.

### NURSING CARE
Fluid and nutritional support is needed. Nutritional support may be difficult to achieve unless the regurgitation or vomiting can be controlled. Inhibition of vomiting and regurgitation using antiemetic drugs is indicated.

### ACTIVITY
No activity restrictions should be needed, unless required by fluid lines or other supportive care. Patients with motion sickness may need premedication before traveling.

### DIET
Prolonged fasting is not practical in most birds. A very bland, easily digested diet should be given. Gavage feeding may be required if the patient is anorectic. If the patient is severely polydipsic, water may have to be restricted or offered intermittently.

### CLIENT EDUCATION
Client education will depend on the specific diagnosis.

### SURGICAL CONSIDERATIONS
Surgery or endoscopy may be indicated for removal of foreign material from the GI tract. Crop biopsy is indicated for definitive diagnosis of PDD.

 **MEDICATIONS**

### DRUG(S) OF CHOICE
Maropitant, ondansetron, metoclopramide may be used as antiemetics. Appropriate antimicrobial therapy should be used to treat any infections identified. Celecoxib, robenicoxib, or other COX-2 selective drug should be used to control inflammation for ABV infections. Sucralfate or histamine-2 blockers should

be used if endoscopy, surgery, or gastric bleeding occurs.

### CONTRAINDICATIONS
None.

### PRECAUTIONS
Drugs that have any GI adverse effects may complicate monitoring of the patient's progress.

### POSSIBLE INTERACTIONS
None.

### ALTERNATIVE DRUGS
N/A

 **FOLLOW-UP**

### PATIENT MONITORING
The frequency and severity of vomiting or regurgitation should be monitored during the course of therapy. Other monitoring depends on the specific diagnosis and any complications encountered during the course of the disease. Abnormal findings on the initial workup should be followed until they reach normal levels.

### PREVENTION/AVOIDANCE
Dependent on the specific etiology. Protection from exposure to infectious disease, access to foreign objects and toxins are the main preventative measures.

### POSSIBLE COMPLICATIONS
Dehydration and weight loss are the primary concerns for birds with regurgitation and vomiting. Aspiration pneumonia or aspiration rhinitis may occur if the regurgitated material is inhaled or extends into the choana. The various causes of this sign have their own potential complications. ABV often results in neurologic signs. *Macrorhabdus* infection often results in gastric bleeding and may predispose to gastric neoplasia.

### EXPECTED COURSE AND PROGNOSIS
The prognosis is highly dependent on the underlying cause of the problem. Prognosis is excellent for behavioral regurgitation and motion sickness. Prognosis is good for simple upper GI infections. Prognosis is fair for ulcers, *Macrorhabdus* infections, and foreign bodies. Prognosis is guarded to poor for ABV, cryptosporidiosis, and koilin dysplasia. Prognosis is grave for neoplasia.

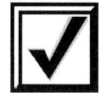 **MISCELLANEOUS**

### ASSOCIATED CONDITIONS
N/A

### AGE-RELATED FACTORS
N/A

### ZOONOTIC POTENTIAL
Most etiologies of vomiting and regurgitation have no zoonotic potential.

### FERTILITY/BREEDING
N/A

### SYNONYMS
N/A

### SEE ALSO
Aspiration Pneumonia
Candidiasis
Cryptosporidiosis
Dehydration
Emaciation
Enteritis and Gastritis
Foreign Bodies (Gastrointestinal)
Ileus (Functional Gastrointestinal, Crop Stasis)
*Macrorhabdus ornithogaster*
Polydipsia
Rhinitis and Sinusitis
Sick-Bird Syndrome
Appendix 8, Algorithm 3: Regurgitation/Vomiting

### ABBREVIATIONS
ABV—avian bornavirus
CBC—complete blood count
COX—cyclooxygenase
CT—computed tomography
GI—gastrointestinal
NSAIDs—non-steroidal anti-inflammatory drugs
PCR—polymerase chain reaction
PDD—proventricular dilatation disease

### INTERNET RESOURCES
N/A

*Suggested Reading*
Welle KR. (2016). Gastrointestinal system. In: *Current Therapy in Exotic Pet Practice* (ed. M.A. Mitchell, T.N. Tully Jr.), 229–276. St. Louis MO, Elsevier.
Denbow, D.M. (2015). Gastrointestinal anatomy and physiology. In: *Sturkie's Avian Physiology*, 6th edn. (ed. G.C. Whittow), 337–366. San Diego, CA: Academic Press.
Fudge, A.M. (2000). Avian liver and gastrointestinal testing In: *Laboratory Medicine: Avian and Exotic Pets*, 47–55. Philadelphia, PA: Saunders.
Girling, S. (2004). Diseases of the digestive tract of psittacine birds. *In Practice*, 26:146–153.
Hadley, T.L. (2005). Disorders of the psittacine gastrointestinal tract. *Veterinary Clinics of North America: Exotic Animal Practice*, 8:329–349.
**Author:** Kenneth R. Welle, DVM, DABVP (Avian)

 **Client Education Handout available online**

**R**

# RENAL DISEASES

## BASICS

### DEFINITION
Renal disease describes any disorder affecting the kidneys. Renal failure is end-stage renal disease severe enough to negatively impact renal function.

### PATHOPHYSIOLOGY
As renal tissue loses function, the remaining nephrons initially increase their performance as a functional adaptation; however, a significant loss of renal tissue reduces GFR. This cumulative loss of nephrons with subsequent loss of renal function can be a slow, insidious process (chronic renal failure) or rapid (acute kidney injury). Renal disease can be caused by anything that compromises renal perfusion (prerenal), structure and function of the nephrons (primary renal disease), or anything that prevents normal renal excretion (postrenal disease).

### SYSTEMS AFFECTED
**Nervous**: Renomegaly can cause compression or impingement on the branches of the lumbosacral plexus that pass through or near the kidneys.
**GI**: Ceca, rectum, cloaca play a role in reabsorption of ureteral water.
**Cardiopulmonary**: Affected when fluid overload occurs.
**Musculoskeletal**: Rare reports of invasion into the synsacrum or secondary osteopenia of long bones in renal tumor case reports. Articular gout.
**Behavioral**: Rare feather-destructive behavior/self-mutilation overlying the synsacrum.

### GENETICS
Genetic problems presumably play a role in some conditions like renal neoplasia in budgerigars (*Melopsittacus undulatus*). Genes expressing multidrug resistance protein have also been identified in African white-backed vultures (*Gyps africanus*), which may explain their sensitivity to diclofenac.

### INCIDENCE/PREVALENCE
Based on retrospective avian pathology studies, renal disease is relatively common in birds.

### GEOGRAPHIC DISTRIBUTION
N/A

### SIGNALMENT
**Species**: Renal disease can be seen in any avian species; reported conditions include the following. Diclofenac nephrotoxicity (Old World *Gyps* vultures). Primary renal tumors (budgerigars). Renal amyloidosis (captive waterfowl, shorebirds, gulls). Renal parasites (waterfowl, marine birds). Urolithiasis (poultry layers).

**Mean age and range**: Juvenile birds: Vitamin $D_3$ toxicosis, excess dietary calcium (psittacine chicks, pigeons), renal coccidiosis (aquatic birds), "perirenal hemorrhage syndrome" (turkey poults), urolithiasis (pullets). Adult birds: Primary renal tumors (young to middle-aged adult budgerigars).
**Predominant sex**: Urolithiasis in hens.

### SIGNS
#### General Comments
Appreciable changes in urinary output are uncommon, but polyuria, anuria, oliguria, or even stranguria and hematuria can be observed. Although many clinical signs are similar to those seen in mammals, there are also signs of renal disease unique to birds—unilateral or bilateral ataxia, lameness, neurologic deficits, paralysis secondary to direct compression or impingement on the branches of the lumbosacral plexus. Constipation due to compression of the rectum.

#### Historical Findings
Nonspecific signs of illness include lethargy, anorexia, generalized weakness. Lameness, paresis, or paralysis with no history of trauma. Change in droppings—volume, color of urine or urates, diarrhea. Regurgitation or vomiting. Inadequate husbandry—nutritional imbalances, poor sanitation. In addition to signs of nephritis, infectious bronchitis virus is characterized by respiratory signs in broilers and decreased egg production, poor egg quality in layers.

#### Physical Examination Findings
**Visual examination**: The affected leg may be held feebly, resting the plantar surface of the tarsometatarsus on the perch or cage floor. Dyspnea may be observed secondary to coelomic distension, ascites. Change in droppings volume or color of urine and/or urates.
**Hands-on examination**: Evidence of weight loss, emaciation (renal lipidosis can be seen in obese birds with hepatic lipidosis). Evidence of dehydration. Crop stasis. Coelomic distention due to a mass lesion, renomegaly, and/or ascites. In larger birds like raptors, the caudal renal division can be palpated with a lubricated gloved finger inserted into the cloaca. Compare reflexes and sensation in birds with evidence of ataxia or lameness. Feather-destructive behavior, self-mutilation over the synsacrum. Evidence of gout in joints.

### CAUSES
**Degenerative**: Age-related end-stage kidney disease is rare in birds. Urate nephrosis.
**Anatomic**: Anomalous inherited defects of the urinary tract are rare. Renal agenesis is most frequently described. Dilated ureter, remnant ureters. Renal aplasia or hypoplasia

are often incidental findings due to compensation by remaining kidney tissue. Solitary or multiple renal cysts.
**Metabolic**: Dehydration—urate nephrosis. Diabetes mellitus. Lipidosis.
**Neoplasia**: Renal carcinoma is the most common tumor of the avian kidney. Other reported renal tumors include renal adenoma, nephroblastoma, cystadenoma, fibrosarcoma, embryonal nephroma. Metastasis to the kidney is uncommon but reports have included multicentric lymphoma/leukemia, seminoma, hemangiosarcoma, bronchial adenocarcinoma, pancreatic adenocarcinoma, fibroma, fibrosarcoma, humeral air sac neoplasm, melanoma, and mast cell tumor.
**Nutrition**: Excess dietary calcium. Excess dietary vitamin $D_3$. Excess dietary protein (but only under specific conditions). Low dietary protein: Renal lipidosis has been associated with starvation, low-protein diets, and biotin deficiency. Biotin deficiency is also a possible cause of fatty liver and kidney disease in turkeys. Vitamin A deficiency—squamous metaplasia can lead to ureteral obstruction and post-renal failure. High cholesterol diets. Pyridoxine hydrochloride (vitamin $B_6$) toxicosis—acute tubular necrosis in falcons.
**Infection**: Bacterial nephritis. Most cases are associated with multisystemic disease or sepsis. Less commonly, nephritis can develop secondary to infection ascending from the cloaca or colon. Gram-negative bacteria: Enterobacteriaceae: *E. coli*, *Klebsiella*, *Salmonella* spp., *Yersinia* spp., *Proteus*, *Pseudomonas*, *Pasteurella multocida*, *Brachyspira alvinipulli*. Gram-positive bacteria: *Staphylococcus* spp., *Streptococcus* spp. (finches, canaries). *Listeria* spp. *Erysiplelothrix rhusiopathatiae* (Coturnix quail). *Mycobacterium* spp. *Chlamydia psittaci*. Viruses known to infect the kidneys are generally part of systemic infection, and include: Adenovirus—can cause renomegaly, but usually an incidental finding, Astrovirus (geese, ducks, chickens), bornavirus, coronavirus, enterovirus, herpesvirus (Marek's disease, psittacid herpesvirus), infectious bronchitis virus, influenza virus, nephritis virus, Newcastle disease virus, orthovirus, paramyxovirus (pigeons), polyomavirus—avian polyomavirus (best known virus affecting kidneys of caged birds), goose hemorrhagic polyomavirus, poxvirus, reovirus, reticuloendotheliosis virus, retrovirus (avian leukosis/lymphoid leukosis), togavirus—West Nile virus, Eastern/Western equine encephalitis viruses. Fungal nephritis is relatively uncommon. Can result from local extension of fungal air sacculitis (*Aspergillus* spp.) or less commonly via fungal thrombosis. *Penicillium chrysogenum*, *Cryptococcus neoformans* (part of systemic

disease). Parasites: Renal coccidiosis (*Eimeria* spp., *Isospora* spp.) in juvenile waterfowl, less commonly raptors. Renal trematodes, cestodes (scattered reports in pigeons, owls, passerines, waterfowl, and a variety of other species). Protozoa: rare reports of *Cryptosporidium* spp., *Encephalitozoon*, Microspiridia (lovebirds, particularly PBFD-positive), sarcocystis (rare to sporadic cases). Hemoparasites: *Plasmodium* (avian malaria), *Leukocytozoon* spp., and *Hemoproteus* spp. have been associated with lymphoplasmacytic inflammation in renal tissue.

**Inflammation**: Amyloidosis: relatively uncommon disease except in gyrfalcons and flamingos, process associated with chronic, systemic inflammatory conditions (e.g., pododermatitis, mycobacteriosis). Interstitial nephritis.

**Immune**: Hemoglobinuric nephrosis is a rare occurrence in caged birds with immune-mediated hemolytic anemia caused by heavy-metal exposure, crude oil ingestion, or garlic ingestion. Immune complex disease (glomerulonephrosis) is an uncommon, often mild to moderate finding at necropsy. Affected birds have a concurrent inflammatory or infectious disease.

**Idiopathic**: Glomerular lipidosis. Fatty liver and kidney syndrome has been described in merlins in the UK. Although significant fatty changes are seen histologically in the kidneys, birds do not exhibit signs of renal disease. Sudden death syndrome or "perirenal hemorrhage syndrome" is the main cause of acute death in large turkey flocks from 8–4 weeks of age.

**Toxic exposure**: Avicide (3-chloro-p-toluidine). Ethylene glycol. Heavy metals—lead, zinc (caged birds, raptors, waterfowl), arsenic, mercury (fish-eating aquatic birds), cadmium. Mycotoxins can contaminate formulated feeds and grains, particularly corn. Nephrotoxic medications. Allopurinol. Antimicrobials: Aminoglycosides, sulphonamides, florfenicol, fenbendazole. Intravenous contrast media. NSAIDs. Birds display a highly variable response to NSAIDs possibly because of differences in protein binding. Nephrotoxicity has been reported with carprofen in the Harris hawk (*Parabuteo unicinctus*), northern saw-whet owl (*Aegolius acadicus*), Maribou stork (*Leptoptilos crumeniferus*). Diclofenac in Old World vultures (*Gyps* spp.), Japanese quail (*Coturnix japonica*), mynah birds (Sturnidae), pigeons (*Columba livia*), broiler chickens. Flunixin meglumine in flamingos, cranes, northern bobwhite quail (*Colinus virginianus*), eiders (*Somateria spectabilis*, *Somateria fischeri*). Ketoprofen in eiders, broiler chickens. Meloxicam in Rhode Island red hens (*Gallus gallus domesticus*).

Historically, meloxicam has been considered one of the safer NSAIDs based on studies in Hispaniolan Amazon parrots (*Amazona ventralis*), gray parrots (*Psittacus erithacus*), budgerigars, zebra finches (*Taeniopygia guttata*), pigeons, Japanese quail, and American kestrels (*Falco sparverius*). Acetaminophen. Oxalate—ingestion of plants containing toxic levels (i.e. rhubarb leaves). Rodenticides (vitamin D$_3$ analogs). Salt toxicosis. Crude oil.

**Traumatic**: Myoglobinuric nephrosis. Capture myopathy. Severe crush injury (wild birds, poultry, birds attacked by dogs or foxes). Muscle necrosis (ostrich unable to stand for any length of time). Urolithiasis (poultry), ureterolithiasis (reported once in a double yellow-headed Amazon, *Amazona oratrix*) partially or completely obstruct the ureters. The underlying cause of uroliths remains unclear, but high dietary calcium, dietary electrolyte imbalances, dehydration, and IBV have been suggested as possible causes. Direct trauma is a very rare cause of renal hemorrhage because the kidneys are protected within the renal fossae of the synsacrum.

## RISK FACTORS

**Medical conditions**: Conditions that reduce glomerular filtration—blood loss, severe dehydration, shock. Chronic inflammation. Immunocompromise. Old age. Systemic hypertension. Uncontrolled diabetes mellitus. Gut dysbiosis: shown to play a role in the development of gout in goslings.

**Medications**: Diuretics, nephrotoxins (see Causes section).

**Environmental factors**: Poor husbandry—adverse conditions that promote dehydration. High moisture conditions that promote the development of moldy feed (mycotoxicosis). Improper nutrition. Overcrowding (renal coccidiosis). Prolonged stress can potentially reduce renal blood flow since the renal portal valve opens under sympathetic nerve stimulation, allowing blood to bypass the kidneys. Amyloidosis is typically associated with prolonged periods of stress and chronic inflammatory disease. Exposure to soil (parasitic intermediate hosts), poisoned rodents (rodenticides), insecticides (arsenic), mining runoff (arsenic, cadmium).

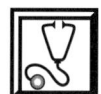

# DIAGNOSIS

## DIFFERENTIAL DIAGNOSIS

Differentials for early renal disease are quite broad since this includes anything that can cause nonspecific signs of illness. Hematuria: Potential sources other than the kidneys include the reproductive tract, cloaca, or distal GI tract. Polyuria: Stressors, including

systemic disease; diabetes mellitus, diabetes insipidus, additional endocrine and metabolic diseases, sepsis, diets with high moisture content, GI diseases. Coelomic distention: Gonadal enlargement, egg binding, as well as other mass lesions. Lameness: orthopedic disease, metabolic disorders, reproductive tumors (budgerigars). Neurologic deficits: reproductive tumors (budgerigars), toxic exposure (particularly heavy metals), trauma, infectious disease.

## CBC/BIOCHEMISTRY/URINALYSIS

CBC: nonspecific, stress-related changes Mild, normocytic-normochromic nonregenerative anemia. Mild-to-marked heterophilia, monocytosis, lymphopenia. Biochemistry panel: UA is an insensitive renal function test. Normal UA values do not mean kidney function is normal since hyperuricemia can be seen when GFR decreases by more than 70–80%. Elevations in BUN can be seen with dehydration in birds, or after high-protein meals in carnivorous birds. Creatinine levels may be elevated in pet birds fed high-protein diets (e.g. parrots on dog chow). Creatinine also increases in significantly dehydrated pigeons. Urea: creatinine and urea: uric acid ratios can be used to better define pre-and postrenal azotemia, as both ratios should be high during dehydration and postrenal obstruction. Low serum protein, hypoalbuminemia has been reported in chickens with advanced tubular nephrosis and interstitial nephritis. Avian kidneys usually cannot concentrate sodium or electrolytes much above normal blood levels, and significant changes are not generally seen, however, hyponatremia, hyperkalemia, hypocalcemia, and hyperphosphatemia have been reported. NAG is a renal tubular marker that has been uncommonly used in birds, but has shown promise in experimental kidney injuries in birds. Urinalysis indicated in birds with hyperuricemia or persistent polyuria. Persistent hematuria has been associated with renal neoplasia, avian polyomavirus, bacterial and viral nephritis, and some forms of toxic nephropathy. Myoglobinuria can cause false positive hematuria. Porphyrinuria, as seen in lead-poisoned Amazon parrots, can result in urine that mimics hemoglobinuria, hematuria. Although proteinuria is the hallmark sign of glomerulonephritis in mammals, voided urine samples are "normally" positive for protein due to fecal contamination in the cloaca. The presence of renal casts can indicate renal pathology.

## OTHER LABORATORY TESTS

Protein electrophoresis. Blood heavy metal levels. Serology. PCR testing as indicated based on history, signalment. Fecal parasite exam.

R

## IMAGING

**Survey radiograph**: Evaluate renal divisions. The cranial lobe of the kidneys is superimposed by the gonads in some birds. Middle and the caudal renal lobes are superimposed by the bony pelvis. Evaluate renal size Loss or compression of the abdominal air sac diverticula. Renal enlargement leads to displacement of the proventriculus, ventriculus, and intestines on the lateral view.

**Radiopacity**: Dehydration, fibrosis, gout, mineralization.

**Contrast studies**: Of the GI tract can help determine the location of the kidneys and the source of organomegaly.

**Sonographic evaluation**: Evaluate renal size, determine location of an abdominal mass, scan for the presence of an obstruction, and evaluate renal vascular status.

**Alternate imaging techniques**: Endoscopy allows direct visualization of renal size, shape, and surface appearance (see renal biopsy below). Nuclear scintigraphy to evaluate renal function. MRI. CT (gold standard for definitive diagnosis of urolithiasis). Do not perform intravenous excretory urography in birds with severe renal compromise. X-ray dark-field radiography (gout).

## DIAGNOSTIC PROCEDURES

**Renal biopsy**: Indication: Definitively diagnose primary renal disease and specific pathologic tissue damage when considering specific therapy. Contraindications: Small kidneys, advanced disease, coagulopathy. Usually performed via endoscopy; however, a dorsal pelvic surgical approach is also described.

**Culture**: Identification of bacteria within renal tissue can be difficult; blood culture preferred. Measure systolic blood pressure. Water deprivation test useful to rule out unknown causes of polyuria/polydipsia including diabetes insipidus and psychogenic polydipsia.

**Cytology**: Murexide text or polarized light to identify UA crystals.

**Histopathology**: Congo red staining method to reveal amyloid.

**GFR**: can be estimated in a laboratory setting by measuring clearance of an exogenous marker like H-inulin, exogenous creatine, or iohexol. This test requires extensive anesthesia and cannulation of the ureters for extended periods of time to obtain uncontaminated urine.

## PATHOLOGIC FINDINGS

### Gross Findings

Enlarged kidneys may bulge out of the renal fossa. Masses: Adenomas and adenocarcinomas are large, somewhat friable, usually focal, nodular swellings that vary from white, tan to red-brown in color.

Renal masses are often located in the cranial pole of the affected kidney. Discolorations: Pallor. Chalky white urate deposits, tubules and ureters distended with urates. Renal coccidiosis: Kidneys are often enlarged with white-to-yellowish nodules containing urates and/or oocysts. Amyloid-infiltrated kidneys may be enlarged, firm, pale, or waxy.

### Histopathology

Renal histologic lesions are rarely pathognomonic for a specific disease process; many different diseases cause similar lesions. Amyloid-infiltrated tissues stain brown with iodine, brown color changes to blue with addition of sulfuric acid. Bacterial or viral nephritis: granulomas, interstitial nephritis, degeneration or nephrosis, glomerulopathy, tubular dilation and impaction with inflammatory cells. As nephritis becomes chronic, tubular necrosis, cyst formation, distortion and interstitial fibrosis with mononuclear cell infiltration become evident. Renal coccidiosis: cytologic smears of renal tissue and ureters often contain different stages of coccidian oocysts. Toxic nephropathy: Proximal tubular necrosis, visceral gout, nephrosis.

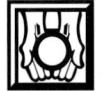

## TREATMENT

### APPROPRIATE HEALTH CARE

Treat the underlying cause of renal disease whenever possible.

### NURSING CARE

Fluid therapy to maintain hydration, treat dehydration (which can rapidly exacerbate renal disease), and/or manage hyperuricemia. Monitor the patient closely for signs of fluid overload. Nutritional support.

### ACTIVITY

Birds with renal tumors or articular gout are likely to have difficult with ambulation and spend more time on the cage floor. Provide low or no perches and other husbandry adaptations to improve quality of life.

### DIET

Gradually transition the bird to a healthy, balanced diet.

### CLIENT EDUCATION

Monitor appetite, body weight, droppings. Stress the importance of keeping the patient hydrated. Long-term prognosis.

### SURGICAL CONSIDERATIONS

Primary renal tumors are extremely difficult to remove successfully—location within renal fossae makes access difficult. Extensive vascular network poses a significant risk of hemorrhage. Close association with the

lumbosacral plexuses means there is a risk of neurologic damage. Removal of postrenal obstruction (e.g., ureterotomy). Lithotripsy has also been described in a Magellanic penguin (*Spheniscus magellanicus*).

## MEDICATIONS

### DRUG(S) OF CHOICE

Systemic antibiotics are indicated in suspected or confirmed cases of bacterial nephritis. Base on culture and sensitivity of blood or biopsy samples whenever possible or select a broad-spectrum agent (e.g. beta-lactams). A course of 4–6 weeks minimum is recommended. Analgesia (e.g. opioids) for renal tumor or articular gout patients. Corticosteroids (e.g. methylprednisolone) may reduce peritumoral inflammation and edema with renal tumors. Parenteral vitamin A for oliguric and anuric renal patients with hyperuricemia. Diuretics (e.g. furosemide, mannitol) to reduce fluid overload and increase urinary output in oliguric and anuric patients.

### CONTRAINDICATIONS

Avoid nephrotoxic drugs and synthetic colloid fluids that could exacerbate renal disease. Steroids can cause general immunosuppression and predispose birds to opportunistic secondary infection.

### PRECAUTIONS

Calcium EDTA: Associated with nephrotoxicosis in mammals, producing an acute but reversible necrotizing nephrosis. Calcium EDTA has been used for weeks with no deleterious effects in birds.

### POSSIBLE INTERACTIONS

Dehydration and renal disease may result in adverse responses to NSAIDs, especially COX inhibitors like meloxicam.

### ALTERNATIVE DRUGS

Chelation therapy to manage heavy metal toxicosis. Colchicine to reduce renal fibrosis. Phosphate binders for hyperphosphatemia. ACE inhibitors to correct hypertension. Omega fatty acids have been used as an adjunct therapy for their anti-inflammatory, lipid-stabilizing, and renal protective properties. Silymarin has been shown to have nephroprotective, antioxidant, anti-inflammatory, immunomodulatory, and anti-fibrotic properties. Chemotherapy: The use of carboplatin has been described in the management of a budgerigar parakeet with renal adenocarcinoma. Cinnamon extract and probiotic supplementation was used in broiler chickens with copper-induced nephrotoxicity.

(CONTINUED)

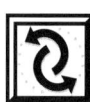

# FOLLOW-UP

## PATIENT MONITORING
Body condition, body weight. Appetite, water intake. Droppings including color and volume of urine and urates. Hydration status. CBC/biochemistry panel to evaluate treatment response and disease progression.

## PREVENTION/AVOIDANCE
Ensure adequate water intake.

## POSSIBLE COMPLICATIONS
Birds can develop articular or visceral gout with severe dehydration or any severe renal dysfunction that results in chronic, moderate to severe hyperuricemia. GI ulcers are rarely reported in birds with renal disease. Ventricular erosions have been associated with naturally occurring urolithiasis in chickens. Hemostatic abnormalities like fibrinous renal vessel thrombi are noted with some forms of renal disease but are rare in birds compared with mammals.

## EXPECTED COURSE AND PROGNOSIS
Renal disease can be a chronic condition that progresses over months to years eventually leading to renal failure. Poor long-term prognosis.

# MISCELLANEOUS

## ASSOCIATED CONDITIONS
Gout, sepsis.

## AGE-RELATED FACTORS
Some causes of renal disease, like renal tumor and amyloidosis, are more common in adult birds. Young birds are more commonly affected by some infectious agents and some nutritional causes of renal disease.

## ZOONOTIC POTENTIAL
Some of the viruses known to infect the kidneys have zoonotic potential: Avian influenza virus, Newcastle disease virus, togaviruses.

## FERTILITY/BREEDING
In addition to signs of nephritis, infectious bronchitis virus is characterized by decreased egg production and poor egg quality in layers.

## SYNONYMS
Renal insufficiency, renal failure, nephritis, nephrosis.

## SEE ALSO
Dehydration
Diabetes Insipidus
Diabetes Mellitus and Hyperglycemia
Diarrhea
Feather-Damaging and Self-Injurious Behavior
Hyperuricemia
Lameness
Nutritional Imbalances
Polydipsia
Polyuria
Neoplasia (Renal)
Toxicosis (Heavy Metals)
Toxicosis (Vitamin D)
Urate and Fecal Discoloration

## ABBREVIATIONS
ACE—angiotensin-converting enzyme
BUN— blood urea nitrogen
CBC—complete blood count
COX—cyclooxygenase
CT—computed tomography
EDTA—ethylenediaminetetraacetic acid
GFR—glomerular filtration rate
IBV—infectious bronchitis virus
MRI—magnetic resonance imaging
NAG—N-acetyl-beta-D-glucosaminidase
NSAIDs—non-steroidal anti-inflammatory drugs
PBFD—psittacine beak and feather disease
PCR—polymerase chain reaction
UA—uric acid

## INTERNET RESOURCES
N/A

*Suggested Reading*
Cojean, O., Larrat, S., Vergneau-Grosset, C. (2020). Clinical management of avian renal disease. *Veterinary Clinics of North America: Exotic Animal Practice*, 23:75–101.

Houck, E.L., Petritz, O.A., Chen, L.R., et al (2022). Clinicopathologic, gross necropsy, and histopathologic effects of high-dose, repeated meloxicam administration in Rhode Island red chickens (*Gallus gallus domesticus*). *Journal of Avian Medicine and Surgery*, 36:128–139.

Nethathe, B., Abera, A., Naidoo, V. (2020). Expression and phylogeny of multidrug resistance protein 2 and 4 in African white backed vulture (*Gyps africanus*). *PeerJ*, 8:e10422.

Phalen, D.N. (2020). Diseases of the avian urinary system. *Veterinary Clinics of North America: Exotic Animal Practice*, 23:21–45.

Pollock, C.G. (ed.). (2020). Renal disease. *Veterinary Clinics of North America: Exotic Animal Practice*, 23(1):1–248.

Scope, A., Schwendenwein, I. (2020). Laboratory evaluation of renal function in birds. *Veterinary Clinics of North America: Exotic Animal Practice*, 23:47–58.

Wang, X., Han, C., Cui, Y., et al (2021). Florfenicol causes excessive lipid peroxidation and apoptosis induced renal injury in broilers. *Ecotoxicology and Environmental Safety*, 207:111282.

Wildmann, A.K., Cushing, A.C., Pfisterer, B.R., Sula, M.M. (2022). Retrospective review of morbidity and mortality in a population of captive budgerigars (*Melopsittacus undulates*). *Journal of Zoo and Wildlife Medicine*, 53:433–441.

**Author**: Christal Pollock, DVM, DABVP (Avian Practice)

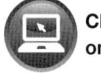

**Client Education Handout available online**

R

# REOVIRUS

## BASICS

### DEFINITION
Reoviruses are common in avian species. Apart from arthritis and tenosynovitis in chickens, turkeys, and geese, clear relationship to other clinical diseases cannot be definitively established. Occasional high mortality with necrotising hepatitis is described in psittacine birds.

### PATHOPHYSIOLOGY
Avian reoviruses are member of the Reoviridae family in the genus Orthoreovirus, characterized by 10 double-stranded RNA segments. Horizontal transmission by fecal–oral route or cutaneous infections via footpads. Infection and replication in enteric epithelia cells of the small intestine. Invasion of multiple organs, resulting in arthritis, tenosynovitis, hepatitis, hydropericardium, osteoporosis, runting–stunting syndrome, malabsorption syndrome.

### SYSTEMS AFFECTED
Gastrointestinal. Hepatobiliary. Musculoskeletal.

### GENETICS
N/A

### INCIDENCE/PREVALENCE
Commonly described in chickens, turkeys, and geese with arthritis/tenosynovitis. Flock morbidity can be high, with no or (usually) low mortality.

### GEOGRAPHIC DISTRIBUTION
Worldwide.

### SIGNALMENT
**Species**: Chickens and turkeys. Ducks and geese. Psittacines. Pigeons.
**Mean age and range**: Younger birds are more susceptible.
**Predominant sex**: None.

### SIGNS
*Historical Findings*
Lameness appears at 4–5 weeks of age in chickens and turkeys, at 2–3 weeks of age in geese. Growth retardation, poor feathering. Diarrhoea with pasty vent in turkey and duck chicks. Sudden death and increased flock mortality in psittacine birds.

*Physical Examination Findings*
Swollen hock joints and enlargement in the area of the gastrocnemius or digital flexor tendon.

### CAUSES
Infectious.

### RISK FACTORS
Co-infections with other pathogens enhances pathogenicity.

## DIAGNOSIS

### DIFFERENTIAL DIAGNOSIS
Enteritis caused by other enteric viruses in poultry, particularly rotavirus, coronavirus, astrovirus, adenovirus. Diarrhoea in poultry caused be clostridia and/or coccidia. Arthritis caused by *Mycoplasma synoviae*. Sudden death and necrotising hepatitis caused by viral pathogens in psittacine birds and pigeons, especially herpesvirus, adenovirus, circovirus, and rotavirus.

### CBC/BIOCHEMISTRY/URINALYSIS
Leucocytosis with lymphocytosis. Elevated glutamate dehydrogenase in liver necrosis.

### OTHER LABORATORY TESTS
rt-PCR of joint lesions, liver or faecal swabs. Serology.

### IMAGING
N/A

### DIAGNOSTIC PROCEDURES
Necropsy including histopathology with immunohistochemistry or in situ hybridization.

### PATHOLOGIC FINDINGS
Marked edema with small amount of straw colored or blood-tinged exudate in the hock joint and petechial haemorrhages in the synovial membranes. Hepatosplenomegaly with multiple white small foci in case of necrotizing hepatitis. Distension of small intestines and ceca with watery contents and gas in case of enteritis. Mononuclear cell infiltrates in the synovial membrane. Necrotizing myocarditis in turkeys. Acute necrosis with infiltration of mononuclear cells in liver and spleen.

## TREATMENT

### APPROPRIATE HEALTH CARE
Inpatient medical management may be required; fluid and nutritional support are indicated if the patient is debilitated and dehydrated, and treatment is ideally administered via gavage.

### NURSING CARE
Fluid support (SQ, IV, IO). Nutritional support via gavage may be indicated if anorexic.

### ACTIVITY
No restrictions indicated.

### DIET
N/A

### CLIENT EDUCATION
Increasing ventilation rate and temperature as well as adding fresh litter may help to reduce transmission risk.

### SURGICAL CONSIDERATIONS
N/A

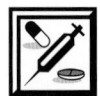

## MEDICATIONS

### DRUG(S) OF CHOICE
No drug treatment available.

### CONTRAINDICATIONS
N/A

### PRECAUTIONS
N/A

### POSSIBLE INTERACTIONS
N/A

### ALTERNATIVE DRUGS
N/A

## FOLLOW-UP

### PATIENT MONITORING
Viral shedding via faeces.

### PREVENTION/AVOIDANCE
Vaccination of chicken and turkey poults with commercially available vaccines in chickens and polyvalent autogenous vaccines in turkey breeders.

### POSSIBLE COMPLICATIONS
N/A

### EXPECTED COURSE AND PROGNOSIS
Course can vary depending from mild to severe. Prognosis depends on several factors, such as virus pathogenicity, age of infection, and the presence of a secondary bacterial infection.

## MISCELLANEOUS

### ASSOCIATED CONDITIONS
Secondary bacterial infection of the gastrointestinal tract. Stunting of growth. Pasted and inflamed vents with increased risk of vent pecking in turkey chicks.

### AGE-RELATED FACTORS
Age-associated resistance is likely.

### ZOONOTIC POTENTIAL
None.

### FERTILITY/BREEDING
N/A

## SYNONYMS

Runting and stunting syndrome.
Malabsorption syndrome.

## SEE ALSO

Adenoviruses
Herpesvirus (Columbid Herpesvirus 1 in
Pigeons and Raptors)
Herpesvirus (Duck Viral Enteritis)
Herpesvirus (Passerine Birds)
Herpesvirus (Psittacid Herpesviruses)
Joint Diseases
Mycoplasmosis
Myocarditis
Liver Disease
Spleen (Diseases of)
Tendinitis and Tenosynovitis

## ABBREVIATIONS

rt-PCR—reverse transcriptase polymerase
chain reaction

## INTERNET RESOURCES

N/A

*Suggested Reading*

Perpiñán, D., Garner, M.M., Wellehan, J.F.,
Armstrong, D.L. (2010). Mixed infection
with reovirus and chlamydophila in a flock
of budgerigars (*Melopsittacus undulatus*).
*Journal of Avian Medicine and Surgery*,
24:316–321.

Pitcovsky, J. Goyal, S.M. (2020). Avian
reovirus infection. In: *Diseases of Poultry*,
14th edn. (ed. D.E. Swayne, M. Boulianne,
C.M. Logue, et al.), 382–401. Oxford,
UK: Blackwell.

Sánchez-Cordón, P.J., Hervás, J., Chacón de
Lara, F., et al. (2002). Reovirus infection in
psittacine birds (*Psittacus erithacus*):
morphologic and immunohistochemical
study. *Avian Diseases*, 46:485–492.

van den Brand, J.M., Manvell, R., Paul, G.,
et al. (2007). Reovirus infections associated
with high mortality in psittaciformes in the
Netherlands. *Avian Pathology*, 36:293–299.

Vindevogel, H., Meulemans, G., Pastoret, P.P.,
et al. (1982). Reovirus infection in the pigeon.
*Annals of Veterinary Research*, 13:149–152.

**Author**: Volker Schmidt, PD Dr Med Vet,
DECZM (Avian and Herpetological)

R

## RESPIRATORY DISTRESS

# BASICS

## DEFINITION
Respiratory distress refers to difficulty in breathing, and the psychological experience associated with such difficulty.

## PATHOPHYSIOLOGY
Respiratory distress most commonly occurs secondary to lower respiratory tract disease. Upper respiratory disease may induce respiratory distress with complete and bilateral nasal obstruction. Non-respiratory diseases (thoracic inlet mass effect, coelomic cavity disease) leading to compression of the airways or air sacs may induce respiratory distress.

## SYSTEMS AFFECTED
**Respiratory**: Lower or upper respiratory diseases.
**Reproductive**: Organomegaly, dystocia, ovarian cyst, egg-related peritonitis.
**Renal/urologic**: Organomegaly, gout.
**Hepatobiliary**: Organomegaly, metabolic disease, ascites.
**Gastrointestinal**: Organomegaly.
**Cardiovascular**: Cardiac disease with pulmonary edema.

## GENETICS
None.

## INCIDENCE/PREVALENCE
Common.

## GEOGRAPHIC DISTRIBUTION
N/A

## SIGNALMENT
Species, age or sex predilection vary with the cause of respiratory distress: Tracheal obstruction—small bird species (lovebirds, cockatiels); hypersensitivity syndrome—macaw species; aspergillosis—grey parrots, Amazon parrots and *Pionus* sp.; dystocia—female; *Sternostoma* sp.—canaries, finches.

## SIGNS

### General Comments
The veterinarian must quickly evaluate whether the patient's condition requires immediate emergency intervention. Physical examination may have to be postponed until the bird is more stable; patient should be held upright without impairing keel movements; consider oxygen administration. Large airway disease—inspiratory stridor, increased rate and effort with open-beak breathing exacerbated by exertion. Gasping occurs with almost complete obstruction. Tracheal transillumination may be helpful to identify *Sternostoma* sp. in passerines and to locate a tracheal foreign body. Small-airway disease (hypersensitivity syndrome)—soft expiratory

wheezes, severe respiratory distress with open-beak breathing, and sometimes collapse with gasping. Parenchymal disease (lungs, air sacs)—increased respiratory rate and/or effort. Poor body condition with a history of lethargy/anorexia is usually present. Moist expiratory sounds may be auscultated with pulmonary disease while clicking noises suggest air sac disease. Coelomic diseases—increased respiratory rate and effort at rest; becomes severely dyspneic with open-beak breathing on handling; history of lethargy/anorexia prior to the development of respiratory signs. Coelomic distension is present in most cases.

### Historical Findings
Exposure to toxic aerosols. Acute onset of respiratory distress while eating. Malnutrition. Suboptimal hygiene, corn cob litter. Macaw with periodic respiratory distress; housed with cockatiel, cockatoo, or grey parrot sp. Hand-fed juvenile bird, severely depressed bird, vomiting/regurgitation. Recent contact with sick bird. Old World parrots kept outdoors with access to dirt ground in Gulf coast area. Recent anesthetic event with tracheal intubation.

### Physical Examination Findings
Lower respiratory involvement—depression, exercise intolerance, open-beak breathing, neck extension, obvious sternal movements, wings held away from the body, inspiratory (large airways) or expiratory (small airways) noise, gasping, coughing, tail bobbing, head shaking, coelomic distension, moving black specks in trachea. Upper respiratory involvement—facial or nasal swelling/asymmetry, nasal discharge, matted feathers around the nares, malformed rhinotheca, sneezing, wheezing, nasal sounds with open-beak breathing, repetitive yawning, nasal or oral cavity scratching, rubbing beak on perches, tachypnea without increased respiratory efforts, papilloma.

## CAUSES
Infectious—bacteria (*Chlamydia* sp., Gram-negative bacteria, *Mycobacterium* sp.), fungi (*Aspergillus* sp., *Candida* sp., etc.), virus (herpesvirus, poxvirus, paramyxovirus, reovirus), parasites (*Sarcocystis* sp., *Sternostoma* sp., *Trichomonas* sp., *Syngamus* sp., *Cyathostoma* sp., *Serratospiculum* sp., etc.). Metabolic—ascites (liver, heart disease), organomegaly. Inflammatory—egg-related peritonitis. Toxic—aerosols (PFTE—Teflon™), self-cleaning ovens, bleach, ammonia, etc.), avocado. Immune mediated—hypersensitivity syndrome. Iatrogenic—aspiration pneumonia, membranous stenosis following tracheal intubation. Traumatic—collision, ruptured air sac, bite wounds. Degenerative—congestive heart failure,

atherosclerosis. Accidental—foreign body aspiration. Neoplastic—respiratory or extra-respiratory tumors impairing breathing.

## RISK FACTORS
Medical conditions—malnutrition may predispose to respiratory diseases. Environmental factors—exposure to toxic aerosols, suboptimal environment (poor hygiene, etc.).

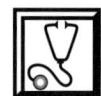

# DIAGNOSIS

## DIFFERENTIAL DIAGNOSIS
See Causes section.

## CBC/BIOCHEMISTRY/URINALYSIS
CBC to identify evidence of inflammation/infection, erythrocytosis in chronic respiratory distress. Biochemistry to evaluate organ function.

## OTHER LABORATORY TESTS
Serum protein electrophoresis to identify and characterize inflammation. Specific pathogen testing to determine possible presence of *Chlamydia*, *Aspergillus*, *Mycobacterium* spp., herpes virus. Sensitivity and specificity vary depending on testing modalities and which pathogen is targeted.

## IMAGING
Skull radiographs to identify upper respiratory disease. Subtle lesions may not be apparent. Whole-body radiographs to identify lower respiratory disease or pathology compressing the air sacs. Subtle or peracute (aspiration pneumonia) lower respiratory disease may not be apparent. Contrast radiographs to outline upper respiratory lesion or tracheal foreign body. Fluoroscopy to outline tracheal foreign body after contrast administration. Pre- and post-contrast CT examination to identify upper or lower respiratory disease. MRI to identify upper or lower respiratory disease. Coelomic ultrasonography to identify and characterize coelomic disease compressing the air sacs; to evaluate large respiratory lesions adjacent to body wall. ECG to identify cardiac disease.

## DIAGNOSTIC PROCEDURES
Endoscopy to directly assess upper and lower respiratory system; to collect cytology, culture, histopathologic samples. Cytology to evaluate cells and microbial population. Choanal swab, nasal, sinus, and transtracheal lavage, and impression smears from biopsy samples may be submitted for evaluation. Fine-needle aspirate of coelomic effusion, enlarged organ or other lesion compressing the air sacs. Best performed guided by ultrasound under mild sedation.

R

Bacterial/fungal culture and sensitivity to evaluate microbial population. See cytology for sample types. Histopathology to characterize lesions in diseased tissue. ECG to investigate cardiac diseases.

## PATHOLOGIC FINDINGS
Gross and histopathologic findings will differ depending on the underlying cause of respiratory distress.

## TREATMENT
### APPROPRIATE HEALTH CARE
Emergency inpatient intensive care management: All birds in respiratory distress require immediate stabilization in a warmed oxygen-enriched incubator. Surgical management once patient is stable: Placement of air sac cannula, tracheotomy, tracheal resection and anastomosis may be performed following initial stabilization.

### NURSING CARE
*Supportive Care*
Oxygen therapy is indicated for all cases of respiratory distress. Ideal method of oxygen delivery is within a cage. Humidification is required if oxygen supplementation is performed for more than a few hours. Humidification is achieved by bubbling the oxygen through a container with sterile saline or distilled water. Fluid therapy may be provided SQ in birds exhibiting mild dehydration (5–7%) or IO/IV in birds with moderate to severe dehydration (> 7%) or critically ill birds exhibiting signs consistent with shock. Avian daily maintenance fluid requirements are 50 ml/kg. In most patients, lactated Ringer's solution or Normosol® (Hospira, Inc., Lake Forest, IL) crystalloid fluids are appropriate. Warmth (85–90°F/27–30°C) to minimize energy spent to maintain body temperature.

*Therapeutic Care*
Nasal flush to remove mucous/discharge and improve breathing. Endoscopy to remove tracheal foreign bodies (medium and large birds) and debulk tracheal granulomatous lesions. Prior placement of an air sac cannula highly recommended. Suction to retrieve tracheal foreign bodies in small birds where the endoscope is too large to be inserted within the small trachea. Prior placement of an air sac cannula is required. An appropriately sized urinary catheter is inserted in the trachea until it reaches the foreign body and suction is applied. Tracheal stent to restore tracheal patency when tracheal resection–anastomosis is not an option. Complications may include tracheitis, deciliation, and tracheomalacia.

Coelomocentesis to aspirate coelomic effusion and drain cystic structures and decrease air sac compression. Best performed guided by ultrasound under mild sedation. May be performed blindly on the right lateral coelom just cranial to the cloaca. Patient should be maintained in an upright position to decrease the likelihood of fluid entering the lungs. Concurrent oxygen therapy recommended.

### ACTIVITY
Patient activity should be minimal to avoid worsening of clinical signs.

### DIET
Birds presenting in respiratory distress may require assisted feeding—must be performed rapidly to minimize stress and worsening of respiratory signs. A smaller volume is typically administered. Enteral nutritional preparation may be administered initially at 20 ml/kg directly in the crop. Volume administered may be progressively increased according to the patient tolerance with the goal to meet the patient's anticipated energy requirements.

### CLIENT EDUCATION
Balancing the need to perform diagnostic tests and administer treatment in light of the patient's condition is critical. Patient clinical condition may worsen despite appropriate care.

### SURGICAL CONSIDERATIONS
Surgical considerations will differ depending upon the underlying cause of respiratory distress. Air sac cannula placement to provide an alternate airway. Emergency placement of an air sac cannula is indicated with large airway obstruction. An air sac tube may partially improve respiration in birds with primary lung and air sac disease. Various types of tubing or standard endotracheal tubing can be modified for cannulation purposes. The diameter of the cannula should approximate the bird's tracheal diameter. Consider sedation or inhalant anesthesia to facilitate placement of the cannula. The patient is positioned in lateral recumbency with the upper leg pulled caudally. Skin incision is performed over the triangle created by the cranial muscle mass of the femur, ventral to the synsacrum and caudal to the last rib. Using a pair of hemostats, the caudal air sac is entered making a popping noise. The air sac cannula is inserted between the last two ribs or just caudal to the last rib. The bird should immediately begin to breathe through the tube if placed correctly. Patency may be evaluated using the end of a laryngoscope (fogging) or a feather may be held in front of the cannula (breath-associated movements). The cannula

is sutured into place using a Chinese finger trap technique. Consider placing a filter, such as the removed inner filter from a respirator mask, over the end of the tube to prevent entry of particulate matter. A brief coelioscopy through the air sac tube can also be performed to confirm placement in the air sac. Endoscopy at removal is recommended to assess the presence of focal aspergillosis and inflammation, common with long treatment with air sac cannula. The cannula may have to be changed after 3–5 days by placing another one in the contra-lateral side. Culture of the tip of the cannula is also recommended at removal.

## MEDICATIONS
### DRUG(S) OF CHOICE
Medication will differ depending upon the underlying cause of respiratory distress. Nebulization therapy within an oxygen cage, through an endotracheal tube or face mask. Antibiotics (enrofloxacin 10 mg/ml saline), antifungals (amphotericin B 7–10 mg/ml sterile water), bronchodilators (aminophylline 3 mg/ml sterile saline) may be nebulized. Jet or ultrasonic nebulization are preferred. Particle size needs to be less than five microns to allow for optimal dispersion. Nebulization sessions typically last 15–30 minutes and may be repeated several times a day depending on the medication delivered and the patient's clinical condition. Bronchodilators (terbutaline 0.01 mg/kg IM q6–8h; aminophylline 10 mg/kg IV q3h then 4 mg/kg PO q6–12h, theophylline 10 mg/kg PO q12h) to address bronchoconstriction. Corner stone treatment for patient with hypersensitivity syndrome. Benzodiazepine (midazolam 0.5–2 mg/kg IM) to decrease anxiety associated with being unable to breathe normally. Analgesic (butorphanol 1–4 mg/kg IM q2–6h) is indicated to address pain. Adverse effects in light of the patient's overall condition need to be considered. Diuretic (furosemide 0.15–2.0 mg/kg PO, IM, IV q8h) to treat pulmonary edema. Critically dyspneic birds often require higher dosages (4–8 mg/kg) to achieve initial stabilization. NSAIDs (meloxicam 0.5–1 mg/kg PO/IM q12h depending on species) to decrease inflammation that may be associated with the disease condition. Adverse effects in light of the patient's overall condition need to be considered. Antiparasitic therapy varies with the specific cause. Antibiotic therapy to treat primary and secondary bacterial infection, which may be associated with the disease condition. Antibiotic selection varies with the specific cause of respiratory distress.

R

# RESPIRATORY DISTRESS (CONTINUED)

Antifungal therapy to treat aspiration pneumonia and fungal disease. Antifungal selection varies with the causative agent, the severity of clinical signs, the location of infection and patient species.

### CONTRAINDICATIONS
None.

### PRECAUTIONS
Fluid deficits should be addressed prior to using NSAIDs.

### POSSIBLE INTERACTIONS
None.

### ALTERNATIVE DRUGS
N/A

 FOLLOW-UP

### PATIENT MONITORING
Varies with the cause of respiratory distress.

### PREVENTION/AVOIDANCE
Avoid exposure to toxic aerosols. Offer a balanced diet according to the bird species.

### POSSIBLE COMPLICATIONS
Varies with the cause of respiratory distress. Suffocation with tracheal obstruction.

### EXPECTED COURSE AND PROGNOSIS
Varies with the cause of respiratory distress. Respiratory distress secondary to upper airway disease carries a better prognosis than respiratory distress secondary to lower airway, coelomic or cardiac disease. The delay between the onset of respiratory distress and time to seeking veterinary care influences prognosis. Death may occur if treatment is delayed. Teflon exposure and severe fungal infections carry a grave prognosis.

 MISCELLANEOUS

### ASSOCIATED CONDITIONS
Varies with the cause of respiratory distress.

### AGE-RELATED FACTORS
Aspiration pneumonia should be ruled out in handfed juvenile birds with respiratory distress.

### ZOONOTIC POTENTIAL
*Chlamydia psittaci* is zoonotic.

### FERTILITY/BREEDING
N/A

### SYNONYMS
Dyspnea

### SEE ALSO
Air Sac Mites
Ascites
Aspergillosis
Aspiration Pneumonia
Atherosclerosis
Chlamydiosis
Coelomic Distention
Congestive Heart Failure
Dehydration
Dystocia and Egg Binding
Egg Yolk and Reproductive Coelomitis
Helminthiasis (Respiratory)
Herpesvirus (Columbid Herpesvirus 1 in Pigeons and Raptors)
Herpesvirus (Duck Viral Enteritis)
Herpesvirus (Passerine Birds)
Herpesvirus (Psittacid Herpesviruses)
Myocardial Diseases
Neoplasia (Respiratory)
Orthoavulaviruses
Ovarian Diseases
Pneumonia
Poxvirus
Rhinitis and Sinusitis
Toxicosis (Airborne)
Tracheal and Syringeal Diseases
Appendix 8, Algorithm 4: Respiratory Distress

### ABBREVIATIONS
CT—computed tomography
ECG—electrocardiogram
MRI—magnetic resonance imaging
NSAIDs—non-steroidal anti-inflammatory drugs

### INTERNET RESOURCES
Brown, C. Air sac cannila placement in birds. *LafeberVet*: https://lafeber.com/vet/air-sac-cannula

*Suggested Reading*
Graham, J.E. (2004). Approach to the dyspneic avian patient. *Seminars in Avian and Exotic Pet Medicine*, 13:154–159.
Mejia-Fava, J., Holmes, S.P, Radlinsky, M., et al. (2015). Use of a nitinol wire stent for management of severe tracheal stenosis in an eclectus parrot (*Eclectus roratus*). *Journal of Avian Medicine and Surgery*, 29:238–249.
Orosz, S. E., Lichtenberger, M. (2011). Avian respiratory distress: etiology, diagnosis, and treatment. *Veterinary Clinics of North America: Exotic Animal Practice*, 14:241–255.
Tell, L.A., Stephens, K., Teague, S.V., et al. (2012). Study of nebulization delivery of aerosolized fluorescent microspheres to the avian respiratory tract. *Avian Diseases*, 56:381–386.
Westerhof, I. (1995). Treatment of tracheal obstruction in psittacine birds using a suction technique: A retrospective study of 19 birds. *Journal of Avian Medicine and Surgery*, 9:45–49.

**Author:** Isabelle Langlois, DMV, DABVP (Avian)

**R**

# RESPIRATORY INFECTIONS OF BACKYARD CHICKENS

## BASICS

### DEFINITION
Respiratory diseases of backyard flocks often originate from numerous causes, most commonly infectious diseases including mycoplasmosis, infectious coryza, fowl cholera, and infectious laryngotracheitis. Less common diseases include infectious bronchitis, pox (diphtheritic, wet form), gape worm (uncommon in poultry, common in game birds), and aspergillosis. Respiratory diseases in backyard poultry are often the consequence of co-infection with more than one primary respiratory pathogen, with secondary bacterial infections.

### PATHOPHYSIOLOGY
Environmental factors such as poor ventilation, high humidity, high environmental pathogen contamination, overcrowding, or lack of pre-existing immunity (inadequate vaccination), or poor biosecurity can predispose to respiratory diseases. Infectious agents enter the respiratory tract most commonly via inhalation (although systemic spread is also possible); production of inflammatory exudate caused by the bird's immune response can result in decreased respiratory function and difficulty breathing.

### SYSTEMS AFFECTED
Respiratory tract.

### GENETICS
N/A

### INCIDENCE/PREVALENCE
Incidence/prevalence is highly variable. In Ontario, Canada, 27% of backyard birds had respiratory clinical signs derived from coinfections of bacteria (e.g., *Mycoplasma gallisepticum* and *Mycoplasma synoviae*, *Escherichia coli*, and *Avibacterium* spp.) and viruses (e.g. IBV and ILTV). In the USA, the prevalence of respiratory diseases was estimated to be as high as 75% for IBV, 73% for *M. synoviae*, and 69% for *M. gallisepticum*, and 45% for ILTV.

### GEOGRAPHIC DISTRIBUTION
Worldwide.

### SIGNALMENT
**Species**: A wide variety of avian species, due to the broad definition of backyard poultry.
**Mean age and range**: Chicken layers are the most common type of backyard poultry. This could skew the average presentation age towards more mature birds, as layers have a longer growout period compared with poultry raised for meat purposes.
**Predominant sex**: N/A

## SIGNS

### Historical Findings
**Non-specific respiratory disease**:
Chickens may exhibit respiratory symptoms like rales, sneezing and coughing; depending on severity, there may be a drop in egg production, flock activity, and feed and water intake.
**Mycoplasmosis**: Affected birds (usually chickens, turkeys and gamefowl) can show snick, sneeze and/or tracheal rales; symptoms tend to be chronic and disease spreads slowly throughout the flock. In turkeys, *M. gallisepticum* can cause severe infraorbital sinusitis. In meat-type chickens and turkeys, *M. synoviae* can lead to lameness, synovitis, and drop in egg production. Infectious coryza (caused by *Avibacterium paragallinuarum*) is typically seen in chickens, pheasants, or guinea fowl; it causes oculonasal discharge, facial edema, and/or swollen infraorbital sinuses.
**Fowl cholera** (caused by *Pasteurella multocida*): Sudden mortality in chickens and turkeys, with septicemic form being more common in turkeys than in chickens; in chickens, subacute and chronic form can be seen, with localized development of granulomas (e.g. chronic cellulitis in wattles, or chronic otitis externa).
**ILT** (caused by Gallid herpesvirus-1 or ILTV): Mortality rate can double daily and typically appears 7–10 days after returning from a poultry exhibition or adding new birds to a flock. This disease mainly affects chickens, but can also affect peafowl and pheasants; turkeys have only been infected in experimentally. In the acute form, birds experience severe fibrinohemorrhagic tracheitis, which may lead to asphyxiation due to accumulation of exudate in the trachea. Birds become infected after visiting fairs or exhibitions, where vaccinated (live attenuated vaccine is most common) or convalescent birds mingle with naïve birds; as any herpesvirus, ILTV can undergo latency and become reactivated when birds experience stressful situation.
**Infectious bronchitis**: Chickens of all ages; birds may show sneezing, snicking, tracheal rales and/or coughing, and may appear sick and reluctant to move, with a puffed-up appearance.
**Pox (diphtheritic, wet form)**: Spreads slowly in a flock; mild increase in mortality; dyspnea is caused by proliferative and necrotic plaques that accumulate in the tracheal lumen; secondary bacterial infections are common.
**Gape worm**: Increased flock mortality in young poultry, especially game birds such as

pheasants, quail, and partridges; it has also been reported in chickens, turkeys, guinea fowl, peafowl, and geese.
**Aspergillosis**: Usually appears when young birds are being brooded in an environment that is excessively warm and moist, which promotes development of fungal spores; after exposure, higher flock mortality is within 2 weeks. Contamination with spores can also occur in the incubator, where large amounts of spores are released when contaminated eggs break. In adult birds, aspergillosis presents as a chronic illness, with weight loss and respiratory signs; geese, turkeys, and ducks are most commonly affected.

### Physical Examination Findings
**Non-specific respiratory disease**: Affected birds may show tracheal rales, snicks, sneezes, and coughing; depending on severity, birds may remain alert, active and still eat and drink.
**Mycoplasmosis from *M. gallisepticum***: Chickens—elevated flock mortality, mucus exuding from the nares, coughing, tracheal rales and/or snicks, sneezes. Turkeys and peafowl—infraorbital sinusitis.
**Mycoplasmosis from *M. synoviae***: Chickens—snick, sneeze, and/or tracheal rale, and if an animal is euthanized, mild airsacculitis with a frothy exudate may be seen. Meat birds—hock joint swelling may be present.
**Infectious coryza**: Oculonasal discharge, facial edema, and/or swollen infraorbital sinuses.
**Fowl cholera**: Death may occur without any premonitory signs. In subacute to chronic forms (mainly in chickens), there may be subcutaneous masses (granulomas) in the periocular region, ear canal, or wattles. Septicemia may manifest as fibrin in multiple body cavities.
**ILT**: In the case of asphyxia due to tracheal plug, death may occur without any premonitory signs; other signs include coughing, head shaking, dyspnea, expectoration of bloody mucous, and blood on feathers and chicken coop walls. Lesions can be blood, fibrin, or a mix of both in the larynx and top third of the trachea. Some cases of ILT may also have conjunctivitis.
Infectious bronchitis: Chickens have tracheitis resulting in rales.
**Pox (diphtheritic, wet form)**: Wet pox can cause lesions on the mucous membranes, usually appearing as exophytic masses at the opening of the larynx and proximal trachea. This mass can suffocate the bird if it blocks the trachea, causing death.
**Gape worm**: Open-beak breathing, head shaking, and/or walking with their open beak

**R**

## RESPIRATORY INFECTIONS OF BACKYARD CHICKENS    (CONTINUED)

on the ground, a reddish nematode parasite attached to the tracheal mucosa.

**Aspergillosis**: Young birds typically show yellow, seed-like granules of granulomatous inflammation in the lungs. In older birds, clinical signs are chronic illness and weight loss before death, with the lesions being fungal airsacculitis. The air sacs (typically cranial thoracic) near the lungs can be filled with large amounts of yellow material that crumbles easily, and may have a gray fuzzy coating (fungal hyphae and fruiting bodies). In birds that die suddenly without warning, a plug of fibrin and fungal mycelia may be detected blocking the tracheal bifurcation (syrinx).

### CAUSES
Mycoplasmosis: *M. gallisepticum, M. synoviae.* Infectious coryza: *Av. (Hemophilus) paragallinarum.* Fowl cholera: *P. multocida.* ILTV: Gallid herpesvirus 1. Infectious bronchitis: Avian coronavirus. Pox (diphtheritic, wet form): Fowl pox. Gape worm: *Syngamus trachea.* Aspergillosis: *Aspergillus fumigatus.* Non-infectious respiratory disease: Changes in the local environment can trigger nonspecific respiratory signs, or predispose to infections; predisposing factors include dust or high levels of ammonia, high humidity levels, overcrowding, poor biosecurity practices.

### RISK FACTORS
Non-specific respiratory diseases can be facilitated by cold weather, poor air quality, or co-infections. Infectious respiratory diseases can spread quickly through direct contact with birds, or indirectly through people, animals, food, water, and the environment. Problems like cold weather, bad air quality, and coinfections can make it easier for the disease to spread. Introducing a new bird into the flock without following proper quarantine procedures can also increase the risk of infection. Presence of multi-age flocks can increase the risk of clinical disease, due to transmission between carrier and naive birds. Poor biosecurity causing contact with wild birds or different species can increase risk of transmission between reservoirs and susceptible poultry (e.g. PPMV-1 from pigeons to chickens) Gape worm: Infection may occur directly by ingestion of infective eggs or larvae; however, severe field infection is associated with ingestion of transport hosts such as earthworms, snails, slugs, and arthropods (e.g. flies). Aspergillosis: Regions with hot and humid seasons are at higher risk of developing a sufficient concentration of mold to cause clinical disease in poultry. Heavily contaminated litter can also be the source of the infection.

## DIAGNOSIS

### DIFFERENTIAL DIAGNOSIS
Depending on the severity, secondary bacterial infections, septicemia, and systemic viral diseases should be included in the list of differential diagnoses. Mycoplasmosis from *M. gallisepticum*: Pathogenic *E. coli*, fowl cholera, infectious bronchitis, *Mycoplasma synoviae*, turkey viral rhinotracheitis, or swollen head syndrome of chickens. Mycoplasmosis from *M. synoviae*: *M. gallisepticum*, infectious bronchitis, or non-virulent OAvV-1. Infectious coryza: Fowl cholera (*P. multocida*), secondary bacterial infections following infections by mycoplasmas, ornithobacteriosis infection, or swollen head syndrome (extremely rare in the United States). Fowl cholera: Septicemias caused by *E. coli* or *A. paragallinarum*, Newcastle disease, avian influenza. ILT: Newcastle disease, avian influenza, septicemic pasteurellosis, acute infectious coryza, or infectious bronchitis. Infectious bronchitis: Mycoplasmosis, non-virulent OAvV-1, low pathogenic avian influenza, or infectious coryza. Pox (diphtheritic, wet form): Infectious laryngotracheitis. Gape worm: Respiratory pathogen causing open mouth breathing (e.g. as wet pox and ILT). Aspergillosis: Fowl cholera and *E. coli* septicemia.

### CBC/BIOCHEMISTRY/URINALYSIS
N/A

### OTHER LABORATORY TESTS
Diagnostic tests depend on the pathogens involved. Most useful for a diagnostic work up are culled birds that present clinical signs representative of the flock problem. Mycoplasmosis from *M. gallisepticum*: Culture, PCR, serology are used to diagnose; regulatory testing (such as NPIP) uses serological methods (such as plate agglutination or ELISA) to screen breeder flocks, and follow-up methods to confirm a suspect positive. Culture is the gold standard for *M. gallisepticum*. Most commercial poultry are *M. gallisepticum*-free, so understanding the source of backyard birds is important for differential diagnosis. Mycoplasmosis from *M. synoviae*: Culture and identification, PCR, and/or serology. Infectious coryza: Culture. *A. paragallinarum* requires V-(NAD) factor for growth. Fowl cholera: Culture. ILT: Histopathology, virus isolation, and PCR. Infectious bronchitis: Serology (nonvaccinated birds), virus isolation, and PCR. Pox (diphtheritic, wet form): Histopathology, virus isolation, and PCR. Gape worm: Gross lesions.

Aspergillosis: Gross lesions and confirmation by histopathology.

### IMAGING
Radiography and computed tomography can be used to diagnose pneumonia and air sacculitis.

### DIAGNOSTIC PROCEDURES
N/A

### PATHOLOGIC FINDINGS
**Nonspecific respiratory disease**: Grossly, tracheal rales, snicks, sneezes, and coughing. The birds remain alert and active and keep eating and drinking.

**Mycoplasmosis from *M. gallisepticum***: Chicken—grossly, cough, tracheal rales, and/or snicks and sneezes. Microscopically uncomplicated *M. gallisepticum*—mild airsacculitis (small to moderate amounts of yellow frothy material). White to yellow material (fibrin) over the surfaces of the pericardial sac, liver, and air sacs (fibrinous polyserositis). Turkeys and peafowl (infectious sinusitis)—grossly, infraorbital sinuses are often greatly distended. Thick stringy mucus exudes from the interior. With secondary bacterial infection, the sinus exudate may change to more caseous.

**Mycoplasmosis from *M. synoviae***: Grossly, a snick, sneeze, and/or tracheal rale. Swollen hock joints. Microscopically, a mild airsacculitis with a frothy exudate within the air sacs.

**Infectious coryza**: Grossly, birds can die suddenly or show respiratory symptoms with oculonasal discharge, facial swelling, and swollen infraorbital sinuses. The sinuses can contain mucus or a hard, yellow, caseous substance. Infected flocks have a characteristic smell.

**Fowl cholera**: Grossly, death without premonitory signs (acute septicemic form) or subcutaneous masses (granulomas) in periocular region ears, or wattles (subacute and chronic forms). Subcutaneous masses and swellings have lots of easily crumbled yellow material when cut into. Turkeys—fibrinous bronchopneumonia.

**ILT**: Grossly lesions may include blood, fibrin, or a combination of both in the larynx and upper trachea, and some cases there may be conjunctivitis. Histological lesions are pathognomonic, and characterized by intranuclear inclusion bodies with development of epithelial syncitia in the trachea.

**Infectious bronchitis**: Gross lesion may include a reddened caudal trachea, rales, and possibly increased mucus. Histologically, non-specific inflammation is observed.

**Pox (diphtheritic, wet form)**: Grossly, there are proliferative lesions on tracheal epithelium. Histologically, proliferating epithelial cells show large intracytoplasmic inclusions that are characteristics (Bollinger bodies).

**Gape worm**: Grossly, red nematode parasites may attach to the tracheal mucosa, showing up as white nodules. These parasites may obstruct the trachea and lead to death. **Aspergillosis**: Yellow granules in the lungs (granulomas) of younger birds. Older birds may present with large amounts of yellow, easily crumbled material and a gray, fuzzy covering of mycelia and fruiting bodies in the air sacs.

## TREATMENT

### APPROPRIATE HEALTH CARE
Depends on the severity of disease. Good hygiene, including proper ventilation of the cage or aviary area, and proper nutrition, should be maintained at all times.

### NURSING CARE
N/A

### ACTIVITY
N/A

### DIET
N/A

### CLIENT EDUCATION
Proper biosecurity measures.

### SURGICAL CONSIDERATIONS
N/A

## MEDICATIONS

### DRUG(S) OF CHOICE
Antimicrobial treatment may resolve clinical signs, although recovered birds often remain shedders or chronically infected for life, presenting a possible source of infection for naïve birds. Mycoplasmosis from *M. gallisepticum*: Tylosin and tetracyclines may reduce infection, but do not eliminate the organism. Clinical signs may reappear after stopping antibiotic treatment. Mycoplasmosis from *M. synoviae*: Tylosin and tetracyclines can lessen effects of infection, but no antibiotic completely eliminates the organism. Infectious coryza: Sulfonamides, tetracycline, or erythromycin may provide relief, but caution must be taken when treating egg-laying chickens due to restrictions on antibiotic use. Vaccination may aid prevention, but serotype-specific (A, B, or C) vaccines must match the infecting bacterial serotype to avoid vaccine failure. Fowl cholera: Tetracyclines and sulfa drugs can be used during disease outbreaks, but antibiotics are ineffective against the chronic form. ILT: There is no medication to treat infectious laryngotracheitis. Antibiotics may

be used to control secondary infections in severe cases. Infectious bronchitis: Tetracycline or sulfa drugs can be used for suspected secondary bacterial infections. Pox (diphtheritic, wet form): There is no medication to treat fowlpox. Gape worm: Fenbendazole has been approved for use in chickens. Off-label medications such as thiabendazole, mebendazole, cambendazole, and levamisole may be effective. Aspergillosis: Treatment of aspergillosis is long and difficult, and may involve 4–6 months of systemic antifungal agents (e.g. itraconazole, voriconazole) and topical application of antifungal agents via endoscopy or nebulization, as well as environmental modification and supportive care.

### CONTRAINDICATIONS
N/A

### PRECAUTIONS
Drugs for food-producing backyard poultry should comply with applicable regulations.

### POSSIBLE INTERACTIONS
N/A

### ALTERNATIVE DRUGS
N/A

## FOLLOW-UP

### PATIENT MONITORING
N/A

### PREVENTION/AVOIDANCE
Proper biosecurity measures. Non-specific respiratory disease: Keep the environment optimal. Infectious coryza: Vaccination may aid prevention, but serotype-specific (A, B, or C) vaccines must match the infecting bacterial serotype to avoid vaccine failure. Fowl cholera: Exclude cats and rats from poultry flocks. Commercial vaccines are available. It is important to determine the serotype of the infecting *P. multocida* for serotype-specific vaccines. Types 1, 3, 4, and 3 × 4 are the most common. ILT: Modified live ILT vaccines can cause latently infected carrier birds. Genetically modified pox or turkey herpes virus (Marek) vaccines, which only contain the protective portion of the ILT virus, are safer alternatives. Modified live ILT vaccines should not be used in backyard chickens. Infectious bronchitis: Future flocks should be vaccinated with a serotype that guards against the field strain. Pox (diphtheritic, wet form): Vaccinating and controlling biting insects is important, as pox virus can be transmitted from bird to bird this way. Gape worm: Controlling earthworms and other insect vectors is essential for preventing the disease and its

transmission between flocks. Aspergillosis: Candling eggs frequently in incubators and setters is important for detecting embryos that may have died from fungal infection. Dust control and providing dry, cool environments can help prevent this condition in older turkeys, ducks, and geese.

### POSSIBLE COMPLICATIONS
Mycoplasmosis from *M. gallisepticum*: Secondary *E. coli* infections may cause increased mortality, known as chronic respiratory disease in broiler chickens, and elevated death loss in turkeys and peafowl. Infectious bronchitis: When complicated by *E. coli*, lesions may include septicemia and fibrin deposits on the pericardial sac, liver capsule, and in the body cavity. Pox (diphtheritic, wet form): Wet pox is often complicated as a result of a co-infection with ILT virus and fowl pox virus.

### EXPECTED COURSE AND PROGNOSIS
The prognosis of respiratory diseases in backyard chickens depends on the severity of the disease and how quickly it is diagnosed and treated.

## MISCELLANEOUS

### ASSOCIATED CONDITIONS
Chickens affected by respiratory diseases may exhibit decreased egg production.

### AGE-RELATED FACTORS
Respiratory disease caused by *M. gallisepticum*, infectious coryza, gapeworm infection, and aspergillosis can all lead to increased mortality in young poultry.

### ZOONOTIC POTENTIAL
Fowl cholera isolates of *P. multocida* are *not* considered to have zoonotic potential as avian isolates are generally non-pathogenic in mammals exposed by the oral or subcutaneous routes, whereas humans are typically only susceptible to mammalian strains of *P. multocida* when bitten by an infected animal. Aspergillosis is not transmitted among birds or between birds and humans, but humans may become infected by inhaling spores when working with infected materials or birds.

### FERTILITY/BREEDING
Overall, non-specific respiratory disease can cause a drop in egg production. Infectious coryza in backyard birds can affect the fertility of poultry by causing a significant (10–40%) drop in egg laying. Infectious bronchitis in backyard birds can cause a reduction in the fertility of poultry, leading to reduced egg production and poorer egg quality.

R

## SYNONYMS
N/A

## SEE ALSO
Aspergillosis
Mycoplasmosis
Pasteurellosis
Pneumonia
Respiratory Distress
Rhinitis and Sinusitis
Also individual named viral diseases

## ABBREVIATIONS
ELISA—enzyme-linked immunosorbent assay
IBV—infectious bronchitis virus
ILT—infectious laryngotracheitis
ILTV—infectious laryngotracheitis virus
NAD—nicotinamide adenine dinucleotide
NPIP—National Poultry Improvement Plan
OAvV—avian orthoavulavirus
PCR—polymerase chain reaction
PPMV-1—pigeon paramyxovirus type 1

## INTERNET RESOURCES
Canadian Food Inspection Agency. How to prevent and detect disease in small flocks and pet birds: https://inspection.canada.ca/animal-health/terrestrial-animals/diseases/backyard-flocks-and-pet-birds/eng/1323643634523/1323644740109
Hartsook, C. Backyard biosecurity for poultry. Iowa State University: https://www.extension.iastate.edu/smallfarms/backyard-biosecurity-poultry
Martin, E., Brouwer, E., Todd, K. Diagnosing respiratory disease in backyard chickens. University of Guelph: https://www.uoguelph.ca/ahl/content/diagnosing-respiratory-disease-backyard-chickens
Williams, Z., Fulton, M. Poultry disease: Infectious coryza. Michigan State University: https://www.canr.msu.edu/resources/poultry-diseases-infectious-coryza

## Suggested Reading
Fulton, M.R. (2021). Respiratory Disease. In: *Backyard Poultry Medicine and Surgery: A guide for veterinary practitioners* (ed. T.Y. Morishita, C.B. Greenacre), 218–228. Ames, IA: Wiley.
Brochu, N.M., Guerin, M.T., Varga, C., et al. (2019). A two-year prospective study of small poultry flocks in Ontario, Canada, part 2: causes of morbidity and mortality. *Journal of Veterinary Diagnostic Investigation*, 31:336–342.
Crispo, M., Blackall, P., Khan, A., et al. (2019). Characterization of an outbreak of infectious coryza (*Avibacterium paragallinarum*) in commercial chickens in central California. *Avian Diseases*, 63:486–494.
Derksen, T., Lampron, R., Hauck, R., et al. (2018). Biosecurity assessment and seroprevalence of respiratory diseases in backyard poultry flocks located close to and far from commercial premises. *Avian Diseases*, 62:1–5.

**Authors:** Sunoh Che, DVM, PhD, DACVPM, and Leonardo Susta, DVM, PhD, DACVP

R

# BASICS

## DEFINITION
Two retroviruses causing lymphoid neoplasia are of clinical importance in Galliformes: the alpharetrovirus of the lymphoid leukosis (LL), and the gammaretrovirus of reticuloendotheliosis (RE). These viruses are common in chicken flocks, and it can be difficult to differentiate between these viral etiologies due to their similar clinical signs.

## PATHOPHYSIOLOGY
**LL**: Caused by lymphoid leukosis virus (LLV), an alpharetrovirus predominantly involving B lymphocytes, vertically (through the egg) or horizontally transmitted (oculonasal, oral, respiratory or skin, via feces, saliva or skin dander). Disease is most commonly from a virus of subgroup A or B, less commonly subgroup J. Can also be transmitted as a contaminant of live vaccines (Marek's disease, fowl pox) produced in chicken embryo cells or tissues. Incubation period from time of infection to time of clinical signs can range from a few weeks to several months.
**RE**: Caused by reticuloendotheliosis virus (REV), a gammaretrovirus involving B or T lymphocytes, vertically or horizontally transmitted. Mosquitoes can transmit REV. Can also be transmitted as a contaminant of live vaccines (Marek's disease, fowl pox) produced in chicken embryo cells or tissues. Incubation period from time of infection to time of clinical signs can range from two weeks to several months.

## SYSTEMS AFFECTED
**Gastrointestinal**: Diarrhea, hepatomegaly.
**Hemic/lymphatic/immune**: LL—leukemia is not typically seen, thus the term "leukosis" is used. Commonly affects the bursa of Fabricius. RE—immunosuppression is considered one of the most important effects of infection; stunted growth can be due to immunosuppression.
**Musculoskeletal**: RE—stunted growth. Neuromuscular.
**Reproductive**: Decreased egg production and quality, reproductive tract tumors.
**Skin/endocrine**: RE—abnormal feathering ("nakanuke").

## GENETICS
N/A

## INCIDENCE/PREVALENCE
LLV is considered to be ubiquitous in chicken flocks, while REV is considered common. LL—incidence of neoplasms in infected flocks is usually only 1–2%, although losses of up to 20% can occur. RE—clinical disease is rare, but losses from mortality or condemnation at slaughter in affected flocks can be as high as 20%.

## GEOGRAPHIC DISTRIBUTION
Worldwide.

## SIGNALMENT
**Species**: Chickens—RE, LL; turkeys, pheasants, partridges, prairie chickens, peafowl, quail, ducks, geese—RE.
**Mean age and range**: LL—≥ 14 weeks of age, with most mortality at 24–40 weeks. Generally, resistance to infection increases with age. RE—stunted growth can be noticed as early as 1 month; lymphomas typically occur at ≥ 15 weeks, depending on bird species.
**Predominant sex**: LL—females are more likely to develop tumors than males.

## SIGNS

### General Comments
Both viruses can cause lethargy, diarrhea, inappetence, emaciation, dehydration, depressed egg laying, stunted growth.

### Historical Findings
Stunted growth: RE.

### Physical Examination Findings
Abnormal feather development, with adhesion of the barbs to a localized section of the shaft ("nakanuke")—RE. Abdominal distention—LL.

## CAUSES
Vertical transmission from hen—LL, RE. Vertical transmission from rooster—RE. Horizontal transmission from infected birds—LL, RE.

## RISK FACTORS
LL: Incidence may be reduced by the presence of infectious bursal disease virus.

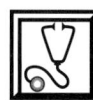

# DIAGNOSIS

## DIFFERENTIAL DIAGNOSIS
Both viruses should be considered in the differential diagnosis list, as well as Marek's disease, herpesvirus, and other neurological or visceral diseases (e.g. ovarian adenocarcinoma).

## CBC/BIOCHEMISTRY/URINALYSIS
RE: Anemia is sometimes seen. LL: Leukemia is rarely seen.

## OTHER LABORATORY TESTS
Antibody titer measurement (ELISA or virus neutralization) is available for both viruses, but since the viruses all occur commonly, evidence of exposure for a particular virus does not necessarily confirm the etiology of observed clinical signs. Viral antibodies present in birds < 4 weeks old are likely to have been maternally derived. Viral antibodies against LLV in day-old chicks indicate the presence of exposure in the hen; therefore, the chick may be congenitally infected and could spread the infection to other chicks. Individual birds without antibodies in a known infected flock may have "tolerant infection" and be viremic shedders of LLV or REV. Samples for antibody detection include plasma, serum, or egg yolk (LLV). Viral detection by virus isolation, PCR or ELISA is available for both viruses but, as above, evidence of infection does not confirm etiology. Samples for testing include buffy coat cells from heparinized whole blood (LLV), oviduct swabs (LLV), cloacal swabs (LLV, REV), egg albumen (LLV, REV), embryo tissue (LLV), meconium (LLV), feces (LLV, REV), oral swabs (LLV), semen (LLV, REV), or suspensions of splenic, feather tip or lymphomatous tissue (LLV).

## IMAGING
N/A

## DIAGNOSTIC PROCEDURES
Antemortem diagnostic tests are unlikely to be informative as to a specific etiologic diagnosis.

## PATHOLOGIC FINDINGS
Various gross findings can be seen, depending on the phase of disease. Swelling and loss of striations in peripheral nerves, especially the sciatic nerves, less frequent in adult birds than in young birds—RE. Hepatomegaly—LL, RE. Diffuse, miliary or nodular tumors in liver—LL, RE. Splenomegaly—LL, RE. Diffuse, miliary or nodular tumors in spleen—LL, RE. Spleen is soft in texture—LL. Bursal enlargement—LL. Bursal atrophy—RE. Nodular tumors in bursa—LL, RE. Thymus atrophy—RE. Diffuse or focal tumors in bone marrow—LL. Intestinal thickening and annular lesions—RE. Kidney involvement—LL. Ovarian involvement—LL. Skin lesions on head and mouth—RE. Abnormal feathering—RE. Leukemia, although uncommon—LL (lymphoblastic). If lymphomas are found in ducks, geese, pheasants or quail, REV is a likely cause rather than Marek's disease virus or LLV. Various microscopic findings can be seen in cytologic or histopathologic examination, depending on the phase of disease. Extravascular infiltrations of lymphoblasts—LL, RE.

# TREATMENT

## APPROPRIATE HEALTH CARE
Treatment has been unsuccessful for birds clinically affected by any of these viruses; symptomatic infections become fatal.

**R**

### NURSING CARE
N/A

### ACTIVITY
N/A

### DIET
N/A

### CLIENT EDUCATION
N/A

### SURGICAL CONSIDERATIONS
N/A

# MEDICATIONS

### DRUG(S) OF CHOICE
Treatment has been unsuccessful for birds clinically affected by any of these viruses; symptomatic infections become fatal. NSAIDs may temporarily improve the quality of life of affected birds.

### CONTRAINDICATIONS
N/A

### PRECAUTIONS
N/A

### POSSIBLE INTERACTIONS
N/A

### ALTERNATIVE DRUGS
See Drug(s) of Choice section.

# FOLLOW-UP

### PATIENT MONITORING
N/A

### PREVENTION/AVOIDANCE
LL, RE: Vaccines are not commercially available, therefore eradication from a flock depends on breaking the vertical transmission cycle from dam to chicks (eliminating dams and roosters that are infected), and prevention of reinfection of chicks. Although roosters do not transmit LLV via semen to embryos, they can be a venereal source of infection for hens. Hatched chicks can be reared in isolation in small groups and tested for viremia and viral antibodies from approximately 8 weeks of age to verify virus-free status. RE: Reduction of insect vectors (mosquitoes). Hygiene, including removal of used litter and disinfection. LLV and REV only survive for a few hours outside a host. The most effective types of disinfectants for these viruses are chlorine-releasing agents and iodophors; chlorhexidine is ineffective. Freezing and thawing will degrade LLV and REV, as will high temperatures (> 122°F/50°C.) or pH extremes (< 5 or > 9). Biosecurity, preventing introduction of new viral strains to a bird enclosure. Minimization of stress, especially in newly-hatched chicks (to encourage development of immunity) and around the time of onset of egg production.

### POSSIBLE COMPLICATIONS
N/A

### EXPECTED COURSE AND PROGNOSIS
Symptomatic infections with any of these two viruses invariably become fatal.

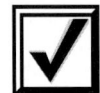

# MISCELLANEOUS

### ASSOCIATED CONDITIONS
LL—fowl glioma.

### AGE-RELATED FACTORS
LL—congenitally infected chicks are an important source of infection for other chicks in the hatchery and during the brooding period.

### ZOONOTIC POTENTIAL
Although seropositivity has been seen in humans, there is no direct evidence of disease potential in humans for LLV or REV.

### FERTILITY/BREEDING
Poor egg production, egg size, fertility, hatchability, and chick growth rate.

### SYNONYMS
LL—big liver disease, lymphatic leukosis, visceral lymphoma, lymphocytoma, lymphomatosis, visceral lymphomatosis.

### SEE ALSO
Dermatitis
Lameness
Neoplasia (Lymphoproliferative)
Neurologic (Non-Traumatic Diseases)
Regurgitation and Vomiting
Respiratory Distress
Also individual named viral diseases

### ABBREVIATIONS
ELISA—enzyme-linked immunosorbent assay
LL—lymphoid leukosis
LLV—lymphoid leukosis virus
NSAIDs—non-steroidal anti-inflammatory drugs
PCR—polymerase chain reaction
RE—reticuloendotheliosis
REV—reticuloendotheliosis virus

### INTERNET RESOURCES
Dinev, I. (2007). Lymphoid leukosis. *Diseases of Poultry: A color atlas*. The Poultry Site: http://www.thepoultrysite.com/publications/6/diseases-of-poultry/202/lymphoid-leukosis
Dunn, J. (2022). Overview of neoplasms in poultry. *Merck Veterinary Manual*: http://www.merckmanuals.com/vet/poultry/neoplasms/overview_of_neoplasms_in_poultry.html

*Suggested Reading*
Nair, V., Gimeno, I., Dunn, J. et al. (2019). Neoplastic diseases. In: *Diseases of Poultry*, 14th edn. (ed. D.E. Swayne, D.E., M. Boulianne, C.M. Logue, et al.), 548–715. Hoboken, NJ: Wiley.
Payne, L.N. (1998). Retrovirus-induced disease in poultry. *Poultry Science*, 77:1204–1212.
Payne, L.N., Venugopal, K. (2000). Neoplastic diseases: Marek's disease, avian leukosis and reticuloendotheliosis. *Revue Scientifique et Technique*, 19:544–564.
**Author**: Marion Desmarchelier, DMV, IPSAV, MSc, DACZM, DECZM (Zoo Health Management), DACVB
**Acknowledgements**: Lisa Harrenstein, DVM, DACZM, and Shannon Ferrell, DVM, DABVP (Avian), DACZM

R

# BASICS

## DEFINITION
Rhinitis is inflammation of one or both nasal cavities. Sinusitis is inflammation of one or more diverticulae of the infraorbital paranasal sinus.

## PATHOPHYSIOLOGY
The upper respiratory system in birds consists of the paired nasal cavities and paired infraorbital paranasal sinuses. Air flows into the nasal cavity through bilateral nares (nostrils). The nasal cavity is divided by the nasal septum, which is incomplete in psittacine birds. Three nasal conchae (rostral, middle, and caudal) serve to warm and moisten inspired air. The middle and caudal conchae communicate with the infraorbital sinus through small dorsal openings. Air exits the nasal cavity ventrally through the choana, a slit-like opening in the palate. The infraorbital sinus is the only true paranasal sinus in birds. It is located ventromedial to the orbit and consists of several diverticulae—rostral, preorbital, infraorbital, postorbital, and mandibular. The right and left infraorbital sinuses communicate in psittacine birds but not in passerine birds. The infraorbital sinus communicates with the cervicocephalic air sac. Most bacterial and fungal infections of the nasal cavity and infraorbital sinus are secondary to other diseases of the nasal cavity or infraorbital sinus, which predispose these structures to infection, such as hypovitaminosis A, foreign bodies, trauma, airborne toxins and irritants, developmental abnormalities, and neoplasia.

## SYSTEMS AFFECTED
Respiratory, ophthalmic, gastrointestinal.

## GENETICS
Choanal atresia and imperforate naris may have a genetic basis.

## INCIDENCE/PREVALENCE
Unknown.

## GEOGRAPHIC DISTRIBUTION
N/A

## SIGNALMENT
**Species**: Variable.
**Mean age and range**: Variable. Congenital diseases such as choanal atresia and imperforate naris are seen in young birds. Neoplastic diseases are generally seen in middle-aged to older birds.
**Predominant sex**: None

## SIGNS
### Historical Findings
Wheezing, sneezing, nasal snuffling, nasal discharge, infraorbital sinus ("cheek") flaring, head shaking, open-beak breathing, lethargy, reduced appetite.

### Physical Examination Findings
**Rhinitis**: Serous to mucopurulent nasal and/or ocular discharge, matted feathers surrounding the affected naris or nares and/or eye(s), redness or swelling of the opening to the affected naris/nares, distortion or erosion of the nasal opening and cavity or distortion along upper beak extending rostrally from affected naris or nares, nasal obstruction, blunting or loss of the choanal papillae, choanal discharge, open mouth breathing.
**Sinusitis**: Periorbital swelling, sneezing, infraorbital sinus ("cheek") flaring with breathing, sunken eyed appearance (reported with Gram-negative bacterial infections in macaws, termed "sunken sinus syndrome"), serous to mucopurulent nasal or ocular discharge.

## CAUSES
**Congenital**: Choanal atresia, most commonly reported in grey parrots. Imperforate naris or nares.
**Nutritional**: Hypovitaminosis A.
**Neoplasia**: Nasal or sinus adenocarcinoma. Squamous cell carcinoma. Lymphoma. Fibroma, fibrosarcoma. Basal cell carcinoma. Malignant melanoma.
**Immune-mediated**: (Allergic) rhinitis and sinusitis.
**Infectious**: Viral—rarely the underlying cause of rhinitis or sinusitis in companion birds. Avian influenza virus, herpesvirus, paramyxovirus (e.g. Newcastle disease virus), poxvirus, reovirus. Primary bacterial agents (may also be considered as secondary or opportunistic agents in some cases)—*Bordetella avium*, *Chlamydia psittaci*, *Enterobacter* spp. (e.g. canaries and finches), *Helicobacter* spp. ("spiral bacteria") in cockatiels, *Mycoplasma* spp. (e.g. finches, budgerigars, cockatiels), *Mycobacterium* spp., *Salmonella* spp., *Yersinia pseudotuberculosis* (e.g. canaries and finches). Secondary (opportunistic) bacterial agents (may also be considered primary agents in certain cases)—*Escherichia coli*, *Haemophilus* spp., ▪ *Klebsiella* spp., ▪ *Nocardia asteroides*, ▪ *Pasteurella* spp., ▪ *Pseudomonas aeruginosa*, ▪ *Staphylococcus* spp., ▪ *Streptococcus* spp. Fungal agents (fungal infections are often considered opportunistic and noncontagious)—*Aspergillus* spp. (particularly in grey parrots), *Candida albicans*, *Cryptococcus* spp., *Mucor* spp. Parasitic agents—*Knemidocoptes pilae* (e.g. canaries), *Trichomonas* spp. (e.g. canaries).
**Foreign bodies**: Food particles, wood shavings, etc.
**Rhinoliths**: Proliferative nasal granulomas—most frequently reported in grey parrots.
**Trauma**

## RISK FACTORS
Poor air quality (e.g. exposure to cigarette smoke, vape aerosols, cooking fumes). Inadequate humidity. Inadequate bathing. Hypovitaminosis A (results in squamous metaplasia of the epithelial lining to the upper respiratory tract).

# DIAGNOSIS

## DIFFERENTIAL DIAGNOSIS
Lower respiratory disease. Diseases of the oral cavity. Ocular disease.

## CBC/BIOCHEMISTRY/URINALYSIS
Hematologic and biochemistry findings are generally non-specific. Infectious and inflammatory diseases may be associated with leukocytosis and heterophilia or monocytosis.

## OTHER LABORATORY TESTS
Cytology is useful to evaluate fluid and tissue samples. Special stains (e.g. Gram, acid-fast) are useful to further evaluate micro-organisms such as bacteria and fungi. Microbiologic C/S is useful for identification of micro-organisms and for determining suitable antibiotics for treatment. Infectious disease screening: Serologic tests are available for a number of infectious agents, such as *C. psittaci* and *Aspergillus* spp. Additional serodiagnostic assays such as gliotoxin and galactomannan biomarker evaluation are available for further screening for aspergillosis in birds. PCR assays are available for a number of infectious agents, such as *C. psittaci* and *Mycobacterium* spp. Additional testing methods are available and may be useful in select cases, such as immunohistochemistry and in situ hybridization on tissue samples. EPH is potentially useful for further evaluating for evidence of an inflammatory response to disease. Histopathology is indicated for tissue samples obtained through biopsy of affected structures.

## IMAGING
### Radiographic Findings
Survey radiographs of the skull can be helpful in evaluating bony and soft tissue structures. Sedation or general anesthesia is recommended for imaging. Superimposition of bony structures can make interpretation of findings difficult. Additional views such as oblique or skyline views may provide additional diagnostic information. Contrast radiographs may be especially helpful in the diagnosis of choanal atresia and other obstructive diseases. Iodinated contrast such as iohexal (e.g. Omnipaque™, GE Healthcare, Marlborough, MA) is diluted to 15–29% in sterile saline and instilled into the naris.

R

Absence of radiographic evidence of flow through the choanal slit into the oral cavity can be diagnostic for choanal atresia.

### Ultrasonographic Findings
Ultrasound waves do not travel efficiently through air such as that normally present within the nasal and infraorbital sinus cavities. However, fluid or tissue masses present within these cavities during disease states may be visible or may enhance visualization. Fluid or masses identified by ultrasonography can often be sampled by ultrasound-guided fine-needle aspirate.

### Advanced Imaging
CT with or without contrast enhancement can be very helpful in further evaluation of the skull and its components. Sedation or general anesthesia is often advisable for imaging. Like CT, MRI can be helpful in further evaluating the skull. MRI is most suitable for diseases affecting soft tissue structures. Both CT and MRI allow for image reconstruction matrices, eliminating problems with superimposition of anatomic structures by conventional radiography.

### DIAGNOSTIC PROCEDURES
#### Sample Collection Methods
**Nasal swab:** A sterile specimen collection swab is placed into the naris or nares. This method is best suited for the collection of serous to mucopurulent nasal discharge. Environmental contamination is common. Syringe aspiration of contents of the nasal cavity through the naris or nares may be useful for collection of fluid samples. Environmental contamination is common. For nasal lavage (nasal irrigation, nasal flush), the bird is positioned with the head down and approximately 5–10 ml/kg of warm sterile saline or water is instilled into the nasal cavity through the naris or nares. The fluid is collected as it flushes through the choanal slit and out the oral cavity. The fluid sample is representative of the nasal cavity but not the infraorbital sinus, except possibly for the preorbital diverticulum. Contamination with oral flora is unavoidable.
**Sinus aspiration and lavage:** Can safely be performed in the awake bird. The preorbital diverticulum of the infraorbital sinus can be sampled through a site halfway between the eye and the external naris under (or over) the jugal arch. The needle is directed perpendicular to the skin. A 25-gauge hypodermic or butterfly needle is suitable in most cases. Fluid within the preorbital diverticulum can be aspirated using this method. The infraorbital diverticulum of the infraorbital sinus can be aspirated directly ventral to the orbit dorsal to the jugal arch. Great care must be taken to avoid the ocular globe. If no fluid is immediately

aspirated, sterile saline can be instilled and aspirated.
**Choanal swab:** A moistened sterile swab is inserted into the rostral diverticulum of the choanal slit. This sample only represents a small portion of the upper respiratory tract. Contamination with oral flora is common.

### Endoscopy
Endoscopy can be used to visualize and obtain diagnostic samples from the upper respiratory tract. Anatomic areas amenable to endoscopy include the rostral choanal sulcus, external naris (in larger birds), and several diverticula of the infraorbital sinus through a surgical approach.

### PATHOLOGIC FINDINGS
Variable.

# TREATMENT
### APPROPRIATE HEALTH CARE
Birds with rhinitis or sinusitis are most often managed on an outpatient basis unless surgery is performed. Lavage of the nasal cavity or the infraorbital sinus using the methods described earlier can be useful to flush these cavities to remove inflammatory and foreign debris and to instill medications. For chronic conditions such as nasal cavity erosion associated with rhinolithiasis, clients can be instructed on performing nasal irrigation at home. Sinus lavage requires the use of a hypodermic needle in a challenging anatomic location and therefore must be performed by a trained veterinary professional. Rhinoliths can be manually removed using bent-tipped hypodermic needles, ear curettes, and other devices. Topical anesthesia and sedation or general anesthesia is advised. The nasal cavity should be lavaged after debridement. Nebulization can be used to deliver medications to the nasal cavity and infraorbital sinus, provided that there is patent air flow through these anatomic structures. Nebulization is unlikely to be successful with obstructive diseases.

### NURSING CARE
Extensive nursing care is generally not required in cases of rhinitis or sinusitis.

### ACTIVITY
Restrictions in activity are generally not required in cases of rhinitis or sinusitis.

### DIET
If rhinitis or sinusitis is believed associated with hypovitaminosis A, dietary modifications should be advised.

### CLIENT EDUCATION
Clients should avoid exposure of their birds to airborne toxins and irritants such as cigarette smoke, vape aerosols, and cooking fumes.

### SURGICAL CONSIDERATIONS
Patients should be assessed for lower respiratory disease, which would increase the risks of general anesthesia needed for surgery. Sinusotomy: Surgical access to the preorbital diverticulum of the infraorbital sinus is approximately midway between the medial canthus of the eye and external naris, below (or sometimes above) the jugal arch. Through this site, the diverticulum can be visually or endoscopically explored. Purulent or caseous debris and sinoliths can then be debrided. The incision can be left open to heal, or drains or stents can be placed, allowing continued lavage and drug delivery. Sinus trephination: If the rostral or preorbital diverticulum of the infraorbital sinus within the frontal bone is involved, bony trephination may be necessary to gain surgical access to the sinus cavity. The bony defect can be left open for continued lavage and drug delivery. Choanal atresia and imperforate naris repair: Several surgical techniques have been described for the repair of choanal atresia and imperforate naris.

# MEDICATIONS
### DRUG(S) OF CHOICE
#### Topical Antimicrobials
Antibiotics: Broad-spectrum ophthalmic antibiotic solutions are often prescribed for topical application to the nasal cavity. Fluoroquinolones—ciprofloxacin ophthalmic solution 3 mg/ml 0.3% (e.g. Ciloxan®, Novartis, Fort Worth, TX), ofloxacin ophthalmic solution 3 mg/ml 0.3% (e.g. Ocuflox®, Allergan, Irvine, CA). Aminoglycosides—gentamicin sulfate ophthalmic solution 3 mg/ml (0.3%). Antifungals—clotrimazole 10 mg/ml (1%) solution; amphotericin B, at dilutions no greater than 0.05 mg/ml. Sinus irrigation using a 50 mg/ml solution was associated with severe granulomatous inflammation and death in a grey parrot in one report.

#### Systemic Antimicrobials
Systemic antibiotics are indicated for more severe or invasive bacterial infections, ideally based on results of culture and sensitivity testing. Bactericidal antibiotics are generally preferred over bacteriostatic antibiotics. Antifungals are indicated for more severe or invasive mycotic infections. Azole antifungals—itraconazole, voriconazole. Terbinafine. Amphotericin B.

*Antimicrobials for Nebulization*

Antibiotics: Enrofloxacin, gentamicin.
Antifungals: Clotrimazole 10 mg/ml 1%
solution; terbinafine. Disinfectants—F10®SC
veterinary disinfectant 1: 250 dilution
(Health and Hygiene Pty. Ltd., Florida Hills,
South Africa).

### CONTRAINDICATIONS
None.

### PRECAUTIONS
None.

### POSSIBLE INTERACTIONS
None.

### ALTERNATIVE DRUGS
None.

## FOLLOW-UP

### PATIENT MONITORING
Birds with rhinitis or sinusitis should be
periodically evaluated until the condition is
resolved. For chronic cases such as
rhinolithiasis with nasal cavity erosion, birds
should be re-evaluated every few months.

### PREVENTION/AVOIDANCE
Airborne toxins and irritants such as cigarette
smoke, vape aerosols, and cooking fumes
should be avoided. Diets should be balanced
and adequate in carotenoids or preformed
vitamin A and other nutrients.

### POSSIBLE COMPLICATIONS
Systemic spread of bacterial or fungal
infections (sepsis) can occur with advanced or
refractory rhinitis or sinusitis. Neoplasms can
be locally aggressive or metastasize to regional
or distant sites.

### EXPECTED COURSE
### AND PROGNOSIS
Complete resolution is achievable in most
cases of uncomplicated bacterial or mycotic
rhinitis or sinusitis, and in cases involving

foreign bodies or trauma. However,
resolution of underlying conditions such as
congenital choanal atresia or neoplasia is
often challenging at best.

## MISCELLANEOUS

### ASSOCIATED CONDITIONS
Hypovitaminosis A is often associated with
other conditions.

### AGE-RELATED FACTORS
None.

### ZOONOTIC POTENTIAL
*C. psittaci*, one cause of rhinitis and sinusitis
in birds, is a zoonotic and reportable disease.
Avian influenza also has zoonotic potential
and is also a reportable disease.

### FERTILITY/BREEDING
N/A

### SYNONYMS
N/A

### SEE ALSO
Aspergillosis
Bordetellosis
Mycoplasmosis
Neoplasia (Respiratory)
Nutritional Imbalances
Respiratory Distress
Toxicosis (Airborne)
Also individual named viral diseases

### ABBREVIATIONS
C/S—culture and sensitivity
CT—computed tomography
EPH—protein electrophoresis
MRI—magnetic resonance imaging
PCR—polymerase chain reaction

### INTERNET RESOURCES
N/A

*Suggested Reading*
Crosta, L. (2021). Respiratory diseases of
parrots: Anatomy, physiology, diagnosis
and treatment. *Veterinary Clinics of North
America: Exotic Animal Practice*,
24:397–418.
King, A.S., McLelland, J. (1984). *Birds, Their
Structure and Function*. Philadelphia, PA:
Baillière Tindall.
Noonan, B.P., de Matos, R., Butler, B.P.,
et al. (2014). Nasal adenocarcinoma and
secondary chronic sinusitis in a hyacinth
macaw (*Anodorhynchus hyacinthinus*).
*Journal of Avian Medicine and Surgery*,
28:143–150.
Pye, G.W. (2022). Surgery of the avian
respiratory system and cranial coelom.
In: *Surgery of Exotic Animals*
(ed. R.A. Bennett, G.W. Pye), 190–203.
Hoboken, NJ: Wiley.
Schmidt, R.E., Reavill, D.R., Phalen, D.N.
(2015). *Pathology of Pet and Aviary Birds*,
2nd edn. Ames, IA: Wiley.
Tully, T.N., Harrison, G.J. (1994).
Pneumonology. In: *Avian Medicine:
Principles and Application* (ed. B.W. Ritchie,
G.J. Harrison, L.R. Harrison), 556–580.
Lake Worth, FL: Wingers Publishing.
Turner, R.C., Graham, J.E., Hahn, S., et al.
(2019). Infraorbital keratin cyst in an
umbrella cockatoo (*Cacatua alba*).
*Journal of Avian Medicine and Surgery*,
33:150–154.
Zwart, P., Samour, J. (2021). The avian
respiratory system and its noninfectious
disorders: A review. *Journal of Exotic Pet
Medicine*, 37:39–50.
**Author**: Lauren V. Powers, DVM, DABVP
(Avian Practice), DABVP (Exotic
Companion Mammal Practice)

 **Client Education Handout available
online**

R

# ROTAVIRUS

 **BASICS**

## DEFINITION
Avian rotavirus group A is a common cause of enteritis and diarrhoea in young poultry, and results in important losses in the poultry industry globally. Pigeon-associated clade of rotavirus A G18P[17] is known to cause fatal outbreaks of disease in juvenile and adult domestic pigeons in Australia, Europe and USA since 2016.

## PATHOPHYSIOLOGY
Avian rotavirus is a member of the Reoviridae family, characterized by 10–12 linear double-stranded RNA segments. Co-infection of cells with different rotavirus strains can result in genetic reassortment. Horizontal transmission by fecal–oral route. Infection and replication in enteric epithelia cells of the small intestine. Infection of liver cells in pigeons.

## SYSTEMS AFFECTED
Gastrointestinal. Hepatobiliary in pigeons.

## GENETICS
N/A

## INCIDENCE/PREVALENCE
Commonly described in poultry and pigeons. Morbidity can reach 100%; usually low mortality.

## GEOGRAPHIC DISTRIBUTION
Worldwide.

## SIGNALMEN
**Species**: Domestic galliform birds. Domestic pigeons.
**Mean age and range**: Galliform birds less than 6 weeks of age. Mainly young pigeons.
**Predominant sex**: None.

## SIGNS
### Historical Findings
Lethargy and depression. Ruffled feathers. Anorexia and weight loss. Diarrhoea. Extreme thirst. Regurgitation of water and seeds in pigeons.

### Physical Examination Findings
Depression. Dehydration. Crop filled with green watery content in pigeons.

## CAUSES
Infectious.

## RISK FACTORS
Fancy pigeon shows; training or races with young pigeons.

 **DIAGNOSIS**

## DIFFERENTIAL DIAGNOSIS
Enteritis caused by other pathogens in poultry, particularly reovirus, coronavirus, astrovirus, adenovirus, *Clostridia*, *Coccidia*. Young pigeon disease syndrome. Adenovirus infection in pigeons. Herpesvirus infection in pigeons.

## CBC/BIOCHEMISTRY/URINALYSIS
N/A

## OTHER LABORATORY TESTS
rt-PCR of cloacal swabs. Serology.

## IMAGING
N/A

## DIAGNOSTIC PROCEDURES
Necropsy.

## PATHOLOGIC FINDINGS
Increased amount of fluid in the small intestine. Watery filled caeca in poultry. Watery green fluid in the crop of pigeons. Mottled, congested, and friable liver in pigeons. Separation and desquamation of enterocytes from the lamina propria, villous atrophy and fusion, infiltration of mixed inflammatory cells. Coalescing hepatocellular necrosis with infiltration of mononuclear cells in pigeons.

 **TREATMENT**

## APPROPRIATE HEALTH CARE
Inpatient medical management may be required; fluid and nutritional support are indicated if the patient is debilitated and dehydrated.

## NURSING CARE
Fluid support (SQ, IV, IO) Nutritional support via gavage may be indicated if anorexic.

## ACTIVITY
No restrictions indicated.

## DIET
N/A

## CLIENT EDUCATION
Increasing ventilation rate and temperature, as well as adding fresh litter, may help to reduce transmission risk.

## SURGICAL CONSIDERATIONS
N/A

 **MEDICATIONS**

## DRUG(S) OF CHOICE
None. Self-limited flock disease with recovery of the birds after 10 days at the latest.

## CONTRAINDICATIONS
N/A

## PRECAUTIONS
N/A

## POSSIBLE INTERACTIONS
N/A

## ALTERNATIVE DRUGS
N/A

 **FOLLOW-UP**

## PATIENT MONITORING
Viral shedding via feces.

## PREVENTION/AVOIDANCE
Vaccine (Colvac® RP, Pharmagal Bio, Czech Republic) is available for pigeons. It is a combined vaccine including pigeon paramyxovirus 1 antigen.

## POSSIBLE COMPLICATIONS
N/A

## EXPECTED COURSE AND PROGNOSIS
High morbidity with risk of stunting.

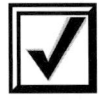 **MISCELLANEOUS**

## ASSOCIATED CONDITIONS
Secondary bacterial infection of the gastrointestinal tract. Stunting of growth. Pasted and inflamed vents with increased risk of vent pecking in poultry chicks. Litter ingestion.

## AGE-RELATED FACTORS
N/A

## ZOONOTIC POTENTIAL
None.

## FERTILITY/BREEDING
N/A

## SYNONYMS
Poult enteritis and mortality syndrome in turkey poults, young pigeon disease syndrome.

## SEE ALSO
Adenoviruses
Circovirus (Psittacines)
Circoviruses (Non-Psittacine Birds)
Coccidiosis (Intestinal)
Colibacillosis
Diarrhea
Flagellate Enteritis
Foreign Bodies (Gastrointestinal)
Helminthiasis (Gastrointestinal)
Herpesvirus (Columbid Herpesvirus 1 in Pigeons and Raptors)
Ileus (Gastrointestinal, Crop Stasis)
Neoplasia (Gastrointestinal)
Toxicosis (Ingested, Gastrointestinal)

## ABBREVIATIONS
rt-PCR—reverse transcriptase polymerase chain reaction

## INTERNET RESOURCES
N/A

*Suggested Reading*

Day, J.M. (2020). Rotavirus infections. In: *Diseases of Poultry*, 14th edn. (ed. D.E. Swayne, M. Boulianne, C.M. Longue, et al.), 409–417. Ames, IA: Blackwell.

McCowan, C., Crameri, S., Kocak, A., et al. (2018). A novel group A rotavirus associated with acute illness and hepatic necrosis in pigeons (*Columba livia*), in Australia. *PLoS One*, 13(9): e0203853.

Rubbenstroth, D., Ulrich, R., Wylezich, C., et al. (2020). First experimental proof of rotavirus A (RVA) genotype G18P[17] inducing the clinical presentation of 'young pigeon disease syndrome' (YPDS) in domestic pigeons (*Columba livia*). *Transboundary and Emerging Diseases*, 67:1507–1516.

Schmidt, V., Kümpel, M., Cramer, K., et al. (2021). Pigeon rotavirus A genotype G18P[17]-associated disease outbreaks after fancy pigeon shows in Germany: A case series. *Tierärztliche Praxis Ausgabe K Kleintiere Heimtiere*, 49:22–27.

Shehata, A.A., Basiouni, S., Sting, R., et al. (2021). Poult enteritis and mortality syndrome in turkey poults: causes, diagnosis and preventive measures. *Animals*, 11:2063.

**Author**: Volker Schmidt, PD Dr Med Vet, DECZM (Avian and Herpetological)

R

# SALMONELLOSIS

## BASICS

### DEFINITION
Salmonellosis is infection with an organism from the genus *Salmonella*, a Gram-negative bacterium. There are two species of *Salmonella*, with *Salmonella enterica* subsp. *enterica* being responsible for most infections in birds. There are over 1000 serotypes of *S. enterica enterica*. Infections can lead to clinical signs but are often asymptomatic in many animals.

### PATHOPHYSIOLOGY
*Salmonella* organisms are most commonly transmitted between animals and/or people by the fecal–oral route, but some serotypes can be transmitted transovarially. Although systemic signs do occur, GI signs such as diarrhea are most common.

### SYSTEMS AFFECTED
GI: Diarrhea due to enteritis. Musculoskeletal: Polyarthritis and osteomyelitis have been reported. Conjunctivitis in pigeons. Acute sepsis, leading to death.

### GENETICS
N/A

### INCIDENCE/PREVALENCE
The prevalence of asymptomatic infections in poultry and waterfowl is high; these types of birds often act as carriers (infected, asymptomatic shedders). The prevalence is lower in other avian species and may be more likely to lead to clinical disease.

### GEOGRAPHIC DISTRIBUTION
*Salmonella* spp. are distributed across the entire world. Wildlife species, such as waterfowl and poultry, often act as asymptomatic reservoirs.

### SIGNALMENT
**Species**: All avian species are susceptible to *Salmonella* infections.
**Mean age and range**: Young, old, or immunocompromised animals are more likely to develop clinical disease.

### SIGNS

#### General Comments
Many animals infected with *Salmonella* will not show any clinical signs.

#### Historical Findings
Exposure to another animal, which was either asymptomatic or sick, that was shedding the organism in its feces. Inappropriate husbandry leading to increased pathogen exposure or increased susceptibility due to immunosuppression.

#### Physical Examination Findings
Diarrhea, which can be hemorrhagic. Non-specific signs, such as lethargy, anorexia, polyuria, and/or conjunctivitis. Swelling of joints.

### CAUSES
Salmonellosis is caused by ingestion of *Salmonella* bacteria.

### RISK FACTORS
Poor husbandry or exposure to asymptomatic birds may increase exposure to *Salmonella*. Immunosuppression may increase risk of developing clinical disease from infection.

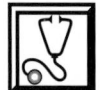

## DIAGNOSIS

### DIFFERENTIAL DIAGNOSIS
Other causes of diarrhea including *Escherichia coli*, *Yersinia*, *Pasteurella*, influenza, *Giardia*, *Coccidia*, toxins, or bacterial septicemias.

### CBC/BIOCHEMISTRY/URINALYSIS
Evidence of dehydration or inflammation, such as increased PCV or total protein, or a leukocytosis may be present, but these tests are not specific for salmonellosis.

### OTHER LABORATORY TESTS
A sample of feces should be submitted for culture to isolate the organism. The diagnostic laboratory should be notified of suspected *Salmonella* as an etiologic agent because special procedures are needed for optimum isolation. Serology can be used as a screening tool in a poultry flock situation but is not typically performed for individual birds. Whole-genome sequencing is used in investigations to determine the source of an outbreak.

### IMAGING
Radiographs can be obtained to examine changes in joints or bones, but a fine-needle aspirate and culture will be needed to isolate the organism.

### DIAGNOSTIC PROCEDURES
Collection of feces or a tissue sample for culture will be needed to definitively diagnose salmonellosis. A fine-needle aspirate may be needed to collect a sample from a joint or bone. Samples from affected tissues can be collected at necropsy.

### PATHOLOGIC FINDINGS
Gross and histopathologic findings will vary with severity and duration of disease but can include dehydration, enteritis, muscle necrosis, hepatomegaly, splenomegaly, pericarditis, epicarditis, granuloma formation in various organs, and diffuse inflammation.

## TREATMENT

### APPROPRIATE HEALTH CARE
Asymptomatic cases are typically not recognized or treated. Symptomatic cases are treated as described below.

### NURSING CARE
Most cases of salmonellosis can be treated only with fluids (PO, SQ, IV) and appropriate nutrition.

### ACTIVITY
Movement of the animal should be limited to reduce fecal contamination and reduce exposure of other animals or people.

### DIET
Although appetite may be decreased, oral intake of normal food and fluids is acceptable.

### CLIENT EDUCATION
Salmonella is zoonotic, and owners must take precautions to eliminate exposure to themselves, other humans, and other animals. Hand washing and cleaning and disinfection of contaminated areas and equipment are essential.

### SURGICAL CONSIDERATIONS
N/A

## MEDICATIONS

### DRUG(S) OF CHOICE
Salmonellosis is not typically treated with antibiotics because infections are typically self-resolving with supportive care and because of the possibility of the development of antibiotic-resistant strains of *Salmonella*. Antibiotics can be used in severe cases, but drug choice must be based on C/S results. Please note that the use of fluoroquinolones is not allowed in poultry in the USA.

### CONTRAINDICATIONS
Antibiotics that have not been shown to be appropriate based on C/S.

### PRECAUTIONS
*Salmonella* can develop antibiotic resistance.

### POSSIBLE INTERACTIONS
N/A

### ALTERNATIVE DRUGS
N/A

S

 FOLLOW-UP

## PATIENT MONITORING
Fecal output and consistency should be monitored and will typically return to normal within 1 week. Attitude should also improve with fluid administration. Repeat cultures can be performed, but shedding of the organism can occur for days to weeks after clinical signs resolve.

## PREVENTION/AVOIDANCE
Avoid exposure to *Salmonella* by keeping environments clean and disinfected and purchasing food from reputable sources.

## POSSIBLE COMPLICATIONS
People can become sick with salmonellosis.

## EXPECTED COURSE AND PROGNOSIS
Most patients that have predominately GI signs will recover without sequelae. More severe or systemic infections that lead to osteomyelitis or sepsis have a poorer prognosis.

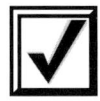 MISCELLANEOUS

## ASSOCIATED CONDITIONS
N/A

## AGE-RELATED FACTORS
Young and old animals are more susceptible to disease.

## ZOONOTIC POTENTIAL
There are approximately 1.35 million cases of human salmonellosis in the USA annually. Most of these cases are foodborne, but some are related to animal exposure.

## FERTILITY/BREEDING
*Salmonella* can infect the testes or ovaries, which could affect breeding potential.

## SYNONYMS
Pullorum disease, fowl typhoid, and paratyphoid are distinct diseases in poultry and are associated with particular serotypes of *Salmonella*. Typhoid and paratyphoid refers to infections in humans with *Salmonella* serotype Typhi and *Salmonella* Paratyphi, respectively, but these serotypes do not typically affect animals.

## SEE ALSO
Cloacal Disease
Colibacillosis
Diarrhea
Enteritis and Gastritis
Regurgitation and Vomiting
Urate and Fecal Discoloration

## ABBREVIATIONS
C/S—culture and sensitivity
GI—gastrointestinal
PCV—packed cell volume

## INTERNET RESOURCES
Centers for Disease Control and Prevention. Salmonella: http://www.cdc.gov/salmonella
Centers for Disease Control and Prevention. Keeping pets healthy keeps people healthy too!: http://www.cdc.gov/healthypets
Food Animal Residue Avoidance Databank: http://www.farad.org
US Department of Agriculture. Defend the flock program: http://healthybirds.aphis.usda.gov
Yeakel, S.D. (2022). Salmonelloses in poultry. *Merck Veterinary Manual*: http://www.merckmanuals.com/vet/poultry/salmonelloses/overview_of_salmonelloses_in_poultry.html

*Suggested Reading*
Basler, C., Nguyen, T.A., Anderson, T.C., et al. (2016). Outbreaks of human *Salmonella* infections associated with live poultry, United States, 1990–2014. *Emerging Infectious Diseases*, 22:1705–1711.
Hernandez, S.M., Keel, K., Sanchez, S.I. (2012). Epidemiology of a *Salmonella enterica* subsp. *enterica* serovar Typhimurium strain associated with a songbird outbreak. *Applied and Environmental Microbiology*, 78:7290–7298.
Marietto-Goncalves, G.A., de Almeida, S.M., de Lima, E.T., et al. (2010). Isolation of *Salmonella enterica* serovar Enteriditis in blue-fronted Amazon parrot (*Amazona aestiva*). *Avian Diseases*, 54:151–155.
**Author**: Marcy J. Souza, DVM, MPH, MPPA, DABVP (Emeritus, Avian), DACVPM

S

## SARCOCYSTOSIS

 **BASICS**

### DEFINITION
Disease is caused by an intracellular protozoan parasite of the genus *Sarcocystis*. *Sarcocystis falcatula* is the most common protozoal parasite that infects psittacines. *Sarcocystis calchasi* is the causative agent of pigeon protozoal encephalitis and causes similar disease in psittacines. *Sarcocystis horvathi* and *Sarcocystis wenzeli* infect chickens, and *Sarcocystis rileyi* infect ducks but are unlikely to cause significant disease.

### PATHOPHYSIOLOGY
The reproductive cycle occurs via two hosts. Sexual reproduction occurs within the intestines of the definitive host and asexual reproduction occurs within various tissues of the intermediate host. Disease can weaken the intermediate host making it more vulnerable to predation/scavenging by the definitive host.

#### Sexual Reproductive Cycle
The definitive host is typically a carnivore or omnivore. The definitive host ingests tissue (from the intermediate host) that contains a sarcocyst (encysted parasite). Once ingested, the sarcocyst releases bradyzoites into the intestines. The bradyzoites develop into a microgamete (male) or macrogamete (female) and fuse to form an oocyst. Oocysts sporulate in the intestinal wall of the definitive host releases the infective sporocysts into the feces. Sporocysts can remain viable for months, but are susceptible to desiccation. The definitive host of *S. falcatula* is the opossum (*Didelphis virginiana* and *Didelphis albiventris*). In North America, the definitive host of *S. calchasi* is the family Accipitridae: Cooper's hawk (*Accipiter cooperii*), red-tailed hawk (*Buteo jamaicensis*), northern goshawk. In Europe, the northern goshawk (*Accipiter gentilis*) and most likely the European sparrowhawk (*Accipiter nisus*) are the definitive hosts.

#### Intermediate Host
The intermediate host becomes infected by directly eating the sporocysts from contaminated soil, water, or food, or after eating a mechanical vector (especially flies and cockroaches and occasionally rodents). The most common intermediate hosts for *S. falcatula* are the brown-headed cowbird (*Molothrus ater*) and grackle (*Quiscalus mexicanus* and *Quiscalus quiscula*). Other birds that can act as intermediate hosts and include Psittaciformes, Passeriformes, Columbiformes, and Strigiformes. Clinical cases have been reported in a great horned owl (*Bubo virginianus*), a golden eagle (*Aquila chrysaetos*), three bald eagles (*Haliaeetus*

*leucocephalus*), psittacines, and wild raptors. Experimentally, pigeons (*Columba livia*) have been infected. The natural intermediate host for *S. calchasi* is the pigeon (*Columba livia*) and it has caused infection in other birds. Experimental infection has occurred in the cockatiel (*Nymphicus hollandicus*) and it has been identified in a free-ranging Eurasian collared dove (*Streptopelia decaocto*) and captive psittacines. An outbreak occurred in wild Brandt's cormorants (*Phalacrocorax penicillatus*) in 2019, despite the lack of a natural avian predator. Aberrant intermediate host: Only immature parasites found within tissues, so it cannot infect the definitive host.

#### Asexual Reproduction
After ingestion, sporozoites are released from the sporocysts, which then penetrate the intestines and spread throughout the body. Sporozoites then undergo schizogony to form merozoites mainly within vessel walls.
**Asexual reproduction of *S. falcatula*:** schizogony occurs within the pulmonary vessels resulting in the acute form of disease. The vessels hypertrophy occluding the lumen and finally resulting in pulmonary edema. Death is due to asphyxiation. In the final asexual phase, merozoites either form more schizonts or enter the cardiac and striated muscles to form cysts. Cysts within the striated muscle are rarely associated with disease. Meront migration within liver, kidney, heart, and brain also result in tissue damage.
**Asexual reproduction of *S. calchasi*:** Acute phase: Approximately 10 days post infection, the pigeon develops polyuria and lethargy. This correlates with asexual replication, which occurs in the liver and spleen. Acute phase in psittacines results in encephalitis and death. Disease either resolves or progresses in the pigeon; 50–60 days post infection, mature sarcocysts are found in skeletal muscle, cardiac muscle and granulomatous, necrotizing encephalitis develops. Histopathological changes occur within the brain prior to the development of neurologic clinical signs. Some hypothesize a delayed-type hypersensitivity response as the cause of the encephalitis.

### SYSTEMS AFFECTED
Respiratory, musculoskeletal and cardiac—myositis; CNS—encephalitis; gastrointestinal, splenitis/hepatitis; renal.

### GENETICS
N/A

### INCIDENCE/PREVALENCE
More common late fall to spring, probably due to the migratory pattern and breeding season of grackles and cowbirds. In one study, 18% of infected opossum were infected with *S. falcatula*.

### GEOGRAPHIC DISTRIBUTION
*S. calchasi* has been reported in North America, Japan, and Europe. Most likely worldwide. *S. falcatula* is common in aviaries along the Gulf Coast of the USA. Range of the opossum occurs over most of the contiguous USA except the Rocky Mountains, the southwest and extreme northern areas. Range of the brown-headed cowbird—contiguous USA. Range of common grackle—east of the Rocky Mountains.

### SIGNALMENT
*S. calchasi*: Pigeon and psittacines, raptors. Typically asymptomatic. Pathogenicity is higher in captive and immature birds.
*S. falcatula*: Old World species (especially cockatoos (*Cacatua alba*), cockatiels (*Nymphicus hollandicus*), grey parrots (*Psittacus erithacus*), and Columbiformes most often present with the acute form of the disease. New World species evolved around the definitive host, so adults are less frequently effected. American and neotropical psittacines species have a greater incident in nestlings because of naive immune systems. It is believed that they become infected when cockroaches enter the nest. Death in an adult neotropical bird is uncommon. Exotic Columbiformes (blue-crowned pigeons (*Goura cristata*) and pheasant pigeons (*Otidiphaps nobilis*) are susceptible to disease and often succumb to acute fatal disease within the lung. Anseriformes and Galliformes appear to be resistant. Can be found incidentally at necropsy especially in Passeriformes. Males are more commonly affected than females which may be associated with care of the nest.

### SIGNS
#### Historical Findings
Outdoor aviary: Acute death of the bird or of some of the flock without previous signs of injury. In the surviving birds, respiratory signs and/or weakness may be first noted.

#### Physical Examination Findings
*S. falcatula*: Acute (death often occurs within 48 hours), dyspnea, increased respiratory rate and effort, lethargy, blood or clear fluid within the mouth, biliverdinuria, good BCS. Chronic: Lethargy, depression, anorexia, mild diarrhea, blood in the mouth. Mild to moderated muscle wasting, weakness in wings and/or legs, ataxia, tremors, paresis, paralysis, torticollis, opisthotonus, seizures. Hepatomegaly, biliverdinuria, SQ hemorrhage, emaciation. Non-suppurative meningoencephalitis in a golden eagle and straw-necked ibis.
*S. calchasi*: Acute: Polyuria, lethargy, death, mild diarrhea. Chronic: Head tilt, torticollis, opisthotonos, paresis, paralysis, nystagmus,

star gazing, recumbency, tremor, ataxia, normal to thin BCS. Recovered: Residual neurologic effects. Signs in pigeons are dose dependent. Low infectious dose (< 102 sporocysts) develop only chronic neurologic signs. Medium infectious dose (103–104 sporocysts) both acute and chronic signs. High infectious dose ($8 \times 10^4$ to $3 \times 10^6$) death during acute phase. Signs in psittacines are independent of dose.
**S. calchasi in raptors**: Emaciation, soiled vent.

## CAUSES
Ingestion of infective form of the *Sarcocystis* spp.

## RISK FACTORS
Contact with opossum, raptors, cockroaches and flies. Outdoor aviaries.

# DIAGNOSIS
## DIFFERENTIAL DIAGNOSIS
**Hepatitis**: See Liver Disease chapter.
**Pneumonia**: Upper airway disease, heart failure, pulmonary hypersensitivity, neoplasia, trauma.
**CNS disease**: Hepatoencephalopathy, CNS neoplasia, CNS abscess, epilepsy, infectious encephalopathy (see below).
**Infectious**: Viral—Avian orthoavulavirus 1, bornavirus, eastern/western equine encephalitis, West Nile virus; bacterial mycobacteriosis, listeriosis, *Chlamydophila*, salmonellosis, listeriosis; fungal *Aspergillus*; parasitic toxoplasmosis, schistosomiasis, bayliascaris.
**Nutritional**: Hypovitaminosis B, vitamin E or selenium deficiency, hypocalcemia.
**Toxin**: Organophosphates, dimetridazole, lead, hypernatremia.
**Vascular**: Arteriosclerosis, infarct, ischemia.
**Trauma**.

## CBC/BIOCHEMISTRY/URINALYSIS
Hemogram: Leukocytosis, heterophilia. Biochemistry panel: Marked elevations in CPK, AST and LDH in muscular form of the disease. Occasionally, elevated TP seen.

## OTHER LABORATORY TESTS
EPH: False negative results commonly occur in acute cases. Hypergammaglobulinemia ± hyperbetagammaglobulinemia in chronic cases. Decreased A/G ratio. IFA for *S. falcatula*. Antibody titers may be seropositive antibodies to species other than *S. falcatula*. False negative results occur in acute cases because the humoral immune response does not have time to react. Rarely, seroconversion may represent exposure or subclinical infection. Combined positive IFA and elevated EPH beta and gamma

fractions increase likelihood of disease. Theoretically the ECG may show changes if the cardiac muscle is compromised.
*S. calchasi*: The definitive raptor host may how sporocysts or oocysts with fecal flotation/centrifugation techniques.

## IMAGING
Survey radiographs: Hepatomegaly, splenomegaly, renomegaly, muscle wasting. Increased lung opacity with pulmonary edema in *S. falculata*. CT: Hepatomegaly, splenomegaly, increased lung density, renomegaly.

## DIAGNOSTIC PROCEDURES
Mucosal scrapings taken at necropsy.

## PATHOLOGIC FINDINGS
The most accurate antemortum diagnosis is made via muscle or lung biopsy. Biopsy of quadriceps muscle obtains better results than pectoral muscle, because sarcocysts persist longer in the quadriceps Muscle squash preparation sand tissue digestion techniques can sometimes be use to release bradyzoites.

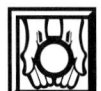

# TREATMENT
## APPROPRIATE HEALTH CARE
Inpatient treatment is required if symptomatic. Outpatient treatment if treatment for a cage mate.

## NURSING CARE
Supportive care. Minimize stress by placing in a quiet area with minimum traffic. Place in warm, humid environment (85–90°F/27–30°C and 70% humidity), unless there is evidence of head trauma. Dyspneic birds place in incubator with 40–80% oxygen supplementation at 5 l/minute.

## ACTIVITY
Activity should be restricted in all dyspneic and neurologic patients. Place in a smaller cage and restrict flight. Pad cage to protect from falls. Remove perches, provide soft bedding and easy access to bowls.

## DIET
Nutritional support via gavage feeding for anorexic patients. Gavage 5% of body weight initially and slowly increase up to 8–10% to avoid aspiration. Crop emptying can take 2–4 hours. Change all birds to a nutritionally complete diet.

## CLIENT EDUCATION
Avoid contact with opossum, raptors, cockroaches, and flies. Consider testing and treatment: (hemogram, blood chemistries, EPH, and IFA) in birds housed with the patient.

## SURGICAL CONSIDERATIONS
Pulmonary edema makes patients high risk for anesthetic complications. Increased risk of hemorrhage and hemoaspiration. Consider furosemide prior to biopsy.

# MEDICATIONS
## DRUG(S) OF CHOICE
*Sarcocystis falcatula*: Birds are sometimes resistant to treatment and relapses are common. Pyrimethamine (0.5 mg/kg PO q12h), trimethoprim-sulfadiazine (30 mg/kg PO q8h) and an antiprotozoal medication. Treatment for 6 weeks or longer. Diclazuril (10 mg/kg PO q24h), ponazuril 20 mg/kg q24hr for 7 days, toltrazuril (25 mg/kg q7d for 3 treatments). Pyrimethamine (0.5–1 mg/kg PO q12h for 2–4 days, then 0.25 mg/kg PO q24h for 30 days) for exposed birds. Anti-inflammatory medication: Meloxicam.
**Dyspnea**: Bronchodilators—beta-agonists relax smooth muscle and decrease airway inflammation; less toxic in aerosolized form. Terbutaline 0.01 mg/kg IM q6h. Followed by nebulization at 0.01 mg/kg in 9 cc of saline. Methylxanthines. Theophylline has been used at a dose of 2 mg/kg PO q12h. Aminophylline are 10 mg/kg IV q6–8h, 4 mg/kg IM q12–24h and 5 mg/kg PO q12h. Adverse effects include CNS excitation, vomiting, and tachycardia. May be less effective at bronchodilation in birds, but clinical improvement has been noted with their use. Use limited to birds that fail to respond to beta-agonist treatment. Anti-anxiety analgesic: Butorphanol 1–2 mg/kg IM q2–3h. Furosemide 0.1–2 mg/kg IM b.i.d. in acute dyspnea. Anti-inflammatory medications. Fluid therapy if unable to maintain hydration and there is no evidence of pulmonary edema. Warm fluids to 100–104°F (38–40°C). Hypotonic fluids contraindicated in birds with salt glands. Subcutaneous or oral fluids indicated for mild levels of blood loss and maintenance. Crystalloids should be sufficient. Contraindicated in hypovolemia, hypothermia, and shock due to peripheral vasoconstriction. Correct for 4–5% of fluid loss ($0.04$–$0.05 \times BW_{kg} \times 1000$) in addition to maintenance. Divide into multiple doses as dictated by volume. SQ fluids: Place up to 10 cc/kg in each SQ injection site. Use the inguinal web, intrascapular and axillary areas. LRS absorbs well. Contraindications: Hypertonic fluids and colloids and fluids containing > 2.5% dextrose, Brown pelicans and turkey vultures. IO/IV fluids indicated for moderate levels of blood loss, surgery or hypothermia. Allow for rapid administration and dissemination of fluids. IV catheter

S

22- to 26-g catheter in jugular, basilic, ulnar, or medial metatarsal vein. May be difficult in birds < 100 g. IO catheter: Distal ulna or proximal tibiotarsus. Contraindicated in the ulna of Cathartiformes. Confirm placement with radiographs. Correct for 4–8% of fluid loss ($0.04$–$0.08 \times BW_{kg} \times 1000$) in addition to maintenance; 80% of fluid deficit should be replaced over 6–8 hours in acute loss and over 12–24 hours in chronic loss. Consider adding a colloid (3–5 ml/kg), especially if hypotensive, hypovolemic, or hypoproteinemic. Contraindicated in coagulopathy, congestive heart failure, renal disease, pneumonia. LRS contraindicated for rapid effusion. Plasmalyte A closest to avian plasma.

## CONTRAINDICATIONS
Corticosteriods. Toltrazuril for *S. calchasi* in pigeons. Fluids if pulmonary effusion is present.

## PRECAUTIONS
N/A

## POSSIBLE INTERACTIONS
N/A

## ALTERNATIVE DRUGS
N/A

## FOLLOW-UP

### PATIENT MONITORING
Diagnostic monitoring: White blood cell count, CPK, AST, LDH, EPH. Muscle biopsy. Monitor for response to treatment and response to clinical signs. Neurologic cases—perform serial neurologic exams to asses patients response to treatment.

### PREVENTION/AVOIDANCE
Aggressive trapping of opossums. Protection with dogs or flightless chickens (silkie chicken). Provide indoor housing. Aggressive cockroach and fly control. Store food in metal containers. Disinfection: Heat to more than 140°F (60°C) for 1 minute, 131°F (55°C) for 15 minutes or 122°F (50°C) for 1 hour. Sodium hypochlorite (bleach) was effective in killing *S. neurona* after 1 hour.

### POSSIBLE COMPLICATIONS
If treatment is initiated early, the progression of the disease may be halted, leaving persistent weakness or neurologic signs.

Progressive neurologic signs. Chronic weight loss. Death.

## EXPECTED COURSE AND PROGNOSIS
*S. calchasi*: Poor prognosis for psittacines. Dose-dependent in pigeon (see Signs section). *S. falcatula*: Generally poor especially in respiratory disease and encephalitis. However, prognosis dependent on state of disease and organ involvement. Affected birds normally die in 48 hours in acute forms of disease. If treatment is initiated early, the progression of the disease may be halted, leaving persistent weakness or neurologic signs.

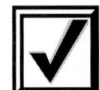

## MISCELLANEOUS

### ASSOCIATED CONDITIONS
Secondary infections from parasites, bacteria, viruses, and/or fungi may be seen.

### AGE-RELATED FACTORS
American and neotropical psittacines species have a greater incident in nestlings because of naïve immune systems.

### ZOONOTIC POTENTIAL
None.

### FERTILITY/BREEDING
Avoid the use of sulfonamides in reproductive animals as they may be teratogenic.

### SYNONYMS
N/A

### SEE ALSO
Aspergillosis
Atherosclerosis
Botulism
Coccidiosis (Systemic)
Hemoparasites
Mycobacteriosis
Neoplasia (Neurological)
Nutritional Imbalances
Orthoavulaviruses
Pneumonia
Salmonellosis
Seizures
Toxicosis (Environmental/Pesticides)
West Nile Virus

### ABBREVIATIONS
A/G—albumin/globulin
AST—aspartate aminotransferase
BCS—body condition score
$BW_{kg}$—body weight in kilograms
CNS—central nervous system
CPK—creatine phosphokinase
CT—computed tomography
ECG—electrocardiogram
EPH—plasma protein electrophoresis
IFA—indirect immunofluorescent assay
LDH—lactate dehydrogenase
LRS—lactated Ringer's solution
PMV-1—paramyxovirus 1

### INTERNET RESOURCES
Center for Food Security and Public Health, Iowa State University. Sarcocystosis technical factsheet: https://www.cfsph.iastate.edu/diseaseinfo/factsheets
Lierz M. (2016). *Sarcocystis calchasi*: A new threat for pigeons and psittacine birds. *Association of Avian Veterinarians Australasian Committee Annual Conference*: https://www.aavac.com.au/files/2016-11.pdf

*Suggested Reading*
Cray, C., Zielezienski-Roberts, K., Bonda, M., et al. (2005). Serologic diagnosis of sarcocystosis in psittacine birds: 16 cases. *Journal of Avian Medicine and Surgery*, 19:208–215.
Mete, A. (2019). *Sarcocystis calchasi* outbreak in feral rock pigeons (*Columbia livia*) in California. *Veterinary Pathology*, 56:317–321.
Rimoldi, G., Speer, B., Wellehan, J.F.X. Jr., et al. (2013). An outbreak of *Sarcocystis calchasi* encephalitis in multiple psittacine species within an enclosed zoological aviary. *Journal of Veterinary Diagnostic Investigation*, 25:775–781.
Olias, P., eMaier, K., Wuenschmann, A., et al. (2014). *Sarcocystis calchasi* has an expanded host range and induces neurological disease in cockatiels (*Nymphicus hollandicus*) and North American rock pigeons (*Columbia livia* f. dom.) *Veterinary Parasitology*, 200:59–65.
Rogers, K.H., Arranz-Solís, D., Saeij, J.P.J., et al. (2021). *Sarcocystis calchasi* and other Sarcocystidae detected in predatory birds in California, USA. *International Journal for Parasitology*, 17:91–99.
Villar, D., Kramer, M., Howard, L., et al. (2008). Clinical presentation and pathology of sarcocystosis in psittaciform birds: 11 cases. *Avian Diseases*, 52:187–194.
**Author:** Erika Cervasio, DVM, DABVP (Avian, Feline, Canine)
**Acknowledgements:** Kristin Vyhnal, DVM, MS, DACVP

**S**

# BASICS

## DEFINITION
A seizure is a sudden disruption of the forebrain's normal neurotransmission, which can result in altered consciousness and/or other neurological and behavioral manifestations. When the seizures are chronic, this is described as epilepsy. Generalized seizures involve both cerebral hemispheres and can have several phases, including tonic (sustained muscle contraction), myoclonic (brief muscle contraction), clonic (rhythmic muscle contraction), or atonic (loss of muscle tone). Focal seizures result in initial activation of only one part of one cerebral hemisphere and can take many forms, including focal motor, focal sensory, or focal autonomic seizures.

## PATHOPHYSIOLOGY
Seizures are caused by increased excitation or decreased inhibition of the electrical activity of the neurons in the forebrain, although the exact events that create and terminate a seizure are unknown.

## SYSTEMS AFFECTED
Nervous.

## GENETICS
N/A

## INCIDENCE/PREVALENCE
N/A

## GEOGRAPHIC DISTRIBUTION
WNV: Reported in parrots in California and Louisiana. Lead toxicity is more prevalent in urban regions that have older housing with lead paint.

## SIGNALMENT
Grey parrots—seizures related to hypocalcemia in parrots 2–15 years of age. Seizures related to hydrocephalus at ages 5 months to 10 years; 5 of 7 reported cases of hydrocephalus in psittacine birds are in grey parrots.

## SIGNS

### Historical Findings
Since the seizure activity is not usually witnessed by the veterinarian, the owner's historical findings are most important to differentiate a seizure from other events (see Differential Diagnosis section). Having the owner video the seizure can be very helpful in differentiation. There are four stages the owner may recognize and describe: (1) Prodromal or pre-ictal period: Behavioral change that precedes a seizure by hours to days; can include restlessness, agitation, decreased interaction/vocalization with owner, fearful behavior, or "clinging" to owner. (2) Aura period: Subjective sensation at onset of seizure usually not noted in animals but can include regurgitation/vomiting and voiding feces/urates. (3) Ictal period or seizure event: Usually lasts 60–90 seconds; signs in birds include loss of consciousness, vocalization, flapping of wings, contraction of limbs, abnormal placement of the head with it thrown backward, and falling. Focal seizures can start in one part of the body and progress to generalized seizures or can stay as a brief cluster of signs. (4) Postictal period: Abnormal behavior immediately following the seizure—restlessness, aggression, lethargy, confusion, vision loss, hunger, thirst, disorientation, ataxia. Once it has been determined that the patient had a seizure, other historical findings can include head trauma, exposure to other sick birds, diet changes, outdoor housing in area with endemic WNV, current medications, exposure to toxins, any recent illnesses, or change in the droppings.

### Physical Examination Findings
Unless the episode is observed, most patients with intracranial disease have normal physical examination findings and are normal between seizures. Signs of trauma such as bruising, bleeding, fractures, corneal ulceration can be seen if the patient fell during the seizure. Rarely, other signs of forebrain disease can be seen such as altered behavior, central blindness, decreased consciousness, circling, and/or a head turn. Animals with seizures caused by hepatic encephalopathy can have other signs of disease, such as depression, ascites, biliverdinuria, and weight loss. Animals with systemic infectious disease such as *Chlamydia psittaci* can have signs of respiratory and GI disease and those with avian bornavirus can have multiple systems affected.

## CAUSES
Causes of seizures are categorized as extracranial and intracranial with intracranial further categorized as structural or functional disorders.

### Extracranial
Toxicities and metabolic disturbances that interfere with CNS function or are directly neurotoxic.
**Metabolic**: Hepatic encephalopathy, hypoglycemia, hypocalcemia, hypomagnesemia.
**Nutritional**: Thiamine deficiency (in piscivorous birds eating frozen fish), hypovitaminosis E, selenium deficiency.
**Trauma**: Head or neck; post-traumatic seizures have been reported in a white-crowned pionus 22 months after traumatic brain injury.
**Toxic**: Lead, zinc, organic mercury, pyrethroids, organophosphates, carbamates, methylxanthines.

### Intracranial
**Structural disorders**: There is gross structural cause within the brain. Degenerative—neuronal ceroid lipfuscinosis reported in one lovebird and one mallard duck. Anatomic—hydrocephalus. Neoplastic—primary (astrocytoma, primitive neuroectodermal tumor, glial cell tumors, choroid plexus papillomas, lymphosarcoma, pituitary adenoma) or metastatic neoplasia. Infectious/inflammatory/auto-immune—*C. psittaci*, WNV, *Clostridium tertium*, and avian bornavirus-associated ganglioneuritis. Vascular—secondary to atherosclerosis; secondary to reproductive activity in egg-laying hens with high estrogen levels leading to blood hyperviscosity, emboli, and hypoxia ("hyperlipidemic syndrome"); secondary to hypertension (seizures were seen in 3/5 psittacine birds presenting with indirect systolic blood pressures of 200–275 mmHg).
**Functional disorders**: No gross structural changes are evident in the brain and the cause is probably neurochemical dysfunction. Idiopathic epilepsy, diagnosis of exclusion when all other causes have been ruled out, has been reported in has been reported peach-faced lovebirds, red-lored Amazon parrots, double yellow-headed Amazon parrots, and greater Indian hill mynahs.

## RISK FACTORS
Exposure to lead containing products (i.e. paint, toys).

# DIAGNOSIS

## DIFFERENTIAL DIAGNOSIS
Differential diagnoses include tremors, involuntary movements, syncope, metabolic collapse (i.e. hypoglycemia), vestibular disease, intermittent claudication-like syndrome, exercise intolerance, peripheral nerve disease (i.e. chronic lead toxicity, sciatic compression from renal tumor), neuromuscular disease. Historical findings: If the episode occurs after exercise/activity, suspect syncope, metabolic collapse, intermittent claudication-like syndrome, exercise intolerance, hypoglycemia, or neuromuscular disease. If the animal is unconscious during the episode, suspect seizure or severe syncope. If the animal has atypical behavior after the episode ("postictal period"), suspect seizure, although short episodes of confusion can be seen with severe syncope. Physical examination findings: Peripheral nerve disease or neuromuscular disease: conscious proprioception deficits, decreased grip/movement of affected limb(s) and/or muscle atrophy of affected limbs.

S

Vestibular disease: Nystagmus, ataxia, head tilt. Syncope: Arrhythmias, murmur, pulse deficits.

### CBC/BIOCHEMISTRY/URINALYSIS

**CBC:** Leukocytosis if there is an infectious disease causing seizures. Heterophilia with or without a left shift can be seen with bacterial or fungal infections. Eosinophilia can be seen with parasitic diseases. As with any chronic disease, anemia of chronic inflammation can be seen.

**Biochemistry:** Elevation in CPK and AST due to muscle exertion or trauma. Hypoglycemia can be seen as a cause of seizures or a result of glucose takeup during prolonged seizure activity. Hypocalcemia and hypomagnesemia have been reported specifically in African grey parrots. Elevation in bile acids and decrease in albumin can be seen with hepatic encephalopathy. Elevation in blood cholesterol and triglycerides in egg-laying hens with reproduction-related hyperlipidemic syndrome; will also see hypercalcemia.

### OTHER LABORATORY TESTS

Blood lead and zinc levels. WNV—rt-PCR. *C. psittaci*—paired antibody titers, culture, and/or PCR. Avian bornavirus—see Bornaviral Disease (Psittaciformes) chapter.

### IMAGING

Metallic densities can be seen in the GI tract if lead toxicity has caused the seizures. Absence of metal does not preclude lead toxicity, as only 25% of birds with lead toxicity have metal noted radiographically. Whole-body radiographs including the skull should be performed to rule out trauma. Echocardiography should be performed in any bird with evidence of heart disease (i.e. arrhythmia, murmur, pulse deficits) to rule out syncope as a cause of collapse versus seizures.

### DIAGNOSTIC PROCEDURES

MRI or CT to look for intracranial disease. Electroencephalography can be performed to confirm seizure activity but is usually nonspecific. May only be effective in larger birds so that the electrodes can be properly placed. Cerebrospinal fluid analysis can be obtained to look for elevations in leukocyte and protein levels, although there are no established reference ranges for avian species.

### PATHOLOGIC FINDINGS

Pathologic findings depend on the underlying cause of the seizures. If there is an intracranial functional cause for the seizures (i.e. idiopathic epilepsy) then no abnormalities will be noted pathologically. Intracranial structural causes could include gross lesions such as hydrocephalus or only

those noted on histopathology such as avian bornavirus. Likewise, extracranial causes such as head trauma may be grossly noted. Samples may also be collected for specific etiology such as virus isolation or immunohistochemistry staining for WNV, PCR for avian bornavirus, and/or PCR or culture for *C. psittaci*.

## TREATMENT

### APPROPRIATE HEALTH CARE

Emergency management: Systemic stabilization of airway, breathing and circulation. Ensure patent airway and administer 100% oxygen therapy, obtain IV or IO access. Stop the seizure activity. Benzodiazepines Diazepam IV/IO/cloacal 0.5–2.0 mg/kg or midazolam administered IV/IO/IM/IN 0.1–2 mg/kg; can repeat 2–3 times; can use a CRI of diazepam 0.1–0.5 mg/kg/hr IV or IO; if 1–2 doses fail to control seizures consider adding longer-acting anticonvulsant such as levetiracetam 20–60 mg/kg IV. If seizures have still not stopped, consider propofol boluses 1–2 mg/kg IV/IO, ketamine boluses 5 mg/kg IV/IO, or inhalant isoflurane. Correct the underlying condition. If hypocalcemic, 10% calcium gluconate IV/IO 0.5–1.5 ml/kg over 10 minutes while monitoring heart rate and rhythm. If hypoglycemic, 25% dextrose IV or IO to effect over 15 minutes or oral glucose solution *with caution* to prevent aspiration. If head trauma and suspect increased intracranial pressure, hypertonic saline 7.5% NaCl 4 ml/kg, 3% NaCl 5.4 ml/kg over 15–20 minutes IV or IO, or mannitol 0.5–1.0 g/kg over 15–20 minutes IV/IO. Outpatient medical management, see Medications section.

### NURSING CARE

A well-padded cage with no perches should be provided to prevent further trauma if another seizure occurs. Eye lubrication should be applied if the patient is obtunded and not blinking properly. The patient's body and cage temperatures should be monitored, as patients with prolonged seizure activity can be hyperthermic and those that are obtunded may not be able to maintain their body temperature. Fluid therapy (SQ, IV, or IO) is required if the patient is not able to eat and drink properly. If the patient is hypoglycemic, 2.5% dextrose should be added to the IV or IO fluids until the patient is able to eat on its own. Oxygen therapy should be administered as needed.

### ACTIVITY

Patients with severe neurologic dysfunction should not be allowed to fly.

### DIET

Food and water should be removed from the patients' cage if they are depressed or obtunded to prevent aspiration and/or drowning in the water dish. Supplementation with oral calcium and/or magnesium as needed if hypocalcemic or hypomagnesemic. Support feeding as needed for patients with hypoglycemia. Specialized low-protein diets may be formulated for birds with hepatic encephalopathy. Dietary thiamine supplementation can be added to piscivore diets lacking vitamin $B_1$.

### CLIENT EDUCATION

Clients need to understand the goals of seizure treatment, which are to reduce the frequency and severity of seizures, to minimize the potential adverse effects, and to maximize the patients' quality of life. It is important for owners to know that the bird may still have seizures even when on the medications. Compliance is very important, and clients need to be prepared that their bird may require lifelong medications 1–3 times daily and that doses cannot ever be skipped. Clients should be made aware that anticonvulsant drug therapy in avian patients is not well studied and, therefore, frequent serum drug monitoring will be required.

### SURGICAL CONSIDERATIONS

Ketamine and inhalant anesthetics should be used with caution if any increase in intracranial pressure is suspected.

## MEDICATIONS

### DRUG(S) OF CHOICE

Underlying diseases causing seizures should be treated appropriately. For example, lead toxicity should be treated with chelating agents and hypocalcemia with oral calcium supplementation. Phenobarbital is generally not recommended in avian patients due to subtherapeutic levels with PO use; suggested serum therapeutic range of 20–30 mg/dl; 2 mg/kg PO q12h in an African grey parrot resulted in non-detectable serum phenobarbital levels; a PK study in African grey parrots using single dose 20 mg/kg PO only reached serum levels of 6.99–8.68 mg/dl, indicating that even high oral doses do not reach therapeutic levels. Potassium bromide: Canine dose is 20–40 mg/kg PO q24h with suggested serum therapeutic range of 1–3 mg/ml; 80 mg/kg PO q24h in a cockatoo kept serum levels between 1.7 and 2.2 mg/ml but in an African grey parrot 50 mg/kg PO q12h and 100 mg/kg PO q12h resulted in subtherapeutic serum levels of 0.6 and 0.7 mg/ml, respectively, and was ineffective at controlling seizures.

Levetiracetam: Suggested serum therapeutic range of 5.5–21 µg/ml; doses of 50 mg/kg and 100 mg/kg PO q8h reached this range in an African grey parrot; doses of 50 mg/kg PO q8h and 100 mg/kg PO q12h has been suggested based on pharmacokinetic studies in Hispaniolan Amazons; a single case report in a white-crowned pionus required 150 mg/kg PO q8h for seizure control. Zonisamide: Suggested serum therapeutic range of 10–40 µg/ml; 20 mg/kg PO q8h reached this range in a grey parrot; a PK study in Hispaniolan Amazon parrots indicated that 20 mg/kg PO q2h over a 10-day period yielded plasma concentrations within the therapeutic range for dogs and humans with no obvious signs of toxicosis. Gabapentin: Suggested serum therapeutic range of 4–16 mg/l; a PK study in Hispaniolan Amazon parrots indicated that 15 mg/kg PO q8h reaches effective plasma concentrations reported for humans (4–8 mg/l); a PK study in great horned owls also suggested q8h PO dosing. Deslorelin 4.7 mg administered SQ q2–6m; this GnRH agonist can be used to suppress reproductive hormones in female birds with seizures to prevent hyperlipidemic syndrome associated with high estrogen concentration, which can trigger seizures.

## CONTRAINDICATIONS
Behavioral medications such as SSRIs, tricyclic antidepressants, and antipsychotics can lower seizure threshold and should not be used with anticonvulsants. Specifically in birds, extrapyramidal adverse effects have been reported in a macaw with clomipramine and haloperidol therapy. Steroids are contraindicated in cases of traumatic brain injury as methylprednisolone use is associated with an increase in mortality 2 weeks and 6 months post injury in humans.

## PRECAUTIONS
Possible adverse effects of anticonvulsant medications include sedation and sometimes ataxia, so patients should be closely monitored when starting these medications. Phenobarbital should not be used in patients with liver disease.

## POSSIBLE INTERACTIONS
There are several drug interactions with phenobarbital; therefore, no other medication should be administered without checking first with a veterinarian.

## ALTERNATIVE DRUGS
N/A

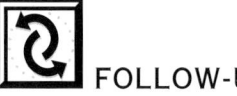

## FOLLOW-UP

### PATIENT MONITORING
Because there are few published doses of anticonvulsant therapies in avian patients, serum drug levels should be checked. If the serum levels are too low, samples should be collected for serum peak and trough measurements so that serum half-life can be calculated. Depending on the half-life of the medication this should be initiated 1–3 weeks after initiating therapy until adequate seizure control is reached.

### PREVENTION/AVOIDANCE
Avoid contact with heavy metals or other toxic substances. Controversial use of off label WNV vaccine in birds. Consider use of levetiracetam for prophylactic management of post-traumatic seizures in patients with traumatic brain injuries.

### POSSIBLE COMPLICATIONS
Any patient with seizures may progress to status epilepticus, which is an emergency.

### EXPECTED COURSE AND PROGNOSIS
Prognosis depends on the underlying cause. If the underlying cause can be diagnosed and cured, permanent CNS damage may have already occurred and may be irreversible or may improve with time. Progressive diseases such as multifocal Avian bornavirus is almost always fatal.

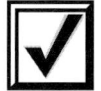

## MISCELLANEOUS

### ASSOCIATED CONDITIONS
N/A

### AGE-RELATED FACTORS
Neoplasia and ischemic stroke are seen more frequently in older animals, whereas degenerative and anatomical causes are seen more frequently in younger animals.

### ZOONOTIC POTENTIAL
If seizures are associated with *C. psittaci*.

### FERTILITY/BREEDING
N/A

### SYNONYMS
Epilepsy

### SEE ALSO
Bornaviral Disease (Psittaciformes)

Hypocalcemia and Hypomagnesemia
Neoplasia (Neurologic)
Neural Larva Migrans
Neurologic (Degenerative)
Neurologic (Trauma)
Nutritional Imbalances
Otitis
Sick-Bird Syndrome
Toxicosis (Heavy Metals)
Trauma
West Nile Virus

### ABBREVIATIONS
AST—aspartate aminotransferase
CNS—central nervous system
CPK—creatinine phosphokinase
CRI—constant rate infusion
CT—computed tomography
GI—gastrointestinal
GnRH—gonadotropin-releasing hormone
MRI—magnetic resonance imaging
rt-PCR—reverse transcriptase polymerase chain reaction
SSRI—selective serotonin reuptake inhibitor
WNV—West Nile virus

### INTERNET RESOURCES
N/A

*Suggested Reading*
Beaufrère, H., Nevarez, J., Gaschen, L., et al. (2011). Diagnosis of presumed acute ischemic stroke and associated seizure management in a Congo African grey parrot. *Journal of the American Veterinary Medical Association*, 239:122–128.
Delk, K. (2012). Clinical management of seizures in avian patients. *Journal of Exotic Pet Medicine*, 21:132–139.
Kabakchiev, C., Laniesse, D., James, F., et al. (2020). Diagnosis and long-term management of post-traumatic seizures in a white-crowned pionus (*Pionus senilis*). *Journal of the American Veterinary Medical Association*, 256:1145–1152.
Keller, K.A., Guzman, D.S.M., Boothe, D.M., et al. (2019). Pharmacokinetics and safety of zonisamide after oral administration of single and multiple doses to Hispaniolan Amazon parrots (*Amazona ventralis*). *American Journal of Veterinary Research*, 80:195–200.
Platt, S. (2012). Seizures. In: *Small Animal Neurologic Emergencies* (ed. S. Platt, L. Garosi), 155–172. London, UK: Manson Publishing.

**Author**: Nicole R. Wyre, DVM, DABVP (Avian and Exotic Companion Mammal), CVA, CTPEP

S

# SEPSIS

## BASICS

### DEFINITION
Sepsis is a life-threatening, overwhelming, and dysregulated host response to a severe infection, which can lead to tissue damage, organ failure, and death. It may be seen with bacterial, viral, fungal, or parasitic infection/infestation, although it is more commonly seen with bacterial diseases. Sepsis should be differentiated from septicemia and bacteremia. Bacteremia is the presence of viable bacterial organisms in the bloodstream, which can clear up without causing illness. When an infection is established, multiplies in the bloodstream, and induces clinical signs, this type of bacteremia is called septicemia.

### PATHOPHYSIOLOGY
The host immune system may react severely to pathogen-associated products, such as LPS, also called endotoxins, present in the cell wall of Gram-negative bacteria, exotoxins produced by Gram-positive bacteria, fungal cell walls; flagellin from protozoans, as well as lipoteichoic acid, peptidoglycan, or bacterial DNA. Endotoxins can damage blood vessels, causing edema, hemorrhage, and coagulation necrosis, especially in the liver. Production of microthrombi and embolism secondary to the activation of the white blood cells and platelets at the inflammation site may lead to decreased tissue oxygen delivery, multiple organ dysfunction, and organ failure. Ability to induce septicemia has been correlated with genomic variation in some bacteria (*Salmonella*, *Escherichia coli*).

### SYSTEMS AFFECTED
All systems can be affected by sepsis via the systemic inflammatory response, septicemic shock, and multiple organ dysfunction.
**Cardiovascular**: Increased vascular permeability. Decreased systemic vascular resistance. Increased/decreased cardiac input. Marked electrocardiographic changes.
**Gastrointestinal**.
**Hemic/lymphatic/immune**: Formation of microthrombi and embolism. Hyper/hypercoagulable state.
**Hepatobiliary**: Liver necrosis.
**Neuromuscular**: Lameness.
**Nervous**: Central nervous system
**Ophthalmic**: Uveitis and conjunctivitis in lovebirds.
**Renal/urologic**: Nephritis.
**Reproductive**: Oophoritis, orchitis, metritis
**Respiratory**: Primary pneumonitis or air sacculitis; secondary to coelomic distension.

### GENETICS
N/A

### INCIDENCE/PREVALENCE
Prevalence or incidence of sepsis is not commonly documented. Prevalence of septicemia by *Erysipelothrix rhusiopathiae* has been reported to reach 7% of adult wild takahe.

### GEOGRAPHIC DISTRIBUTION
Worldwide.

### SIGNALMENT
**Species**: All bird species.
**Mean age and range**: Neonates are more prone to bacterial sepsis. However, sepsis can occur in birds of all age.
**Predominant sex**: No sex predilection.

### SIGNS

#### General Comments
Most birds with sepsis present with unspecific severe systemic clinical signs. Variable specific clinical signs may be present, depending on the primary site of infection or secondary organ dysfunction.

#### Historical Findings
Acute or peracute presentation.

#### Physical Examination Findings
Profound lethargy, unable to stand. Anorexia. Ruffled plumage. Dyspnea. Diarrhea. Death. Neurological deficit—primary or secondary to hypoglycemia or hypotension. Polyuria and/or polydipsia. Heart murmur with endocarditis. Acute occurrence of necrosis to the distal digits or adnexa of the head and neck—*Staphylococcus* septicemia. Serofibrinous arthritis—*E. coli* septicemia. Conjunctivitis/uveitis—lovebirds. Lameness.

### CAUSES
Sepsis may result from bacterial (most common), viral, fungal, or parasitic infection. Although all bacteria may induce sepsis, the most commonly associated bacteria are listed here. *E. coli*, referred to as colibacillosis or colisepticemia; most commonly serotypes 01, 02, or 078 in poultry, passerines (canaries, finches). *Pasteurella multocida* (avian cholera), especially turkey. *Pseudomonas/Aeromonas* spp. *Klebsiella pneumoniae*. *Clostridium*, especially in lories and lorikeets due to high sugar content in their food. *Salmonella* spp. in lories and lorikeets. *Chlamydia psittaci*. *Borrelia anserina*—avian spirochetosis. *Staphylococcus* spp. *Streptococcus* spp. *Yersinia pseudotuberculosis*—canaries. *Erysipelothrix rhusiopathiae*, especially in ducks and geese, occasionally occurs in other avian species including Psittaciformes; wild and captive birds. *Citrobacter* spp. (passerines—finches and waxbills). *Enterococcus hirae*. *Listeria*

*monocytogenes*. *Salmonella* spp., *E. coli*, *Pseudomonas* spp., *Streptococcus* spp., and *Erysipelas* spp. are frequently implicated in neonate septicemia. *Burkholderia cepacian*. Other frequent pathogens include avian poxvirus—septicemic form in passerines (canaries, finches). Coccidiosis—poultry. Mixed infection with fungi (*Candida* spp., *Aspergillus* spp.) and Gram-negative bacteria. Specific causes reported in birds include predator wounds—*Klebsiella* spp., *Pasteurella* spp., and *Haemophilus* spp. are frequent in wild birds secondary to cat bite wounds. Reproductive tract infection. Septic coelomitis. Crop burn and fistula, crop stasis, esophageal perforation. Chronic cloacal prolapse. Neoplasia with bacterial surinfection. Open fractures. Hepatic lipidosis. Feather-damaging behavior for septicemia with *Staphylococcus* and *Streptococcus* spp. Iatrogenic—benzimidazole toxicity, chemotherapy, bacterial contamination through surgery or endoscopy.

### RISK FACTORS
Stress related to inappropriate environment, transport, mixing or crowding, inadequate heat, or poor nutrition. Inappropriate breeding or neonate care practice. Untreated underlying diseases. Immunosuppressed birds. Inappropriate asepsis during surgical procedures, vascular access port or IV/IO catheter. Surgical implants. Diabetes mellitus. Exposure to reptiles (salmonellosis).

## DIAGNOSIS

### DIFFERENTIAL DIAGNOSIS
Any causes of profound lethargy. Any causes of hypotension. Liver disease. Neoplasia. Metabolic disorders. Cardiac failure, atherosclerosis. Infectious diseases without sepsis (West Nile virus, bornavirus, polyomavirus, herpesvirus, reovirus, adenovirus *Coxiella*-like disease).

### CBC/BIOCHEMISTRY/URINALYSIS
Hematology: Leukocytosis or leukopenia. Absolute heteropenia. Left shift (immature heterophilia). Presence of heterophil toxicity. Hemolytic anemia—salmonellosis, spirochetosis. Thrombocytopenia. Biochemistry: Hypoglycemia. Ionized hypocalcemia. Decreased albumin (negative acute phase protein). Increased creatine kinase with damaged muscles and nerves. Increased creatinine. Urinalysis: (although not routinely done due to fecal contamination)—increased protein levels.

**S**

**(CONTINUED)**

## OTHER LABORATORY TESTS
Other tests may apply depending on suspected causative agents. PCR or serology for organisms of interested (e.g. *C. psittaci*, *B. anserina*). Coagulation parameters if available.

## IMAGING
Most septicemic birds are not stable enough to perform imaging for diagnosis during the first 24 hours of presentation. Imaging may reveal splenomegaly, hepatomegaly, and uniformed distension of the digestive tract. Cardiac ultrasound may be recommended with heart murmur or arrythmias.

## DIAGNOSTIC PROCEDURES
**Antemortem**: Aerobic bacterial culture with antibiogram and anaerobic culture are recommended. Blood culture is privileged if not contraindicated with bird size. Ultrasound-guided needle aspiration of organs (livers, kidney, spleen) for cytology and culture may be used. Biopsies of organs (liver, kidney) via coelomic endoscopy may be taken, although difficult to obtain with an ill bird. Marked changes can be detected on ECG before the onset of gross lesions—elevated P-, T-, S-, R-waves.
**Postmortem**: Culture on heart blood should be performed. Sampling the liver for culture should be avoided due the postmortem invasion of the liver by bacteria. Direct smear of heart blood stained with methylene blue may show typical bipolar stained rods in case of pasteurellosis.

## PATHOLOGIC FINDINGS
Gross and microscopic lesions of septicemia are often subtle. Splenomegaly with pale coloration. Hepatomegaly with focal necrosis. Multifocal hepatic white spots with colibacillosis. Multifocal petechial hemorrhage on the heart. Hyperemia and petechiation of internal organs, especially lung, gastrointestinal serosa, pleura, pericardial fat, skeletal muscles. Pericardial effusion—*Pasteurella* spp.

 TREATMENT

## APPROPRIATE HEALTH CARE
Emergency inpatient intensive care management. A broad-spectrum antibiotic with wide tissue distribution should be started within 1 hour of identifying sepsis via IV or IO route, pending culture results. Fluid therapy with IO or IV access should be rapidly initiated. Correction of electrolyte abnormalities should be planned and monitored. Supplementation with dextrose

should be added in case of hypoglycemia. IV bolus crystalloids should be repeated until blood pressure increases within normal range for the species, if blood pressure measurements are available.

## NURSING CARE
Hypothermic patients may be warmed externally and via infusion of warmed fluids. Oxygen therapy should be provided. Coelomocenthesis should be performed in case of coelomic effusion.

## ACTIVITY
Patient should be restrained from any activity.

## DIET
Sepsis increases patient's energy requirements from 1.2–3 times the minimum basal energy requirements. Nutritional support should be calculated based on the patient's current condition. Although rarely needed in birds, total parenteral nutrition may be offered if the bird is too weak for crop/proventricular gavage.

## CLIENT EDUCATION
Owners should be aware of the poor prognosis associated with sepsis in birds and the need of intensive care hospitalization for at least 4–5 days.

## SURGICAL CONSIDERATIONS
Birds with sepsis are usually not stable enough for general anesthesia. If a surgery is necessary, patient should be stabilized beforehand.

 MEDICATIONS

## DRUG(S) OF CHOICE
IV/IO antibiotics should be started within 1 hour of recognizing sepsis. Pending culture results, selected antibiotic should cover the suspected etiologic bacteria, based on history and physical exam, or covered empirically Gram-negative, -positive, aerobic, and anaerobic bacteria. Mixed bacterial infections of Gram-positive, Gram-negative, aerobic, and anaerobic bacteria: Piperacillin/tazobactam 100 mg/kg IV q4–8h—antibiotic of choice with bite wounds, cefotaxime 75–100 mg/kg IM, IV q4–8h. Gram-negative bacteria: Enrofloxacin 5–15 mg/kg SQ, IM, slow IV over 30 minutes q12–24h—active against *Chlamydia* spp., amikacin 10–20 mg/kg IV, IM q8–12h, ceftazidime 50–100 mg/kg IM, IV q4–8h. Gram-positive bacteria: Amoxicillin 100–150 mg/kg q4h (IM) or q8h (IV), ampicillin sodium 100–150 mg/kg IM q4–24h. If sepsis related to fungal or

protozoal infection, the specific treatment should be initiated to the antibiotherapy.

## CONTRAINDICATIONS
Amikacin is contraindicated with renal disease. IV enrofloxacin administration should be best avoided in raptors. Antibiotic should be selected according to the state/country law regulation in food animal species. Because of sodium content, high dosages of piperacillin/tazobactam may adversely affect patients with cardiac failure or hypernatremic conditions.

## PRECAUTIONS
Enrofloxacin: Slow IV administration over 30 minutes are recommended to limit adverse effects. Enrofloxacin should be used with caution in patients with seizure disorders as it may cause central nervous system stimulation. Dose should be adjusted with patients with severe renal or hepatic diseases to prevent drug accumulation. Best to avoid repeated IM administration. Best to dilute with sterile NaCl. Patients should be rehydrated before using enrofloxacin (crystalluria) and amikacin (potential nephrotoxicity). In case of significantly impaired renal function, ceftazidime dose should be adjust to avoid accumulation as this drug is primarily excreted via glomerular filtration.

## POSSIBLE INTERACTIONS
Amikacin can interact with beta-lactam antibiotics and should be avoided with furosemide, NSAIDs and nephrotoxins drugs. Concomitant use of cefotazime or ceftazidime and amynoglycosides or nephrotoxic drugs should be avoided. It is best to avoid the use of bacteriostatic and bactericidal antibiotics in association. Sucralfate and antacids should be given 2 hours before or after oral enrofloxacin when patient is stable as they may prevent enrofloxacin absorption.

## ALTERNATIVE DRUGS
N/A

 FOLLOW-UP

## PATIENT MONITORING
Patients should receive constant monitoring day and night until stable as septicemic patient status may change rapidly. Hematology may be repeated after 48 hours to monitor response to treatment. Biochemistry may be repeated depending on the severity of the abnormal parameters. Maximal blood sampling usually the

S

limitations in blood work follow-up. Imaging may be repeated after 7–14 days in case of splenomegaly or hepatomegaly to monitor the evolution.

### PREVENTION/AVOIDANCE
Avoid untreated chronic diseases with no medical follow-up. In neonates, the incidence of bacterial septicemia can be reduced through brooder hygiene and by identifying and controlling infections in subclinical parent.

### POSSIBLE COMPLICATIONS
Septicemic shock: Predominately with Gram-negative bacteria as they possess LPS, but also with Gram-positive bacteria and fungi. Free LPS from dead bacteria attach to circulating binding proteins. These complex bind to monocytes, macrophages, and heterophils, which triggers the production of cytokines (IL1, IL6, tumor necrosis factor). These latter in combination with the acute phase proteins produced by the liver eradicate the pathogens via the innate immune system. If a high level of LPS is released, the number of produced cytokines increases drastically inducing systemic vasodilation, diminished myocardial contractility, widespread endothelial injury, and increased vascular permeability. This can lead to severe hypotension and subsequent organ failure. Disseminated intravascular coagulation, although not proven in birds. Half of the birds with systemic bacterial infections have been reported to have kidney involvement, suggesting that any bacterial septicemia can potentially result in nephritis.

### EXPECTED COURSE AND PROGNOSIS
Septicemic birds rarely survive even when treated intensively.

## MISCELLANEOUS

### ASSOCIATED CONDITIONS
Reproductive diseases: Bacterial oophoritis and orchitis are often associated with septicemia and hematogenous delivery to the ovary/testes, especially in poultry. Septic egg-yolk peritonitis. Yolk sac infections. Cardia diseases: Fibrinous pericarditis. Pericardial effusion. Myocarditis. Endocarditis. Viral diseases: Avian influenza. Newcastle disease. Infectious bronchitis.

### AGE-RELATED FACTORS
Neonates are prone to sepsis. Young birds may be more prone to colisepticemia.

### ZOONOTIC POTENTIAL
Some etiologic agent associated with sepsis may be zoonotic (e.g. *Chlamydia*, *Salmonella*).

### FERTILITY/BREEDING
Sepsis with primary or secondary infectious of the reproductive may impair the bird fertility.

### SYNONYMS
N/A

### SEE ALSO
Ascites
Aspergillosis
Atheroclerosis
Avian Influenza
Bornaviral Diseases
Candidiasis
Congestive Heart Failure
Chlamydiosis
Clostridiosis
Coccidiosis (Systemic)
Colibacillosis
Dermatitis
Egg Yolk and Reproductive Coelomitis

Feather-Damaging and Self-Injurious Behavior
Fractures
Hepatic Lipidosis
Ileus (Functional Gastrointestinal, Crop Stasis)
Luxations
Myocardial Diseases
Poxvirus
Renal Disease
Salmonellosis
Spirochete Infection
Spleen (Diseases of)
Wounds (Including Bite Wounds, Predator Attacks)

### ABBREVIATIONS
IL—interleukin
LPS—lipopolysaccharide
NSAIDs—non-steroidal anti-inflammatory drugs
PCR—polymerase chain reaction

### INTERNET RESOURCES
N/A

*Suggested Reading*
Galindo-Cardiel, I., Opriessnig, T., Molina, L., Juan-Salles, C. (2012). Outbreak of mortality in psittacine birds in a mixed-species aviary associated with *Erysipelothrix rhusiopathiae* infection. *Veterinary Pathology*, 49:498–502.
Ward, M.P., Ramer, J.C., Proudfoot, J., et al. (2003). Outbreak of salmonellosis in a zoologic collection of lorikeets and lories (*Trichoglossus*, *Lorius*, and *Eos* spp.). *Avian Diseases*, 47:493–498.
Lierz, M. (2005). Systemic infectious disease. *BSAVA Manual of Psittacine Birds*, 2nd edn. (ed. N. Harcourt-Brown J. Chitty), 155–169. Ames, IA: Blackwell.
**Author**: Noémie Summa, DMV, IPSAV (Zoological Medicine), DACZM

# BASICS

## DEFINITION
Sick-bird syndrome is a term used to describe a group of clinical signs and symptoms that are exhibited by birds suffering from various illnesses. These clinical signs include lethargy, weakness, loss of appetite, weight loss, decreased activity, depression, respiratory distress, and increased susceptibility to other infections. Sick-bird syndrome is not a specific disease, but rather a collection of signs that may be indicative of underlying diseases, such as bacterial, viral, fungal, or parasitic infections, nutritional deficiencies, or other health conditions such as injury or toxicity. In some cases, birds suffering from sick-bird syndrome may also exhibit neurological signs such as tremors or seizures. Treatment involves identifying and addressing the underlying cause of the symptoms, which may require diagnostic testing and medical intervention by a veterinarian with experience in avian medicine.

## PATHOPHYSIOLOGY
Many birds have evolved to hide signs of illness as a survival mechanism, making early detection and intervention challenging. When the bird becomes sick enough to develop obvious symptoms, the client often thinks the bird is acutely ill. The pathophysiology of sick-bird syndrome can vary depending on the underlying cause of the symptoms. However, there are some common mechanisms that may contribute to the development of this condition. These include septicemia, toxemia, cardiovascular collapse, anemia, dehydration, hypoxemia, electrolyte abnormalities, acid–base imbalances, and caloric deficits/hypoglycemia.

## SYSTEMS AFFECTED
Any of the organ systems could be affected when a bird presents in this state. Disease of any one organ system could be the primary problem, but multiple organ systems could be involved initially or as a secondary problem.

## GENETICS
Color mutations in birds can affect their immune function and make them more susceptible to certain diseases. Genetic mutations that cause changes in pigmentation can also impact other physiological processes, such as vitamin D metabolism. These factors can contribute to the development of sick-bird syndrome in color-mutated birds.

## INCIDENCE/PREVALENCE
Because this is a non-specific disease presentation, almost any cause of illness in birds can present in a similar way.

## GEOGRAPHIC DISTRIBUTION
N/A

## SIGNALMENT
Sick-bird syndrome can affect a wide range of avian species, including both wild and domestic birds. However, some species may be more susceptible to certain illnesses, and specific husbandry practices may increase the risk of developing the syndrome. All ages and both sexes are susceptible.

## SIGNS
### General Comments
If a bird presents with non-specific clinical signs, a quick check of the body weight on the way to a warmed incubator with oxygen helps to stabilize the bird, while a thorough history is taken and a plan for exam, testing, and treatment is made, so handling of the bird is kept to a minimum.

### Historical Findings
Owners may report vague clinical signs, including lethargy, weakness, decreased appetite, fluffed up at the bottom of the cage, eyes closed, or respiratory distress. A detailed history and diagnostic testing can aid in identifying and treating the underlying cause of the bird's symptoms. Many owners surmise that the pet was ill acutely. With questioning, signs that occurred before the bird became obviously ill may be more notable with the benefit of hindsight. Behavior changes or reduction in vocalization several days to weeks prior may indicate chronicity.

### Physical Examination Findings
Physical exam findings are non-specific and vary depending on the cause of illness and body systems affected. Lethargy or weakness, sitting on the bottom of the cage, depressed mentation, eyes closed, fluffed feathers, poor muscle mass, dehydration, respiratory distress, abnormal feathering, diarrhea, polyuria, tremors, or seizures may be present.

## CAUSES
Many avian illnesses could result in non-specific clinical signs and eventual presentation in an advanced state. An incomplete list includes: Bacterial infections—Gram-negatives and a few Gram-positives. Chlamydiosis. Mycobacteriosis. Viral infections—herpesvirus, polyomavirus, circovirus, bornavirus, other. Fungal infections—candidiasis, aspergillosis, macrorhabdosis. Parasitic infections—flagellates, cryptosporidiosis, helminthiasis. Toxicologic conditions—lead, zinc, inhaled, other.

Neoplastic conditions. Metabolic disorders. Malnutrition and related/secondary diseases. Other non-infectious disorders—reproductive diseases, atherosclerosis.

## RISK FACTORS
Species predispositions, poor husbandry practices, malnutrition, exposure to toxins, uncontrolled exposure to other birds or animals, and stressors such as overcrowding can make birds more susceptible to disease.

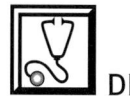

# DIAGNOSIS

## DIFFERENTIAL DIAGNOSIS
Possible diagnoses are listed in the Causes section.

## CBC/BIOCHEMISTRY/URINALYSIS
Note: A delay in obtaining samples may be necessary for critically ill birds until they are more stable. For acutely or critically ill birds, in-house chemistry analysers that are able to obtain values without diluting samples are needed for accurate and timely results. An estimated CBC and differential review in-house is also ideal. Urinalysis is not typically performed on acutely ill birds, because of contamination of urine in the cloaca and reflux to the colon for water reabsorption. Findings will vary depending on the pathologic process causing the clinical signs.

## OTHER LABORATORY TESTS
Specific tests indicated will be based on physical exam findings, history, and size or condition of the patient. Potential for zoonotic disease should be considered and risk factors screened from owner history. Smaller birds will reduce the available sample volume. Prioritize tests by patient status and tolerance for handling. Results from initial tests may indicate the direction for the next step.

## IMAGING
Radiographs might be part of the diagnostic plan, depending on the patient, the client's finances, and the risk of performing the procedure and the likelihood of getting good positioning. If radiographs can be taken quickly and safely, there is often valuable information that can be gained. There is considerable debate in the veterinary community as to how to best perform radiographs in a critically ill bird. Some advocate for the use of, and routinely administer gas anesthesia; others will manually restrain without it; a third option would be to consider butorphanol (IM) and/or midazolam (IM or intranasal) for these instances. A quick dorsoventral standing

S

radiograph can be done if looking for metallic foreign bodies (heavy-metal poisoning). This minimizes the risk in the critically ill patient, but would otherwise be considered a non-diagnostic radiograph. Ultrasound of the coelom is a minimally invasive method to assess for free fluid or location of intracoelomic masses, especially if coelomic distension is present. CT or MRI allows a more detailed evaluation of many areas, especially detailed structures such as the skull and sinuses.

### DIAGNOSTIC PROCEDURES
Visible or accessible lesions may have testing by fine needle aspirates, cytology swab samples, or biopsy techniques. Cardiac symptoms can be further evaluated with ECG and blood pressure. Endoscopy is another option to both diagnose and treat many birds.

### PATHOLOGIC FINDINGS
Depending on the underlying disease process and organ system involved, these can vary widely.

## TREATMENT

### APPROPRIATE HEALTH CARE
All critical patients should be hospitalized with supportive care or any specific treatment indicated. However, the stability of the patient dictates the need for caution in handling or delaying indicated testing or treatment.

### NURSING CARE
Oxygen therapy. Thermal support (80–90°F/26.6–32°C). Fluid therapy. Nutritional support. It is important to warm the patient and ensure hydration before gavage feeding. Also, ensure the patient has adequate mentation and can remain upright to reduce risk of aspiration.

### ACTIVITY
Sick birds should be limited in their activity and prevent flying. In some cases, they should also be restricted from climbing. An incubator setup in the hospital or at home is often needed.

### DIET
Depending on the underlying health issue, diet should be assessed and frequently improved. Supportive hand feeding with elemental type diets may be helpful in the initial stages of treatment.

### CLIENT EDUCATION
In all cases, it is important to outline the course of action with the client, including the diagnostic and treatment plan and the prognosis. Emphasize the likelihood that the

bird is usually more sick than the owner may have thought. It should be stressed with all clients, during annual or post-purchase examinations that they need to look for changes in their bird's behavior, demeanor, appetite, droppings, breathing, or anything else at all times. The key word is changes. If it is different from the usual state of the bird, then it is worth investigating as opposed to taking a "wait and see" approach.

### SURGICAL CONSIDERATIONS
Depending on the underlying disease process and organ system involved, surgery may be necessary.

## MEDICATIONS

### DRUG(S) OF CHOICE
Primary care involves stabilization of the patient. Testing, if possible, should be the main guide for therapy choices. Empirical therapy based on specific history or examination findings may be reasonable if testing is not possible. Evidence-based reasoning for choice of medications is preferred. Responsible use of antibiotics or antifungals is important to avoid development of resistance. Some species have specific sensitivities to certain drugs. Other species such as food animals may have restrictions on the use of certain drugs (www.farad.org).

### CONTRAINDICATIONS
N/A

### PRECAUTIONS
N/A

### POSSIBLE INTERACTIONS
N/A

### ALTERNATIVE DRUGS
N/A

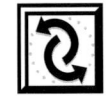

## FOLLOW-UP

### PATIENT MONITORING
Trained veterinary staff should closely monitor hospitalized patients. Once released from the hospital, each patient should be monitored as needed, depending on the severity of the condition and the specific disorder. This should include examinations as well as specific laboratory testing as indicated.

### PREVENTION/AVOIDANCE
Education of every client is essential to prevent birds from being presented in an advanced state of illness.

### POSSIBLE COMPLICATIONS
N/A

### EXPECTED COURSE AND PROGNOSIS
Prognosis is extremely variable, depending upon the specific diagnosis.

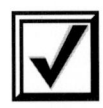

## MISCELLANEOUS

### ASSOCIATED CONDITIONS
N/A

### AGE-RELATED FACTORS
N/A

### ZOONOTIC POTENTIAL
N/A

### FERTILITY/BREEDING
N/A

### SYNONYMS
N/A

### SEE ALSO
Anemia
Anorexia
Dehydration
Dystocia and Egg Binding
Nutritional Imbalances
Regurgitation and Vomiting
Respiratory Distress
Toxicosis (Airborne)
Trauma
Appendix 8, Algorithm 1: Sick-Bird Syndrome

### ABBREVIATIONS
CT—computed tomography
ECG—electrocardiogram
MRI—magnetic resonance imaging

### INTERNET RESOURCES
Food Animal Residue Avoidance Databank: www.farad.org

*Suggested Reading*
Doneley, B., Harrison, G., Lightfoot, T. (2006). Maximizing information from the physical examination. In: *Clinical Avian Medicine* (ed. G.J. Harrison, T.L. Lightfoot), 153–211. Palm Beach, FL: Spix Publishing.
**Author:** Hillary G. Frank, DVM, DABVP (Avian)
**Acknowledgements:** George A. Messenger, DVM, DABVP (Avian), first edition author.

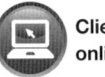 **Client Education Handout available online**

# BASICS

## DEFINITION
Two main types of spirochete infections have been described in birds: Avian (fowl) spirochetosis is an acute septicemic disease caused by the spirochete *Borrelia anserina*, affecting mainly poultry with anecdotal reports in other bird species. Avian intestinal spirochetosis (AIS) is a spirochaete colonization by *Brachyspira* spp. of the caecum and/or rectum of breeder chickens. Spiral bacteria have also been associated with upper respiratory tract and oral cavity infections in cockatiels.

## PATHOPHYSIOLOGY
*B. anserina*: The main transmission is through ticks, especially the soft tick *Argus persicus*, with mosquitoes and mites to a lesser extent. *B. anserina* can survive over 1 year in ticks and can be passed transovarially. Transmission can also occur through infectious droppings, ingestion of infected ticks, or cannibalism of infected carcasses. The organism is not resistant outside hosts/ vectors. AIS: Some of these spirochetes may induce a mild chronic disease; others are non-pathogenic.

## SYSTEMS AFFECTED
*B. anserina*: Cardiovascular—pericarditis. GI—enteritis with diarrhea. Hemic/ lymphatic/immune—splenomegaly. Hepatobiliary—hepatomegaly. Nervous— ataxia and paralysis. Renal/urologic— nephromegaly. Respiratory—dyspnea and cyanosis. AIS: GI—enteritis and typhlitis with diarrhea. Reproductive—delayed and/or decreased egg production by 5%.

## GENETICS
*B. anserina*: Dwarf chickens appear to be more resistant than white leghorns and synthetic broilers.

## INCIDENCE/PREVALENCE
High rates of infection (> 40%) have been reported with AIS.

## GEOGRAPHIC DISTRIBUTION
*B. anserina*: Present in tropical and temperate regions. Described in California, New Mexico, Texas, and Arizona. AIS: Worldwide.

## SIGNALMENT
**Species**: *B. anserina*—geese, ducks, turkeys, chickens, pheasants, grouse, partridges, pigeons, crows, magpies, house sparrows, canaries, starlings, African grey parrots. AIS—commercial layer and meat breeder chickens. Spiral bacteria in cockatiels. **Mean age and range**. *B. anserina*—all age groups are susceptible if not previously exposed. AIS—young chicks (1–3 weeks of age) are particularly susceptible.
**Predominant sex**: None.

## SIGNS
### General Comments
*B. anserina* is usually acute presentation with high morbidity and mortality, 10–100% depending upon the susceptibility of the host. AIS—mild and chronic disease.

### Historical Findings
*B. anserina*: Droopy blue heads, weakness, paralysis, wet feces, increased thirst. AIS: Chronic decreased egg production, wet feces.

### Physical Examination Findings
*B. anserina*: Depression, general weakness, anorexia, cyanosis of the comb, greenish diarrhea, ataxia and paralysis, high fever, death from embolism due to agglutinating borrelias, anemia. AIS: Chronic diarrhea. Reduced growth rates.

## CAUSES
*B. anserina*: Gram-negative, helical motile spirochete. AIS: *Brachyspira (Serpulina) intermedia*, *Brachyspira (Serpulina) pilosicoli*, *Brachyspira (Serpulina) alvinipulli*.

## RISK FACTORS
*B. anserina*: Exposure to arthropod vectors or infected birds in endemic area. AIS: Stress may precipitate clinical disease and increase its severity.

# DIAGNOSIS

## DIFFERENTIAL DIAGNOSIS
Salmonellosis, collibacillosis.

## CBC/BIOCHEMISTRY/URINALYSIS
Hemolytic anemia. Decreased albumin, alkaline phosphatase, and cholesterol levels. Increased AST levels.

## OTHER LABORATORY TESTS
*B. anserina*: Spirochetes can be identified in Giemsa-stained blood smears or darkfield microscopy of blood and other fluids. It is present in the peripheral blood of infected birds from 4th to 9th day post infection, and then in parenchymal organs for 30 days. Thus, spirochetes may not be observed during late stages of the disease. The organism can be concentrated in the buffy coat of centrifuged blood to facilitate diagnosis in case of low spirochetemia. Culturing *B. anserina* is very difficult. Antibodies (agglutination, fluorescence techniques, immunodiffusion) can be tested from 4th to 30th day post infection.
**AIS**: Although not sensitive, spirochetes may be observed in wet mount preparations of feces or cecal droppings. Diagnosis is based on spirochete-specific antigens through direct or indirect fluorescent antibody tests, visualization of characteristic periplasmic flagella by electron microscopy, isolation, culture, and identification, multilocus enzyme electrophoresis, and PCR on intestinal biopsy material.

## IMAGING
*B. anserina*: Hepatomegaly and splenomegaly may be seen.

## DIAGNOSTIC PROCEDURES
*B. anserina*: Spirochetosis should be suspected if the tick *Argas persicus* is found on typical sick birds. However, nymphs and adult ticks live in the house and feed mostly at night.

## PATHOLOGIC FINDINGS
***B. anserina***: Gross lesions—severely enlarged liver with hemorrhages and necrotic foci are characteristic in most species except in pheasants. Mucoid hemorrhagic enteritis. Serofibrinous pericarditis. Swollen kidneys. Splenomegaly with ecchymotic hemorrhages. Histology— multiple necrotic foci without usually inflammatory reactions.
**AIS**: Pale-colored, foul-smelling, foamy cecal contents with no gross lesions. Histologic examination of ceca shows from no abnormalities to necrosis.

# TREATMENT

## APPROPRIATE HEALTH CARE
Inpatient or outpatient medical management and emergency inpatient intensive care management may be needed, depending on the severity of the clinical signs.

## NURSING CARE
Supportive care, including fluid therapy, nutritional support, and oxygen therapy is recommended in debilitated birds with anorexia and dyspnea. Additional padding and adaptation of the environment may be needed with paralyzed birds.

## ACTIVITY
Restricted activity during the first month post infection may be recommended to limit transmission bird to bird or to arthropod vector.

## DIET
N/A

## CLIENT EDUCATION
Modalities of transmission should be discussed with the owners to limit the spread of the disease.

## SURGICAL CONSIDERATIONS
N/A

S

## SPIROCHETE INFECTION

# MEDICATIONS

## DRUG(S) OF CHOICE
***B. anserina***: Penicillin, streptomycin, tylosin, oxytetracyclines, aureomycin, and dihydrostreptomycin HCl have been used successfully for treatment of *B. anserina*. A single intramuscular dose is usually effective.
**AIS**: Sensitivity to lincomycin, carbadox and tiamulin has been reported. Tiamulin was shown to be the most active. Lincomycin is the drug of choice in the USA since it is registered for use in broilers.
**Cockatiel spiral bacteria**: Doxycycline in drinking water (400 mg/l) has been shown to be an effective treatment in cockatiels.

## CONTRAINDICATIONS
Food animal law regulations should be followed in poultry species.

## PRECAUTIONS
N/A

## POSSIBLE INTERACTIONS
Bacteriostatic antibacterials such as the tetracyclines should not be used with bactericidal drugs such as penicillin.

## ALTERNATIVE DRUGS
N/A

# FOLLOW-UP

## PATIENT MONITORING
*B. anserina*: Recheck blood smears or buffy coat evaluation may be done 7–10 days post infection to monitor the presence of the spirochetes. Hematology and biochemistry may be controlled 7–10 days after initial presentation if abnormalities were observed on blood work. Follow-up imaging evaluation may be needed to evaluate the liver and spleen 7–14 days post initial presentation.

## PREVENTION/AVOIDANCE
Control or eradication all the vectors and transmitters of *B. anserina*. Bacterins and vaccines have been used to produce a shorter and weaker immunity than natural infection but are not available in the USA. AIS: Careful attention to biosecurity to prevent the introduction of spirochetes on fomites.

## POSSIBLE COMPLICATIONS
*B. anserina*: Mortalities and recurrence may occur in endemic area.

## EXPECTED COURSE AND PROGNOSIS
*B. anserina*: Spontaneous recovery may occur around the 6th day post infection. A strain-specific immunity develops in survivors. Recovered birds clear the infection completely and do not become carriers. AIS: The exact outcome may vary depending on the species, the strain of spirochete involved, the age at infection, and the nutritional status of the birds. Reduced level of infection over several months may be expected. Reinfestation may occur.

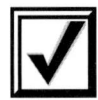

# MISCELLANEOUS

## ASSOCIATED CONDITIONS
N/A

## AGE-RELATED FACTORS
Young chicks (1–3 weeks of age) are particularly susceptible to AIS.

## ZOONOTIC POTENTIAL
N/A

## FERTILITY/BREEDING
N/A

## SYNONYMS
*B. anserina*: Spirochaeta gallinarum, avian borreliosis, avian spirochetosis, fowl spirochetosis, spirochetosis

## SEE ALSO
Sepsis

## ABBREVIATIONS
AIS—avian intestinal spirochetosis
AST—aspartate aminotransferase
GI—gastrointestinal
PCR—polymerase chain reaction

## INTERNET RESOURCES
Behboudi, S. (2022). Avian intestinal spirochaetosis. *CABI Compendium*: https://doi.org/10.1079/cabicompendium.64098
Behboudi, S. (2022). Borrelia anserina infections. *CABI Compendium*: https://doi.org/10.1079/cabicompendium.9163

*Suggested Reading*
Evans, E.E., Wade, L.L., Flammer, K. (2008). Administration of doxycycline in drinking water for treatment of spiral bacterial infection in cockatiels. *Journal of the American Veterinary Medical Association*, 3:389–393.
Stephens, C.P., Hampson, D.J. (2001). Intestinal spirochete infections of chickens: a review of disease associations, epidemiology and control. *Animal Health Research Reviews*, 2:83–91.
**Author**: Noémie Summa, DMV, IPSAV (Zoological Medicine), DACZM

# BASICS

## DEFINITION
The avian spleen is located dorsal to the right liver lobe and to the isthmus between the proventriculus and ventriculus in the intestinal peritoneal cavity. Accessory spleens adjacent to the main spleen may be presents in some species such as chickens but have not been described in psittacines. The splenic shape varies from oval (psittacines), triangular (duck, goose), or tubular or comma-shaped (passerines) and its normal color from pink to red-brown. The spleen is frequently involved in systemic diseases in birds and can be the primary site of specific pathologies.

## PATHOPHYSIOLOGY
The avian spleen serves as the principal organ of systemic immunity in birds through blood filtration, antigen processing, and plasma cell proliferation. Unlike mammals, the spleen does not function as a blood reservoir or hematopoietic site in adult birds. Its importance in disease resistance is most likely accentuated by the presence of rudimentary lymph nodes (cervicothoracic and lumbar nodes in some waterfowls) or lack of lymph nodes in most avian species. The avian spleen is a sensitive indicator of primary and secondary diseases, but its response is usually non-specific.

## SYSTEMS AFFECTED
Hemic/lymphatic/immune: Change in splenic size (splenomegaly or splenic atrophy) is most often seen.

## GENETICS
Toucans, birds of paradise, quetzals, tanagers, hornbills, manakans, mynahs, and starlings are predisposed to ISD supposedly secondary to little ability to downregulate iron uptake when dietary supply is abundant.

## INCIDENCE/PREVALENCE
Specific prevalence or incidence of splenic diseases in avian patients has not been yet described. Spleen has been reported to be a frequent site of neoplasia in budgerigar and is the second most common site of lymphoma in psittacines after the liver. As the spleen is often involved with secondary diseases, splenic changes are frequent in birds.

## GEOGRAPHIC DISTRIBUTION
Diseases of the spleen can be found worldwide.

## SIGNALMENT
**Species**: All avian species are susceptible to splenic diseases. Most viruses target specific avian species.

**Mean age and range**: Splenic atrophy is most commonly seen in young birds with bursal disease or with older birds.
**Predominant sex**: None.

## SIGNS

### General Comments
Clinical signs may vary, depending on the etiologic cause of the splenic disease.

### Historical Findings
Owners may report acute or chronic progression of the disease.

### Physical Examination Findings
Non-specific systemic clinical signs such as lethargy, dysorexia, behavior changes, low posture, or fluffed appearance may be seen. Severe splenomegaly may be suspected when palpating a firm mass effect in the right caudodorsal coelomic cavity.

## CAUSES
Chlamydiosis and mycobacteriosis are the most frequent causes of splenomegaly in psittacines.

### Infectious
**Viral**: Polyomavirus, adenovirus, herpesvirus (Pacheco's disease, Marek's disease, inclusion body disease of cranes virus), retrovirus (avian leukosis virus), togavirus, paramyxovirus, reovirus, coronavirus, parvovirus, picornavirus.
**Bacterial**: Chlamydiosis, mycobacteriosis, colisepticemia, salmonellosis, spirochetes, *Yersinia, Erysipelas.*
**Parasitic**: Sarcocystosis, toxoplasmosis, systemic coccidiosis, spirochetosis, atoxoplasmosis, *Plasmodium*, Leukocytozoon.
**Fungal**: Disseminated aspergillosus, zygomycosis, candidiasis.

### Non-Infectious
**Toxic**: mycotoxins (ochratoxin A), polychlorinated biphenyls, selenium, aflatoxin B1, T-2 toxin.
**Degenerative**: aging, glucocorticoids.
**Auto-immune**: immune-mediated hemolytic anemia.
**Metabolic**: lipidosis, hemosiderosis, hemochromatosis, amyloidosis, lysosomal storage disease, visceral gout.
**Neoplastic**: lymphoma, lymphosarcoma, hemangiosarcoma, fibrosarcoma, leiomyosarcoma, myeloid neoplasia, myelocytoma, metastatic neoplasia (leiomyosarcoma, malignant melanoma, squamous cell carcinoma, intestinal carcinoma).
**Nutritional**: ISD, lipidosis.
**Physiologic**: Seasonal variations in association with migration in some species.

## RISK FACTORS
Suboptimal environments may play a role (inappropriate diet, exposition to parasite vectors or toxins) or exposure to other infected birds or animals. Stress and

immunosuppression have been associated with some of the cited infectious diseases (aspergillosis, mycobacteriosis).

# DIAGNOSIS

## DIFFERENTIAL DIAGNOSIS
Granuloma, hematoma (liver laceration), other mass effects.

## CBC/BIOCHEMISTRY/URINALYSIS
Marked leucocytosis (> 30 000 10⁹ cells/l) with heterophilia is usually seen with chlamydiosis, mycobacteriosis, aspergillosis and salmonellosis. Leukocytosis can also be seen with neoplasia and toxins (aflatoxicosis). Leukocytosis without heterophilia, leucopenia, lymphocytosis or lymphopenia have been described with viral infection. Hemoparasites may be seen on blood smears. Biochemistry abnormality may vary depending on the etiology of the splenic disease and its targeted organs.

## OTHER LABORATORY TESTS
Specific tests for chlamydiosis and mycobacteriosis is usually recommended with splenomegaly in psittacines.

## IMAGING
The spleen can be visualized on the lateral survey radiographs in approximatively one-third of normal large psittacines, and is not seen on the ventrodorsal radiograph unless abnormal. Spleen diameter in psittacines is supposed to be < 1.5 times the width of the mid-diaphyseal femur, although this reference is controversial for some authors (Table 1). Splenomegaly is best assessed on the lateral radiograph and can displace the ventriculus caudodorsally. On the ventrodorsal radiograph, splenomegaly can be seen as a mass effect superposed with the cranial division of the right kidney. The spleen is usually difficult to detect via ultrasound, unless significantly enlarged. Advanced imaging (MRI, CT) offers a better visualization of the spleen in avian species.

## DIAGNOSTIC PROCEDURES
Coelomic endoscopy through a left coelomic air sac approach is indicated in case of persistent splenomegaly unresponsive to attempted treatments. Splenic biopsies with a 5 Fr elliptical cup or FNA during endoscopy or during ultrasonographic examination may be attempted while being prepared for possible severe hemorrhages. Cytologic examination, histopathology, microbiologic culture, virus isolation, specific stains such as acid-fast, and PCR can be performed on spleen samples, depending on the suspected condition.

**Table 1**

| Suggested normal spleen sizes. | |
| --- | --- |
| *Species* | *Size (mm)* |
| Budgerigar | 1 |
| African grey parrot, Amazon parrot | 5–6 |
| Umbrella cockatoo | 8 |

## PATHOLOGIC FINDINGS

The gross and histopathologic appearance of the avian spleen may be similar for many diseases and additional testing is usually recommended to reach a diagnosis. Splenomegaly, splenic atrophy, splenic congestion, necrosis, or infiltration can be seen. Splenic congestion in frequently seen with bacterial or viral infections, and necrosis with viral infections. Splenic infarcti have been associated with bacterial endocarditis in chicken. Splenomegaly and airsacculitis is highly suggestive of chlamydiosis. Marked splenomegaly, with well-demarcated tan to yellow laminated caseous nodules, is frequently associated with mycobacteriosis. Fibrin deposition and splenic autolysis is seen with colibacillosis in chickens. The presence of hemosiderin in splenic tissues is common in chronic diseases and ISD. Excessive amount of iron accumulation with erythrophagocytosis has been associated with hemolytic anemias.

 TREATMENT

### APPROPRIATE HEALTH CARE

Most avian patients with splenic diseases present with significant clinical disease, implying emergency inpatient intensive care management or hospitalization during diagnostic testing.

### NURSING CARE

Supportive care (nutritional support, fluid and oxygen therapy) is often needed, no matter the etiology of the splenic disease.

### ACTIVITY

Activity should be restricted until a final diagnosis is reached.

### DIET

Diet should be modified immediately if related to the splenic disease (ISD, lipidosis).

## CLIENT EDUCATION

Prognosis with splenic diseases is usually reserved and owners should be informed of the severity of the disease, as well as the potential zoonotic risks.

## SURGICAL CONSIDERATIONS

Birds with splenic diseases should not undergo surgical procedures unless necessary to reach a final diagnosis or as part of the therapeutic treatment plan. Stabilization prior to general anesthesia is highly recommended.

 MEDICATIONS

### DRUG(S) OF CHOICE

Therapeutic treatment should be adapted based on the suspected or diagnosed causes of the splenic disease. Broad-spectrum antibiotic therapy should be considered if diagnostic testing is delayed or while waiting for the test results. In psittacines with marked splenomegaly, antibiotics effective against *Chlamydia* sp. (doxycycline, azithromycin) should be considered.

### CONTRAINDICATIONS

Oral treatment may be contraindicated depending on the bird's general status (digestive stasis, general profound weakness).

### PRECAUTIONS

As some of the possible etiologies of splenic diseases may induce hepatic diseases, drugs with hepatic metabolism should be used with caution and adverse effects should be monitored.

### POSSIBLE INTERACTIONS

Contraindications may apply depending on the drugs used and their interactions.

### ALTERNATIVE DRUGS

N/A

 FOLLOW-UP

### PATIENT MONITORING

Hematology should be repeated 2–7 days after the initial result, depending on the severity of the hematologic abnormalities to monitor the response to the current therapy. Imaging (recheck radiographs, ultrasound or advanced imaging) is usually recommended 7–14 days following the first survey to evaluate the evolution of the spleen size.

### PREVENTION/AVOIDANCE

Guidelines to prevent recurrence may be offered, depending on the etiology (contact with other animal, exposure to vectors).

### POSSIBLE COMPLICATIONS

Splenic diseases encompass many etiologies, some of which are life threatening or untreatable conditions.

### EXPECTED COURSE AND PROGNOSIS

Prognosis is highly variable, depending on the etiology, severity, or stage of the disease.

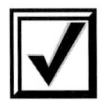 MISCELLANEOUS

### ASSOCIATED CONDITIONS

None.

### AGE-RELATED FACTORS

Prognosis may be influenced by the age of the birds and may be worse in very old and young birds

### ZOONOTIC POTENTIAL

Chlamydiosis, mycobacteriosis, and salmonellosis may be potential zoonotic diseases.

### FERTILITY/BREEDING

Depending of the etiology, suitability of the avian patient for breeding may be impacted.

## SYNONYMS
Splenomegaly, splenic atrophy.

## SEE ALSO
Amyloidosis
Aspergillosis
Chlamydiosis
Collibacillosis
Iron Storage Disease
Mycobacteriosis
Mycotoxicosis
Neoplasia (Lymphoproliferative)
Neoplasia (Gastrointestinal and Hepatic)
Salmonellosis
Sarcocystosis
Toxoplasmosis

## ABBREVIATIONS
CT—computed tomography
FNA—fine-needle aspiration
ISD—iron storage disease
MRI—magnetic resonance imaging
PCR—polymerase chain reaction

## INTERNET RESOURCES
N/A

*Suggested Reading*
John, J.L. (1994). The avian spleen: A neglected organ. *Quarterly Review of Biology* 69:327–351.
Powers, L.V. (2000). The avian spleen: Anatomy, physiology and diagnostics. *Compendium on Continuing Education for the Practising Veterinarian North American Edition: Small Animal/Exotics* 22:838–880.
Powers, L.V. (2000). Diseases of the avian spleen. *Compendium on Continuing Education for the Practising Veterinarian North American Edition: Small Animal/Exotics* 22:925–933.
Boyer, C. (2013). *Etude rétrospective de la taille de la rate sur des radiographies chez les Gris du Gabon (Psittacus erithacus).* Doctoral dissertation, École Nationale Vétérinaire D'Alfort, Chambray-les-Tours, France.
**Author**: Noémie Summa, DMV, IPSAV (Zoological Medicine), DACZM

S

# TENDINITIS AND TENOSYNOVITIS

## BASICS

### DEFINITION
Tendinitis is inflammation of a tendon, typically associated with acute injury and usually accompanied by pain and swelling. Tenosynovitis is inflammation of a tendon sheath. This term has also been used in the poultry literature synonymously with viral arthritis, and is used to define the changes in the tendons and tendon sheaths associated with a condition considered different from that caused by *Mycoplasma synoviae*. Tendon rupture is traumatic breakage of a tendon secondary to acute trauma, or advanced pathology compromising tendon integrity.

### PATHOPHYSIOLOGY
Tendinitis and tenosynovitis can occur secondary to infectious, traumatic, nutritional, genetic, or environmental causes.

#### Infectious
*M. synoviae* and avian reovirus are the main infectious causative agents in chickens and turkeys. Infections can occur together or as single isolate. Bacterial infections such as *Staphylococcus, Streptococcus, Salmonella, Riemerella anatipestifer*, and *Escherichia coli* are also reported in cases of tenosynovitis in poultry. Bacteria close to the joint or footpad may become introduced with trauma and enter through compromised epithelium or mucosal surfaces, such as bumblefoot. Infection can occur secondary to systemic infection. Staphylococcus is a common isolate with bumblefoot lesions. In avian reovirus, early infection causes inflammation and scarring of the gastrocnemius and flexor tendons and subsequent arthritis/synovitis. Virulence can vary greatly among isolates within different hosts. Disease presentation in individual affected depends on immune status, pathogenicity of the virus, and route of exposure. Transmission is both horizontally via fecal–oral contamination and vertically. Hens can be asymptomatic and transmit to chicks. Transmission in adult poultry is enhanced with pododermatitis lesions. Respiratory transmission is possible, especially in young chicks (1 day old). Chickens develop an age-associated resistance beginning as early as 2 weeks. Shedding can be prolonged and persistence in the environment can be lengthy. Incubation period varied, but at least 1 day. *M. synoviae*—chickens, joint swellings, airsacculitis, and/or upper respiratory disease. Vertical transmission plays a major role in spread of *Mycoplasma* in chickens and turkeys. Horizontal transmission occurs readily by direct contact via the respiratory tract. Often, 100% of birds become infected, although none, or only a few, develop joint lesions.

Low level of concurrent respiratory clinical signs. The route of *M. synoviae* infection may play a role in the resulting disease. Incubation period is 11–21 days. Other *Mycoplasma* spp: *Mycoplasma iowae*—turkeys, acute tenosynovitis, *Mycoplasma meleagridis*—turkeys, airsacculitis, and developmental skeletal deformities. *Pasteurella multocidia*—lameness and purulent arthritis with swollen joints. *Enterococcus*—fibrinous arthritis and tenosynovitis with osteomyelitis and necrotic myocarditis.

#### Traumatic
Tendon ruptures are often associated with advanced cases of infectious tendinitis. Gastrocnemius tendon injury is characterized by swelling, accumulation of blood, and fibrous tissue developed in the gastrocnemius muscle tendon and the hock, developing a synovitis. It can be associated with an infectious cause (viral or bacterial) as disease compromises tendon integrity. Rupture can also occur from a non-inflammatory origin. Rupture often is located at the non-vascular part of the tendon. Spontaneous gastrocnemius tendon rupture can happen in fast-growing heavy-bodied birds, with one or both legs being affected. Cruciate ligament rupture has been reported to occur in captive birds with routine handling (e.g. nail trim and capture for restraint).

#### Raptor Tendon Injuries
In raptors, ring injuries can occur due to the metal band compressing the thin soft tissue of the tarsus. Similar injury results with aylmeri anklets in falconer birds if the brass ring is rubbing against the ankle. Animal bites associated with falconer hunting. Plantar infection (usually associated with trapped prey in the foot pad) can cause infection and subsequent necrosis of the tendon attachment. Furniture damage- entanglement in the jesses on the perch causing friction burns.

#### Nutritional
Separation of the gastrocnemius tendons from the hypotarsus has been seen in birds with angular limb deformities that developed secondary to nutritional deficiencies.

### SYSTEMS AFFECTED
Musculoskeletal.

### GENETICS
Poor genetics leading to abnormal development of the pelvic limb structures can give predisposition to tendinitis.

### INCIDENCE/PREVALENCE
Backyard poultry are not often affected by *M. synoviae* or reoviral infections, more common in production poultry, especially those in commercial meat production. Reovirus causes a significant economic impact on poultry. In chickens with reovirus, morbidity can be as high as 100% and mortality generally less than 6%. In turkeys

with reovirus, morbidity is 5–7% and mortality, including culling, 2–30%. *M. synoviae* morbidity in chicken flocks with clinical synovitis varies from 2% to 75%, morbidity 5–15%. Morbidity in turkey flocks is usually low (1–20%) but mortality from trampling and cannibalism may be significant. Gastrocnemius tendon rupture is not common in backyard poultry, but occurs in meat-type breeds in birds > 12 weeks. Tendon injuries can be common in birds of prey.

### GEOGRAPHIC DISTRIBUTION
Worldwide distribution.

### SIGNALMENT
**Species**: Infectious tenosynovitis—chickens, turkeys, ducks, other fowl, raptors. Traumatic—raptors, captive birds undergoing handling. Infectious causes (*Mycoplasma* and reovirus) more associated with broiler chickens and industry birds.

**Mean age and range**: Reovirus infects young chickens, but joint lesions develop in birds 4–7 weeks or older with clinical signs typically seen in birds > 12 weeks. Turkeys are typically 14 weeks or older. In chickens, signs of lameness are unlikely to be seen before 4–7 weeks or older. *Mycoplasma* infection in chickens can occur as early as 1 week, but acute infection is generally seen at 4–16 weeks. Acute infection occasionally occurs in adult chickens. Chronic infection follows the acute phase and may persist for the life of the flock. Turkeys with Mycoplasma-associated infectious synovitis are usually between 10 and 24 weeks.

**Predominant sex**: There are no reported sex predilections for chickens with infectious tenosynovitis. Avian reovirus affects male turkeys with a higher prevalence.

### SIGNS
#### Historical Findings
Limping, lameness, poor doer.

#### Physical Examination Findings
Lameness with limping with varied severity, progressing to non-weight-bearing. Inflammation and swelling of one or multiple joints (hock joints, foot pads, interphalangeal joints) and/or swelling of gastrocnemius tendon. Affected joints usually feel warm. Joints can appear reddish-purple with or without green areas, indicating hemorrhage (> 3 days), in gastrocnemius tendon rupture. To determine the lesion location, observe the bird in both a standing position and when ambulating. Assess the grip of both feet. Manipulation of the muscles to extend and flex digits can help to reveal which tendons are affected. Inspect the legs for wounds, scabs, and swellings to give insight into the bird's proprioception. Exams can be performed in both conscious birds and under anesthesia.

T

**Infectious**: In cases of infectious tenosynovitis the presence of a gray, white, or yellow caseous exudate in synovium and surrounding tissues can be seen. *Mycoplasma*—swelling over hock joints and foot pads predominately, but swelling can be in numerous joints. In chickens, the first observable signs can be a pale comb, lameness, emaciation, leg weakness, and retarded growth. Breast blisters are common as this infection affects the sternal bursa. Respiratory clinical signs may or may not be present. Reovirus—swollen hock joints, in conjunction with visible swellings in the gastrocnemius, metatarsal extensor, or digital flexor tendons. The gastrocnemius tendon may rupture. Swelling of the footpads is less common. Chickens with reovirus can develop hydropericardium, chronic respiratory clinical signs, stunted growth, and malabsorptive syndrome.

**Tendon rupture**: Non-weight-bearing lameness and swelling over the affected joint. Loose ends of the tendon can be palpated bunched up on the posterior surface of the leg cranial to the hock. Cranial drawer sign with ruptured cruciate tendons. Ruptured gastrocnemius tendon—dropped hock, inability to move and palpable swelling associated with the tendon. Birds sit on their hocks with toes pointed ventrally.

## CAUSES
Infectious (*M. synoviae*, avian reovirus, *Staphylococcus*, *Streptococcus*, *Salmonella*, *R. anatipestifer*, *E. coli*), traumatic, nutritional, genetic.

## RISK FACTORS
Genetics, nutrition, and environment can increase the risk of tendon disease and injuries. Poor management practices, such inadequate feeding, poor litter quality (wet), inefficient lighting or perching, extreme temperature (lower temperatures and higher humidity in the winter), improper ventilation, and chronically debilitating diseases (e.g. *Coccidia*) can lead to stress and immunocompromization. Inadequate skeletal growth during first 6 weeks of life can lead to poor conformation, resulting in inappropriate load on the legs and tendons. This happens secondary to inadequate space for required physical activity and proper tendon development, or malnutrition.

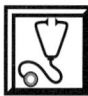

## DIAGNOSIS
### DIFFERENTIAL DIAGNOSIS
Wooden breast syndrome in gastrocnemius muscle, slipped tendon of the gastrocnemius (perosis), osteoarthritis, neoplasia of the synovium or bone, *Salmonella* (swollen joints secondary to arthritis).

## CBC/BIOCHEMISTRY/URINALYSIS
No biochemistry abnormalities expected other than elevated CK and possibly elevated AST. CBC may have an elevated total white blood cell count in response to inflammation and/or infection. Anemia of chronic disease.

## OTHER LABORATORY TESTS
In cases of suspected infection, aerobic and anerobic bacterial C/S can help guide antimicrobial selection and treatment duration. Avian reovirus—gold standard diagnosis is viral isolation of synovial fluid. Commercially available ELISA is used to assess antibodies induced by vaccination, but also can be used for field exposure in clinical animals. It should be noted that reoviruses can be found normally in the respiratory and GI tracts in 80% of chickens and is non-pathogenic. The presence of the virus is therefore not significant for diagnosis, and diagnosis must be in conjunction with associated clinical signs. rt-PCR and IFA are other testing modalities, but often not practical to use in large-scale testing. *M. synoviae*: Isolation of organism from infected fluids or tissue (more sensitive in acute infections). Detection via PCR (more sensitive), fluorescent antibody staining, and serology. Culture requires specific medium and can be challenging, as growth is lengthy and can yield negative results with chronic infections.

## IMAGING
Radiographs: Soft tissue swelling surrounding the affected joints. Bone defects can be seen with advanced and chronic cases. Typically, do not see osteomyelitis with *M. synoviae* lesions. Cranial displacement of the tibiotarsus is seen with cruciate ligament rupture. Ultrasound or CT can be used to evaluate tendon sheath and intraarticular fluid and abscess.

## DIAGNOSTIC PROCEDURES
N/A

## PATHOLOGIC FINDINGS
### Gross Pathology Findings
Swelling and edema of the digital flexor tendon ± gastrocnemius tendon rupture at the level of the hock. Small amount of straw-colored blood-tinged exudate can be present in joints. Purulent exudate in the hock may be present with either reoviral or *Mycoplasma* infections. In reoviral infections, small pitted erosions can develop in the articular cartilage of the distal tibiotarsus and the lesions can coalesce and go into the underlying bone. Osteomyelitis is typically absent with *Mycoplasma* infections.

### Microscopic Findings
Histopathological findings include intense and diffuse lymphohistiocytic inflammatory

infiltrate with accumulation of heterophils primarily in the synovial capsule. Reovirus: Similar inflammatory changes develop in the tarsometatarsal and hock joint areas. Acute phase—edema, coagulation necrosis, heterophil accumulation, and perivascular infiltration; Hypertrophy and hyperplasia of synovial cells, infiltration of lymphocytes and macrophages, and a proliferation of reticular cells. Chronic phase—synovial membrane develops villous processes, and lymphoid nodules are seen; increase in fibrous connective tissue and a pronounced infiltration or proliferation of reticular cells, lymphocytes, macrophages, and plasma cells; some tendons are replaced completely by irregular granulation and fibrous tissues, resulting in ankylosis and immobility. *Mycoplasma*: Heterophils and fibrin infiltrates into joint spaces and along tendon sheaths; villous formation and lymphocytic and macrophagic subsynovial infiltrate occurs in synovial membranes.

## TREATMENT
### APPROPRIATE HEALTH CARE
Tendon sheath infections are stubborn to treat and almost always require irrigation of sheath to drain purulent material as well as systemic antibiotics based on C/S results. Adequate pain medication (anti-inflammatories and/or opiates) should be provided in these cases, as tendon sheath inflammation and associated pathology can be painful. Supportive care is likely needed in cases of debilitated birds. Frequent wound care to address infections with mechanical debridement and flushing as well as bandaging to keep sites clean. Regional limb perfusion with appropriate antimicrobial therapy may be used for treatment of the bacterial component. No treatment is currently described for ruptures gastrocnemius tendons. *M. synoviae* vaccination is not routinely used. Antimicrobials targeted to treat *Mycoplasma* can be used, but their use is controversial as, despite treatment birds will remain carriers for life. No treatment is currently described for avian reovirus. Reoviral vaccinations in hens provide maternal antibodies and day-1 immunity to chicks. Maternal antibodies are best achieved by the use of inactivated vaccines administered by SQ injection at ≥ 12 weeks. If a live vaccine is used, it should be administered prior to the onset of egg production to prevent transovarian transmission of the vaccine virus. It is unlikely that non-commercial birds will be vaccinated, so quarantine of young birds is important. Age-related immunity develops in chicks at 2 weeks. It should be

T

noted that the vaccines of today are not as efficacious, as emerging reoviruses are mutating and the vaccines are not providing adequate coverage.

## NURSING CARE
Gavage feeding and fluid therapy may be needed in debilitated birds. Warm compresses over affected joints may help with associated pain and inflammation. Physical therapy post tendon surgery is important to prevent adhesions.

## ACTIVITY
Normal use of the limb needs restriction post tendon surgery. With tenosynovitis and tendinitis, activity restriction may be helpful to allow inflammation to resolve.

## DIET
N/A

## CLIENT EDUCATION
Preventive measures are the best way to control infectious tendinitis and tenosynovitis in poultry. Prevent trauma to birds to prevent introduction of infectious agents through cuts. Reduce immunosuppression in birds. Improve hygiene to reduce bacterial load. Prevention of pododermatitis and traumatic injury to the joints. *Mycoplasma* does not stay readily in the environment, so obtaining *Mycoplasma*-free stock and biosecurity is important in management.

## SURGICAL CONSIDERATIONS
Surgical correction of cruciate ligament ruptures can be achieved with extracapsular stabilization techniques via a lateral suture technique, or via ridged external or internal stabilization, with the goal of arthrodesis. Caution to avoid damaging the fibular nerve intraoperatively, as damage can lead to prolonged recovery and reduced function of the limb.

### Tendon Repair
Tendon ruptures are routinely repaired in raptors. In general, gentle handing of tendons and tendon sheaths is advised to prevent postoperative adhesions. Use atraumatic instruments and magnification. To begin, often there is need to transect the inappropriately adhered pedicle of one end of the severed tendon from the adjacent soft tissue. Once you have two free ends of the tendon, join the ends together using a modified Kessler suture pattern. The goal is to get tendons in as close proximity as possible, but direct contact is not mandatory. Joining tendons with an end-to-end anastomosis can fail surgically if there is no healing response at those ends. This likely occurs due to poor vascular, which is why closure of the tendon sheath in a manor to not disrupt the blood supply is paramount. Postoperatively, immobilizing the limb in a manner that will

remove tension from the tendon is important, but controlled passive range of motion may be important to prevent unwanted adhesions. Tendon autografts are also described in raptors.

# MEDICATIONS

## DRUG(S) OF CHOICE
Response to antibiotic treatment in cases of bacterial tenosynovitis has a variable to poor response. From a flock management standpoint, it is often suggested to cull affected birds that are transmitting disease. When treating bacterial arthritis, antimicrobial selection should ideally be made based on C/S results. Antimicrobials can be administered systemically, topically, and through regional limb perfusion. *Staphylococcus*—penicillins, tetracyclines, sulfonamides, lincomycin, spectinomycin. *Mycoplasma*—tylosin, tetracycline, spectinomycin, lincomycin, erythromycin. Birds remain carriers for life. Analgesia should be included in treatment plan, including NSAIDs or opioids.

## CONTRAINDICATIONS
Considering that many birds affected are food animals, proper use of antimicrobials not on the prohibited drug list is mandatory. It should be noted that clinical signs of *Mycoplasma* infection can resolve but birds are carriers for life.

## PRECAUTIONS
N/A

## POSSIBLE INTERACTIONS
N/A

## ALTERNATIVE DRUGS
N/A

# FOLLOW-UP

## PATIENT MONITORING
Continued monitoring of the affected joint in initial cause (e.g. pododermatitis wound) should be carefully monitored.

## PREVENTION/AVOIDANCE
See above environmental recommendations and client education.

## POSSIBLE COMPLICATIONS
N/A

## EXPECTED COURSE AND PROGNOSIS
Prognosis is fair to poor. In birds that do recover, joint changes are often advanced with arthrodesis of the affected joint and limited

range of motion. However, ambulation is usually sufficient enough that walking does not put excessive stress on the contra limb. In *Mycoplasma* infection, acute signs can be followed by slow recovery with appropriate antimicrobial selection; however, synovitis may persist for the life of the flock.

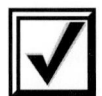

# MISCELLANEOUS

## ASSOCIATED CONDITIONS
N/A

## AGE-RELATED FACTORS
Outlined above.

## ZOONOTIC POTENTIAL
None.

## FERTILITY/BREEDING
N/A

## SYNONYMS
Tenosynovitis is often referred to synonymously as viral tendinitis in the poultry literature; tendonitis.

## SEE ALSO
Joint Diseases
Pododermatitis

## ABBREVIATIONS
AST—aspartate aminotransferase
C/S—culture and sensitivity
CK—creatine kinase
ELISA—enzyme-linked immunosorbent assay
GI—gastrointestinal
IFA—immunofluorescence assay
NSAIDs—non-steroidal anti-inflammatory drugs
PCR—polymerase chain reaction
rt-PCR—reverse transcriptase polymerase chain reaction

## INTERNET RESOURCES
US Department of Agriculture, Animal and Plant Health Inspection Service. (2021). Defend the Flock: Biosecruity 101: https://www.aphis.usda.gov/aphis/ourfocus/animalhealth/animal-disease-information/avian/defend-the-flock-program/dtf-biosecurity

*Suggested Reading*
Chinnadurai, S.K., Spodnick, G., Degernes, L., et al. (2009) Use of an extracapsular stabilization technique to repair cruciate ligament ruptures in two avian species. *Journal of Avian Medicine and Surgery*, 4:307–313.
Ferguson-Noel, N., Noormohammadi A.H. (2019). *Mycoplasma synoviae* infection. In: *Diseases of Poultry*, 14th edn. (ed. D.E. Swayne), 924–965. Hoboken, NJ: Wiley-Blackwell.
Greenacre, C.B. (2021). Musculoskeletal Diseases. In: *Backyard Poultry Medicine and Surgery: A Guide for Veterinary Practitioners*,

T

2nd edn. (ed. C.B. Greenacre, T.Y. Morishita), 234–258. J Hoboken, NJ: Wiley.

Harcourt-Brown, N.H. (2000). Tendon repair in the pelvic limb of birds of prey. Part II: Surgical techniques. In: *Raptor Biomedicine* III. (ed. J.T. Lumeij, J.D.

Remple, P.T. Redig, et al.), 217–231. Lake Worth, FL: Zoological Education Network.

Pitcovski, J., Sagar M., Goyal S.M. (2019). Avian reovirus infections. In: *Diseases of Poultry*, 14th edn. (ed. D.E. Swayne), 382–400. Hoboken, NJ: Wiley-Blackwell.

Thorp, B.H. (2008). Diseases of the musculoskeletal system. In: *Poultry Diseases*, 6th edn. (ed. M. Pattison, P.F., McMullin, J.M. Bradbury, D.J. Alexander), 470–489. Philadelphia, PA: Elsevier.

**Author**: Lauren Thielen DVM, ABVP (Avian Practice)

T

# THYMUS (DISEASES OF)

## BASICS

### DEFINITION
The avian thymus is one of the avian immune system's primary lymphoid organs, including the bone marrow, bursa of Fabricius, and yolk sac. It lies along the vagus nerve and internal jugular veins. It usually comprises 7–8 separate lobes on either side of the neck. These lobes extended from around the caudal aspect of the ramus of the mandible to the thoracic inlet. Each thymic lobe is divided into lobules, which are further indistinctly divided into a cortex and a medulla. The cortex of the thymus contains densely packed small lymphocytes and a few medium-sized lymphocytes. During T cell maturation, the cells migrate toward the corticomedullary border, where macrophages select thymocytes (immature T cells) before entering the medulla and circulation. The medulla contains larger but much fewer lymphocytic cells and is thought to have more of an endocrine function. The septae of the thymus also consist of a dense cellular composition consisting of fibroblasts, plasma cells, lymphocytes, and, occasionally, a few granulocytes. The thymus's primary role is the development and maturation of T cells which then populates secondary lymphoid tissues. These immature lymphoid cells are derived from immigrating embryonic stem cells that colonize the thymus during early development. Overall, depending on the species, the thymus reaches its greatest size about 2–3 weeks after hatching and then slowly regresses as the bird ages. The thymus also contains some B lymphocytes, and in older birds, it contains germinal centers. Thu,s the thymus also acts as a peripheral lymphoid organ and, in times of stress, can also become erythropoietic. The thymus also has a role in the development of NK cells. The main function of the thymus is to support the cell-mediated immune response, which is mediated by T cells and NK cells. In birds, T cells constitute between 60% and 70% of blood lymphocytes. These T cells consist of many different specialized subpopulations with different functions. Any malfunctions of the immune system can result in an inappropriate, excessive, or insufficient immune response. Thus, any diseases that compromise the thymus can lead to immunodeficiency (increases in inflammation, defective immune responses, and increases in susceptibility to cancer), resulting in significant systemic disease.

### PATHOPHYSIOLOGY
Any infection causing clinical disease may result in immunosuppression or immune cell depletion. Some diseases specifically target the thymus, and T and NK cells.

#### Viral Induced
Many common viral diseases of pet and backyard birds will result in thymic lesions and decreased T and NK cell function. As a result, animals will become immunocompromised, leading to secondary infections. Some of the common viral infections include circovirus, parvovirus of ducks and geese, Marek's disease, avian influenza, paramyxoviruses, and adenovirus infections.
**Circovirus**: All avian circoviruses, such as PBFD virus, pigeon circovirus, chicken anemia virus, and goose circovirus, can infect and lead to depletion and deficiency of T cells.
**PBFD virus**: All parrots are considered to be susceptible, but it is primarily observed in psittacines from Africa and Australia. It is most commonly observed in younger animals, <3 years of age. The virus primarily replicates in these intestinal lymphoid organs and then spreads to the thymus and other tissues. The virus causes atrophy at both the bursa and the thymus leading to immunosuppression with subsequent fatal secondary infections.
**Duck enteritis virus**: Causes massive depletion of bursal and thymic lymphocytes resulting in thymic and bursal atrophy, leading to secondary infections and sepsis.
**Avian leukosis and reticoendotheliosis virus**: Targets T cells (early stages) and B cells and leads to atrophy of the thymus and bursa of fabricius.
**Infectious bursal diseases virus**: Targets T cells and GALT (early-stage B cells) and can lead to thymic and bursal atrophy.
**Avian influenza virus**: Depending on the strain of influenza, the body responses with the release of IFN-α, IFN-β, TLR-6, triggering a dysregulation in the immune response cause atrophy of the thymus.
**Marek's disease (alphaherpesvirus)**: The virus infects thymic cells, leading to thymic and bursa of Fabricius apoptosis and atrophy. Marek's virus will also cause latency in T cells, transforming them into T cell lymphomas.

#### Bacterial
Infections with pathogen bacteria are also unknown to result in thymic atrophy. The exact mechanism depends on the type of bacteria. *Salmonella* spp. cause a decreased number of thymocytes and an increase in glucocorticoids leading to thymic atrophy. One study in chicks showed that the release of lipopolysaccharides could be the main pathogenic factor for thymic atrophy of chicks infected with *Salmonella typhimurium*. *Mycobacterium avium* infections have been shown to cause elevations glucocorticoids, IFN, and disruption of the bird's endocrine system, leading to thymic atrophy. *Mycoplasma gallisepticum* infections have been shown to induce immune dysregulation leading to thymic damage and atrophy.

#### Fungal
Mycotoxins and secondary metabolites frequently cause immune suppression. Toxins such as alfatoxin, T-2 toxin, and ochratoxin have been reported to lead to bursa and thymic lymphoid depletion.

#### Other
**Stress-associated immune depression**: Increases in long-term glucocorticoids can lead to apoptosis of lymphoid cells, inhibition of inflammatory proteins, and thymic atrophy.
**Neoplasia (thymomas)**: Tumors can appear cystic and hemorrhagic; they are locally invasive and usually are found along the neck. Surgical correction is typically curative.
**Toxins**: Prolonged exposure to lead and other toxins, such as petrochemicals, can result in the depression of lymphocytes, particularly T lymphocytes, leading to thymic atrophy.
**Nutritional**: Malnutrition and zinc deficiencies have been shown to cause thymic atrophy.

### SYSTEMS AFFECTED
Immune system (thymus).

### GENETICS
Underlying genetics may predispose certain species or breeds of birds, making them more venerable certain diseases leading to thymic disorders (e.g. leghorn and silkie chickens are more susceptible to Marek's disease).

### INCIDENCE/PREVALENCE
Dependent on underlying causes.

### GEOGRAPHIC DISTRIBUTION
Dependent on underlying causes.

### SIGNALMENT
Young birds: infectious diseases. Older birds: neoplastic conditions.

### SIGNS
Diseases of the thymus usually result in immunosuppression that leads to sepsis and death. Most birds will initially show signs of ill thrift, lethargy, and wasting. In later stages, birds will show signs of sepsis and shock.

### CAUSES
Malfunction of the thymus and the depletion of T and NK cells due to underlying pathologies.

## RISK FACTORS
For infection-induced causes, stress-associated immune depression (poor nutrition and captive conditions), contact with latent or chronically infected birds, lack of vaccination (etc Marek's vaccine), or non-adherence to quarantine periods.

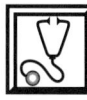

## DIAGNOSIS
### DIFFERENTIAL DIAGNOSIS
Any diseases that focuses on the avian primary lymphoid organs (bursa of Fabricius, bone marrow, and yolk sac) and secondary lymphoid organs (spleen, disseminated or mucosal associated lymphoid tissue) can show similar clinical signs and disease.

### CBC/BIOCHEMISTRY/URINALYSIS
CBC: Possible leukopenia may be seen with diseases of the thymus in young birds.

### OTHER LABORATORY TESTS
Determining underlying cause. Necropsy usually provides definitive diagnosis. Investigation of serological, PCR, and immunofluorescent assays for infectious diseases (viral and fungal). Blood test for heavy metals.

### IMAGING
Radiographs and advance imaging techniques can be useful in determining thymic masses.

### DIAGNOSTIC PROCEDURES
Biospies for thymic masses.

### PATHOLOGIC FINDINGS
Immunosuppression and dysfunction of the thymus.

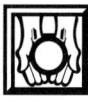

## TREATMENT
### APPROPRIATE HEALTH CARE
Limit systemic and local inflammatory reactions. Treat any secondary bacterial infections.

### NURSING CARE
Supportive care (supplemental heat, fluid replacement, assist feeding).

### ACTIVITY
N/A

### DIET
Supplementation of antioxidants such as carotenoids, vitamin E, and selenium to the diets of chicks has been shown to exert a positive effect on the development of lymphoid organs and cell-mediated and humoral immune responses in both commercial and non-commercial bird species.

### CLIENT EDUCATION
N/A

### SURGICAL CONSIDERATIONS
Complete surgical removal of thymic masses, such as thymonas, is usually considered curative.

## MEDICATIONS
### DRUG(S) OF CHOICE
Antibiotics based on culture and sensitivity.

### CONTRAINDICATIONS
N/A

### PRECAUTIONS
N/A

### POSSIBLE INTERACTIONS
N/A

### ALTERNATIVE DRUGS
N/A

## FOLLOW-UP
### PATIENT MONITORING
N/A

### PREVENTION/AVOIDANCE
All infectious diseases that affect the thymus have specific virulence and modes of transmissions. Proper hygiene and quarantine are essential in prevention. Some viral diseases have vaccinations (e.g. Marek's disease vaccine).

### POSSIBLE COMPLICATIONS
N/A

### EXPECTED COURSE AND PROGNOSIS
Depends on the course to the disease and the susceptibility of the species. May result in death, recovery, latent infection, or chronic infections.

## MISCELLANEOUS
### ASSOCIATED CONDITIONS
N/A

### AGE-RELATED FACTORS
The thymus regresses as the bird ages.

### ZOONOTIC POTENTIAL
N/A

### FERTILITY/BREEDING
N/A

### SYNONYMS
N/A

### SEE ALSO
Mycobacteriosis
Mycotoxicosis
Neoplasia (Lymphoproliferative)
Nutritional Imbalances
Salmonellosis
Toxicosis (Heavy Metals)
Also individual named viral diseases

### ABBREVIATIONS
GALT—gut-associated lymphoid tissue
IFN—interferon
NK—natural killer
PBFD—psittacine beak and feather disease
PCR—polymerase chain reaction
TLR—Toll-like receptor

### INTERNET RESOURCES
N/A

*Suggested Reading*
Altimeter, K.S., Rakich, P.M., Weis, R. (2001). Thymoma in a finch. *Journal of Avian Medicine and Surgery*, 15:37–39.
Ciriaco, E., Pinera, P.P., Diaz-Esnal, B., Laurà, R. (2003). Age-related changes in the avian primary lymphoid organs (thymus and bursa of Fabricius). *Microscopy Research and Technique*, 62:482–487.
Kendall, M.D. (1980). Avian thymus glands: a review. *Developmental and Comparative Immunolology*, 4:191–209.
Luo, M., Xu, L., Qian, Z., Sun, X. (2021). Infection-associated thymic atrophy. *Frontiers in Immunology*, 12:652538.
Pendl, H., Tizard, I. (2016). Immunology. In: *Current Therapy in Avian Medicine and Surgery*, (ed. B.L. Speer), 400–432. St. Louis, MO: Elsevier.
Schmidt, R.E., Pendl, H. (2013). The avian immune system. In: *Proceedings of the First International Conference on Avian, Herpetological, and Exotic Mammal Medicine*, Wiesbaden, Germany, 11–14.
Umar, S., Munir, M.T., Ahsan, U., et al. (2017). Immunosuppressive interactions of viral diseases in poultry. *World's Poultry Science Journal*, 73:121–135.
Zuvaidy, A.J. (1980). An epithets thymoma in a budgerigar (*Melopsittacus undulates*). *Avian Pathology*, 9:575–581.
**Author:** Rodney W. Schnellbacher DVM, DACZM

T

# THYROID DISEASES

## BASICS

### DEFINITION
The thyroid glands produce thyroxine, which has numerous effects on metabolism. Any disease state of the thyroids is included here, including hypothyroidism, thyroid hyperplasia (goiter), and thyroid neoplasia. Diseases of the thyroid are uncommon in birds. They may include endocrine changes, or the thyroids may enlarge, creating a space-occupying mass which is responsible for the clinical signs.

### PATHOPHYSIOLOGY
Hypothyroidism in pet birds is uncommon enough in the literature that the mechanism responsible for its development is not known. In chickens, humans, and dogs, autoimmune thyroiditis is often responsible for the destruction of the thyroid cells. This has not been documented in other birds. Iodine deficiency can result in thyroid hyperplasia. Without iodine, functional thyroid hormone cannot be produced. This in turn fails to activate the negative feedback to the pituitary and excessive TSH is produced, resulting in hyperplasia of the thyroid glands. The enlarged glands may compress the esophagus and trachea. The etiology of thyroid neoplasia is not known.

### SYSTEMS AFFECTED
GI changes may occur if the coelomic esophagus is compressed by enlarged thyroid glands. Hemic changes may include mild nonregenerative anemia. Respiratory effects of thyroid disease are common. With goiter or thyroid neoplasia, the trachea may be displaced or compressed leading to vocal changes, wheezing, or dyspnea. Skin conditions are the most prominent aspect of hypothyroidism. Poor feather development, delayed molt, excess subcutaneous fat deposition, and hyperkeratosis.

### GENETICS
These conditions are not known to be genetic.

### INCIDENCE/PREVALENCE
Thyroid hyperplasia was once very common in budgerigars. With improved diets, it is now uncommonly seen. It occurs most commonly in macaws and budgerigars. Thyroid neoplasia is an uncommonly encountered tumor in pet birds. There is only a single confirmed report of hypothyroidism in parrots. However, this condition is frequently suspected but not confirmed by appropriate diagnostics.

### GEOGRAPHIC DISTRIBUTION
There appears to be no specific geographic distribution.

### SIGNALMENT
Thyroid diseases can occur in any species. Macaws and budgerigars are predisposed to goiter.

### SIGNS
#### General Comments
Thyroid hyperplasia usually presents as a respiratory or GI problem.

#### Historical Findings
Owners may note skin and feather problems, vocal changes, or breathing abnormalities.

#### Physical Examination Findings
Hypothyroidism is associated with feather hypoplasia, feather loss, and epidermal atrophy. Obesity may be seen in hypothyroid birds. Hypothyroidism may be associated with lipemia, nonregenerative anemia, and hypercholesterolemia. Recurrent skin infections may be encountered in hypothyroid birds. Birds with goiter or thyroid neoplasia may exhibit respiratory wheezes or squeaks, due to the pressure placed on the syrinx. Severe cases may result in overt dyspnea. The thyroid may also compress the coelomic esophagus, resulting in crop stasis.

### CAUSES
The cause of hypothyroidism in pet birds is not usually determined. In chickens, there is a genetically influenced autoimmune thyroiditis that results in hypothyroidism. However, this has not been demonstrated in other birds. Iodine deficiency is usually thought to be the cause of goiter. The ingestion of goitrogenic food items may also contribute. The cause of thyroid neoplasia is not generally determined. It could be speculated that it may result from chronic hyperplasia, but this has not been documented.

### RISK FACTORS
Dietary iodine deficiency is the main risk factor for thyroid hyperplasia. Ingestion of goitrogenic foods such as cruciferous vegetables (kale, Brussels sprouts, mustard greens), soy-based foods, and some fruits can exacerbate the problem by inhibiting iodine metabolism.

## DIAGNOSIS

### DIFFERENTIAL DIAGNOSIS
Hypothyroidism should be distinguished from viral feather diseases such as PBFD and polyomavirus, as well as other skin disorders. Thyroid neoplasia and hyperplasia should be differentiated from respiratory or upper GI disorders as well as other masses in the coelomic inlet.

### CBC/BIOCHEMISTRY/URINALYSIS
Mild anemia, gross lipemia, and hypercholesterolemia may be seen with hypothyroidism.

### OTHER LABORATORY TESTS
Hypothyroidism must be diagnosed using a TSH stimulation test. The thyroxine (T4) level should at least double 4–6 hours after administration of TSH.

### IMAGING
Very large thyroids may be seen radiographically. However, the thyroids are located just inside the coelomic inlet in birds. Definitive diagnosis of thyroid hyperplasia or neoplasia may require advanced imaging such as computed tomography.

### DIAGNOSTIC PROCEDURES
Endoscopy using a coelomic inlet approach will allow visualization of the thyroid. Biopsy techniques should be carefully applied since the thyroids are very closely associated with the vasculature.

### PATHOLOGIC FINDINGS
Gross enlargement of both thyroids may be seen with thyroid hyperplasia. Enlargement of one thyroid occurs with neoplasia. Most are not functional tumors, so atrophy of the contralateral thyroid is not common. Pathology of hypothyroidism may include skin changes such as ortho- and parakeratotic hyperkeratosis of the epidermis and moderate, widespread vacuolar degeneration and necrosis in the follicular epithelium.

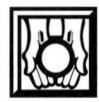

## TREATMENT

### APPROPRIATE HEALTH CARE
Most patients would be treated as outpatients. Exceptions would be severely enlarged thyroids resulting in dyspnea or esophageal compression with nutritional deficits resulting from crop stasis.

### NURSING CARE
Oxygen therapy is indicated for dyspneic patients. Fluid and nutritional support should be provided as needed. A liquid diet may pass through easier than a solid diet in patients with external esophageal compression.

### ACTIVITY
Unless dyspneic, activity levels need not be altered.

### DIET
As many hypothyroid birds are obese, a review of the diet to assure a balanced diet is provided is warranted. Additional caloric restriction may be indicated, but should be carefully monitored during thyroid supplementation to prevent excessive weight

loss. In addition to iodine supplementation, goitrogenic items should be restricted in the diet of birds with thyroid hyperplasia.

## CLIENT EDUCATION
Dietary counseling.

## SURGICAL CONSIDERATIONS
Although not reported, surgical removal of a neoplastic thyroid gland may be possible. The close association of the gland with the carotid artery makes this a very delicate and risky procedure. Access to the site is very restricted as well.

# MEDICATIONS

## DRUG(S) OF CHOICE
Hypothyroidism: Synthetic thyroid hormone is used as replacement therapy in cases of hypothyroidism. A starting dose of 0.2 µg/kg can be used, and then adjusted based on monitoring blood levels. Thyroid hyperplasia: Lugol's iodine solution can be used by making a stock solution of 1 ml per 30 ml water. A single drop (0.05 ml) can be added to 250 ml drinking water. Radioactive iodine therapy could be considered in cases of thyroid neoplasia.

## CONTRAINDICATIONS
None.

## PRECAUTIONS
None.

## POSSIBLE INTERACTIONS
None known.

## ALTERNATIVE DRUGS
There are some commercial supplements containing iodine for birds. These may be used as alternatives to Lugol's iodine.

# FOLLOW-UP

## PATIENT MONITORING
Patients receiving thyroid supplementation should be monitored every 3–6 months. A general examination, hematology, chemistries, and thyroid levels should be evaluated at these visits.

## PREVENTION/AVOIDANCE
Balanced nutrition may prevent thyroid hyperplasia.

## POSSIBLE COMPLICATIONS
Iatrogenic hyperthyroidism could occur with excess supplementation of thyroxine. Dyspnea, weight loss, or regurgitation may occur with very large thyroid glands.

## EXPECTED COURSE AND PROGNOSIS
Hypothyroid birds can be managed long term with supplementation. Birds with goiter generally respond well to therapy. Thyroid neoplasia carries a poor to grave prognosis.

# MISCELLANEOUS

## ASSOCIATED CONDITIONS
None known.

## AGE-RELATED FACTORS
None known.

## ZOONOTIC POTENTIAL
None.

## FERTILITY/BREEDING
Hypothyroidism could affect breeding success, although there are few data supporting this.

## SYNONYMS
N/A

## SEE ALSO
Circoviruses
Feather-Damaging Behavior
Feather Disorders
Neoplasia (Respiratory)
Nutritional Imbalances
Obesity
Polyomavirus
Tracheal and Syringeal Diseases

## ABBREVIATIONS
GI—gastrointestinal
PBFD—psittacine beak and feather disease
TSH—thyroid stimulating hormone

## INTERNET RESOURCES
N/A

*Suggested Reading*
Schmidt, R.E., Reavill, D.R. (2008). The avian thyroid gland. *Veterinary Clinics of North America: Exotic Animal Practice*, 11:15–23.
van Zeeland, Y., Shoemaker, N. (2022). Avian endocrinology. *Proceedings, ExoticsCon 2022*, 84–90.
**Author:** Kenneth R. Welle, DVM, DABVP (Avian)

T

# TOE AND NAIL DISEASES

## BASICS

### DEFINITION
Most birds possess 4 digits with varying number of phalanges (except ratites). Typically, each digit has one more phalanx than the number of the digit: Digit I has 2 phalanges, digit II has 3 phalanges, etc. Digit I, often referred to as the hallux, projects caudally and is rudimentary in ground-dwelling birds. The main action of the digits and nails is flexion and extension. When perching, a bird's tendons are flexed and small sprocket-like projections extend from their tendons and interdigitate to hold them in place. This reduces the energy expenditure for perching. Toes have different configuration depending on the bird species and include anisodactyl (3 toes forward, 1 toe backward, in most perching birds), zygodactyl (2 toes forward, 2 toes backward, as in parrots and woodpeckers), pamprodactyl (all toes facing forward, as in swifts or mousebirds), and syndactyl (fused toes, as in kingfishers and hornbills). Nails are made of keratin and cover the terminal phalanx of each digit. Nails are used for digging, scratching, grooming, perching, climbing, fighting, and grasping prey. In some species such as the barn owl, one nail or claw/talon is modified into a comblike structure known as the pectinate claw. In aquatic species, feet are webbed with various webbing configuration between toes (lobate, palmate, semipalmate).

### PATHOPHYSIOLOGY
Articular gout may develop secondary to hyperuricemia. Accumulation of monosodium urate crystals within the synovial capsule and tendon sheaths results in inflammation. Hypovitaminosis A may lead to skin hyperkeratosis. Hyperviscosity syndrome may be related to pulmonary hypertension secondary to chronic pulmonary interstitial fibrosis, which may lead to right ventricular hypertrophy and failure in many cases. Birds with inadequate cardiac output related to a left ventricle decreased in size or with poor systolic function may also develop pulmonary hypertension and hypoxemia. Atherosclerosis is commonly involved. In these birds, polycythemia develops as a consequence of chronic hypoxemia, creating resistance to blood flow by increasing blood viscosity and rendering erythrocytes larger and less deformable. Leukemia may also lead to hyperviscosity syndrome. Avascular necrosis of digits may occur secondary to circumferential constriction caused by fibres or other foreign material, scabs, necrotic tissue, or inappropriately sized leg band. Older passerines may develop prominent scaling with age, which can lead to a constriction effect by a ring that was previously of adequate size. Avascular necrosis may also occur as sequelae to frostbite. Certain cardiovascular conditions may predispose birds to distal extremity necrosis by causing deficiencies in the peripheral circulation. A constricted toe syndrome, potentially associated with humidity issues, has been described in chicks of certain species, whereby an annular band of fibrous tissue leads to avascular necrosis of a digit. Trauma may lead to various lesions of the toes and nails including wounds, fractures, luxation, tendon ruptures, arthritis, necrosis, thrombosis of peripheral vessels, and toe and nail avulsions and amputations. Self-trauma is also seen in some species of psittacines (quaker mutilation syndrome, Amazon foot necrosis). Infectious agents (e.g. poxvirus) may lead to toe lesions secondarily infected by opportunistic bacteria. Pododermatitis may extend to the digital pads on the plantar surface of the toes.

### SYSTEMS AFFECTED
**Skin/exocrine:** Skin puncture, laceration, abrasion, ulceration, hyperkeratosis or necrosis; proliferative lesions. Breaking, crushing or avulsion of nails.
**Musculoskeletal:** Lameness, abnormal posture, perching issues, visible swellings involving joints, bones or soft tissue, muscle atrophy.
**Cardiovascular:** Change in skin color.
**Neuromuscular:** Altered neuromuscular function of the digits.
**Behavioral:** Change in activity; any disease process altering the function of the digits and nails may impact on bird behavior when perching or moving as well as its capacity to position itself correctly during courtship and mating.
**Gastrointestinal:** Decreased appetite due to discomfort/pain or inability to maneuver to access food and water.

### GENETICS
N/A

### INCIDENCE/PREVALENCE
Unknown. Variable according to the disease condition.

### GEOGRAPHIC DISTRIBUTION
N/A

### SIGNALMENT
No specific species, age, or sex predilection for diseases of toes and nails in general. Degenerative disease—middle-aged to geriatric birds of all species and both sexes. *Knemidocoptes* sp. is most commonly diagnosed in budgerigars (*Melopsittacus undulatus*) and Passeriformes. Papillomatous lesions—papillomaviruses in European finches. Cutaneous papillomas affecting the feet have been described in macaws and cockatoos, and an uncharacterized herpesvirus was suspected. Constricted toe syndrome is seen most commonly in eclectus, macaws, and grey parrots. Amazon foot necrosis—females are more represented than males. Most commonly seen in yellow-napped Amazons (*Amazona auropalliata*) and double yellow-headed Amazons (*Amazona oratrix*), but is also described in conures and quakers (*Myiopsitta monachus*). Hyperviscosity syndrome—older birds, female sex; Amazon parrots, grey parrots, followed by cockatiels, lovebirds, eclectus, cockatoos, and macaws are more commonly affected with atherosclerosis. Traumatic injuries to talons, in particular avulsion, are more common in raptors because of their long talons and use in predation. Tendon ruptures are more common in birds of prey secondary to trauma or prey bites.

### SIGNS
#### General Comments
Severity of clinical signs depends on the location and extent of the lesion.

#### Historical Findings
Contact with other birds (infectious diseases). White/yellow nodules associated with any joint (articular gout). Falling or dysfunction of one foot (kidney or gonadal enlargement). Traumatic event. Exposure to extreme temperature (thermal burns, frostbite). Swelling of one or more digits in one or several chicks within a clutch (constricted toe syndrome). Inability to flex a toe in case of flexor tendon rupture. Obesity, chronic malnutrition (Amazon foot necrosis, hyperviscosity syndrome). Oestrogenic cyclicity prior to the mutilatory behaviors (Amazon foot necrosis). Collapsing, transient or intermittent weakness and dysfunction of one or both feet with or without altered mentation, disorientation, confusion, intermittent extension/rigidity of one or both feet, clenching of digits, difficulty perching, tremors claudication (hyperviscosity syndrome).

#### Physical Examination Findings
Proliferative lesions may be seen with papillomaviruses, poxvirus, *Knemidocoptes* sp., neoplasia. A fine honeycomb-shaped pattern is characteristic of *Knemidocoptes* infection. White/yellow nodular enlargement of any joint or tendon sheaths. Altered skin integrity or skin discoloration—traumatic or thermal injury (frostbite and burn), infectious diseases, constricted toe syndrome, avascular necrosis. An annular constricting band of fibrous tissue at a joint on one or more digits with constricted toe syndrome.

Swelling may be seen distal to the constriction band that prevents venous drainage with constricted toe syndrome; traumatic, metabolic (gout), or infectious processes. Tendon rupture may also lead to swelling at the site of the rupture. Muscular atrophy of the affected limb and asymmetrical wear pattern/pododermatitis on the plantar surface of the contralateral foot. Inability to flex a toe may be evidenced in case of flexor tendon rupture. Flexor muscles may be compressed manually to induce flexion by squeezing the tigh and toes should flex. Toe flexion that does not include the last phalanx is indicative of deep flexor tendon rupture. Distended veins (basilic, jugular, etc.), cardiac arrhythmias, heart murmur, increased breath sounds or crackles on pulmonary auscultation—hyperviscosity syndrome.

## CAUSES
Degenerative—osteoarthritis. Infectious—parasitic (*Knemidocoptes* spp., *Pelecitus* spp.), bacterial, fungal, viral (poxvirus, herpesvirus, papillomavirus), pododermatitis. Metabolic—articular gout may develop secondary to hyperuricemia associated with primary renal disease or causes of prerenal or postrenal origin. Nutritional—hypovitaminosis A, nutritional secondary hyperparathyroidism. Neoplastic—hemangiosarcoma of the metatarsal pad reported in a Java sparrow (*Lonchura oryzivora*), squamous cell carcinoma involving a digit reported in an American flamingo (*Phoenicopterus ruber*); kidney or gonadal tumors may impede innervation to the ipsilateral leg, altering neuromuscular function of the feet. Traumatic—subluxation, luxation, fracture; laceration, constricting or crushing injury; overgrown nails becoming trapped or entangled leading to breaking, crushing or avulsion; thermal injury (burn or frostbite); electrocution; self-mutilation; sprains or strain; pododermatitis. Unknown—constricted toe syndrome is suspected to be related to rearing in an environment with low humidity; Amazon foot necrosis may result from delayed hypersensitivity reaction following staphylococcal dermatitis. Circumstantial evidences suggest this might be a contact dermatitis (nicotine or tobacco smoke, crack-cocaine exposure). The possibility of a hepatocutaneous-like syndrome has also been described. Vascular—hyperviscosity syndrome related to pulmonary or cardiovascular disease (atherosclerosis), avascular necrosis secondary to circumferential constriction, trauma, or complication of constricted toe syndrome. Thrombosis of extremities related to hypercoagulability or systemic infection.

## RISK FACTORS
Obesity may predispose to osteoarthritis and cardiovascular diseases. Frostbite—sudden exposure to low temperatures during the winter months (bird escaping outside) or persistent exposure to low and wet temperature in birds housed outside during the winter months. Hyperuricemia should be considered a risk factor for development of articular gout. Constricted toe syndrome—poor environmental humidity is suspected to play a role in this condition. Amazon foot necrosis—pre-existing hepatic diseases is not uncommon to find, although this is not a clear nor documented predictor. Hyperviscosity syndrome—high-calorie and fat diets, dyslipidemia, limited physical activity are predisposing factors. Environmental factors such as high altitude (reduced oxygen–hemoglobin binding affinity and pulmonary vasoconstriction with hypoxemia) and extreme temperatures (hot, cold), which increase oxygen demands may exacerbate the symptoms.

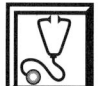

# DIAGNOSIS

## DIFFERENTIAL DIAGNOSIS
Proliferative lesions—herpesvirus, papillomaviruses, poxvirus, *Knemidocoptes* spp., neoplasia. Frostbite—contact dermatitis, pododermatitis, cellulitis, avascular necrosis. Ulcerative lesions—bacterial, fungal or parasitic infection, neoplasia. Articular gout—infectious arthritis, granuloma, cyst. Constricted toe syndrome—constriction by filaments of fibrous material.

## CBC/BIOCHEMISTRY/URINALYSIS
CBC to characterize the inflammation/infection. Biochemistry to evaluate organ function.

## OTHER LABORATORY TESTS
Cytology to evaluate cells, microbial population, the presence of pathogen (such as *Knemidocoptes* sp., poxviral inclusions), urate crystals, inflammatory, and neoplastic lesions. Cytology of joint aspirates may confirm septic arthritis or articular gout. Polarized light will highlight uric acid deposits. Murexide test to confirm the presence of urate crystals. A drop a nitric acid is mixed with a small amount of suspected material on a slid and dried by evaporation in a Bunsen flame. Once the preparation is cooled, a drop of concentrated ammonia is added. In the presence of urates, a mauve color with appear. Bacterial/fungal culture and sensitivity to evaluate microbial population. Histopathological evaluation to evaluate cells and tissue organization/ architecture as well as the presence of infectious organisms. Molecular diagnostic—PCR-based DNA probe for poxvirus.

## IMAGING
Whole-body radiographs to evaluate for orthopedic injury and soft tissue modification (muscle atrophy, swelling); size, contour, and radiodensity of the heart and great vessels; organomegaly (liver, kidney), pulmonary parenchyma, serosal detail. Echocardiography to evaluate heart chambers and great vessels. Computed tomography with contrast administration to evaluate orthopedic injury, vasculature, organomegaly, pulmonary parenchyma. Magnetic resonance imaging to evaluate soft tissue. Thermal imaging—infrared thermography of the toes and feet may highlight inflamed areas of increased heat or thrombotic/necrotic areas of decreased heat.

## DIAGNOSTIC PROCEDURES
Orthopedic and neurological examination when the patient is stable. Sedation and analgesia may be considered for orthopedic evaluation only. Blood pressure measurement is indicated when vascular disease is suspected. Indirect measurement is more practical with a Doppler ultrasonic flow detector placed on the wing or leg (over the superficial ulnar artery or cranial tibial artery, respectively), a cuff measuring 30–40% of the limb circumference, and a sphygmomanometer. Of note, this technique does not allow accurate and repeatable arterial blood pressure measurements in the clinical setting. Electrocardiography can provide information to suggest certain cardiac abnormalities, including chamber enlargement. Must be used with other modalities as severe pathology and mechanical dysfunction can exist in the absence of ECG changes. Arthrocentesis to confirm the presence of urate crystals. Do not fix with alcohol as it will dissolve the uric acid crystals.

## PATHOLOGIC FINDINGS
**Papillomas**: Frondlike projections of hyperplastic epithelium supported by thin, inflamed, fibrovascular stromal stalks. The fibrovascular stroma will have varying infiltrates of plasma cells, lymphocytes, and heterophils. Mitotic activity is primarily in the polygonal basal cells.
**Poxvirus**: Marked epithelial hyperplasia and vacuolar degeneration. Scattered areas of coagulative necrosis may be present. The virus forms eosinophilic intracytoplasmic inclusion bodies (called Bollinger bodies in histological sections and Borrel bodies in impression smears).
**Traumatic injury**: Skin puncture, laceration, tearing with associated injury (bruising, crushing, contusion, oedema, laceration, necrosis) to adjacent tissues.

T

## TOE AND NAIL DISEASES                                    (CONTINUED)

**Frostbite:** Coagulative necrosis with a peripheral inflammatory infiltrate of heterophils and macrophages. Well-defined inflammatory margin between affected and unaffected tissue.

## TREATMENT

### APPROPRIATE HEALTH CARE

Papillomas, minor skin trauma or infection (such as *Knemidocoptes* sp.), nail avulsion. Outpatient medical management is appropriate in most cases.

**Subluxation, luxation, fracture:** Outpatient medical management in most cases. Brief hospitalization may be appropriate for initiation of analgesic therapy and collection of baseline diagnostic data such as radiographs. Orthopedic injury is best treated with external coaptation. Plantar splint is applicable using light casting material. Splint may be reinforced using Steinmann pin, Kirschner wire, thermoplastic or dental acrylic materials. Ball bandage, which involves placing a ball of gauze in the grasp of the bird's foot and immobilizing the toes around the surface of the ball with conforming gauze, tape or other bandage material, may also be considered. Ball bandage are well tolerated in birds of prey. In small passerine species, a splint can be made by cutting a piece of flat material such as x-ray film to the shape of the foot. The plantar surface of the foot is placed on the splint and the digits are secured with tape. Regardless of the technique chosen, it is important to immobilize the joints proximal and distal to the injury. Because of the large flexor tendons of birds of prey, it may provide sufficient stability to closed digital fracture in some instances without the need to bandage. Applying bandages or bangaging for extended period of time to immobilize some phalangeal fractures in raptors may lead to the boney callous enclosing the flexor tendons and restricting flexion in the future.

**Frostbite, thermal burn, major trauma, hyperviscosity syndrome, articular gout:** Inpatient medical management. For cases of articular gout, surgery to remove the uric acid crystal deposits will not be feasible in most cases. This condition is severely painful and the primary cause should be determined. Likewise, hyperviscosity syndrome requires in depth medical investigations.

**Avascular necrosis:** Outpatient medical management is indicated as long as there is not a clear definition between healthy and necrotic tissue. Constricting fibers may be removed with a bent 25- to 30-gauge needle under magnification. The tip can be used to elevate the fiber, which can then be cut by gently rolling the needle such that the beveled edge severs the fiber. A hydroactive dressing should be placed to protect the injured tissues to prevent desiccation and the formation of a constricting scab. Scabs should be monitored and debrided or incised to prevent further vascular compromise prior to application of a hydroactive dressing.

**Constricted toe syndrome:** Outpatient surgical management (see surgical considerations) is preferred for neonatal patients. If needed, the patient may be briefly hospitalized.

### NURSING CARE

**Wound management, cleansing and staged debridement:** Lesions must be managed as part of the overall patient assessment. All wounds should be flushed copiously to mechanically dislodge non-viable tissue and bacteria from the wound surface. Topical antiseptic or sterile saline may be used. Clotting powder may be beneficial to control bleeding following nail avulsion. Consider sedation and analgesia. If debris or necrotic tissues persist within the wound after wound cleansing, staged debridement is indicated. Consider local anesthetic, sedation, or anesthesia to minimize stress and to have optimal control of hemostasis and tissue handling.

**Hydrotherapy:** Consider to increase blood flow to traumatic wound or frostbite and decrease inflammation. Water temperature should be warm (98–102°F/37–39°C). Bandage must be adapted to the exact nature of the wound, its location, the patient, and its functional needs. Temporary bandaging indicated if patient requires medical stabilization until more thorough wound treatment can be performed. Application of few layers of flexible collodion to the nail bed may be considered to serve as a barrier to water and infection instead of a bandage.

**Fluid therapy:** May be provided SQ in birds exhibiting mild dehydration (5–7%) or IO/IV in birds with moderate to severe dehydration (> 7%) or critically ill birds exhibiting signs consistent with shock. Fluid therapy is indicated if articular gout is present, especially in the presence of hyperuricemia. Avian daily maintenance fluid requirements are 50 ml/kg. Typically, maintenance plus half the fluid deficit is administered during the first 12 hours, with the remainder of the deficit replaced over the following 24–48 hours. In most patients, lactated Ringer's solution or Normosol®-R (Hospira, Inc., Lake Forest, IL) crystalloid fluids are appropriate. For birds with hypotensive shock, a colloidal solution may be administered concurrently with crystalloids. Blood transfusion should be considered with severe blood loss.

**Oxygen therapy:** Indicated if anemia is present; beneficial for any sick avian patient. All methods of oxygen supplementation require humidification if used for more than a few hours.

**Other:** Warmth (85–90°F/27–30°C) to minimize energy spent to maintain body temperature. Nutritional support with assisted feeding is indicated in an anorectic patient or if weight loss superior to 5% body weight is documented. Elizabethan collar should be reserved for birds that insist on self-traumatizing their feet or nails. Physical therapy indicated if the healing process may alter the range of motion of any joint; to begin in the maturation phase to avoid delayed healing process.

### ACTIVITY

Cage adaptation to prevent falling, facilitate access to food and water (multiple stations, ramp for access), and improve feet comfort (padded perch or plateform, padded substrate). Plastic, plexiglass, or glass enclosures may be more appropriate with horizontal space preferred over vertical space. Cage rest following orthopedic or soft-tissue injury to allow appropriate healing. Exercise restriction, minimization of stress with judicious, limited handling, and restraint should be part of the longer-term management plan for hyperviscosity syndrome.

### DIET

Dietary modification—conversion to a lower-calorie or fat diet to minimize fat stores, especially in obese patient (hyperviscosity syndrome, Amazon foot necrosis, osteoarthritis); conversion to a diet restricted in proteins (purines) may slow down the progression of articular gout, although this has not been objectively evaluated in birds.

### CLIENT EDUCATION

Frostbite, constricted toe syndrome, thermal burn, electrocution—educate owners on proper housing requirements. Appropriate housing modifications to accommodate and protect the birds with persistent deficits. Maintain proper nail length to reduce the risk of entanglement while maintaining adequate grip. Operant learning methods should be employed to facilitate low-stress medication administration when long-term medication is required. Weight monitoring is indicated if modifications have been made to the cage, a bandage has been placed or if the bird is wearing an Elizabethan collar. Bandages and splints must be kept dry and clean. Daily assessment is required to minimize complications.

### SURGICAL CONSIDERATIONS

Surgical fixation of fracture with intramedullary pins, external fixators, and/or plates may be necessary in larger bird species.

It should be determined whether surgical fixation is the best treatment strategy for some digital fractures, as cage rest and/or bandages may be enough. Amputation should be considered in severe trauma to the digits and asvascular necrosis, but only after medical management has failed. Flexor tendon ruptures have to be surgically repaired once infection is resolved, if present. Surgery should be delayed for 3–4 weeks with tendon immobilization. The tendon will develop a highly vascular adhesion to the tendon sheath during that time. Then the skin and tendon sheath should be opened and the tendon ends mildly debrided taking care to dissect and preserve a vascularized pedicle from the adhesion to the tendon sheath that developed post-rupture. The tendon ends are then joined using a Kessler's knot for tendon repair. The tendon sheath and skin are closed routinely. For deep flexor tendon avulsion from the terminal phalanx, the tendon end should be split in half and attached on either side of the distal phalanx boney prominence using a suture passed through a hole drilled within the prominence using a hypodermic needle. A ball bandage is then applied to immobilize all toes for 3–4 weeks. Articular gout—in rare instances, urate tophi may be surgically removed to improve the patient's comfort. Constricted toe syndrome—the affected digit should be surgically prepared. Then, with an 11-scalpel blade or edge of a hypodermic needle, four longitudinal incisions in respect to the digit alignment should be performed at 90, 180, 270 and 360 degrees, avoiding the lateral veins and arteries. The digit(s) should then be protected with a light bandage. A hydrocolloidal dressing is preferred as the first bandage layer.

## MEDICATIONS

### DRUG(S) OF CHOICE
Medication will differ depending upon the underlying cause of digit or nail disease. Peroperative antibiotics should be provided for infected lesions and during surgical procedures, as appropriate. Analgesic therapy (butorphanol 1–4 mg/kg IM q2–4h in Galliformes, Psittaciformes, Passeriformes; buprenorphine or hydromorphone 0.1–0.6 mg/kg IM q3–6h in birds of prey, tramadol 30 mg/kg PO q8–12h in Psittaciformes, 7.5 mg/kg PO q12–24h in Galliformes, 5–10 mg/kg PO q4–12h in birds of prey, depending on the species) is indicated to alleviate pain. NSAIDs (meloxicam 0.5–1.0 mg/kg PO/SQ q12–24h) are indicated postoperatively for constricted toe syndrome, traumatic injuries and with any painful condition. Adverse

effects in light of the patient's overall condition need to be considered (contraindication in cases of articular gout or renal disease). GABA analogue (gabapentin 11–15 mg/kg q8–12h) to treat neuropathic pain. Peripheral vasodilator (isoxsuprine 10 mg/kg PO q12–24h) to manage edema in cases of frostbite and to improve peripheral circulation in cases of hyperviscosity syndrome. Improve peripheral perfusion (pentoxifylline 15–25 mg/kg PO q8–12h) through promoting passage of erythrocytes in damaged microvasculature by increasing their flexibility in cases of hyperviscosity syndrome or frostbite. Reduce urid acid production. Allopurinol (10–30 mg/kg PO q12–24h) is a competitive xanthine oxidase inhibitor that prevents the conversion of xanthine into urid acid in some species. In birds of prey, pigeons and grey parrots, its use has actually been associated with increased uric acid concentration. Colchicine (0.01–0.04 mg/kg q24h, then progressively increased to q12h) reversibly inhibits xanthine dehydrogenase and has been used anecdotally in some species. Of note, none of these medications will decrease monosodium urate crystals already deposited in the joints and tendon sheaths. Their use may not be beneficial or worsen the bird's status. Rasburicase 0.5–mg/kg IM is a recombinant urate-oxidase (from *Sacharomyces cerevisae*); it shows promise in lowering uric acid levels in psittacines. Control reproductive activity (leuprolide acetate 800 µg/kg IM q2–3w, 4.7 mg deslorelin acetate implant SQ interscapulary) of females with hyperviscosity syndrome. Improve lipid metabolism, reduce inflammation, and minimize the development of atherosclerosis with omega 3 fatty acids (0.1–0.2 ml/kg of flaxseed oil to corn oil mixed at a ratio of 1:4 PO or added to food) with hyperviscosity syndrome. Antiparasitic agent (ivermectin 200 µg/kg topically over right jugular or PO (repeat in 3–4 weeks); selamectin 23 mg/kg topically, repeat in 3–4 weeks) for *Knemidocoptes* sp. infection. Propylene glycol may be used to dilute ivermectin. All in-contact birds must be treated as subclinical carriers are documented. Vitamin A is indicated if hypovitaminosis A is suspected in addition to dietary modifications (1000–20,000 iu/bird IM once or PO q12h).

### CONTRAINDICATIONS
NSAIDs in clinical cases where articular gout or renal disease has been diagnosed.

### PRECAUTIONS
Fluid deficits should be addressed prior to using NSAIDs. Parenteral fluid administration must be carefully considered

in case of hyperviscosity syndrome since this may reflect severe cardiovascular disease.

### POSSIBLE INTERACTIONS
When gabapentin and tramadol are used simultaneously, lower dosage should be used to prevent sedative effect.

### ALTERNATIVE DRUGS
None.

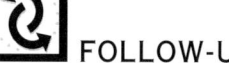

## FOLLOW-UP

### PATIENT MONITORING
Varies with the type and severity of injuries/disease and the patient's status. Monitoring for renal dysfunction or gastrointestinal disturbances are indicated with long-term administration of NSAIDs q3–4m. Any bird with a persistent support deficit due to its condition or damage will benefit from a bi- or triannual follow-up to ensure early prevention and control of possible pododermatitis. Monitoring of ischemic and inflammatory lesions may be performed with infrared thermography.

### PREVENTION/AVOIDANCE
Quarantine new birds to prevent infectious diseases. Control mosquito to prevent dissemination of poxvirus. Exposure to cold temperature and hot liquid/appliances must be mitigated in such way that the bird can't suffer from thermal injury. Cage furniture must be carefully evaluated to prevent injury. Leg band removal to prevent avascular necrosis from circumferential compression. Constricted toe syndrome—The rearing environment humidity should be increased in an attempt to prevent reoccurrence with subsequent chicks.

### POSSIBLE COMPLICATIONS
Open fracture and severely contaminated or traumatized lesions are at higher risk of bacterial contamination and osteomyelitis. Malunion or non-union can occur with suboptimal reduction of a fracture. Disruption of damaged tissues, dressing or bandage materials—some birds may focus their attention on the injured tissue site/dressing/bandage materials. Decreased mobility may occur with external coaptation, fracture misalignment or during the maturation process of healing. Hyperviscosity syndrome may be a consequence of severe pulmonary or cardiovascular disease. Therefore, congestive heart failure and death may occur. Vascular compromise and peripheral neuropathy are possible complications due to the paucity of soft tissue of the feet. Pododermatitis may develop on the contralateral leg if only one foot is affected by a pathological process. Tendon infection, rupture, or decrease in function may occur.

# TOE AND NAIL DISEASES

## EXPECTED COURSE AND PROGNOSIS
Varies with the severity of injuries and their cause. Nerve and vascular damage—poor prognosis for healing and return to function when the extremities are involved. Prognosis is guarded for articular gout and hyperviscosity syndrome. Excellent for most nail avulsion as the sheath will regrow normally or almost normally. Well-aligned, properly reduced fractures will have sufficient endosteal callus to be stabilized at 3 weeks, with complete healing occurring within 6 weeks.

 **MISCELLANEOUS**

## ASSOCIATED CONDITIONS
Articular gout may occur concurrently with visceral gout. Renal disease may or may not be involved. Hyperviscosity syndrome may be associated with atherosclerosis, cardiomyopathy, congestive heart failures, pulmonary and/or systemic hypertension, as well as pulmonary diseases. Neurologic deficit affecting a single foot may be associated with a coelomic mass involving the kidney or gonad.

## AGE-RELATED FACTORS
See Signalment section.

## ZOONOTIC POTENTIAL
None.

## FERTILITY/BREEDING
Bird with persistent anatomic anomaly or mobility deficit may be unable to copulate successfully.

## SYNONYMS
Osteoarthritis and degenerative joint disease are used interchangeably. Nail, claw, talon.

## SEE ALSO
Arthritis
Atherosclerosis
Congestive Heart Failure
Cere and Skin Color Changes
Dermatitis
Dyslipidemia/Hyperlipidemia
Ectoparasites (Mites)
Ectoparasites (Ticks, Lice, Dipterans)
Electrocution
Fractures
Herpesvirus (Psittacid Herpesviruses)
Hyperuricemia
Joint Diseases
Liver Disease
Luxations
Metabolic Bone Disease
Myocardial Diseases
Neoplasia (Integument)
Neoplasia (Lymphoproliferative)
Nutritional Imbalances
Obesity
Papillomatosis (Cutaneous)
Pneumonia
Pododermatitis
Poxvirus
Renal Diseases
Tendinitis and Tenosynovitis
Wounds (Including Bite Wounds, Predator Attacks)

## ABBREVIATIONS
GABA—gamma-aminobutyric acid
NSAIDs—non-steroidal anti-inflammatory drugs

## INTERNET RESOURCES
Higbie, C. (2017). External Coaptation in Birds: Bandages and Splints. *LafeberVet*: https://lafeber.com/vet/external-coaptation-birds-bandages-splints
Pollock, C. (2007). Band removal in birds. *LafeberVet*: https://lafeber.com/vet/band-removal

*Suggested Reading*
Calle, P.P., Montali, R.J., Janssen, D.L., et al. (1982). Distal extremity necrosis in captive birds. *Journal of Wildlife Disease*, Oct;18(4):473–9. https://doi:10.7589/0090-3558-18.4.473
Montesinos, A., Ardiaca, M., Bonvehi, C., et al. (2022). Effects of treatment with allopurinol and rasburicase on plasma uric acid levels of African grey parrots (*Psittacus erithacus*). *Proceedings of the 5th Virtual International Conference of Avian, Herpetological and Exotic Mammal Medicine*, 2022, 131.
Martel-Arquette, A., Mans, C., Sladky, K. (2016). Management of severe frostbite in a grey-headed parrot (*Poicephalus fuscicollis suahelicus*). *Journal of Avian Medicine and Surgery*, 30:39–45.
Harcourt-Brown NH. (2000). Tendon repair in the pelvic limb of birds of prey. Part II. Surgical techniques. In: *Raptor Biomedicine III* (ed. J.T. Lumeij, D. Remple, P.T. Redig et al.), 217–238. Lake Worth, FL: Zoological Education Network.

**Author**: Isabelle Langlois, DMV, DABVP (Avian)

# BASICS

## DEFINITION
Nutritional, infectious, and traumatic diseases most commonly affect the avian tongue. This highly diverse organ can be used for collecting, manipulating, and swallowing food, depending on the species. The tongue of finches, canaries, and other passerine birds is long, slender, flat, and cornified. Psittacine birds have a thick, round, and muscular tongue. The tongue of lories and lorikeets is densely covered with fimbria that evert when the tongue is protruded. These fimbriae are used to gather pollen and nectar. Piscivores and carnivores possess a non-protrusible tongue with rasp-like surface composed of keratinized papillae. The tongue is used to filter food particles from water in some aquatic bird species, such as flamingos and ducks. The tongue is rudimentary in species that swallow whole prey, like the pelican. The tongue can be very long in some species like woodpeckers, with the hyobranchial apparatus wrapping around the brain case.

## PATHOPHYSIOLOGY
Hypovitaminosis A can lead to squamous metaplasia of the epithelial lining of the small compound tubular mandibular or lingual salivary glands. The small mucus glands in the oral cavity fill with keratin and expand to form submucosal nodules containing yellow-white and friable material. These lesions may become secondarily infected, leading to the development of abscesses. Bird tongues are filled with tactile sensory corpuscles, especially at the tip. These corpuscles are best developed in the spoon-tipped tongues of the seed-eating songbirds and in the strong club-shaped muscular tongue of parrots. The tongue plays a crucial role in the three stages of swallowing: (1) The tongue moves the food pellets to the palate where it is held by mucous secretions while the choanal opening is reflexively closed. (2) The tongue rakes the bolus caudally in a rostral–caudal movement, while the infundibular cleft and glottis are reflexively closed. (3) The laryngeal mound carries the food bolus towards the esophagus in a rostral-caudal movement. Consequently, any disease processes involving the tongue may hinder the bird's capacity to prehend and consume food items. Submandibular lingual entrapment is hypothesized to be secondary to unsuitable forage that forms a sublingual ball of grass or other food materials. When not dislodged, food and debris will continue to accumulate, leading to stretching of the intermandibular skin. In extreme or chronic cases, this may cause the tongue to slip ventrally, with the incapacity for the bird to reposition its tongue. Tongue entrapment may also occur with string foreign bodies such as fishing lines in aquatic bird species. Infectious agents affecting the mouth typically also spread to glossal tissue.

## SYSTEMS AFFECTED
**GI**: The tongue is situated within the oral cavity as a component of the digestive system.
**Behavioral**: Disease processes may prevent the bird from exhibiting normal behaviour or may lead to development of abnormal behaviour (continuous tongue movement may be a sign of discomfort).
**Musculoskeletal**: The tongue is supported by the hyobranchial apparatus, which consists of a rostral rod, the entoglossal bone, and a caudal rod, the rostral basibranchial bone. Psittacines are unique in having paired entoglossal hyoid bones. They also have intrinsic muscles in the anterior regions of their tongues, independent of the hyobranchial apparatus that adds flexibility. Any injury to the hyobranchial apparatus may result in abnormal tongue movement/mobility.
**Nervous**: Neurological diseases may lead to tongue paresis or paralysis through the hypoglossal nerve (XII).

## GENETICS
None.

## INCIDENCE/PREVALENCE
Unknown. Variable according to the disease's origin. Vitamin A deficiency is becoming less common in caged birds with the development and use of pelleted diets. Goose parvovirus is an important cause of oral lesions in goose farming countries in Asia and Europe.

## GEOGRAPHIC DISTRIBUTION
N/A

## SIGNALMENT
No specific species, age or sex predilection for tongue diseases in general. Trichomoniasis is most common in Columbiformes, some wild passerines, and free-ranging ornithophagous raptors such as northern goshawk and falcons feeding on pigeons. Handraised psittacines and nectarivous birds such as hummingbirds are susceptible to tongue candidiasis. Oral papillomatosis is most common in New World psittacines (macaws, conures, Amazon parrots and hawk-headed parrots). Goose parvovirus is a highly contagious and fatal disease of gosling and Muscovy ducks. *Clinostomum complanatum* is a pathogen causing few clinical signs in pelicans but severe debilitation in related species (herons and egrets) with acute inflammation of the submucosa. Granular cell tumors are reported to arise from the tongue of psittacines (Amazon parrots, cockatiels).

## SIGNS

### Historical Findings
Suboptimal diet, nodular lesions around or under the tongue, bleeding from the tongue, mass and/or ulceration of the tongue, laceration, tongue discoloration.

### Physical Examination Findings
Hypovitaminosis A, trichomoniasis, candidiasis—whitish, well-circumscribed, nodular lesion or plaques. Neoplastic, infectious—mucosal proliferation and/or formation of masses that may be partially necrotic. Grossly, the oral mucosa may be ulcerated and covered with caseous debris. Extensive destruction of oral structures with severe neoplastic process. Trauma, acute viral infection with polyomavirus or Psittacid herpesviruses (PsHV)—abrasion, laceration, ulceration, with variable hemorrhage (often overlooked due to the severity of the systemic disease process with viral infections). Papillomatosis—white to pink, raised, focal or locally extensive cauliflower-like lesions are most commonly found at the base of the tongue. They may also be found along the margins of the choanal fissure and the glottis.

## CAUSES
**Nutritional**: Hypovitaminosis A, feeding of dry mashes of fine physical consistency during the first few weeks after hatching may lead to the so-called syndrome "curled tongue". Niacin nutritional deficiency can result in sloughing of the distal aspect of a young chick's tongue (black tongue). Unsuitable forage may lead to submandibular lingual entrapment in herbivorous Australian waterfowl and flamingos, among others.
**Neoplastic**: Epithelial (papillomatosis, squamous cell carcinoma, salivary gland carcinoma) or mesenchymal (fibroma, fibrosarcoma, lymphosarcoma) origin, granular cell tumors.
**Infectious**: Parasites (*Trichomonas* spp., *Capillaria* sp., *Clinostomum complanatum*, *Contracaecum* sp.), virus (poxvirus, columbid herpesvirus 1, goose parvovirus or Derzsy's disease or goose hepatitis, polyomavirus, gallid alphaherpesvirus 2, Marek's disease virus, (PsHV-1, -2, and -3, poxvirus), bacteria (Gram-negative bacteria, *Mycobacterium* spp.), fungi (*Candida* sp.).
**Traumatic**: Self-inflicted trauma with toys or other object, intraspecific or interspecific aggression, foreign body (hooks, parts of toys, ingested bones, seed fragments, string foreign body—most common in pigeons and doves), chemical (silver nitrate sticks) or thermal (overheated foods) burns, electrocution. Fishing line may lead to tongue entrapment and lesions.
**Toxic**: Plants containing oxalate crystals may lead to swelling/oedema of oral mucous membranes. Protoanemonin and phorbol

**T**

ester may lead to GI irritation. Cationic detergents can cause tissue necrosis and inflammation of the mouth, tongue, pharynx, and oesophagus. In Galliformes, ingestion of trichothecenes (T-2) toxin produced by *Fusarium* spp. can cause caustic injury to the GI mucosa.

### RISK FACTORS
Nutritional deficiencies (vitamin A, niacin) and inadequate diet (fine dry mashes fed to juveniles, unsuitable forage in Anseriformes) may predispose to tongue diseases. Hand feeding, feeding spoiled, stale or sour foods may predispose to candidiasis. Feeding raptors freshly killed pigeons and doves may predispose to trichomoniasis as they are often inapparent carriers of *Trichomonas* spp. Environmental factors—exposure to toxic or traumatic items; lack of hygiene may predispose to secondary infection. Immunosuppresion may predispose to oral candidiasis.

## DIAGNOSIS

### DIFFERENTIAL DIAGNOSIS
See Causes section.

### CBC/BIOCHEMISTRY/URINALYSIS
CBC to identify evidence of inflammation/infection. Biochemistry to evaluate organ function.

### OTHER LABORATORY TESTS
Serum protein electrophoresis—to identify and characterize inflammation. Specific pathogen testing—to determine for *Mycobacterium* sp., polyomavirus, herpes virus. Sensitivity and specificity vary depending on testing modalities and which pathogen is targeted.

### IMAGING
Skull radiographs or CT to evaluate for orthopedic injury and to characterize the extent of the lesion.

### DIAGNOSTIC PROCEDURES
Cytology to evaluate cells and microbial population. Hypovitaminosis A is characterized by sheets or aggregates of cornified squamous epithelial cells with little background debris unless secondary infection is present. Inflammatory cells and increased numbers of yeast (> 1/hpf) is diagnostic for a candida infection. Wet-mount preparations have proven to be a more sensitive and specific means for diagnosis of trichomoniasis. Bacterial/fungal C/S to evaluate microbial population. Histopathological evaluation to evaluate cells and tissue organization/architecture.

### PATHOLOGIC FINDINGS
See Signs section. Variable, depending on the origin of lingual disease. Hypovitaminosis A—squamous metaplasia of oral glands with subsequent hyperkeratosis. Secondary bacterial infections leading to necrosis and an inflammatory infiltrate that is primarily heterophilic may be seen. Columbid herpesvirus 1—ulcerations and diphteric plaques on the oropharynx, cere, rictus, and/or trachea as part of systemic infection. Intranuclear inclusion bodies in epithelial cells adjacent to the necrotic foci. Goose parvovirus—fibrinous material on the tongue, pericarditis, pulmonary edema, liver dystrophy, catarrhal enteritis. Polyomavirus—oral hemorrhage and necrosis with karyomegalic nuclei and intranuclear inclusion bodies in epithelial and endothelial cells. Bacterial infection—acute infections are hemorrhagic whereas chronic infections will lead to granuloma formation. Histologically, there is necrosis and an infiltrate of heterophils, macrophages, and plasma cells. Organisms may be seen but special stains are generally required. Candidiasis—histologically, numerous organisms are present in the mucosa and keratin. There may be excessive keratinization. Inflammation is variable and primarily comprises lymphocytes, plasma cells, and macrophages. Trichomoniasis—histologically, the mucosa may be moderately proliferative with some superficial necrosis. Macrophages and plasma cells are the predominant inflammatory responses, except when organisms invade tissue (marked heterophilic response). Trichomonads must be distinguished from large pleomorphic macrophages. They stain readily with silver stains. Capillariasis—inflammation with hemorrhage may be seen. Histologically, nematodes fragments are found in the mucosa. Sometimes an incidental finding. Papillomatosis—highly vascular connective tissue core covered by a proliferative mucosal epithelium. Lymphoplasmacytic infiltration into the connective tissue core is a variable feature of this disease.

## TREATMENT

### APPROPRIATE HEALTH CARE
Outpatient medical management—stable patient with minor wounds that can be closed primarily or do not require closure. Stable patient with hypovitaminosis A. Inpatient medical management—patient with acute wounds for which delayed primary closure and/or assisted feeding is required. Emergency inpatient intensive care management—patient with severe wounds requiring immediate assessment of the "ABCs" (airway, breathing, and circulation); patient with hemorrhagic wounds requiring immediate intervention to stop blood loss and prevent hypotensive shock; patient with chronic lesion reaching the point of decompensation. Surgical management once patient is stable—patient with wounds requiring primary closure, delayed primary closure or secondary closure; patient requiring biopsy of the lesion or correction of a intermandibular sublingual entrapment.

### NURSING CARE
Oxygen therapy is indicated for all cases with a history of blood loss, respiratory impairment or lethargy. Ideal method of oxygen delivery is within a cage. Humidification is required if oxygen supplementation is performed for more than a few hours. Humidification is achieved by bubbling the oxygen through a container with sterile saline or distilled water. Fluid therapy may be provided SQ in birds exhibiting mild dehydration (5–7%) or IO/IV in birds with moderate to severe dehydration (> 7%), or critically ill birds exhibiting signs consistent with shock. Avian daily maintenance fluid requirements are 50 ml/kg. In most patients, lactated Ringer's solution or Normosol® (Hospira, Inc., Lake Forest, IL) crystalloid fluids are appropriate. Warmth (85–90°F/27–30°C) to minimize energy spent to maintain body temperature. All wound management needs to be done as part of the overall patient assessment.

### ACTIVITY
Patient's activity should be altered according to the patient's general status and the origin of tongue disease. Feeding activities should be adapted to the patient's condition.

### DIET
Assisted feeding may be required for a patient unable to prehend or swallow food. Enteral nutritional preparations may be administered initially at 20–30 ml/kg directly in the crop and the volume administered may be progressively increased according to patient tolerance with the goal to meet the patient's anticipated energy requirements during the healing process. Oesophagosomy tube may be considered if long-term assisted feeding is deemed to be required to allow healing of the tongue. Diet may need to be altered to softer and smaller items to facilitate prehension, mastication, and swallowing.

### CLIENT EDUCATION
Keys to treatment success are in large part dependent on the cause of the tongue lesions and their severity, and the ultimate probability of the bird regaining ability to feed on its own. Many birds, but not all, will adapt and progressively learn to feed on their own. The ability of the bird to eat and drink on its own is necessary prior to outpatient management.

### SURGICAL CONSIDERATIONS
Salivary gland impaction/abscess—lancing and curetting abscesses involving the tongue may be indicated to restore tongue function, enhance healing and relieve discomfort associated with the lesion(s). Care should be

T

exercised not to injure any of the vital structures of the tongue. Laceration of the tongue (mainly in psittacine birds)—a simple interrupted suture using 5-0 to 6-0 absorbable suture material may be performed after careful debridement of the epithelial margins. It is crucial to conserve as much tissue as possible after severe trauma. Glossal tissue tends to bleed a lot. Gular/subglossal impaction may need to be surgically approached by incising ventrally between the mandibular rami.

## MEDICATIONS
### DRUG(S) OF CHOICE
Medication will differ depending upon the underlying cause of tongue disease. Antiparasitic therapy to treat nematodes. Antibiotic therapy to treat primary and secondary bacterial infection which may be associated with the disease condition. Antibiotic selection should be based on C/S. Antifungal therapy to treat fungal disease. Antifungal selection varies with the causative agent and should be based on culture. Vitamin A is indicated if hypovitaminosis A is suspected in addition to dietary modifications (1000–20,000 iu/bird IM once or PO q12h). Analgesic therapy: Butorphanol 1–4 mg/kg q2–4h in Galliformes, Psittaciformes, Passeriformes; buprenorphine or hydromorphone in birds of prey; tramadol 30 mg/kg q8–12h in Psittaciformes, 7.5 mg/kg q12–24h in Galliformes, 5–10 mg/kg q4–12h in birds of prey, depending on the species, is indicated to alleviate pain. NSAIDs (meloxicam 0.5–1.0 mg/kg PO/SQ q12–24h) indicated in most cases of ulcerated, infected, extensive lesions. Adverse effects in light of the patient's overall condition need to be considered.

### CONTRAINDICATIONS
None.

### PRECAUTIONS
Fluid deficits should be addressed prior to using NSAIDs. Chemotherapeutic agent—if neoplastic disease is confirmed, apply biosecurity measures for chemotherapy.

### POSSIBLE INTERACTIONS
Interactions are described for many chemotherapeutic agents. Carefully review possible interactions prior to initiating any chemotherapy.

### ALTERNATIVE DRUGS
N/A

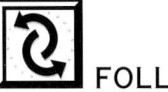

## FOLLOW-UP
### PATIENT MONITORING
Varies with the severity of disease and patient's general status. Critical assessment of the patient's comfort level on a daily basis for inpatients. Biweekly to weekly re-evaluation to monitor form and function, and to monitor the healing process.

### PREVENTION/AVOIDANCE
Ensure appropriate nutrition for the species. Maintain proper hygiene and apply biosecurity measures to prevent infections. Household dangers must be mitigated in such way that the bird cannot get injured. Birds should never be left unsupervised in the presence of a predator species. Only indirect contact with predators should be permitted. Only indirect contact between birds not tolerating each other should be permitted. Do not allow a bird to land on another bird's cage.

### POSSIBLE COMPLICATIONS
In acute injury, anorexia without proper nutritional support may lead to starvation and death; severe hemorrhage may lead to anemia, exsanguination, blood aspiration, asphyxiation, and death. Inability to eat a normal diet for the species once the healing process is completed; pellet size and texture may need to be adjusted permanently, or the bird may need to be offered hand-feeding formula. Permanent loss of the bird's ability to eat on its own.

### EXPECTED COURSE AND PROGNOSIS
Varies according to the origin of lingual disease. Minor laceration involving the distal third of the tongue are typically associated with a fair prognosis. Neoplasia involving the tongue carries a guarded prognosis. Bacterial, parasitic, and fungal diseases treated early in the course of the disease carry a better prognosis.

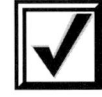

## MISCELLANEOUS
### ASSOCIATED CONDITIONS
None.

### AGE-RELATED FACTORS
"Clubbed tongue" and "black tongue" secondary to nutritional deficiencies are seen in chicks. Juvenile birds are more susceptible

to candidiasis. Neoplastic disease is more frequent in older birds.

### ZOONOTIC POTENTIAL
None.

### FERTILITY/BREEDING
N/A

### SYNONYMS
Glossitis for any tongue-related inflammatory processes.

### SEE ALSO
Candidiasis
Electrocution
Helminthiasis (Gastrointestinal)
Herpesvirus (Psittacid Herpesviruses)
Neoplasia (Gastrointestinal and Hepatic)
Oral Plaques
Polyomavirus
Poxvirus
Trichomoniasis
Wounds (Including Bite Wounds, Predator Attacks)

### ABBREVIATIONS
C/S—culture and sensitivity
CT—computed tomography
GI—gastrointestinal
hpf—high power field
NSAIDs—non-steroidal anti-inflammatory drugs
PsHV—Psittacid herpesvirus

### INTERNET RESOURCES
Schmidt, R.E., Reavill, D.R. (2003). *A Practitioner's Guide to Avian Necropsy.* VetBooks: https://vetbooks.ir/a-practitioners-guide-to-avian-necropsy-cd

*Suggested Reading*
Anderson, N.L. (1997). Recurrent deep foreign body granuloma in the tongue of an african grey parrot (*Psittacus erithacus timneh*). *Journal of Avian Medicine and Surgery*, 11:105–109.
Grosset, C., Guzman, D.S.M., Waymire, A., et al. (2013). Extraoral surgical correction of lingual entrapment in a Chinese goose (*Anser cygnoides*). *Journal of Avian Medicine and Surgery*, 27:301–308.
Schmidt, R.E., Reavill, D.R., Phalen, D.N. (2015). Gastrointestinal system and pancreas. *Pathology of Pet and Aviary Birds*, 2nd edn. (ed. R.E. Schmidt, D.R. Reavill, D.N. Phalen), 55–94. Ames, IA: Wiley.
**Author**: Isabelle Langlois, DMV, DABVP (Avian)

T

# TOXICOSIS (AIRBORNE)

## BASICS

### DEFINITION
Airborne toxins are defined as particles or chemicals that are inspired and cause damage to various tissues of the body.

### PATHOPHYSIOLOGY
The avian respiratory tract is particularly sensitive to airborne toxins because of specific anatomic and physiologic features that allow them to absorb oxygen more efficiently than can mammals. These include a crosscurrent flow of air and blood that allows the potential for blood oxygen levels to be higher than the oxygen levels in the expired breath. With this ability also comes the risk of absorbing higher amounts of toxins from the air, causing them to reach toxic levels sooner than would mammals.

### SYSTEMS AFFECTED
Respiratory system—direct exposure to the toxin. Nervous system—secondary to hypoxia. Cardiovascular system—secondary to a compromised respiratory system. Ocular and upper gastrointestinal—inflammation and irritation.

### GENETICS
N/A

### INCIDENCE/PREVALENCE
N/A

### GEOGRAPHIC DISTRIBUTION
N/A

### SIGNALMENT
No sex or age predilections have been described. PTFE—smaller birds like budgerigars may be more susceptible than larger birds. COPD (hypersensitivity syndrome)—macaws are more susceptible than other species.

### SIGNS

#### General Comments
Increased respiratory effort, open mouth breathing, exercise intolerance, cyanosis of facial skin, depression, ataxia, weakness, tail bobbing. CO toxicity—cherry red mucus membranes. Acute death or coma. Weight loss, sneezing and coughing may occur with COPD of macaws. The onset clinical signs of acute smoke inhalation may be delayed several hours after the exposure.

#### Historical Findings
Recent toxin exposure. Acute death or coma may occur after PTFE or CO poisoning. Sneezing and nasal discharge. Smoking habit of the owner. Multiple species of birds housed nearby (COPD).

#### Physical Examination Findings
Open mouth breathing. Cyanosis. Sneezing and/or coughing. Increased respiratory effort. Ataxia, incoordination. Cherry red mucus membranes. Dyspnea. Lethargy, depression. Nasal discharge on nares and feathers of the face. Weight loss.

### CAUSES
Many types of toxins may be encountered and include the following: PTFE found on the surface of nonstick cookware, irons and ironing boards, heat lamps and self-cleaning ovens produce acidic fluorinated gases and particles. Feather dander and dust from powder down-producing birds like cockatoos (*Cacatua* spp.), cockatiels (*Nymphicus hollandicus*), and African grey parrots (*Psittacus erithacus*), which can cause hypersensitivity reactions known as COPD of macaws or macaw hypersensitivity syndrome. Smoke—solid or liquid material released into the air by pyrolysis (combustion). $CO$, $CO_2$. Nicotine, butadiene, and other chemicals released in cigarette smoke. Many other airborne toxins can have variable effects on birds, including air fresheners, scented candles, aerosols, methane, gasoline fumes, glues, paint fumes, self-cleaning ovens, solvents, bleach, ammonia, propellants, and grooming products (nail polish, hair products). More recently, airborne volatile toxicants present in crude oil spills on beaches are being investigated as potential contributors to morbidity in exposed wild birds.

### RISK FACTORS
Presence and use of non-stick cookware or other source of PTFE. Presence of powder down-producing birds in the immediate environment of a macaw. Cigarette smoking by the owner. Housework involving painting or cleaning with aerosol producing chemicals. Recent fire or other event releasing smoke into the environment.

## DIAGNOSIS

### DIFFERENTIAL DIAGNOSIS
Respiratory compromise caused by trauma and secondary air sac rupture, bacterial, fungal, or viral infections, neoplasia, ascites, or hypovitaminosis A with secondary sinusitis. Primary heart disease, atherosclerosis causing left-heart failure, congenital heart disease. Avocado toxicity. Ataxia and weakness secondary to other neurologic disease, metabolic derangements, or systemic disease.

### CBC/BIOCHEMISTRY/URINALYSIS
In most cases, the hemogram will not show any consistent changes, except with polycythemia of COPD. PCV can be as high as 80%. Biochemistry profile varied based on the systems affected.

### OTHER LABORATORY TESTS
N/A

### IMAGING
Radiographs may be useful in ruling out causes of respiratory disease and to evaluate the heart and lungs for secondary complications. Radiographic changes are often not apparent until the disease is advanced. COPD—often unremarkable. Occasionally, right-sided heart failure is seen due to chronic polycythemia. CT or MRI may show smaller lesions not readily identifiable on radiographs, particularly in the sinuses.

### DIAGNOSTIC PROCEDURES
Coelomic endoscopic examination and lung biopsy may reveal consistent histologic changes associated with damage to the lungs caused by airborne toxin (see Pathologic Findings section). It may also help to elucidate the presence of other secondary diseases such as aspergillosis or bacterial infections that may require specific treatment.

### PATHOLOGIC FINDINGS
PTFE toxicity—grossly, red, wet lungs, eosinophilic fluid-filled bronchi, and multifocal to confluent hemorrhage. Microscopic changes include air capillary collapse, congestion, hemorrhage and edema. Chronic smoke inhalation may cause tertiary bronchi obliterans. COPD of macaws—grossly, firm and "rubbery" lungs. Microscopic changes include eosinophilic infiltration of the interstitium, proliferative fibrous connective tissue, and a mixed cellular infiltrate. Tertiary bronchi may be obstructed due to hypertrophy of smooth muscle. These lesions are usually well advanced by the time that polycythemia has occurred. Atherosclerotic plaques may results from chronic exposure to butadiene in cigarette smoke.

## TREATMENT

### APPROPRIATE HEALTH CARE
Inpatient intensive care management is often required. Administer bronchodilators and antianxiety analgesic, then place in oxygen. Administer diuretics if heart failure is present and antimicrobials for potential secondary

infections. NSAIDs may also be helpful in mild cases of PTFE toxicosis.

## NURSING CARE
Oxygen therapy 78–85% $O_2$ at a flow rate of 5 l/minute. HEPA filtration. Fluid therapy to maintain hydration or correct dehydration. Nebulization with saline can be beneficial.

## ACTIVITY
Acute—exercise restriction until symptoms have resolved. Chronic—lifelong exercise restriction due to permanent respiratory system damage.

## DIET
Ingluvial gavage for anorectic patients.

## CLIENT EDUCATION
Prognosis varies based on the level of exposure and chronicity of disease. Educate owners on the sources of airborne toxins and their role in removing these toxins from the environment. Separate macaws from powder down-producing bird species. HEPA filtration can be helpful.

## SURGICAL CONSIDERATIONS
Caution in patients with chronic respiratory system damage.

## MEDICATIONS

## DRUG(S) OF CHOICE
Anti-anxiety analgesic—butorphanol at 0.5–2 mg/kg IM. Terbutaline 0.01 mg/kg IM q6–12h or 0.1 mg/kg PO q12–24h or via nebulization. Eye ointment if ocular irritation is present. NSAIDs—meloxicam at 0.5 mg/kg PO q12–24h. Short-acting corticosteroid use is controversial but some will use for smoke inhalation and COPD. Dexamethasone may be considered at a dose of 0.2–1.0 mg/kg IM once or q12–24h; dexamethasone sodium phosphate at 2 mg/kg once or q6–12h during the acute phase.

## CONTRAINDICATIONS
Housing New World and Old World species in the same space without adequate ventilation and filtration.

## PRECAUTIONS
Use caution if using corticosteroids in birds; consider concurrent antibiotic and antifungal therapy.

## POSSIBLE INTERACTIONS
N/A

## ALTERNATIVE DRUGS
Midazolam 0.5–1.0 mg/kg IM may be used to reduce anxiety if butorphanol is not sufficient. Other bronchodilators include theophylline or aminophylline. These may be less effective at bronchodilation in birds, but clinical improvement has been noted with their use: Theophylline 2 mg/kg PO q12h; aminophylline 10 mg/kg IV q3h, 4 mg/kg IM q12 2.5 mg in 3 cc saline q4–6h during acute clinical signs.

## FOLLOW-UP

## PATIENT MONITORING
COPD—frequent monitoring of PCV to assess treatment effectiveness. Imaging (radiographs, CT or MRI) to evaluate lungs and air sacs, heart size, and to check for the presence of atherosclerotic plaques.

## PREVENTION/AVOIDANCE
Airborne toxicosis is a complication of captivity. Elimination of the potential toxins before exposure is often possible and carries the best prognosis.

## POSSIBLE COMPLICATIONS
Heart failure can result if polycythemia or pulmonary fibrosis if significant.

## EXPECTED COURSE AND PROGNOSIS
In the case of exposure to PTFE and clinical signs are present, the prognosis is usually very poor. In the case of COPD, the condition can be improved with medication, HEPA filtration, and elimination of allergens from the environment, but even with good control, the condition will often shorten the normal lifespan of the patient.

## MISCELLANEOUS

## ASSOCIATED CONDITIONS
N/A

## AGE-RELATED FACTORS
N/A

## ZOONOTIC POTENTIAL
N/A

## FERTILITY/BREEDING
Birds with COPD may have decreased breeding success.

## SYNONYMS
COPD of macaws, macaw hypersensitivity syndrome.

## SEE ALSO
Air Sac Rupture
Aspergillosis
Hemorrhage
Pneumonia
Respiratory Distress
Toxins (Ingested, Gastrointestinal)
Tracheal and Syringeal Diseases
Appendix 6: Common Avian Toxins

## ABBREVIATIONS
CO—carbon monoxide
$CO_2$—carbon dioxide
COPD—chronic obstructive pulmonary disease
CT—computed tomography
HEPA—high-efficiency particulate air
MRI—magnetic resonance imaging
NSAIDs—non-steroidal anti-inflammatory drugs
$O_2$—oxygen
PCV—packed cell volume
PTFE—polytetrafluoroethylene

## INTERNET RESOURCES
N/A

*Suggested Reading*
Dubansky, B., Verbeck, G., Mach, P., Burggren, W. (2018). Methodology for exposing avian embryos to quantified levels of airborne aromatic compounds associated with crude oil spills. *Environ Toxicol Pharmacol.* 58:163–169.
Graham, J. (2017). Avian respiratory emergencies. *Proceedings of the International Veterinary Emergency and Critical Care Symposium,* Nashville, TN.
Lightfoot, T.L., Yeager, J.M. (2008). Pet bird toxicity and related environmental concerns. *Veterinary Clinics of North America: Exotic Animal Practice,* 11:229–259.
Orosz, S.E., Lichtenberger, M. (2011). Avian respiratory distress: Etiology, diagnosis and treatment. *Veterinary Clinics of North America: Exotic Animal Practice,* 14:241–255.
Phalen, D.N. (2000). Respiratory medicine in cage and aviary birds. *Veterinary Clinics of North America: Exotic Animal Practice,* 3:423–452.
Schmidt, R.E. (2013). The Avian Respiratory System. *Proceedings of the Western Veterinary Conference,* Las Vegas, NV.
**Author:** Stephen M. Dyer, DVM, DABVP (Avian)

**T**

 **Client Education Handout available online**

# TOXICOSIS (ANTICOAGULANT RODENTICIDE)

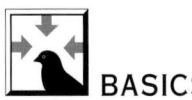 **BASICS**

## DEFINITION

An impairment of coagulation resulting in life-threatening hemorrhage caused by ingestion of rodent poison bait (primary poisoning) or ingestion of a poisoned prey item (secondary poisoning). Anticoagulant rodenticides (ARs) are divided into two groups that share the same mechanism of action but differ in their potencies and half-lives. First-generation anticoagulant rodenticides (FGARs) include warfarin, diphacinone, and chlorophacinone. The FGARs are less potent and have shorter half-lives. Second-generation anticoagulant rodenticides (SGARs) include brodifacoum, difethialone, and bromadiolone. The SGARs are more potent and have longer half-lives.

## PATHOPHYSIOLOGY

ARs interfere with blood clotting by inhibiting the enzyme vitamin K epoxide reductase. This inhibition results in the accumulation of an inactive (oxidized) form of vitamin K, which in turn is unable to activate the vitamin K dependent clotting factors (II, VII, IX, and X). The depletion of these activated clotting factors causes a coagulopathy and hemorrhage. Although it was previously thought that birds lacked factors VII and X, these conclusions were drawn from studies that used non-avian tissue thromboplastin in their laboratory assays; tests using mammalian reagents are recognized to produce inaccurate results. Clinical signs resulting from AR toxicosis will not be apparent for 2–5 days following ingestion of a toxic dose, owing to the presence of activated clotting factors in the circulation at the time the AR is consumed. When these activated clotting factors are depleted, which is dependent upon the half-lives of the factors, coagulopathy occurs.

## SYSTEMS AFFECTED

**Cardiovascular**: Anemia, hypoproteinemia, hypovolemic shock (pallor of mucus membranes, poor capillary refill time).
**Musculoskeletal**: Intramuscular bleeding, weakness, massive swelling in the absence of fractures.
**Skin**: Bruising, subcutaneous hemorrhage, severe bleeding from minor lacerations.
**Nervous**: Dull mentation secondary to hypovolemic shock, neurologic signs possible if hemorrhage occurs within the CNS or surrounding spinal cord.
**Respiratory**: Dyspnea possible if pulmonary hemorrhage occurs.
**Urologic/reproductive/GI**: Bleeding from the vent possible if hemorrhage from renal, reproductive, or GI systems occurs.

## GENETICS
N/A

## INCIDENCE/PREVALENCE

The avian species most commonly affected by AR exposure and toxicosis are free-living birds of prey. Studies in the USA published in 2020 and 2021 found exposure, primarily to SGARs, among multiple species of free-living birds of prey in 100% and 89% of tested populations, respectively. Poisonings have occurred in avian species housed in zoos. Poisoning in psittacine birds kept as pets is not commonly reported.

## GEOGRAPHIC DISTRIBUTION

Mortalities and exposures have been documented in free-living birds of prey in multiple regions worldwide where ARs are used, including the USA, Canada, and Europe.

## SIGNALMENT

There appear to be differences in sensitivity to ARs among avian species, with evidence that birds of prey may be more sensitive than other species that have been studied.

## SIGNS

### General Comments

Bleeding can be spontaneous or induced by traumatic injury. If the bleeding is initiated by a traumatic event, however, the amount of hemorrhage will be in excess of what would be expected with uncomplicated trauma. Signs are in part dependent on the location of the hemorrhage.

### Historical Findings

Free-living birds of prey are often found on the ground, unable to fly due to weakness and hypovolemic shock. Captive or pet birds may have a known exposure to AR bait.

### Physical Examination Findings

Dull mentation. Weakness. Profound pallor of the mucous membranes. Collapse of the cutaneous ulnar vein. Bleeding may or may not be obvious. In many cases, extensive SQ hemorrhage and IM bruising will be present but can only be appreciated if the clinician parts the feathers with isopropyl alcohol and looks for these signs. In other instances, a traumatically induced injury may be present but the extent of hemorrhage will be disproportionate to the injury; for example, severe external hemorrhage from a minor laceration or formation of an excessively large hematoma at a point of possible traumatic impact. Increased respiratory rate and/or effort can indicate hemorrhage involving the respiratory system. Bleeding from the vent can indicate hemorrhage involving the GI, renal, or reproductive systems. Neurologic abnormalities can be associated with hemorrhage involving the CNS or spinal cord.

## CAUSES

Primary poisoning—ingestion of AR bait. Secondary poisoning—ingestion of poisoned prey.

## RISK FACTORS

Free-living birds hunting in areas of AR use. Accessibility of AR baits or contaminated food to captive or pet birds.

 **DIAGNOSIS**

## DIFFERENTIAL DIAGNOSIS

**Blood loss anemia secondary to trauma**: Traumatic blood loss will be accompanied by other obvious signs of trauma, such as fractures, ocular injury (which may only affect the posterior segment of the eye with the anterior chamber appearing normal), or large wounds. Traumatic blood loss in birds will generally not result in anemia as severe as that seen with AR toxicosis. Profound anemia with or without visible massive bruising or with an externally bleeding wound that does not clot should raise the index of suspicion for AR toxicosis.
**Anemia secondary to malnutrition**: Malnourished birds will lack subcutaneous fat deposits, will show muscle wasting with a prominent keel, and will have normal coagulation.
**Disseminated intravascular coagulation**: Birds may show other signs of systemic illness. Other causes of coagulopathy. Not well described in birds; liver dysfunction may result in coagulopathy.

## CBC/BIOCHEMISTRY/URINALYSIS

Anemia is often profound (PCV may be < 10%). Hypoproteinemia.

## OTHER LABORATORY TESTS

Assessment of coagulation: Commercial coagulation profiles are not available for avian species and tests run with mammalian thromboplastin will provide inaccurate results. Viscoelastic coagulation testing has been investigated in some avian species, but its accuracy remains uncertain. However, the lack of clotting in birds suffering AR toxicosis is usually quite evident if 0.1–0.2 ml blood placed in a serum collection tube, which is then inverted occasionally and observed for clotting. In normal birds, signs of clot formation in the tube should be obvious within 5–10 minutes. In many AR poisoned birds, no signs of clotting are seen after several hours. AR testing: Identification of the rodenticide from a plasma sample can be done by many diagnostic laboratories. False negatives are possible, however, as the half-lives of ARs in blood are short. The need to pursue AR identification should be weighed against the drawbacks of taking

T

additional blood for testing from an anemic and shocky bird. AR screens can be performed on liver tissue postmortem.

## IMAGING
Radiographs may help rule in or rule out trauma. Radiography and/or ultrasonography may aid in visualizing blood within the coelom, if present. However, these procedures should be performed cautiously in critical patients.

## DIAGNOSTIC PROCEDURES
N/A

## PATHOLOGIC FINDINGS
Findings on gross necropsy vary with the location of hemorrhage. Common lesions include extensive SQ and IM bruising, coelomic hemorrhage, generalized bruising of the sternum, and pallor of internal organs. Focal, limited hemorrhage or bruising is more consistent with trauma. Histopathology may corroborate a gross diagnosis of AR toxicosis with findings of marked, acute hemorrhage of multiple tissues, hypoxic insult of organs such as liver, or possibly extramedullary hematopoiesis.

## TREATMENT

### APPROPRIATE HEALTH CARE
Emergency inpatient intensive care management for birds with active hemorrhage and severe blood loss. Inpatient medical management: free-living birds of prey require admission to a wildlife clinic or rehabilitation center for the duration of medical management; may be required for captive or pet birds if treatment cannot be reliably administered by caretaker or owner. Outpatient medical management: Can be considered for captive or pet birds once condition is stable.

### NURSING CARE
Fluid therapy. Repeated subcutaneous crystalloid fluid therapy can be a very effective means of volume replacement in hypovolemic birds. Although conspecific whole-blood or plasma transfusions can provide red blood cells and/or clotting factors, suitable blood donors and appropriate volumes for transfusion are often unavailable. The stress to the patient of IV or IO catheter placement should be carefully considered. Thermal support. Anemic, hypovolemic birds will benefit from supplemental heat. Oxygen therapy. Beneficial for anemic birds and important therapy for birds in respiratory distress.

### ACTIVITY
Activity should be restricted until medical management restores normal coagulation.

## DIET
Once patient condition is stable, proper nutritional intake should be ensured. If patient will not self-feed, nutritional support in the form of hand feeding or gavage feeding should be considered.

## CLIENT EDUCATION
For captive or pet birds, caretakers or owners should be counseled regarding preventing future exposure to AR products.

## SURGICAL CONSIDERATIONS
N/A

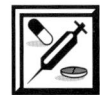

## MEDICATIONS

### DRUG(S) OF CHOICE
Vitamin $K_1$: 2.5–5 mg/kg SQ q8h while active hemorrhage is occurring. Once patient is stable, 2.5 mg/kg PO once daily. Bioavailability is enhanced if given with food. Duration of treatment depends on type of AR due to the difference in the half-lives of FGARs and SGARs; 4 weeks of vitamin $K_1$ therapy has been successful in the treatment of birds of prey with SGAR toxicosis. Shorter treatment may be adequate for FGAR toxicosis but has not been documented in birds. If the type of AR is unknown, treatment should be continued for four weeks due to the difficulty of accurately assessing coagulation.

### CONTRAINDICATIONS
None.

### PRECAUTIONS
IV administration of vitamin $K_1$ may result in anaphylaxis. This route should not be used. IM administration in actively bleeding birds can result in the formation of a large hematoma and is best avoided. Jugular venipuncture can result in life-threatening hemorrhage.

### POSSIBLE INTERACTIONS
None.

### ALTERNATIVE DRUGS
None. Vitamin $K_3$ is not an effective antidote for AR toxicosis.

## FOLLOW-UP

### PATIENT MONITORING
Normal coagulation is restored following the synthesis and activation of new clotting factors, which occurs following administration of vitamin $K_1$. Response to vitamin $K_1$ therapy may be seen within 12–36 hours, depending on the extent of factor depletion. PCV may

show marked increase within 3–5 days as birds regenerate red blood cells quickly. Reassessment of coagulation via the method described in the Diagnosis section 3–4 days should be performed after discontinuation of vitamin $K_1$ to ensure normal clotting factor activation in the absence of vitamin $K_1$ therapy. Because of the lack of accurate avian coagulation tests, patients should be closely observed during this time.

## PREVENTION/AVOIDANCE
Consumer education regarding the risks of ARs to free-living birds of prey is an important factor in decreasing exposure in these species. Avian clinicians that treat free-living birds can play a role in public education on this subject. In the USA, confirmed or suspected cases of AR toxicosis can be reported to the US Environmental Protection Agency via the National Pesticide Information Center at http://npic.orst.edu/eco. For captive or pet birds, prevent access to AR baits or contaminated food.

## POSSIBLE COMPLICATIONS
Hemorrhage can recur if vitamin $K_1$ therapy is interrupted or discontinued too soon. Vitamin $K_1$ must be administered for the duration of the toxic effects of the AR, which is dependent upon the type of AR. If the patient survives the initial acute crisis and appropriate therapy is maintained for the proper duration, adverse sequelae should not be expected.

## EXPECTED COURSE AND PROGNOSIS
Successful treatment, rehabilitation, and release of even severely anemic free-living birds of prey with AR toxicosis is possible. Birds appear able to recover from severe blood loss, quickly regenerate red blood cells, and respond well to treatment consisting of crystalloid or other fluid replacement and vitamin $K_1$ therapy. Prognosis largely depends on the location of hemorrhage. Birds with external, IM, or SQ hemorrhage have a better prognosis for survival than birds that bleed internally, such as into the respiratory tract, the pericardial sac, or the central nervous system.

## MISCELLANEOUS

### ASSOCIATED CONDITIONS
None.

### AGE-RELATED FACTORS
None.

### ZOONOTIC POTENTIAL
None.

### FERTILITY/BREEDING
None.

T

# TOXICOSIS (ANTICOAGULANT RODENTICIDE) (CONTINUED)

## SYNONYMS
None.

## SEE ALSO
Anemia
Coagulopathies and Coagulation
Hemorrhage
Sick-Bird Syndrome
Toxicosis (Heavy Metals)
Trauma
Appendix 3: Laboratory Testing (USA)
Appendix 6: Common Avian Toxins

## ABBREVIATIONS
AR—anticoagulant rodenticide
CNS—central nervous system
FGAR—first-generation anticoagulant rodenticide
GI—gastrointestinal
PCV—packed cell volume
SGAR—second-generation anticoagulant rodenticide

## INTERNET RESOURCES
LafeberVet: https://lafeber.com/vet/presenting-problem-anticoagulant-rodenticide-toxicosis-in-free-living-birds-of-prey

Murray, M. (2013). Anticoagulant rodenticide toxicosis in free-living birds of prey. *LafeberVet*: https://lafeber.com/vet/presenting-problem-anticoagulant-rodenticide-toxicosis-in-free-living-birds-of-prey
National Pesticide Information Center. Ecological Pesticide Incident Reporting: http://npic.orst.edu/eco
US Environmental Protection Agency. Controlling rodents and regulating rodenticides: http://www2.epa.gov/rodenticides

*Suggested Reading*
Murray, M. (2020). Continued anticoagulant rodenticide exposure of red-tailed hawks (*Buteo jamaicensis*) in the northeastern United States with an evaluation of serum for biomonitoring. *Environmental Toxicology and Chemistry*, 39:2325–2335.
Murray, M. (2011). Anticoagulant rodenticide exposure and toxicosis in four species of birds of prey presented to a wildlife clinic in Massachusetts, 2006–2010. *Journal of Zoo and Wildlife Medicine*, 42:88–97.
Murray, M., Tseng, F. (2008). Diagnosis and treatment of secondary anticoagulant rodenticide toxicosis in a red-tailed hawk (*Buteo jamaicensis*). *Journal of Avian Medicine and Surgery*, 22:41–46.
Nevill, H. (2009). Diagnosis of nontraumatic blood loss in birds and reptiles. *Journal of Exotic Pet Medicine*, 18(2):140–145.
Okoniewski J.C., VanPatten C., Ableman A.E., (2021). Anticoagulant rodenticides in red-tailed hawks (*Buteo jamaicensis*) from New York City, New York, USA 2012-18. *Journal of Wildlife Diseases*, 57(1):162–167.
Wernick, M.B., Steinmetz, H.W., Martin-Jurado, O., et al. (2013). Comparison of fluid types for resuscitation in acute hemorrhagic shock and evaluation of gastric luminal and transcutaneous PCO2 in leghorn chickens. *Journal of Avian Medicine and Surgery*, 27(2):109–119.

**Author**: Maureen Murray, DVM, DABVP (Avian)

**Acknowledgements**: Portions adapted from Murray, M. (2013). Presenting problem: Anticoagulant rodenticide toxicosis in free-living birds of prey. LafeberVet.

T

# BASICS

## DEFINITION

### Organophosphates and Carbamates
Pesticides are used every day in every part of the world in agricultural applications. Organophosphates (OP) and carbamates (CA) are common components of many pesticides used in a variety of agricultural, urban, and suburban applications. They are used for lawn and crop pest control, topical parasite control in livestock, and as avicides for control of perceived bird pests. OP and CA use has largely replaced the use of organochlorine compounds, such as DDT, as the former do not accumulate in the environment and tend to break down rapidly. Because OPs and CAs do not persist in the environment, intoxications seen clinically are typically acute and localized to a specific area where pesticide application has recently occurred.

### Neonicotinoids
Neonicotinoids (NEOs) are a class of insecticide related to nicotine and include compounds frequently used in veterinary medicine, such as imidacloprid and nitenpyram. They are currently one of the most widely used classes of insecticide in the world. They are considered to be broad spectrum insecticides, particularly effective against chewing and sucking insects. These compounds can be applied to seeds or soil, after which NEOs will be systemically distributed throughout the tissues of the treated plants. These compounds are generally thought to be less toxic to birds and mammals than OPs or CAs, but their use has still raised concerns regarding their effects on honeybee populations and those of insectivorous birds. Ingestion of NEO-treated seeds is the most likely route of intoxication for terrestrial avian species. It has been demonstrated that a single seed coated with NEO contains enough toxin to kill a passerine bird. Residues on plants, soil, and in water are other potential sources of exposure. In the 2000s, more restrictions have gone into place in the USA and Europe regarding the use of these compounds because of these effects.

### Polychlorinated Biphenyls
Polychlorinated biphenyls (PCBs) and polybrominated biphenyls (PBBs) are highly toxic, carcinogenic compounds that have been used historically in numerous consumer and industry applications (e.g. plastics production, paints, carbonless copy paper, and insecticides). These compounds can be grouped together as persistent halogenated pollutants or PHPs. Because of their highly toxic properties, manufacture of PCBs has decreased significantly over the past several decades and their use has been banned in the USA since 1979. Because of their persistence in the environment, PCBs remain a potential source of intoxication for humans and non-human animals. These compounds are resistant to degradation and have a tendency to bioaccumulate within the food chain. Despite the cessation of production and use of these compounds, it is estimated that as much as 370,000 tons of PCBs still are present in the environment, globally.

## PATHOPHYSIOLOGY

**OPs and COs**: The activities of OP and CA are as cholinesterase inhibitors. Toxic effects are a result of the toxin binding the enzyme AChE in the peripheral and central nervous system. AChE breaks down the neurotransmitter ACh at synaptic junctions. Therefore, inhibition of the enzyme that breaks down the neurotransmitter leads to potentiation of that neurotransmitter's effects. Increased ACh activity results in hyperstimulation of the parasympathetic nervous system and resulting clinical signs can be classified as muscarinic, nicotinic, or central. Muscarinic signs are usually the first to appear and include ptyalism, decreased upper GI motility/crop stasis, diarrhea, and dyspnea caused by constriction of airways and increased airway secretions. Nicotinic and central signs are primarily neurologic and include generalized weakness, tremors, and seizures. The most clinically significant effects are typically seen in the cardiovascular and respiratory systems. This persistent stimulation leads ultimately to paralysis of the muscles involved in respiration, which is the cause of death in intoxicated birds.

**NEOs**: The activity of NEOs is at the nicotinic acetylcholine receptors of cells in the peripheral and central nervous systems. NEOs block the postsynaptic binding of acetylcholine in cells of the central and peripheral nervous systems, causing excitation and eventual paralysis and death. Much like OPs and CAs, NEOs mimic the effects of acetylcholinesterase on these receptors, binding them irreversibly. Clinical signs of NEO intoxication can include ataxia, muscle tremors, and generalized weakness. In addition to affecting bird populations through direct intoxication/death, NEOs have also been shown to have negative affects on the reproductive cycle of avian species, affecting shell quality and fertilization success rates.

**PHPs**: Because PHPs are persistent in the environment, exposure is often in low doses and chronic. These toxins are absorbed via the GI, integumentary, and respiratory tracts. PHPs accumulate in lipids and can be translocated from females to offspring through egg production. Presence and severity of clinical signs is dose dependent and can include endocrine and reproductive dysfunction, metabolic changes, and neurotoxicity. Acute exposure is uncommon, but could cause nausea, vomiting, respiratory, and skin irritation.

## SYSTEMS AFFECTED
GI signs resulting from toxins that inhibit AChE activity (OP, CA, NEO) include increased saliva production, crop stasis, delayed gastric emptying, vomiting, and diarrhea. Neuromuscular effects of OP, CA, or NEO intoxication include muscle tremors, seizures, and generalized weakness. The primary cardiovascular effect of OP or CA intoxication is bradycardia, which can be pronounced, and associated hypotension. Respiratory distress due to increased secretions within the respiratory tract is a significant sequela of OP and CA intoxication. Continued cholinergic stimulation will ultimately lead to respiratory failure from exhaustion of respiratory muscles. NEO exposure may also progress to paralysis of the muscles of respiration and death. OP or CA exposure may inhibit aquatic birds' abilities to regulate electrolytes by decreasing the activity of $Na^+,K^+$-ATPase in salt glands. PHP exposure can result in a wide variety of symptoms affecting various organ systems, depending on route of exposure and dose encountered. GI symptoms can include decreased appetite. Integumentary abnormalities, such as hyperkeratosis, are also observed, especially when exposure is via the skin. A syndrome termed "chick edema disease" has been described in birds, where PCB intoxication results in fluid accumulation in the subcutaneous tissues and coelomic cavity. Significant hepatic changes can be observed, including enlargement, lipid deposition, and hepatocellular necrosis. Disruptions of normal endocrine, reproductive, and immune function are also possible sequelae of PHP exposure. Neoplasia may also result.

## GENETICS
N/A

## INCIDENCE/PREVALENCE
OP and CA intoxications occur across the USA and worldwide. In a retrospective study of the National Wildlife Health Center's mortality database, it was found that 335 avian mortality events occurred in 42 states between 1980 and 2000, with the greatest number of events occurring in Washington, Virginia, and Ohio. Areas with a high percentage of agricultural activity may have a higher incidence of intoxication events. The use of NEOs has increased greatly in recent

T

years. NEOs are the currently the most widely used pesticides in the world. A study performed by Auburn University found that a 100-kg increase in the amount of NEO applied resulted in a 2.2% decrease in grassland bird populations and a 1.4% decrease in non-grassland bird population at the county level. A 0.5% decrease in species diversity was also recorded for both groups of birds.

## GEOGRAPHIC DISTRIBUTION
Intoxications with all of the compounds described here occur across the USA and the world, wherever these toxins have used for pest control or in other applications.

## SIGNALMENT
Waterfowl, raptors, and passerines are the groups most commonly affected by anticholinesterase inhibitor intoxication. Geese and dabbling ducks, which congregate in large numbers in agricultural areas, may be affected by OP/CA by either ingesting treated vegetation or invertebrate prey items or from contact with agricultural run-off. Because these birds often feed together in large flocks, large numbers of waterfowl may be affected at one site. Raptors, especially eagles and hawks, which scavenge as a normal part of their feeding strategy, are most commonly affected by feeding on carcasses that have been treated with OP/CA. However, raptor species that feed on insect prey (such as kestrels and Swainson's hawks) may become intoxicated via this route. Passerine species most commonly affected are those commonly found in agricultural areas, such as blackbirds, grackles, and starlings. These species may also be targeted for intentional poisoning due to their perceived nuisance to agricultural sites. Species most commonly affected by NEO intoxication are those that would ingest NEO-treated seeds, such as ground foraging, granivorous birds. Insectivorous bird species may also be exposed through ingestion of contaminated prey items. Any species of bird could potentially be exposed to PHP toxins, given their history of widespread use and their persistence in the environment. Because of the tendency of PHP compounds to bioaccumulate within the food chain, it would be expected that predatory species would be more susceptible to developing clinical signs of PHP intoxication.

## SIGNS
Affected birds typically in good body condition. Ataxia. Convulsions/tremors. Lethargy. Nictitans prolapse. Respiratory distress. Clenched feet. Ptyalism. Upper GI hypomotility. Bradycardia.

## CAUSES
Birds may become intoxicated by OP/CA by the following routes: Ingestion of prey items that have been treated with these toxins. Invertebrate prey. Carcasses of larger vertebrates that are scavenged. Consumption of treated seed. Intentional baiting of nuisance birds. Vegetation with pesticide residue. Water runoff. Inhalation. Absorption through skin. Seeds treated with insecticide.

## RISK FACTORS
Risk factors for OP/CA intoxication are primarily related to feeding strategy and environment. Birds who congregate in agricultural areas to feed, such as dabbling ducks and geese, are more likely to be affected in greater numbers. Bird species that feed on carrion or grain also have a higher likelihood of intoxication that other species. Bird species that forage in agricultural fields are more likely to come in contact w/NEO treated seed, plants, and insect prey items. Granivorous and insectivorous birds, such as blackbird species, would be good examples of a species at high risk for NEO exposure. PHPs are found everywhere in the environment and are persistent in many scenarios. Since PHPs bioaccumulate in the food chain, predatory avian species, such as raptors, scavengers, and piscivores, would be most likely to develop clinical signs related to exposure.

## DIAGNOSIS

### DIFFERENTIAL DIAGNOSIS
Heavy metal toxicosis. Hypocalcemia. Algal toxicosis/avian vacuolar. Myelinopathy. Botulism.

### CBC/BIOCHEMISTRY/URINALYSIS
Usually unremarkable.

### OTHER LABORATORY TESTS
N/A

### IMAGING
Usually unremarkable, although there may be ingesta present in the GI tract in acutely intoxicated birds or increased density of the lung tissue associated with increased respiratory secretions.

### DIAGNOSTIC PROCEDURES
Definitive diagnosis of OP/CA intoxication is by assessment of AChE activity in the plasma (sublethal intoxications) or brain tissue (lethal intoxications). A decrease of greater than 20% AChE activity is indicative of exposure to OP/CA toxins; a decrease greater than 50% decrease is indicative of

lethal exposure. As there are not established normal values for brain or plasma AChE activity for most species of birds, the AChE activity of the patient must be compared with the AChE activity of a normal conspecific. Assessment of AChE activity will confirm exposure to OP/CA toxins, but will not determine a specific toxin. GI contents may be assayed for specific toxins. Fat, liver, and kidney samples may also be analyzed for the presence of toxins. However, because OP/CA break down quickly, this is often unrewarding.

## PATHOLOGIC FINDINGS
There are no specific gross lesions associated with OP/CA intoxication. Affected birds are typically in good body condition and may have food material present in the upper GI tract, indicative of acute intoxication. Fluid accumulation in lungs consistent with respiratory failure may be found on postmortem examination.

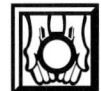

## TREATMENT

### APPROPRIATE HEALTH CARE
There are no specific treatments for the environmental toxins described. Evacuate crop contents to prevent further absorption of ingested toxin. Respiratory support, including supplemental oxygen therapy and/or assisted ventilation may be necessary in patients demonstrating severe respiratory signs. Prognosis in these cases is poor.

### NURSING CARE
Nutritional and fluid support should be provided to patients too debilitated to eat and drink on their own. Thermal support may also be necessary but should be monitored closely as patients having muscle fasiculations may have a tendency to overheat. Basic cleanliness should be maintained in patients who are recumbent and unable to preen. Large waterfowl, such as geese, who are sternally recumbent, should be housed on heavily padded substrate or on a cushion that elevates the keel off of the substrate to avoid development of decubital ulcers along the keel.

### ACTIVITY
N/A

### DIET
N/A

### CLIENT EDUCATION
N/A

### SURGICAL CONSIDERATIONS
N/A

## MEDICATIONS

### DRUG(S) OF CHOICE
Atropine 0.5 mg/kg IM or SQ t.i.d.–q.i.d. until symptoms subside. Pralidoxime iodide (2-PAM) 20–100 mg/kg IM. Activated charcoal 2–8 mg/kg PO b.i.d. until GI tract cleared.

### CONTRAINDICATIONS
Pralidoxime iodide treatment may be contraindicated in cases of CA intoxication as some CA inhibit AChE activity.

### PRECAUTIONS
N/A

### POSSIBLE INTERACTIONS
N/A

### ALTERNATIVE DRUGS
N/A

 ## FOLLOW-UP

### PATIENT MONITORING
N/A

### PREVENTION/AVOIDANCE
N/A

### POSSIBLE COMPLICATIONS
Sublethal doses of OP/CA have been shown to result in an inability to thermoregulate, changes in breeding and nesting behavior, and increased susceptibility to traumatic injury. NEO exposure has been shown to decrease reproductive success, immunosuppression, and genotoxic effects at sublethal doses. Reductions in the numbers of invertebrate prey items can also have deleterious effects on populations of insectivorous birds. PCB or PBB exposure has been shown to decrease male fertility by decreasing spermatogenesis.

### EXPECTED COURSE AND PROGNOSIS
Prognosis is generally poor without therapy and supportive care. Course and prognosis are related to degree of intoxication.

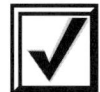 ## MISCELLANEOUS

### ASSOCIATED CONDITIONS
Sublethal intoxications may result in impairments in mentation and reaction ability that could predispose affected birds to traumatic injuries, such as vehicular trauma or predation.

### AGE-RELATED FACTORS
Immature birds are more severely affected by the activities of anticholinesterase toxins.

### ZOONOTIC POTENTIAL
N/A

### FERTILITY/BREEDING
Direct effects of OP/CA exposure on breeding are not well described. However, loss of invertebrate prey items in an area treated with these toxins may result in increased instances in nest abandonment and changes in incubation behavior. Decreased nest attentiveness and changes in song character have been observed in passerines. A variety of reproductive abnormalities in avian species have been attributed to exposure to NEO pesticides. Reproductive success may be affected by abnormal testicle morphology, reduced fertilization, decreased thickness of eggshells, and decreased embryo size. Chick survival can be diminished due to impaired hatching and developmental abnormalities. Hatchlings may experience poor weight gain or decreased feeding behaviors. PHP exposure has been shown to have negative effects on reproductive success in both males and females. Decreased testicular size and reduced spermatogenesis are both potential sequelae of PHP exposure in many species, including chickens. Effects of PHPs on reproductive success in female birds is not well described. However, females of mammalian species exposed to PHPs demonstrate decreased mating, altered estrous, and decreased weight gain of pregnant females. Exposure to these toxins have also been shown to cause abortion, as well as many tertatogenic and developmental abnormalities.

### SYNONYMS
Anticholinesterase toxicity.

### SEE ALSO
Anticoagulant Rodenticide
Botulism
Diarrhea
Hypocalcemia and Hypomagnesemia
Ileus (Functional Gastrointestinal, Crop Stasis)
Neurologic (Non-Traumatic Diseases)
Neoplasia (Neurologic)
Neurologic (Trauma)
Respiratory Distress
Seizures
Toxicosis (Anticoagulant Rodenticides)
Toxicosis (Heavy Metals)
Toxicosis (Iatrogenic)
Toxicosis (Ingested, Gastrointestinal)
Trauma

### ABBREVIATIONS
Ach—acetylcholine
AChE—acetylcholinesterase
CA—carbamate
DDT—dichlorodiphenyltrichloroethane
GI—gastrointestinal
NEO—neonicotinoid
OP—organophosphate
PBB—polybrominated biphenyl
PCB—polychlorinated biphenyl
PHP—persistent halogenated pollutant

### INTERNET RESOURCES
American Bird Conservancy. (2013). birds, bees, and aquatic life threatened by gross underestimate of toxicity of world's most widely used pesticide: https://abcbirds.org/news/birds-bees-and-aquatic-life-threatened-by-gross-underestimate-of-toxicity-of-worlds-most-widely-used-pesticide-2
Coppock, R.W. (2022). Halogenated aromatic poinoning (PCB and others). *MSD Veterinary Manual*: https://www.merckvetmanual.com/special-pet-topics/poisoning/halogenated-aromatic-poisoning-pcb-and-others
Gupta, R.C., Doss, R.B. (2022). Carbamate toxicosis in animals. *MSD Veterinary Manual*: http://www.merckmanuals.com/vet/toxicology/insecticide_and_acaricide_organic_toxicity/carbamate_insecticides_toxicity.html

*Suggested Reading*
Addy-Orduna, L.M., Brodeur, J.C., Mateo, R. (2019). Oral toxicity of imidacloprid, thiamethoxam, and clothianidin in eared doves: A contribution for the risk assessment of neonicotinoids in birds. *Science of the Total Environment*. 650:1216–1223.
Ensley, S.M. (2018). Neonicotinoids. In: *Veterinary Toxicology: Basic and Clinical Principals* (ed. R.C. Gupta), 521–524. New York, NY: Academic Press.
Fleischli, M.A., Franson, J.C., Thomas, N.J., et al. (2004). Avian mortality events in the United States caused by anticholinestersase pesticides: A retrospective summary of National Wildlife Health Center records from 1980 to 2000. *Archives of Environmental Contamination and Toxicology*, 46:542–550.
Glasier, L.C. (1999). Organophosphorous and carbamate pesticides. In: *USGS Field Manual of Wildlife Diseases: General Field Procedures and Diseases of Birds* (ed. J.C. Franson, M. Friend), pp. 287–293. Reston, VA: US Geological Survey.
Grue, C.E., Hart, A.D.M., Mineau, P. (1991). Biological consequences of depressed brain cholinesterase activity in wildlife. In: *Cholinesterase-Inhibiting Insecticides: Their impact on wildlife and the environment* (ed. P. Mineau), 151–209. St. Louis, MO: Elsevier.

T

# TOXICOSIS (ENVIRONMENTAL, PESTICIDES)

Hallman, C.A., Foppen, R.P.B., van Turnhout, C.A.M., et al. (2014). Declines in insectivorous birds are associated with high neonicotinoid concentrations. *Nature*, 511:341–343.

Henry, C.J., Kolby, E.J., Hill, E.F., et al. (1987). Case history of bald eagles and other raptors killed by organophosphorous insecticides topically applied to livestock. *Journal of Wildlife Diseases*, 23:292–295.

Hill, E.F. (1997). Organophosphorous and carbamate pesticides. In: *Handbook of Ecotoxicology* (ed. D.J. Hoffman, B.A. Rattner, G.A. Burton Jr., J. Cairnes Jr. (eds), 243–274. Boca Raton, FL: Blackwell Science.

Kimbrough, R., Buckley, J., Fishbein, G.F., et al. (1978). Animal toxicology. *Environmental Health Perspectives*, 24:173–184.

Kodavanti, P.R.S., Valdez, M.C., Yang, J., Curras-Collazo, M. (2018). Polychlorinated biphenyls, polybrominated biphenyls, polychlorinated dibenzo-p-dioxins, and polychlorinated dibenzofurnas. In: *Veterinary Toxicology: Basic and Clinical Principles*, 3rd edn. (ed. R.C. Gupta), 675–690. St. Louis, MO: Elsevier.

Li, Y., Miao, R., Khanna, M. (2020). Neonicotinoids and decline in bird biodiversity in the United States. *Nature Sustainability*, 3:1027–1035.

Vos, J.G. (1972). Toxicology of PCBs for mammals and for birds. *Environmental Health Perspectives*, 1:105–117.

**Author**: Author Shannon M. Riggs, DVM

T

# TOXICICOSIS (HEAVY METALS)

## BASICS

### DEFINITION
Toxicities induced by the ingestion of certain forms and doses of metals. Lead and zinc poisonings frequently occur in pet and wild birds, while copper and mercury toxicities are mainly seen in the wild.

### PATHOPHYSIOLOGY
Heavy metals are absorbed mainly by the GI tract (rarely by the lungs after inhalation). Due to the poor rate of absorption, lead shot embedded in muscles does not usually induce toxicity. Lead is widely distributed in soft tissues, and bones serve as the long-term storage site for the metal. Lead is toxic to multiple enzymatic systems and interferes with the numerous cellular functions that require calcium. In particular, lead will affect the red blood cells (microcytic anemia and/or porphyrinuria), the renal tubules (Fanconi syndrome nephropathy), and the central and peripheral nervous systems (encephalopathy and polyneuropathy by demyelination and neuronal necrosis). Both the immune and reproductive systems can also be impaired (infertility, embryonic mortality, and teratogenicity). Although the exact mechanism of zinc toxicity is not completely understood, zinc has a high affinity for the pancreas, liver, and the kidneys. Through both its direct and indirect effects, zinc can cause anemia, pancreatitis, hepatic failure, and renal failure. Zinc salts have direct irritant and corrosive effects on tissue, interfere with the metabolism of other ions such as copper, calcium, and iron, and inhibit erythrocyte production and function.

### SYSTEMS AFFECTED
GI, nervous, neuromuscular, hemic/lymphatic/immune, renal/urologic, behavioral, hepatobiliary, reproductive.

### GENETICS
N/A

### INCIDENCE/PREVALENCE
Lead and zinc poisonings are both common in pet birds. Lead toxicity is very common in wild birds, while mercury poisoning occurs less frequently.

### GEOGRAPHIC DISTRIBUTION
Worldwide.

### SIGNALMENT
**Species**: All pet birds, wild and captive waterfowl, poultry, raptors.
**Mean age and range**: Lead will accumulate throughout life in wild birds, so adults are more at risk for chronic toxicity.
**Predominant sex**: No known sex predilection.

## SIGNS

### General Comments
Subacute toxicosis can impair flight capacity and affect the behavior. Wild raptors with chronic lead exposure may therefore present for trauma and may not display the typical signs of acute toxicity. The severity of clinical signs does not always correlate well with blood metal concentration. Signs of lead toxicosis are generally more severe than those seen with zinc poisoning.

### Historical Findings
Non-specific signs—lethargy, anorexia, depression. GI signs—regurgitation, diarrhea. Neurologic signs—seizures, weakness, head down posture. Urologic signs—polyuria/polydipsia, red urine. Sudden death.

### Physical Examination Findings
Abnormal mentation. Ataxia, twitching, circling, paresis, paralysis, blindness. Crop stasis. Green staining around the cloaca. Hemoglobinuria, porphyrinuria. Weight loss (chronic). Polyuria/polydipsia.

### CAUSES
Ingestion of particles of heavy metals, either directly (i.e. parts of toys, galvanized cages, lead-based paints, fishing weights, lead-coated seeds, US pennies 1982 and later) or indirectly (i.e. ingestion of a prey shot with lead pellets).

### RISK FACTORS
Inappropriate supervision, exposure to old lead paints, drapery weights, jewelry, galvanized wires, and so on (pet birds). Presence of lead in the environment, hunting season (wild birds).

## DIAGNOSIS

### DIFFERENTIAL DIAGNOSIS
Meningoencephalitis: Viruses (bornavirus, West Nile virus, paramyxovirus, reovirus), bacteria (*Chlamydia psittaci*, *Salmonella*), fungal (*Aspergillus* spp.), parasites (*Baylisascaris*, *Toxoplasma*, *Sarcocystis*). Other toxicoses: Pesticides, cannabis, iatrogenic (itraconazole in African grey parrots), toxins (botulism). Metabolic disorders: Hepatic and renal failure, diabetes mellitus, hypocalcemia. Trauma. Pancreatitis. Foreign body ingestion. Neoplasia: Central nervous system, digestive system, lymphoma. Atherosclerosis.

### CBC/BIOCHEMISTRY/URINALYSIS
Regenerative microcytic hypochromic anemia. Greater number of immature red blood cells, poikilocytosis, and nuclear abnormalities (fusiform, elongated, and irregular nuclei) are seen with zinc toxicosis in birds). Elevation of uric acid, AST, LDH and

CK. Hemoglobinuria and porphyrinuria (Amazon parrots).

### OTHER LABORATORY TESTS
Reference ranges vary with species.
**Lead**: Collect whole blood on EDTA or heparin. Do not submit serum or plasma. Blood levels: As a general rule, intoxication is confirmed if the lead concentration in whole blood is > 0.2 ppm (20 μg/dl). Subclinical toxicosis occurs at lower levels. Some species (pigeons, waterfowl) seem to be able to tolerate higher levels before showing clinical signs of acute toxicity. Tissue levels > 3–6 ppm in liver or kidneys. Decreased ALAD activity.
**Zinc**: Collect blood on serum tubes without rubber components. Most pet birds have normal zinc levels below 3.5 ppm (0.35 mg/dl). Zinc toxicity is suspected when liver concentrations > 75 ppm (mg/kg) wet weight.

### IMAGING
Metal particles can be visualized on radiographs. However, their absence does not rule out heavy metal toxicity.

### DIAGNOSTIC PROCEDURES
None.

### PATHOLOGIC FINDINGS

#### Gross lesions
Non-specific and not commonly reported (bile stasis, swollen kidneys, mottled pancreas, pectoral atrophy).

#### Microscopic findings
**Lead**: Acute tubular necrosis (sometimes associated with characteristic acid-fast intranuclear inclusion bodies), myocardial and hepatocellular necrosis, brain edema, peripheral nerve degeneration, and necrosis of the ventriculus muscles.
**Zinc**: Pancreatic necrosis and vacuolation/degranulation of acinar cells, hepatic biliary retention and hemosiderosis to multifocal necrotizing hepatitis, acute tubular necrosis, enteritis, erosive ventriculitis with koilin degeneration.

## TREATMENT

### APPROPRIATE HEALTH CARE
Patients with acute heavy metal poisoning should be hospitalized and require intensive medical care.

### NURSING CARE
Aggressive fluid therapy (renal failure), IV/IO if possible. Nutritional support adapted to the species. Keep the bird in an environment appropriate to its neurologic condition (padded cage, if having seizures; comfortable bedding, if sternally recumbent; etc.).

# TOXICICOSIS (HEAVY METALS) (CONTINUED)

## ACTIVITY
Birds with neurologic signs should not be allowed to fly.

## DIET
Fine or coarse grit, as well as cathartic emollients (peanut butter) may be added to the diet to hasten the passage of any metallic particles in the GI tract.

## CLIENT EDUCATION
If oral chelation therapy is administered at home, put an emphasis on the potential for drug toxicity.

## SURGICAL CONSIDERATIONS
Proventricular and ventricular saline lavages have been used to remove lead particles in birds. In rare cases, endoscopic or surgical removal of the metallic particles may be warranted.

## MEDICATIONS

### DRUG(S) OF CHOICE
Edetate calcium disodium (CaNa$_2$EDTA, injectable sterile solution) 35 mg/kg q12h IV or IM for 5 days, followed by a "rest" period of 3–5 days to allow a redistribution of tissue and fluid lead concentrations and to prevent excessive chelation of endogenous minerals. Assessment of blood concentrations after the rest period will indicate if the protocol needs to be repeated. Drug of choice for lead, zinc, and mercury intoxications. Midazolam 0.1–0.2 mg/kg IM can be used to control seizures. Antibiotics (amoxicillin/clavulanic acid 125 mg/kg q12h PO, enrofloxacin 15 mg/kg q12h PO) might be indicated due to the immunosuppressive effects of lead and in cases with a severe enteritis.

### CONTRAINDICATIONS
Previous history of acute renal failure (not associated with the current toxicity).

### PRECAUTIONS
Potential nephrotoxicity. Chelation of other minerals such as zinc, magnesium, and copper with long-term use. Might require additional dilutions for IV injections (if concentration is ≥ 150 mg/ml).

### POSSIBLE INTERACTIONS
Use with caution with other nephrotoxic compounds.

### ALTERNATIVE DRUGS
DMSA acid (succimer, needs to be compounded) 20–35 mg/kg q12h PO for 5–7 days. Reassessment of metal concentrations is recommended. Not as effective for zinc chelation. Does not chelate other essential minerals. Not nephrotoxic. Narrow margin of safety (80 mg/kg can be lethal in cockatiels). D-penicillamine 55 mg/kg PO q12h for 1–2 weeks, followed by a "rest" week before reassessing the blood concentrations. Not recommended if metallic particles still present in the GI tract as could increase their absorption. Dimercaprol has a very narrow margin of safety and should not be used in birds.

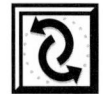

## FOLLOW-UP

### PATIENT MONITORING
Heavy metal blood concentration should be reassessed a few days after chelation therapy is discontinued. If still high, the protocol is repeated until blood levels are considered within an acceptable range.

### PREVENTION/AVOIDANCE
Prevent access to any source of lead and zinc. Birds should be under close supervision when free in the house.

### POSSIBLE COMPLICATIONS
Seizures can lead to severe trauma in birds. Dehydration can be secondary to renal and GI losses.

### EXPECTED COURSE AND PROGNOSIS
Prognosis is poor without chelation therapy and supportive care. Birds respond generally very rapidly to chelation therapy with neurologic status being back to normal within 24–36 hours. Medical intensive care and nutritional support in the hospital can be expected to be required for 3–5 days. Outcome is usually positive if the bird is diagnosed and treated in a timely and appropriate manner.

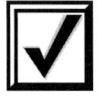

## MISCELLANEOUS

### ASSOCIATED CONDITIONS
None.

### AGE-RELATED FACTORS
N/A

### ZOONOTIC POTENTIAL
N/A

### FERTILITY/BREEDING
Lead and mercury have been shown to reduce fertility and cause embryonic deaths. Chelation therapy might be considered in breeding birds, even with subclinical blood lead concentrations.

### SYNONYMS
Plumbism, saturnism (lead), new wire disease (zinc), hydrargyria (mercury).

## SEE ALSO
Anemia
Anorexia
Bornaviral Disease (Aquatic Birds)
Bornaviral Disease (Psittaciformes)
Diarrhea
Enteritis and Gastritis
Foreign Bodies (Gastrointestinal)
Ileus (Functional Gastrointestinal, Crop Stasis)
Liver Disease
Neurologic (Non-traumatic Diseases)
Regurgitation and Vomiting
Seizures
Sick-Bird Syndrome
Urate and Fecal Discoloration

## ABBREVIATIONS
ALAD—delta-aminolevulinic acid dehydratase
AST—aspartate aminotransferase
CK—creatine kinase
DMSA—meso-2,3-dimercaptosuccinic acid
EDTA—ethylenediaminetetraacetic acid
GI—gastrointestinal
LDH—lactate dehydrogenase

## INTERNET RESOURCES
N/A

*Suggested Reading*
Fallon, J.A., Redig, P., Miller, T.A., et al. (2017). Guidelines for evaluation and treatment of lead poisoning of wild raptors. *Wildlife Society Bulletin*, 41:205–211.
Friend, M., Franson, J.C. (1999). Chemical toxins. In: *Field Manual of Wildlife Diseases. General Field Procedures and Diseases of Birds*, 284–353. Madison, WI: Biological Resources Division, US Geological Survey, Department of Interior.
Lightfoot, T.L., Yeager, J.M. (2008). Pet bird toxicity and related environmental concerns. *Veterinary Clinics of North America. Exotic Animal Practice*, 11: 229–259.
Puschner, B., Poppenga, R.H. (2009). Lead and zinc intoxication in companion birds. *Compendium: Continuing Education for Veterinarians*, 31(1):E1–E12.
Richardson, J.A. (2006). Implication of toxic substances in clinical disorders. In *Clinical Avian Medicine* (ed. G.J. Harrison, T.L. Lightfoot), 711–719. Palm Beach, FL: Spix Publishing.
**Author:** Marion Desmarchelier, DMV, MSc, DACZM, DECZM (Zoo Health Management), DACVB
**Acknowledgements:** Shannon Ferrell, DVM, DABVP (Avian), DACZM

**Client Education Handout available online**

# BASICS

## DEFINITION
Iatrogenic toxicosis is an adverse effect that is unintentionally induced by a diagnostic, treatment, or procedure. These are most often undesirable effects of treatments prescribed by a healthcare provider but may also occur as a result of the exposure to medications or supplements administered by an owner, or incorrect administration of medications by an owner. While there are many drugs that may lead to iatrogenic toxicoses, the following drugs are discussed in this chapter: Ivermectin/avermectins, itraconazole, vitamin A, benzimidazoles, steroids, gabapentin, cannabis. Chemotherapeutic drugs are not addressed, as the risk of toxicosis is inherent with the use of any chemotherapeutic agent.

## PATHOPHYSIOLOGY

### Ivermectin/avermectins
Ivermectin is a macrocyclic lactone antiparasitic which binds to glutamate-gated chloride channels of the nervous system of invertebrates, causing paralysis of somatic muscles. It is administered topically or subcutaneously. The therapeutic dosage range in birds is relatively narrow, and miscalculations in either dose or dilution for administration can easily lead to overdosage and toxicity. Correct dosage is 0.2–0.4 mg/kg and may be administered topically or subcutaneously. Topical administration in small birds is generally one drop from an insulin syringe on the back of the head or over the jugular vein. The recommended dosage of selamectin is 18 mg/kg topically; topical doses of up to 92 mg/kg were evaluated in zebra finches with no reported adverse effects.

### Benzimidazoles
Benzimidazoles are antiparasitic drugs that bind preferentially to the tubulin of parasitic microtubules. Multiple cellular functions are disrupted, including shape, division, absorption and transport, motility, and secretion. Benzimidazoles have a higher affinity for invertebrates than vertebrate tubules. They are not highly protein bound but have high volumes of distribution, especially to GI mucosa, bile ducts, and lungs. They are administered orally in a single high dose or daily for a period of several days.

### Vitamin A
Vitamin A is a vital fat-soluble vitamin that helps promote and maintain epithelial cells, and is important in vision, maintaining immune system function, and reproduction. The majority of vitamin A is stored in the liver. The active form of vitamin A is preformed vitamin A. Ingested beta carotenoids are converted into vitamin A in the intestine and stored in the liver in the inactive forms of retinol and retinol esters. Once liver storage capacity is exceeded, vitamin A esters and retinol are released into the bloodstream.

### Itraconazole
Itraconazole is an azole antifungal with fungicidal against *Aspergillus* spp. and fungistatic against many other types of fungal organisms. It works by inhibiting cytochrome P450 and disrupting the fungal cell membrane. It requires an acid environment for absorption and is 99% absorbed when taken with food. Compounded formulations are less bioavailable and therefore less effective.

### Glucocorticoids
Glucocorticoids are a class of drugs that have potent immunosuppressive and anti-inflammatory effects. They bind to glucocorticoid receptors and play an important role in carbohydrate, lipid and protein metabolism. They are also important in response to stress and the immune system. They suppress interleukin and cytokine synthesis and cell mediated immunity, and decrease leukocyte production and function. Gluconeogenesis and hepatic glycogen storage in the liver accompanied by decreased cellular glucose uptake serve to elevate blood glucose levels. It also depletes calcium stores by decreasing intestinal calcium absorption and increasing renal calcium excretion. Reduces collagen synthesis leading to thinning of skin. However, the most severe adverse effects in birds are due to the immunosuppressive effects of steroids.

### Gabapentin
Gabapentin is used as an anticonvulsant and analgesic. Its mechanism of action is not entirely known but acts in part via blockage of voltage gated ion channels, decreasing calcium influx into cells and effecting glutamate, norepinephrine and substance P. Although high doses can be used, dosing must start low and may be gradually increased. Sedation may occur with increasing dosage, but patients adapt within a few days; the maximum dosage is variable among individuals and is the dose at which a patient does not adapt to the current dosage.

### Cannabinoids
All parts of the cannabis plant contain cannabinoids, although the concentration is less in seeds than the plant. Once dried, cannabinoids are concentrated and plants are often prepared along with hemp. Birds may accidentally ingest plant matter in the form of dried plants or in resin from being smoked in a household. It is unknown whether birds may become intoxicated from inhaling cannabis when smoked in the same room. The use of cannabis has been investigated in poultry with regard to weight gain and was found to increase weight gain when added to feed at 5% and 10% but decrease weight gain at 20% of feed. While there are currently no published case reports on cannabinoid toxicity in birds, there are clinical discussions on veterinary forums.

## SYSTEMS AFFECTED
**Behavioral**: Ivermectin/avermectins: ataxia, abnormal behaviors, vocalization, lethargy. Gabapentin: ataxia, decreased alertness, agitation.
**Endocrine/metabolic**: Glucocorticoids—thinning of skin; feather changes or loss due to excessive steroid; decreased calcium due to increased renal excretion; increased chance of hyperglycemia, diabetes.
**Gastrointestinal**: Benzimidazoles—stomatitis, diarrhea, melena. Vitamin A, itraconazole: decreased appetite. Glucocorticoids—melena, diarrhea. Gabapentin—diarrhea.
**Hemic/lymphatic/immune**: Benzimidazoles—myelosuppression, anemia and thrombocytopenia may all occur depending on the medication. Glucocorticoids—severe immunosuppression, sepsis.
**Hepatobiliary**: Vitamin A—hepatomegaly. Itraconazole—hepatotoxicity. Glucocorticoids—hepatic lipidosis.
**Musculoskeletal**: Vitamin A—bone resorption, osteoporosis.
**Nervous**: Ivermectin/avermectins—ataxia, incoordination. Gabapentin—ataxia, agitation, hyperesthesia, body tremors. Cannabinoids—weakness, ataxia, tremors, seizures.
**Ophthalmic**: Vitamin A—conjunctivitis.
**Renal/urologic**: Vitamin A—epithelial thickening of renal tubules, possibly PU/PD; glucocorticoids—PU/PD.
**Reproductive**: Vitamin A—poor reproduction.
**Respiratory**: Vitamin A— thickening of epithelial linings can lead to respiratory infections; Glucocorticoids—bacterial or fungal respiratory infections.
**Skin/exocrine**: Vitamin A—dry skin, cracked mucus membranes and mucosal regions. Glucocorticoids—thinning of skin, cutaneous bacterial or fungal infections.

## GENETICS
None.

## INCIDENCE/PREVALENCE
Worldwide.

## GEOGRAPHIC DISTRIBUTION
Worldwide.

T

## SIGNALMENT

All species, age, and range of birds are susceptible. For benzimidazoles, certain species such as pigeons, doves, cockatiels, and storks may be more susceptible, even at published doses.

## SIGNS

### General Comments

Clinical signs will vary according to the organ system affected.

### Historical Findings

A medication or treatment has been prescribed by a veterinarian or administered by an owner. The medication or treatment may be administered correctly and have an adverse effect, or may be incorrectly administered or dosed. The medication or treatment should be evaluated, along with directions provided and owners administration routes, and any compounding that may have occurred should be assessed.

### Physical Examination Findings

Variable, according to systems affected.
**Ivermectin/avermectins:** Signs of toxicity are associated with the central nervous system and usually occur within hours of dosing. These include ataxia, inappetence/anorexia, depression, blindness, mydriasis, muscle tremors, bradycardia, respiratory depression, and death.
**Benzimidazoles:** Signs of toxicity are radiomimetic. It causes bone marrow suppression characterized by anemia and thrombocytopenia. Intestinal crypt necrosis also occurs leading to GI signs such as stomatitis, diarrhea, and melena.
**Vitamin A:** Clinical signs of vitamin A toxicosis are similar to those of vitamin A deficiency, so history of administration is an important factor in making the diagnosis. Dry skin, cracking of mucus membranes and mucosal regions (nares, sinuses, commissures of the mouth, palate, renal tubules), decreased appetite, hepatomegaly, bone resorption and osteoporosis, and poor reproduction. In one flock of lorikeets, initial clinical signs were conjunctivitis and crusting of the eyelids, followed by respiratory signs, diarrhea, and death. All remaining birds recovered once vitamin A supplementation was discontinued.
**Glucocorticoids:** PU/PD, hyperglycemia, fungal or bacterial infections, thinning of skin, melena, diarrhea, sepsis, hepatic lipidosis, cutaneous lesions, feather loss, lethargy, weakness, death.
**Gabapentin:** diarrhea, ataxia, tremors, hyperesthesia.
**Cannabinoids:** weakness, ataxia, tremors, seizures.

## CAUSES

See Definition section.

## RISK FACTORS

**Ivermectin/avermectins:** Contraindicated in birds with suspected or confirmed abnormalities of the blood–brain barrier.
**Benzimidazoles:** Certain species of birds may be more susceptible, even at published doses, such as pigeons and doves, cockatiels, and storks.
**Vitamin A:** Seed-based diets are deficient in vitamin A, so supplementation may be necessary. Commercially available injectable formulations of vitamin A are extremely concentrated and require dilution for administration. Incorrect dilution, failure to dilute, or more commonly, repeat administration of a correct dose can all lead to overdose, accumulation in liver and fat, and vitamin A toxicosis. Dietary consumption of vitamin A toxicosis in birds has not been documented.
**Itraconazole:** Animals with impaired renal or hepatic function are at increased risk of toxicity. Absorption in some species is variable; grey parrots are known to experience toxicity at doses that are therapeutic in other birds.
**Glucocorticoids:** Birds are extremely susceptible to the adverse effects of steroids, and toxicity may occur with doses that may be therapeutic in other species. The immunosuppressive effects leave birds highly susceptible to infection, particularly fungal diseases such as aspergillus. Even topical or ophthalmic steroids can be absorbed in toxic amounts through the thin skin of birds.
**Gabapentin:** Although high uses can be used, dosages should begin low and be gradually increased to allow the patient to adapt to dosage increases.
**Cannabinoids:** The increased usage of cannabinoid products in households increases the availability of these drugs to birds.

## DIAGNOSIS

### DIFFERENTIAL DIAGNOSIS

**Ivermectin/avermectins:** Cardiovascular event, infectious diseases of the central nervous system, sepsis, other toxins that may cause neurologic signs.
**Benzimidazoles:** Neoplastic myelosuppression, rodenticide toxicity, GI infection.
Itraconazole: Infectious or neoplastic causes of hepatic enzyme elevation, GI infection.
**Vitamin A:** Any dermatologic disorder, respiratory disease, renal disease.
**Gabapentin:** Lead, zinc, metabolic disorders, or any other toxin that may cause neurologic abnormalities.

## CBC/BIOCHEMISTRY/URINALYSIS

**Benzimidazoles:** Anemia, thrombocytopenia.
**Itraconazole:** Elevation of bile acids, AST.
**Glucocorticoids:** Elevation of bile acids, AST, uric acid, glucose; decreases of calcium, lymphopenia.

## OTHER LABORATORY TESTS

**Vitamin A:** Analysis of liver vitamin A levels remains the most accurate means of diagnosis. Blood vitamin A levels correlate poorly but very high levels support a diagnosis.
**Cannabinoids:** Urine or fecal THC testing. The volume of urine in birds is too small to test alone but urine can be mixed with feces and water to allow enough volume for sampling. Even with a negative test, toxicity is still possible, especially with a history of ingestion or contact.

## IMAGING

Radiographs are necessary for evaluation of organ size but are a non-specific diagnostic. Ultrasound and CT are unlikely to be beneficial in cases of iatrogenic toxicosis.

## DIAGNOSTIC PROCEDURES

N/A

## PATHOLOGIC FINDINGS

N/A

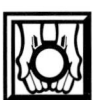

## TREATMENT

### APPROPRIATE HEALTH CARE

Discontinue the medication under the direction of a veterinarian. Some medications still require weaning or tapering.
**Ivermectin/avermectins:** Crop lavage within 1–2 hours if ingested, followed by administration of activated charcoal. Rinsing/bathing with dish soap if applied topically. Methocarbamol and/or midazolam/diazepam if muscle tremors present (22–50 mg/kg IV q12h, followed by 32.5 mg/kg PO). Atropine can be used for bradycardias. IV lipid emulsion 20% bolus then CRI for 1–3 hours. Generalized supportive care—heat, fluid therapy, nutritional support.
**Benzimidazoles:** In acute cases of known overdosing (1–3 hours depending upon species), crop and gastric lavage and activated charcoal can be administered. Unfortunately, most cases are identified after administration. Standard supportive care can be initiated, such as fluid therapy, transfusions. Hematopoietic agents such as erythropoietin or darbopoietin, or leucocyte stimulating agents such as granulocyte colony-stimulating factor or granulocyte/macrophage colony-stimulating factor, can be considered. Prognosis is guarded.

T

**Vitamin A**: Discontinuation of supplementation of vitamin A, along with appropriate general supportive care is usually curative. Secondary infection or other underlying diseases should be addressed concurrently.

**Itraconazole**: Discontinue administration and provide supportive care including fluids and hepatoprotectants. If a single large dose is inadvertently administered, perform crop lavage and follow with activated charcoal. This is only effective within a few hours of ingestion, depending on crop emptying time for the individual species.

**Glucocorticoids**: It is crucial that doses of steroids administered for longer than 10–14 days are tapered rather than stopped abruptly. Use of steroids leads to suppression of normal cortisol production from the adrenal glands and stopping steroids without tapering can lead to iatrogenic hypoadrenocorticism. Supportive care and appropriate antimicrobial therapy may be necessary. Prophylactic antifungal therapy may be indicated in some species, including penguins, raptors and waterfowl.

**Gabapentin**: Treatment is supportive. Activated charcoal can be used if administered immediately after ingestion.

**Cannabinoids**: Supportive care and fluid therapy. Crop lavage if performed immediately after ingestion. Intravenous lipid therapy can be used in severe cases. Midazolam can be administered to control seizures.

### NURSING CARE
Fluid therapy, feeding, and maintaining patient in an appropriate position to enable respiration. If neurologic status is impaired, consider propping up the head and using a 'donut' in the enclosure to keep the bird in an appropriate position with the head elevated. If the bird is unable to move, passive range of motion exercises can be performed.

### ACTIVITY
Restrict activity to a small cage or crate if neurologic status or mentation is impaired. If severely impaired, provide a padded enclosure with no perching materials to keep patient safe from injury or falls.

### DIET
Modification of the diet should is generally not necessary unless the diet is the source of the toxicity. However, supplemental feeding may be required through the illness and recovery. Measures to prevent aspiration, such as small volumes and propping of the head, may be necessary.

### CLIENT EDUCATION
Evaluate all medications used and administered. Always provide appropriately marked syringes and go over the use of all medications at home. Use licensed compounding pharmacies.

### SURGICAL CONSIDERATIONS
N/A

## MEDICATIONS
### DRUG(S) OF CHOICE
Ivermectin/avermectins: Methocarbamol and/or midazolam/diazepam if muscle tremors present (22–50 mg/kg IV q12h, followed by 32.5 mg/kg PO). Atropine can be used for bradycardias. Intravenous lipid emulsion 20% bolus then CRI for 1–3 hours.

### CONTRAINDICATIONS
N/A

### PRECAUTIONS
Ivermectin/avermectins: Avoid concurrent use with drugs that alter p-glycoprotein function; examples that may be used in birds include amiodarone, clarithromycin, doxycycline, fluoxetine, itraconazole, ketoconazole, omeprazole/pantoprazole.

### POSSIBLE INTERACTIONS
N/A

### ALTERNATIVE DRUGS
N/A

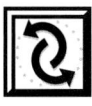

## FOLLOW-UP
### PATIENT MONITORING
N/A

### PREVENTION/AVOIDANCE
N/A

### POSSIBLE COMPLICATIONS
N/A

### EXPECTED COURSE AND PROGNOSIS
N/A

## MISCELLANEOUS
### ASSOCIATED CONDITIONS
N/A

### AGE-RELATED FACTORS
None.

### ZOONOTIC POTENTIAL
None.

### FERTILITY/BREEDING
Avoid ingestion of eggs in poultry or food producing animals during treatment and for appropriate withdrawal periods.

### SYNONYMS
N/A

### SEE ALSO
N/A

### ABBREVIATIONS
AST—aspartate aminotransferase
CRI—constant rate infusion
CT—computed tomography
GI—gastrointestinal
PD—polydipsia
PU—polyuria
THC—tetrahydrocannabinol

### INTERNET RESOURCES
N/A

*Suggested Reading*
Done, L., Ialeggio, D. (2015). Therapeutic use of methocarbamol in a demoiselle crane (*Anthropoides virgo*) with severe ataxia and lateroflexion of the neck. *Veterinary Record Case Reports* 3(1):e000172.
Gozalo, A.S., Schwiebert, R.S., Lawson, G.W. (2006). Mortality associated with fenbendazole administration in pigeons. *Journal of the American Association for Laboratory Animal Science* 45:63–66.
Heggem, B. (2008). Therapeutic review: fenbendazole. *Journal of Exotic Pet Medicine* 17:307–310.
Khan, R.U., Durrani, F.R., Chand, N., Anwar, H. (2010). Influence of feed supplementation with *Cannabis sativa* on quality of broilers carcass. *Pakistan Veterinary Journal* 30:34–38.
Martel A. (2016). Aspergellosis. In: *Current Therapy in Avian Medicine and Surgery* (ed. B.L. Speer), 63–73. St. Louis, MO: Elsevier.
Park, F. (2006). Vitamin A toxicosis in a Lorikeet flock. *Veterinary Clinics: Exotic Animal Practice* 9:495–502.
Shaver, S.L., Robinson, N.G., Wright, B.D., et al. (2009). A multimodal approach to management of suspected neuropathic pain in a prairie falcon (*Falco mexicanis*). *Journal of Avian Medicine and Surgery* 23:209–213.
**Author**: Natalie Antinoff, DVM, DABVP (Avian)

T

# TOXICOSIS (INGESTED, GASTROINTESTINAL)

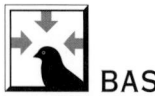

## BASICS

### DEFINITION
Plants, human food items, cleaning products, tobacco products, medicines, and food supplements can be a source of ingested toxins for avian species. Many plants commonly found in and around a home environment are potentially toxic to birds (Table 1). However, there are many other plants considered to be toxic for birds and this list is not comprehensive. Among human food items, avocado toxicosis is associated with a wide range of clinical signs in birds.

### PATHOPHYSIOLOGY
Avocado toxicosis is caused by persin, a fungicidal toxin found in all parts of the avocado. Chocolate contains theobromine and caffeine, both methylxanthines acting as adenosine receptor antagonists resulting in cardiovascular, neurological, and renal signs. Cardiac glycosides affect heart contractility and rhythm. Oxalate crystals cause inflammation of the oropharyngeal mucosa. Protoanemonin, phorbol esters, and cationic detergents are GI irritants. Nitrotoxins are believed to inhibit succinate dehydrogenase and fumarase, resulting in failure of the tricarboxilic acid cycle. Grayanotoxins and dry stems and leaves of *Nicotiana* sp. (tobacco products) are alkaloids inhibiting inactivation of calcium channels, resulting in prolonged depolarization and excitation. They are also significant GI irritants. Sulfur-containing alkaloids are oxidizing agents activated by mechanical manipulation (cutting and crushing of the plant) and affecting erythrocytes resulting in hemolytic anemia. Xylitol may cause hypoglycaemia in some bird species such as nectarivorous species with rudimentary ceca.

## SYSTEMS AFFECTED
**Cardiovascular:** Myocardial necrosis (avocado); altered heart contractility and rhythm (cardiac glycosides, grayanotoxins, tobacco products, theobromine, caffeine); hypo/hypertension (tobacco products); tachycardia, pale mucous membranes, collapse (*Allium*).
**Respiratory:** Related to heart failure (avocado, cardiac glycosides).
**GI:** Swelling/edema of oral mucous membranes (oxalate crystals), GI irritation (protoanemonin, phorbol ester), tissue necrosis and inflammation of the mouth, tongue, pharynx, and esophagus (cationic detergents); nausea, vomiting, diarrhea (theobromine, caffeine, nicotine products).
**Nervous:** Weakness, ataxia, paralysis, seizures and coma (cardiac glycosides, nitrotoxin, grayanotoxins, tobacco products); hyperactivity, muscle tremors, seizures (theobromine, caffeine).

### Table 1

| Common plant toxins, sources and effects. | | | |
|---|---|---|---|
| *Toxins* | *Plant sources* | *Systems affected* | *Clinical signs* |
| Persin | *Persea americana* (avocado) | Cardiovascular | Weakness, depression, dyspnea, shock |
| Cardiac glycosides | *Convallaria majalis* (lily of the valley) *Digitalis purpurea* (foxgloves) Rhododendron sp. *Nerium oleander* (oleander) *Taxus* sp. (yew) *Kalanchoe* sp. | Cardiovascular Nervous | Arrhythmias, cardiac arrest Tremors, ataxia, seizures, coma |
| Oxalate crystals | *Schefflera* sp. (umbrella plant) *Spathephyllum* sp. (peace lily) *Dieffenbachia* sp. (dumb cane) *Philodendron* sp. *Epiprenum* sp. (pothos) *Alocasia* sp. (Elephant's ear) | GI | Swelling/edema of oral mucous membranes, dysphagia, ptyalism, regurgitation, inappetence |
| | *Rheum* (rhubarb) | Renal/urinary GI | Vomiting, swelling/edema of oral mucous membranes, clinical signs of renal failure such as lethargy, polyuria, polydipsia, anorexia, anuria, coma |
| Protoanemonin | *Montana rubens* (clematis) | GI | Diarrhea, ptyalism, vomiting |
| Phorbol ester | *Euphorbia* sp. (poinsettia) | GI | Diarrhea, vomiting |
| Nitrotoxin | *Coronilla varia* (crown vetch) | Nervous | Tachypnea, weakness, ataxia, tremors, collapse |
| Grayanotoxin | Ericaceae family: rhododendron, pieris *Menziesia, Leucothoe, Ledum, Kalmia* | Nervous Cardiovascular GI | Weakness, ataxia, paralysis, coma Bradycardia, hypotension Mucosal irritation, ptyalism, vomiting |
| Sulfur-containing alkaloids | *Allium cepa* (domesticated onion) *Allium porrum* (leek) *Allium schoenoprasum* (chives) *Allium sativum* (garlic) | Hemic Renal/urinary | Lethargy, weakness, tachycardia, pale mucous membranes, collapse, death |

T

**Hemic/lymphatic/immune**: Hemolytic anemia (*Allium*).
**Renal/urologic**: Renal failure (rhubarb, *Allium*), hemoglobinuria and hemoglobinuric nephrosis (*Allium*), polyuria (theobromine, caffeine).

## GENETICS
N/A

## INCIDENCE/PREVALENCE
Between January 2019 and December 2022, the American Society for the Prevention of Cruelty to Animals Animal Poison Control Center managed 2066 calls regarding exotic birds. Avocado exposure represented 8.5% of those calls, chocolate 7.5%, and plants 14.9%.

## GEOGRAPHIC DISTRIBUTION
N/A

## SIGNALMENT
No specific species, age or sex predilection.

## SIGNS
### General Comments
Clinical signs associated with toxic plant ingestion are variable depending on the plant species and quantity consumed. Not all species of birds are equally affected by persin, the toxin of avocado. Median lethal dose (LD50) in budgerigars is approximately 2 g. The adverse effects of avocado may occur as quickly as 15–30 minutes following ingestion, but may also be delayed up to 30 hours. Weakness and depression are usually noted initially, followed by respiratory distress secondary to heart failure. The toxic dose of theobromine and caffeine in avian species is unknown. In dogs, the LD50 of theobromine and caffeine are both reported to be 100–200 mg/kg. In one case, 250 mg/kg theobromine and 20 mg/kg caffeine were retrieved from the crop at necropsy.

### Historical Findings
Potential exposure to plants, human food items, or other ingestible household dangers. Time spent outside of the cage without supervision. Healthy bird in good body condition becoming acutely ill.

### Physical Examination Findings
Weakness, depression, lethargy. Cardiac arrhythmias, tachycardia, bradycardia, hypertension, increased capillary refill time, pale mucous membranes. Tachypnea, dyspnea. Erythematous oropharyngeal mucous membranes, ptyalism, repetitive head-shaking, regurgitation and vomiting, mucoid feces (chocolate), diarrhea. Ataxia, paralysis, tremors, seizures, coma. Discolored urine and urates.

## CAUSES
Toxins affecting the cardiovascular system—persin (avocado), cardiac glycosides (lily of the valley, foxgloves, rhododendron, oleander, yew, *Kalanchoe* sp.), tobacco products, theobromine, caffeine, and, to a lesser degree, grayanotoxin. Toxins affecting the GI system—oxalate crystals (umbrella plant, peace lily, dumb cane, *Philodendron* sp., pothos, elephant's ear, rhubarb), protoanemonin (clematis), phorbol ester (poinsettia), products containing cationic detergents (liquid potpourri, fabric softeners, germicides, sanitizers, etc.), xylitol, theobromine, caffeine. Toxins affecting the nervous system—nitrotoxin (crown vetch), grayanotoxin (Ericaceae family: rhododendron, pieris, menziesia, leucothoe, ledum, kalmia), tobacco products, theobromine, caffeine, and, to a lesser degree, cardiac glycosides. Toxins affecting the hemic system—sulfur-containing alkaloids (allium). Toxins affecting the renal/urinary system—oxalate crystals (rhubarb), sulfur-containing alkaloids (allium).

## RISK FACTORS
The presence of consumable toxic elements in and around the house renders toxic exposure possible. Birds allowed to roam freely out of their cage in the house without supervision or birds that are taken outside to the garden without being directly supervised are at higher risk of ingesting toxic items.

 **DIAGNOSIS**

## DIFFERENTIAL DIAGNOSIS
Degenerative (cardiomyopathy)—history of exercise intolerance, distended coelom. Metabolic (hepatic lipidosis, atherosclerosis)—inappropriate diet, obesity, distended abdomen, palpable liver lobes, liver lobes visualized through the abdominal skin by wetting the feathers, yellow-discolored urates, biliverdinuria, intermittent lameness. Infectious (*Chlamydia*, herpesvirus, reovirus, adenovirus, paramyxovirus, bornavirus)—history of recent exposure to other birds, (*Trichomonas*, *Helicobacter* sp)—stomatitis in cockatiels. Immune–mediated anemia. Traumatic (head trauma)—ecchymosis, skin wound, ocular lesions, ear bleeding, palpable fracture. Toxic (heavy metal toxicosis, mycotoxins, iatrogenic toxins)—GI, urinary, and neurological signs. Other signs may be observed depending on the toxin.

## CBC/BIOCHEMISTRY/URINALYSIS
Indicated to assess evidence of infection, inflammation, and organ function, especially if toxin exposure is not documented. No specific abnormalities reported with most toxins. Electrolyte imbalances and hemoconcentration due to vomiting and diarrhea. Hemolysis, hemolytic anemia, occasional Heinz bodies and hemoglobinuria with allium toxicosis. Hypoglycemia (xylitol).

## OTHER LABORATORY TESTS
None.

## IMAGING
Whole-body radiographs—to evaluate internal organs for abnormalities. Echocardiography—to evaluate the heart for cardiac abnormalities.

## DIAGNOSTIC PROCEDURES
ECG—to evaluate cardiac arrhythmias.

## PATHOLOGIC FINDINGS
Gross and pathological findings will differ depending upon the toxin ingested. Avocado—myocardial necrosis, subcutaneous edema, hydropericardium, generalized congestion. Oxalate crystals—oropharyngeal erythema and edema, renal tubular damage. Allium—hemoglobinuric nephrosis, hepatosplenic erythrophagocytosis. Chocolate—hepatic, renal, and pulmonary congestion; degeneration of hepatocytes, renal tubular cells, and cerebrocortical cells.

 **TREATMENT**

## APPROPRIATE HEALTH CARE
Emergency inpatient intensive care management—patient exhibiting severe depression, cardiac, neurologic, respiratory abnormalities, anemia, and shock. Inpatient medical management—patient vomiting with/without moderate to severe oropharyngeal erythema and edema. Outpatient medical management—patient otherwise normal; therapeutic approach may require brief hospitalization.

## NURSING CARE
Crop lavage—if early decontamination is possible (i.e. within 1–2 hours of ingestion). If clinical signs have already started, decontamination is no longer indicated. Sedation or general anesthesia with endotracheal intubation may be considered to perform crop lavage. Contraindications to crop lavage are ingestion of corrosive substances or petroleum distillates. Stainless steel ball-tipped feeding tube or red rubber feeding tube may be used. The crop is instilled with 20 ml/kg warm saline solution, massaged gently and emptied by aspirating its content. This process is repeated as needed 3–4 times until the crop content has been removed. Proventricular lavage may be considered along with crop lavage. Sedation or general anesthesia with endotracheal

**T**

## TOXICOSIS (INGESTED, GASTROINTESTINAL)    (CONTINUED)

intubation is recommended to perform proventricular lavage. Contraindications to proventricular lavage are ingestion of corrosive substances or petroleum distillates. Red rubber feeding tube may be used. The proventriculus is instilled with 5 ml/kg of warm saline solution, and emptied by aspirating its content. This process is repeated as needed 3–4 times until the proventriculus content has been removed. Fluid therapy may be provided SQ in birds exhibiting mild dehydration (5–7%) or OI/IV in birds with moderate to severe dehydration (> 7%) or critically ill birds exhibiting clinical signs consistent with shock. Oral fluids are contraindicated in birds severely depressed or birds exhibiting GI/neurological signs. In most patients, lactated Ringer's solution, Plasmalyte-A® (Baxter Healthcare, Deerfield, IL), or Normosol®-R (Hospira, Inc., Lake Forest, IL) crystalloid fluids are appropriate. For birds with hypotensive shock, a colloidal solution may be administered concurrently with crystalloids. Blood transfusion should be considered with severe anemia. Oxygen therapy is indicated if respiratory distress or anemia is present; beneficial for any sick avian patient. Warmth (85–90°F/27–30°C) to minimize energy spent to maintain body temperature. Pericardiocentesis may be considered if pericardial tamponade is diagnosed on ECG. Best performed guided by ultrasound under mild sedation.

### ACTIVITY
Patient activity level should be adjusted according to its general status. Birds exhibiting severe illness should be kept in a small, warm environment. Birds showing neurological deficits may require an adapted environment with lower perches and padded surfaces to prevent injury.

### DIET
Birds reluctant to eat may require assisted feeding. Neurological impairment and severe depression increase the risk of aspiration pneumonia. Enteral nutritional preparations may be administered initially at 20–30 ml/kg directly in the crop and the volume administered may be progressively increased according to the patient's tolerance.

### CLIENT EDUCATION
The prognosis of birds following avocado ingestion depends on how quickly treatment is administered. Death may occur if no treatment is provided. This is also true for birds exposed to cardiac glycosides, neurotoxins and sulfur-containing alkaloids. Birds suffering from erythema or edema following ingestion of clematis, poinsettia, or a plant containing calcium oxalates typically recover with symptomatic and supportive therapy.

### SURGICAL CONSIDERATIONS
N/A

## MEDICATIONS
### DRUG(S) OF CHOICE
Activated charcoal (2–8 g/kg of body weight); administer with a gavage tube; not very effective in adsorbing petroleum distillates and corrosive agents; may be repeated q6–8 h on a case-by-case basis to counteract the enterohepatic circulation. Cathartics—magnesium hydroxide may be mixed with activated charcoal (10–12 ml MgOH with 5 ml of activated charcoal PO once); sodium sulfate 2000 mg/kg PO q24h for 2 days. Bulking cathartics—psyllium 2.5 ml mixed with 60 ml water or enteral feeding formula q12–24h, or peanut butter diluted in mineral oil (2 : 1) added to the diet daily until clinical signs resolve (less effective than psyllium). Sucralfate (25 mg/kg PO q8h) indicated to treat oropharyngeal irritation from calcium oxalate ingestion. Diuretics (furosemide 1.0–5.0 mg/kg IM q2–12h for acute treatment and 1–10 mg/kg PO q 8–12h for maintenance once initial stabilization is achieved) may be indicated for pulmonary edema and pericardial effusion. ACE inhibitor (enalapril 1.25 mg/kg PO q 8–12h) may be indicated for heart failure. Bronchodilator (aminophylline 10 mg/kg IV q3h then 4 mg/kg PO q6–12h; 3 mg/ml water or sterile saline for nebulization) may be indicated if respiratory compromise is present. Benzodiazepine may be indicated to control seizures (diazepam 0.5–1.5 mg/kg IV/IO/IN/IM q8–12h; 1 mg/kg/h CRI IV) or sedate anxious or hyperactive patients (midazolam 1–2 mg/kg IM/IN). NSAIDs (meloxicam 0.5–1.0 mg/kg PO/SQ q12–24h in most species) may be considered to alleviate pain from oropharyngeal inflammation. Antioxidants (vitamin E 0.06 mg/kg IM q7d; vitamin C 20–50 mg/kg IM q1–7d) have been suggested with allium toxicity to reduce oxidative erythrocyte damage. However, they have not been shown to be beneficial in cats with onion toxicity.

### CONTRAINDICATIONS
Emesis—emetic medications typically used in mammals are ineffective in birds.

### PRECAUTIONS
Fluid deficits should be addressed prior to using cathartics, diuretics, and NSAIDs. Cathartics may lead to diarrhea and worsen dehydration. All medications used to treat toxic plant or human food items ingestion are off-label use.

### POSSIBLE INTERACTIONS
Activated charcoal may affect drug absorption. Combination of high-dose diuretics and ACE inhibitors may alter renal perfusion.

### ALTERNATIVE DRUGS
None.

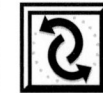

## FOLLOW-UP
### PATIENT MONITORING
Varies with the toxin ingested and the severity of clinical signs.

### PREVENTION/AVOIDANCE
Birds should never have access to toxic plant or human food items in their surroundings.

### POSSIBLE COMPLICATIONS
If the ingested toxin is already absorbed from the GI tract, treatment may be unrewarding. Aspiration pneumonia may occur if a bird vomits and is unable to hold its head upright or swallow properly. Depending on the organ system affected and the toxin involved, chronic changes (cardiac disease, renal disease, liver disease) may persist following recovery.

### EXPECTED COURSE AND PROGNOSIS
Varies with the toxin ingested, the quantity consumed by the bird and the delay between the ingestion and presentation to a veterinarian. Once respiratory signs develop following avocado ingestion, death usually follows quickly. Ingestion of chocolate or cigarette butts left in the household ashtrays have resulted in death. Ingestion of calcium oxalate containing plants is generally associated with a good prognosis with no reported deaths in the avian literature.

## MISCELLANEOUS
### ASSOCIATED CONDITIONS
Heart disease. GI disease. Neurologic disease. Renal/urinary disease.

### AGE-RELATED FACTORS
N/A

### ZOONOTIC POTENTIAL
N/A

### FERTILITY/BREEDING
N/A

### SYNONYMS
N/A

### SEE ALSO
Congestive Heart Failure
Dehydration
Diarrhea

Myocardial Diseases
Mycotoxicosis
Regurgitation and Vomiting
Toxicosis (Airborne)
Toxicosis (Environmental, Pesticides)
Toxicosis (Heavy Metals)
Toxicosis (Iatrogenic)

## ABBREVIATIONS
ACE—angiotensin-converting enzyme
CRI—constant rate infusion
ECG—electrocardiogram
GI—gastrointestinal
IN—intranasal
LD50—median lethal dose
NSAIDs—non-steroidal anti-inflammatory drugs

## INTERNET RESOURCES
N/A

*Suggested Reading*
Gardner, B.R., Mitchell, E.P. (2017). Acute, fatal, presumptive xylitol toxicosis in Cape sugarbirds (*Promerops cafer*). *Journal of Avian Medicine and Surgery*, 31:356–358.
Hargis A.M., Stauber, E., Casteel, S., Eitner, D. (1989). Avocado (*Persea americana*) intoxication in caged birds. *Journal of the American Veterinary Medical Association*, 194:64–66.
Lightfoot, T.L., Yeager, J.M. (2008). Pet bird toxicity and related environmental concerns. *Veterinary Clinics of North America: Exotic Animal Practice*, 11:229–259.
Richardson, J. (2006). Implications of toxic substances in clinical disorders. In: *Clinical Avian Medicine* (ed. G.J. Harrison, T. Lightfoot), 711–719. Palm Beach, FL: Spix Publishing.

Richardson, J.A., Murphy, L.A., Khan, S.A., Means, C. (2001). Managing pet bird toxicoses. *Clinician's Notebook*, 3:23–27.
Wade, L.L., Newman, S.J. (2004). Hemoglobinuric nephrosis and hepatosplenic erythrophagocytosis in a dusky-headed conure (*Aratinga weddelli*) after ingestion of garlic (*Allium sativum*). *Journal of Avian Medicine and Surgery*, 18:155–161.
Wismer T. (2016). Advancements in diagnosis and management of toxicologic problems. In: *Current Therapy in Avian Medicine and Surgery* (ed. B. Speer), 589–599. Saint Louis, MO: Elsevier.

**Author**: Isabelle Langlois, DMV, DABVP (Avian)

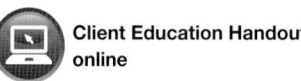 **Client Education Handout available online**

T

# TOXICOSIS (VITAMIN D)

## BASICS

### DEFINITION
Excessive levels of vitamin $D_3$ in the body resulting in hypercalcinosis and associated clinical signs.

### PATHOPHYSIOLOGY
Excessive oral supplementation or parenteral administration of vitamin D, results in increased vitamin D levels in the body. The vitamin D is then converted in the liver to 25-hydroxycholecalciferol and further hydroxylated to 1,25-dihydroxycholecalciferol (cholecalciferol, vitamin $D_3$) in the kidney. There is a negative feedback system attached to this process, while excess dietary supply is absorbed without restraint. Hypervitaminosis D results in excessive uptake of calcium (and phosphate) in the GI tract, thereby mimicking toxic changes seen in hypercalcinosis, such as visceral calcinosis, nephrocalcinosis, visceral gout and urate nephrosis.

### SYSTEMS AFFECTED
**Renal/urologic**: Calcium deposits formed in the kidney (nephrocalcinosis), resulting in polyuria and polydipsia as a result of renal failure and gout.
**Endocrine/metabolic**: Disruption of the calcium homeostasis as the excessive levels of vitamin D result in increased calcium levels in the blood (hypercalcemia).
**Behavioral**: Birds may become disoriented.
**Cardiovascular**: Calcium and uric acid deposits may be formed in the pericardium and/or arterial walls, thereby resulting in acute death. Hypercalcemia may also result in cardiac arrhythmias.
**GI**: Anorexia, nausea, and vomiting may be seen resulting from hypercalcemia and/or hyperuricemia.
**Musculoskeletal**: Painful joints (due to articular gout) and/or muscle weakness may be seen; demineralization of bones may also occur.
**Skin/exocrine**: Accumulation of whitish colored material (calcium deposits) may be present in the skin.
**Reproductive**: Reduced productivity and embryonic mortality may occur in hens that are fed high levels of vitamin D.

### GENETICS
There are currently no indications for an underlying genetic basis.

### INCIDENCE/PREVALENCE
An exact incidence is not known, but the disease is nowadays considered rare due to the increased knowledge regarding commercial hand-feeding formulas for chicks.

### GEOGRAPHIC DISTRIBUTION
N/A

### SIGNALMENT
**Species predilections**: Macaws, particularly blue-and-gold (*Ara ararauna*) and hyacinth (*Anodorrhynchus hyacinthinus*) macaws appear highly sensitive, but the condition may also be found in other species (e.g. cockatiels, grey parrots, cockatoos).
**Mean age and range**: The condition is particularly common in young, developing chicks.
**Predominant sex**: No sex predilection is known.

### SIGNS
#### Historical Findings
Polyuria, polydipsia, anorexia, depression, crop stasis, and weight loss (or poor weight gain); most often involves growing psittacine neonates which are fed a homemade diet or commercially prepared diet to which a vitamin and/or mineral supplement has been added. Single or multiple members of the same clutch may be affected.

#### Physical Examination Findings
Clinical examination may reveal birds in poor condition that appear weak and/or disoriented. Birds may also present with a distended crop, poly- and/or hematuria. Upon physical examination swollen, painful joints (articular gout) and accumulation of whitish colored calcium deposits in the subcutis may also be noted.

### CAUSES
Vitamin D toxicosis may occur when feeding developing birds vitamin D containing supplements and/or by parenteral administration of vitamin D containing supplements. Toxicity is suggested to occur at levels as low as 4–10 times the recommended dose and may be exacerbated by high dietary levels of calcium and/or phosphorus. Toxicity can vary highly between different species (e.g. chickens can tolerate up to 100 times the recommended dose), suggesting different needs and sensitivities to vitamin $D_3$ in the different bird species.

### RISK FACTORS
Neonatal birds fed homemade diets or regular diets supplemented with vitamin D and/or calcium supplements.

## DIAGNOSIS

### DIFFERENTIAL DIAGNOSIS
Pathologic hypercalcemia resulting from other causes, predominantly prolonged and excessive dietary calcium intake. Other causes of hypercalcemia may include primary hyperparathyroidism, pseudohyperparathyroidism (i.e. hypercalcemia associated with neoplasia), and cholecalciferol rodenticide ingestion, but these have not or rarely been reported in birds. Other causes of polyuria and/or polydipsia. Other causes of visceral and/or articular gout, including kidney failure and dehydration. Diagnosis is usually based on the (dietary) history combined with typical radiographic and biochemical changes.

### CBC/BIOCHEMISTRY/URINALYSIS
Blood biochemistry will usually reveal hypercalcemia, hyperphosphatemia and/or hyperuricemia; eucalcemia, however, does not necessarily rule out the condition. Elevated plasma creatine kinase levels have also been noted in affected birds.

### OTHER LABORATORY TESTS
Measurement of vitamin D metabolites in the blood may potentially aid in the diagnosis, although this is not routinely done.

### IMAGING
Radiographic findings include renomegaly and (extensive) mineralization of the kidneys and other organs (e.g. proventriculus, lungs).

### DIAGNOSTIC PROCEDURES
N/A

### PATHOLOGIC FINDINGS
Upon gross pathology, widespread soft-tissue calcification and damage, especially to the kidneys, are the most noticeable findings. Visceral and/or articular gout may also be observed. Special calcium stains are needed to clearly separate urate deposition from calcium deposition.

## TREATMENT

### APPROPRIATE HEALTH CARE
Treatment includes diuresis with crystalloid fluids (e.g. 0.9% NaCl) via the SQ, IV or IO route, in combination with correction of the diet. Diuretics (e.g. furosemide) are added to the treatment in cases of persistent hypercalcemia following diuresis with crystalloid fluids.

### NURSING CARE
Treatment is mostly symptomatic and aimed at promoting forced diuresis, combined with nutritional support (force-feeding) in anorectic patients.

### ACTIVITY
N/A

### DIET
Provision of a well-balanced diet and discontinue use of all supplements immediately. Vitamin $D_3$ concentrations

present in various hand-feeding formulas and formulated diets for adults range from 400 to 2970 iu/kg, thereby following the current recommendations for parrot species (500–2000 iu/kg feed) and therefore need no further supplementation.

### CLIENT EDUCATION
Clients should be aware of the potential risks associated with feeding home-made diets and/or supplementation with vitamins and/or minerals, particularly in breeds such as macaws, as this may result in deficiencies and/or over dosages.

### SURGICAL CONSIDERATIONS
Hypercalcemia may be associated with cardiac arrhythmias. Close anesthetic monitoring is warranted. In addition, provide sufficient fluid support to prevent further renal damage.

## MEDICATIONS
### DRUG(S) OF CHOICE
Furosemide is recommended in cases of persistent hypercalcemia and can be administered in doses of up to 10 mg/kg q12h PO/SQ/IM/IV. In mammals, treatment with calcitonin is advocated for cases of severe and/or persistent hypercalcemia to rapidly decrease the magnitude of hypercalcemia and reduce the resulting tissue damage. No reports, however, exist on the use of calcitonin in birds. Allopurinol can be used in patients with elevated plasma uric acid concentrations, although its use is controversial. In case of nausea, regurgitation and/or crop stasis, the motility-enhancing and anti-emetic drug metoclopramide (0.5 mg/kg q8–12h PO/SQ/IM) may be administered.

### CONTRAINDICATIONS
NSAIDs and other drugs that may impair renal function should be used with caution and their use omitted, if possible. Also omit the use of calcium- and/or vitamin D containing drugs, as these may exacerbate the condition.

### PRECAUTIONS
Caution is warranted when administering drugs for which the kidneys form the main route of excretion, since renal function may be impaired in these patients, thereby resulting in a decreased elimination.

### POSSIBLE INTERACTIONS
N/A

### ALTERNATIVE DRUGS
N/A

## FOLLOW-UP
### PATIENT MONITORING
Closely monitor calcium and phosphate levels as well as renal function (uric acid levels) throughout the therapy.

### PREVENTION/AVOIDANCE
Avoid the use of homemade diets (particularly in neonates), as well as the use of vitamin and/or mineral supplements (including those containing vitamin D precursors) in birds that are fed commercial diets, especially in species prone to hypervitaminosis D.

### POSSIBLE COMPLICATIONS
Renal failure with subsequent hyperuricemia and visceral or articular gout are common.

### EXPECTED COURSE AND PROGNOSIS
Prognosis is usually poor in patients that demonstrate signs of (extensive) tissue calcification and visceral or articular gout.

## MISCELLANEOUS
### ASSOCIATED CONDITIONS
Vitamin D toxicosis is often accompanied by hypercalcemia and hyperuricemia, the latter resulting from renal failure due to nephrocalcinosis.

### AGE-RELATED FACTORS
N/A

### ZOONOTIC POTENTIAL
N/A

### FERTILITY/BREEDING
Hypervitaminosis D in a hen may result in poor reproductive performance and/or embryonic mortality (high levels of vitamin D$_3$ and calcium are transferred to the embryo).

### SYNONYMS
Hypervitaminosis D, vitamin D toxicity.

### SEE ALSO
Dehydration
Hyperuricemia
Hypocalcemia
Polydipsia
Polyuria
Renal Diseases
Thyroid Diseases
Toxicosis (Anticoagulant Rodenticide)

### ABBREVIATIONS
GI—gastrointestinal
NSAIDs—non-steroidal anti-inflammatory drugs

### INTERNET RESOURCES
N/A

*Suggested Reading*
Brue, R.N. (1994). Nutrition. In: *Avian Medicine: Principles and Application* (ed. B.W. Ritchie, G.J. Harrison, L.R. Harrison), 63–95. Lake Worth, FL: Wingers Publishing.
De Matos, R. (2008). Calcium metabolism in birds. *Veterinary Clinics of North America: Exotic Animal Practice*, 11:59–82.
Schoemaker, N.J., Lumeij, J.T., Beynen, A.C. (1997). Polyuria and polydipsia due to vitamin and mineral oversupplementation of the diet of a salmon crested cockatoo (*Cacatua moluccensis*) and a blue and gold macaw (*Ara ararauna*). *Avian Pathology*, 26:201–209.
Takeshita, K., Graham, D.L., Silverman, S. (1986). Hypervitaminosis D in baby macaws. In: *Proceedings of the Annual Meeting of the Association of Avian Veterinarians*, Miami, FL, 341–346.
**Authors:** Yvonne R. A. van Zeeland, DVM, MVR, PhD, DECZM (Avian, Small Mammal), Nico Schoemaker, DVM, PhD, DECZM (Small Mammal, Avian), DABVP (Avian), and Petra Zsivanovis, DrMedVet, DECZM (Avian)

**T**

# TOXOPLASMOSIS

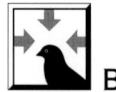 BASICS

## DEFINITION
*Toxoplasma gondii* is an intracellular protozoan parasite of the subphylum Apicomplexa.

## PATHOPHYSIOLOGY
The definitive host is the Felidae family, which includes the domestic cat. Cats become infected from the feces of other cats or from eating birds and rodents. The role of mechanical insect vectors is unknown. Sexual reproduction occurs spontaneously in Felidae, forming unsporulated oocysts. Oocysts are the environmentally resistant stage. Defecated oocysts then sporulate in the environment. *T. gondii* rarely causes clinical disease in most avian species, however potentially all birds can act as an intermediate host. Birds can be infected by ingesting a sporulated oocyte, tissue cysts in prey and contaminated water. Asexual reproduction in the intermediate host. After ingestion of an oocyst or tissue cyst, sporozoites or bradyzoites are released (respectively). Sporozoites or bradyzoites then enter the lamina propria of the small intestines and multiply as tachyzoites. The tachyzoites disseminate via the blood and lymph. After the immune system is activated the tachyzoites form bradyzoites within tissue cyst. Tissue cysts are most common in the CNS, myocardium, and skeletal muscles.

## SYSTEMS AFFECTED
CNS, ophthalmic, renal, musculoskeletal, hepatic, splenic, respiratory.

## GENETICS
N/A

## INCIDENCE/PREVALENCE
All birds can become intermediate hosts and have positive serology results. High seropositivity does not always correlate with clinical disease. Clinical disease has been reported in Passeriformes, Psittaciformes, Strigiformes, Galliformes, Anseriformes, Struthioniformes, Rheiformes, Casuariformes, Sphenisciformes and Pelecaniformes. Prevalence varies, depending on geographical areas and avian species. The seroprevalence is often in the range of 10–40% in wild birds in the USA.

## GEOGRAPHIC DISTRIBUTION
Worldwide including aquatic environments, especially warm, humid climates. Feral cats significantly hinder reproductive programs in Hawaiian birds.

## SIGNALMENT
Canaries and mynahs have unique presentations of toxoplasmosis. Partridges, especially rock partridges (*Alectoris graeca*) and gray partridges (*Perdix perdix*), are more susceptible than other gallinaceous birds. Columbiformes are highly susceptible to disease and barred doves (*Geopelia maugeus*) are the most susceptible. Compared with other passerines, budgerigars (*M. undulatus*) are relatively resistant. Raptors are considered to be resistant to infection, but subclinical disease has been associated with increased vehicular trauma and human perceived behavior changes. Piscivores become exposed to oocysts via contaminated water. Higher trophic levels of terrestrial species had higher exposure to *T. gondii*. Seropositivity in Strigiformes is higher than in Falconiformes and Ciconiiformes. Barred owls (*Strix varia*) had the highest seropositivity in Strigiformes. The acidic stomach of Ciconiiformes is protective of disease and seropositivity was significantly lower (3.8%).

## SIGNS
### General Comments
Clinical signs depend on the number of tachyzoites released, the immune system's ability to prevent the spread of the tachyzoites, and the organs damaged by the tachyzoites.

### Historical Findings
Acute death, and blindness, lethargy, anorexia, weight loss, depression, vague respiratory signs, fluffed feathers.

### Physical Examination Findings
Conjunctivitis, ocular exudates, fever. Respiratory signs—tachypnea, dyspnea. GI ± diarrhea. Myocarditis. Neurologic signs: Blindness, head tilt, torticollis, circling, ataxia, seizure. Columbiformes experimentally infected pigeons showed rapidly progressive renal disease. Canaries (*Serinus canaria*) Birds that do not exhibit or survive the acute phase of the disease will present with the ocular disease (uveitis, conjunctivitis, blepharitis, choroiditis, unilateral ocular atrophy, eyeball collapse, cataracts, optic neuritis, retinal detachment) and neurologic signs from encephalitis (torticollis, circling, twitching, seizures). In one study of canaries with ocular disease, half had encephalitis. Rock partridges (*Alectoris graeca*) succumb primarily from fibrinonecrotic enteritis and occasional desquamation of entire mucosa. If birds survived enteritis, most became clinically normal. Hawaiian crow (*Corvus hawaiiensis*) had involvement in liver, spleen, adrenal gland, and skeletal muscle. Blindness and chorioretinitis have been reported in raptors. Mynahs show acute respiratory signs followed by hepatosplenomegaly, catarrhal pneumonia, myositis. One author believes that this was misdiagnosed atoxoplasmosis.

## CAUSES
Ingestion of infected oocysts.

## RISK FACTORS
Birds fed raw meat. Immune suppression hypothesized (i.e. PBFD). Sedentary birds. Genotype of *T. gondii*. Environment—cat and rodent density; soil contamination rates; mild winters and wet, cool summers; pet birds housed with cats; backyard chickens (vs. free-range organic). Raptors: Higher tropic level in terrestrial species. Close proximity to urban and rural environments. > 1 year of age. Diet higher trophic level for terrestrial species, groundfeeder seropositivity.

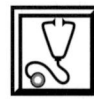 DIAGNOSIS

## DIFFERENTIAL DIAGNOSIS
Histopathology differentials—atoxoplasma and sarcocystis. Infectious—*Chlamydia psittaci*, fungal infections, PMV-1, mycobacteriosis, listeriosis, *Apergillus* sp., sarcocystis, *Baylisascaris*, West Nile virus, eastern equine encephalitis, duck plague, leukocytozoon infection, avian malaria, botulism. Nutritional—hypovitaminosis B, vitamin E or selenium deficiency, hypocalcemia. Vascular—arteriosclerosis, infarct. Trauma. Toxins and medications adverse effects—organophosphates, dimetridazole, heavy metals. CNS disease—hepatoencephalopathy, CNS neoplasia, CNS abscess, epilepsy, avian vacuolar myelinopathy.

## CBC/BIOCHEMISTRY/URINALYSIS
Hemogram: Non-specific changes. Leukopenia or leukocytosis, monocytosis, heterophilia. Biochemistry panel: Results are variable based on the organ affected. Liver: Elevated bile acids, AST. Muscle: Elevated AST, CK. Renal: Elevated uric acid. Hyperproteinemia.

## OTHER LABORATORY TESTS
Sabin–Feldman dye test on pigeon serum. Not effective in sparrows and chickens. Serology (not all tests used in mammals work on avian serum). Modified agglutination test is most sensitive and specific. PCR with *T. gondii*-specific primers. Cerebrospinal fluid tap to diagnose encephalitis.

## IMAGING
Survey radiographs: Hepatomegaly, splenomegaly, pneumonia. CT: Hepatomegaly, splenomegaly, pneumonia, encephalitis.

## DIAGNOSTIC PROCEDURES
Antemortem diagnosis is difficult. Most diagnoses are made on histologic examination. Immunohistochemistry on

brain tissue slides. PCR on brain tissue slides or other infected tissues.

## PATHOLOGIC FINDINGS
**Gross lesions**: Dark red, mottled, edematous lungs; pale and swollen liver, spleen and kidneys, with variable numbers of small pale or dark red foci; sometimes mild multifocal pectoral muscle hemorrhage; sometimes multiple pale foci in the myocardium; sometimes injected meninges or ocular hyperemia.
**Histology**: Mild lymphohistiocytic meningoencephalitis with mild necrosis and parenchymal hemorrhage, and rare tachyzoites or bradyzoites. Non-suppurative chorioretinitis and iridocyclitis, often with subretinal organisms. Lymphohistiocytic to granulomatous and necrotizing hepatitis, splenitis, and interstitial nephritis. Granulomatous to eosinophilic myositis; both skeletal and cardiac muscle can be affected. Granulomatous and necrotizing interstitial pneumonia. Definitive diagnosis of *T. gondii* is made via immunohistochemical analysis or electron microscopy of the shizonts, as standard histology may appear very similar to sarcocystosis.

## TREATMENT

### APPROPRIATE HEALTH CARE
Outpatient care is possible if symptoms are minimal. Inpatient care is necessary for symptomatic birds.

### NURSING CARE
Nutritional support via gavage feeding. Dyspneic birds placed in incubator with 78–85% oxygen supplementation at 5 l/minute. Minimize stress by placing in a quiet, dark cage. Place in warm, humid environment (85°F/27°C and 70% humidity), unless there is evidence of head trauma. Fluid therapy if dehydrated and there is no pulmonary edema: Warm fluids to 100–104°F (38–40°C). Hypotonic fluids contraindicated in birds with salt glands. SQ, IO, or IV, depending on level of dehydration and vascular access. 60–150 ml/day maintenance depending on species plus any additional fluids to correct for dehydration and ongoing losses.

### ACTIVITY
If clinical for disease, activity should be restricted until the patient has made a full recovery.

### DIET
No diet modification is necessary unless anorexic. Nutritional support via gavage feeding for anorexic patients. Gavage 5% of body weight initially and slowly increase

to 8–10% to avoid aspiration. Crop emptying can take 2–4 hours. Change all birds to a nutritionally complete diet.

### CLIENT EDUCATION
Eliminate direct and indirect contact with cats and cat feces.

### SURGICAL CONSIDERATIONS
Pulmonary edema makes patients high risk for anesthetic complications. Consider furosemide prior to biopsy.

## MEDICATIONS

### DRUG(S) OF CHOICE
Pyrimethamine 0.5 mg/kg PO q12 h and trimethoprim-sulfamethoxazole (30 mg/kg PO q8h) for 14–28 days. Diclazuril 10 mg/kg PO q24 h on day 0, 1, 2, 6, 8 and 10 (Passerines). Furosemide 0.1–2 mg/kg PO, SQ, IM, or IV q6–24h to counteract edema. Meloxicam 0.35–1.0 mg/kg PO q12–24h to treat inflammation. One case of infected canaries was successfully treated with trimethoprim/sulfadiazine in the water.

### CONTRAINDICATIONS
N/A

### PRECAUTIONS
N/A

### POSSIBLE INTERACTIONS
N/A

### ALTERNATIVE DRUGS
N/A

## FOLLOW-UP

### PATIENT MONITORING
Monitor for response to treatment and resolution of clinical signs. Monitor the patient's weight once to twice daily to assess nutritional status. Hemocytology—monitor for resolution of leukocytosis or leukopenia. Neurologic cases—perform serial neurologic exams to assess the patient's response to treatment.

### PREVENTION/AVOIDANCE
Prevent access to cat feces. Prevent feral cat access to aviary/zoo collections. Use boot covers to prevent fomite transmission in aviaries. In situations where cats live with birds, scoop litter daily prior to sporulation. Do not feed birds raw meat. Disinfectants: Oocyst inactivated by ammonia, formalin and temperatures > 151°F. Tachyzoites and tissue cysts are susceptible to most disinfectants and pH < 4.0.

### POSSIBLE COMPLICATIONS
Ocular atrophy, blindness, persistent neurologic signs, death.

### EXPECTED COURSE AND PROGNOSIS
Persistent neurologic signs. Death. Experimentally infected pigeons show rapidly progressive renal disease. Asymptomatic infections are common in chickens, ducks, sparrows, and many wild birds. Course and prognosis depend on the number of tachyzoites released, the immune system's ability to prevent the spread of the tachyzoites, and the organs damaged by the tachyzoites. Parasite genotype may also be a factor, but more research is needed.

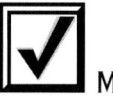

## MISCELLANEOUS

### ASSOCIATED CONDITIONS
Secondary infections from parasites, bacteria, viruses, and/or fungi may be seen.

### AGE-RELATED FACTORS
Clinical disease: none. Raptors > 1 year of age had higher seropositivity rates.

### ZOONOTIC POTENTIAL
Most infections cause no illness to mild clinical signs (flu-like symptoms and lymphadenopathy). Infection in immunocompromised individuals can cause serious, life-threatening disease and can cause mild to severe congenital defects in a fetus. Immunocompromised people: Ataxia, seizures, headache, tuberculosis-like lung disease, seizures, chorioretinitis, weakness, coma, and encephalitis. Pregnancy: Miscarriage, stillbirth, seizure, hepatosplenomegaly, jaundice, chorioretinitis, hydrocephalus, microcephaly, fever, cerebral calcifications, hearing loss, and mental disabilities. Epidemiological studies show a higher infection of *T. gondi* in individuals with schizophrenia, and other psychiatric and behavioral disorders.

### FERTILITY/BREEDING
Avoid the use of sulfonamides in reproductive animals as they may be teratogenic.

### SYNONYMS
N/A

### SEE ALSO
Aspergillosis
Atherosclerosis
Botulism
Hemoparasites
Coccidiosis (Systemic)
Mycobacteriosis

T

# TOXOPLASMOSIS

Nutritional Imbalances
Orthoavulaviruses
Pneumonia
Seizures
Toxicosis (Environmental/Pesticides)
West Nile Virus

## ABBREVIATIONS

AST—aspartate aminotransferase
CK—creatine kinase
CNS—central nervous system
GI—gastrointestinal
PBFD—psittacine beak and feather disease
PCR—polymerase chain reaction
PMV-1—Newcastle disease

## INTERNET RESOURCES

Center for Food Security and Public Health.
Toxoplasmosis: https://www.cfsph.iastate.
edu/diseaseinfo/factsheets

*Suggested Reading*
Ammar S., Wood, L., Su, C., et al. (2021).
   *Toxoplasma gondii* prevalence in carnivorous
   wild birds in the eastern United States.
   *International Journal for Parasitology:
   Parasites and Wildlife*, 15:153–157.
Calton, W.W., McGavin, M.D. (1995).
   *Thomson's Special Veterinary
   Pathology*, 2nd edn. St. Louis, MO: Mosby.
Doneley, R.J.T. (2009). Bacterial and parasitic
   diseases of parrots. *Veterinary Clinics of North
   America: Exotic Animal Practice*, 12:417–432.
Dorrenstein, G.M. (2002). Avian pathology
   challenge. *Journal of Avian Medicine and
   Surgery*, 16:240–244.
Dubey J.P. (2002). A review of toxoplasmosis
   in wild birds. *Veterinary Parasitology*,
   106:121–153.

Harrison, G.J., Lightfoot, T.L. (eds.) (2006).
   *Clinical Avian Medicine*. Palm Beach, FL:
   Spix Publishing.
Lopes, C., Brandao, R., Lopes, A.F., et al.
   (2021). Prevalence of antibodies to
   *Toxoplasma gondii* in different wild bird
   species admitted to rehabilitation centres in
   Portugal. *Pathogens*, 10)1144.
Wilson, A.G., Lapen, D.R., Mitchell,
   G.W., et. al. (2019). Interaction of diet
   and habits predicts *Toxoplasma gondii*
   infection rates in wild birds at a global
   scale. *Global Ecology and Biogeography*,
   29:1189–1198.

**Author**: Erika Cervasio, DVM, DABVP
(Avian, Feline, Canine)
**Acknowledgements**: Kristin Vyhnal, DVM,
MS, DACVP

T

# TRACHEAL AND SYRINGEAL DISEASES

## BASICS

### DEFINITION
Conditions or diseases affecting the larynx, trachea, or the syrinx. The trachea in birds has complete tracheal rings and may show species-specific features, such as the presence of a tracheal sac, diverticulum, bulb, long septum, or extreme coiling and elongation. The syrinx is an organ located at the caudal bifurcation of the trachea, responsible for production of the voice in birds, which involves the vibration of tympaniform membranes within the syringeal tympanum, during the expiratory phase of respiration (in most birds). The syrinx is a particularly complex organ in singing passerines. In passerines and psittacines, syringeal intrinsic muscles are present. In Anseriformes, a syringeal bulla may be present in males.

### PATHOPHYSIOLOGY
Clinical signs are usually caused by the reduction of the tracheal or syringeal lumen caused by tissue proliferation, exudate, foreign bodies, traumatic tracheal collapse, or external compression. In viral diseases (e.g. herpesviruses, poxviruses), tracheal lesions may be part of a systemic disease process. Coughing is a reflex associated with tracheal irritation. Birds rarely cough with cardiomegaly.

### SYSTEMS AFFECTED
Respiratory.

### GENETICS
N/A

### INCIDENCE/PREVALENCE
N/A

### GEOGRAPHIC DISTRIBUTION
N/A

### SIGNALMENT
**Species**: Among Psittaciformes, blue-and-gold macaws are suspected to be at greater risk of post-intubation tracheal stenosis. A variety of other species have been reported with this condition. Tracheal foreign bodies are encountered in small Psittaciformes, especially cockatiels. Certain species (pelagic birds, arctic birds, juvenile birds) may be more prone to respiratory fungal infections.
**Mean age and range**: Any age.
**Predominant sex**: Both.

### SIGNS
#### Historical Findings
Increased amplitude of respiratory movements. Tail bobbing. Respiratory distress, open-beak breathing. Respiratory noises. Coughing. Shaking the head. Voice changes. Voice loss. Lethargy. Anorexia,

weight loss. Collapse. Decreased flight and hunting performance in falconry birds.

#### Physical Examination Findings
Inspiratory dyspnea, or inspiratory + expiratory dyspnea. Increased inspiratory noises upon auscultation. Open-beak breathing. Rhythmic overinflation of the infraorbital sinus. Cyanosis. Abnormal body posture. Inflamed glottis. Mass on the glottis. Foreign body, mites, or tracheal lesions may be visible upon tracheal transillumination.

### CAUSES
**Tracheal stenosis following intubation**: Occurs about 1–2 weeks after an intubation event. The exact causative event is unknown—possibly physical or chemical irritation of the mucosa by the endotracheal tube itself, constant flow of air responsible for focal mucosal desiccation may cause inflammation and promote infection locally in the trachea, which progresses in stenosis of the trachea due to excessive fibrous tissue or granuloma formation. Foreign body (e.g. millet seed, insect part).
**Infectious causes**: Bacterial—various bacterial agents have been implicated in tracheitis, which may lead to tracheal stenosis either by fibrous tissue or granuloma formation: *Chlamydia psittaci* in turkeys. *Bordetella avium* in turkeys. *Mycoplasma* spp. are commonly found in tracheas of birds of prey and are considered commensals. *Enterococcus faecalis* is associated with chronic tracheitis in canaries. *Mycobacterium genavense* has been reported in an Amazon parrot with granulomatous tracheitis. Viral—herpesvirus infections; infectious laryngotracheitis in chickens, *Amazon laryngotracheitis* in Amazon parrots and a few other psittacine species (in recently imported birds), psittacid herpesvirus 1 (glottal lesions, mainly in green-winged macaws), cytomegalovirus in Australian finches, and psittacid herpesvirus-3 or -5 infection in eclectus parrots and Bourke's parakeets. Poxvirus (diphtheric or wet form) in passerine birds, various parakeets, lovebirds, and mynahs. Fungal—*Aspergillus* infection can be responsible for granulomas in the trachea. The syrinx seems to be a site of predilection. Commonly diagnosed in Amazon parrots, grey parrots, macaws, and falcons. Parasitic—*Syngamus* spp. (mainly *Syngamus trachea*), *Cyathostoma* spp. (mainly *Cyathostoma bronchialis*), and acarids such as *Sternostoma tracheacolum* (tracheal, air sac mites). Tracheal worms infest mainly Anseriformes, birds of prey, and poultry, whereas tracheal mites infest primarily canaries and Australian finches.
**Toxic**: Inhaled toxins and smoke-inhalation injuries may cause severe necrotizing tracheitis.

**Trauma**: Attack by a predator or a conspecific may lead to tracheal trauma. Damage to the crista ventralis during intubation in species with this anatomical feature in the glottis, damage to the bronchial bifurcation in certain species (e.g. *Spheniscus* spp. in penguins). Tracheal rupture of unknown cause was also described once in a mallard duck with no history of trauma.
**Nutritional deficiencies**: Hypovitaminosis A has been associated with epithelial changes in the trachea and notably in the syrinx. It is also a risk factor for infectious diseases of the trachea by altering the mucosal defenses and increasing air turbulence. Goiter has been associated with respiratory signs in budgerigars.
**Neoplasia**: Uncommon. Tracheal osteochondroma has been reported in parrots. Masses in the thoracic inlets have been associated with syringeal and bronchial compressions (e.g. tracheal myelolipoma). There is one report of a syringeal melanoma in a grey parrot.
**Tracheal collapse**: Described once in a Pekin duck.

### RISK FACTORS
Post-intubation tracheal stenosis and tracheal trauma—repeated intubation. Intubation too distal in the trachea, where it narrows significantly. Use of cuffed endotracheal tubes. Poor diet, especially lacking in vitamin A or iodine (budgerigars). Previous surgery of the trachea (e.g. tracheotomy). Infectious tracheal diseases may originate from a conspecific (lack of quarantine, persistently infected bird, especially with herpesviruses). Tracheal mites are transmitted from contaminated feces. Exposure to inhalants (polytetrafluoroethylene, smoke, air fresheners, other toxic aerosols). Exposure to intermediate or paratenic hosts for tracheal worms (e.g. earthworms). Exposure to contaminated feces for species with direct life cycle.

## DIAGNOSIS

### DIFFERENTIAL DIAGNOSIS
Nasal and sinus diseases. Lower respiratory diseases (expiratory dyspnea). Cardiovascular diseases with respiratory signs. Iodine deficiency (frequent in budgies) can be responsible for goiter disease that may cause a partial external obstruction of the trachea. Overheating may cause panting and open mouth breathing. Cough mimicking.

### CBC/BIOCHEMISTRY/URINALYSIS
Inflammatory leukogram: Heterophilic leukocytosis and/or monocytosis may be present if an infectious or inflammatory

**T**

process is ongoing. Marked leukocytosis is usually encountered with avian chlamydiosis and aspergillosis, although some cases of aspergillosis may show a normal leukogram. Erythrocytosis may be seen with chronic hypoxemia (more common in chronic lower respiratory diseases).

## OTHER LABORATORY TESTS

Arterial blood gas is the gold standard to assess oxygenation and ventilation. $PaO_2$ ≤ 80 mmHg indicates hypoxemia. Cytology of tracheal/syringeal lesion may help to identify *Aspergillus* hyphae. Bacterial culture and sensitivity of a tracheal swab. Biopsy of lesions, if possible, more sensitive for bacterial and fungal cultures, histopathology. Protein electrophoresis—decreased albumin to globulin ratio, increased concentration of beta and gamma globulins, and decreased concentration of albumin reported with aspergillosis. In falcons with aspergillosis, there can be increased prealbumin concentrations and increased concentration of alpha 2 globulins. Acute phase proteins—possible increase of serum amyloid A and haptoglobin in granulomatous aspergillosis. PCR is Commercially available for *C. psittaci* (conjunctival, choanal, cloacal swab), *Mycobacterium genavense*, *Mycobacterium avium*, *Mycobacterium intracellulare*, *Mycoplasma* spp., psittacid herpesvirus, other viruses. Serology is available for *C. psittaci*—elementary agglutination antibody test (IgM), indirect fluorescent antibody, complement fixation, or ELISA (IgY). Recommended to pair with a PCR test. Serology for aspergillosis is also available but may be of low sensitivity and specificity. Serum galactomannan assay to test and ELISA for anti-*Aspergillus* antibodies to test for aspergillosis seems to be associated with low sensitivity.

## IMAGING

### Radiography

Can be useful in the diagnosis of tracheal stenosis. The affected part of the trachea becomes more radio-opaque, and the tracheal rings, readily visualized, can be irregular or collapsed. The syrinx is more difficult to visualize, due to surperimposition of structures, but syringeal granulomas can usually be identified. Overinflation of caudal air sacs may be appreciated with syringeal diseases causing a valve-like effect resulting in air trapping into these air sacs. The tracheal and syringeal cartilages become calcified with aging and a radiographic conspicuous syrinx is not unusual in older birds. In many male ducks, a large syringeal bulla is also present.

### Computed Tomography

CT had a much increased sensitivity in diagnosing respiratory disorders than radiography and is especially indicated for

perisyringeal diseases, which can be difficult to interpret on radiographs.

### Tracheoscopy

The gold standard to investigate tracheal and syringeal diseases. The procedure must be performed with care not to induce further lesions of the trachea. This is facilitated by the use of a 0-degree scope. The diameter of the scope will depend on the size of the bird (common used diameters are 1.9 and 2.7 mm). Limits of this examination include tracheal length and size of the bird. Psittaciformes lack a pessulus (median syringeal cartilage) in the syrinx.

### Endoscopy

Endoscopy of the interclavicular air sac may be useful to visualize tissues and organs adjacent to the trachea, syrinx, and possible lesions or masses in the thoracic inlet.

## DIAGNOSTIC PROCEDURES

Pulse oximetry measures the hemoglobin saturation in oxygen (likely underestimated by mammalian pulse oximeters). Capnometry measures the end-tidal $CO_2$ in the expired gas: should not be affected in upper respiratory diseases.

## PATHOLOGIC FINDINGS

Pathologic findings will depend on the cause of the disease.

 # TREATMENT

## APPROPRIATE HEALTH CARE

An air sac tube should be placed either in the caudal thoracic or abdominal air sac if tracheal obstruction is suspected. It is also indicated during tracheal surgery for gas anesthesia administration. A tracheoscopy can be performed under anesthesia if the bird is stable or when the air sac tube has been placed. If a lesion partially or completely obstructing the trachea is visualized, endoscopically guided surgical debriding can be performed (e.g. aspergilloma). An endoscopic radiosurgical electrode or $CO_2$ laser may be used. Samples may be taken for diagnostic tests during this same procedure for cytology and culture. Topical administration of an antimicrobial may be performed during the tracheoscopy and is indicated for fungal tracheitis. Removal of foreign body can also be attempted during a tracheoscopy. Endoscopic removal of tracheal worms may be indicated if tracheal obstruction is an issue. Nebulization allows high local concentration of therapeutics, maximizing its efficacy, while minimizing systemic absorption, reducing potential for toxicity, and reducing drug biotransformation. Humidification of the

mucociliary escalator may also improve its efficiency. Because of the trachea and bronchi large diameters, even large particle size (e.g. humidification, vaporization) should be deposited in these locations. Nebulization time is typically 15–30 minutes and frequency is typically once to twice daily. In birds, the respiratory surface and functional efficiency of avian lungs may lead to greater systemic absorption of the drugs being nebulized than in other species.

## NURSING CARE

Oxygen therapy if the patient is dyspneic. Gavage feeding in case of anorexia. Fluid replacement or maintenance therapy. Sedation may be useful to reduce the distress associated with severe dyspnea. Midazolam or midazolam-butorphanol are usually the drugs of choice for mild to marked sedation.

## ACTIVITY

N/A

## DIET

Provide a well-balanced diet.

## CLIENT EDUCATION

Inform the clients of the risk of tracheal stenosis secondary to intubation.

## SURGICAL CONSIDERATIONS

Seed tracheal foreign bodies may be removed with the help of a needle inserted in the trachea just below the seed. The seed is slightly dislodged cranially by the needle's bevel. Then, a syringe should be connected to the needle and air pushed in an attempt to force the seed out through the glottis. Tracheotomy is indicated for removal of foreign objects or surgical debriding for which endoscopic treatment was unsuccessful. In small birds (e.g. cockatiels), tracheoscopy may be challenging and a tracheotomy may be the only option. Tracheotomy of approximately 50% of tracheal circumference is performed between tracheal rings. Once the procedure is completed, the tracheotomy is repaired with absorbable simple sutures comprising at least one ring on each side of the incision with the knots outside of the tracheal lumen. Tracheostomy has been described in parrots and birds of prey. Long-term survival may be poor. Tracheal resection and anastomosis—surgical treatment is necessary in almost all cases of tracheal stenosis; 5–10 tracheal rings or 10% of the tracheal length can usually be removed safely, but up to 12–15 rings have been removed in extreme cases. The anastomosis is performed with absorbable simple sutures comprising at least one ring on each side of the incision. Two additional sutures to counteract tension may be placed when more than 10% of the trachea is removed. Stenting of the trachea has been described using a custom-made nitinol stent

**(CONTINUED)**

in an eclectus parrot, placed by tracheoscopy and fluoroscopy.

## MEDICATIONS

### DRUG(S) OF CHOICE

**Tracheal stenosis**: Dexamethasone 0.05–0.1 mg/kg locally on the affected area in the trachea during tracheoscopy to reduce inflammation. Antibiotics according to results of bacterial culture and sensitivity. A broad-spectrum antibiotic may be used while waiting for the results or if the owner declines the culture (e.g. amoxicilline/clavulanic acid 125 mg/kg PO q12h, enrofloxacin 10–15 mg/kg q12–24h).
**Avian chlamydiosis**: Doxycycline 25–50 mg/kg PO q12h for 21–45 days, long-lasting injectable may be given at 70 mg/kg IM q1w, water-based medication in cockatiels 200–400 mg/l. Azithromycin 10–40 mg/kg PO q24–48h for 21–45 days.
**Aspergillosis**: A combination of antifungal is recommended in confirmed cases. Amphotericin B 1.5 mg/kg IV q12h or voriconazole 10–20 mg/kg IV q12h for 1–3 days. Amphotericin B 0.1–5 mg/ml sterile water intratracheal. Voriconazole 10–20 mg/kg PO q12h. Terbinafine 15–25 mg/kg PO q12h. Antifungals frequently need to be given for several months.
**Parasites**: Ivermectin 0.2–0.4 mg/kg IM, SQ, PO, topical. Repeat for 10–14 days in most cases. Fenbendazole 20–50 mg/kg PO q24h for 5 days. Nebulization: Antibiotics—amikacin 5–6 mg/ml sterile water, enrofloxacin 10 mg/ml sterile water, piperacillin 10 mg/ml sterile water. Antifungals—amphotericin B 0.1–5 mg/ml sterile water, terbinafine 0.01 mg/kg in 5–10 ml sterile saline, voriconazole 10 mg/ml sterile saline. Mucolytic—N-acetyl-cysteine 22 mg/ml sterile water; may induce bronchospasm and may be combined with bronchodilators.

### CONTRAINDICATIONS

Although corticosteroids can be beneficial in the treatment of tracheal stenosis, they are contraindicated if an infection is suspected. Birds are corticoid-sensitive species, so the overall condition of the bird should be carefully evaluated before using steroid medications. Stenotic lesions also frequently harbor secondary pathogens. Systemic adverse effects may also be encountered in birds. Systemic enilconazole and ketoconazole are highly toxic in birds and should not be employed through this route. Triazoles may cause hepatotoxicity in cytochrome P450 sensitive species such as grey parrots. Itraconazole frequently causes anorexia in birds of prey.

### PRECAUTIONS
N/A

### POSSIBLE INTERACTIONS
N/A

### ALTERNATIVE DRUGS
N/A

## FOLLOW-UP

### PATIENT MONITORING

Progression of clinical signs. Regular tracheoscopy to monitor progression of tracheal stenosis and resolution of fungal granuloma or postoperatively to monitor for recurrence (can happen up to several years after the procedure).

### PREVENTION/AVOIDANCE

Intubate with great care, and ensure the endotracheal tube is not inserted too deep inside the trachea. Move the head and neck of intubated birds carefully. Use well-lubricated uncuffed endotracheal tubes. Humidification of oxygen may be performed under anesthesia using humidifiers for inhalant gas. Provide a well-balanced diet. Quarantine any new bird to limit the risk of contagious infectious disease. Reduce access to intermediate parasite host (e.g. limiting access to the ground—earthworms). Limit exposure to household toxic inhalants.

### POSSIBLE COMPLICATIONS

Severe dyspnea, cyanosis, death if not treated. Complications of surgery—bleeding, dehiscence, subcutaneous emphysema, recurrence of stenosis over time. Voice changes may also be encountered due to neurologic and muscular trauma on syringeal muscles and modification of tracheal airflow.

### EXPECTED COURSE AND PROGNOSIS

Medical therapy has not been associated with good results in tracheal stenosis and recurrence and postoperative complications have been reported commonly after tracheal resection and anastomosis. The prognosis for tracheal stenosis is therefore guarded. Aspergillosis is associated with a guarded prognosis as treatment is long and difficult. Other causes of tracheal disease are usually associated with a good prognosis after adequate treatment is given.

## MISCELLANEOUS

### ASSOCIATED CONDITIONS

Associated conditions may be associated with the etiology of the tracheal disease (e.g. aspergillosis granulomas, if present in the trachea, can also be found elsewhere),

so imaging of the whole body is recommended. *C. psittaci* can also be responsible for hepatitis, pneumonia and airsacculitis. *Mycoplasma* infection is often responsible for conjunctivitis and sinusitis in Columbiformes, Passeriformes, and Galliformes.

### AGE-RELATED FACTORS
None.

### ZOONOTIC POTENTIAL
Avian chlamydiosis is a zoonotic disease.

### FERTILITY/BREEDING
N/A

### SYNONYMS
N/A

### SEE ALSO
Air Sac Mites
Air Sac Rupture
Aspergillosis
Aspiration Pneumonia
Avian Influenza
Chlamydiosis
Herpesvirus (Columbid Herpesvirus 1 in Pigeons and Raptors)
Herpesvirus (Duck Viral Enteritis)
Herpesvirus (Passerine Birds)
Herpesvirus (Psittacid Herpesviruses)
Mycoplasmosis
Neoplasia (Respiratory)
Nutritional Imbalances
Orthoavulaviruses
Poxvirus
Respiratory Distress
Thyroid Diseases
Toxicosis (Airborne)
Trauma

### ABBREVIATIONS
CT—computed tomography
ELISA—enzyme-linked immunosorbent assay
IgM—immunoglobulin M
IgY—immunoglobulin Y
$PaO_2$—partial pressure of arterial oxygen
PCR—polymerase chain reaction

### INTERNET RESOURCES
N/A

*Suggested Reading*
Adair J.E., Riggs G.L. (2022). Surgical repair of a complete transverse tracheal rupture in a mallard duck (*Anas platyrhynchos*). *Journal of Avian Medicine and Surgery*, 35:451–456.
Clippinger, T.L., Bennett, R.A. (1998). Successful treatment of a traumatic tracheal stenosis in a goose by surgical resection and anastomosis. *Journal of Avian Medicine and Surgery*, 12:243–247.
Dennis, P.M., Avery Bennett, R.A., Newell, S.M., Heard, D.J. (1999). Diagnosis and treatment of tracheal obstruction in a cockatiel (*Nymphicus hollandicus*). *Journal of Avian Medicine and Surgery*, 13:275–278.

T

Henry-Guyot E., Langlois I., Lanthier I. (2016). Tracheal collapse in a pekin duck (*Anas platyrhynchos domestica*). *Journal of Avian Medicine and Surgery*, 30:364–367.

Jankowski, G., Nevarez, J.G., Beaufrère, H., et al. (2010). Multiple tracheal resections and anastomoses in a blue and gold macaw (*Ara ararauna*). *Journal of Avian Medicine and Surgery*, 24:322–329.

McLelland, J. (1965). The anatomy of the rings and muscles of the trachea of *Gallus domesticus*. *Journal of Anatomy*, 99:651–656.

Passarelli M.E., Antinoff N., Hudson C., et al. (2020). Removal of a tracheal myelolipoma in a cockatiel (*Nymphicus hollandicus*) by surgical resection and anastomosis. *Journal of Avian Medicine and Surgery*, 34:181–185.

Sanchez-Migallon Guzman, D., Mitchell, M., Hedlund, C.S., et al. (2007). Tracheal resection and anastomosis in a mallard duck (*Anas platyrhynchos*) with traumatic segmental tracheal collapse. *Journal of Avian Medicine and Surgery*, 21:1500–1157.

Yaw, T.J., Doss, G.A., Colopy, S.A., et al. (2020). Emergency tracheotomy and subsequent tracheal resection and anastomosis in a blue crane (*Anthropoides paradiseus*), *Journal of the American Veterinary Medical Association*, 256:1262–1267.

**Authors**: Delphine Laniesse, DVM, DVSc, DECZM (Avian), and Hugues Beaufrère, DrMedVet, PhD, DABVP (Avian), DECZM (Avian), DACZM

T

# BASICS

## DEFINITION
A wound or injury to any body system.

## PATHOPHYSIOLOGY
Blunt force resulting in injury to the body or head. Laceration, abrasion, or puncture wound to the skin or musculature. Self-mutilation secondary to behavioral abnormalities, pain, or discomfort. Edema or subcutaneous hemorrhage secondary to electrical shock. Head trauma results in direct damage to the intracranial structures, disturbance of autoregulatory mechanisms, (depletion of ATP, electrical gradient damage, and glutamine release), failure of pressure autoregulation of arteries and damage to the cerebral ischemic response. Ocular trauma can affect behavior, flight, breeding, and feeding. Wounds heal by primary or secondary intention. Spine of the birds is susceptible to injury at the junction of the thoracolumbar spine and the fixed synsacrum. There are 3 phases of wound healing: (1) Inflammatory phase occurs in first 0–36 hours. Clot formation. Leukocyte, monocyte, plasma cell, and macrophage infiltration. Necrotic material, bacteria, and debris phagocytized. (2) Proliferative/collagen phase occurs from 3–4 days; microfibril aggregates form and capillaries bud into the wound area. (3) Remodeling/maturation phase occurs from weeks to months; there is remodeling of collagen to achieve normal strength. Delay in wound healing can be due to foreign material, necrosis, poor blood supply, excessive tension, motion, malnutrition, dehydration, hypoproteinemia, anemia, sepsis, and location (keel, extremities).

## SYSTEMS AFFECTED
Skin/exocrine, musculoskeletal, cardiovascular, behavioral—as primary cause of self-induced trauma, neuromuscular, neurologic, ophthalmic, respiratory.

## GENETICS
N/A

## INCIDENCE/PREVALENCE
Trauma is a common avian emergency.

## GEOGRAPHIC DISTRIBUTION
Worldwide.

## SIGNALMENT
Paired cockatoos—the male often attacks the female mate (especially in hand-reared Moluccan cockatoos). Paired eclectus parrots: the female often attacks the male mate. Wildlife. Birds with flight or allowed unsupervised activity outside the cage. Bustards, storks and cranes—keel injuries

from charging enclosures. Cockatoos have a higher incident of self-mutilation. Quaker parakeets have a severe and sometimes fatal self-mutilation syndrome. Macaws—palatine bone avulsion. Wildlife—predation, fishing gear injuries, window strikes, traumatic brain injuries, and vehicular, windmill, and power-line impact.

## SIGNS

### Historical Findings
Recent blunt force trauma. Fight with another animal. Pair-bonded birds. Active bleeding. History of behavioral abnormalities/self mutilation. History of night fright. Unsupervised activity.

### Physical Examination Findings
Abnormal posturing. Beak fractures, avulsions, depressions, luxation, luxation of palatine bone in macaws. Bleeding of broken blood feather. Bradycardia. Brachial plexus, pelvic nerve avulsion. Cranial nerve or peripheral nerve deficits. Cold distal extremities. Collapse. Coma. Damaged or missing feathers. Death. Dehydration and hypovolemia. Dyspnea. Ecchymosis, green discoloration in later stages. Fracture(s) or malposition of a limb. Hemorrhage. Horner syndrome. Hypermetria. Hypothermia (measure cloacal temperature in birds > 150 g). Laceration, abrasion or puncture wound to the body or head. Laceration caudal to vent secondary to a fall. Lens luxation. Lethargy. Muscle atrophy. Recumbency. Seizures. Shock. Tachycardia. Tachypnea. Wing droop.

## CAUSES
Cannibalism in chickens and quail—environment, overcrowding, diarrhea. Behavioral/self-mutilation—anxiety, attention seeking behavior, boredom, compulsion disorders, displacement behaviors, overcrowding, pain. Gunshot wound. Iatrogenic—aggressive nail or wing trims, blood oversampling, laceration of blood vessels during venipuncture, recent surgery and failure to use proper hemostatic techniques, bursitis in tethered birds of prey, gavage feeding. Vehicular and windmill impact. Flying into a window or other stationary objects. Interaction with another pet or predatory species. Electrical shock from power-line impact. Chemical exposure. Recent fall—aggressive wing trim, cardiac disease, neuromuscular disease, night fright. Neuromusculoskeletal disease that causes weakness. Poultry—predators, cannibalism, cage entrapment/injury, self trauma (nails, beaks, spurs).

## RISK FACTORS
Aggressive cage mate. Birds with flight. Housing with a cage mate. Unsupervised activity.

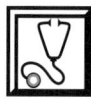

# DIAGNOSIS

## DIFFERENTIAL DIAGNOSIS
Coagulopathies. Dermatopathy. Nutritional deficiencies. Infection. Systemic disease. Neoplasia. Neurologic disease.

## CBC/BIOCHEMISTRY/URINALYSIS
Caution must be used in birds with excessive hemorrhage. Only 1% of the bird's weight in grams is recommended for blood work. (i.e. 1 ml blood for every 100 g body weight). Therefore, all blood loss from hemorrhage and bruising must be taken into account.

## OTHER LABORATORY TESTS
**Biochemistry panel**: Liver enzyme abnormalities (elevated AST, LDH, GGT and ALT). Elevated CK and potassium.
**Hemogram**: Anemia, typically defined as a PCV < 3–5%; however, normals can vary with different species. PCV will normalize in 2–7 days after acute blood loss. Will show as non-regenerative in acute hemorrhage (< 2 days). May show signs of regeneration between 2 and 7 days. Polychromasia, reticulocytosis, macrocytosis, anisocytosis. Polychromasia is noted in mallard ducks 12 hours post-hemorrhagic event. Decreased hemoglobin levels. Hypoproteinemia. Thrombocytopenia secondary to consumption.
**Biochemistry panel**: Muscle and liver enzyme abnormalities. Electrolyte abnormalities.
**Urinalysis**: Hematuria. Blood in stools.

## IMAGING
**Survey radiographs**: May identify fractures, luxation, subluxation of the spine, air sac rupture, SQ emphysema, visceral damage, loss of serosal detail, separation of liver from sternum (air sac rupture), microcardia, or bullet fragments. Survey radiographs of passerines for window strike.
**MRI/CT/scintigraphy**: Fractures, luxation, subluxation, and visceral damage. Spinal injury and brain injury. Ruptured intervertebral disc. Thrombus.

## DIAGNOSTIC PROCEDURES
Blood pressure measurement can be considered to access cardiovascular status. Intraocular pressure to identify uveitis and glaucoma (varies with species of bird).

## PATHOLOGIC FINDINGS
Hemorrhage, bruising, and tissue necrosis from a laceration or puncture wound. Edema, subcutaneous hemorrhage, and burned feathers are possible as a result of electrical shock. Fractures or malposition of any bone. Damaged and missing feathers as a result of feather damaging behavior.

T

Head trauma: Hemorrhage in the epidural, subdural and/or leptomeningeal areas and in the brain parenchyma, cerebral edema, extracerebral haemorrhage. In animals, the margin of error in a concussive injury that results in unconsciousness or death is small due to the small size of the patient's brain. Spinal trauma: Bony changes sufficient to cause severe spinal trauma may not be visible radiographically. Spinal edema, necrosis, microvascular injury. Non-specific histologic findings may include evidence of digestion chambers, Wallerian degeneration, and/or neuronal loss.

# TREATMENT

## APPROPRIATE HEALTH CARE
Outpatient medical management is possible if the hemorrhage is minimal, the laceration or abrasion is small, or in broken blood feathers that have not resulted in excessive blood loss. Inpatient medical management is required in cases of excessive blood loss. USFWS regulates possession and treatment of wildlife. States may also regulate care.
**Address active hemorrhage**: Hemostasis, silver nitrate, styptic powder, potassium permanganate, electrocautery, emergency surgery as indicated, compression or pressure wrap application (apply compression for 30–60 seconds; avoid compression of the keel).
**Beak injuries**: Collision injury, bite wounds, and falls. Provide nutritional and fluid support. Loss of greater than one-third of the rostral beak leads to permanent deformity. Medically manage superficial puncture wounds. Cement plugs in deeper puncture wounds. Fractures and luxations—debride necrotic tissue, pin placement, cerclage wires, and PMMA bone cement.
**Bursitis**: Antibiotics, anti-inflammatory medications, bandaging.
**Broken blood feather**: Remove broken blood feather (can result in damage to the feather follicle). Surgical closure if indicated.
**Bleeding/avulsed nail**: Trim/file rough edges of nail. Apply bandage. Amputation if indicated.
**Imping**: For birds that fall due to excessive wing trims.
**Fracture repair**: Correct bending, axial and rotational forces. External coaptation—body wrap for coracoid fractures and humeral fractures. Do not constrict respirations. Figure of eight bandage for fractures distal to elbow. Ball bandage and snowshoe splints for digit fractures; birds < 80–150 g—tape splints of tibiotarsus and tarsometatarsus; combined tape splints with thermoplastic bandage for birds up to 600 g. Internal fixation—IM pins, cerclage wires, and plates.

Implant removal necessary due to weight. Plate placement high risk for iatrogenic fracture. External fixation—monitor for pin loosening and osteomyelitis.

### Wound Care
Bite wounds from other birds most often occur on head, digits, and feet. Falls most often result in keel and ventral coccygeal injuries. Trim tail feathers to prevent repeat trauma. Clean and remove feathers 2–3 cm from wound and clean. Remove devitalized tissue and foreign material. Lavage with 0.9% saline, LRS, dilute chlorhexidene or dilute povidone iodine. Use drains only with active flushing systems. Endoscopic or surgical removal of bullet fragment. Wound closure with primary or secondary intention. Primary closure: Debride and suture wounds. Minimize tension in wound closure. Secondary closure: Apply topical ointments and occlusive dressing with 90% water. (1% silver sulfadiazine cream, triple antibiotic cream). Use absorbable sutures. Give broad-spectrum antibiotics and pain management. Prevent access with a wrap or Elizabethan collar. Physical therapy to minimize fibrosis. Remove sutures when completely healed.

### Head Trauma
Treat to maintain cerebral perfusion, decrease edema, and control intracranial pressure. Treat hemorrhage. Oxygen supplementation. Start at 40% and wean to 21% over 3 days. Avoid respiratory compromise with over-supplementation of $O_2$. Budgerigars developed oxydative stress at 95% $O_2$ within 3 hours. Keep at lower end of preferred body temperature. Treat hypovolemia and cerebral edema with low-volume resuscitation with HSS (3 ml/kg) over 10 minutes. ± HES at 3 ml/kg IV/IO. If unavailable, decreased IVF rate by 33–50%. Mannitol: Secondary choice to HSS, 0.25–1.0 g/kg over 15–20 minutes. Repeat q4–6h for a total of 3 doses within 24-hour period. Contraindicated in hypovolemia. Use in patients with hypernatremia. Maintain normoglycemia and avoid hyperglycemia. Jugular venipuncture is contraindicated. Keep quiet and in low light and padded cage. Elevate head 25–30 degrees if recumbent. Perform serial neurological exams q30–60 m. Pain management—butorphanol 1–2 mg/kg IM q2–4h. Use caution with opiods due to respiratory depression. Steroids contraindicated. Once hydrated, meloxicam 0.5–1 mg/kg IM q12h. Control seizures with a propofol CRI, benzodiazepines, or antiepileptics.

## NURSING CARE
Minimize stress by placing in a quiet area with minimum traffic. Place in warm, humid environment (85–90°F/27–30°C and 70% humidity), unless there is evidence of head

trauma. Dyspneic birds place in incubator with 78–85% oxygen supplementation at 5L/minute. Stop access to feathers in self-mutilation cases with a collar designed for birds, wraps, or bandaging.

## ACTIVITY
Activity should be restricted until the wound has healed, PCV normalizes, and the patient has made a full recovery. Place in a smaller cage and restrict flight. Pad bird to prevent all movement in spinal injury. Remove perches, provide soft bedding and easy access to bowls.

## DIET
No diet modification is necessary unless anorexic. Correct hydration before correcting nutrition. Nutritional support via gavage feeding for anorexic patients. Gavage 5% of body weight initially and slowly increase up to 8–10% to avoid aspiration. Crop emptying can take 2–4 hours. Esophagotomy tube placement for beak injuries. Change all birds to a nutritionally complete diet.

## CLIENT EDUCATION
Debilitated birds have a poor prognosis despite treatment. Discuss the importance of avian enrichment. Discuss the potential risks in the birds every day environment.

## SURGICAL CONSIDERATIONS
Necessary if bleeding cannot be stopped with pressure. Electrocautery should be used to minimize blood loss. Prior to surgery, patients with hypotension, excessive blood loss, or hypovolemic shock should be stabilized. Electrocautery should be used to minimize blood loss.

# MEDICATIONS

## DRUG(S) OF CHOICE

### Fluid Therapy
Warm fluids to 100–104°F (38–40°C) and monitor for hyperthermia. Hypotonic fluids contraindicated in birds with salt glands. Subcutaneous or oral fluids indicated for mild levels of blood loss and maintenance. Crystalloids should be sufficient. Contraindicated in hypovolemia, hypothermia, and shock due to peripheral vasoconstriction. Correct for 4–5% of fluid loss (0.04–0.05 × body weight/kg × 1000) in addition to maintenance. Divide into multiple doses as dictated by volume. SQ fluids: Place up to 10 cc/kg in each SQ injection site. Use the inguinal web, intrascapular and axillary areas. LRS absorb well. Contraindications: Hypertonic fluids and colloids and fluids containing > 2.5% dextrose, brown pelicans and turkey vultures. IO/IV fluids indicated for moderate levels of blood loss, surgery, or hypothermia. Allow for rapid administration and dissemination of

fluids. IV catheter 22–26 gauge in jugular, basophilic, ulnar, or medial metatarsal vein; may be difficult in birds < 100 g. IO catheter in distal ulna or proximal tibiotarsus. Contraindicated in the ulna of Cathartiformes. Confirm placement with radiographs. Higher risk of joint complications and infections. Avoid puematic bones. Correct for 4–8% of fluid loss (0.04–0.08 × body weight/kg × 1000) in addition to maintenance; 80% of fluid deficit should be replaced over 6–8 hours in acute loss and over 12–24 hours in chronic loss. Consider adding a colloid (3–5 ml/kg), especially if hypotensive, hypovolemic, or hypoproteinemic. Contraindicated in coagulopathy, congestive heart failure, renal disease, pneumonia. LRS contraindicated for rapid effusion. Plasmalyte-A® (Baxter Healthcare, Deerfield, IL) closest to avian plasma.

### Management of Hypovolemic Shock
Management of hypovolemic shock due to blood loss: TP <1 g/dl and no anemia, consider plasma transfusion. Replace via IO/IV catheter. Assess blood pressure, heart rate, mucus membranes, and CRT to assess response to treatment. Repeat fluid boluses until the blood pressure is greater than 90 mmHg. Treat in the following order: HSS (3–5 ml/kg) over 10 minutes ± HES (3 ml/kg) bolus, 09% NaCl (3 ml/kg) and HES (5 ml/kg) bolus over 10 minutes, 10–25 ml/kg crystalloid boluses over 5–7 minutes. Replace 10% body weight. Once stable, place on crystalloids for maintenance, deficits, and ongoing losses. If there is no response to above treatments, check blood glucose, PCV/TP and ECG. If hypoglycemic, give 50% dextrose 50–100 mg/kg IV slow to effect; dilute 1:1 with 0.9% saline.

### Additional Medications
Additional medications may be needed based on the disease process. Blood transfusion. Psychotropic drugs for self-mutilation. Erythropoietin/iron dextran (anemia). Vitamin B supplementation (anemia).

### Pain Management
Butorphanol: dosing varies on species. Meloxicam may be contraindicated in active hemorrhage. Nutritional support via gavage feeding. Ocular trauma: Anti-inflammatory drugs, systemic and topical antibiotics. Chose broad-spectrum antibiotics for lacerations and abrasions; for bites, choose piperacillin or a fluoroquinolone.

### CONTRAINDICATIONS
Corticosteroids weaken the immune system and complicate head trauma due to fluid retention and hyperglycemia. Jugular phlebotomy and supplemental heat in patients with head trauma. Phlebotomy if greater than 1% of blood loss has occurred. Jugular venipuncture in head trauma. Hemorrhage: Avoid drugs with anticoagulant of anti-platelet effects. (NSAIDs, clopidogrel, sulfonamindes, heparin, warfarin, plasma expanders, estrogens, cytotoxic drugs). Adequan® (American Regent Animal Health, Shirley, NY; polysulfated glycosaminoglycan) hss been associated with fatal hemorrhage/bleeding diathesis in multiple avian species. Avoid over-heparinization.

### PRECAUTIONS
Indirect blood pressure measurement does not always correlate with direct arterial measurement but it can provide information about blood pressure trends.

### POSSIBLE INTERACTIONS
N/A

### ALTERNATIVE DRUGS
N/A

## FOLLOW-UP

### PATIENT MONITORING
Monitor for response to treatment and resolution of clinical signs (heart rate, CRT, mucus membrane quality). Perform serial blood pressure measurements until normalized. Head trauma—perform serial neurologic exams to assess patient's response to treatment. Monitor the patient's weight once to twice daily to assess nutritional status. Fractures—splints should be assessed weekly until removal and surgical stabilization should be monitored once to twice weekly. Monitor for cessation of active bleeding and petechiation formation. Stabilization/normalization of hematocrit/PCV and total solids, typically occurs within 2–7 days. Hemorrhagic/hypovolemic shock—resolution of tachycardia, bradycardia, hyper or hypertension. Normalization of PCV/TS typically occurs within 3–6 days. Monitor PCV/total solids daily in the acute phase and CBC routinely.

### PREVENTION/AVOIDANCE
Perform routine wing trimming if the bird cannot be kept safely in the environment. Provide enrichment and behavior modification for self-mutilating patients. Discuss risk of unsupervised interaction with another animal or unsupervised activity. Use appropriate wing trimming techniques. Discontinue reinforcement behavior. Cannibalism: Decrease light, provide proper nutrition, decrease bird density, keep vents clean, red spectacles for individual aggressive poultry.

### POSSIBLE COMPLICATIONS
N/A

### EXPECTED COURSE AND PROGNOSIS
Varies with the severity of traumatic injuries. Nerve and vascular damage may have poor prognosis for healing and return to function, especially if the extremities are involved. Spinal fractures and loss of deep pain have a poor prognosis. Leg amputation carries a poor prognosis and is contraindicated in raptors. USFWS prohibits amputation above the elbow, release of blind birds, amputation of leg or foot, and inability to feed, perch, or ambulate. Treatment and release of wildlife should be based on age, species, hunting style, and degree of impairment.

## MISCELLANEOUS

### ASSOCIATED CONDITIONS
Myiasis; 30–75% of raptors with traumatic injuries have concurrent ocular lesions.

### AGE-RELATED FACTORS
Young more prone to trauma from improper wing trimming.

### ZOONOTIC POTENTIAL
N/A

### FERTILITY/BREEDING
Avoid teratogenic antibiotics in laying hen. Traumatic injury can result from a conspecific, particularly with breeding pairs of cockatoos and eclectic parrots.

### SYNONYMS
Injury, wounds, contusion abrasions.

### SEE ALSO
Anemia
Beak Injury
Beak Malocclusion (Lateral Beak Deformity)
Beak Malocclusion (Mandibular Prognathism)
Feather Cyst
Feather Damaging and Self-Injurious Behavior
Feather Disorders
Fractures
Hemorrhage
Joint Diseases
Lameness
Luxations
Neurologic (Trauma)
Ocular Lesions
Phallus Prolapse
Pododermatitis
Problem Behaviors: Aggression, Biting and Screaming
Seizures
Toe and Nail Diseases
Wounds (Including Bite Wounds, Predator Attacks)

T

# TRAUMA

## ABBREVIATIONS
ALT—alanine transverse
AST—aspartate aminotransferase
ATP—adenosine triphosphate
CBC—complete blood count
CK—creatine kinase
CRI—constant rate infusion
CRT—capillary refill time
CT—computed tomography
ECG—electrocardiogram
GGT—gamma-glutamyl transferase
GI—gastrointestinal
HES—hetastarch
HSS—hypertonic saline solution
LDH—Lactate Dehydrogenase
LRS—lactated Ringer's solution
MRI—magentic resonance imaging
NSAIDs—non-steroidal anti-inflammatory drugs

PCV—packed cell volume
PMMA—polymethyl methacrylate
TP—total protein
USFWS—United States Federal Wildlife Service

## INTERNET RESOURCES
N/A

*Suggested Reading*
Fordham, M., Roberts, B.K. (eds.) (2016). Emergency and critical case (special issue). *Veterinary Clinics of North America: Exotic Animal Practice.* 19(2):i–xiv, 325–668.
Graham, J.E., Doss, G.A., Beaufrère, H. (2021). Part II: Avian. In: *Exotic Animal Emergency and Critical Care Medicine*, 431–694. Hoboken, NJ: Wiley Blackwell.

Lichtenberger, M., Lennox, A. (2016). Critical care. In: Current Therapy in Avian Medicine and Surgery (ed. B Speer), 582–588. St. Louis, MO: Elsevier.
**Author**: Erika Cervasio, DVM, DABVP (Avian, Canine, Feline)
**Acknowledgements**: Heather W. Barron, DVM, DABVP (Avian), DECZM (Avian), Rebecca Duerr, DVM, MPVM, PhD, Marla Lichtenberger, DVM, DACVECC, Kristin Vyhnal, DVM, MS, DACVP, Jorg Mayer, DVM, MS, DABVP (ECM), DECZM (Small Mammal)

 **Client Education Handout available online**

# BASICS

## DEFINITION
Trichomoniasis is disease due to infection with a trichomonad protozoan: usually *Trichomonas gallinae*, *Trichomonas columbae* (usually affecting the upper digestive tract), or *Tetratrichomonas gallinarum* (usually affecting the lower digestive tract and ceca but occasionally found in livers and other sites). There are other *Trichomonas* species, and other trichomonads, that have been identified in birds, with fewer data on pathogenicity.

## PATHOPHYSIOLOGY
Infection occurs with a virulent organism from a contaminated environment or direct contact with infected birds, after a 4- to 18-day incubation period; *T. gallinae* and *T. columbae* damage and cause caseated material and adherent plaque buildup on the mucosa of the oropharynx, the digestive tract down to and including the proventriculus, and to the upper and sometimes lower respiratory system (sinuses, trachea, and even air sacs). There is also pathology from invading visceral tissue especially the liver. *T. gallinarum* affects the intestines and the ceca. There are less-virulent strains and infection with these strains may provide cross-protection from more virulent strains. Birds can be co-infected with multiple species of trichomonads.

## SYSTEMS AFFECTED
**Gastrointestinal**: Via damage by the organism and a foreign body effect by the space-occupying lesion (caseated mass) production.
**Neurologic**: Via intracranial and ocular or periocular tissue invasion.
**Respiratory**: Blockage with caseated material.
**Behavioral**: Especially in reaction to the general irritation from the parasite, and overall lethargy.
**Hepatobiliary**: Due to invasion into liver.

## GENETICS
N/A

## INCIDENCE/PREVALENCE
Common.

## GEOGRAPHIC DISTRIBUTION
Worldwide, found in captive and wild species. Significant conservation concern.

## SIGNALMENT
**Species**: *T. gallinae*, *T. columbae*: pigeons (and other doves), raptors, passerines (including canaries), budgerigars, cockatiels, other parrots, mynahs, poultry. *T gallinarum*: poultry and other gallinaceous birds, sea birds, and waterfowl. Trichomonads are suspected to have caused disease in fossilized relatives of birds, demonstrating broad species involvement.

**Mean age and range**: Found in all ages but does tend to cause higher morbidity and mortality in juveniles.
**Predominant sex**: None.

## SIGNS

### Historical Findings
May be reported as normal, with no signs noted by owner, or sudden death. Decreased activity, lethargy, weak flight, or being unwilling to fly. Decreased appetite and weight loss, and increased water consumption. Gagging, neck stretching, regurgitation, head flicking (ejecting bits of food as well), difficulty swallowing. Nasal discharge and difficulty breathing, malodor, "blowing bubbles." Green diarrhea, as well as polyuria and green urates.

### Physical Examination Findings
May be asymptomatic. Lethargy, reduced body condition, or failure to thrive. Caseated, diphtheric plaques (white, yellow, tan, or brown) at commissure of beak, oral cavity, oropharynx, laryngeal mound, sinuses, and choana. Plaques can progress to large proliferative or invasive masses. Plaques can usually be easily removed without bleeding. Greenish fluid accumulation within oropharynx. Regurgitation or crop and gut atony with fluid distention. Dyspnea, nasal discharge, sneezing, sialorrhea, dysphagia. Non-specific neurologic signs. Ocular and periocular lesions, conjunctivitis. Thickened esophagus and crop wall. Hepatomegaly. Polyuria and/or biliverdinuria. Diarrhea (may be sour smelling) with pericloacal fecourate soiling. Umbilical swelling in juveniles.

## CAUSES
*Trichomonas* organisms are labile and do not have a stable cyst. There is no intermediate host. They can be transmitted via contamination of food, water, and wet bedding, parental feeding of chicks, and eating infected birds.

## RISK FACTORS
Overcrowding, lack of quarantine of newly introduced birds, poor hygiene (especially wet seeds, contaminated with organic debris), compromised immune system. Infected parents. Feeding on potentially infected species (in the case of raptors feeding on pigeons for example). Pigeon herpesvirus co-infections may make the bird more susceptible to worse lesions.

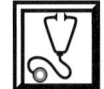

# DIAGNOSIS

## DIFFERENTIAL DIAGNOSIS
Squamous metaplasia from hypovitaminosis A. Candidiasis. Poxvirus. Herpesvirus. Bacterial stomatitis. Neoplasia. Capillaria.

Nodules in the pigeon choanal area can be due to harmless sialoliths. Digestive tract malfunction caused by: hepatic disease, GI tract foreign bodies, neoplasia, other parasites, viruses, yeast and bacteria, proventricular dilatation disease, and heavy metal toxicity. Causes of respiratory distress include other parasites (tracheal mites), viral, fungal (aspergillosis) or bacterial disease, respiratory foreign bodies, or toxic/irritating inhalants (PTFE). Diarrhea: Other enteritis-causing organisms, toxicants, diet sensitivities, and others. Liver lesions can resemble those of bacterial infections (including *Mycobacterium*), *Aspergillus*, neoplasia, or histomoniasis. Plaque lesions due to pigeon herpesvirus are generally more voluminous, located more rostrally, and the sites bleed when the plaques are removed.

## CBC/BIOCHEMISTRY/URINALYSIS
The hemogram would likely show a varying leukocytosis depending on progression of disease. Eosinophilia has been reported to be associated with infection. Biochemistry might show hypoalbuminemia and might show changes with the liver-associated values if the organism has invaded the liver. Inflammatory proteins might also be elevated.

## OTHER LABORATORY TESTS
For *T. gallinae* and T. *columbae*, wet mount of an esophageal swab or of the plaques might show flagellated protozoa (teardrop to round shape), 3–5 long anterior flagella and a tailing flagella attached to an undulating membrane (8–14 μm in size). It may slowly turn in one spot, or have irregular back and forth forward motion. For *T. gallinarum*, a wet mount of fecal material can show a similar organism. The organism dies very quickly after the sample cools down, so the direct evaluation must be immediate. In the absence of a wet mount, the organisms may stay intact to be seen on a sample smear stained with a "quick" cytological stain, Giemsa, or trichrome stain. A bovine *Trichomonas* culture medium (InPouch™ LF, BioMed Diagnostics, White City, OR) has been reported to successfully isolate avian strains. PCR tests are also available for the more common *Trichomonas* species. Parrots may not have organisms visible on a wet mount or cytology. Consider cultures for bacterial and fungal co-infections.

## IMAGING
Radiology might show a thickened crop/esophageal wall. The hepatic silhouette may be widened and irregular radiopacities within. Contrast GI radiology might show ingluvial or gastric stasis and mural thickening. There might be opacities noted in the air sacs as well. Lesions involving bone can show lytic change and erosion. Coelomic linear

T

radiopaque densities might be visible if cecal cores are sufficiently solid and inspissated.

## DIAGNOSTIC PROCEDURES
Upper GI endoscopy can allow evaluation of mucosal surfaces for lesions. Laparoscopy might be required to visibly evaluate the serosa of liver and other viscera, and air sacs (biopsies as needed) might be useful in cases where lesions are not present in more accessible locations.

## PATHOLOGIC FINDINGS
Ulcerative and proliferative lesions, plaques and caseated material found in potentially many places. Intracranial involvement, the digestive tract from the beak to the proventriculus, and the respiratory system from the sinuses through the trachea and into the air sacs. The crop wall may be thickened and opaque otherwise. The liver may have discolored lesions present. Organisms may not be visible with histopathology. *T gallinarum* may cause lower intestinal/cecal lesions, such as caseated cores. The general body condition will likely be poor.

## TREATMENT

### APPROPRIATE HEALTH CARE
For milder cases, the patient can get home care, assuming the caretaker is able to properly medicate and monitor food and fluid intake. For seriously ill birds, hospital care may be required to provide supportive care and debriding as needed of caseous material.

### NURSING CARE
Supportive care needed may include fluid therapy (SQ or IV crystalloids; with sufficient debilitation and/or hypoalbuminemia, IV colloidal fluids may be indicated); supplemental warmth and humidity; oxygen therapy if patient is dyspneic; assisted feeding.

### ACTIVITY
Activity should be reduced until signs resolve.

### DIET
There may be maldigestion and significant weight loss; hyperalimentation may be required during recovery once digestive function resumes. The use of liquified or other easily digested foods and added digestive enzymes to assist assimilation can also be helpful.

### CLIENT EDUCATION
The treatment will likely be successful if there is no significant damage caused by the organism; however, in some cases the prognosis will be poor. The overall predisposing factors that led to the disease need to be addressed including new bird

quarantine and testing. Some protocols advocate regular flock treatments to reduce the burden of organisms before it causes too many birds in a flock to become ill.

## SURGICAL CONSIDERATIONS
Surgical curettage of larger pockets such as in the sinuses or within the trachea can allow airway conservation, help limit the damage, and resolve infection. With sufficient plaque buildup blocking the tracheal lumen, surgical placement of an air sac cannula might be helpful. Otherwise, this is a medically managed condition.

## MEDICATIONS

### DRUG(S) OF CHOICE
Members of the nitroimidazole class are generally effective. Drugs include metronidazole at 25–50 mg/kg PO q12–24h, as well as ronidazole, and carnidazole.

### CONTRAINDICATIONS
Some references report metronidazole toxicity in some types of birds such as finches. At this time, the USA prohibits the use of nitroimidazoles in poultry produced for food; confirm any legal restrictions at your location.

### PRECAUTIONS
The nitroimidazoles are known to have neurologic adverse effects and dose may vary between individuals, so observe for signs of reactions.

### POSSIBLE INTERACTIONS
None.

### ALTERNATIVE DRUGS
Copper sulfate.

## FOLLOW-UP

### PATIENT MONITORING
The patient should be continually monitored to make sure food intake is adequate, that any indication of a secondary infection is not present, and to make sure plaques are fully resolved within weeks. A follow-up esophageal swab and wet mount may be required to confirm success of therapy.

### PREVENTION/AVOIDANCE
Quarantine and testing of new birds into groups, and regular testing of birds during annual or semiannual health examinations via esophageal swab and wet mount. In the case of raptors, not feeding prey of susceptible species. The organisms are sensitive to drying and die soon after elimination from the host, so control of the

organism in the environment is straightforward. Routine cleaning of water supply surfaces with a 10% bleach solution will also control transmission.

## POSSIBLE COMPLICATIONS
Permanent damage to the beak, oropharyngeal tissues, sinuses, and liver may occur. A plaque may slough and obstruct the airway. Secondary bacterial and fungal infections may require separate identification and therapy.

## EXPECTED COURSE AND PROGNOSIS
Signs after infection can advance quickly. Prognosis is good for mild to moderately affected cases. Improvement of general clinical signs after treatment initiation can start occurring within a few days and all lesions will likely disappear within weeks. Cases with deep tissue or visceral migration have a more guarded to poor prognosis and may take longer to return to normal.

## MISCELLANEOUS

### ASSOCIATED CONDITIONS
The many other diseases and infectious agents that are associated with the risk factors of this disease (lack of quarantine, overcrowding, immune system compromise) often exacerbate this condition. Pigeon herpesvirus lesions are often made worse with *Trichomonas*.

### AGE-RELATED FACTORS
Nestlings are often more severely affected than adults. Adults are more likely to be infected without signs.

### ZOONOTIC POTENTIAL
*T. gallinarum* has been found rarely in human disease.

### FERTILITY/BREEDING
Birds should be cleared of this organism before breeding as chicks can be severely affected.

### SYNONYMS
Canker, trich, roup, frounce.

### SEE ALSO
Air Sac Mites
Aspergillosis
Candidiasis
Diarrhea
Enteritis
Flagellate Enteritis
*Macrorhabdus ornithogaster*
Nutritional Imbalances
Oral Plaques
Poxvirus

## ABBREVIATIONS
GI—gastrointestinal
PCR—polymerase chain reaction
PTFE—polytetrafluoroethylene

## INTERNET RESOURCES
N/A

*Suggested Reading*
Gómez-Muñoz, M., Gómez-Molinero, Á., González, F. et al. (2022). Avian oropharyngeal trichomonosis : treatment, failures and alternatives, a systematic review. *Microorganisms*, 10:2297.

Forrester, D.J., Foster, G.W. (2008). Trichomonosis. In *Parasitic Diseases of Wild Birds* (ed: C.T. Atkinson, N.J. Thomas, D.B. Hunter), 120–153. Hoboken, NJ: Wiley-Blackwell.
**Author**: Vanessa Rolfe, DVM, ABVP (Avian)

T

# UNDIGESTED FOOD IN DROPPINGS

 **BASICS**

## DEFINITION
The presence of undigested food in droppings is a clinical sign that can be associated with multiple avian disease processes; this chapter discusses some of the more commonly seen causes for this sign. Undigested food in droppings is most often noticed in birds that are eating seed. It may be more difficult to detect the presence of undigested food in the stool of a bird that is eating a formulated diet or other non-seed items; in those cases, there might be bulky or loose stools without obvious undigested food. Diarrhea is defined as an increased frequency and liquidity of the fecal discharges; in the avian patient, one can also add fecal consistency and the presence of undigested food.

## PATHOPHYSIOLOGY
Formation of a proper fecal portion is dependent on proper intestinal, hepatic, and pancreatic function, as well as the mechanical functions of the coprodeum, urodeum, and vent. Alterations in any of these organ systems or structures may alter the avian patient's ability to create a formed, consistent fecal movement. There are a few mechanisms by which a bird can develop the presence of undigested food in the stool. In the normal bird, there is back and forth movement of ingesta between the proventriculus and the ventriculus. Disease of either or both organs can interfere with this process, resulting in the passage of poorly prepared digesta into the small intestine and eventually into the stool. Disease of the small intestines can result in this clinical sign due to decreased mucosal secretion, malabsorption or hypermotility. Pancreatic disease with resultant exocrine deficiency can result in inadequate digestion. Coelomic disorders can also interfere with GI function, resulting in clinical signs of such.

## SYSTEMS AFFECTED
While in most cases the cause of undigested food in the droppings is going to be related to disease of the GI tract or the pancreas, there might be other organ systems affected, either secondarily or concomitantly with the GI tract.
**GI**: Disease of the proventriculus, ventriculus, small intestine, pancreas.
**Hepatobiliary**: Any liver disorder in theory, but undigested food is not commonly seen with liver disease.
**Musculoskeletal**: Muscle wasting due to negative energy balance.
**Nervous**: CNS signs; muscle weakness and seizures seen with lead toxicosis, bornaviral disease.

**Renal/urologic**: Renal disease seen with zinc and lead, kidneys secondarily affected with many disorders.
**Reproductive**: Disorders involving the female reproductive tract could secondarily affect the GI tract and pancreas.
**Skin**: May see feather picking secondary to giardiasis, poor general feather condition with severe GI or any chronic disease.

## GENETICS
N/A

## INCIDENCE/PREVALENCE
The incidence and prevalence are dependent upon each specific etiology. It is important to recognize the myriad etiologies and pathophysiologies that could cause this clinical sign and consider them during the diagnostic process. While some of the etiologies may be rare, if all else is ruled out, they should be included in the differential diagnosis and ultimately ruled out.

## GEOGRAPHIC DISTRIBUTION
This clinical sign has no geographic boundaries. Some of the disorders might be more common in certain parts of the world.

## SIGNALMENT
**Species**: Any species of birds could develop this clinical sign. Some species are known for certain disorders. *Macrorhabdus ornithogaster* (avian gastric yeast): Budgerigars, cockatiels, lovebirds, finches, parrotlets. Giardiasis: Budgerigars, cockatiels, lovebirds, rarely other parrots, finches. *Spironucleus* spp: Pigeons, turkeys, budgerigars, cockatiels, Australian king Parrots. Cochlosomiasis (flagellated protozoan): Cockatiels, finches, especially Gouldians, poultry. Candidiasis: Cockatiels, finches. Proventricular, ventricular nematodes: *Synhimantus* (*Dispharynx*) spp., *Acuaria* spp. (finches and galliformes). Bornaviral disease: Grey parrots, Amazon parrots, cockatoos, macaws, and others. Proventricular/ventricular neoplasia: Budgerigars, grey-cheeked parakeets, lovebirds, and Amazon parrots. Mycobacteriosis: Grey-cheeked parakeets, cockatiels, Amazon parrots, waterfowl, and zoo collections. Internal papillomatosis: Macaws, Amazon parrots, and conures.
**Mean age and range**: Many infectious disorders, such as flagellate enteritis, bacterial infection, and macrorhabdosis are seen more commonly in the young; neoplastic processes are more likely in the elderly patient.
**Predominant sex**: Both sexes are susceptible.

## SIGNS
### General Comments
Signs and findings include those that may be seen in conjunction with this clinical sign and those that occur concurrently as a result of the underlying etiology.

### Physical Examination Findings
Undigested food in droppings—seeds or other food items seen; if not eating seeds, often seen as bulky or voluminous feces. Malodorous feces. Diarrhea (not to be confused with polyuria). Anorexia or, in some cases, increased appetite. Poor body condition with loss of body fat and muscle wasting. Distended crop; delayed crop emptying. Regurgitation or vomiting. Weakness, depression due to lack of nutrient assimilation. True diarrhea—liquid frequent stools. Biliverdinuria due to hepatic disease. Hemoglobinuria in lead poisoning cases. Hematochezia and/or melena in some cases of enteritis, zinc toxicosis. GI stasis—lead poisoning, grit impaction. Seizures and other neurologic signs—lead poisoning. Coelomic distention due to fluid, enlarged liver, mass, reproductive disease.

## CAUSES
A comprehensive list of potential causes is listed below. In general, disorders of the proventriculus, ventriculus, and pancreas are arguably the most common causes for this clinical sign, yet a number of small intestinal, hepatic and systemic disorders should be included for the sake of thoroughness.
**Proventricular disease**: Gastric foreign bodies or impaction. Avian ganglioneuritis—proventricular dilation, avian bornavirus. Macrorhabdosis. Poxvirus, mucosal/systemic form. Herpesvirus, specifically Psittacid herpesvirus 1, causing mucosal papillomas. Bacterial infections, primary or secondary. Mycobacterial disease. Candidiasis; report of *Candida glabrata* causing proventriculitis in an eclectus parrot. Zygomycete fungal infection. Cryptosporidiosis. Nematodes: *Spiroptera* sp., *Synhimantus* (*Dispharynx*) sp. *Tetrameres* sp., others. Proventricular carcinomas at the isthmus (common in budgerigars).
**Ventricular disease**: Foreign bodies—damaged koilin, can perforate and cause coelomitis (traumatic gastritis is common in ground dwelling birds, ratites, and pigeons). Grit impaction. Mineralization. Zinc toxicosis—ventricular erosion and pancreatic damage. Avian ganglioneuritis. Adenoviral infection. Bacterial infection. Mycobacterial infection. Ventricular mycosis—*Candida*; Zygomycetes. Nematodes. Neoplasia—carcinomas.
**Small intestinal disease**: Candidiasis. Coccidial infections. Flagellate enteritis—giardiasis, spironucleosis, and cochlosomiasis. Bacterial enteritis—*Escherichia coli*, *Klebsiella*, *Salmonella*, and *Enterobacter* spp. *Clostridium*, *Campylobacter*, *Enterococcus* spp., others. Mycobacterial infection. Chlamydiosis. Nematodes. Intestinal neoplasia. Viral disease—avian bornavirus, paramyxovirus, herpesvirus, adenovirus, reovirus, rotavirus.

**Pancreatic diseases**: Pancreatitis. Pancreatic atrophy or fibrosis. Chlamydiosis. Zinc toxicosis.

**Hepatic disease**: Numerous etiologies and disorders but probably unlikely to result in undigested food in droppings.

**Coelomic disease**: Coelomitis—perforated GI tract, reproductive-related. Coelomic neoplasia.

### RISK FACTORS
Poor sanitation, poor food quality, malnutrition, stress, overcrowding, exposure to other birds with contagious diseases, age, concurrent diseases, long-term antibiotic use (candidiasis), allowing birds to roam throughout the home (lead, zinc, other toxins) are predisposing factors.

## DIAGNOSIS

### DIFFERENTIAL DIAGNOSIS
Covered under causes of this clinical sign.

### CBC/BIOCHEMISTRY/URINALYSIS
CBC may show anemia in lead poisoning cases. Leukocytosis may be seen in cases of significant inflammation/infection (mycobacteriosis, chlamydiosis, other). Eosinophilia seen sometimes with giardiasis and other flagellates. Hypoproteinemia is seen in cases where there is significant malabsorption. There may be other electrophoretic changes associated with infection, protein loss, liver diseases, egg-laying disorders and other conditions. Elevated bile acids and liver enzymes will be seen in cases of liver disease.

### OTHER LABORATORY TESTS
Direct fecal smears—can see yeasts, several types of parasites including flagellates, macro suspension technique for avian gastric yeast. Fecal parasite testing, zinc sulfate centrifugation—helminths. Fecal Gram staining (trying to match with culture results and not overinterpret results). Fecal cytology, several stains—Diff-Quik™ (Siemens Healthineers, Malvern, PA), fungal stains, other. Fecal acid fast staining—*Cryptosporidium* spp. and *Mycobacterium* spp. Fecal culture—aerobic and anaerobic. Fecal occult blood testing. Lead and zinc blood testing. Fecal PCR testing—*Chlamydia, Cryptosporidium* sp., *Macrhorhabdus ornithogaster*, bornavirus and other viral testing.

### IMAGING
CT and radiography can be very useful in determining the cause of this clinical sign. Contrast radiographs might be helpful to delineate lesions such as coelomic masses, organomegaly, or to properly outline the GI tract and to see the lining and the lumen of the organs. Heavy-metal foreign bodies might be visible in the ventriculus; the proventriculus could be dilated in cases of avian ganglioneuritis and in lead toxicosis, internal papillomatosis, and other conditions. It is best to do a contrast study to further clarify. A dilated, thin-walled proventriculus and ventriculus is suggestive of avian ganglioneuritis but is not pathognomonic. Fluoroscopy could further examine the GI tract and especially its motility.

### DIAGNOSTIC PROCEDURES
Endoscopy of the proventriculus or ventriculus or the coelomic cavity to obtain mucosal samples for cytology and culture. Laparoscopy to obtain biopsy specimens of internal organs such as liver, pancreas, small intestine. Biopsy of the crop (or less commonly, the proventriculus, ventriculus or small intestine), generally in an attempt to confirm avian ganglioneuritis.

### PATHOLOGIC FINDINGS
Gross pathological findings for the more common causes of this clinical sign are as follows. Avian ganglioneuritis—enlarged, dilated thin-walled proventriculus and/or ventriculus with potential dilation of the small intestine; histologically, lymphoplasmacytic ganglioneuritis; lesions also in CNS, heart, adrenals. Macrorhabdosis, minimal gross findings—excess mucus production; histologically, organisms seen in the proventricular mucosa, mononuclear inflammation. Lead toxicosis—hemoglobinuria, may see enlarged dilated proventriculus or other areas of the GI tract; histologically, renal and hepatic pathology. Zinc toxicosis—grossly may see melena due to erosive ventriculitis; histologically, pancreatic lesions, vacuolation and degranulation of acinar cells. Proventricular or ventricular carcinomas—infiltrative to proliferative mass, usually located at the isthmus. Flagellate enteritis—distended intestines with excess mucous or gas or fluid, or no lesion; histologic evidence of organisms along the villi. Proventricular, ventricular, intestinal bacterial or fungal or yeast infection—redness, exudation, erosions, degeneration of koilin layer, organisms present in koilin or deeper into the tissues. Clostridial overgrowth in intestines—focal to diffuse hemorrhage, necrosis and fibrin deposition; presence of large Gram-positive spore-forming rods. Mycobacteriosis—diffuse and/or nodular thickening and opacification of the intestinal wall; histologically, diffuse infiltration of lamina propria with large macrophages that contain acid-fast bacteria. Pancreatic atrophy/fibrosis—pale, small firm pancreas; histologically normal acini replaced by interstitial fibrosis.

## TREATMENT

### APPROPRIATE HEALTH CARE
A definitive diagnosis will dictate next steps for an appropriate therapy, supportive care, and symptomatic treatment may be initiated to provide comfort until the diagnosis is confirmed. Patients with mild to moderate disease without other, more serious clinical signs can be treated as outpatients, pending results of testing. Patients with severe disease need to be hospitalized to stabilize while a thorough diagnostic workup is performed.

### NURSING CARE
Nursing care must be done in the sicker patients. This might include incubation, gavage feeding, fluid therapy, and possibly oxygen therapy.

### ACTIVITY
N/A

### DIET
It makes sense that dietary manipulation could be beneficial for these patients, especially while diagnostic testing results are pending and also if the patient is weakened or otherwise doing poorly. Formulated diets should be more digestible for these patients.

### CLIENT EDUCATION
Proper administration of medications should be explained. Clients should be advised to watch for worsening of the patient's condition and to return to the hospital as needed. Monitoring of the droppings by the owner should be emphasized. Counsel client in biosecurity and hygiene practice to avoid spread of infectious diseases. Preventative medicine with regular health exams and routine fecal testing can be recommended.

### SURGICAL CONSIDERATIONS
For inpatients with foreign bodies, including lead and zinc and other heavy metals, surgical intervention might be necessary.

## MEDICATIONS

### DRUG(S) OF CHOICE
For candidiasis, nystatin (300,000 IU/kg PO q12h) may be used for mild infection. Azole antifungals (fluconazole, terbinafine, voriconazole) are indicated for severely invasive and systemic infection. For *Macrorhabdus* infection, amphotericin B (compounded) at 100 mg/kg PO or gavage q12h for up to 30 days or via drinking water at 0.1 mg/ml for 28 days; recent literature suggests that this dose via drinking water proved to be effective in more than 50% of

**U**

cases. Treatment with sodium benzoate in drinking water at 1 tbs/L. For giardiasis, cochlosomiasis and spironucleosis, various nitroimidazoles can be used, including metronidazole. For cryptosporidiosis, ponazuril might be successful. For lead and zinc toxicosis, 35 mg/kg calcium disodium EDTA IM/SQ q12h, usually done 5 days on and 2–5 days off, then repeated; it is unclear if this is a necessary precaution. For avian ganglioneuritis, no effective treatment has been found. COX-2 inhibitors such as celecoxib at 10 mg/kg q24h PO and meloxicam 1 mg/kg PO q24h have been investigated. For bacterial infections, selection of the appropriate antibiotic should be based upon the results of C/S testing. Note that there is a degree of clinical judgment needed when faced with the results of a fecal or cloacal culture; the presence of a Gram-negative organism does not equate with disease of the GI tract. For clostridial infections, and amoxicillin/clavulanate (125 mg/kg PO q12h) have been suggested. For mycobacteriosis, several multiple-drug protocols have been recommended. For pancreatic insufficiency, pancreatic enzymes can be supplemented.

## CONTRAINDICATIONS
N/A

## PRECAUTIONS
N/A

## POSSIBLE INTERACTIONS
N/A

## ALTERNATIVE DRUGS
N/A

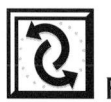

# FOLLOW-UP

## PATIENT MONITORING
The owner at home should monitor all patients, either during the diagnostic workup phase, and during and after treatment, or by the veterinary team in the hospital. Follow-up examinations, including laboratory testing should be done as needed.

## PREVENTION/AVOIDANCE
Prevent further access to heavy metals and foreign bodies. Avoid exposure to or housing with individuals that have been proven to have infectious or contagious diseases.

## POSSIBLE COMPLICATIONS
N/A

## EXPECTED COURSE AND PROGNOSIS
The presence of seed in the droppings is generally a fairly grave sign. Determining a prognosis is dependent upon arriving at a proper diagnosis. In theory, the sooner the diagnosis is achieved, the better the prognosis. For bacterial, flagellate, fungal, and chlamydial infections, the prognosis with treatment should be good. Cryptosporidiosis is difficult to treat and the prognosis is fairly poor. Birds with clinical avian ganglioneuritis generally do not survive very long, but there are exceptions. Lead and zinc toxicosis cases can be cured with chelation therapy for the proper length of time. Mycobacterial infections are very tedious and difficult to treat and treatment is controversial.

# MISCELLANEOUS

## ASSOCIATED CONDITIONS
N/A

## AGE-RELATED FACTORS
The very young are most affected in all of these protozoal diseases; parents/adults are often asymptomatic carriers.

## ZOONOTIC POTENTIAL
There is some question about the zoonotic potential of cryptosporidiosis, although it seems to be very rare or unlikely; mycobacterial infections are potentially zoonotic but rarely reported; *Giardia* might be zoonotic but this is not well documented; some bacterial infections such as chlamydiosis and salmonellosis could cause disease in people.

## FERTILITY/BREEDING
Several of these conditions could adversely affect future fertility, especially egg-related coelomitis, neoplasia, mycobacteriosis.

## SYNONYMS
N/A

## SEE ALSO
Aspergillosis
Bornaviral Disease (Aquatic Birds)
Bornaviral Disease (Psittaciformes)
Chlamydiosis
Cryptosporidiosis
Diarrhea
Emaciation
Enteritis and Gastritis
Herpesvirus
Flagellate Enteritis
Foreign Bodies (Gastrointestinal)

Ileus (Functional Gastrointestinal, Crop Stasis)
*Macrorhabdus ornithogaster*
Mycobacteriosis
Neoplasia (Gastrointestinal and Hepatic)
Pancreatic Diseases
Regurgitation and Vomiting
Sick-Bird Syndrome
Toxicosis (Heavy Metals)
Urate and Fecal Discoloration

## ABBREVIATIONS
AGY—avian gastric yeast
C/S—culture and sensitivity
CNS—central nervous system
CT—computed tomography
GI—gastrointestinal

## INTERNET RESOURCES
VIN searches and PubMed searches are useful to learn more detail about any of these individual topics.
National Library of Medicine. PubMed: https://pubmed.ncbi.nlm.nih.gov
Veterinary Information Network: https://www.vin.com

*Suggested Reading*
Baron, H.R., Stevenson, B.C., Phalen, D.N. (2021). Comparison of in-clinic diagnostic testing methods for *Macrorhabdus ornithogaster*. *Journal of Avian Medicine and Surgery*, 35:37–44.
Brandão, J., Beaufrère, H. (2013). Clinical update and treatment of selected infectious gastrointestinal diseases in avian species. *Journal of Exotic Pet Medicine*, 22:101–117.
Hoppes, S.M., Tizard, I., Shivaprasad, H.L. (2013). Avian bornavirus and proventricular dilatation disease: Diagnostics, pathology, prevalence, and control. *Veterinary Clinics of North America: Exotic Animal Practice*, 16:339–355.
Phalen, D.N. (2014). Update on the diagnosis and management of *Macrorhabdus ornithogaster* (formerly megabacteria) in avian patients. *Veterinary Clinics of North America: Exotic Animal Practice*, 17:203–210.
Reavill, D.R., Schmidt, R.E., Phalen D.N. (2015). Gastrointestinal system and pancreas. In: *Pathology of Pet and Aviary Birds*, 2nd edn., 55–94. Ames, IA: Wiley.
Summa, N.M., Guzman, D.S.M. (2017). Evidence-based advances in avian medicine. *Veterinary Clinics of North America: Exotic Animal Practice*, 20: 817–837.
**Author**: Mariana Sosa-Higareda, DVM
**Acknowledgements**: updated from first edition chapter authored by George Messenger, DVM, DABVP (Avian)

U

# URATE AND FECAL DISCOLORATION

## BASICS

### DEFINITION
The avian dropping consists of three portions: the feces, the urates, and liquid urine. The normal color of the stool of most birds on a seed diet is either brown or a rich dark green, due to the presence of biliverdin. The urates are normally a chalky white color. Birds may be presented for evaluation of abnormal urate/urine or fecal color, or these abnormalities may be discovered during the examination of the patient. The evaluation of bird droppings is an essential component of the overall exam. Abnormal coloration of the fecal or urate/urine portion of the dropping can help to reveal very valuable information about the health of the avian patient.

### PATHOPHYSIOLOGY
Fecal color can be strongly influenced by diet, bile pigments, and potentially blood from the GI tract. Bile pigments are a strong, dark-green color. This color presents in comparatively increased amount when there is inadequate food intake, but also can be often visible in the droppings from patients who eat primarily seed. Some pelleted food diets contain colored pellets, and birds may preferentially eat one color over another. These may change the color of the feces. Darkly colored fruits such as blueberries and cherries may also change the color of the feces and create a false appearance of melena. Birds with lead poisoning have increased destruction of red blood cells, resulting in intravascular hemolysis. This, combined with nephrosis, contributes to hemoglobinuria and/or hematuria. Birds with upper GI lesions or bleeding diathesis (due to vitamin K antagonist toxins and other causes) can have black stools indicative of melena. In the presence of hepatic disease, biliverdinuria may occur, causing the urates to turn green or yellow. This occurs because of the accumulation of biliverdin, which is normally removed by the liver. Birds produce small amounts of bilirubin because of the decreased production of an enzyme (biliverdin reductase) that converts biliverdin into bilirubin. Renal or reproductive pathology may lead to the presence of frank blood in the urine or pink-tinged urine and/or urate staining, due to mixing with urine in the cloaca.

### SYSTEMS AFFECTED
**GI**: Upper GI bleeding (black stools – melena).
**Hemic/lymphatic/immune**: Intravascular hemolysis with lead toxicosis (red, pink, brown urine or urates).
**Hepatobiliary**: Liver disease of all types (yellow, golden, mustard, or green urates).

**Renal/urinary**: Lead toxicosis—renal tubular necrosis, hemoglobinuria (red, pink, brown urates/urine); renal disease can result in hematuria also.
**Musculoskeletal**: Muscle damage after intramuscular injection.

### GENETICS
N/A

### INCIDENCE/PREVALENCE
Discoloration of the urates or feces is a fairly common finding in birds.

### GEOGRAPHIC DISTRIBUTION
Any of these diseases can be seen anywhere in the world.

### SIGNALMENT
**Species**: Amazon parrots, conures, and eclectus parrots are more likely to develop hemoglobinuria secondary to lead poisoning. All birds otherwise susceptible to most disease processes that cause any of these clinical signs.
**Mean age and range**: All ages are susceptible.
**Predominant sex**: Both sexes are susceptible.

### SIGNS
#### General Comments
Historical findings and physical findings will vary depending on the specific problem.

#### Historical Findings
It is important to get a good dietary history as well as to question the introduction of new toys into the bird's cage. Inquire about time out of the cage and potential for foreign material ingestion.

#### Physical Examination Findings
**Lead toxicosis**: General non-specific signs. polyuria/polydipsia. Hemoglobinuria. Weakness. Seizures; occasionally other neurologic signs. Anemia.
**Liver disease**: General non-specific signs. Vomiting or regurgitation. Diarrhea. Lethargy. Biliverdinuria. Yellow to orange urates. Enlarged liver. Possible abdominal pain. Possible coelomic effusion.
Intestinal diseases: Non-specific signs. Diarrhea. Undigested food in droppings. Possible melena or frank blood (rare, usually cloacal), or clay-colored stools.

### CAUSES
Leaching of dyes from colored newspaper can retroactively discolor the stool or urine part of a bird's dropping (when it is dropped onto the paper) and this should not be misconstrued as an abnormality associated with the patient.

#### Urate and/or Urine Discoloration
**Green**: Biliverdinura due to liver disease or (rarely) hemolytic anemia; GI stasis in anorexic birds or in stools that are not fresh, bile pigments may leach into urine/urates.

**Yellow**: Liver disease; anorexia; muscle injury such as IM injection; use of B complex vitamins.
**Brown or reddish brown**: Hemoglobinuria secondary to lead poisoning (see causes for red).
**Red**: Hematuria/hemoglobinuria most often due to lead toxicosis (also described as "tomato soup," port wine, or chocolate) and rarely mercury or zinc toxicosis; hematuria can also result from kidney, cloacal, or reproductive disease.
**Pink**: Hematuria or hemoglobinuria (same causes as for red).
**Orange**: Vitamin B injection in last few hours.
**Blue, yellow, red, green, purple, orange (bright colors)**: From blueberries, blackberries, beets, pomegranates, other fruits or vegetables, or from artificial dyes or food coloring in some toys or foods (including some formulated diets). This will usually be seen in the clear urine, and perhaps in the stool, and generally will not discolor the urates.

#### Fecal Discoloration
**Brown**: Often normal in birds eating mainly formulated diet; normal in finches, canaries, quail and others. Coliform infections may produce a distinct brown color change and liquidity in certain species. May have an odor, as will viral diseases with secondary bacterial infection.
**Green (more than normal)**: This color can often present in comparatively increased amount when there is inadequate food intake. Budgerigars with macrorhabdosis will classically have a slightly paler green and looser stool.
**Clay**: Malabsorption or maldigestion; intestinal disease, pancreatic and possibly liver disease.
**Black (melena)**: Caused by upper GI bleeding due to a variety of stomach (including ulcerative ventriculitis due to zinc toxicosis) or intestinal lesions, or a bleeding disorder. Anorexia or moribund states commonly result in this change, especially in smaller birds. Budgerigar stools often look black after they have dried out, but upon close exam of a fresh stool, they are dark green.
**Red**: Hematuria (frank blood) due to lower GI disease (often cloacal), but also possibly from reproductive or urinary disease.
**Orange, yellow, blue, red, orange, purple**: As with urine/urate discoloration, these can be due to ingestion of beets, berries, and other fruits and vegetables, as well as artificial dyes or food coloring in food or toys.

### RISK FACTORS
Birds allowed to roam the house are more likely to develop heavy-metal toxicosis. Poor diets and inactivity can very often lead to hepatic lipidosis in some species. Exposure to other ill birds (herpesvirus, *Chlamydia*, etc.) increases the likelihood of acquiring infections.

**U**

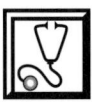

## DIAGNOSIS

### DIFFERENTIAL DIAGNOSIS
Differentials for all forms of urate and fecal discoloration are listed under causes.

### CBC/BIOCHEMISTRY/URINALYSIS
Findings will vary depending on the pathologic process causing the clinical sign. Lead toxicosis—hypochromic regenerative anemia; ballooning degeneration in RBCs. Liver disease—elevated bile acids; often see AST elevations, but this is not specific for liver.

### OTHER LABORATORY TESTS
In most cases, the nature of the urine or fecal color change will determine the direction of the diagnostic workup. Some additional tests that might be necessary include gross examination of droppings—make sure to carefully and critically examine and evaluate each portion. Roll out feces on a piece of white paper to look for undigested food and blood clots and to differentiate urates from feces. Fecal direct smear in the case of potential flagellates or helminths or avian gastric yeasts. Fecal cytology—WBCs, RBCs, and occasionally other findings. Fecal flotation for parasite ova and *Giardia* cysts. Fecal Gram stains if patient has diarrhea. Beware of overinterpreting the results. Fecal acid-fast stain—mycobacteria and cryptosporidia. Fecal C/S—in cases of suspected bacterial infection, or to corroborate Gram stain results. Blood lead (and occasionally zinc) testing.

### IMAGING
Hepatomegaly or decreased liver size with some liver diseases. Heavy-metal objects can sometimes be seen in the ventriculus or other parts of the GI tract with lead and/or zinc poisoning.

### DIAGNOSTIC PROCEDURES
Laparoscopic or surgical biopsy of the liver, kidney, or pancreas in some cases. Exploratory laparotomy to evaluate organs in cases of suspected reproductive and other conditions. Cloacoscopy in the case of lower GI bleeding (frank blood). Upper GI endoscopy in the case of melena enables visualization of the esophagus, crop, proventriculus, and ventriculus in most species. For larger birds, ingluviotomy may be necessary. Barium GI series may identify areas of intestinal wall thickening or dilation, foreign body, or intussusception. Ultrasound may identify intestinal wall thickening. CT can identify intestinal wall thickening as well as pathology of organs such as liver, kidney, or reproductive tract.

### PATHOLOGIC FINDINGS
There could be a wide variety of lesions associated with discolored feces and urates. Some of the more common ones include any form of liver disease and associated pathology—hepatic lipidosis, chlamydiosis, mycobacteriosis, viral disease (herpesvirus and other), biliary carcinomas, bacterial disease, inflammatory and immune mediated conditions, toxins, aspergillosis, and cirrhosis. In macrorhabdosis, increased mucous or mild changes in the proventriculus near or at the isthmus, presence of organisms microscopically. In zinc toxicosis, erosive ventriculitis and pancreatic lesions may be seen. In small intestinal or pancreatic disease resulting in malabsorption/maldigestion or melena, numerous pathologic processes could be present, including chronic pancreatitis with fibrosis, pancreatic neoplasia, chronic zinc poisoning (pancreas), GI parasites (helminths or flagellates), bacterial enteritis, mycobacteriosis, chlamydiosis, neoplasia, and other lesions.

## TREATMENT

### APPROPRIATE HEALTH CARE
During the examination, the severity of the bird's condition is determined. Birds that are seriously ill need to be hospitalized and subjected to an appropriate diagnostic workup and treatments as deemed necessary.

### NURSING CARE
Fluid, thermal, and nutritional support may be necessary in birds that are hospitalized.

### ACTIVITY
N/A

### DIET
N/A

### CLIENT EDUCATION
In all cases, it is important to outline the course of action with the client, including the diagnostic and treatment plan and the prognosis. Explanation of the normal and abnormal appearance of avian droppings is always useful with all bird owners.

### SURGICAL CONSIDERATIONS
N/A

## MEDICATIONS

### DRUG(S) OF CHOICE
For lead and zinc toxicosis, calcium EDTA 35 mg/kg IM q12h for 5–10 days; DMSA 15–40 mg/kg PO q12h for 5–10 days; penicillamine 55 mg/kg PO q12h for 5–10 days; might need to be repeated or

continued for longer periods. For liver diseases, many possible therapies, depending on the underlying cause. If underlying cause is not known, alcohol-free silymarin products are often used; lactulose has been historically used but this might be of questionable efficacy. For bacterial infections, antibiotics should be based upon the results of C/S testing. For macrorhabdosis, amphotericin B at 25–100 mg/kg PO q12h for 10–30 days. The lower dosage might be efficacious. For GI diseases, sucralfate 25–100 mg/kg PO q8–12h may be used as a gastroprotectant. Other gastroprotectants, such as famotidine or pantoprazole, may be used.

### CONTRAINDICATIONS
N/A

### PRECAUTIONS
N/A

### POSSIBLE INTERACTIONS
N/A

### ALTERNATIVE DRUGS
N/A

## FOLLOW-UP

### PATIENT MONITORING
Each patient should be monitored as needed, depending on the severity of the condition and the specific disorder. This should include examinations, as well as specific laboratory testing and examination of the droppings.

### PREVENTION/AVOIDANCE
N/A

### POSSIBLE COMPLICATIONS
N/A

### EXPECTED COURSE AND PROGNOSIS
Prognosis is extremely variable, depending upon the specific diagnosis. Cases of lead poisoning carry a favorable prognosis if the condition is diagnosed and treated promptly.

## MISCELLANEOUS

### ASSOCIATED CONDITIONS
N/A

### AGE-RELATED FACTORS
N/A

### ZOONOTIC POTENTIAL
N/A

### FERTILITY/BREEDING
N/A

### SYNONYMS
N/A

## SEE ALSO
Anorexia
Bornaviral Disease (Aquatic Birds)
Bornaviral Disease (Psittaciformes)
Campylobacteriosis
Chlamydiosis
Cloacal Diseases
Clostridiosis
Coccidiosis (Intestinal)
Colibacillosis
Cryptosporidiosis
Diarrhea
Enteritis and Gastritis
Flagellate Enteritis
Helminthiasis (Gastrointestinal)
Herpesvirus (Columbid Herpesvirus 1 in
Pigeons and Raptors)
Herpesvirus (Duck Viral Enteritis)
Herpesvirus (Passerine Birds)
Herpesvirus (Psittacid Herpesviruses)
Liver Disease
*Macrorhabdus ornithogaster*
Pancreatic Diseases
Polyuria

Salmonellosis
Sick-Bird Syndrome
Toxicity (Heavy Metals)
Undigested Food in Droppings

## ABBREVIATIONS
AST—aspartate aminotransferase
C/S—culture and sensitivity
CT—computed tomography
DMSA—meso-2,3-dimercaptosuccinic acid
EDTA—ethylenediaminetetraacetic acid
GI—gastrointestinal
RBC—red blood cell
WBC—white blood cell

## INTERNET RESOURCES
N/A

*Suggested Reading*

Bauck, L. (2000). Abnormal droppings. In:
*Manual of Avian Medicine* (ed. G.H. Olsen,
S.E. Orosz), 62–69. St. Louis, MO: Mosby.
Denver, M.C., Tell, L.A., Galey, F.D. et al.
(2000). Comparison of two heavy metal
chelators for treatment of lead toxicosis
in cockatiels. *American Journal of Veterinary
Research*, 61:935–940.
Doneley, B., Harrison, G., Lightfoot, T. (2006).
Maximizing information from the physical
examination. In: *Clinical Avian Medicine*,
153–211. Palm Beach, FL: Spix Publishing.
Ferrell, S.T., Tell, L.A. (2001). *Clostridium
tertium* infection in a rainbow lorikeet with
enteritis. *Journal of Avian Medicine and
Surgery*, 15(3):204–208.
Fudge, A.M. (2000). Avian liver and
gastrointestinal testing. In: *Laboratory
Medicine: Avian and Exotic Pets*, 47–55.
Philadelphia, PA: Saunders.
Wismer, T. (2016). Advancements in diagnosis
and management of toxicologic problems.
In: Speer BL, ed. *Current Therapy in
Avian Medicine and Surgery*. St. Louis, MO:
Elsevier, pp 589–599.

**Author**: Natalie Antinoff DVM, DABVP
(Avian)

**Acknowledgements**: Revised from previous
edition authored by George A. Messenger,
DVM, DABVP (Avian)

U

# UROPYGIAL GLAND DISEASE

## BASICS

### DEFINITION
Disease or condition affecting the uropygial gland. The uropygial gland is a bilobed gland found dorsally at the base of the tail, secreting a lipoid sebaceous material that is suspected to have several roles: Plumage waterproofing in some species, antimicrobial activity, protection against certain ectoparasites (e.g. feather lice), anti-abrasive effects during preening, conversion of provitamin D to vitamin D, which is then ingested during preening, production of pheromones, sex-related changes in the ultraviolet appearance of the plumage, and excretion of some pesticides and pollutants.

### PATHOPHYSIOLOGY
Trauma, neoplasia, impaction or infection of the gland, responsible for its increase in size, possible loss of function, and further infiltration or damage to adjacent uropygial structures.

### SYSTEMS AFFECTED
Skin/exocrine.

### GENETICS
N/A

### INCIDENCE/PREVALENCE
N/A

### GEOGRAPHIC DISTRIBUTION
N/A

### SIGNALMENT
**Species**: All species of birds that have a uropygial gland (except Amazon parrots, hyacinth macaws, Pionus parrots, some Columbiformes, ratites, bustards, frogmouths, and woodpeckers, which do not have a uropygial gland).
**Mean age and range**: Any age.
**Predominant sex**: Both.

### SIGNS

#### Historical Findings
Poor feather quality. Mass dorsally at the base of the tail. Overpreening at the base of the tail. Bleeding dorsally at the base of the tail. Water birds—disruption of feather waterproofing in some instances.

#### Physical Examination Findings
Increased size of the uropygial gland. Asymmetry of the gland. Ulceration or necrosis of the gland, which can be associated with localized hemorrhage. Feather loss around the gland.

### CAUSES
Nutritional: Hypovitaminosis A, responsible for glandular metaplasia and hyperkeratosis of the gland and possible impaction. Neoplasia: Adenoma, adenocarcinoma, squamous cell carcinoma, papilloma, intraluminal epithelioma. Inflammation: Adenitis, chronic dermatitis. Infection: Bacterial abscess, fungal granuloma. Impaction. Foreign body. Trauma: Rupture of the gland causing inflammation and scar tissue formation.

### RISK FACTORS
Trauma: Self-mutilation or trauma to the area of the gland. Improper diet (hypovitaminosis A).

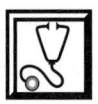

## DIAGNOSIS

### DIFFERENTIAL DIAGNOSIS
See Causes section.

### CBC/BIOCHEMISTRY/URINALYSIS
Unremarkable in most cases. A mild leukocytosis and monocytosis may be present in inflammatory and infectious processes.

### OTHER LABORATORY TESTS
Cytology (on gland secretion or impression smear of ulcers): May be useful in differentiating between an infectious process (bacteria, yeasts, and inflammatory cells may be visible) and neoplasia (neoplastic cells may be observed). Histopathology: In case of poor response to initial therapy or an obvious mass, a biopsy may be collected. Bacteriology: Bacterial culture and sensitivity is recommended in suspected cases of infection of the gland (a swab of the secretions or ulcers can be performed). Fungal culture.

### IMAGING
Not indicated as a diagnostic tool for this condition.

### DIAGNOSTIC PROCEDURES
Biopsy for histology (essential to confirm a neoplastic process).

### PATHOLOGIC FINDINGS
Findings specific to the various causes (abscess, neoplasia, squamous metaplasia).

## TREATMENT

### APPROPRIATE HEALTH CARE
Digital pressure may be applied on the gland to express its content in cases of impaction. Hot compresses can be applied on the gland prior to this procedure to soften the content and facilitate the expulsion. If ulcerations or wounds secondary to trauma are noted, wound care should be performed: disinfection (e.g. diluted chlorhexidine), debridement of necrotic tissues if necessary, topical ointment if indicated (e.g. medical honey, silver sulfadiazine cream), dressing. If digital pressure cannot resolve the impaction, an incision over the affected lobe of the gland can be performed. Expulsion of the material should follow, and the gland may be flushed with sterile saline or diluted chlorhexidine.

The wound should then be allowed to heal by secondary intention. A culture swab or the impacted material may be submitted for bacterial culture and sensitivity. Cytology should be performed on the removed materials. Surgery: Excision of the uropygial gland can be performed without adverse consequences in most species of birds (may cause feather abnormalities in water birds). The surgery is recommended in suspected cases of neoplasia, and may be recommended in extensive infections or severe trauma. Recurrent impaction or infiltrative processes may also justify an excisional surgery that may involve the entire uropygium.

### NURSING CARE
Supportive care.

### ACTIVITY
N/A

### DIET
Provide a well-balanced diet. In case of birds reluctant to switch to a pelletized diet, all-seed diet should be supplemented with multivitamin powder.

### CLIENT EDUCATION
The client should be informed of the localization and normal aspect of the uropygial gland. Normal behavior (preening in the area of the gland) can be discussed.

### SURGICAL CONSIDERATIONS
Uropygial gland excision: The uropygial gland is very vascular and, therefore, surgical excision should be performed with care as to limit the risk of hemorrhage. A fusiform incision is made over the uropygial gland and the gland is dissected with blunt and radiosurgical dissection. The gland may greatly extend cranially. The blood supply is typically located at different levels along the cranial, middle, and caudal portions of the gland. The follicles of the rectrices should be spared during dissection and coagulation if possible. The skin closure is routine, however if significant tension is encountered secondary intention healing may be selected using bandages. Uropygium amputation: In case of significant infiltration of cancerous tissue, excision of the whole uropygium may be indicated to obtain clear margins. CT of the affected area is indicated to better delineate the tumor. Significant hemorrhage may be encountered during the surgery.

## MEDICATIONS

### DRUG(S) OF CHOICE
Neoplasia: Systemic chemotherapy. Topical chemotherapy (e.g. 5-fluorouracil). Intratumoral chemotherapy (e.g. carboplatin, cisplatin). Radiation therapy (strontium-90

therapy). Cryotherapy. Electrochemotherapy (with cisplatin and bleomycin). Bacterial infection: Antibiotic therapy according to the results of culture and sensitivity. Anti-inflammatory/analgesics may be indicated (e.g. meloxicam).

## CONTRAINDICATIONS
None.

## PRECAUTIONS
Chemotherapy and radiation therapy should be performed by specialists in oncology as they represent a serious health hazard.

## POSSIBLE INTERACTIONS
None.

## ALTERNATIVE DRUGS
N/A

 FOLLOW-UP

## PATIENT MONITORING
Monitor the size of the gland/area of surgery (using calipers). Regular CBC and biochemistry panels are indicated in birds receiving chemotherapy.

## PREVENTION/AVOIDANCE
Annual health checks during which the uropygial gland should be evaluated. Provide a well-balanced diet.

## POSSIBLE COMPLICATIONS
Lack of response to treatment. Recurrence after treatment. Bleeding during treatment/ surgery. Permanent injury to the gland.

## EXPECTED COURSE AND PROGNOSIS
Impaction: Good, although recurrence is possible. Abscess, granuloma, adenitis: Usually good after treatment. Trauma: Good except if severe trauma. Neoplasia: Guarded, may not respond to treatment or may recur.

 MISCELLANEOUS

## ASSOCIATED CONDITIONS
Poor feather condition. Disruption of the waterproof property of the plumage in some aquatic bird species. Self-mutilation in the uropygial area.

## AGE-RELATED FACTORS
None.

## ZOONOTIC POTENTIAL
None.

## FERTILITY/BREEDING
N/A

## SYNONYMS
N/A

## SEE ALSO
Neoplasia (Gastrointestinal and Hepatic)
Neoplasia (Integument)
Neoplasia (Lymphoproliferative)
Neoplasia (Neurologic)
Neoplasia (Renal)
Neoplasia (Reproductive)
Neoplasia (Respiratory)

## ABBREVIATIONS
CBC—complete blood count
CT—computed tomography

## INTERNET RESOURCES
N/A

*Suggested Reading*
Atlman, R.B. (1997). Soft tissue surgical procedures. In: *Avian Medicine and Surgery* (ed. R.B. Altman, S.L. Clubb, G.M. Dorrestein, K. Quesenberry), 704–732. Philadelphia, PA: Saunders.
Lucas, A.M., Stettenheim, P.R. (1972). *Avian Anatomy: Integument, Part II*. Agriculture Handbook 362, 613–626. Washington, DC: US Government Printing Office.
Nemetz, L.P., Broome, M. (2004). Strontium-90 therapy for uropygial neoplasia. *Proceedings of the Association of Avian Veterinarians Annual Conference*, 15–20.
Racnik, J., Svara, T., Zadravec, M., et al. (2019). Electrochemotherapy with bleomycin in the treatment of squamous cell carcinoma of the uropygial gland in a cockatiel (*Nymphicus Hollandicus*). *Journal of Exotic Pet Medicine*, 29:217–221.
Robertson, J., Sanchez-Migallon Guzman, D., Sinnott, D., et al. (2020). Modified tail amputation technique in a blue and gold macaw (*Ara ararauna*) with uropygial gland adenocarcinoma. *Journal of Avian Medicine and Surgery*, 34:57–64.
Ambar, N., Eshar, D., Njaa, B.L. (2022). Intraluminal uropygial gland epithelioma in an african grey parrot (*Psittacus erithacus*). *Journal of Avian Medicine and Surgery*, 35:433–439.
**Authors**: Delphine Laniesse, DVM, DVSc, DECZM (Avian), and Hugues Beaufrère, DrMedVet, PhD, DABVP (Avian), DECZM (Avian), DACZM

**U**

# USUTU VIRUS

## BASICS

### DEFINITION
Usutu virus (USUV) is an emerging mosquito-borne flavivirus, which has been circulating in the European passerine bird population since 2001, although retrospective analyses suggest first introductions from Africa in 1996. The virus can induce mass mortality in avian hosts and due to its neuroinvasive potential, reflected by several clinical human cases, USUV has been anticipated as a risk for public health.

### PATHOPHYSIOLOGY
Usutu virus is an arbovirus of the family Flaviviridae and genus Flavivirus, first discovered in South Africa in 1959. Passerine birds are a reservoir for this virus, which is mainly transmitted by blood-feeding mosquitos of *Culex* species. Direct transmission via excreta may be possible. The genomic RNA is enclosed by a small capsid protein, which is surrounded by a double lipid membrane including the two viral envelope proteins, designated M and E, in which E serves as the primary attachment protein for receptor-mediated endocytosis. In infected cells, 7 non-structural proteins (NS1, NS2A, NS2B, NS3, NS4A, NS4B and NS5) are synthesized and play an important role for viral replication, assembly, and immune evasion.

### SYSTEMS AFFECTED
Neuromuscular, hepatobiliary.

### GENETICS
N/A

### INCIDENCE/PREVALENCE
Blackbirds, magpies, and great gray owls play a dominant role as amplifying hosts, although it has been shown that at least 58 bird species belonging to 26 taxonomic families and 13 orders are susceptible to the virus. To date, 8 lineages of USUV can be characterized based on phylogenetic analyses. Based on their geographical distribution, they are designated as Africa 1–3 and Europe 1–5. In some European countries, several different USUV lineages circulate simultaneously. Endemic mass fatalities, are common in late summer, particularly in blackbirds.

### GEOGRAPHIC DISTRIBUTION
Europe.

### SIGNALMENT
**Species**: Wide species distribution, but most often reported in wild blackbirds, passerine birds kept in aviaries, and great gray owls kept in captivity. Domestic geese and chickens are less affected.
**Mean age and range**: None.
**Predominant sex**: None.

## SIGNS

### Historical Findings
Lethargy and depression. Ruffled feathers. Anorexia and weight loss. Sudden death with no clinical signs. Rarely, ataxia, abnormal head movements, disorientation, tremors, and uncoordinated flight.

### Physical Examination Findings
Depression. Enlarged liver. Tremors.

### CAUSES
Infectious.

### RISK FACTORS
Ponds. High bird density.

## DIAGNOSIS

### DIFFERENTIAL DIAGNOSIS
West Nile virus, avian malaria, trauma.

### CBC/BIOCHEMISTRY/URINALYSIS
N/A

### OTHER LABORATORY TESTS
Blood rt-PCR, serology.

### IMAGING
Enlarged liver and spleen.

### DIAGNOSTIC PROCEDURES
Necropsy.

### PATHOLOGIC FINDINGS
Haemorrhages. Hepatosplenomegaly. Pale mottling of heart, liver, kidney, and spleen. Necrosis and haemorrhages with mononuclear cell infiltrations in the brain, cardiac and skeletal muscle, liver, spleen, kidney.

## TREATMENT

### APPROPRIATE HEALTH CARE
Inpatient medical management may be required.

### NURSING CARE
Fluid support (SQ, IV, IO) may be indicated if the bird is debilitated. Nutritional support via gavage may be indicated if anorexic.

### ACTIVITY
No restrictions indicated.

### DIET
N/A

### CLIENT EDUCATION
Necropsy in case of mass fatalities. Use of mosquito net for the aviaries. Reducing of mosquito burden in water/ponds. Wearing repellents to protect against mosquitos.

### SURGICAL CONSIDERATIONS
N/A

## MEDICATIONS

### DRUG(S) OF CHOICE
Ivermectin—0.2 mg/kg PO, SQ, IM once, may have an effect on the viral load.

### CONTRAINDICATIONS
N/A

### PRECAUTIONS
N/A

### POSSIBLE INTERACTIONS
None reported.

### ALTERNATIVE DRUGS
N/A

## FOLLOW-UP

### PATIENT MONITORING
Serology. Viral shedding via urine and faeces.

### PREVENTION/AVOIDANCE
Avoid transmission via mosquito feeding.

### POSSIBLE COMPLICATIONS
N/A

### EXPECTED COURSE AND PROGNOSIS
Birds that are treated earlier in the course of disease tend to have a better prognosis. Mass fatalities in aviary birds are common.

## MISCELLANEOUS

### ASSOCIATED CONDITIONS
Co-infection with avian malaria is occasionally seen.

### AGE-RELATED FACTORS
N/A

### ZOONOTIC POTENTIAL
Yes.

### FERTILITY/BREEDING
N/A

### SYNONYMS
N/A

### SEE ALSO
Eastern and Western Equine Encephalitis
Neurologic (Non-Traumatic Diseases)
Neurologic (Trauma)
Neoplasia (Neurological)
Toxicosis (Heavy Metals)
Toxicosis (Environmental, Pesticides)
West Nile Virus

### ABBREVIATIONS
rt-PCR—reverse transcriptase polymerase chain reaction
USUV—usutu virus

## INTERNET RESOURCES
N/A

*Suggested Reading*
Folly, A.J., Lawson, B., Lean, F.Z., et al. (2020). Detection of usutu virus infection in wild birds in the United Kingdom, 2020. *Eurosurveillance*, 25(41):2001732.

Giglia, G., Agliani, G., Munnink, B.B.O., et al. (2021). Pathology and pathogenesis of Eurasian blackbirds (*Turdus merula*) naturally infected with usutu virus. *Viruses*, 13:1481.
Schmidt, V., Cramer, K., Böttcher, D., et al. (2021). Usutu virus infection in aviary birds during the cold season. *Avian Pathology*, 50:427–435.

Vilibic-Cavlek, T., Petrovic, T., Savic, V., et al. (2020). Epidemiology of usutu virus: The European scenario. *Pathogens*, 9:699.
Wald, M.E., Claus, C., Konrath, A., et al. (2022). Ivermectin inhibits the replication of usutu virus in vitro. *Viruses*, 14:1641.
**Author**: Volker Schmidt, PD DrMedVet, DECZM (Avian, Herpetological)

U

# WEST NILE VIRUS

## BASICS

### DEFINITION
West Nile virus (WNV) is an RNA arbovirus in the family *Flaviviridae*, and the genus *Flavivirus*, transmitted by female mosquitoes, which causes neurological disease and potentially death in multiple bird species, horses, humans, and certain other individual mammal and reptile species. As of 2019, 8 distinct lineages have been identified, but only 2 are widespread and are the primary concerns. Lineage 1 contains those emerging and most concerning for disease–lineage 1a (Europe, Middle East, Asia, North/Central/South America), lineage 1b (Australasia, Oceania), and lineage 1c (India). Lineage 2 had been less concerning and limited to Southern Africa, but became more virulent there and spread to Europe. A concerning finding in a 2010 Arizona outbreak was cocirculation of three distinct genetic variants, including strains with novel envelope protein mutations, which adds to the complexity and perhaps explains why this virus continues to do so much damage in endemic areas.

### PATHOPHYSIOLOGY
Usually, the bird is bitten by an infected mosquito; however, other arthropods such as ticks, hippoboscid flies, and other fly species may be rare sources of transmission. *Culex* spp. (*Culex pipens*) and *Aedes* spp. are primary vector species. In some cases, less efficient methods of acquiring WNV include ingestion of infected bird carcasses (reported in alligators fed WNV-infected horsemeat and virus directly in the water) or contaminated fluids (blood, feces, urine, saliva, crop milk). In mammals, maternal transmission has been suggested and a variant considered by some in birds.

### SYSTEMS AFFECTED
**Nervous**: Torticollis, opisthotonos, nystagmus, ataxia, clenched feet, upper motor neuron signs, head tilt, uncoordinated flight, paralysis, tremors, and seizures.
**Behavioral**: Depression, ruffled feathers, decreased activity to lethargy.
**Ophthalmic**: Chorioretinitis, cortical blindness.
**Musculoskeletal**: Drooping wings, clenched feet, neck muscle rigidity.
**Cardiovascular**: Bradycardia, murmurs, cardiac arrest (death).
**Gastrointestinal**: Anorexia, rapid weight loss, diarrhea, regurgitation.
**Endocrine/metabolic**: Hyperthermia or hypothermia.
**Renal/urologic**: Polyuria to hypouria, green staining of urates.
**Respiratory**: Nasal discharge, labored breathing, aspiration.

**Skin/exocrine**: Urate/fecal matting by vent, wounds over pressure points from thrashing, possible keel region feather loss, some raptors have had feather abnormalities, including stunted growth and pinched-off feathers (at the quill).
**Immune**: In humans, immunosuppression is reported.
**General**: Weight loss, dehydration.

### GENETICS
In mammals, morbidity and mortality is often not related to virulence, but instead to host genetics and the reaction or perhaps overreaction of the host's immune system to the presence of the virus. It is unknown whether this reaction occurs in avian species, but it may also be the case.

### INCIDENCE/PREVALENCE
In many places, WNV is considered endemic, but seasonal patterns occur based upon mosquito activity (late summer). The infection in the individual bird is usually acute and lasts up to 1 week, with a very high but short viremic period. There also appear to be periodic "spikes." Likely similar patterns emerge based upon a myriad of factors in birds. However, isolated cases outside mosquito season have been documented in birds. Incubation period is 4–14 days in birds. Some birds become detectably viremic 1 day post inoculation. While most clinical birds progress rapidly or improve, there has been a subset with clinical signs for weeks to months.

### GEOGRAPHIC DISTRIBUTION
WNV is firmly established in avian and mosquito populations worldwide. The virus is endemic and transmission is reinitiated annually in the summer within temperate areas of North America and Europe.

### SIGNALMENT
**Species**: All bird species are likely susceptible and serve as reservoirs, amplifiers, and infection source for dead end hosts; most cases are likely subclinical. As a group, passerines are reported most affected and gallinaceous birds the least, but there are exceptions (greater sage grouse are heavily impacted, and see passerine carrier species below). Species most likely to be clinical include corvids (crows, ravens, jays, magpies) and raptors (owls, eagles, falcons, hawks). Other birds have been documented with WNV infection, including pelicans, flamingos, penguins, emus, wild turkeys, cormorants, kori bustards, bronze-winged ducks, sandhill cranes, common coots, red-legged partridges, Australian psittacines. American robins and house sparrows may be significant, nonclinical reservoirs for WNV; and passerines, shorebirds, and gulls are highly competent hosts.
**Mean age and range**: Young of the year seem more susceptible.
**Predominant sex**: None.

## SIGNS

### Historical Findings
Usually seen in the summer in the USA and Europe, but year-round occurrence seems to be increasing due to climate change. Exposure and transmission in overwintering regions is an issue; drought seems to contribute to severity, also areas where there is no aggressive mosquito mitigation.

### Physical Examination Findings
See Systems Affected section.

### CAUSES
West Nile virus.

### RISK FACTORS
Immunosuppression, age, species predilection, lack of previous exposure, mutation of virus, drought, poor regional mosquito mitigation, ± lack of vaccination.

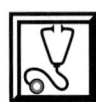

## DIAGNOSIS

### DIFFERENTIAL DIAGNOSIS
Other arboviruses (EEE, WEE, VEE, St. Louis encephalitis, LaCrosse, Powassan, Buggy Creek), trauma, heavy-metal toxicity, bacterial meningitis, fungal meningitis, protozoal meningitis, baylisascariasis, hepatoencephalopathy, neoplasia, other toxins, vascular disease (stroke, aneurysm, athlerosclerosis), avian vacuolar myelinopathy, nutritional deficiency or excess (Vitamin E, $B_6$, $B_{12}$ deficiencies).

### CBC/BIOCHEMISTRY/URINALYSIS
Generally unremarkable, most abnormalities secondary to issues like dehydration, anorexia. Elevated CPK is not uncommon.

### OTHER LABORATORY TESTS
Two- to fourfold increase in paired WNV-specific antibodies in acute and convalescent sera, IgM in CSF, or IgM in serum (suggestive) via ELISA, with confirmation of results by plaque reduction neutralization test. Preferred sample is serum. Can be done with plasma, but toxicity due to the presence of anticoagulant may prevent accurate antibody titer determination. Virus isolation from serum, CSF, tissues (brain, heart, kidneys, spleen), oral or cloacal swabs. Avian viremia peaks quickly, and can be especially difficult in animals with low viremic levels to start. rt-PCR can be more sensitive than virus isolation. IHC is best during active infection. Bodily fluids such as blood (centrifuged for separation of serum or plasma), CSF, saliva, or swabs of body cavities (oropharyngeal or cloacal cavities), or tissues (heart, kidney, and spleen have been consistently useful for virus isolation), IHC, and PCR testing in birds; feather pulp, non-vascular feathers, brain, eye, spinal cord,

liver, and other tissues can be pooled to possibly increase sensitivity. Testing maggots from carcasses for RNA may be useful in decomposed birds. Most state public health laboratories conduct WNV testing; however, virus isolation and plaque reduction neutralization tests are time and labor intensive and require BSL-3 conditions.

## IMAGING
Only useful to rule out other etiologies.

## DIAGNOSTIC PROCEDURES
N/A

## PATHOLOGIC FINDINGS
Gross lesions are often absent, but can be non-specific, including white–tan mottling or streaking of the myocardium, splenomegaly, congested cerebral vessels, and poor nutritional condition. Histologic lesions can be minimal to severe, and can include heterophilic to lymphoplasmacytic myocarditis, encephalitis, ganglionitis, hepatitis, and nephritis. Vasculitis can also occur.

# TREATMENT
## APPROPRIATE HEALTH CARE
Patients should be isolated separately from other susceptible avian species. Birds with respiratory viral infections initially will benefit from intensive care with oxygen supplementation. Debilitated patients may not be able to thermoregulate and would benefit from placement into a heated intensive care unit or, for larger patients, a cage with added subfloor heating or heat lamp. Mild cases may resolve without treatment.

## NURSING CARE
The bird may need to be stabilized to keep from thrashing and self-traumatizing, regurgitating, and aspirating. Large birds may benefit from hay bales or a sling. Smaller birds may require towels and removal from a wire cage to prevent falls. Padding may be needed to minimize pressure sores or rub wounds. Consider a tail feather protector. Some may swallow with orally placed food; others require supportive feeding or esophageal tube placement. Patients who are not eating need to have caloric supplementation with one of the commercial powdered or liquid enteric formulations per label instructions. If the patient is dehydrated, supplemental fluid administration is warranted. Warm fluids to 100–103°F (38–39°C), 50–60 ml/kg q24h subcutaneously. IV or IO catheter may be placed in severely debilitated patients with 10 ml/kg slow bolus over 5–10 minutes. L-lysine supplements and homeopathic

treatments have had some success in raptors. Regular cleaning/plucking of fecal/urate contaminated feathers should be assessed. Cold laser therapy to minimize edema and ligament contracture may be warranted.

## ACTIVITY
Minimize exposure to sound, light, and tactile stimulation early on. However, over time increasing exposure to stimulus seems to encourage the bird to help with management. If the bird is not standing on its own, initiate physical therapy.

## DIET
Assisted nutritional support is usually required early on and essential for the extended temporal component of recovery from this disease. Watch closely, especially early on, for aspiration from regurgitation.

## CLIENT EDUCATION
Birds clinically affected by WNV may recover over a few weeks, but most severely affected cases carry a guarded prognosis and require a commitment of supportive care for 45–90 days. There may also be permanent damage to the neurologic, ophthalmic, and cardiac systems.

## SURGICAL CONSIDERATIONS
Potential placement of feeding tubes.

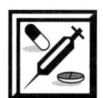

# MEDICATIONS
## DRUG(S) OF CHOICE
Most treatments are supplemental, as mentioned in Nursing Care section. The use of broad-spectrum or synergistic use of antimicrobials may be helpful, but do not address the primary problem. The use of anti-inflammatories such as NSAIDs, corticosteroids, and/or IV DMSO may also be warranted. In cases of seizures or disorientation, IM midazolam may help in the short term and gabapentin may be useful. Maropitant as an appetite stimulant could be another tool. For birds previously and currently on a good balanced diet, vitamin E injections to prevent captive capture myopathy are generally not needed or helpful.

## CONTRAINDICATIONS
Remember that if the bird is considered a food animal or wildlife being released that could enter the human food chain, all applicable laws should be considered and severely limit the use of medications.

## PRECAUTIONS
Despite previous mention, it is important to remember that corticosteroids are 4–8 times more potent in birds compared with mammals; so repeated use should be carefully evaluated. They also likely suppress the immune system which may or not be helpful.

## POSSIBLE INTERACTIONS
N/A

## ALTERNATIVE DRUGS
N/A

# FOLLOW-UP
## PATIENT MONITORING
Follow-up WNV plaque neutralization serology may help track; repeat CBCs and chemistries may help monitor for organ failure, hydration issues, and secondary infections.

## PREVENTION/AVOIDANCE
Mosquito control measures should be implemented: Screened housing, fans, avoiding stagnant water, larvicides, and stocking mosquito fish in ponds. Insect repellents create toxicity concerns with birds and are *not* recommended at this time. Isolate infected individuals and quarantine new animals. Avoid feeding potentially contaminated meat or carcasses. Currently, there are several vaccines developed for use in horses that are available in the USA. Many zoological facilities vaccinate sensitive avian species with this vaccine. Caution should be exercised in the extra-label use of vaccines or use of vaccines that have not been adequately assessed in the target animal (i.e. controlled challenge studies) and vaccination should not be assumed to be protective. While not common, anaphylactic reactions to these vaccines, up to and including death, have been seen in various avian species including lorikeets and roseate spoonbills. Seroconversion studies using one vaccine product in birds have occurred but are species limited. WNV does not persist for long periods in the environment. 70% ethanol and bleach are sufficient for general cleaning. Viricides such as Virkon® S (Lanxess, Cologne, Germany) are highly effective when concern is high but can be damaging to skin and mucus membranes.

## POSSIBLE COMPLICATIONS
Death and chronic debilitation can occur.

## EXPECTED COURSE AND PROGNOSIS
Even with intense management, the short- and long-term prognosis for the individual bird should be considered guarded.

**W**

# MISCELLANEOUS
## ASSOCIATED CONDITIONS
N/A

## AGE-RELATED FACTORS
Juvenile birds seem more susceptible; however, naive geriatric birds may also be at risk.

## ZOONOTIC POTENTIAL
Generally, not considered a direct zoonotic disease because of the mosquito involvement; however, risk during handling tissues and fluids, inhalation, mucous membrane contact, open cuts and puncture wounds from a needle stick or contaminated equipment. Gloves should be worn when handling suspect animals and bedding.

## FERTILITY/BREEDING
In mammals, there are reported effects on reproductive organs, but these effects have not been reported in avian species. The level of mortality from the disease can have significant effects on the populations and genetic diversity of endangered species and sensitive species such as corvids and raptors.

## SYNONYMS
N/A

## SEE ALSO
Atherosclerosis
Eastern and Western Equine Encephalitis Viruses
Liver Disease
Neoplasia (Gastrointestinal and Hepatic)
Neoplasia (Integument)
Neoplasia (Lymphoproliferative)
Neoplasia (Neurologic)
Neoplasia (Renal)
Neoplasia (Reproductive)
Neoplasia (Respiratory)
Neurologic (Non-Traumatic Diseases)
Nutritional Imbalances
Ocular Lesions
Seizures
Toxicity (Heavy Metals)
Trauma
Also individual named viral diseases

## ABBREVIATIONS
BSL—biosecurity level
CBC—complete blood count
CPK—creatinine phosphokinase
CSF—cerebrospinal fluid
DMSO—dimethyl sulfoxide
EEE—eastern equine encephalitis
ELISA—enzyme-linked immunosorbent assay
Ig—immunoglobulin
IHC—immunohistochemistry
NSAIDs—nonsteroidal anti-inflammatory drugs
PCR—polymerase chain reaction
rt-PCR—reverse transcriptase polymerase chain reaction
VEE—Venezuelan equine encephalitis
WNV—West Nile virus
WEE—Western equine encephalitis

## INTERNET RESOURCES
Centers for Disease Control and Prevention. West Nile virus: http://www.cdc.gov/westnile
Cornall Uniuversity College of Veterinary Medicine, Animal Health Diagnostic Center: West Nile virus diagnostic testing: https://www.vet.cornell.edu/animal-health-diagnostic-center/testing/protocols/west-nile-virus
Wikipedia. West Nile virus: http://en.wikipedia.org/wiki/West_Nile_virus

*Suggested Reading*
Fiacre, L., Pagès, N., Albina, E., et al. (2020). Molecular determinants of West Nile virus virulence and pathogenesis in vertebrate and invertebrate hosts. *International Journal of Molecular Sciences*, 21:9117.
Habarugira, G., Suen, W.W., Hobson-Peters, J., et al. (2020). West Nile virus: An update on pathobiology, epidemiology, diagnostics, control and "one health" implications. *Pathogens*, 9:589.
Weaver, G.V. (2018). West Nile virus. In: *Infectious Disease Manual* (ed. R.R. Sim, R. Sadler, M. Thurber), 436–441. Jacksonville, FL: American Association of Zoo Veterinarians.

**Author**: Eric Klaphake, DVM, DACZM

W

# WOUNDS (INCLUDING BITE WOUNDS, PREDATOR ATTACKS)

## BASICS

### DEFINITION
A wound may be open (skin disruption) or closed (skin crushed). Wounds most often are the result of trauma, with laceration and bite wounds being very common. Bite wounds are considered contaminated with a microbial population representative of the biter's oral flora, the victim's skin, and the environment. Crushing injuries are common with bite wounds and damage to the underlying tissues is often more extensive than the often minor-appearing skin lesions.

### PATHOPHYSIOLOGY
Devitalized tissue, dead space, compromised blood supply, and body fluid accumulation create a prime environment for bacterial growth. Wound infection may occur if treatment is delayed. Bite wounds typically lead to mixed aerobic and anaerobic infections. Cat bites are more likely to become infected than dog bites. Common aerobic isolates from dog and cat bite wounds include *Pasteurella*, *Streptococcus*, *Staphylococcus*, *Neisseria*, *Corynebacterium*, and *Moraxella* spp. Common anaerobic isolates include *Fusobacterium*, *Bacteroides*, *Porphyromonas*, *Prevotella*, *Propionibacterium*, and *Peptostreptococcus* spp. Beta-lactamase production is a common feature among anaerobes isolated from infected bites. Multiple or severe bite wound injuries may lead to SIRS.

### SYSTEMS AFFECTED
**Skin/exocrine**: Wound, bruising, infection, cellulitis, abscess, subcutaneous emphysema.
**Musculoskeletal**: Crushing, tearing, laceration, avulsion, necrosis of muscles, tendons and ligaments, luxation, fracture.
**Renal/urologic**: Polyuria (stress, gastrointestinal infection, sepsis, SIRS).
**Cardiovascular**: Hemorrhage, hypotension, shock, vascular compromise.
**Nervous**: Nerve damage, head trauma.
**Respiratory**: Hemorrhage, edema, pulmonary contusion, perforated air sac, trachea, or sinus, tachypnea, dyspnea (sepsis, SIRS).
**Ophthalmic**: Traumatic ocular lesions.
**Gastrointestinal**: Perforated esophagus or crop, vomiting, diarrhea, delayed crop emptying (bacterial infection from preening feathers soiled by mammalian saliva, sepsis).

### GENETICS
N/A

### INCIDENCE/PREVALENCE
Common.

### GEOGRAPHIC DISTRIBUTION
N/A

### SIGNALMENT
No specific species, age or sex predilection.

### SIGNS

#### General Comments
If there is significant injury or long delay between the time of the injury and presentation to the veterinarian, the patient may require stabilization therapy before physical examination and/or therapeutic management can be performed. Sedation or anesthesia, local or systemic analgesics may be indicated for birds that do not tolerate restraint or have very painful injuries.

#### Historical Findings
Exposure to potential harmful material/equipment (chemicals, electrical cord, etc.) or cold weather. Traumatic event witnessed by the owner. Direct contact with a predator species or another bird. Biting event witnessed by the owner. Documented feather-damaging behaviour. Recent stress reported by the owner. Skin mass previously observed.

#### Physical Examination Findings
Skin—single or multiple wounds. After hemoglobin is broken down, biliverdin pigment accumulates giving bird bruises a greenish discoloration within 2–3 days post injury. Puncture wounds caused by feline predators are often very fine and difficult to see, with the only outward sign of attack being moist or clumped feathers. Discolored skin (black or blanched white), absence of skin bleeding, no capillary refill time, cold to the touch, and absence of bleeding from a cut toe nail are consistent with vascular compromise. Presence of a mass in the vicinity of the wound. Muscle, ligament, tendon—crushing, laceration, tearing; palpable fracture or luxation; lameness, inability to fly. Polyuria. Lethargy, depression, pale mucus membranes, prolonged capillary refill time, tachycardia, hypotension, hemorrhage. Tachypnea, dyspnea. Nerve damage, peripheral or central neurologic deficit, cranial nerve deficits. Vomiting, diarrhea, delayed crop emptying. Palpebral, conjunctival, and corneal lesions; uveitis.

### CAUSES
Traumatic (most common). Predator or conspecific bites. Self-mutilation. Cutaneous neoplasia. Chemical or thermal burns. Electrocution. Frostbite.

### RISK FACTORS
Environmental factors—cohabitation with another bird or predator species, exposure to harmful material or equipment; living in the northern hemisphere during the winter season.

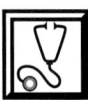

## DIAGNOSIS

### DIFFERENTIAL DIAGNOSIS
Cutaneous neoplastic lesions, dermatitis, dermatomycosis, cutaneous xanthomatosis.

### CBC/BIOCHEMISTRY/URINALYSIS
CBC to characterize the inflammation/infection. Biochemistry to evaluate organ function.

### OTHER LABORATORY TESTS
Culture—aerobic and anaerobic; indicated for all bite wounds or chronic wounds to identify organisms present and their antimicrobial susceptibility; do not culture fresh bite wounds, since infectious agents will most likely not be recovered during this time; growth and identification of anaerobic organisms are frequently a difficult task and should not be misinterpreted as absence of these organisms in infected wounds. Blood culture may be indicated in case of sepsis or suspected bacteremia.

### IMAGING
Whole-body radiographs to evaluate for internal or orthopedic injury. Infrared thermal imaging may help in remotely detecting and monitoring wounds in unfeathered areas.

### DIAGNOSTIC PROCEDURES
Orthopedic and neurological examination when the patient is stable. Sedation and analgesia may be considered for orthopedic evaluation only. In-depth wound assessment when the patient is stable to determine the extent of the injury and remove any debris or devitalized tissue. Wound communication with body cavities must be determined. Sterile instruments and aseptic technique should be used. Consider sedation or anesthesia and analgesia.

### PATHOLOGIC FINDINGS
Skin puncture, laceration, tearing with associated injury (bruising, crushing, contusion, edema, laceration, necrosis) to adjacent tissues. Abscess. Pulmonary contusion. Generalized changes compatible with sepsis.

## TREATMENT

### APPROPRIATE HEALTH CARE
Outpatient medical management—stable patient with minor wounds that can be closed primarily or do not require closure. Inpatient medical management—patient with acute wounds for which delayed primary closure is required. Emergency inpatient intensive care

**W**

# WOUNDS (INCLUDING BITE WOUNDS, PREDATOR ATTACKS) (CONTINUED)

management—patient with severe wounds requiring immediate assessment of ABCs; patient with hemorrhagic wounds requiring application of a pressure bandage immediately to stop blood loss and prevent hypotensive shock. Surgical management once patient is stable—patient with wounds requiring primary closure, delayed primary closure, or secondary closure.

## NURSING CARE

**Wound management**: All wound management needs to be done as part of the overall patient assessment.

**Feather cutting/removal**: Create a 2- to 3-cm circumferential featherless zone around the wound. Plucking may cause tearing of the skin. Consider applying sterile water-soluble gel within the wound to keep down feathers from adhering to the wound.

**Wound cleansing**: All wounds should be flushed copiously to dislodge non-viable tissue and bacteria from the wound surface mechanically. Topical antiseptic may be used initially. Sterile saline may be used once bacterial balance has been restored using topical antiseptic. Appropriate pressure can be obtained using a 20-ml syringe fitted with an 18-gauge needle. Consider sedation and analgesia.

**Staged wound debridement**: Indicated if debris or necrotic tissues persist within the wound after wound cleansing; facilitates identification of non-viable tissue while preserving potentially viable tissue; continued until all non-viable tissue has been removed from the wound. Consider local anesthetic on the wound. Consider sedation or anesthesia to minimize stress and to have optimal control of hemostasis and tissue handling.

**Hydrotherapy**: Consider whether mechanical non-selective debridement is indicated and to stimulate formation of granulation tissue, increase blood flow to the wound and decrease inflammation.

**Bandage**: Must be adapted to the exact nature of the wound, its location, the patient and its functional needs. Temporary bandaging indicated if patient requires medical stabilization until more thorough wound treatment can be performed. Consider a distracting device consisting of a tape tag over the bandage that the bird can reach and damage while preserving the actual bandage until the patient gets used to the bandage. The primary layer of the bandage comprises a dressing that must be adapted to the phase of wound healing; numerous products available to enhance various phases (inflammation, proliferation, remodeling, or maturation) of wound healing. Adherent bandages, and honey or sugar, are used during the initial inflammatory stage of healing, Non-adherent bandages are applied for the proliferative and remodeling stages of healing. Dressings can be occlusive or nonocclusive. The secondary and tertiary layers of the bandage serve to further

immobilize and protect the wound. The secondary layer is usually composed of an absorptive material, such as cast padding. The tertiary layer consists of adhesive material, such as elastic wrap.

**Fluid therapy**: May be provided SQ in birds exhibiting mild dehydration (5–7%) or IO/IV in birds with moderate to severe dehydration (> 7%) or critically ill birds exhibiting signs consistent with shock. Avian daily maintenance fluid requirements are 50 ml/kg. Typically, maintenance plus half the fluid deficit is administered during the first 12 hours, with the remainder of the deficit replaced over the following 24–48 hours. In most patients, lactated Ringer's solution or Normosol®-R (Hospira, Inc., Lake Forest, IL) crystalloid fluids are appropriate. For birds with hypotensive shock, a colloidal solution may be administered concurrently with crystalloids. Blood transfusion should be considered with severe blood loss.

**Oxygen therapy**: Indicated if respiratory distress or anemia is present; beneficial for any sick avian patient. All methods of oxygen supplementation require humidification if used for more than a few hours.

**Warmth**: (85–90°F/27–30°C) To minimize energy spent to maintain body temperature.

**Elizabethan collar**: Should be reserved for birds that insist on self-traumatizing their wounds; may suggest pain and the cause should be investigated.

**Physical therapy**: Indicated if the healing process of a wound may alter the range of motion of any joint; to begin in the maturation phase to avoid delayed healing process.

## ACTIVITY

Patient's activity should be altered according to its injuries.

## DIET

Birds suffering severe injury may require assisted feeding. Enteral nutritional preparations may be administered initially at 20–30 ml/kg directly in the crop. The volume administered may be progressively increased according to patient tolerance with the goal to meet the patient's anticipated energy requirements during the healing process.

## CLIENT EDUCATION

Any actively bleeding wound or a wound secondary to a bite, exposure to chemicals, cold weather or hot liquid, or electrocution, is considered an emergency and requires immediate veterinary care. Appropriate housing modifications may be indicated to facilitate access to food and water. Weight monitoring is indicated if modifications have been made to the cage, a bandage has been placed or if the bird is wearing an Elizabethan collar. Bandages and splints must be kept dry and clean. Daily assessment is required to minimize complications.

## SURGICAL CONSIDERATIONS

Emergency management may be indicated before surgical debridement under anesthesia. Surgical debridement—if performed within 24 hours of a bird sustaining a severe biting injury or clinically significant hemorrhage, it might be placing the patient at unnecessary risk, especially if a more aggressive procedure is required later. Level of tissue damage and surgical risk can usually be assessed adequately 24 hours post injury. Initial wound cleaning, minor debridement, and temporary wound dressing may be preferred over any aggressive surgical wound debridement to allow time for better assessment of tissue damage and patient stabilization. Severed tendons, ligaments, or major nerves—attempt aggressive surgical debridement of the wound and primary reanastomosis of these structures as soon as possible, since tissue contraction may result in the impossibility to affix the ends without tension. Penetration of the coelomic cavity may require surgical exploration to identify and treat concurrent injury. Negative pressure wound treatment may be considered for any wound that require surgical debridement, such as burns, degloving injuries, infected wounds, wounds involving the extremities, and chronic wounds (keel wound and self-mutilation wound). Primary closure indicated for birds presented within 6–8 hours of injury with minimal contamination and tissue trauma. Delayed primary closure—most acute wounds will be healthy enough for closure after 3–5 days of wound management with hydrophilic dressings. Secondary closure, second-intention healing—extensive wounds may require wound management for longer periods. These wounds are closed once a healthy bed of granulation tissue is present, or left to heal by second intention. Primary wound-healing time is 10–14 days for cutaneous healing in most avian patients. Vascularised skin flap, mesh graft, skin graft, extracellular matrices—to be considered in the absence of available skin to close the skin defect without undesirable tension. Stents may also be used to decrease tension while reducing dead space and speed up secondary intention healing in large wounds.

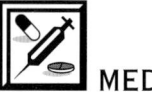

## MEDICATIONS

### DRUG(S) OF CHOICE

*Topical Medications*

Medications used to enhance wound healing function in a variety of different ways. There is no one medication that is essential or best for every wound. Topical antiseptic—chlorhexidine (0.05%), dilute povidone iodine (≤ 1%), hydrogen

# (CONTINUED) WOUNDS (INCLUDING BITE WOUNDS, PREDATOR ATTACKS)

peroxide (3%). Chlorhexidine solution has minimal deleterious effects on wound healing and sustained residual activity. Povidone iodine at a concentration as low as 1–5% and hydrogen peroxide are toxic to fibroblasts and should be used as a single lavage. Topical antimicrobial—use water-soluble topicals such as silver sulfadiazine cream. Silver sulfadiazine promotes epithelialization and penetrates necrotic tissues, but may impede wound contraction. Oil-based ointments should be avoided because when preened into the feathers, they inhibit normal thermoregulatory function.

### Systemic Medications
Antibiotic therapy indicated when infection is confirmed (Gram stain and/or C/S) or might be life-threatening such as bite wounds. Factors such as the ability of the antimicrobial to reach the wound at appropriate concentrations, bacterial resistance patterns, patient status, and the existence of published pharmacokinetics in birds may dictate antibiotic choices. Must be efficacious against aerobic and anaerobic bacteria when treating bite wounds. Examples of antibiotic therapy in such clinical case include amoxicillin-clavulanic acid 125 mg/kg PO q12h for stable patients, piperacillin 100 mg/kg IM/IV q8–12h for unstable patients. Analgesic therapy (butorphanol 1–4 mg/kg q2–4h in Galliformes, Psittaciformes, Passeriformes; buprenorphine or hydromorphone in birds of prey) is indicated in most cases of severe wounds. NSAIDs (meloxicam 0.5–2.0 mg/kg PO/SQ q12–24h) indicated in most cases of severe/extensive wounds. Adverse effects in light of the patient's overall condition need to be considered.

## CONTRAINDICATIONS
Do not flush wounds that could connect to the air sacs or lungs.

## PRECAUTIONS
Fluid deficits should be addressed prior to using NSAIDs.

## POSSIBLE INTERACTIONS
None.

## ALTERNATIVE DRUGS
N/A

# FOLLOW-UP

## PATIENT MONITORING
Varies with the severity of wound injuries and the patient's status.

## PREVENTION/AVOIDANCE
Household dangers must be mitigated in such a way that the bird cannot get injured. Birds should never be left unsupervised in the presence of a predator species. Only indirect contact with predators should be permitted. Only indirect contact between birds not tolerating each other should be permitted. Do not allow a bird to land on another one's cage.

## POSSIBLE COMPLICATIONS
Abscess, septicemia—often secondary to closure of severely contaminated, infected, or traumatized wounds; also occurs following healing of puncture wounds. Mortality—generally due to either infection or concurrent trauma. Disruption of the wound, dressing, or bandage materials—some birds may focus their attention on the wound site, dressing, or bandage materials. Decreased mobility—wound contraction that occurs during the maturation process may decrease the range of motion of the joints.

## EXPECTED COURSE AND PROGNOSIS
Varies with the severity of wound injuries and their cause. Nerve and vascular damage—poor prognosis for healing and return to function, especially if the extremities are involved.

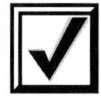

# MISCELLANEOUS

## ASSOCIATED CONDITIONS
None.

## AGE-RELATED FACTORS
N/A

## ZOONOTIC POTENTIAL
N/A

## FERTILITY/BREEDING
Avoid teratogenic antibiotics in laying hen.

## SYNONYMS
None.

## SEE ALSO
Dehydration
Diarrhea
Fractures
Ileus (Functional Gastrointestinal, Crop Stasis)
Lameness
Luxations
Pain
Polyuria
Regurgitation and Vomiting
Trauma

## ABBREVIATIONS
ABC—airway, breathing, and circulation
C/S—culture and sensitivity
CBC—complete blood count
NSAIDs—non-steroidal anti-inflammatory drugs
SIRS—systemic inflammatory response syndrome

## INTERNET RESOURCES
Winkler, K.P. (2022). Wound management. *MSD Veterinary Manual*: http://www.merckmanuals.com/pethealth/special_subjects/emergencies/wound_management.html

### Suggested Reading
Abrahamiam, F.M., Goldstein, E.J.C. (2011). Microbiology of animal bite wound infections. *Clinical Microbiology Reviews*, 24:231–246.
Ferrell, S.T., Cock, H.E.D., Graham, J.E., et al. (2004). Assessment of a caudal external thoracic artery axial pattern flap for treatment of sternal cutaneous wounds in birds, *American Journal of Veterinary Research*, 65:497–502.
Knapp-Hoch, H., de Matos, R. (2014). Clinical technique: Negative pressure wound therapy-general principles and use in avian species. *Journal of Exotic Pet Medicine*, 23:56–66.
Mickelson, M.A., Mans, C., Colopy, S.A. (2016) Principles of wound management and wound healing in exotic pets. *Veterinary Clinics of North America: Exotic Animal Practice*, 19:33–53.
Ritzman, T.K. (2004). Wound healing and management in psittacine birds. *Veterinary Clinics of North America: Exotic Animal Practice*, 7:87–104.
**Author**: Isabelle Langlois, DMV, DABVP (Avian)

**W**

# XANTHOMA/XANTHOGRANULOMAMATOSIS

## BASICS

### DEFINITION
Xanthomas are benign dermal masses or thickenings, often yellow-orange to white in color. The subcutaneous or deeper tissues may also be affected. Disseminated xanthogranulomatosis is rare but has been reported in eclectus parrots and budgerigars with intracoelomic lesions.

### PATHOPHYSIOLOGY
The exact pathophysiology is unclear; however, there does appear to be an association with high-fat or high-cholesterol diets and hypovitaminosis A. Abnormal lipoprotein metabolism has been suggested, as lesions such as atherosclerosis reported concurrently. Other proposed factors include trauma to the affected area, prior or ongoing inflammation of the involved tissues, and psittacine adenovirus-2 infection (red-crowned parakeets).

### SYSTEMS AFFECTED
**Skin**: Masses and yellow dermal changes.
**Musculoskeletal**: Dermal lesions may invade underlying tissues.
**Hepatobiliary**: Disseminated disease.
**Cardiovascular**: Association with atherosclerosis.
**Respiratory**: Dyspnea reported secondary to coelomic mass effect.

### GENETICS
None identified.

### INCIDENCE/PREVALENCE
The prevalence in all psittacine birds on postmortem examination is around 0.5%.

### GEOGRAPHIC DISTRIBUTION
Reported worldwide.

### SIGNALMENT
**Species**: Any species may develop a xanthoma; however, cockatiels and budgerigars are overrepresented. Disseminated xanthogranulomatosis has been reported in eclectus parrots and budgerigars.
**Mean age and range**: Older birds are more commonly affected, though a xanthoma may develop at any age.
**Predominant sex**: Females may be more prone to developing xanthomas.

### SIGNS
#### Historical Findings
**Cutaneous xanthoma**: Mass, often on the wing or sternum, bleeding, self-mutilation.
**Disseminated xanthogranulomatosis**: Weight loss, inappetence, beak overgrowth, regurgitation, dyspnea.

#### Physical Examination Findings
**Cutaneous xanthoma**: Lesions are often found on the wing or sternum, although other locations are reported. Discrete yellow

dermal mass, may be broad based or pedunculated. May also present as a diffuse thickening of the skin with yellow discoloration. Overlying skin is featherless, friable, and yellow to yellow-tan in color. Masses may be ulcerated or hemorrhaging. The bird may be otherwise healthy on examination, or may be obese.
**Xanthogranulomatosis**: Coelomic distension and ascites may be seen.

### CAUSES
Unclear. See Pathophysiology.

### RISK FACTORS
Obesity, hypovitaminosis A, seed diet (high in fat and cholesterol), offering table foods, elevated serum cholesterol, prior trauma to the location of the cutaneous xanthoma. History of coelomitis.

## DIAGNOSIS

### DIFFERENTIAL DIAGNOSIS
Lipoma. Articular gout may mimic the gross appearance of lesions over joints. Granuloma. Other dermal, connective tissue, or intracoelomic neoplasm. Histopathology is required for diagnosis, especially for intracoelomic lesions, although gross appearance of cutaneous lesions is often pathognomonic.

### CBC/BIOCHEMISTRY/URINALYSIS
CBC and biochemistry profile results may be within reference ranges. Leukocytosis reported with xanthogranulomatosis. Inflammatory leukogram may be noted if there is trauma or inflammation associated with the mass. Hypercholesterolemia and hypertriglyceridemia may be noted. Elevated bile acids may be seen with xanthogranulomatosis.

### OTHER LABORATORY TESTS
N/A

### IMAGING
#### Radiography
While this is not directly useful in the diagnosis of a cutaneous xanthoma, it can be used to evaluate underlying structures for evidence of infiltration (e.g. body wall herniation). Disseminated xanthogranulomatosis may present as decreased serosal detail, coelomic distension, and coelomic masses with or without extensive calcification.

#### Coelomic Ultrasound
Anechoic to hypoechoic coelomic effusion, foci of mineralization, hepatic nodules and irregular hepatic margins reported.

#### Computed Tomography
Coelomic effusion and mineralized foci reported, along with diffuse hepatopathy and hepatomegaly, gastrointestinal masses, fluid

and gas dilatation of the proventriculus and intestine, and atherosclerosis.

### DIAGNOSTIC PROCEDURES
The gross appearance of a cutaneous xanthoma is often pathognomonic. However, confirmation by biopsy and histopathology is the gold standard. Intracoelomic lesions require histopathology for diagnosis.

### PATHOLOGIC FINDINGS
The mass or affected portion of skin is soft or firm, yellow to tan in color, and may be friable. With disseminated disease, soft, irregular, yellow or tan lesions can be identified, covering the coelomic viscera and body wall. Ascites is frequently present. Histologically, there are aggregates of macrophages with foamy appearing cytoplasm and lipid vacuoles, together with focal or diffuse aggregates of giant cells around or containing cholesterol clefts. Necrotic debris may be present, along with mixed inflammation, fibrosis, or mineralization. Concurrent atherosclerosis, cholangiohepatitis, cholangitis, and hepatic lipidosis may be identified.

## TREATMENT

### APPROPRIATE HEALTH CARE
Surgical removal of cutaneous xanthomas is preferred. Dietary management may be successful with some individuals. Successful management of xanthogranulomatosis has not been described.

### NURSING CARE
Temporary bandaging may be required to prevent trauma to the site of a cutaneous lesion. An Elizabethan collar may be indicated if the bird is self-mutilating. Antibiotics and analgesics should be used as indicated if the mass is traumatized. Various supportive treatments have reported for xanthogranulomatosis to limited success. Coelomocentesis may improve comfort if significant effusion present.

### ACTIVITY
If the size or presence of a dermal lesion impede the bird's ability to ambulate or fly, these activities should be avoided (flight) or modified (perching, ambulating) to limit the risk of falling. This may entail removing higher perches from the cage, padding the cage bottom in case of falls, and keeping food and water within easy reach of the cage bottom.

### DIET
Converting the bird to a low-fat pelleted diet may help prevent further xanthomatous tissue from developing, but may or may not induce regression of a xanthoma already present. Less severe lesions may respond to dietary improvement as a sole therapy.

## CLIENT EDUCATION

While diet may not cause cutaneous lesions to completely regress, it is an important step in preventing recurrence and can improve the bird's overall health.

## SURGICAL CONSIDERATIONS

Care should be taken to completely excise a cutaneous xanthoma with a margin of healthy tissue; xanthomatous tissues are prone to dehiscence postoperatively. Consider the use of radiosurgery to limit blood loss, as xanthogranulomas tend to be vascular. A larger mass may require second intention healing of the site. Infiltrative masses may necessitate amputation (distal wing) or resection of deeper tissues. As obesity is a risk factor for the development of xanthomas, it is important to ensure adequate ventilation of the anesthetized patient. Cryosurgery may also be used.

# MEDICATIONS

## DRUG(S) OF CHOICE

Corticosteroids (prednisolone) have been used to treat disseminated xanthogranulomatosis.

## CONTRAINDICATIONS

N/A

## PRECAUTIONS

N/A

## POSSIBLE INTERACTIONS

N/A

## ALTERNATIVE DRUGS

N/A

# FOLLOW-UP

## PATIENT MONITORING

If excision is performed, the surgical site should be monitored daily for evidence of dehiscence. Surgical incisions left to heal by second intention should be monitored at the surgeon's discretion. Routine weighing of the patient should be performed when dietary management is employed, to ensure there are no rapid drops in weight and that the patient achieves a healthy weight.

## PREVENTION/AVOIDANCE

Limit the bird's fat intake to prevent development of lesions. Avoid trauma to the distal limbs. Illness of any sort should be addressed promptly, as there may be an association with chronic or ongoing coelomic inflammation and disseminated disease.

## POSSIBLE COMPLICATIONS

Dehiscence of a cutaneous surgical site may be seen, especially if complete excision was not possible. This may necessitate a second surgery or the wound may be allowed to heal by second intention. If left in place, a cutaneous mass may become abraded or otherwise traumatized by the bird's normal activities (flight, grooming, play). This can lead to infection of the lesion, bleeding, and pain. A large mass may also impede movement. Reported cases of disseminated xanthogranulomatosis tend to be significantly ill on presentation, and may die within hours despite supportive care.

## EXPECTED COURSE AND PROGNOSIS

With complete excision, the prognosis for a specific cutaneous lesion is good. This cannot always be accomplished, however, as xanthomas can be extensive and infiltrative. A sizable xanthoma located on the distal wing may require amputation of the distal wing for complete excision. Without addressing the diet and other predisposing factors, there is a risk for reoccurrence in the same area or elsewhere. In reported cases of disseminated xanthogranulomatosis, the prognosis is poor, with affected birds either euthanized or dying within days to nearly 2 years.

# MISCELLANEOUS

## ASSOCIATED CONDITIONS

Obesity, lipomas, atherosclerosis, cholangiohepatitis, and cholangitis.

## AGE-RELATED FACTORS

It has been reported that older birds tend to be more commonly affected by cutaneous lesions, and disseminated lesions have been reported in a wide age range. Thus, there may be other concurrent age-related disease present. This may affect the decision to pursue treatment as opposed to palliative care.

## ZOONOTIC POTENTIAL

None.

## FERTILITY/BREEDING

N/A

## SYNONYMS

N/A

## SEE ALSO

N/A

## ABBREVIATIONS

N/A

## INTERNET RESOURCES

Rich, G. (2023). Tumors: Xanthomas in birds. *VCA Animal Hospital*: http://www.vcahospitals.com/main/pet-health-information/article/animal-health/tumors-xanthomas-in-birds/965

*Suggested Reading*

Donovan, T.A., Garner, M.M., Quesenberry, K., et al. (2022). Disseminated coelomic xanthogranulomatosis in eclectus parrots (*Eclectus roratus*) and budgerigars (*Melopsittacus undulatus*). *Veterinary Pathology*, 59:143–151.

Hanson, M.E., Donovan, T.A., Quesenberry, K., et al. (2020). Imaging features of disseminated xanthogranulomatous inflammation in electus parrots (*Eclectus roratus*). *Veterinary Radiology & Ultrasound*, 61:409–416.

Lightfoot, T.L. (2010). Geriatric psittacine medicine. *Veterinary Clinics of North America: Exotic Animal Practice*, 13:27–49.

Pass, D.A. (2007). The pathology of the avian integument: A review. *Avian Pathology*, 18:1–72.

**Author**: Kristin M. Sinclair DVM, DABVP (Avian Practice, Exotic Companion Mammal Practice)

X

# YERSINIOSIS

## BASICS

### DEFINITION
*Yersinia pseudotuberculosis* is a Gram-negative, non-spore-forming, facultative anaerobic coccobacillus of the family Enterobacteriaceae, which causes acute septicemic and systemic infection in various bird species. The latter is also known as pseudotuberculosis.

### PATHOPHYSIOLOGY
Replication and motility in the environment at low temperatures (39.2°F/4°C), so infections are particularly common during the cold season. Rodents and wild passerines often appear to be subclinically infected and therefore spread the bacterium. Enteric infection after oral ingestion, following by invasion and septicaemia. Chronic stage is characterized by formation of granulomas.

### SYSTEMS AFFECTED
Gastrointestinal, hepatobiliary.

### GENETICS
N/A

### INCIDENCE/PREVALENCE
Most common in finches, toucans, and turacos kept in outdoor aviaries. Less common in psittacine birds, pigeons, backyard poultry. Morbidity and mortality are usually high.

### GEOGRAPHIC DISTRIBUTION
Worldwide.

### SIGNALMENT
**Species**: Passeriformes, Piciformes, Psittaciformes, backyard poultry.
**Mean age and range**: None.
**Predominant sex**: None.

### SIGNS
*Historical Findings*
Lethargy and depression. Ruffled feathers. Diarrhoea. Dyspnoea. Weight loss and wasting in the chronic stage.

*Physical Examination Findings*
Depression. Dehydration. Sudden death. Emaciation in the chronic stage.

### CAUSES
Infection with *Yersinia pseudotuberculosis*.

### RISK FACTORS
Cold season. Outdoor aviaries with contact to wild birds and rodents.

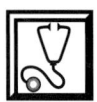

## DIAGNOSIS

### DIFFERENTIAL DIAGNOSIS
Salmonellosis, mycobacteriosis.

### CBC/BIOCHEMISTRY/URINALYSIS
Leucocytosis with increased heterophils and monocytes. Increased GLDH.

### OTHER LABORATORY TESTS
Fecal cultivation with cold temperature enrichment.

### IMAGING
Hepatosplenomegaly. Multifocal spots with increased radiodensity in the visceral organs and bones in the chronic stage.

### DIAGNOSTIC PROCEDURES
Necropsy.

### PATHOLOGIC FINDINGS
Hepatosplenomegaly. Bloody to fibrinous exudate into the body cavity. Submiliary to miliary, sharply demarcated grayish foci within visceral organs. Chronic infections are characterized by granuloma formation in organs, bones, and the skeletal musculature. Coagulation necrosis and thrombophlebitis with multiple coccoid rods. Inflammatory cells infiltrate the necrotic areas and formation of granulomas in a later stage.

## TREATMENT

### APPROPRIATE HEALTH CARE
Inpatient medical management may be required; fluid and nutritional support are indicated if the patient is debilitated and dehydrated.

### NURSING CARE
Fluid support (SQ, IV, IO). Nutritional support via gavage may be indicated if anorexic.

### ACTIVITY
No restrictions indicated.

### DIET
N/A

### CLIENT EDUCATION
Prevent rodents and wild passerine birds from entering the aviaries. Cleaning and disinfecting washable surfaces. The removal or digging of natural soil areas may help to reduce transmission risk.

### SURGICAL CONSIDERATIONS
N/A

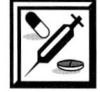

## MEDICATIONS

### DRUG(S) OF CHOICE
Flock should be treated based on culture and sensitivity. Enrofloxacin 200 mg/l drinking water.

### CONTRAINDICATIONS
N/A

### PRECAUTIONS
N/A

### POSSIBLE INTERACTIONS
N/A

### ALTERNATIVE DRUGS
Amoxicillin trihydrate 200–400 mg/l drinking water.

## FOLLOW-UP

### PATIENT MONITORING
Flock control with repeated fecal culture using cold enrichment.

### PREVENTION/AVOIDANCE
Autogenous vaccines of flock specific isolates.

### POSSIBLE COMPLICATIONS
N/A

### EXPECTED COURSE AND PROGNOSIS
Birds with peracute to acute stages of yersiniosis usually die.

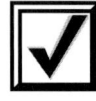

## MISCELLANEOUS

### ASSOCIATED CONDITIONS
N/A

### AGE-RELATED FACTORS
N/A

### ZOONOTIC POTENTIAL
Yes.

### FERTILITY/BREEDING
N/A

### SYNONYMS
Pseudotuberculosis.

### SEE ALSO
Clostridiosis
Colibacillosis
Liver Diseases
Mycobacteriosis
Salmonellosis
Sepsis

### ABBREVIATIONS
GLDH—glutamate dehydrogenase

### INTERNET RESOURCES
N/A

*Suggested Reading*
Ceccolini, M.E., Macgregor, S.K., Spiro, S., et al. (2020). *Yersinia pseudotuberculosis* infections in primates, artiodactyls, and birds within a zoological facility in the United Kingdom. *Journal of Zoo and Wildlife Medicine*, 51:527–538.
Haesebrouck, F., Vanrobaeys, M., De Herdt, P., Ducatelle, R. (1995). Effect of antimicrobial treatment on the course of an experimental *Yersinia pseudotuberculosis* infection in canaries. *Avian Pathology*, 24:273–283.
Gerlach, H. (1994). Bacteria. In: *Avian Medicine: Principles and Application*

(ed. B. Ritchie, G. Harrison, L. Harrison), 949–983. Lake Worth, FL: Wingers Publishing.

Nakamura, S., Hayashidani, H., Sotohira, Y., Une, Y. (2016). Yersiniosis caused by *Yersinia pseudotuberculosis* in captive toucans (Ramphastidae) and a Japanese squirrel (*Sciurus lis*) in zoological gardens in Japan. *Journal of Veterinary Medicine and Science*, 78:297–299.

Stoute, S.T., Cooper, G.L., Bickford, A.A., et al. (2016). *Yersinia pseudotuberculosis* in Eurasian collared doves (*Streptopelia decaocto*) and retrospective study of avian yersiniosis at the California Animal Health and Food Safety Laboratory System (1990–2015). *Avian Diseases*, 60:82–86.

**Author**: Volker Schmidt, PD, DrMedVet., DECZM (Avian, Herpetological)

Y

# YOLK SAC RETENTION AND INFECTION

## BASICS

### DEFINITION
The failure of the yolk content, in neonate chicks, to be reabsorbed in the normal time (typically within 1 week in most species) by the small intestine.

### PATHOPHYSIOLOGY
The pathophysiology of the absorption failure is not clear. The risk factors prevent the yolk sac from being retracted into the abdominal wall and finally absorbed. The presence of yolk sac in an ostrich chick beyond day 13 post hatch should considered as retained.

### SYSTEMS AFFECTED
Gastrointestinal, reproductive, skin.

### GENETICS
N/A

### INCIDENCE/PREVALENCE
Most common cause of neonatal mortality: 5–30% in poultry, 20% in turkeys, 16 % in quails, 7.2% in goslings, 92% in ducklings, 42% in canaries, 15–30% in Asian McQueen's bustard, 50–81% in Humboldt penguins, 53% in tufted puffins with 90% septicaemia due to omphalitis, 97% in zoo ratites (ostrich, rhea, emu), 4.2% in kiwis, 21% in farmed ostriches.

### GEOGRAPHIC DISTRIBUTION
N/A

### SIGNALMENT
**Species**: All avian species. Seen in Galliformes, Anseriformes, Ratites, Falconiformes, Sphenisciformes.
**Mean age and range**: Neonates 1–7 days; in Humboldt penguin to 40 days.
**Predominant sex**: None.

### SIGNS
#### Historical Findings
Anorexia. Reduced activity, depression. Coelomic distension. Progressive torticollis. Head tilt. Inability to stand. Inflamed umbilicus. Sudden anorexia after weight gain.

#### Physical Examination Findings
Loss of weight. Tachycardia. Non-painful abdomen.

### CAUSES
Infection of the umbilicus or the yolk sac. Ground corn as initial feeding/starvation. High ambient temperatures of 95°F (35°C) reduce food intake and body weight. Increased diencephalic oxidative damage 48 hours post hatch. Low brooding temperature (around 68°F/20°C) during the first 7 days post hatch, decreased broiler bone development and reduced chick's body weight due to stress.

### RISK FACTORS
Fluctuation in brooding temperature. Cold or lower than normal brooding temperature. Omphalitis. First chick of the clutch, poor gut fill, prominent bursa of Fabricius (Humboldt penguins). Prolonged or difficult hatch, assisted hatch, presence of external yolk at hatching, external or protuberant umbilicus (kiwis). High incubation temperature, high humidity, high-energy diets, lack of exercise (ostrich). Corn feeding in early life (poultry).

## DIAGNOSIS

### DIFFERENTIAL DIAGNOSIS
Omphalitis, yolk sac rupture. Any condition to cause abdominal distension in neonates (parasitosis, foreign body, liver enlargement due to polyomavirus, enteritis).

### CBC/BIOCHEMISTRY/URINALYSIS
Usually within normal limits except in omphalitis. Marked hyperuricemia (1764 μml/l; reference 0–600 μmol/l) in a brown kiwi.

### OTHER LABORATORY TESTS
Bacteriologic culture of the yolk sac. *Plesiomonas shigelloides* and *Staphylococcus* spp. (Humboldt penguins). *Escherichia coli* in 57% cases, *Pseudomonas* in 19% cases of neonate zoo ratites (ostrich, emu, rhea); 22% infection percentage in farmed ostrich with *E. coli* the most common.

### IMAGING
Radiographs should be performed to rule out any underlying pathology, omphalitis, retained yolk sac. CT was helpful to diagnose a mineralized retained yolk sac in a kiwi. Abdominal ultrasound might help diagnosis.

### DIAGNOSTIC PROCEDURES
None.

### PATHOLOGIC FINDINGS
Retained yolk sacs consist primarily of cords of vacuolated endodermal cells supported by a vascular lamina propria. The yolk sacs are connected to the jejunum by a stalk composed mainly of large vessels, mesenchyme, and melanocyte. Occasionally, small globules of homogeneous eosinophilic material (protein) and rare small foci of hematopoietic cells are observed within the yolk sac lumen. Retained sacs from older birds are not significantly different from retained sacs in relatively younger birds.

## TREATMENT

### APPROPRIATE HEALTH CARE
Emergency inpatient care. Stabilization until possible surgery. Post-surgical inpatient care until 2 weeks old.

### NURSING CARE
Neonatal care includes warm environment, strict hygiene, fluid administration, assisted feeding, careful drug allometric scaling and dosing.

### ACTIVITY
Restricted after possible surgery.

### DIET
Forced feeding in anorectic chicks. Balanced growth diet to avoid other nutritional neonatal diseases.

### CLIENT EDUCATION
Normally postmortem recognition. Recommendation of surgical resolution in ratites.

### SURGICAL CONSIDERATIONS
Surgical removal of yolk sac in kiwis. High (86%) success rate. Circumferential skin incision around the umbilicus laterally extended. Enough length of incision to exteriorize the yolk sac. Traction on the umbilicus with cotton swabs. Caution not to rupture the yolk sac. Peritoneal lavage in case of rupture.

## MEDICATIONS

### DRUG(S) OF CHOICE
Antibiotics for 5–7 days preferably after culture and sensitivity test. NSAIDs may be used in management of the pain and inflammation.

### CONTRAINDICATIONS
None.

### PRECAUTIONS
None.

### POSSIBLE INTERACTIONS
None.

### ALTERNATIVE DRUGS
None.

## FOLLOW-UP

### PATIENT MONITORING
Daily for post-surgical complications and weight gain. Overall growth monitoring.

### PREVENTION/AVOIDANCE
Supplementation of a small quantity of drinking water soon after hatching facilitates the use of the yolk as well as the digestive transit. Brooding temperature at 84.2°F (29°C) could promote the absorption of fatty acids in yolk sac in goslings.

### POSSIBLE COMPLICATIONS
Mineralization of retained yolk sac. Peritonitis after intraoperative rupture. Irregular growth. Death.

Y

## EXPECTED COURSE AND PROGNOSIS

In kiwis, postoperative prognosis is guarded to good.

 MISCELLANEOUS

### ASSOCIATED CONDITIONS

Omphalitis, retained intra-abdominal yolk sac, dead in shell mortality.

### AGE-RELATED FACTORS

Neonates (1–7 days).

### ZOONOTIC POTENTIAL

N/A

### FERTILITY/BREEDING

N/A

### SYNONYMS

N/A

### SEE ALSO

Coelomic Distension
Egg Abnormalities
Egg Yolk and Reproductive Coelomitis
Enteritis and Gastritis

### ABBREVIATIONS

CT—computed tomography
NSAIDs—non-steroidal anti-inflammatory drugs

### INTERNET RESOURCES

N/A

*Suggested Reading*
Bassett, S., Kelly, T., Gartrell, B. (2006). Yolk sac retention and removal in the North Island Brown Kiwi (*Apteryx mantelli*). *Proceedings of the Association of Avian Veterinarians, Australian Committee,* 131–138.

Dzoma, B.M., Dorrestein, G.M. (2001). Yolk sac retention in the ostrich (*Struthio camelus*): histopathologic, anatomic, and physiologic considerations. *Journal of Avian Medicine and Surgery,* 15:81–89.
Khan, K.A., Khan, S.A., Hamid, S., et al. (2002). A study on the pathogenesis of yolk retention in broiler chicks. *Pakistan Veterinary Journal,* 22:175–180.
Samour, J. (2015). *Avian Medicine.* St. Louis, MO: Elsevier Health Sciences.
Taylor, E.L., Flach, E.J., Strike, T., et al. (2021). Risk factors associated with yolk sac retention in captive-bred Humboldt penguin (*Spheniscus humboldti*) chicks. *Journal of Zoo and Wildlife Medicine,* 52:660–670.

**Author:** Panagiotis Azmanis DVM, PhD, DECZM (Avian)

Y

## APPENDIX I

### COMMON DOSAGES FOR BIRDS

| Drug | Dosage | Indication/Comments |
|------|--------|---------------------|
| Acetic acid (vinegar) | 16 ml/l drinking water | May be useful for non-invasive gastrointestinal yeast infections |
| Acyclovir | 10–40 mg/kg IM q12–24h<br>29–330 mg/kg PO q8–12h | Antiviral agent; active against herpesvirus and cytomegalovirus |
| Albendazole | 5.2–50 mg/kg PO q12–24h | Broad-spectrum anthelmintic; toxic in some species |
| Albuterol | 2.5 mg in 3 cc saline q4–6h for nebulization | Bronchodilator |
| Alfaxalone | 2–20 mg/kg IM, IV | Neuroactive steroid used for anesthetic induction and anesthesia |
| Allopurinol | 10–30 mg/kg PO q4–24h | Xanthine oxidase inhibitor; use in treatment of gout controversial |
| Aloe vera | Topical | Anti-inflammatory, antithromboxane activity |
| Aluminum hydroxide | 30–90 mg/kg PO q12h | Phosphate binder; antacid |
| Amikacin | 5–6 mg/ml sterile water or saline for nebulization | Discontinue if renal disease or polyuria develops |
| Aminophylline | 4–10 mg/kg PO, IV; 3 mg/ml sterile water or saline for nebulization | Bronchial and pulmonary vasculature smooth muscle relaxation, pulmonary edema |
| Amitriptyline | 1–5 mg/kg PO q12–24h | Tricyclic antidepressant; inhibits serotonin reuptake; antihistamine |
| Amoxicillin/clavulanate | 125 mg/kg PO q12h | Beta-lactamase inhibitor |
| Amphotericin B | 1.5 mg/kg IV q8h × 3–7 days; 1 mg/kg intratracheal q8–12h, dilute to 1 ml with sterile water; 100 mg/kg PO q12–24h × 10–30 days for *Macrorhabdus ornithogaster*; 0.1–7 mg/ml saline q12h for nebulization | Fungicidal; intratracheal administration may cause tracheitis; nephrotoxic, lipid-based product less toxic |
| Amprolium | 2.2–30 mg/kg PO q24h<br>50–575 mg/ml drinking water | Pyrimidine derivative coccidiostat; some coccidial organisms show resistance |
| Asparaginase | 400–1650 IU/kg SQ, IM | Lymphosarcoma; premedicate with diphenhydramine; higher dosage associated with bone marrow suppression in some species |
| Aspirin (acetylsalicylic acid) | 5–150 mg/kg PO<br>325 mg/250 ml drinking water | Contraindicated with tetracycline, insulin, or allopurinol therapy |
| Atipamezole | 0.25–0.5 mg/kg IM | $\alpha_2$-adrenergic antagonist; 1:1 volume reversal of dexmedetomidine |
| Atorvastatin | 20 mg/kg PO q12–24h | Lipid lowering agent; therapeutic plasma levels in Amazon parrots and cockatiels; do not give with grapefruit or azole antifungals |
| Atropine sulfate | 0.01–0.5 mg/kg SQ, IM, IV | Anticholinergic agent; antidote for organophosphate toxicosis |
| Azithromycin | 40 mg/kg PO q24–48h | Macrolide antibiotic |
| Barium sulfate | 20–50 ml/kg PO via gavage | Radiopaque contrast media; dilute 72% suspension 1:1 with water; dilute 92% suspension 1:2 with water; more dilute concentrations can be used. |
| Benazepril | 0.5 mg/kg PO q24h | ACE inhibitor; heart failure, hypertension |
| Bismuth sulfate | 1–2 ml/kg PO | Weak adsorbent; may be useful for toxin removal |

COMMON DOSAGES FOR BIRDS (CONTINUED)

| Drug | Dosage | Indication/Comments |
|---|---|---|
| Bupivacaine HCl | 2–10 mg/kg SQ, perineurally, into incision site, intra-articular; 50:50 mixture with DMSO for topical application | Local anesthetic agent; minimize dose to limit toxic effects |
| Buprenorphine HCl | 0.05–6 mg/kg IM, IV | Opioid agonist–antagonist |
| Buspirone HCl | 0.5 mg/kg PO q12h | Anxiolytic |
| Butorphanol tartrate | 0.05–6 mg/kg IM, IV q1–4h | Opioid agonist–antagonist; PO bioavailability <10% |
| Calcitonin | 4 IU/kg IM q12h | Hypercalcemia reduction caused by cholecalciferol rodenticide toxicity |
| Calcium EDTA (edetate calcium disodium) | 10–50 mg/kg IM, IV q12h | Preferred initial chelator for lead and zinc toxicosis; maintain hydration |
| Calcium glubionate | 23–150 mg/kg PO q12–24h; 750 mg/ml drinking water | Hypocalcemia, calcium supplementation |
| Calcium gluconate (10%) | 5–500 mg/kg SQ, IM, IV 1 ml/30 ml (3300 mg/L) drinking water | Hypocalcemia; dilute 1:1 with saline or sterile water for IM or IV injections |
| Carboplatin | 5 mg/kg IV, IO, intralesional 125 mg/m² IV | Osteosarcoma, carcinoma, other sarcomas |
| Carnidazole | 5–10 mg/bird PO 12.5–50 mg/kg PO once, repeat in 10–14 days | May be effective against *Trichomonas, Hexamita, Histomonas* |
| Carprofen | 1–40 mg/kg PO, SQ, IM, IV, in feed | Non-steroidal anti-inflammatory; use caution in some species |
| Celecoxib | 10 mg/kg PO q24h | Psittacines/avian ganglioneuritis |
| Cephalexin | 40–100 mg/kg PO, IM q6–8h | First-generation cephalosporin |
| Charcoal, activated | 52–8000 mg/kg PO | Adsorbs toxins from gastrointestinal tract |
| Chlorambucil | 1 mg/bird PO twice weekly, ducks; 2 mg/kg PO twice weekly | Lymphocytic leukemia or lymphosarcoma |
| Chloramphenicol palmitate | 30–100 mg/kg PO q6-12h | Broad spectrum; can cause blood dyscrasias in humans. Used with primaquine for *Plasmodium, Haemoproteus, Leucocytozoon* |
| Chloroquine phosphate | 5–60 mg/kg PO repeated q12h–7d | |
| Cimetidine | 3–10 mg/kg PO, IM, IV q8–12h | Histamine-2 blocker |
| Ciprofloxacin (cipro) | 15–20 mg/kg PO, IM q12h | Broad-spectrum quinolone; do not use in food animals |
| Ciprofloxacin HCl 0.3% | Apply topically | Antibiotic; corneal ulcers, conjunctivitis |
| Cisapride | 0.25–1.5 mg/kg PO q8–12h | Gastrointestinal prokinetic agent; not commercially available, can be compounded |
| Cisplatin | 1 mg/kg IV over 1 hour | Osteosarcoma, carcinoma, other sarcomas |
| Clindamycin | 25–100 mg/kg PO q8–24h | Lincosamide antibiotic; indicated for bone/joint infections |
| Clomipramine | 0.5–8 mg/kg PO q12–24h | Tricyclic antidepressant; antihistamine; extrapyramidal signs and death reported in some species |
| Colchicine | 0.01–0.2 mg/kg PO q12–24h | Anti-inflammatory used to treat gout or hepatic fibrosis/cirrhosis; may potentiate gout formation |
| Cyclophosphamide | 200–300 mg/m² PO, IO | Lymphosarcoma, sarcoma |
| Cyclosporine | 10 mg/kg PO q12h | Immunosuppressive agent; may help prevent avian bornaviral signs |
| Deferoxamine mesylate | 20–100 mg/kg PO, SQ, IM | Preferred iron chelator for hemochromatosis |
| Deslorelin | 4.7-mg or 9.4-mg implant placed SQ intrascapularly | GnRH agonist available as long-term implant |

COMMON DOSAGES FOR BIRDS (CONTINUED)

| Drug | Dosage | Indication/Comments |
|---|---|---|
| Dexmedetomidine HCl | 25–80 µg/kg IM | α₂-agonist; variable results, often used in combination with other drugs |
| Dexamethasone | 0.2–8 mg/kg SQ, IM, IV | Steroidal anti-inflammatory; use with caution |
| Dextrose (50%) | 50–1000 mg/kg IV (slow bolus) | Hypoglycemia; can dilute with fluids |
| Diazepam | 0.05–15.6 mg/kg PO, IM, IV, intranasally | Benzodiazepine; IM administration may cause muscle irritation; reversal with flumazenil |
| Dimercaprol (BAL in oil) | 2.5–35 mg/kg PO, IM | Heavy-metal toxicosis; arsenical compound toxicosis |
| Dimercaptosuccinic acid (DMSA or succimer) | 25–40 mg/kg PO q12h | Oral chelator for lead or zinc; may be effective for mercury toxicosis |
| Diphenhydramine | 2–4 mg/kg PO, IM | Antihistamine |
| Doxorubicin | 2 mg/kg IV<br>30–60 mg/m² IO, IV | Osteosarcoma, mesenchymal, and epithelial tumors, and lymphoproliferative disease |
| Doxycycline | 25–50 mg/kg PO q12–24h | Antibiotic of choice for *Chlamydia* and *Mycoplasma*; may cause regurgitation in some species; wide variation in dosage recommendations for food/water treatment |
| Doxycycline (Vibravenos) | 25–100 mg/kg IM q5–7 days | Not available in the USA without FDA permission; injectable doxycycline of choice for use in birds |
| Enalapril | 0.2–5 mg/kg PO q8–24h | ACE inhibitor; heart failure |
| Enrofloxacin | 5–20 mg/kg PO, SQ, IM q12–24h | Broad-spectrum quinolone; IM formulation extremely painful for repeated injection; best to avoid IV use in birds |
| Epinephrine (1:1000) | 0.5–1 ml/kg IM, IO, IV, intratracheal | Cardiopulmonary resuscitation; bradycardia |
| Fatty acids (omega-3, omega-6) | 0.1–0.2 ml/kg of flaxseed oil to corn oil mixed at a ratio of 1:4 PO or added to food | Glomerular disease; pancreatitis; use to reduce thromboxane A₂ synthesis |
| Fenbendazole | 1.5–50 mg/kg PO q24h | Effective against cestodes, nematodes, trematodes, *Giardia*, acanthocephalans; toxic in many species; can cause feather abnormalities |
| Fentanyl citrate | 20 µg bolus + 0.2–6 µg/kg/min IV CRI | Short acting µ-opioid agonist; reduces isoflurane MAC in some species but variable results and significant adverse effects, including hyperactivity, reported |
| Fipronil | 7.5 mg/kg; spray on skin once, repeat in 30 days | Ectoparasite treatment; apply via pad to base of neck, tail base, under wings; avoid plumage during application to minimize feather damage |
| Fluids | 10–25 ml/kg IO, IV<br>50–90 ml/kg SQ, IO, IV | Fluid therapy; dehydration; hypovolemic shock |
| Fluconazole | 2–15 mg/kg PO q12–24h | Fungistatic; penetrates CNS and eyes; may be ineffective against aspergillosis; can cause death in some species at higher doses |
| Flumazenil | 0.013–0.31 mg/kg IM, IV, intranasally | Benzodiazepine antagonist |
| Fluoxetine | 0.4–4 mg/kg PO q12–24h | Selective serotonin reuptake inhibitor; antidepressant |
| Furosemide | 0.1–10 mg/kg PO, SQ, IM, IV | Diuretic; some species extremely sensitive |
| Gabapentin | 3–25 mg/kg PO q12–24h | GABA analogue; indicated for neuropathic pain |
| Gemfibrozil | 30 mg/kg PO q8h | Lipid-regulating agent; yolk emboli; give with niacin |
| Gentamicin sulfate | 1 drop topical q4–8h | Antibiotic; corneal ulcers; causes irritation |
| Glipizide | 0.5–1.25 mg/kg PO q12–24h | Sulfonylurea antidiabetic; diabetes mellitus |

COMMON DOSAGES FOR BIRDS (CONTINUED)

| Drug | Dosage | Indication/Comments |
|---|---|---|
| Glucosamine/chondroitin sulfate | 20 mg/kg PO (of the chondroitin component) q12h | Nutraceutical used as an adjunctive treatment for osteoarthritis or other painful conditions |
| Glycopyrrolate | 0.01–0.04 mg/kg IM, IV | Anticholinergic agent; slower onset than atropine |
| Guaifenesin | 0.8 mg/kg PO q12h | Expectorant; bronchodilation |
| Haloperidol | 0.1–2 mg/kg PO q12–24h | Butyrophenone dopamine antagonist tranquilizer; extrapyramidal effects and death reported in some species |
| Hetastarch | 10–15 ml/kg IV slowly | Hypovolemia; hypoproteinemia; may be associated with coagulopathy or acute renal disease in mammals |
| Hyaluronidase | 5 IU/kg IV q12h<br>75–150 IU/l fluids | Egg-yolk related disease; increase absorption rate of fluids |
| Hydroxyzine | 2–2.2 mg/kg PO q8–12h<br>30–40 mg/L drinking water | Antihistamine with mild sedative effects |
| Insulin | 0.5–3 IU/kg IM q12–48h | NPH insulin |
| Iodine (Lugol's iodine) | 0.2 ml/L drinking water daily<br>3 drops into 100 ml drinking water | Thyroid hyperplasia |
| Iohexol | 2–3 ml/kg IV over 3–5 seconds; 20–50 ml/kg PO | Iodinated contrast media |
| Iron dextran | 10 mg/kg IM, repeat in 7–10 days | Iron-deficiency anemia |
| Isoflurane | 0.5–4% (usually 1.5–2%) | Inhalant anesthetic of choice in birds |
| Isoxsuprine | 5–10 mg/kg PO q12–24h | Peripheral vasodilator; wing-tip edema; atherosclerosis |
| Itraconazole | 2.5–10 mg/kg PO q12–24h | Fungistatic; effective for systemic and superficial mycosis; use caution in African grey parrots |
| Ivermectin | 0.2–2 mg/kg PO, SQ, topical on skin, IM once, repeat in 7–14 days | Effective against nematodes, acanthocephalans, leeches, most ectoparasites; toxicity reported |
| Kaolin/pectin | 2–15 ml/kg PO q6–12h | Intestinal protectant; antidiarrheal |
| Ketamine HCl | 2–50 mg/kg SQ, IM, IV | Dissociative anesthetic; seldom used as sole agent |
| L-carnitine | 1000 mg/kg feed | Budgerigars; lipomas |
| Lactulose | 0.3 ml/kg PO q12h<br>150–650 mg/kg PO q8–12h | Prophylactic laxative |
| Leuprolide acetate | 100–1250 µg/kg IM | Synthetic GnRH agonist depot drug |
| Levetiracetam | 20–100 mg/kg PO q8h | Anticonvulsant; measure drug levels since metabolism may vary between species |
| Levothyroxine (l-thyroxine) | 0.02 mg/kg PO<br>1–1000 µg/kg PO | May induce molt; use with caution |
| Lidocaine | 1–3 mg/kg<br>15–20 mg/kg perineurally | Local anesthetic agent; toxic doses reported at 2.7–3.3 mg/kg in some species |
| Lorazepam | 0.1 mg/kg PO q12h | Benzodiazepine with anxiolytic and sedative effects |
| Magnesium sulfate | 500–1000 mg/kg PO q12–24h | Cathartic used in lead toxicosis to reduce lead absorption; give 30 minutes after activated charcoal |
| Mannitol | 0.2–2 g/kg IV (slow) | Cerebral edema; anuric renal failure |
| Marbofloxacin | 2–15 mg/kg PO IM, IV q24h | Fluoroquinolone; broad spectrum |
| Maropitant | 1 mg/kg SQ, IM | Antiemetic |
| Meloxicam | 0.1–2 mg/kg PO, IM, IV | Non-steroidal anti-inflammatory |
| Methocarbamol | 32.5–50 mg/kg PO, IV | Capture myopathy; muscle relaxation |

COMMON DOSAGES FOR BIRDS (CONTINUED)

| Drug | Dosage | Indication/Comments |
|------|--------|---------------------|
| Metoclopramide | 0.1–2 mg/kg PO, IM, IV | Gastrointestinal motility disorders |
| Metronidazole | 10–50 mg/kg PO, IM q12–24h | Effective against most anaerobic bacteria; antiprotozoal (*Giardia, Histomonas, Spironucleus, Trichomonas*) |
| Miconazole | Topical | Antifungal; IV formulation and cream can be used topically |
| Midazolam HCl | 0.1–15.6 mg/kg SQ, IM, IV, intranasally | Benzodiazepine with shorter duration than diazepam |
| Mineral oil | 5–15 mg/kg via gavage | Cathartic; foreign body passage; administer directly into crop to avoid aspiration |
| Monensin | 53–108 mg/kg in feed × 8–10 weeks | Ionophore antibiotic anticoccidial feed additive |
| Moxidectin | 0.2–1 mg/kg PO, IM<br>1 mg/bird topically in budgerigars | Treatment for *Serratospiculum, Capillaria*, acanthocephalans, *Paraspiralatus, Physaloptera* |
| N-acetyl-L-cysteine 10–20% | 22 mg/ml sterile water for nebulization | Mucolytic agent; tracheal irritation and bronchoconstriction reported in mammals |
| Naloxone HCl | 2 mg/kg IV | Opioid antagonist |
| Naltrexone HCl | 1.5 mg/kg PO q8–12h | Opioid antagonist; feather picking; self-mutilation |
| Neomycin/polymyxin B/ gramicidin | 1 drop topical q2–8h | Antibiotic; corneal ulcers, conjunctivitis |
| Niacin (nicotinic acid) | 50 mg/kg PO q8h | Yolk emboli; give with gemfibrozil |
| Nystatin | 100,000–600,000 IU/kg PO q8–12h | Candidiasis; not systemically absorbed; lesions must be treated with direct contact |
| Oxytocin | 0.5–10 IU/kg IM | For egg binding and dystocia; use should be preceded by calcium administration |
| Pancreatic enzyme powder | 2–5 g/kg<br>1/8 tsp/kg feed | Exocrine pancreatic insufficiency; maldigestion; mix with food and let stand 30 minutes |
| Paromomycin | 100 mg/kg PO q12h × 7 days; 1000 mg/kg food | *Cryptosporidium*; may cause secondary bacterial or fungal infection |
| Paroxetine | 1–3 mg/kg PO q24h | Selective serotonin reuptake inhibitor |
| Penicillamine | 30–55 mg/kg PO q12h | Preferred chelator for copper toxicosis; may be used for lead, zinc, and mercury toxicosis |
| Pentoxifylline | 15–30 mg/kg PO q8–24h | Anti-inflammatory and vasodilator; useful in frostbite and peripheral arterial disease |
| Permethrin | Dust plumage lightly | Lice, fleas |
| Phenobarbital sodium | 1–7 mg/kg PO, IV<br>50–80 mg/L drinking water | Barbiturate anticonvulsant; may not reach therapeutic levels with oral dosing in African grey parrots |
| Pimobendan | 0.25–10 mg/kg PO q12h | Inodilator for management of congestive heart failure |
| Piperacillin/tazobactam | 100 mg/kg IM, IV q6–12h | Extended-spectrum penicillin |
| Policosanol | 0.3–2 mg PO | Hyperlipidemia |
| Polysulfated aminoglycosaminoglycan | N/A | Hemorrhagic diathesis reported in multiple avian species |
| Potassium bromide | 25–80 mg/kg PO q24h | Long-term seizure management |
| Pralidoxime (2-PAM) | 10–100 mg/kg IM q24–48h | Administer within 24–36 hours of organophosphate intoxication; use lower dose in combination with atropine |
| Praziquantel | 1–10 mg/kg PO, SQ, IM, repeat in 10–14 days | Cestodes, trematodes; toxicity and death in some species |
| Prednisolone (prednisone) | 0.5–4 mg/kg PO, IM, IV | Steroidal anti-inflammatory; use with caution |

COMMON DOSAGES FOR BIRDS (CONTINUED)

| Drug | Dosage | Indication/Comments |
| --- | --- | --- |
| Prednisolone sodium succinate | 0.5–30 mg/kg IM, IV | Steroidal anti-inflammatory; use with caution |
| Primaquine | 0.03–1.25 mg/kg PO q24h | Used with chloroquine for *Plasmodium, Haemoproteus, Leucocytozoon* |
| Propranolol | 0.04–0.2 mg/kg IM, IV | Supraventricular arrhythmia; atrial flutter; fibrillation |
| Propofol | 1–15 mg/kg IV | IV sedative–hypnotic agent; intubation, ventilation, and supplemental oxygen recommended |
| Prostaglandin E$_2$ (dinoprostone) | 0.02–0.1 mg/kg applied topically to uterovaginal sphincter; 1 ml/kg applied topically to uterovaginal sphincter | Dystocia; relaxes uterovaginal sphincter |
| Psyllium | 0.5 tsp/60 ml hand feeding formula or gruel 1 tbs/60 ml water q24h | Bulk diet; delay absorption of ingested toxin |
| Pyrantel pamoate | 4.5–70 mg/kg PO | Intestinal nematodes |
| Pyrethrins (0.15%) | Dust plumage lightly to moderately prn | Ectoparasites |
| Pyrimethamine | 0.25–1 mg/kg q12h | *Toxoplasma, Atoxoplasma, Sarcocystis*; may be effective for *Leucocytozoon* |
| Ronidazole | 2.5–20 mg/kg PO; 100–1000 mg/L drinking water × 5–7 days | *Trichomonas, Cochlosoma* |
| Robenacoxib | 2–10 mg/kg IM weekly for 4 weeks, then monthly | Non-steroidal anti-inflammatory |
| Selamectin | 23 mg/kg topically; repeat in 3–4 weeks | Ectoparasites including *Knemidokoptes* |
| Selenium | 0.05–0.1 mg Se/kg IM q14d | Neuromuscular diseases |
| Sevoflurane | 2.35–7% (usually 2.35–3.6%) | Inhalant anesthetic; higher % used for induction, then decreased |
| Silver sulfadiazine | Topical q12–24h | Useful for treatment of burns and ulcers |
| Silymarin (milk thistle) | 100–150 mg/kg PO divided q8–12h | Hepatic antioxidant; used in patients with liver disease and as ancillary to chemotherapy |
| Sucralfate | 25 mg/kg PO q8h | Esophageal, gastric, duodenal ulcers; give 1 hour before food or other drugs |
| Sulfachlorpyridazine | 150–500 mg/L drinking water | Coccidiostat |
| Sulfadimethoxine | 25–55 mg/kg PO q24h 250–500 mg/L drinking water | Coccidiostat |
| Tamoxifen citrate | 2 mg/kg PO; 40 mg/kg IM to induce molt | Nonsteroidal antiestrogen; may cause leukopenia |
| Tea (black tea leaves, decaffeinated) | 8 g/kg diet | Add to food to decrease iron absorption |
| Terbinafine | 10–30 mg/kg PO q12–24h; 1 mg/ml solution via nebulization | Fungicidal; questionable efficacy for treatment of aspergillosis; may be more effective at higher doses or in combination with itraconazole |
| Terbutaline | 0.01–0.1 mg/kg PO, IM; 0.01 mg/kg with 9 ml saline, nebulize | Bronchodilation |
| Testosterone | 2–8.5 mg/kg IM | Anabolic steroid; contraindicated with hepatic or renal disease; stimulate sexual behavior |
| Theophylline | 2 mg/kg PO q12h | Bronchodilation |

COMMON DOSAGES FOR BIRDS (CONTINUED)

| Drug | Dosage | Indication/Comments |
|---|---|---|
| Thyroid-stimulating hormone (thyrotropin; TSH) | 0.1 IU IM in cockatiels; 0.2–2 IU/kg IM | Obtain blood at 0 hours, then 4–6 hours after TSH stimulation |
| Toltrazuril | 7–35 mg/kg PO q24h; 2–125 mg/L drinking water | Coccidiocidal |
| Tramadol HCl | 5–30 mg/kg PO, IV | Synthetic analogue of codeine with opioid, alpha-adrenergic, and serotonergic receptor activity |
| Trimethoprim/ sulfamethoxazole (Bactrim) | 10–100 mg/kg PO, IM q12–24h | Broad-spectrum sulfonamide; may cause regurgitation |
| Urate oxidase | 100–200 IU/kg IM | Lowers plasma uric acid |
| Vincristine sulfate | 0.1 mg/kg IV q7–14d; 0.5–0.75 mg/m$^2$ IV q7d | Lymphoma and other lymphoid tumors, mast cell tumors, some sarcomas |
| Vitamin A | 200–50,000 IU/kg IM | Hypovitaminosis A |
| Vitamin B$_1$ (thiamine) | 1–50 mg/kg PO, IM | Thiamine deficiency |
| Vitamin B$_{12}$ (cyanocobalamin) | 0.25–0.5 mg/kg IM; 2–5 mg/bird SQ, pigeons | Vitamin B$_{12}$ deficiency; anemia |
| Vitamin C (ascorbic acid) | 20–150 mg/kg PO, IM | Nutritional support; supplemental therapy for pox infection |
| Vitamin D$_3$ | 3300–6600 iu/kg IM | Hypovitaminosis D$_3$ |
| Vitamin E | 0.06–400 mg/kg PO, IM | Hypovitaminosis E |
| Vitamin K$_1$ | 0.2–2.5 mg/kg PO, SQ, IM | Rodenticide anticoagulant toxicosis |
| Voriconazole | 10–20 mg/kg PO, IV q8–24h | Most active drug against aspergillosis |
| Zonisamide | 20–80 mg/kg PO q8–12h | Anticonvulsant; can be used in combination with levetiracetam |

Adapted from: Guzman D., Beaufrère H., Speer B., et al. (2023). Birds. In: Carpenter J., Harms C. (eds.), *Exotic Animal Formulary*, 6th edn., 222–443. St. Louis, MO: Elsevier.

ACE, angiotensin-converting enzyme; BAL, British anti-Lewisite; CNS, central nervous system; DMSO, dimethyl sulfoxide; FDA, Food and Drug Administration; GABA, gamma-aminobutyric acid; GnRH, gonadotropin-releasing hormone; MAC, minimum alveolar concentration; NPH, Neutral Protamine Hagedorn.

Note: Dosing recommendations vary drastically between species; see above reference for most complete information.

# APPENDIX II

## AVIAN HEMATOLOGY REFERENCE VALUES

### Table II-A

| Parameter | Hematological and serum biochemical reference ranges for select parrots | | | | | |
|---|---|---|---|---|---|---|
| | *African grey parrot* (Psittacus erithacus) | *Budgerigar parakeet* (Melopsittacus undulates) | *Cockatiel* (Nymphicus hollandicus) | *Amazon parrots* (Amazona spp.) | *Cockatoos* (Cacatua spp.) | *Conures* |
| WBC ($10^3$/μl) | 5–15[a] | 3–8.5[a,b] | 5–13[a] | 6–17[a] | 5–13[a] | 4–13[a] |
| | 5–11[b] | | 5–10[b] | 6–11[b] | 5–11[b] | 4–11[b] |
| Heterophils (%) | 45–75[a] | 40–75[a] | 40–70[a] | 30–80[a] | 15–64[a] | 40–70[a] |
| | 55–75[b] | 50–75[b] | 55–80[b] | 55–80[b] | 55–80[b] | 55–75[b] |
| Lymphocytes (%) | 20–50[a] | 20–45[a] | 25–55[a] | 20–65[a] | 29–83[a] | 20–50[a] |
| | 25–45[b] | 25–45[b] | 20–45[b] | 20–45[b] | 20–45[b] | 25–45[b] |
| Monocytes (%) | 0–3[a,b] | 0–2[a,b] | 0–2[a,b] | 0–3[a,b] | 0–9[a] | 0–3[a] |
| | | | | | 0–1[b] | 0–2[b] |
| Basophils (%) | 0–5[a] | 0–1[a,b] | 0–6[a] | 0–5[a] | 0–3[a] | 0–5[a] |
| | 0–1[b] | | 0–2[b] | 0–1[b] | 0–1[b] | 0–1[b] |
| Eosinophils (%) | 0–2[a,b] | 0–1[a] | 0–2[a,b] | 0–1[a,b] | 0[a] | 0–3[a] |
| | | 0–2[b] | | | 0–2[b] | 0–2[b] |
| PCV (%) | 40–55[a] | 44–58[a] | 45–54[a] | 40–55[a] | 42–54[a] | 42–54[a] |
| | 42–50[b] | 42–53[b] | 45–57[b] | 44–49[b] | 38–48[b] | 42–49[b] |
| Total protein (g/dl) | 3–5[a] | 2–3[a] | 2.4–4.1[a,b] | 3–5[a,b] | 3–5[a,b] | 2.5–4.5[a] |
| | 3–4.6[b] | 2.5–4.5[b] | | | | 3–4.2[b] |
| Albumin (g/dl) | 1.57–3.23[a,b] | 0.79–1.35[b] | 0.7–1.8[a,b] | 1.9–3.5[a,b] | 1–1.6[a] | 1.9–2.6[a,b] |
| | | | | | 1.8–3.1[b] | |
| Uric acid (mg/dl) | 4–10[a] | 3–8.6[a] | 3.5–11[a] | 2–10[a] | 2–8.5[a] | 2.5–10.5[a] |
| | 4.5–9.5[b] | 4.5–14[b] | 3.5–10.5[b] | 2.3–10[b] | 3.5–10.5[b] | 2.5–11[b] |
| Bile acid (μmol/l) | 18–71[a] | 20–65[a] | 25–85[a] | 19–144[a] | 20–70[a] | 20–45[a] |
| | 13–90[b] | 15–70[b] | 20–85[b] | 18–60[b] | 25–87[b] | 15–55[b] |
| RIA colorimetric | 12–96[a] | 32–117[a] | 15–139[a] | 33–154[a] | 34–112[a] | 32–105[a] |
| AST (iu/l) | 100–350[a] | 55–154[a] | 100–396[a] | 130–350[a,b] | 120–360[a] | 125–378[a] |
| | 100–365[b] | 145–350[b] | 95–345[b] | | 145–355[b] | 125–345[b] |
| GGT (iu/l) | 1–10[a,b] | 1–10[a,b] | 0–5[a] | NA[a] | 0–4[a] | 1–15[a,b] |
| | | | 1–30[b] | 1–12[b] | 1–45[b] | |
| Creatine kinase (iu/l) | 123–875[a] | 54–252[a] | 30–245[a,b] | 45–265[a] | 140–410[a] | 35–355[a,b] |
| | 165–412[b] | 90–300[b] | | 55–345[b] | 95–305[b] | |
| Ca (mg/dl) | 8–13[a] | 6.4–11.2[a] | 8.5–13[a] | 8–13[a] | 8–11[a] | 8–15[a] |
| | 8.5–13[b] | 6.5–11[b] | 8–13[b] | 8.5–14[b] | 8–13[b] | 7–15[b] |
| P (mg/dl) | 3.2–5.4[a,b] | 3–5.2[a,b] | 3.2–4.8[a,b] | 3.1–5.5[a,b] | 3.5–6.5[a] | 2–10[a,b] |
| | | | | | 2.5–5.5[b] | |

AST, aspartate aminotransferase; GGT, gamma-glutamyl transferase; PCV, packed cell volume; RIA, reaction-based indicator displacement assay; WBC, white blood cell.

[a] Carpenter, J. (ed.) (2013). *Exotic Animal Formulary*, 4th edn. St. Louis, MO: Elsevier.

[b] Harrison, G.J., Lightfoot, T.L. (eds) (2006). *Clinical Avian Medicine*, Vol. 2. Palm Beach, FL: Spix Publishing.

**Table II-B**

| | Hematological and serum biochemical reference ranges for select avian species | | | | | |
|---|---|---|---|---|---|---|
| Parameter | Canary (Serinus canaria) | Chicken (Gallus gallus) | Turkey (Meleagridis gallopavo) | Wood duck (Aix sponsa) | Red tailed hawk (Buteo jamaicensis) | Great horned owl (Bubo virginianus) |
| WBC ($10^3/\mu l$) | 4–9[a,b] | 9–32[a] | 16–25.5[a] | 19.9–31.3[a] | 19.1–33.4[a] | 6–8[a] |
| Heterophils (%) | 50–80[a,b] | 15–50[a] | 29–52[a] | | 24–46[a] | 36–58[a] |
| Lymphocytes (%) | 20–45[a,b] | 29–84[a] | 35–48[a] | | 35–53[a] | 20–34[a] |
| Monocytes (%) | 0–1[a,b] | 0.1–7[a] | 3–10[a] | | 3–9[a] | 5.4–12.6[a] |
| Basophils (%) | 0–1[a,b] | 0–8 | 1–9 | | Rare | Rare |
| Eosinophils (%) | 0–2[a,b] | 0–16 | 0–5 | | 9–17 | 0–2.2 |
| PCV (%) | 37–49[a] | 23–55[a] | 30.4–45.6[a] | 42.1–48.9[a] | 31–43[a] | 40–46[a] |
| Total protein (g/dl) | 2.8–4.5[a,b] | 3.3–5.5[a] | 4.9–7.6[a] | 2.1–3.3[a] | 3.9–6.7[a] | 4.3[a] |
| Albumin (g/dl) | 0.81–1.23[b] | 1.3–2.8[a] | 3–5.9[a] | 1.5–2.1[a] | | 1.3[a] |
| Uric acid (mg/dl) | 4–12[a,b] | 2.5–8.1[a] | 3.4–5.2[a] | 2.5–12.9[a] | 8.1–16.8[a] | 13.7[a] |
| Bile acid ($\mu mol/l$) | 23–90[a,b] | | | 22–60[a] | 8.4–10.2[a] | |
| AST (iu/l) | 145–345[a,b] | | | 45–123[a] | 76–492[a] | 287[a] |
| GGT (iu/l) | 1–14[a,b] | | | 0–2.9[a] | 0–20[a] | |
| Creatine kinase (iu/l) | 55–350[a,b] | | | 110–480[a] | | |
| Ca (mg/dl) | 5.5–13.5[a,b] | 13.2–23.7[a] | 11.7–38.7[a] | 7.6–10.4[a] | 10–12.8[a] | 10.2[a] |
| P (mg/dl) | 2.9–4.9[a,b] | 6.2–7.9[a] | 5.4–7.1[a] | 1.8–4.1[a] | 1.9–4[a] | 4.3[a] |

AST, aspartate aminotransferase; GGT, gamma-glutamyl transferase; PCV, packed cell volume; WBC, white blood cell.

[a] Carpenter, J. (ed.) (2013). *Exotic Animal Formulary*, 4th edn. St. Louis, MO: Elsevier.

[b] Harrison, G.J., Lightfoot, T.L. (eds) (2006). *Clinical Avian Medicine*, Vol. 2. Palm Beach, FL: Spix Publishing.

**AUTHORS**
Laura Kleinschmidt, BS, DVM, and J. Jill Heatley, DVM MS DABVP (Avian, Reptile & Amphibian) DACZM

# APPENDIX III

## LABORATORY TESTING (USA)

| Test | Laboratory |
| --- | --- |
| Adenovirus | 2, 9, 16, 18 |
| Anticoagulants (blood or tissue) | 11, 20 |
| Avian encephalomyelitis virus | 16 |
| Avian influenza virus | 6, 13, 16 |
| Avian leucosis/sarcoma virus | 6 |
| Avian nephritis virus | 16 |
| Bacterial culture and sensitivity (aerobic) | Most microbiology laboratories |
| Bacterial culture and sensitivity (anaerobic) | 3 |
| Bacterial and fungal next-generation DNA sequencing | 12 |
| *Bordetella* | 10, 23 |
| Bornavirus | 9 |
| Botulism | 14 |
| *Campylobacter* | 6, 23 |
| *Candida* (cytology) | Most clinical pathology laboratories |
| *Candida* (identification) | 6 |
| Chicken anemia virus | 6, 18 |
| *Chlamydia psittaci* | 9, 21 |
| Cholinesterase | 11 |
| Circovirus | 11, 21 |
| *Clostridium* | 17, 23 |
| *Cryptosporidium* (feces) | 20 |
| Cytology | Most clinical pathology laboratories |
| Drug levels: | |
| Amikacin, bromide (potassium/sodium), cannabinoids (cbd, thc), cyclosporine, digoxin, gabapentin, gentamicin, leflunomide (teriflunomide), levetiracetam, lidocaine, phenobarbital, phenytoin, procainamide, theophylline, valproic acid, vancomycin, zonisamide | 4 |
| Voriconazole, posaconazole, itraconazole, fluconazole, isavuconazole, amphotericin B | 8 |
| Duck enteritis virus | 18 |
| Eastern equine encephalitis virus | 16 |
| Fungal culture | Most mycology laboratories |
| Fungal identification | 8 |
| **Heavy metals** | |
| Lead, zinc, copper | 11 |
| Lead, arsenic, cadmium, zinc, and thallium | 18 |
| Herpesvirus | 9, 21 |
| Infectious bronchitis virus | 1, 6, 16 |
| Infectious bursal disease virus | 1, 6, 18 |
| Infectious laryngotracheitis virus | 6 |
| Insecticide (crop/gastric content) | 11 |
| *Macrorhabdus ornithogaster* (cytology) | Most clinical pathology laboratories |

## LABORATORY TESTING (USA) (CONTINUED)

| Test | Laboratory |
| --- | --- |
| *M. ornithogaster* (polymerase chain reaction) | 18, 19 |
| Marek's disease virus | 6, 16 |
| Metapneumovirus | 16 |
| Mycobacterium | 15 |
| *Mycoplasma* | 1, 6, 13 |
| Mycotoxins (feed) | 5 |
| Mycotoxins quantification (feed and gastric content) | 20 |
| Newcastle disease virus (avian orthoavulavirus 1; formerly Paramyxovirus-1) | 1 |
| Organophosphate/carbamate | 11, 18 |
| Other hormones | 7, 20 |
| Paramyxovirus | 16 |
| Parasites (multiple specific groups such as Acanthocephala, Cestode, *Coccidia*, *Cryptosporidium*, *Entamoeba*, nematodes, trematodes) | 22 |
| Parathyroid hormone | 20 |
| *Pasteurella* (serotyping) | 6 |
| Polyomavirus | 9, 21 |
| Poxvirus (fowl pox) | 6 |
| Reovirus | 16 |
| Reticuloendotheliosis virus | 18 |
| Rotavirus | 16 |
| Salmonella (culture and serogrouping) | 6 |
| Thyroid hormones | 20 |
| | 7 |
| Toxin quantitation (gas chromatography–mass spectrometry) | 18 |
| Tremorgenic mycotoxins (bromethalin, penitrem A, roquefortine, and strychnine) | 20 |
| Vitamin D | 20 |
| West Nile virus | 1 |

LABORATORIES

1 **Animal Health Diagnostic Center, Cornell University College of Veterinary Medicine**
240 Farrier Road
Ithaca, NY 14853
607 253 3943
https://ahdc.vet.cornell.edu/

2 **Charles River Avian Vaccine Services**
Franklin Commons, 106 Route 32
North Franklin, CT 06254
800 772 3271
http://www.criver.com/products-services/avian-vaccine-services

3 **Clinical Laboratory, UC Davis Veterinary Medicine Teaching Hospital**
Central Laboratory Receiving, Room 1033
1 Garrod Drive
Davis, CA 95616-8747
530 752 8684
https://www.vetmed.ucdavis.edu/hospital/support-services/lab-services/clinical-laboratory-services

4 **Clinical Pharmacology Laboratory, College of Veterinary Medicine, Auburn University**
1500 Wire Rd, 214 SRRC
Auburn University, AL 36849
334 844 7187
http://www.vetmed.auburn.edu/veterinarians/clinical-labs

5 **Department of Agricultural Chemistry, Louisiana State University AgCenter**
Room 102 Ag Chemistry Building
110 LSU Union Square
Baton Rouge, LA 70803
225 342 5812
https://www.lsuagcenter.com/portals/our_offices/departments/ag-chemistry

6 **Diagnostic Services and Teaching Laboratory, Poultry Diagnostic & Research Center**
953 College Station Road
Athens, GA 30605
706 542 1904
https://vet.uga.edu/education/academic-departments/population-health/poultry-diagnostic-and-research-center

7 **Endocrinology Service Biomedical and Diagnostic Sciences, University of Tennessee College of Veterinary Medicine**
2407 River Drive, Room A105
Knoxville, TN 37996-4543
865 974 5638
https://vetmed.tennessee.edu/vmc/dls/endocrinology/#:~:text=The%20Diagnostic%20Endocrinology%20Service%20at,as%20for%20several%20other%20species.

8 **Fungus Testing Laboratory**
Department of Pathology and Laboratory Medicine
Room 329E. Mail Code 7750
University of Texas Health Science Center at San Antonio
San Antonio, Texas 78229-3900
210 567 4131
http://strl.uthscsa.edu/fungus

LABORATORIES (CONTINUED)

**9** **Infectious Diseases Laboratory, University of Georgia**
110 Riverbend Road
Riverbend North, Room 150
University of Georgia, Athens, GA 30602
706 542 8092
https://vet.uga.edu/diagnostic-service-labs/infectious-diseases-lab

**10** **Kansas State Veterinary Diagnostic Laboratory**
Kansas State University
1800 Denison Avenue
Manhattan, KS 66506
785 532 5650
http://www.ksvdl.org

**11** **Louisiana Animal Disease Diagnostic Laboratory**
Louisiana State University
River Road Room 1043
Baton Rouge, LA 70803
225 578 9777
https://www.lsu.edu/vetmed/laddl/index.php

**12** **MiDog LLC**
14762 Bentley Cir.
Tustin CA 92780
833 456 4364
https://www.midogtest.com

**13** **Mississippi State Veterinary Research and Diagnostic Laboratory System**
College of Veterinary Medicine, Mississippi State University
3137 Highway 468, West Pearl, MS 39208
601 420 4700
https://www.vetmed.msstate.edu/clinics-locations/lab-system/mississippi-veterinary-research-diagnostic-lab

**14** **National Botulism Reference Laboratory**
School of Veterinary Medicine, University of Pennsylvania
New Bolton Center
382 West Street Road
Kennett Square, PA 19348
610 925 6383
https://www.vet.upenn.edu/veterinary-hospitals/NBC-hospital/diagnostic-laboratories

**15** **National Jewish Health Mycobacteriology Laboratory**
1400 Jackson Street, Room K422
Denver, CO 80206
800 550 6227
https://www.nationaljewish.org/for-professionals/diagnostic-testing/advanced-diagnostic-laboratories/overview

**16** **National Veterinary Services Laboratories, United States Department of Agriculture**
USDA-APHIS-VS-NVSL
1920 Dayton Avenue
Ames, IA 50010
515 337 7266
http://www.aphis.usda.gov/wps/portal/aphis/ourfocus/animalhealth

## LABORATORIES (CONTINUED)

**17     North Carolina Veterinary Diagnostic Laboratory System**
North Carolina State Laboratory of Public Health
4312 District Drive
Raleigh, N.C. 27611
919 733 3986
https://cvm.ncsu.edu/research/labs

**18     Texas A&M Veterinary Medical Diagnostic Laboratory**
483 Agronomy Road
College Station, TX 77843-4471
979 845 3414
https://tvmdl.tamu.edu

**19     UC Davis Real-time PCR Lab**
1275 Med Science Drive
3110 Tupper Hall
UC Davis, SVM
Davis, CA 95616-8737
530 752 7991
https://pcrlab.vetmed.ucdavis.edu/

**20     Veterinary Diagnostic Laboratory, Michigan State University**
4125 Beaumont Road
Lansing, MI 48910-8104
517 353 1683
http://www.animalhealth.msu.edu

**21     Veterinary Diagnostic Laboratory – Wildlife Epidemiology Laboratory**
1224 Veterinary Medicine Basic Sciences Building
College of Veterinary Medicine, University of Illinois – Urbana-Champaign, Urbana, IL 61802
217-333-1620
https://vdl.vetmed.illinois.edu/wildlife-epidemiology

**22     Zoo Medicine Infectious Disease, University of Florida College of Veterinary Medicine**
2015 SW 16th Ave Building 1017, Room V2-186
Gainesville, FL 32608
352 294 4420
https://idi.vetmed.ufl.edu

**23     Zoologix Inc.**
9811 Owensmouth Avenue Suite 4
Chatsworth, CA 91311-3800
818 717 8880
http://zoologix.com

**AUTHOR**
João Brandão, LMV, MS, DECZM (Avian), DACZM

## APPENDIX IV

### VIRAL DISEASES OF CONCERN

| Virus | Characteristics | Species | Lesions: clinical and gross/histopathology | Transmission/ testing | Testing | AKA Disease |
|---|---|---|---|---|---|---|
| Adenovirus | Aviadenoviruses, non-enveloped dsDNA | Falcons | Acute death; hepatic, splenic necrosis; large intranuclear basophilic to amphophilic inclusion bodies | Horizontally, fecal–oral | VN, PCR | Falcon adenovirus |
| Adenovirus | Aviadenoviruses, non-enveloped dsDNA | Hawks | Acute death; hepatic, splenic, proventricular and ventricular necrosis; large intranuclear basophilic to amphophilic inclusion bodies | Horizontally fecal–oral | PCR | Raptor adenovirus |
| Adenovirus | Aviadenoviruses, non-enveloped dsDNA | Chicken | Sudden mortality; nephritis; necrotic focal hepatic lesions with basophilic intranuclear inclusion bodies | Vertically; horizontally, fecal–oral; | ELISA, IIF, HI, PCR | Fowl adenoviruses |
| Adenovirus | Aviadenoviruses, non-enveloped dsDNA | Duck | Asymptomatic infection; may cause mortality in ducklings, hepatitis, tracheitis with eosinophilic intranuclear inclusions | Vertically; Horizontally, fecal–oral | PCR | Duck hepatitis |
| Adenovirus | Aviadenoviruses, non-enveloped dsDNA | Chicken | Decreased/abnormal egg production; severe inflammation of shell gland with intranuclear inclusion bodies in the epithelial cells; epithelial sloughing in GI tract, duodenum lesions most severe | Vertically; Horizontally, fecal–oral | ELISA, HI, virus isolation, PCR | Egg drop syndrome |
| Adenovirus | Aviadenoviruses, non-enveloped dsDNA | Ostrich | High mortality in chicks under 1 month, gray chalky stools, ascites, proventricular impaction, chalky or wrinkled eggs | Vertically; Horizontally, fecal–oral | PCR | Ostrich adenovirus |
| Adenovirus | Aviadenoviruses, non-enveloped dsDNA; two clinical disease presentations | Pigeon | Intranuclear viral inclusions: hepatocytes, renal tubular epithelium, enterocytes of the small intestine | Horizontally, fecal–oral | PCR | Inclusion body hepatitis and viral enteritis |

## VIRAL DISEASES OF CONCERN (CONTINUED)

| Virus | Characteristics | Species | Lesions: clinical and gross/histopathology | Transmission/ testing | Testing | AKA Disease |
|---|---|---|---|---|---|---|
| Adenovirus | Aviadenoviruses, non-enveloped dsDNA | Poultry | Myocardial and hepatic necrosis; lymphoid depletion of spleen, thymus and bursa of Fabricius; basophilic inclusions in hepatocytes | Vertically; Horizontally, fecal–oral | ELISA, HI, PCR | Hydropericardium syndrome |
| Adenovirus | Aviadenoviruses, non-enveloped dsDNA | Psittacines | Basophilic intranuclear inclusion bodies in hepatocytes, enterocytes, pancreas, renal tubular epithelium; may be no disease in some species | Horizontally, fecal–oral | PCR | Psittacine adenovirus |
| Adenovirus | Aviadenoviruses, non-enveloped dsDNA | Quail | Exudate in nasal passages, trachea, mainstem bronchi; necrosis of tracheal epithelium with intranuclear inclusion bodies; multifocal hepatic necrosis | Horizontally, fecal–oral | ELISA, PCR | Quail bronchitis |
| Adenovirus | Group 2 aviadenoviruses, non-enveloped dsDNA | Turkey | Acute death; hepatomegaly, splenomegaly; lesions similar to chicken but do not involve GI | Horizontally, fecal–oral | ELISA, PCR | Hemorrhagic enteritis virus of turkeys |
| Adenovirus | Group 2 aviadenoviruses, non-enveloped dsDNA | Pheasant | Pulmonary edema, enlarged mottled spleens; lesions resemble those of seen in the chicken but do not involve GI | Horizontally, fecal–oral | ELISA, PCR | Marble spleen disease |
| Adenovirus | Siadenovirus aviadenoviruses, non-enveloped dsDNA | Gouldian finch | Large clear to basophilic intranuclear inclusion bodies in renal tubular epithelial cells, maybe no disease | Suspected to be oral or respiratory transmission | PCR | Gouldian finch adenovirus 1 |
| Avian bornavirus | Parrot bornavirus (PaBV) 1–8, enveloped ssRNA | Psittacines (variable susceptibility) | Lymphoplasmacytic ganglioneuritis and leiomyositis, no viral inclusions; anorexia, passage of whole seed in stool, maldigested excrement, abnormal frequency of defecation or regurgitation | Horizontally, fecal–oral or respiratory | Western blot, ELISA, IFA, IHC, antiganglioside antibody, rt-PCR | AG is term preferred over proventricular dilatation disease |

## VIRAL DISEASES OF CONCERN (CONTINUED)

| Virus | Characteristics | Species | Lesions: clinical and gross/histopathology | Transmission/ testing | Testing | AKA Disease |
|---|---|---|---|---|---|---|
| Avian bornavirus | Aquatic bird bornavirus (AABV) 1-2 enveloped ssRNA | Waterfowl and shorebirds | Mononuclear infiltrations in the CNS and PNS (encephalitis, myelitis, ganglioneuritis) | Horizontally, fecal–oral or respiratory | rt-qPCR on tissues, virus isolation, or immunohistochemistry for N protein | AG |
| Avian encephalomyelitis(AE) | Picornavirus nonenveloped ssRNA | Chickens, pheasant, turkeys | Lenticular cataract, neurologic signs (muscular tremors in chicks), drop in egg production, degeneration and necrosis of neurons, perivascular lymphocytic cuffing, and gliosis with formation of glial nodules | Horizontally, fecal–oral, vertically | Serologic testing of paired serum samples, using virus neutralization or ELISA tests | Tremovirus |
| Avian influenza | Orthomyxoviridae, enveloped, RNA; classified by subtypes based on hemagglutinin and neuraminidase and pathogenicity to domestic chickens (high or low pathogenicity) | All birds | No viral inclusions, lesions vary | Horizontally, fecal–oral route, aerosol | Specific rt-PCR tests, serology | Common reservoirs: waterfowl and shorebirds |
| Avian retrovirus | Alpharetrovirus, enveloped | Chickens, ubiquitous in chicken flocks | Lymphoid neoplasia, bursa of Fabricius enlargement | Horizontally and vertically | ELISA, PCR | Lymphoid leukosis |
| Avian retrovirus | Gammaretrovirus, enveloped | Chickens | Lymphoid neoplasia, immunosuppression | Horizontally and vertically | ELISA, PCR | Reticuloendotheliosis |
| Birnavirus | Birnavirus, non-enveloped dsRNA | Chickens | Immunosuppression, cloacitis, bursal necrosis | Horizontally, fecal–oral, aerosol | AGID | Infectious bursal disease (Gumboro disease) |
| Circovirus | Non-enveloped circular ssDNA | Psittacines, Rare in Neotropical parrots | Intracytoplasmic botryoid IB in growing feathers and the bursa of Fabricius. *African grey*: anorexia, weight loss, vomiting, weakness, and crop stasis. *Cockatoos*: chronic form, retained feather sheaths, blood in shafts, short clubbed feathers, deformed curled feathers, stress | Horizontally, fecal–oral, vertical | PCR, HI | Psittacine beak and feather disease |

## VIRAL DISEASES OF CONCERN (CONTINUED)

| Virus | Characteristics | Species | Lesions: clinical and gross/histopathology | Transmission/ testing | Testing | AKA Disease |
|-------|-----------------|---------|--------------------------------------------|-----------------------|---------|-------------|
| | | | lines in vanes, circumferential constrictions. Beak: progressive elongation, transverse or longitudinal fractures, palatine necrosis, oral ulceration | | | |
| Circovirus | Non-enveloped, circular ssDNA | Chicken | Intracytoplasmic botryoid inclusion bodies in bone marrow and lymphoid tissue | Horizontally, fecal–oral, vertically | PCR, ELISA | Chicken anemia virus |
| Circovirus | Non-enveloped, circular ssDNA | Pigeon | Intracytoplasmic botryoid inclusion bodies in the bursa of Fabricius | Horizontally, fecal–oral; vertically | PCR | Pigeon circovirus |
| Circovirus | Non-enveloped, circular ssDNA | Finch, canary | Intracytoplasmic botryoid inclusion bodies in monocytes | Horizontally, fecal–oral; vertically | PCR | "Blackspot disease" |
| Circovirus | Non-enveloped, circular ssDNA | Goose | Intracytoplasmic botryoid inclusion bodies in the bursa of Fabricius and lymphohistiocytic depletion, slow growth and some feather deformities | Horizontally, fecal–oral; vertically | PCR | Goose circovirus |
| Duck viral hepatitis | Picornavirus non-enveloped ssRNA | Ducklings, not pathogenic for goslings | High mortality, enlarged liver with hemorrhagic foci | Horizontally – fecal oral | IFA, rt-PCR | Duck viral hepatitis |
| Eastern equine encephalitis | Alphavirus enveloped ssRNA | Emus, pheasant, whooping crane | High mortality, depression, anorexia, hemorrhagic gastroenteritis | Mechanical – mosquito transmission | HI, CF, ELISA, VN, rt-PCR | EEE, triple E, sleeping sickness, Usutu virus |
| Herpesvirus | Alphaherpesvirus enveloped dsDNA | New World psittacines | Mucosal papillomas, no viral inclusions | Horizontally, fecal–oral | PCR | Mucosal papillomatosis |
| Herpesvirus | Alphaherpesvirus, dsDNA | Chickens over age 3–4 weeks, ubiquitous in chicken flocks | Lymphoid neoplasia, enlarged peripheral nerves, diffuse or nodular lymphoid tumors in various organs and enlarged feather follicles, no viral inclusions | Horizontally, fecal–oral | PCR | Marek's disease, MD |

**VIRAL DISEASES OF CONCERN (CONTINUED)**

| Virus | Characteristics | Species | Lesions: clinical and gross/histopathology | Transmission/ testing | Testing | AKA Disease |
|---|---|---|---|---|---|---|
| Herpesvirus | Alphaherpesvirus dsDNA | Chickens, pheasants | Hemorrhagic, necrotizing tracheitis, intranuclear inclusion bodies in tracheal epithelium | Horizontally, fecal–oral; respiratory | ELISA, PCR | Infectious laryngotracheitis (ILT) |
| Herpesvirus | Psittacid Herpesvirus-2, Alphaherpesvirus, dsDNA | African grey parrots | Cutaneous papillomas, no viral inclusions | Horizontally, fecal–oral | PCR | Cutaneous papillomatosis |
| Herpesvirus in hawks | Herpesvirus, Columbid Herpesvirus-1 (Previously falconid and strigid herpesvirus-1), dsDNA | Hawks | Splenic and hepatic necrosis with eosinophilic intranuclear inclusions, high mortality | Horizontally, transmitted to raptors from rock pigeons | PCR | Inclusion body disease |
| Infectious bronchitis virus | Coronavirus, enveloped ssRNA | Chickens | Abnormal eggs, sinusitis, nephritis, air sacculitis | Horizontally, fecal–oral; respiratory | Virus isolation, HI, ELISA, rt-PCR | Infectious bronchitis virus |
| Orthoavulavirus | Avian metapneumovirus (aMPV), enveloped ssRNA | Primarily turkeys and chickens | Signs generally more severe in turkeys vs chickens; edema, tracheal deciliation, coelomitis | Horizontally, direct contact, respiratory | ELISA, IFA, rt-PCR | Turkey rhinotracheitis, swollen head syndrome |
| | Orthoavulavirus 1 (OAvV-1), (previously paramyxovirus), enveloped ssRNA | Primarily poultry, can affect all birds | Variable depending on system affected, virulent strains cause hemorrhage through visceral organs | Horizontally, fecal–oral; aerosol | ELISA, rt-PCR | Newcastle disease, NDV/VVND, paramyxovirus |
| | | Pigeon, can affect other avian species | No clinical disease to polydipsia, ataxia, poor balance, torticollis, head tremors, inability to fly, and diarrhea: Interstitial nephritis, lymphoplasmacytic hepatitis and pancreatitis, with nonsuppurative encephalitis | | rt-PCR | Pigeon paramyxovirus type I, PPMV-I |
| Papillomavirus, suspected | Papillomavirus, dsDNA | Finches, chaffinches | Cutaneous papillomas, no viral inclusions | Horizontally | PCR | Cutaneous papillomatosis |
| Parvovirus | Parvovirus, non-enveloped ssDNA | Goslings and Muscovy ducklings | Hemorrhagic nephritis and enteritis, perihepatitis, pericarditis, Cowdry type-A intranuclear inclusion bodies B | Horizontall,– fecal–oral; vertical | Clinical signs, histology, virus isolation, PCR, serology | Goose parvovirus (Derzsy disease), goose hepatitis, goose plague |

VIRAL DISEASES OF CONCERN (CONTINUED)

| Virus | Characteristics | Species | Lesions: clinical and gross/histopathology | Transmission/ testing | Testing | AKA Disease |
|---|---|---|---|---|---|---|
| Polyomavirus | Polyomavirus, non-enveloped dsDNA | Finches | Acute mortality in 2- to 3-day-olds, fledglings, and adults; survivors have poor feather development, long tubular misshapen beaks | Horizontally, fecal–oral; vertical transmission suspected | Histopathology, PCR | APV |
| Polyomavirus | Polyomavirus, non-enveloped dsDNA | Psittacines | Peracute death in nestlings and adult Eclectus, Painted conure, White-bellied caiques

*Clinical signs*: depression, anorexia, weight loss, delayed crop emptying, regurgitation, diarrhea, dehydration, SQ hemorrhages, dyspnea, posterior paresis and paralysis, polyuria | Horizontally, fecal–oral; vertical transmission suspected | Histopathology, PCR | Budgerigar fledgling disease, APV |
| Poxvirus | Avipoxvirus, enveloped dsDNA | 16 have been described and named after the species they infect | Hyperplastic, ballooning degenerative epithelium with IC inclusion bodies (Bollinger bodies); three forms: cutaneous (dry form), diphtheroid (wet or mucosal form), and septicemia or systemic poxvirus | Mechanically with insect vectors, direct contact with fomites | Histopathology, PCR, serology | Psittacinepox, canarypox, pigeonpox, etc. |
| Poxvirus | *Chordopoxvirinae* subfamily, large, dsDNA, enveloped | Chickens, turkeys, waterfowl | Proliferative skin lesions, laryngotracheitis, eosinophilic cytoplasmic IB | Mechanically with insect vectors, direct contact with fomites | Histopathology, FA, IHC, PCR | Fowlpox |
| Reovirus | Non-enveloped dsRNA | Chicken | Arthritis, tenosynovitis, runting-stunting syndrome, atrophy of spleen and bursa of Fabricius | Horizontally – fecal oral, respiratory and vertical transmission; serology, PCR | | Viral arthritis |

## VIRAL DISEASES OF CONCERN (CONTINUED)

| Virus | Characteristics | Species | Lesions: clinical and gross/histopathology | Transmission/ testing | Testing | AKA Disease |
|---|---|---|---|---|---|---|
| Usutu virus | Flaviviridae, enveloped ssRNA | Passerines; can affect other avian species | Hepatosplenomegaly, necrosis and haemorrhages with mononuclear cell infiltrations in the brain, cardiac and skeletal muscle, liver, spleen, kidney | Mechanically, arthropod borne | rt-PCR, serology | USUV |
| West Nile virus | Flaviviridae, enveloped ssRNA | All birds susceptible, most cases subclinical as birds are a natural reservoir host | Heterophilic to lymphoplasmacytic myocarditis, encephalitis, ganglionitis, hepatitis, and nephritis, no viral inclusions (high mortality in corvids and select raptors) | Mechanically, arthropod borne | PCR, IHC | WNV |
| Western equine encephalitis | Alphavirus, enveloped ssRNA | Emus and rheas | High morbidity, low mortality, anorexia, weight loss, weakness, depression, drowsiness, stupor, ataxia, incoordination. Histologic lesions minimal to severe, and can include heterophilic to lymphoplasmacytic myocarditis, encephalitis, ganglionitis, hepatitis, and nephritis (inapparent infection in native birds as virus cycles between mosquitoes and passerines) | Mechanically, mosquito transmission, may be transmitted by ticks | HI, CF, ELISA, VN, PCR | WEE |

**Abbreviations:** AG, avian ganglioneuritis; AGID, agar gel immunodiffusion; CF, complement fixation; dsDNA, double-stranded DNA; ELISA, enzyme-linked immunosorbent assay; FA, fluorescent antibody; GI, gastrointestinal; HI, hemagglutination inhibition; IFA, immunofluorescence assay; IIF, indirect immunofluorescence; PCR, polymerase chain reaction; rt-PCR, reverse transcription polymerase chain reaction; rt-qPCR, reverse transcription quantitative polymerase chain reaction; ssDNA, single-stranded DNA; VN, virus neutralization.

## AUTHORS

Drury R. Reavill, DVM, DABVP (Avian/Reptile & Amphibian), DACVP (deceased); Jennifer E. Graham, DVM, DABVP (Avian/ECM), DACZM

# APPENDIX V

## SELECTED ZOONOTIC DISEASES OF CONCERN AND PERSONAL PROTECTION*

| Infectious agent | Mode of transmission | Disease in humans |
| --- | --- | --- |
| **Viruses** | | |
| Avian influenza | Aerosol | Respiratory |
| Avian paramyxovirus – 1 (Newcastle disease) | Direct contact | Mild, self-resolving conjunctivitis |
| Arboviruses: West Nile virus, Eastern equine encephalitis virus, Western equine encephalitis virus | Arthropod-borne (mosquitoes) | Fever, flu-like symptoms, encephalitis |
| **Bacteria** | | |
| *Campylobacter* spp. | Fecal–Oral, food-borne | Gastrointestinal, Guillain–Barré syndrome |
| *Chlamydia psittaci* | Aerosol | Respiratory |
| *Escherichia coli* | Fecal–oral, food-borne | Gastrointestinal, hemolytic uremic syndrome |
| *Mycobacterium* spp. | Aerosol | Possibly respiratory but no confirmed cases |
| *Salmonella* spp. | Fecal–oral, food-borne | Gastrointestinal |
| **Fungi** | | |
| *Cryptococcus neoformans* | Passed in feces and then aerosolized | Respiratory, meningoencephalitis |
| *Histoplasma capsulatum* | Passed in feces and then aerosolized; most commonly associated with pigeons | Respiratory |
| **Parasite** | | |
| Fowl mites: *Ornithonyssus sylviarum, Dermanyssus gallinae* | Direct contact | Pruritus, papules |

**STEPS TO REDUCE ZOONOTIC DISEASE TRANSMISSION**

A more extensive description of preventive measures can be found in the *Compendium of Veterinary Standard Precautions for Zoonotic Disease Prevention in Veterinary Personnel*, which is written and distributed by the National Association of State Public Health Veterinarians and can be found at: http://www.nasphv.org/documentsCompendiaVet.html

*Hand hygiene*

Hand hygiene can greatly reduce the risk of disease transmission and should be performed after handling each animal and prior to taking breaks where food or drink will be consumed. Warm water and soap are necessary to clean hands if organic material is present, but alcohol-based hand sanitizers are effective against many bacteria and viruses.

*Gloves and sleeves*

Gloves and sleeves provide a protective barrier and should always be worn with handling feces, vomitus, exudates or if breaks in one's skin are present. Gloves should also be worn when cleaning cages or handling dirty laundry.

*Facial protection*

Facial protection, such as goggles or face shields, protects the mucous membranes of the eyes, nose and mouth and may reduce exposure to infectious agents. Facial protection should be worn whenever splashes or sprays are likely to occur, such as flushing wounds or abscesses, or performing a necropsy.

*Respiratory protection*

Masks and respirators can be worn to reduce or eliminate the possibility of inhaling an infectious agent. Masks typically worn in surgery are not adequate protection against inhaled pathogens. Respiratory protection must be fitted to the individual and filters in most (reusable) masks must be replaced periodically.

*Additional information on zoonoses associated with birds can be found in: Souza, M.J. (2011). Zoonoses, public health, and the exotic animal practitioner. *Veterinary Clinics of North America: Exotic Animal Practice*, **14**(3):xi-xii, and Gupta, K.A., Sharma, D., and Kumar, R. (2018). Zoonoses at the human–avian interface: A review. *BAOJ Veterinary Science*, **2**:005.

SELECTED ZOONOTIC DISEASES OF CONCERN AND PERSONAL PROTECTION (CONTINUED)

*Protective outerwear*

Garments such as laboratory coats, smocks, aprons, and coveralls can be worn to reduce contamination but are typically not fluid proof; these items should be laundered daily in hot water. Footwear that can be easily disinfected, such as rubber boots, can be useful, especially if the veterinarian is making house or farm calls.

*Animal handling*

Although injuries from birds are not as common as those associated with dogs, proper handling and communication between the veterinarian and assistant can reduce the likelihood of trauma. It is important to know what part of the bird is "dangerous". For example, the beak of parrots is of most concern, but the feet and talons of raptors are of most concern. Any wounds from trauma inflicted by an animal should be cleaned immediately. Depending on severity, a physician should be contacted.

*Disinfection*

Appropriate disinfection of areas where animals have been housed or examined will reduce contamination. Most bacteria and viruses are killed with commonly used disinfectants, but some organisms, such as *Mycobacterium* spp., may need special disinfectants to be effective.

*Education*

Staff training is essential to eliminate disease transmission. Established protocols should outline specific steps to be taken for disinfection and disease prevention.

**AUTHOR**

Marcy J. Souza, DVM, MPH, MPPA, DABVP (Emeritus, Avian), DACVPM

## APPENDIX VI

### COMMON AVIAN TOXINS AND THEIR CLINICAL SIGNS

| Plants | Lesions | Clinical signs | Treatment/Antidotes |
|--------|---------|----------------|---------------------|
| Avocado (*Persea americana*) | Myocardial degeneration with subcutaneous edema of the neck, chest, and pulmonary system | Listless, ruffled feathers, cessation of perching, dyspnea | Anti-inflammatory agents, oxygen, and antimicrobials |
| Azalea/rhododendron (*Rhododendron* spp.) | Edema of lungs, renal tubular and hepatocellular necrosis | Weakness, dyspnea, weight loss | Supportive care |
| Black locust (*Robinia pseudoacacia*) | Hemorrhagic inflammation of GI tract | Diarrhea, regurgitation/vomiting, dyspnea | Supportive care |
| Castor bean (*Ricinus communis*) | GI tract inflammation, edema, necrosis | Weakness, severe diarrhea, hypotension, collapse | Aggressive fluid replacement replacing electrolytes and glucose as indicated |
| Dieffenbachia (*Dieffenbachia maculata*) | Lingual inflammation, laryngeal inflammation | Anorexia, hypersalivation | Oral fluids as tolerated, IV fluids |
| English ivy (*Hedera helix*) | GI tract irritation/inflammation | Anorexia, regurgitation/vomiting, diarrhea | Fluid replacement, supportive care |
| Foxglove (*Digitalis purpurea*) | Myocardial degeneration, fibrosis and necrosis | Marked weakness, crop stasis, anorexia, arrhythmias, seizures | IV fluids, atropine and/or propranolol depending on arrhythmias, supportive care |
| Lily of the valley (*Convallaria majalis*) | GI hemorrhages and inflammation, myocardial degeneration | Weakness, anorexia, arrhythmias | IV fluids, atropine for arrhythmias |
| Marijuana (*Cannabis sativa*) | None | Behavior changes, disorientation, hyperactivity, tremors | Supportive care |
| Mistletoe (*Phoradendron leucarpum*) | GI tract irritation | Anorexia, regurgitation/vomiting, diarrhea | Correct fluid and electrolyte imbalances |
| Oleander (*Nerium oleander*) | GI hemorrhages and inflammation, myocardial degeneration, fibrosis and necrosis | Marked weakness, crop stasis, anorexia, arrhythmias, seizures | IV fluids, atropine and/or propranolol depending on arrhythmias, supportive care |
| Pothos (*Epipremnum aureum*) | Oral mucosa, crop, and upper GI tract irritation/inflammation | Anorexia, dysphonia, regurgitation, hypersalivation | Oral fluid gavage, milk, supportive care |
| Peace lily (*Spathiphyllum* spp.) | Oral mucosa, crop, and upper GI tract irritation/inflammation | Anorexia, dysphonia, regurgitation, hypersalivation | Oral fluid gavage, milk, supportive care |
| Philodendron (*Philodendron* spp.) | Oral mucosa, crop, and upper GI tract irritation/inflammation | Anorexia, dysphonia, regurgitation, hypersalivation | Oral fluid gavage, milk, supportive care |
| Poinsettia (*Euphorbia pulcherrima*) | Localized irritation of oral mucosa | Anorexia | Supportive care |
| Pokeweed (*Phytolacca americana*) | GI tract inflammation | Diarrhea | Supportive care |
| Virginia creeper (*Pathenocissus quinquefolia*) | GI tract irritation | Regurgitation/vomiting | Supportive care |
| Yew (*Taxus* spp.) | Pulmonary congestion and edema | Bradycardia, weakness, sudden death | Atropine, fluids, supportive care |

COMMON AVIAN TOXINS AND THEIR CLINICAL SIGNS (CONTINUED)

| Common drugs at toxic doses | Clinical signs | Treatment/antidotes |
| --- | --- | --- |
| Acetaminophen | Vomiting, weakness, anorexia | Fluids and supportive care; possibly N-acetylcysteine as antidote |
| Non-steroidal anti-inflammatory drugs | Anorexia, dullness, ruffled feathers, lethargy, depression, recumbence, sunken eyes, watery droppings; elevations in serum uric acid and creatinine | Fluids, GI protectant, supportive care |
| Topical vitamin D analogs and oral vitamin $D_3$ in excess | Increased thirst, dystrophic mineralization, renal failure | Fluids, phosphate binders, calcitonin |
| Ivermectin | Seizures | Steroids, fluids, supportive care |
| Aminoglycosides | Polydipsia, weakness, increased concentrations of uric acid and creatinine | Fluids, supportive care |
| Vitamin A in excess | Osteodystrophy | Supportive care |

| Heavy metals | Clinical signs | Treatment/Antidotes |
| --- | --- | --- |
| Arsenic | Fluffed feathers, pruritis, drooped eyelid, weight loss, feather picking, loss of righting reflex, immobility, seizures | Vitamin $D_3$, chelation (dimercaprol), fluids and supportive care |
| Iron | Lethargy, emaciation, anorexia | Chelation (deferoxamine or calcium disodium EDTA), restrict sources, supportive care |
| Lead | Depression, weakness, crop stasis, regurgitation, polydipsia, seizures, blindness, hemoglobinuria, diarrhea | Removal of source, fluids, nutritional support, chelation (calcium disodium EDTA), supportive care |
| Mercury | Depression, hematuria, weakness, collapse | Fluids, chelation (dimercaprol), supportive care |
| Zinc | Feather loss/picking, depression, polydipsia, GI tract irritation, crop stasis, regurgitation, weight loss, weakness, anemia, seizures | Removal of source, fluids, nutritional support, chelation (calcium disodium EDTA), supportive care |

| Inhaled toxins | Clinical signs | Treatment/Antidotes |
| --- | --- | --- |
| Ammonia | Respiratory tract irritation, immunosuppression with secondary infections | Fresh air, oxygen, supportive care, antimicrobials for infections |
| Carbon monoxide | Respiratory depression, weakness, collapse, seizures | Fresh air, oxygen, supportive care |
| Polytetrafluoroethylene (PTFE) | Respiratory failure, dyspnea, hemorrhage, collapse and death | Fresh air, oxygen, bronchodilators, NSAIDs, supportive care |
| Smoke (marijuana) | Depression or hyperactivity, behavior changes | Fresh air, oxygen, supportive care |
| Smoke (tobacco) | Dyspnea, coughing, tachycardia, pulmonary irritation, ocular irritation | Fresh air, oxygen, supportive care |
| Smoke (wood) | Dyspnea, coughing, sneezing, pulmonary and ocular irritation | Fresh air, oxygen, supportive care |

COMMON AVIAN TOXINS AND THEIR CLINICAL SIGNS (CONTINUED)

| Household | Clinical signs | Treatment/Antidotes |
|---|---|---|
| Alcohol | Lethargy, regurgitation, ataxia, impaired motor coordination, vomiting | Fluids with dextrose, supportive care |
| Aluminum chloride | Oral irritation, GI tract inflammation | Oral gavage/fluids, supportive care |
| Ammonia | Respiratory tract irritation | Fresh air, oxygen, supportive care |
| Chlorine (bleach) | Respiratory tract irritation, photophobia, coughing, sneezing, hyperventilation, GI irritation if ingested | Fluids, milk, GI protectant, supportive care |
| Cigarettes/cigars/tobacco | Vomiting, depression, dyspnea, tachycardia, seizures | Fluids, supportive care |
| Methylene chloride | Respiratory depression, weakness, collapse, seizures | Fresh air, oxygen, supportive care |
| Petroleum products | Depression, respiratory tract irritation, pneumonia | Fluids, oxygen, supportive care |
| Salt (table salt and salty foods) | GI tract irritation, polydipsia, dehydration, weakness and depression | Fluids replaced slowly, supportive care |
| Soaps/detergents | GI tract irritation, vomiting/regurgitation, diarrhea | Fluids, supportive care |
| Yeast dough | Crop stasis, depression | Crop gavage, fluids, supportive care |

| Pesticides | Clinical signs | Treatment/Antidotes |
|---|---|---|
| Anticoagulant rodenticides | Hemorrhage, weakness, collapse, dyspnea | Vitamin $K_1$, supportive care |
| Bromethalin | Depression, seizures | Mannitol, fluids, supportive care |
| Carbamates/organophosphorus insecticides | Ataxia, spastic nictitans, seizures | Fluids, atropine, pralidoxime, steroids, supportive care |
| Pyrethrins/pyrethroids | Incoordination, weakness, muscle tremors, diarrhea | Fluids, supportive care |

| Mycotoxins | Clinical signs | Treatment/Antidotes |
|---|---|---|
| Aflatoxin | Hemorrhage, icterus, anemia, depression, ruffled feathers, anorexia, and other signs of severe hepatic damage, immunosuppression | Removal of suspected feed source, increase high quality protein, supportive care |
| Trichothecenes (i.e. diacetoxyscirpenol) | Enteritis, dehydration, weight loss, malformed feathers, immunosuppression and secondary infections | Removal of suspected feed source, nutritional support, antimicrobials, supportive care |
| Ochratoxin | Anorexia, polydipsia, depression, elevations in serum uric acid and creatinine | Removal of suspected feed source, fluids, supportive care |

**AUTHOR**
John H Tegzes, MA, VMD, DABVT

## APPENDIX VII

**AVIAN TAXONOMY**

| Order | Family | Number of species | Common names |
|---|---|---|---|
| Struthioniformes | Struthionidae | 2 | Ostriches |
| Rheiformes | Rheidae | 2 | Rheas |
| Tinamiformes | Tinamidae | 46 | Tinamous |
| Casuariiformes | Casuariidae | 4 | Cassowaries and emu |
| Apterygiformes | Apterygidae | 5 | Kiwis |
| Anseriformes | Anhimidae | 3 | Screamers |
| | Anseranatidae | 1 | Magpie goose |
| | Anatidae | 174 | Ducks, swans, and geese |
| Galliformes | Megapodiidae | 21 | Megapodes |
| | Cracidae | 57 | Guans, chachalacas, and curassows |
| | Numididae | 8 | Guineafowls |
| | Odontophoridae | 33 | New World quails |
| | Phasianidae | 186 | Pheasants, grouse, partridges, quails |
| Phoenicopteriformes | Phoenicopteridae | 6 | Flamingos |
| Podicipediformes | Podicipedidae | 22 | Grebes |
| Columbiformes | Columbidae | 353 | Pigeons and doves |
| Mesitornithiformes | Mesitornithidae | 3 | Mesites |
| Pterocliformes | Pteroclidae | 16 | Sandgrouse |
| Otidiformes | Otididae | 26 | Bustards |
| Musophagiformes | Musophagidae | 23 | Turacos |
| Cuculiformes | Cuculidae | 147 | Cuckoos |
| Caprimulgiformes | Podargidae | 16 | Frogmouths |
| | Caprimulgidae | 97 | Nightjars |
| | Nyctibiidae | 7 | Potoos |
| | Steatornithidae | 1 | Oilbird |
| | Aegothelidae | 9 | Owlet-nightjars |
| | Apodidae | 112 | Swifts |
| | Hemiprocnidae | 4 | Treeswifts |
| | Trochilidae | 363 | Hummingbirds |
| Opisthocomiformes | Opisthocomidae | 1 | Hoatzin |
| Gruiformes | Sarothruridae | 15 | Flufftails |
| | Rallidae | 155 | Rails and coots |
| | Heliornithidae | 3 | Finfoots |
| | Aramidae | 1 | Limpkin |
| | Psophiidae | 3 | Trumpeters |
| | Gruidae | 15 | Cranes |

AVIAN TAXONOMY (CONTINUED)

| Order | Family | Number of species | Common names |
|-------|--------|-------------------|--------------|
| Charadriiformes | Pluvianellidae | 1 | Magellanic plover |
| | Chionidae | 2 | Sheathbills |
| | Burhinidae | 10 | Thick-knees |
| | Pluvianidae | 1 | Egyptian plover |
| | Recurvirostridae | 9 | Stilts and avocets |
| | Ibidorhynchidae | 1 | Ibisbill |
| | Haematopodidae | 12 | Oystercatchers |
| | Charadriidae | 69 | Plovers and lapwings |
| | Pedionomidae | 1 | Plains-wanderer |
| | Thinocoridae | 4 | Seedsnipes |
| | Rostratulidae | 3 | Painted-snipes |
| | Jacanidae | 8 | Jacanas |
| | Scolopacidae | 97 | Sandpipers and curlews |
| | Turnicidae | 18 | Buttonquails |
| | Dromadidae | 1 | Crab plover |
| | Glareolidae | 17 | Pratincoles and coursers |
| | Stercorariidae | 7 | Skuas and jaegers |
| | Alcidae | 25 | Auks, murres, and puffins |
| | Laridae | 100 | Gulls, terns, and skimmers |
| Eurypygiformes | Rhynochetidae | 1 | Kagu |
| | Eurypygidae | 1 | Sunbittern |
| Phaethontiformes | Phaethontidae | 3 | Tropicbirds |
| Gaviiformes | Gaviidae | 5 | Loons |
| Sphenisciformes | Spheniscidae | 18 | Penguins |
| Procellariformes | Diomedeidae | 20 | Albatrosses |
| | Oceanitidae | 10 | Southern storm-petrels |
| | Hydrobatidae | 18 | Northern storm-petrels |
| | Procellariidae | 98 | Shearwaters and petrels |
| Ciconiiformes | Ciconiidae | 20 | Storks |
| Suliformes | Fregatidae | 5 | Frigatebirds |
| | Sulidae | 10 | Gannets and boobies |
| | Anhingidae | 4 | Anhingas |
| | Phalacrocoracidae | 40 | Cormorants and shags |
| Pelecaniformes | Pelecanidae | 8 | Pelicans |
| | Balaenicipitidae | 1 | Shoebill |
| | Scopidae | 1 | Hamerkop |
| | Ardeidae | 71 | Herons, egrets, and bitterns |
| | Threskiornithidae | 36 | Ibises and spoonbills |
| Cathartiformes | Cathartidae | 7 | New World vultures |

AVIAN TAXONOMY (CONTINUED)

| Order | Family | Number of species | Common names |
|---|---|---|---|
| Accipitriformes | Sagittariidae | 1 | Secretarybird |
| | Pandionidae | 1 | Osprey |
| | Accipitridae | 250 | Hawks, eagles, vultures, kites |
| Strigiformes | Tytonidae | 18 | Barn owls |
| | Strigidae | 229 | Typical owls |
| Coliiformes | Coliidae | 6 | Mousebirds |
| Leptosomiformes | Leptosomidae | 1 | Cuckoo-roller |
| Trogoniformes | Trogonidae | 46 | Trogons |
| Bucerotiformes | Upupidae | 3 | Hoopoes |
| | Phoeniculidae | 8 | Wood hoopoes |
| | Bucorvidae | 2 | Ground hornbills |
| | Bucerotidae | 62 | Hornbills |
| Coraciiformes | Todidae | 5 | Todies |
| | Momotidae | 14 | Motmots |
| | Alcedinidae | 117 | Kingfishers |
| | Meropidae | 31 | Bee-eaters |
| | Coraciidae | 13 | Rollers |
| | Brachypteraciidae | 5 | Ground-rollers |
| Galbuliformes | Bucconidae | 37 | Puffbirds |
| | Galbulidae | 18 | Jacamars |
| Piciformes | Lybiidae | 41 | African barbets |
| | Megalaimidae | 35 | Asian barbets |
| | Capitonidae | 15 | New World barbets |
| | Semnornithidae | 2 | Toucan-barbets |
| | Ramphastidae | 36 | Toucans |
| | Indicatoridae | 16 | Honeyguides |
| | Picidae | 235 | Woodpeckers |
| Cariamiformes | Cariamidae | 2 | Seriemas |
| Falconiformes | Falconidae | 65 | Falcons, caracaras |
| Psittaciformes | Strigopidae | 3 | New Zealand parrots |
| | Cacatuidae | 22 | Cockatoos |
| | Psittaculidae | 202 | Old World parrots |
| | Psittacidae | 177 | New World and African parrots |

AVIAN TAXONOMY (CONTINUED)

| Order | Family | Number of species | Common names |
|---|---|---|---|
| Passeriformes | Acanthisittidae | 4 | New Zealand wrens |
| | Calyptomenidae | 6 | African and green broadbills |
| | Eurylaimidae | 10 | Asian and Grauer's broadbills |
| | Sapayoidae | 1 | Sapayoa |
| | Philepittidae | 4 | Asities |
| | Pittidae | 47 | Pittas |
| | Thamnophilidae | 237 | Antbirds |
| | Melanopareiidae | 4 | Crescentchests |
| | Conopophagidae | 12 | Gnateaters |
| | Grallariidae | 70 | Antpittas |
| | Rhinocryptidae | 65 | Tapaculos |
| | Formicariidae | 12 | Antthrushes |
| | Furnariidae | 314 | Ovenbirds, woodcreepers |
| | Pipridae | 55 | Manakins |
| | Cotingidae | 65 | Cotingas |
| | Tityridae | 35 | Tityras |
| | Oxyruncidae | 8 | Sharpbills, royal flycatchers |
| | Tyrannidae | 441 | Tyrant flycatchers |
| | Menuridae | 2 | Lyrebirds |
| | Atrichornithidae | 2 | Scrubbirds |
| | Ptilonorhynchidae | 27 | Bower birds |
| | Climacteridae | 7 | Australasian treecreepers |
| | Maluridae | 32 | Fairywrens |
| | Meliphagidae | 191 | Honeyeaters |
| | Dasyornithidae | 3 | Bristlebirds |
| | Pardalotidae | 4 | Pardalotes |
| | Acanthizidae | 66 | Thornbills |
| | Pomatostomidae | 5 | Australasian babblers |
| | Orthonychidae | 3 | Logrunners |
| | Cinclosomatidae | 12 | Quail-thrushes, jewel-babblers |
| | Campephagidae | 89 | Cuckooshrikes |
| | Mohouidae | 3 | Whiteheads |
| | Neosittidae | 3 | Sittellas |
| | Psophodidae | 5 | Whipbirds, wedgebills |
| | Eulacestomatidae | 1 | Ploughbill |
| | Oreoicidae | 3 | Australo-Papuan bellbirds |
| | Falcunculidae | 3 | Shriketits |
| | Paramythiidae | 3 | Painted berrypeckers |
| | Vireonidae | 61 | Vireos, greenlets, shrike-babblers |
| | Pachycephalidae | 63 | Whistlers |

AVIAN TAXONOMY (CONTINUED)

| Order | Family | Number of species | Common names |
|---|---|---|---|
| | Oriolidae | 41 | Figbirds, Old World orioles, piopios |
| | Machaerirhynchidae | 2 | Boatbills |
| | Artamidae | 24 | Woodswallows, bellmagpies |
| | Rhagologidae | 1 | Mottled berryhunter |
| | Platysteiridae | 32 | Wattle-eyes, batises |
| | Vangidae | 40 | Vangas, helmetshrikes |
| | Pityriasidae | 1 | Bristlehead |
| | Aegithinidae | 4 | Loras |
| | Malaconotidae | 50 | Bushshrikes |
| | Rhipiduridae | 64 | Fantails |
| | Dicruridae | 28 | Drongos |
| | Paradisaeidae | 44 | Birds-of-paradise |
| | Ifritidae | 1 | Blue-capped ifrit |
| | Monarchidae | 100 | Monarchs |
| | Corcoracidae | 2 | White-winged chough, apostlebird |
| | Melampittidae | 2 | Melampittas |
| | Platylophidae | 1 | Crested jayshrike |
| | Laniidae | 34 | Shrikes |
| | Corvidae | 130 | Crows, jays, magpies |
| | Cnemophilidae | 3 | Satinbirds |
| | Melanocharitidae | 12 | Berrypeckers, longbills |
| | Callaeidae | 5 | Wattlebirds |
| | Notiomystidae | 1 | Stitchbird |
| | Petroicidae | 50 | Australasian robins |
| | Picathartidae | 2 | Rockfowl |
| | Chaetopidae | 2 | Rockjumpers |
| | Eupetidae | 1 | Rail-babbler |
| | Hyliotidae | 4 | Hyliotas |
| | Stenostiridae | 9 | Fairy flycatchers |
| | Paridae | 63 | Tits, chickadees, titmice |
| | Remizidae | 11 | Penduline-tits |
| | Alaudidae | 93 | Larks |
| | Panuridae | 1 | Bearded reedling |
| | Nicatoridae | 3 | Nicators |
| | Macrosphenidae | 18 | African warblers, crombecs |
| | Cisticolidae | 162 | Cisticolas, jerys |
| | Acrocephalidae | 60 | Reed warblers |
| | Locustellidae | 67 | Grassbirds |
| | Donacobiidae | 1 | Black-capped donacobius |
| | Bernieridae | 11 | Malagasy warblers |

AVIAN TAXONOMY (CONTINUED)

| Order | Family | Number of species | Common names |
|---|---|---|---|
| | Propidine | 4 | Cupwings |
| | Hirundinidae | 88 | Swallows |
| | Pycnonotidae | 156 | Bulbuls |
| | Phylloscopidae | 80 | Leaf warblers |
| | Hyliidae | 2 | Hylias |
| | Scotocercidae | 35 | Bush warblers |
| | Aegithalidae | 11 | Bush tits, long-tailed tits |
| | Sylviidae | 32 | Sylviid warblers, babblers |
| | Paradoxornithidae | 38 | Parrotbills, fulvettas |
| | Zosteropidae | 148 | White-eyes, yuhinas |
| | Timaliidae | 58 | Tree-babblers, scimitar-babblers |
| | Pellorneidae | 65 | Ground babblers |
| | Leiothrichidae | 143 | Laughingthrushes |
| | Regulidae | 6 | Kinglets, goldcrests |
| | Tichodromidae | 1 | Wallcreeper |
| | Sittidae | 29 | Nuthatches |
| | Certhiidae | 11 | Treecreepers |
| | Polioptilidae | 21 | Gnatcatchers |
| | Troglodytidae | 86 | Wrens |
| | Elachuridae | 1 | Spotted elachura |
| | Cinclidae | 5 | Dippers |
| | Buphagidae | 2 | Oxpeckers |
| | Sturnidae | 125 | Starlings |
| | Mimidae | 34 | Mockingbirds, thrashers |
| | Turdidae | 175 | Thrushes |
| | Muscicapidae | 345 | Old World flycatchers |
| | Bombycillidae | 3 | Waxwings |
| | Mohoidae | 5 | Hawaiian honeyeaters, oos |
| | Ptiliogonatidae | 4 | Silky-flycatchers |
| | Dulidae | 1 | Palmchat |
| | Hylocitreidae | 1 | Hylocitrea |
| | Hypocoliidae | 1 | Hypocolius |
| | Promeropidae | 2 | Sugarbirds |
| | Modulatricidae | 3 | Dapple-throat, spot-throat |
| | Dicaeidae | 53 | Flowerpeckers |
| | Nectariniidae | 148 | Sunbirds, spiderhunters |
| | Irenidae | 3 | Fairy-bluebirds |
| | Chloropseidae | 12 | Leafbirds |
| | Peucedramidae | 1 | Olive warbler |
| | Urocynchramidae | 1 | Przevalski's finch |

AVIAN TAXONOMY (CONTINUED)

| Order | Family | Number of species | Common names |
|---|---|---|---|
| | Ploceidae | 123 | Weavers, widowbirds |
| | Estrildidae | 138 | Waxbills, munias |
| | Viduidae | 20 | Indigobirds, whydahs |
| | Prunellidae | 12 | Accentors |
| | Passeridae | 43 | Old World sparrows, snowfinches |
| | Motacillidae | 69 | Wagtails, pipits |
| | Fringillidae | 235 | Finches |
| | Calcariidae | 6 | Longspurs, snow buntings |
| | Rhodinocichlidae | 1 | Thrush-tanager |
| | Emberizidae | 44 | Old World buntings |
| | Passerellidae | 132 | New World sparrows |
| | Calyptophilidae | 2 | Chat-tanagers |
| | Phaenicophilidae | 4 | Hispaniolan tanagers |
| | Nesospingidae | 1 | Puerto Rican tanager |
| | Spindalidae | 4 | Spindalises |
| | Zeledoniidae | 1 | Wrenthrush |
| | Teretistridae | 2 | Cuban warblers |
| | Icteriidae | 1 | Yellow-breasted chat |
| | Icteridae | 106 | Oropendolas, New World orioles, blackbirds |
| | Parulidae | 115 | New World warblers |
| | Mitrospingidae | 4 | Mitrospingid tanagers |
| | Cardinalidae | 51 | Cardinals, tanagers, grosbeaks |
| | Thraupidae | 384 | Tanagers |

**AUTHOR**
Hugues Beaufrère, DVM, PhD, DACZM, DABVP, DECZM

CLINICAL ALGORITHMS

## Algorithm 1: Sick-Bird Syndrome

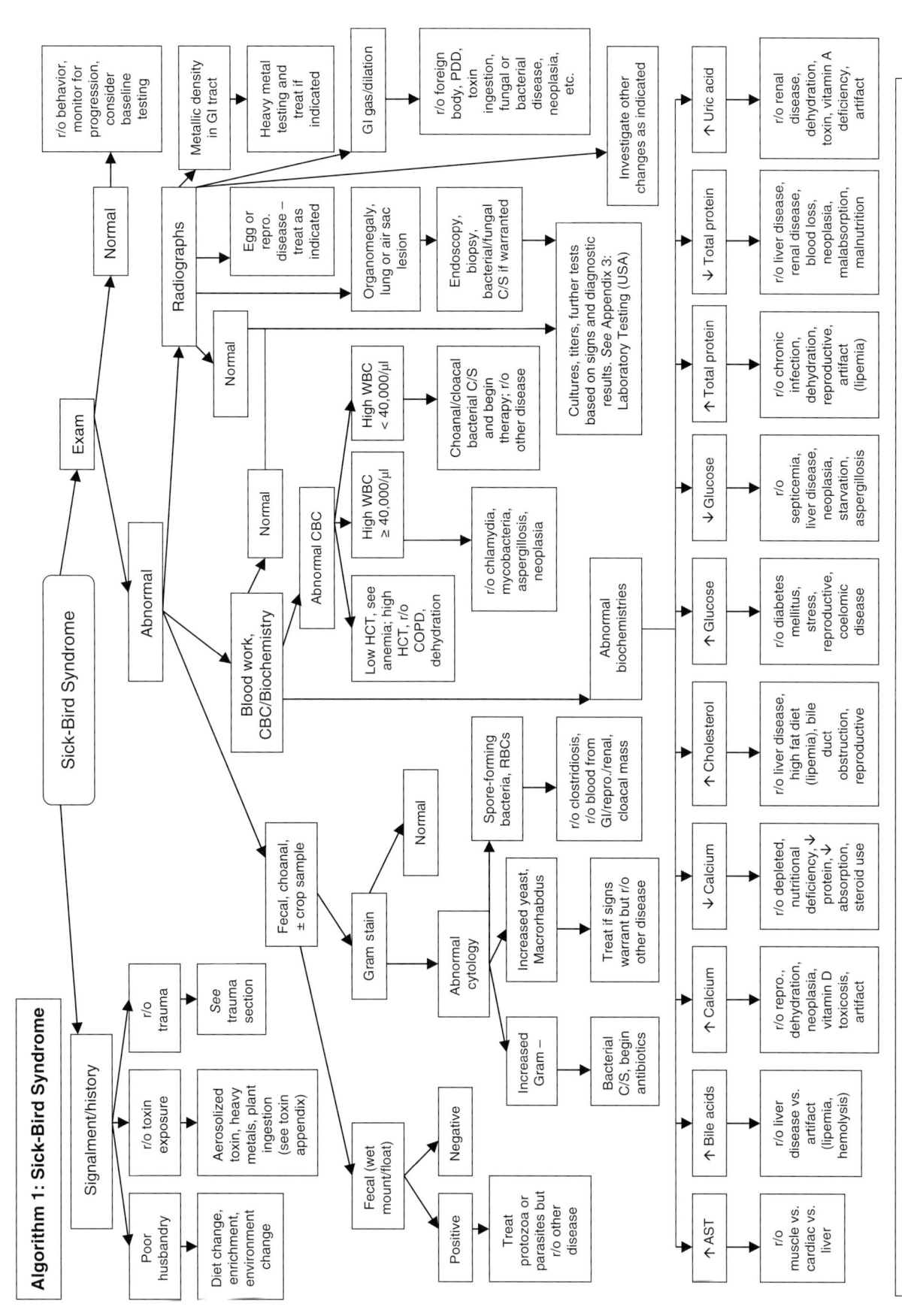

**Abbreviations:** AST, aspartate aminotransferase; C/S, culture and sensitivity; CBC, complete blood count; COPD, chronic obstructive pulmonary disease; GI, gastrointestinal; HCT, hematocrit; PDD, proventricular dilatation disease; r/o, rule out; RBCs, red blood cells; repro., reproduction; WBC, white blood cell.

**Algorithm 2: Diarrhea**

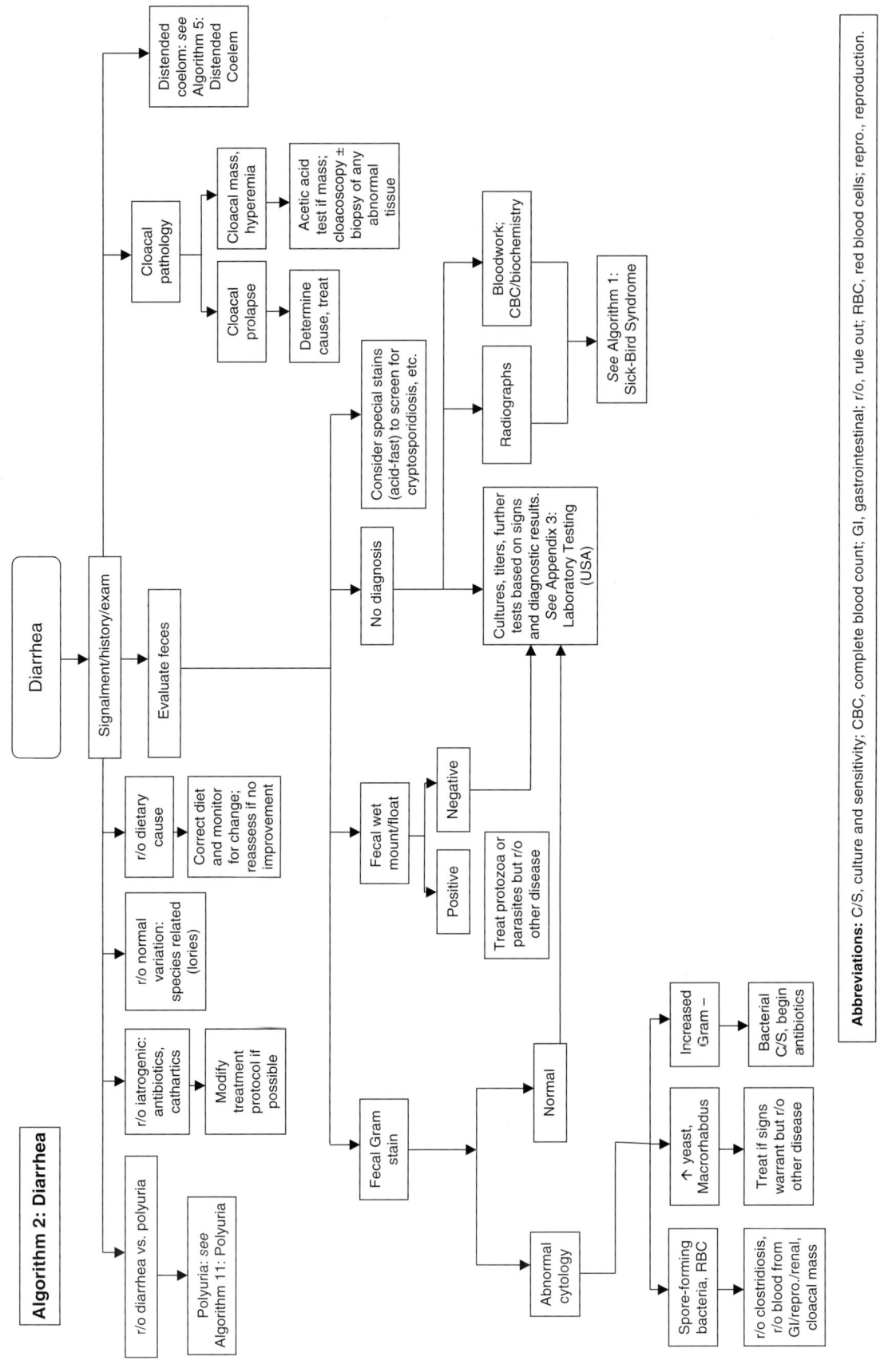

**Abbreviations:** C/S, culture and sensitivity; CBC, complete blood count; GI, gastrointestinal; r/o, rule out; RBC, red blood cells; repro., reproduction.

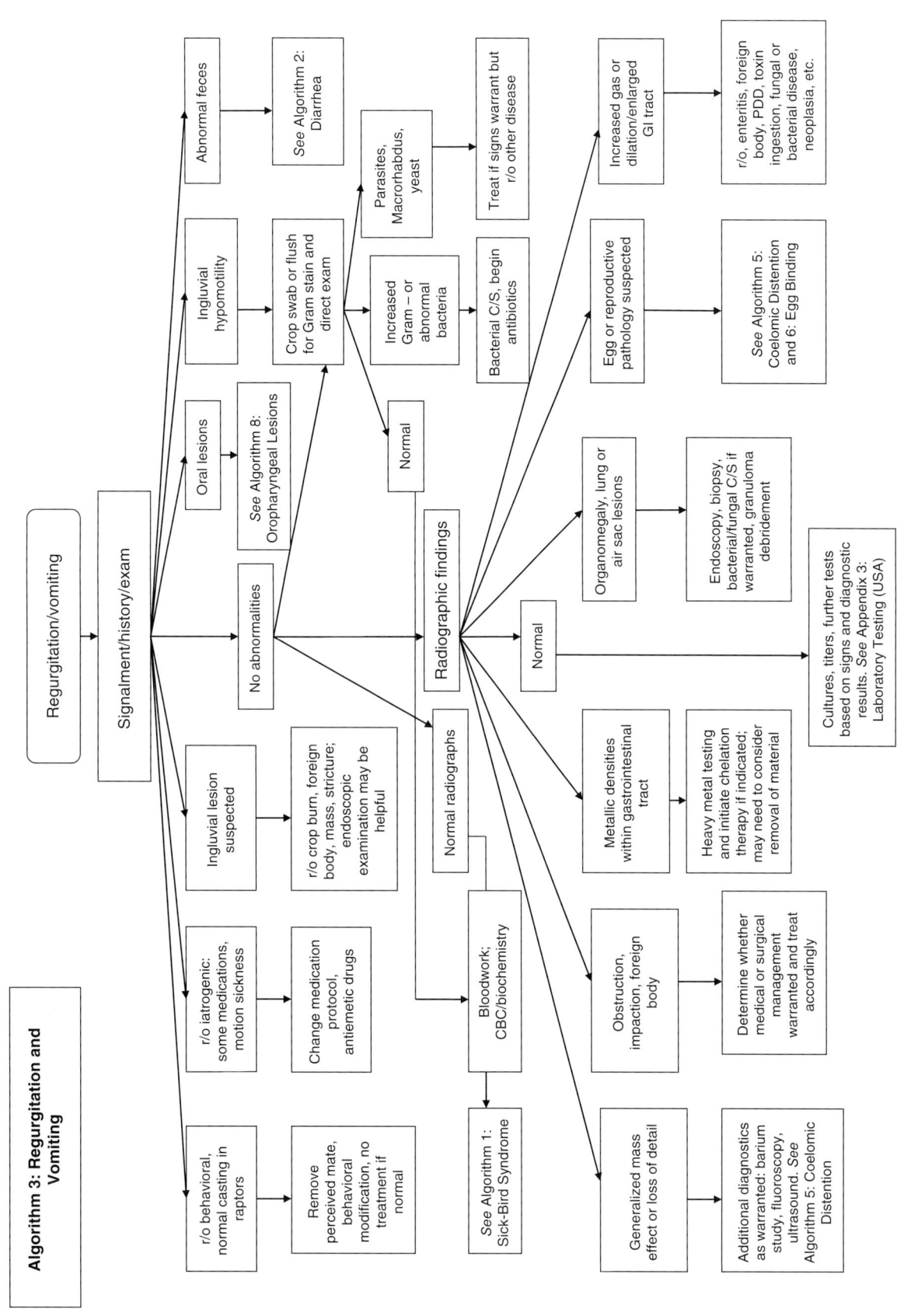

**Algorithm 3: Regurgitation and Vomiting**

Regurgitation/vomiting → Signalment/history/exam

- r/o behavioral, normal casting in raptors → Remove perceived mate, behavioral modification, no treatment if normal
- r/o iatrogenic: some medications, motion sickness → Change medication protocol, antiemetic drugs
- Ingluvial lesion suspected → r/o crop burn, foreign body, mass, stricture; endoscopic examination may be helpful
- No abnormalities
- Oral lesions → See Algorithm 8: Oropharyngeal Lesions
- Ingluvial hypomotility → Crop swab or flush for Gram stain and direct exam
- Abnormal feces → See Algorithm 2: Diarrhea

Crop swab or flush for Gram stain and direct exam:
- Parasites, Macrorhabdus, yeast → Treat if signs warrant but r/o other disease
- Increased Gram – or abnormal bacteria → Bacterial C/S, begin antibiotics
- Normal

No abnormalities → Bloodwork; CBC/biochemistry → See Algorithm 1: Sick-Bird Syndrome

Normal radiographs

Radiographic findings:
- Increased gas or dilation/enlarged GI tract → r/o, enteritis, foreign body, PDD, toxin ingestion, fungal or bacterial disease, neoplasia, etc.
- Egg or reproductive pathology suspected → See Algorithm 5: Coelomic Distention and 6: Egg Binding
- Organomegaly, lung or air sac lesions → Endoscopy, biopsy, bacterial/fungal C/S if warranted, granuloma debridement
- Normal → Cultures, titers, further tests based on signs and diagnostic results. See Appendix 3: Laboratory Testing (USA)
- Metallic densities within gastrointestinal tract → Heavy metal testing and initiate chelation therapy if indicated; may need to consider removal of material
- Obstruction, impaction, foreign body → Determine whether medical or surgical management warranted and treat accordingly
- Generalized mass effect or loss of detail → Additional diagnostics as warranted: barium study, fluoroscopy, ultrasound. See Algorithm 5: Coelomic Distention

**Abbreviations:** C/S, culture and sensitivity; CBC, complete blood count; GI, gastrointestinal; PDD, proventricular dilatation disease; r/o, risk of.

**Algorithm 4: Respiratory Distress**

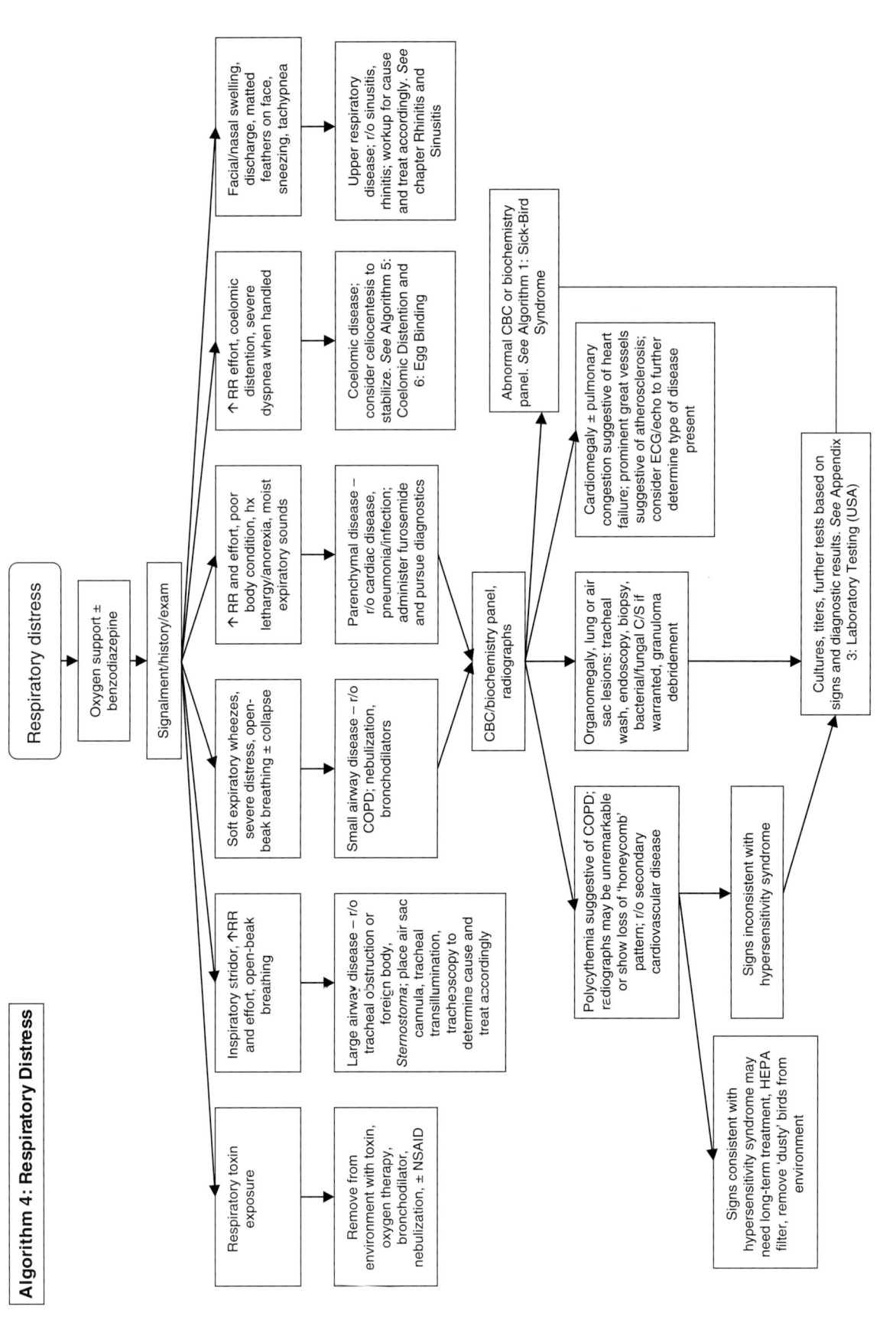

**Abbreviations:** CBC, complete blood count; COPD, chronic obstructive pulmonary disease; ECG, electrocardiogram; HEPA, high-efficiency particulate air; hx, medical history; NSAID, non-steroidal anti-inflammatory drug; r/o, rule out; RR, respiratory rate.

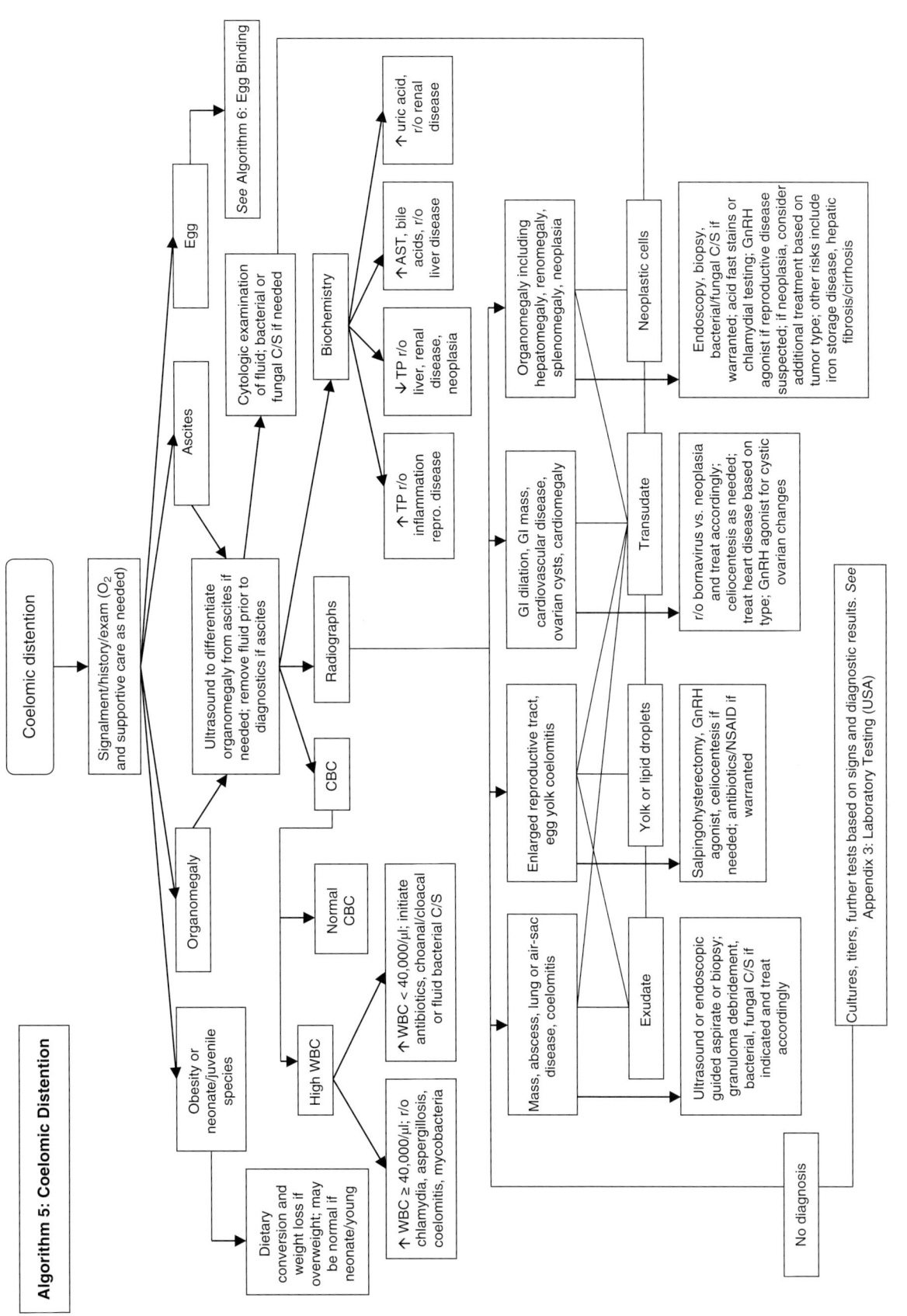

**Algorithm 5: Coelomic Distention**

Coelomic distention

Signalment/history/exam ($O_2$ and supportive care as needed)

Obesity or neonate/juvenile species

Organomegaly

Ascites

Egg → *See Algorithm 6: Egg Binding*

Dietary conversion and weight loss if overweight; may be normal if neonate/young

Ultrasound to differentiate organomegaly from ascites if needed; remove fluid prior to diagnostics if ascites

Cytologic examination of fluid; bacterial or fungal C/S if needed

CBC

High WBC

Normal CBC

↑WBC ≥ 40,000/µl; r/o chlamydia, aspergillosis, coelomitis, mycobacteria

↑WBC < 40,000/µl; initiate antibiotics, choanal/cloacal or fluid bacterial C/S

Radiographs

Biochemistry

↑TP r/o inflammation repro. disease

↓TP r/o liver, renal disease, neoplasia

↑AST, bile acids, r/o liver disease

↑ uric acid, r/o renal disease

Mass, abscess, lung or air-sac disease, coelomitis

Enlarged reproductive tract, egg yolk coelomitis

GI dilation, GI mass, cardiovascular disease, ovarian cysts, cardiomegaly

Organomegaly including hepatomegaly, renomegaly, splenomegaly, neoplasia

Exudate

Yolk or lipid droplets

Transudate

Neoplastic cells

Ultrasound or endoscopic guided aspirate or biopsy; granuloma debridement, bacterial, fungal C/S if indicated and treat accordingly

Salpingohysterectomy, GnRH agonist, celiocentesis if needed; antibiotics/NSAID if warranted

r/o bornavirus vs. neoplasia and treat accordingly; celiocentesis as needed; treat heart disease based on type; GnRH agonist for cystic ovarian changes

Endoscopy, biopsy, bacterial/fungal C/S if warranted; acid fast stains or chlamydial testing; GnRH agonist if reproductive disease suspected; if neoplasia, consider additional treatment based on tumor type; other risks include iron storage disease, hepatic fibrosis/cirrhosis

No diagnosis → Cultures, titers, further tests based on signs and diagnostic results. See Appendix 3: Laboratory Testing (USA)

**Abbreviations:** AST, aspartate aminotransferase; C/S, culture and sensitivity; CBC, complete blood count; GI, gastrointestinal; GnRH, gonadotropin-releasing hormone; NSAID, non-steroidal anti-inflammatory drug; r/o, rule out; repro., reproductive; TP, total protein; WBC, white blood cell.

**Algorithm 6: Egg Binding**

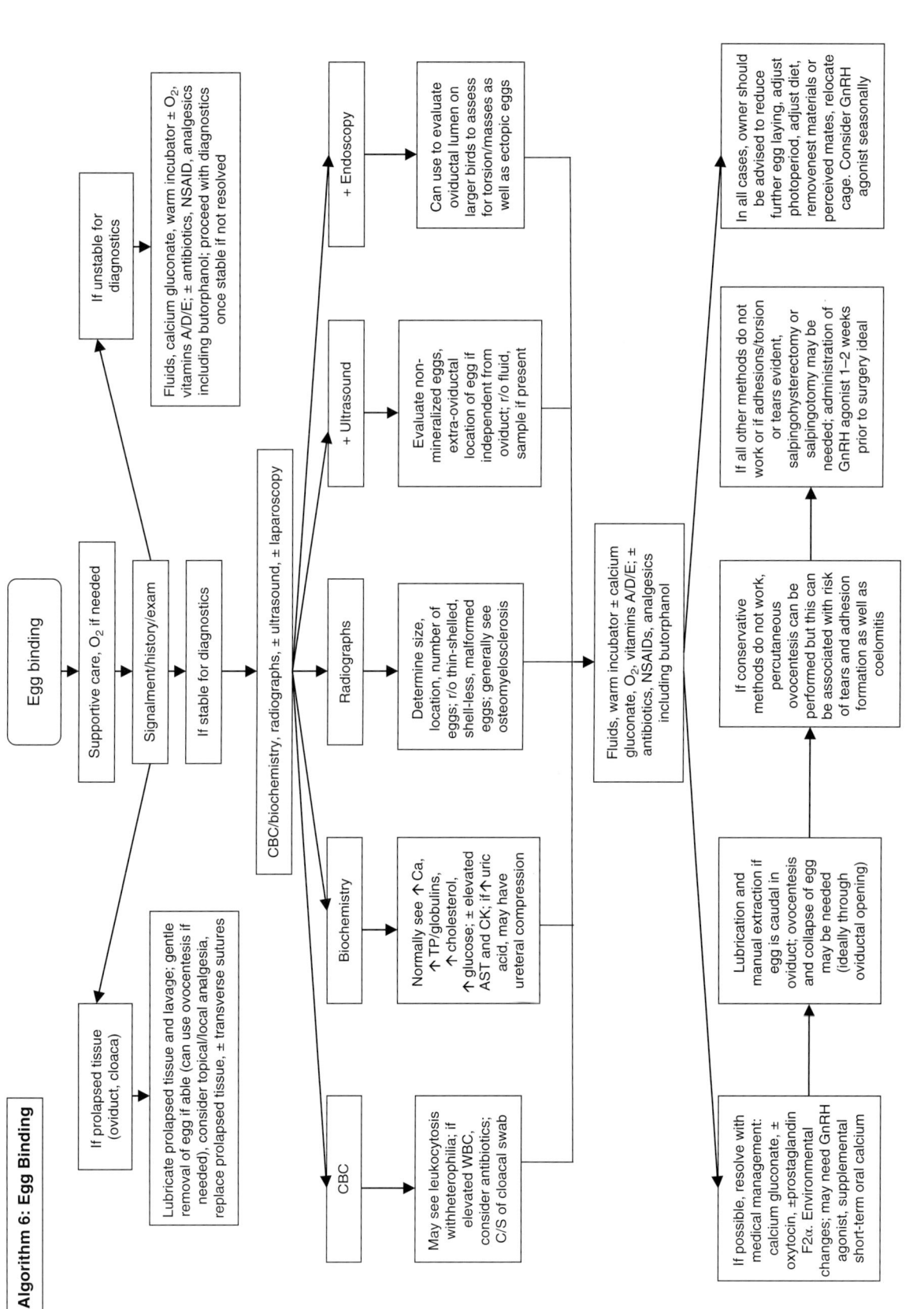

Egg binding

Supportive care, O₂ if needed

Signalment/history/exam

If stable for diagnostics

If unstable for diagnostics

Fluids, calcium gluconate, warm incubator ± O₂; vitamins A/D/E; ± antibiotics, NSAID, analgesics including butorphanol; proceed with diagnostics once stable if not resolved

If prolapsed tissue (oviduct, cloaca)

Lubricate prolapsed tissue and lavage; gentle removal of egg if able (can use ovocentesis if needed), consider topical/local analgesia; replace prolapsed tissue, ± transverse sutures

CBC/biochemistry, radiographs, ± ultrasound, ± laparoscopy

CBC

May see leukocytosis with heterophilia; if elevated WBC, consider antibiotics; C/S of cloacal swab

Biochemistry

Normally see ↑Ca, ↑TP/globulins, ↑cholesterol, ↑glucose; ± elevated AST and CK; if↑uric acid, may have ureteral compression

Radiographs

Determine size, location, number of eggs; r/o thin-shelled, shell-less, malformed eggs; generally see osteomyelosclerosis

+ Ultrasound

Evaluate non-mineralized eggs, extra-oviductal location of egg if independent from oviduct; r/o fluid, sample if present

+ Endoscopy

Can use to evaluate oviductal lumen on larger birds to assess for torsion/masses as well as ectopic eggs

Fluids, warm incubator ± calcium gluconate, O₂, vitamins A/D/E; ± antibiotics, NSAIDs, analgesics including butorphanol

If possible, resolve with medical management: calcium gluconate, ± oxytocin, ±prostaglandin F2α. Environmental changes; may need GnRH agonist, supplemental short-term oral calcium

Lubrication and manual extraction if egg is caudal in oviduct; ovocentesis and collapse of egg may be needed (ideally through oviductal opening)

If conservative methods do not work, percutaneous ovocentesis can be performed but this can be associated with risk of tears and adhesion formation as well as coelomitis

If all other methods do not work or if adhesions/torsion or tears evident, salpingohysterectomy or salpingotomy may be needed; administration of GnRH agonist 1–2 weeks prior to surgery ideal

In all cases, owner should be advised to reduce further egg laying, adjust photoperiod, adjust diet, remove nest materials or perceived mates, relocate cage. Consider GnRH agonist seasonally

**Abbreviations:** AST, aspartate aminotransferase; C/S, culture and sensitivity; Ca, calcium; CBC, complete blood count; CK, creatine kinase; COPD, chronic obstructive pulmonary disease; GI, gastrointestinal; GnRH, gonadotropin- releasing hormone; HCT, hematocrit; PDD, proventricular dilatation disease; NSAID, non-steroidal anti-inflammatory drug; r/o, rule out; RBCs, red blood cells; repro., reproduction; TP, total protein; WBC, white blood cell.

**Algorithm 7: Anemia**

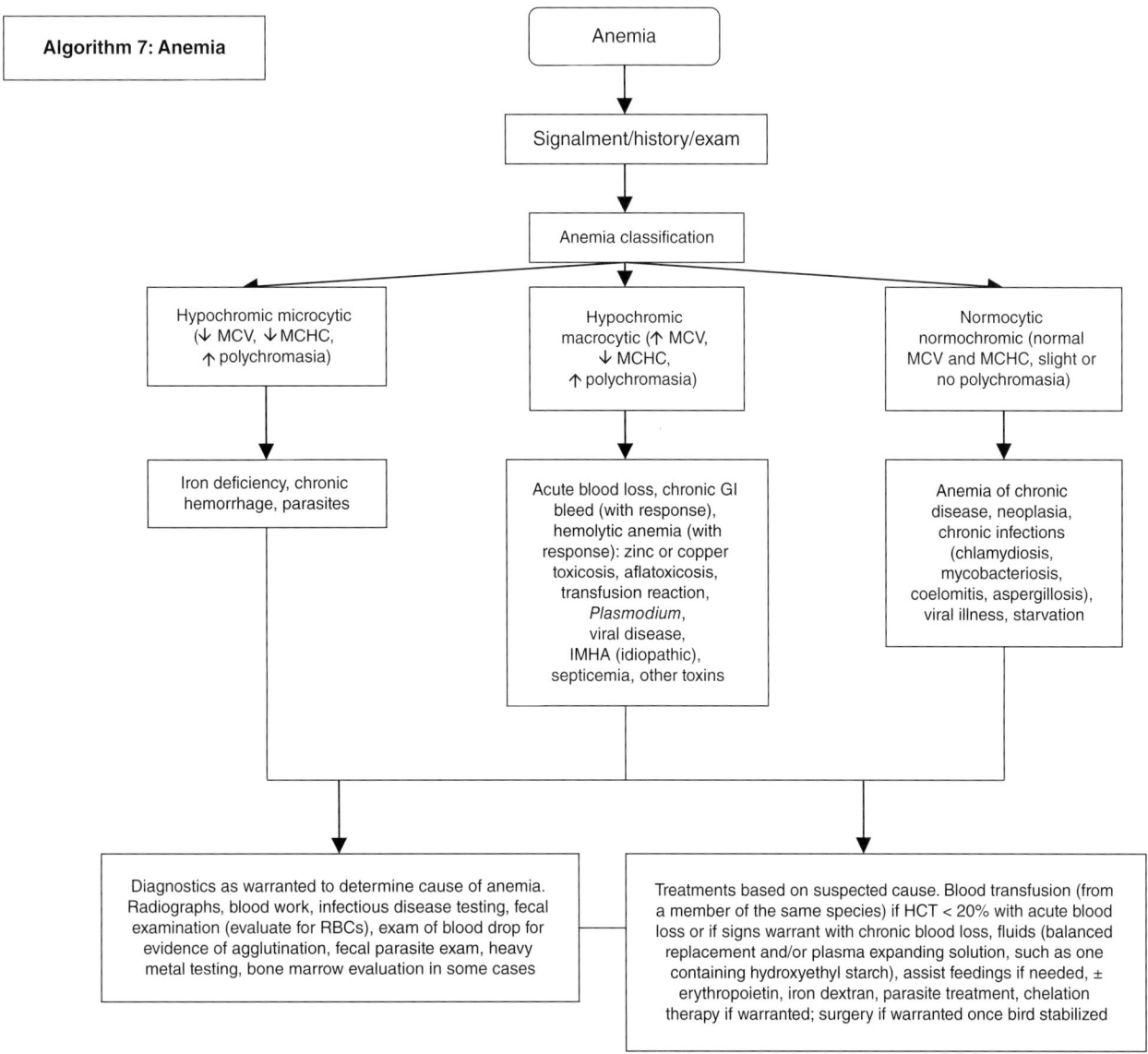

Anemia

Signalment/history/exam

Anemia classification

Hypochromic microcytic (↓ MCV, ↓ MCHC, ↑ polychromasia)

Hypochromic macrocytic (↑ MCV, ↓ MCHC, ↑ polychromasia)

Normocytic normochromic (normal MCV and MCHC, slight or no polychromasia)

Iron deficiency, chronic hemorrhage, parasites

Acute blood loss, chronic GI bleed (with response), hemolytic anemia (with response): zinc or copper toxicosis, aflatoxicosis, transfusion reaction, *Plasmodium*, viral disease, IMHA (idiopathic), septicemia, other toxins

Anemia of chronic disease, neoplasia, chronic infections (chlamydiosis, mycobacteriosis, coelomitis, aspergillosis), viral illness, starvation

Diagnostics as warranted to determine cause of anemia. Radiographs, blood work, infectious disease testing, fecal examination (evaluate for RBCs), exam of blood drop for evidence of agglutination, fecal parasite exam, heavy metal testing, bone marrow evaluation in some cases

Treatments based on suspected cause. Blood transfusion (from a member of the same species) if HCT < 20% with acute blood loss or if signs warrant with chronic blood loss, fluids (balanced replacement and/or plasma expanding solution, such as one containing hydroxyethyl starch), assist feedings if needed, ± erythropoietin, iron dextran, parasite treatment, chelation therapy if warranted; surgery if warranted once bird stabilized

**Abbreviations:** GI, gastrointestinal; HCT, hematocrit; IMHA, immune-mediated haemolytic anemia; MCHC, mean corpuscular hemoglobin concentration; MCV, mean corpuscular volume; RBCs, red blood cells.

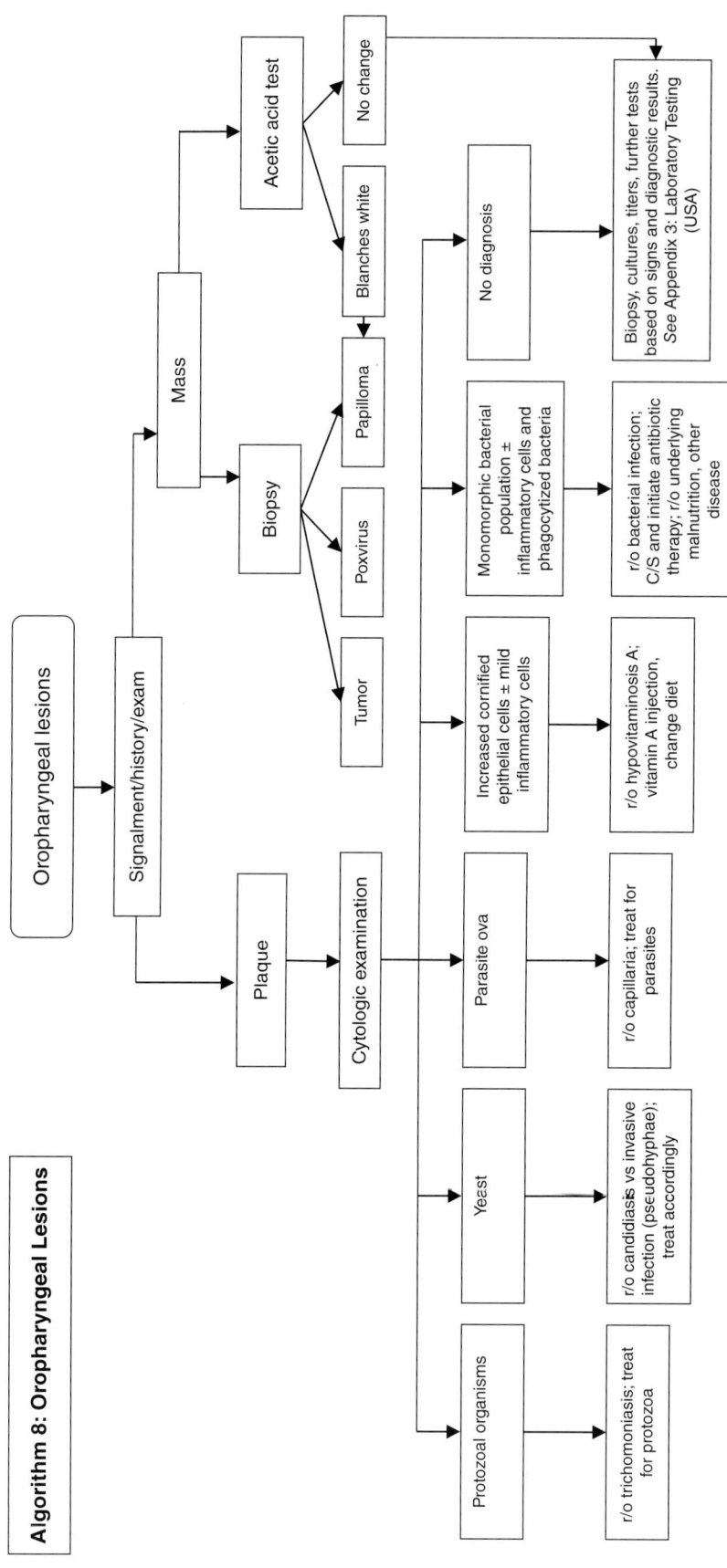

**Algorithm 8: Oropharyngeal Lesions**

**Abbreviations:** C/S, culture and sensitivity; r/o, rule out.

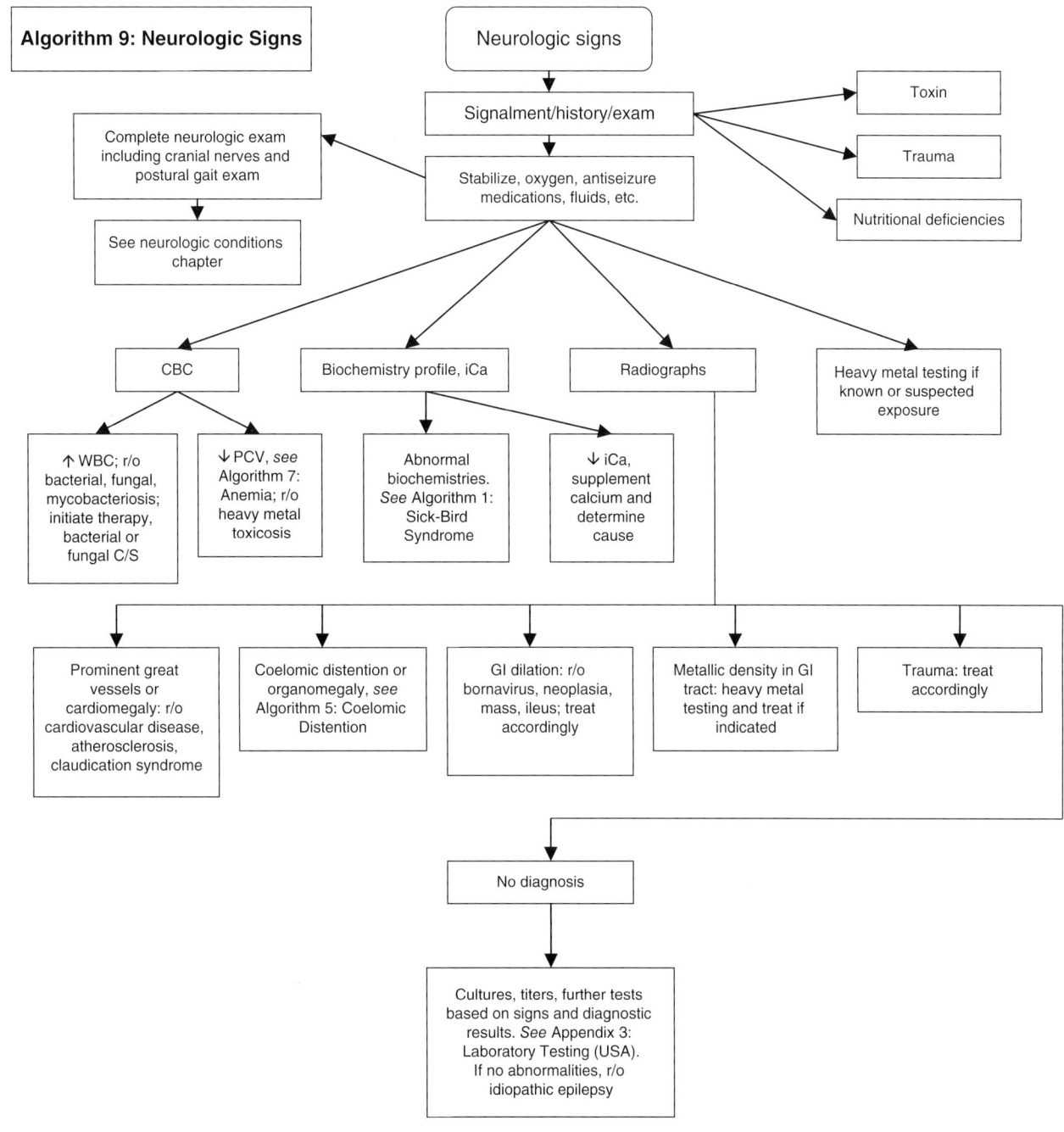

**Algorithm 9: Neurologic Signs**

Neurologic signs

Signalment/history/exam

→ Toxin

→ Trauma

→ Nutritional deficiencies

Complete neurologic exam including cranial nerves and postural gait exam

See neurologic conditions chapter

Stabilize, oxygen, antiseizure medications, fluids, etc.

CBC

Biochemistry profile, iCa

Radiographs

Heavy metal testing if known or suspected exposure

↑ WBC; r/o bacterial, fungal, mycobacteriosis; initiate therapy, bacterial or fungal C/S

↓ PCV, *see* Algorithm 7: Anemia; r/o heavy metal toxicosis

Abnormal biochemistries. *See* Algorithm 1: Sick-Bird Syndrome

↓ iCa, supplement calcium and determine cause

Prominent great vessels or cardiomegaly: r/o cardiovascular disease, atherosclerosis, claudication syndrome

Coelomic distention or organomegaly, *see* Algorithm 5: Coelomic Distention

GI dilation: r/o bornavirus, neoplasia, mass, ileus; treat accordingly

Metallic density in GI tract: heavy metal testing and treat if indicated

Trauma: treat accordingly

No diagnosis

Cultures, titers, further tests based on signs and diagnostic results. *See* Appendix 3: Laboratory Testing (USA). If no abnormalities, r/o idiopathic epilepsy

**Abbreviations:** C/S, culture and sensitivity; CBC, complete blood count; GI, gastrointestinal; iCA, ionized calcium; PCV, packed cell volume; r/o, rule out; WBC, white blood cell.

**Algorithm 10: Polydipsia**

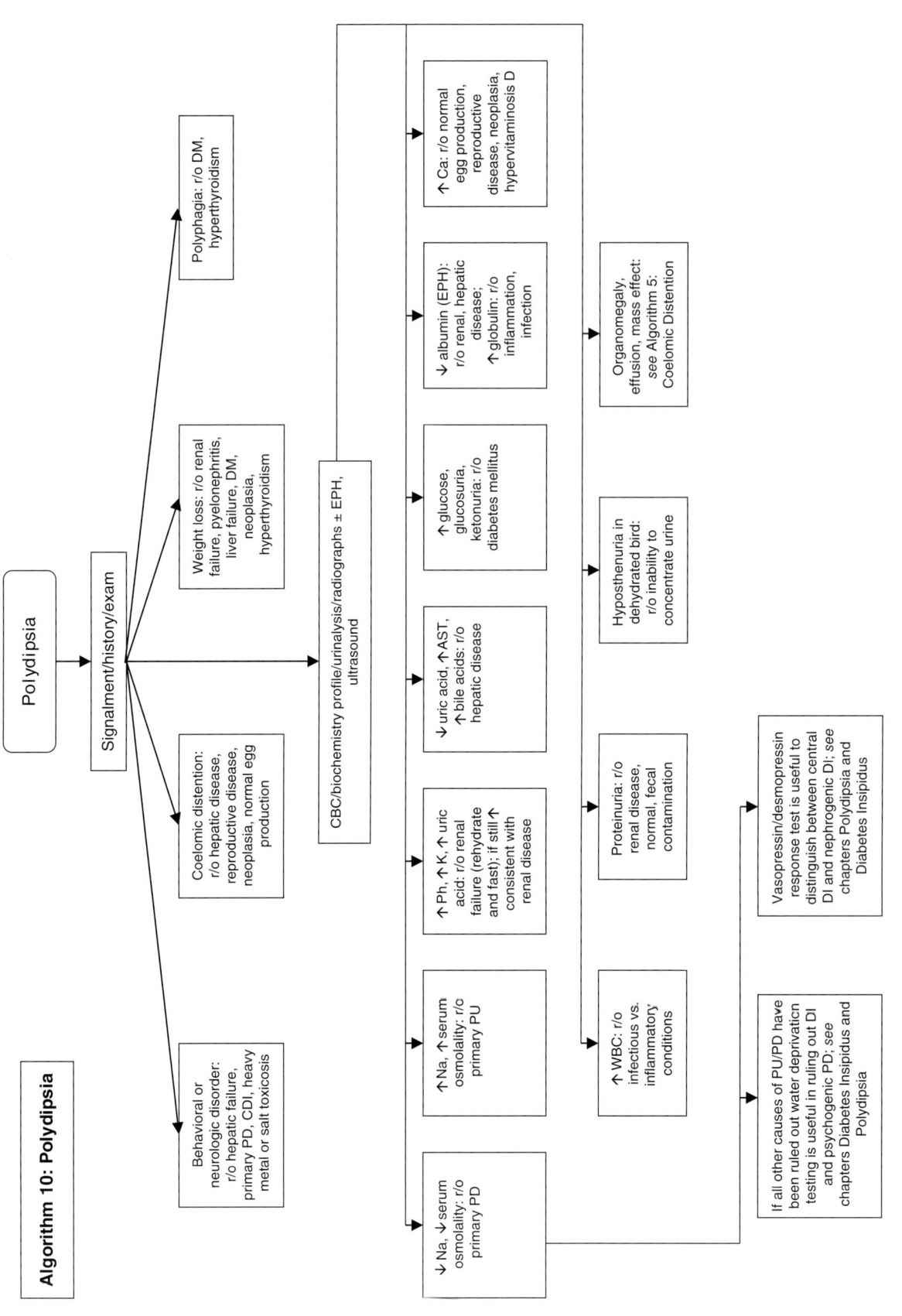

**Abbreviations:** AST, aspartate aminotransferase; CBC, complete blood count; CDI, central diabetes insipidus; DI, diabetes insipidus; DM, diabetes mellitus; EPH, electrophoresis; PD, polydipsia; PU, polyuria; r/o, rule out; WBC, white blood cell.

**Algorithm 11: Polyuria**

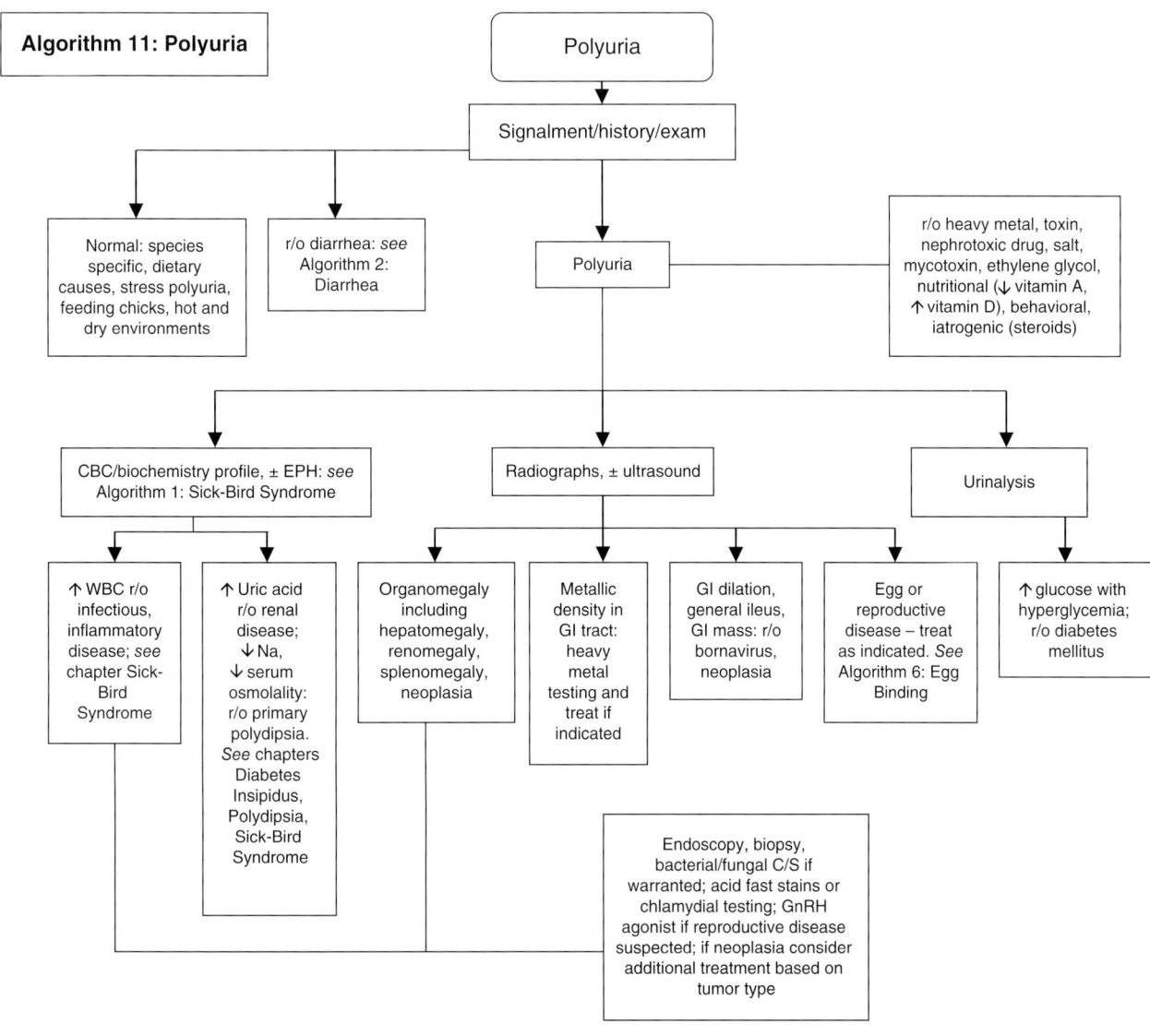

Polyuria

Signalment/history/exam

Normal: species specific, dietary causes, stress polyuria, feeding chicks, hot and dry environments

r/o diarrhea: *see* Algorithm 2: Diarrhea

Polyuria

r/o heavy metal, toxin, nephrotoxic drug, salt, mycotoxin, ethylene glycol, nutritional (↓ vitamin A, ↑ vitamin D), behavioral, iatrogenic (steroids)

CBC/biochemistry profile, ± EPH: *see* Algorithm 1: Sick-Bird Syndrome

Radiographs, ± ultrasound

Urinalysis

↑ WBC r/o infectious, inflammatory disease; *see* chapter Sick-Bird Syndrome

↑ Uric acid r/o renal disease; ↓ Na, ↓ serum osmolality: r/o primary polydipsia. *See* chapters Diabetes Insipidus, Polydipsia, Sick-Bird Syndrome

Organomegaly including hepatomegaly, renomegaly, splenomegaly, neoplasia

Metallic density in GI tract: heavy metal testing and treat if indicated

GI dilation, general ileus, GI mass: r/o bornavirus, neoplasia

Egg or reproductive disease – treat as indicated. *See* Algorithm 6: Egg Binding

↑ glucose with hyperglycemia; r/o diabetes mellitus

Endoscopy, biopsy, bacterial/fungal C/S if warranted; acid fast stains or chlamydial testing; GnRH agonist if reproductive disease suspected; if neoplasia consider additional treatment based on tumor type

**Abbreviations:** C/S, culture and sensitivity; CBC, complete blood count; EPH, electrophoresis; GI, gastrointestinal; GnRH, gonadotropic-releasing hormone; r/o, rule out; WBC, white blood cell.

# Algorithm 12: Feather Loss

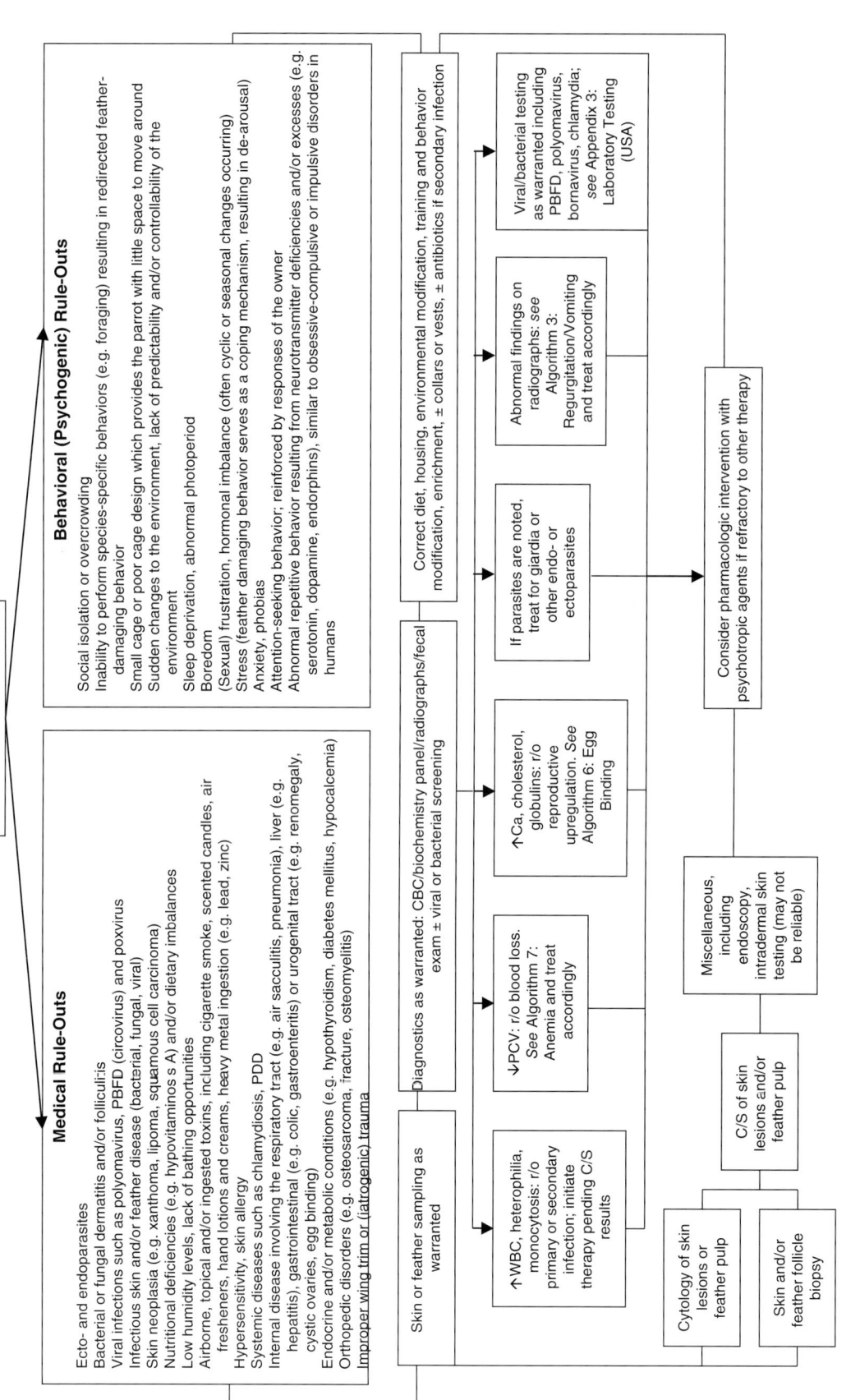

**Feather loss**

**Signalment/history/exam**

## Medical Rule-Outs

Ecto- and endoparasites
Bacterial or fungal dermatitis and/or folliculitis
Viral infections such as polyomavirus, PBFD (circovirus) and poxvirus
Infectious skin and/or feather disease (bacterial, fungal, viral)
Skin neoplasia (e.g. xanthoma, lipoma, squamous cell carcinoma)
Nutritional deficiencies (e.g. hypovitaminos s A) and/or dietary imbalances
Low humidity levels, lack of bathing opportunities
Airborne, topical and/or ingested toxins, including cigarette smoke, scented candles, air
  fresheners, hand lotions and creams, heavy metal ingestion (e.g. lead, zinc)
Hypersensitivity, skin allergy
Systemic diseases such as chlamydiosis, PDD
Internal disease involving the respiratory tract (e.g. air sacculitis, pneumonia), liver (e.g.
  hepatitis), gastrointestinal (e.g. colic, gastroenteritis) or urogenital tract (e.g. renomegaly,
  cystic ovaries, egg binding)
Endocrine and/or metabolic conditions (e.g. hypothyroidism, diabetes mellitus, hypocalcemia)
Orthopedic disorders (e.g. osteosarcoma, fracture, osteomyelitis)
Improper wing trim or (iatrogenic) trauma

## Behavioral (Psychogenic) Rule-Outs

Social isolation or overcrowding
Inability to perform species-specific behaviors (e.g. foraging) resulting in redirected feather-
  damaging behavior
Small cage or poor cage design which provides the parrot with little space to move around
Sudden changes to the environment, lack of predictability and/or controllability of the
  environment
Sleep deprivation, abnormal photoperiod
Boredom
(Sexual) frustration, hormonal imbalance (often cyclic or seasonal changes occurring)
Stress (feather damaging behavior serves as a coping mechanism, resulting in de-arousal)
Anxiety, phobias
Attention-seeking behavior; reinforced by responses of the owner
Abnormal repetitive behavior resulting from neurotransmitter deficiencies and/or excesses (e.g.
  serotonin, dopamine, endorphins), similar to obsessive-compulsive or impulsive disorders in
  humans

**Skin or feather sampling as warranted**

Cytology of skin lesions or feather pulp

C/S of skin lesions and/or feather pulp

Skin and/or feather follicle biopsy

Miscellaneous, including endoscopy, intradermal skin testing (may not be reliable)

**Diagnostics as warranted: CBC/biochemistry panel/radiographs/fecal exam ± viral or bacterial screening**

↓PCV: r/o blood loss. *See Algorithm 7: Anemia* and treat accordingly

↑WBC, heterophilia, monocytosis: r/o primary or secondary infection; initiate therapy pending C/S results

↑Ca, cholesterol, globulins: r/o reproductive upregulation. *See Algorithm 6: Egg Binding*

If parasites are noted, treat for giardia or other endo- or ectoparasites

Abnormal findings on radiographs: *see Algorithm 3: Regurgitation/Vomiting* and treat accordingly

Viral/bacterial testing as warranted including PBFD, polyomavirus, bornavirus, chlamydia; *see Appendix 3: Laboratory Testing* (USA)

**Correct diet, housing, environmental modification, training and behavior modification, enrichment, ± collars or vests, ± antibiotics if secondary infection**

**Consider pharmacologic intervention with psychotropic agents if refractory to other therapy**

**Abbreviations:** C/S, culture and sensitivity; CBC, complete blood count; PBFD, psittacine beak and feather disease; PCV, packed cell volume; r/o, rule out; WBC, white blood cell.

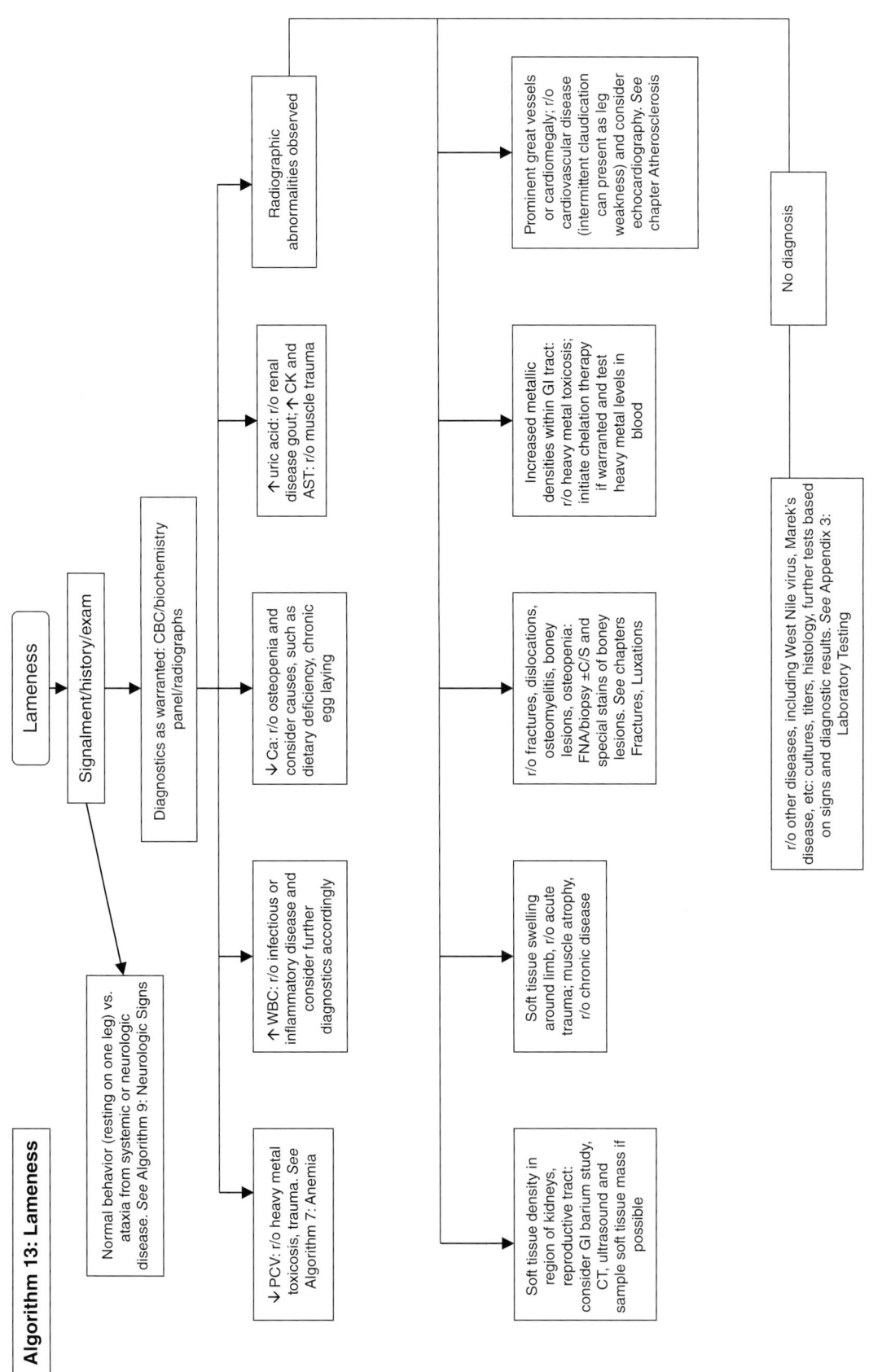

**Algorithm 13: Lameness**

Lameness

Signalment/history/exam

Normal behavior (resting on one leg) vs. ataxia from systemic or neurologic disease. See Algorithm 9: Neurologic Signs

Diagnostics as warranted: CBC/biochemistry panel/radiographs

↓PCV: r/o heavy metal toxicosis, trauma. See Algorithm 7: Anemia

↑WBC: r/o infectious or inflammatory disease and consider further diagnostics accordingly

↓Ca: r/o osteopenia and consider causes, such as dietary deficiency, chronic egg laying

↑uric acid: r/o renal disease gout; ↑CK and AST: r/o muscle trauma

Radiographic abnormalities observed

Soft tissue density in region of kidneys, reproductive tract: consider GI barium study, CT, ultrasound and sample soft tissue mass if possible

Soft tissue swelling around limb, r/o acute trauma; muscle atrophy, r/o chronic disease

r/o fractures, dislocations, osteomyelitis, boney lesions, osteopenia: FNA/biopsy ±C/S and special stains of boney lesions. *See* chapters Fractures, Luxations

Increased metallic densities within GI tract: r/o heavy metal toxicosis; initiate chelation therapy if warranted and test heavy metal levels in blood

Prominent great vessels or cardiomegaly: r/o cardiovascular disease (intermittent claudication can present as leg weakness) and consider echocardiography. See chapter Atherosclerosis

No diagnosis

r/o other diseases, including West Nile virus, Marek's disease, etc: cultures, titers, histology, further tests based on signs and diagnostic results. *See* Appendix 3: Laboratory Testing

**Abbreviations:** AST, aspartate aminotransferase; C/S, culture and sensitivity; CBC, complete blood count; CK, creatine kinase; CT, computed tomography; GI, gastrointestinal; FNA, fine-needle aspiration; PCV, packed cell volume; r/o, rule out; WBC, white blood cell.

**Algorithm 14: Hyperuricemia**

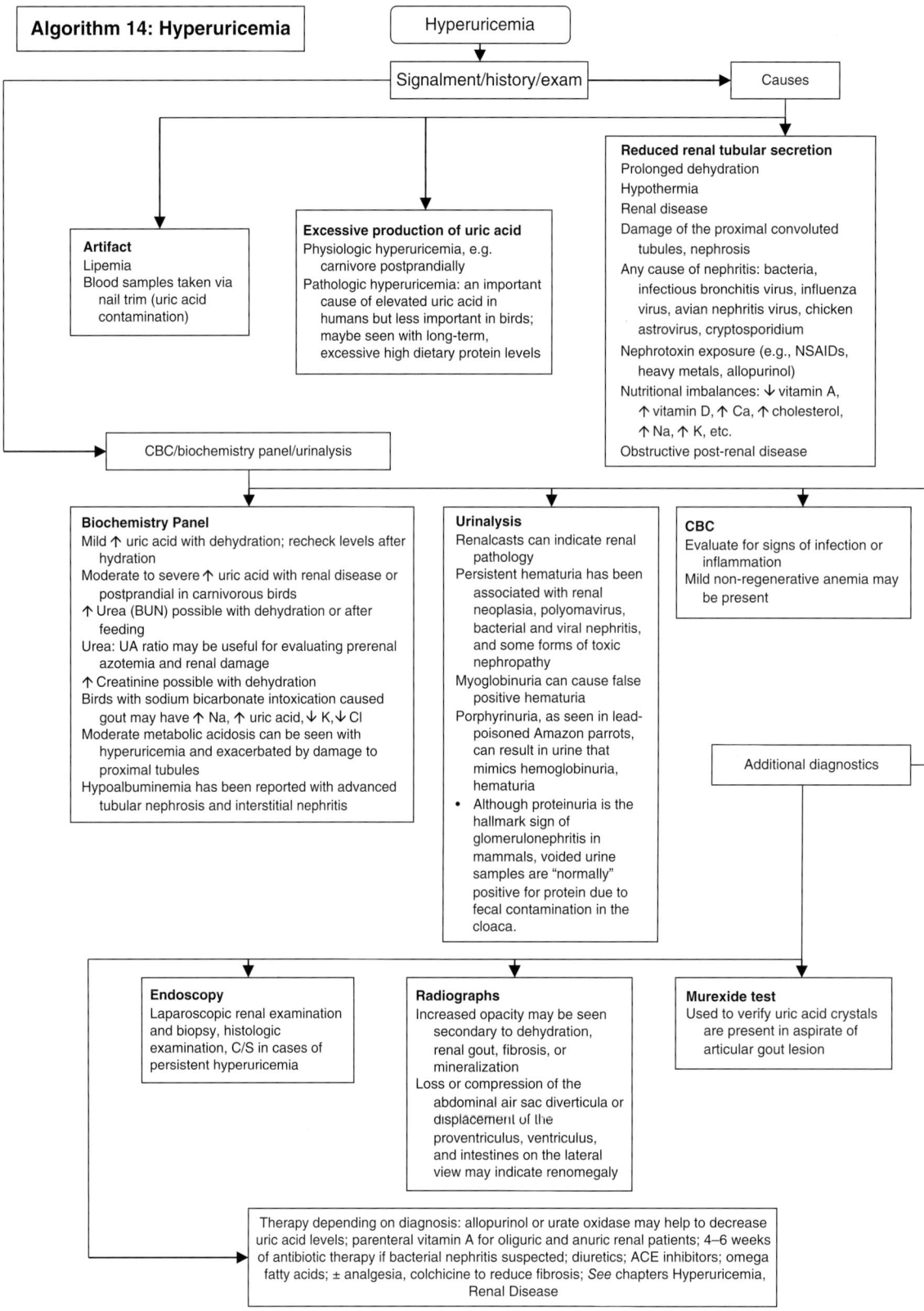

Hyperuricemia

Signalment/history/exam → Causes

**Reduced renal tubular secretion**
Prolonged dehydration
Hypothermia
Renal disease
Damage of the proximal convoluted tubules, nephrosis
Any cause of nephritis: bacteria, infectious bronchitis virus, influenza virus, avian nephritis virus, chicken astrovirus, cryptosporidium
Nephrotoxin exposure (e.g., NSAIDs, heavy metals, allopurinol)
Nutritional imbalances: ↓ vitamin A, ↑ vitamin D, ↑ Ca, ↑ cholesterol, ↑ Na, ↑ K, etc.
Obstructive post-renal disease

**Artifact**
Lipemia
Blood samples taken via nail trim (uric acid contamination)

**Excessive production of uric acid**
Physiologic hyperuricemia, e.g. carnivore postprandially
Pathologic hyperuricemia: an important cause of elevated uric acid in humans but less important in birds; maybe seen with long-term, excessive high dietary protein levels

CBC/biochemistry panel/urinalysis

**Biochemistry Panel**
Mild ↑ uric acid with dehydration; recheck levels after hydration
Moderate to severe ↑ uric acid with renal disease or postprandial in carnivorous birds
↑ Urea (BUN) possible with dehydration or after feeding
Urea: UA ratio may be useful for evaluating prerenal azotemia and renal damage
↑ Creatinine possible with dehydration
Birds with sodium bicarbonate intoxication caused gout may have ↑ Na, ↑ uric acid, ↓ K, ↓ Cl
Moderate metabolic acidosis can be seen with hyperuricemia and exacerbated by damage to proximal tubules
Hypoalbuminemia has been reported with advanced tubular nephrosis and interstitial nephritis

**Urinalysis**
Renal casts can indicate renal pathology
Persistent hematuria has been associated with renal neoplasia, polyomavirus, bacterial and viral nephritis, and some forms of toxic nephropathy
Myoglobinuria can cause false positive hematuria
Porphyrinuria, as seen in lead-poisoned Amazon parrots, can result in urine that mimics hemoglobinuria, hematuria
• Although proteinuria is the hallmark sign of glomerulonephritis in mammals, voided urine samples are "normally" positive for protein due to fecal contamination in the cloaca.

**CBC**
Evaluate for signs of infection or inflammation
Mild non-regenerative anemia may be present

Additional diagnostics

**Endoscopy**
Laparoscopic renal examination and biopsy, histologic examination, C/S in cases of persistent hyperuricemia

**Radiographs**
Increased opacity may be seen secondary to dehydration, renal gout, fibrosis, or mineralization
Loss or compression of the abdominal air sac diverticula or displacement of the proventriculus, ventriculus, and intestines on the lateral view may indicate renomegaly

**Murexide test**
Used to verify uric acid crystals are present in aspirate of articular gout lesion

Therapy depending on diagnosis: allopurinol or urate oxidase may help to decrease uric acid levels; parenteral vitamin A for oliguric and anuric renal patients; 4–6 weeks of antibiotic therapy if bacterial nephritis suspected; diuretics; ACE inhibitors; omega fatty acids; ± analgesia, colchicine to reduce fibrosis; *See* chapters Hyperuricemia, Renal Disease

**Abbreviations:** ACE, angiotensin-converting enzyme; BUN, blood, urea, nitrogen; C/S, culture and sensitivity; CBC, complete blood count; NSAIDs, non-steroidal anti-inflammatory drugs; UA, uric acid.

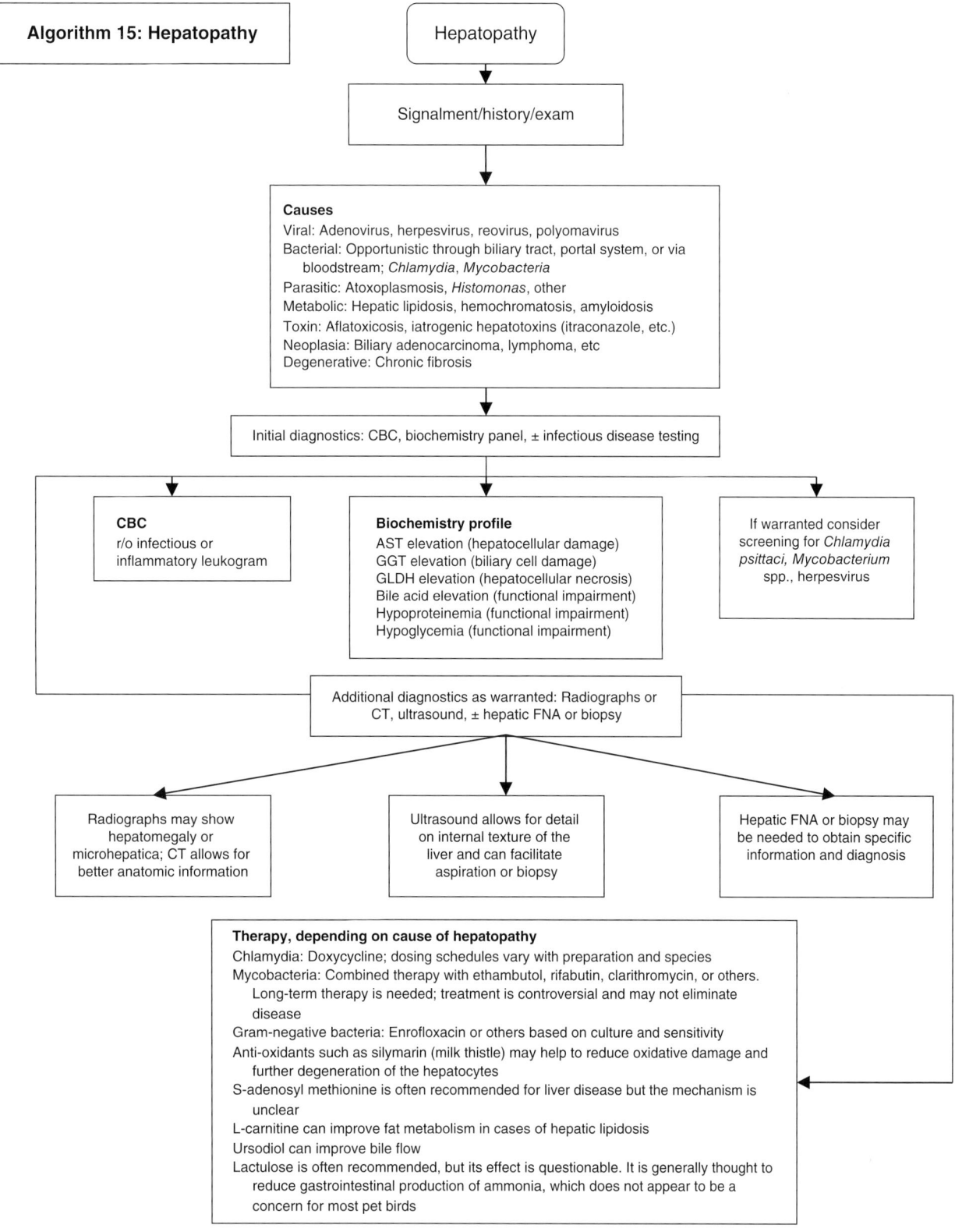

**Algorithm 15: Hepatopathy**

Hepatopathy

↓

Signalment/history/exam

↓

**Causes**
Viral: Adenovirus, herpesvirus, reovirus, polyomavirus
Bacterial: Opportunistic through biliary tract, portal system, or via bloodstream; *Chlamydia, Mycobacteria*
Parasitic: Atoxoplasmosis, *Histomonas*, other
Metabolic: Hepatic lipidosis, hemochromatosis, amyloidosis
Toxin: Aflatoxicosis, iatrogenic hepatotoxins (itraconazole, etc.)
Neoplasia: Biliary adenocarcinoma, lymphoma, etc
Degenerative: Chronic fibrosis

↓

Initial diagnostics: CBC, biochemistry panel, ± infectious disease testing

**CBC**
r/o infectious or inflammatory leukogram

**Biochemistry profile**
AST elevation (hepatocellular damage)
GGT elevation (biliary cell damage)
GLDH elevation (hepatocellular necrosis)
Bile acid elevation (functional impairment)
Hypoproteinemia (functional impairment)
Hypoglycemia (functional impairment)

If warranted consider screening for *Chlamydia psittaci, Mycobacterium* spp., herpesvirus

↓

Additional diagnostics as warranted: Radiographs or CT, ultrasound, ± hepatic FNA or biopsy

Radiographs may show hepatomegaly or microhepatica; CT allows for better anatomic information

Ultrasound allows for detail on internal texture of the liver and can facilitate aspiration or biopsy

Hepatic FNA or biopsy may be needed to obtain specific information and diagnosis

**Therapy, depending on cause of hepatopathy**
Chlamydia: Doxycycline; dosing schedules vary with preparation and species
Mycobacteria: Combined therapy with ethambutol, rifabutin, clarithromycin, or others. Long-term therapy is needed; treatment is controversial and may not eliminate disease
Gram-negative bacteria: Enrofloxacin or others based on culture and sensitivity
Anti-oxidants such as silymarin (milk thistle) may help to reduce oxidative damage and further degeneration of the hepatocytes
S-adenosyl methionine is often recommended for liver disease but the mechanism is unclear
L-carnitine can improve fat metabolism in cases of hepatic lipidosis
Ursodiol can improve bile flow
Lactulose is often recommended, but its effect is questionable. It is generally thought to reduce gastrointestinal production of ammonia, which does not appear to be a concern for most pet birds

**Abbreviations:** AST, aspartate aminotransferase; CBC, complete blood count; CT, computed tomography; FNA, fine-needle aspiration; GGT, gamma-glutamyl transferase; GLDH, glutamate dehydrogenase; r/o, rule out.

**Algorithm 16: Wing Droop**

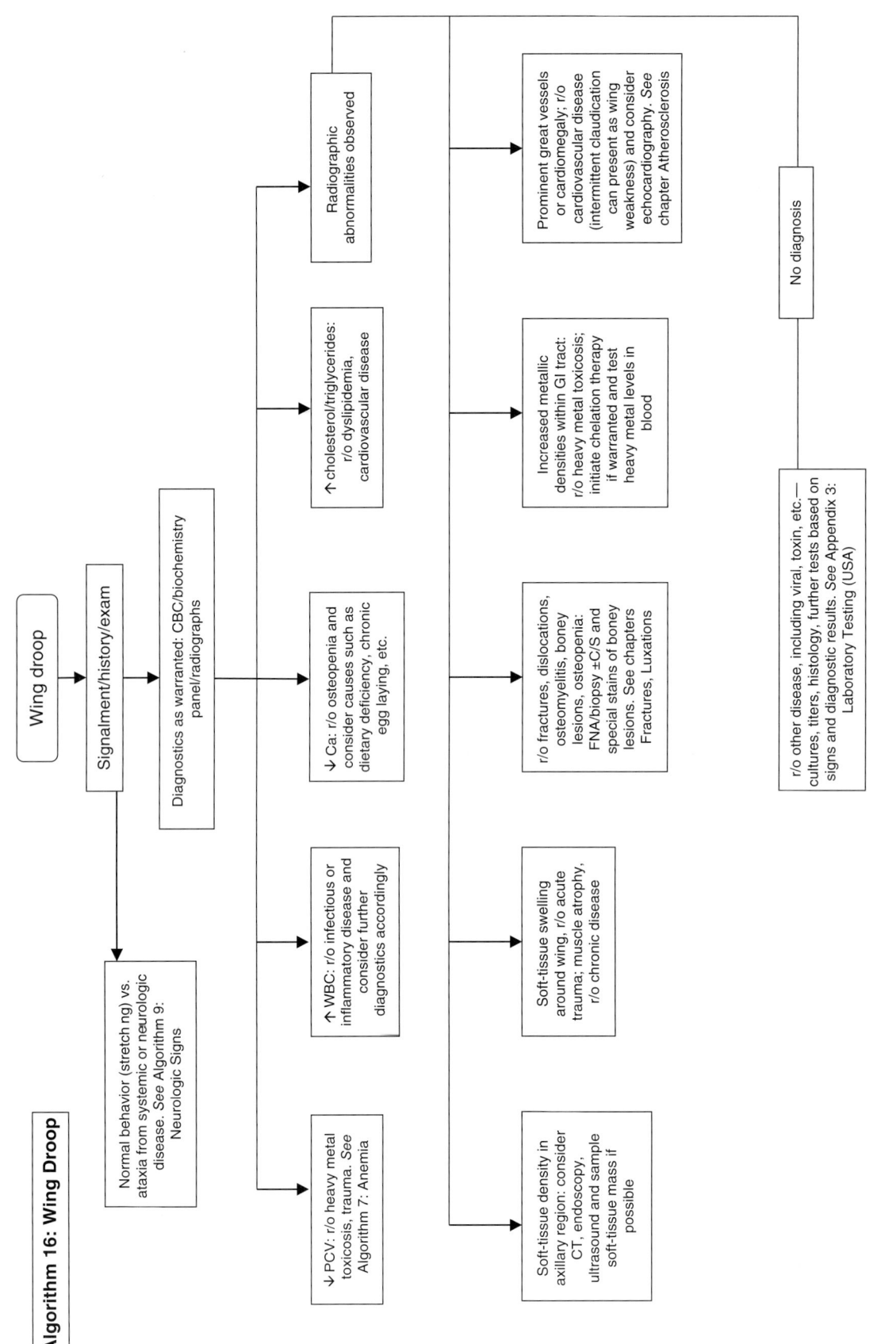

**Abbreviations:** C/S, culture and sensitivity; CBC, complete blood count; FNA, fine-needle aspiration; PCV, packed cell volume; r/o, rule out.

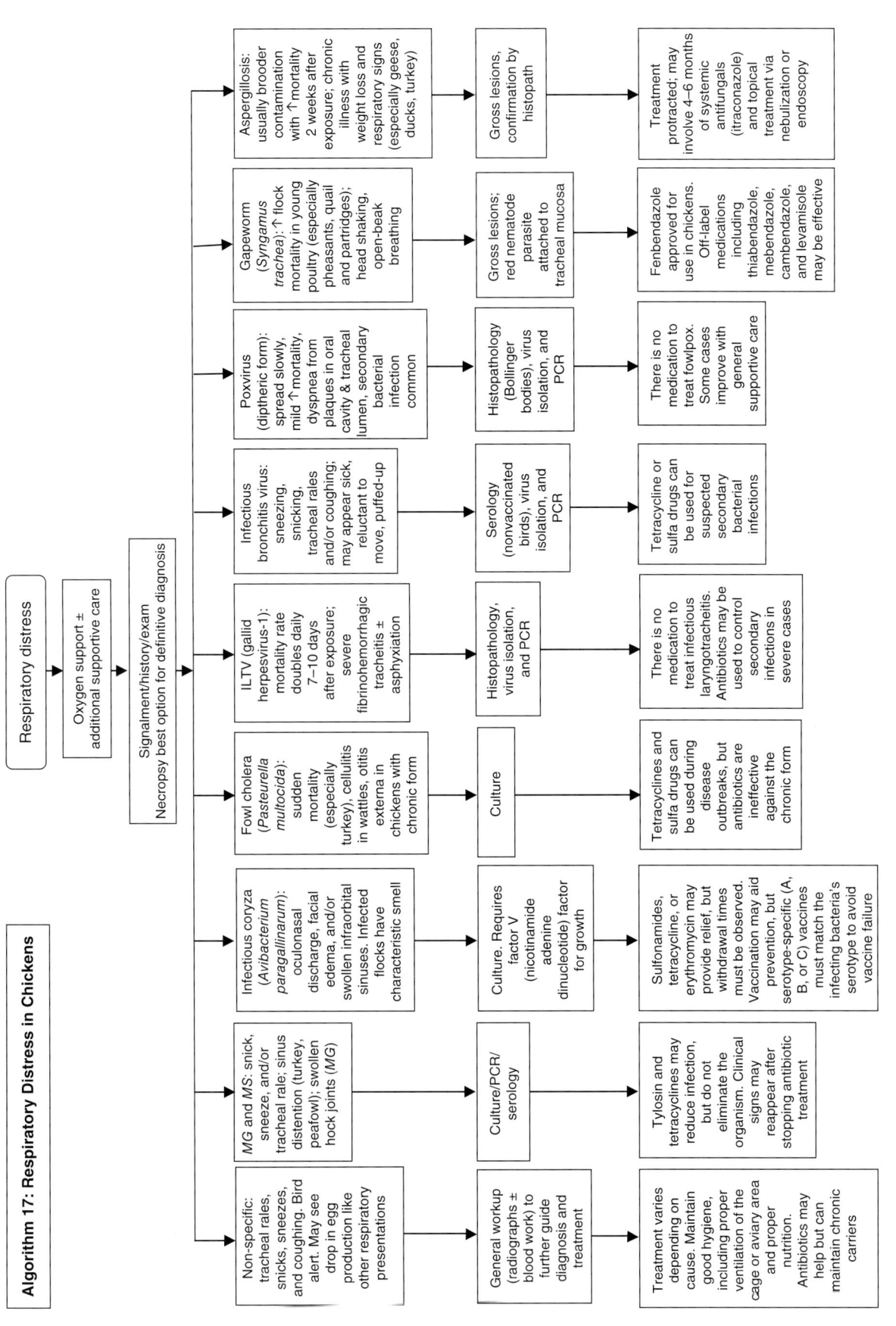

**Algorithm 17: Respiratory Distress in Chickens**

Respiratory distress

↓

Oxygen support ± additional supportive care

↓

Signalment/history/exam
Necropsy best option for definitive diagnosis

**Non-specific:** tracheal rales, snicks, sneezes, and coughing. Bird may see drop in egg production like other respiratory presentations

↓

General workup (radiographs ± blood work) to further guide diagnosis and treatment

↓

Treatment varies depending on cause. Maintain good hygiene, including proper ventilation of the cage or aviary area and proper nutrition. Antibiotics may help but can maintain chronic carriers

**MG and MS:** snick, sneeze, and/or tracheal rale; sinus distention (turkey, peafowl); swollen hock joints (MG)

↓

Culture/PCR/serology

↓

Tylosin and tetracyclines may reduce infection, but do not eliminate the organism. Clinical signs may reappear after stopping antibiotic treatment

**Infectious coryza (Avibacterium paragallinarum):** oculonasal discharge, facial edema, and/or swollen infraorbital sinuses. Infected flocks have characteristic smell

↓

Culture. Requires factor V (nicotinamide adenine dinucleotide) factor for growth

↓

Sulfonamides, tetracycline, or erythromycin may provide relief, but withdrawal times must be observed. Vaccination may aid prevention, but serotype-specific (A, B, or C) vaccines must match the infecting bacteria's serotype to avoid vaccine failure

**Fowl cholera (Pasteurella multocida):** sudden mortality (especially turkey), cellulitis in wattles, otitis externa in chickens with chronic form

↓

Culture

↓

Tetracyclines and sulfa drugs can be used during disease outbreaks, but antibiotics are ineffective against the chronic form

**ILTV (gallid herpesvirus-1):** mortality rate doubles daily 7–10 days after exposure; severe fibrinohemorrhagic tracheitis ± asphyxiation

↓

Histopathology, virus isolation, and PCR

↓

There is no medication to treat infectious laryngotracheitis. Antibiotics may be used to control secondary infections in severe cases

**Infectious bronchitis virus:** sneezing, snicking, tracheal rales and/or coughing; may appear sick, reluctant to move, puffed-up

↓

Serology (nonvaccinated birds), virus isolation, and PCR

↓

Tetracycline or sulfa drugs can be used for suspected secondary bacterial infections

**Poxvirus (diptheric form):** spread slowly, mild ↑mortality, dyspnea from plaques in oral cavity & tracheal lumen, secondary bacterial infection common

↓

Histopathology (Bollinger bodies), virus isolation, and PCR

↓

There is no medication to treat fowlpox. Some cases improve with general supportive care

**Gapeworm (Syngamus trachea):** ↑flock mortality in young poultry (especially pheasants, quail and partridges); head shaking, open-beak breathing

↓

Gross lesions; red nematode parasite attached to tracheal mucosa

↓

Fenbendazole approved for use in chickens. Off-label medications including thiabendazole, mebendazole, cambendazole, and levamisole may be effective

**Aspergillosis:** usually brooder contamination with ↑mortality 2 weeks after exposure; chronic illness with weight loss and respiratory signs (especially geese, ducks, turkey)

↓

Gross lesions, confirmation by histopath

↓

Treatment protracted; may involve 4–6 months of systemic antifungals (itraconazole) and topical treatment via nebulization or endoscopy

**Abbreviations:** MG, Mycoplasma gallisepticum; MS, Mycoplasma synoviae; PCR, polymerase chain reaction.

**Algorithm 18: Cloacal Prolapse**

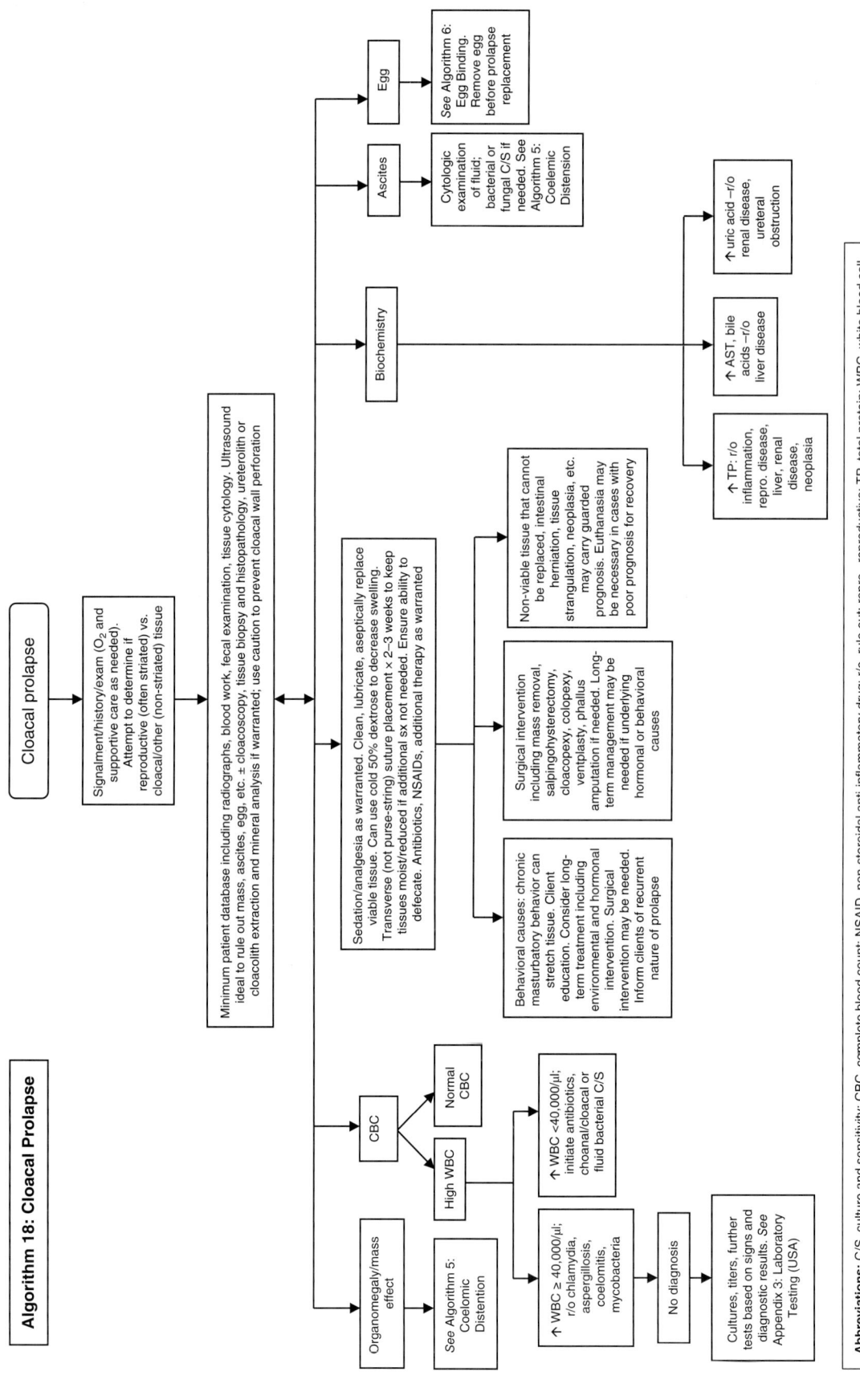

**Abbreviations:** C/S, culture and sensitivity; CBC, complete blood count; NSAID, non-steroidal anti-inflammatory drug; r/o, rule out; repro., reproductive; TP, total protein; WBC, white blood cell.

# INDEX

Page locators in **bold** indicate main articles.

## A

abdominal distension, 330
abdominal herniation, 330
activated charcoal, 450
activated clotting time, 99
acute tubular necrosis, 443
Addison's disease, 4–7
adenoviruses, **1–3**
adrenal gland diseases, **4–7**
adrenal neoplasia, 4–7
adrenocorticotropic hormone (ACTH), 4
*Aetokthonos hydrillicola*, 43
aflatoxicosis
    liver disease, 250
    mycotoxicosis, 274–275
    thymus diseases, 422
aggression, **374–377**
air aspiration, 10–11
airborne toxicosis, **434–435**
air sacculitis, 31, 33
air sac mites, **8–9**
air sac rupture, **10–12**
algal biotoxins, **13–14**
alopecia, 172
Amazon foot necrosis, 426–427
Amazon tracheitis disease (ATD), 215–216
amphotericins, 31–32, 259
amputation
    hypothermia, 232
    myiasis, 277
    phallus prolapse, 352
    salvage wing amputation, 64–65
    toe and nail diseases, 429
    uropygial gland disease, 474
    xanthoma/xanthogranulomatosis, 485
amyloidosis, **15–16**
    pancreatic diseases, 340
    pododermatitis, 360
    renal diseases, 381
anabolic steroids, 203–204
analgesia *see* pain management
anemia, **17–19**
    clinical algorithm, 529
    emaciation, 162
    enteritis and gastritis, 167
    gastrointestinal foreign bodies, 180
    heavy metal toxicosis, 443
    hemoparasites, 197
    hemorrhage, 199, 201
    histomoniasis, 218
    lymphoproliferative neoplasia, 286

    pneumonia, 355
    polyostotic hyperostosis, 367
    retroviruses in Galliformes, 393
    rodenticide toxicosis, 436–437
    sepsis, 408
    thyroid diseases, 424
    urate and fecal discoloration, 471
anemia–dermatis syndrome, 87–88
anesthesia
    hypothermia, 231
    ingested toxicosis, 450
    pain, 338
    seizures, 406
aneurysm, 199
angel wing, **20–21**
angular limb deformity, **22–23**
    angel wing, 21
anorexia, **24–26**
    cryptosporidiosis, 122–123
    duck enteritis virus, 210–211
    Eastern and Western equine encephalitis
        virus, 145–146
    egg yolk coelomitis, 159
    emaciation, 162
    enteritis and gastritis, 165
    gastrointestinal helminthiasis, 190
    hepatic lipidosis, 203
    myocardial diseases, 279
    oral plaques, 320
    ovarian diseases, 332
    oviductal diseases, 334
    renal diseases, 380
    respiratory helminthiasis, 193
    undigested food in droppings, 468
    urate and fecal discoloration, 471
    usutu virus, 476
    vitamin D toxicosis, 452
antecedent–behavior–consequence (ABC),
    374–376
anticoagulant rodenticide toxicosis, **436–438**
    coagulopathies and coagulation,
        98, 100
    hemorrhage, 200
anticonvulsants, 303–304, 306, 406–407
antidiuretic hormone response
    test, 130
anti-inflammatories
    angel wing, 21
    ascites, 28
    cutaneous papillomatosis, 344
    Eastern and Western equine encephalitis
        virus, 146

    joint diseases, 241–242
    lung diseases, 254
    patagium diseases, 347
    renal diseases, 382
    toxoplasmosis, 455
    West Nile virus, 479
antimicrobials
    algal biotoxins, 14
    ascites, 28
    aspergillosis, 31–32
    aspiration pneumonia, 34
    avian influenza, 41
    beak injuries, 46
    body cavity and cardiovascular
        helminthiasis, 189
    bordetellosis, 54
    bornaviral disease, 59–60
    botulism, 63
    bursa of Fabricius diseases, 68
    campylobacteriosis, 70
    candidiasis, 73
    cere and skin color changes, 78
    chlamydiosis, 80
    cloacal diseases, 90–91
    cloacal prolapse, 93
    clostridiosis, 96
    coccidiosis, 102
    coelomic distension, 108
    colibacillosis, 112–113
    columbid herpesvirus 1, 208
    coxiellosis, 117
    cryptosporidiosis, 123
    cutaneous papillomatosis, 344
    dermatitis, 128–129
    diarrhea, 135
    discospondylitis, 138
    duck enteritis virus, 211
    Eastern and Western equine encephalitis
        virus, 146
    egg abnormalities, 156
    egg yolk coelomitis, 159
    enteritis and gastritis, 167
    flagellate enteritis, 178
    fractures, 184
    gastrointestinal helminthiasis, 191
    heat stroke, 186–187
    heavy metal toxicosis, 444
    hemoparasites, 198
    histomoniasis, 218
    hypotension and hypovolemia, 229
    infertility, 237
    integumental neoplasia, 285

antimicrobials (*Continued*)
  joint diseases, 241
  liver disease, 251
  lung diseases, 254
  luxations, 257
  *Macrorhabdus ornithogaster*,
    259–260
  microsporidiosis, 267
  mites, 149
  mycobacteriosis, 269
  mycoplasmosis, 272–273
  mycotoxicosis, 275
  myiasis, 277–278
  neural larva migrans, 300
  ocular lesions, 314
  oil exposure, 317–318
  orthoavulaviruses, 325
  otitis, 328
  oviductal diseases, 335
  pancreatic diseases, 341–342
  passerid herpesvirus-1, 213
  pasteurellosis, 346
  patagium diseases, 347
  pneumonia, 355–356
  pododermatitis, 360
  polyuria, 370
  regurgitation and vomiting, 379
  renal diseases, 382
  respiratory distress, 387–388
  respiratory helminthiasis, 194
  respiratory infections of backyard
    chickens, 391
  rhinusitis and sinusitis, 396–397
  salmonellosis, 400
  sarcocystosis, 403–404
  sepsis, 409
  spirochete infection, 414
  spleen diseases, 416
  tendinitis and tenosynovitis, 419–420
  ticks, lice, dipterans, 152
  toe and nail diseases, 429
  tongue diseases, 433
  tracheal and syringeal diseases, 458–459
  trichomoniasis, 466
  urate and fecal discoloration, 472
  uropygial gland disease, 475
  West Nile virus, 479
  wound management, 483
  yersiniosis, 486
  yolk sac retention/infection, 488
antiotensin-converting enzyme (ACE)
    inhibitors, 281
antioxidants
  liver disease, 251
  thymus diseases, 423
antiseptic medications, 482–483
antithrombotic medications, 39
antitoxins, 63
antivirals
  avian influenza, 41
  orthoavulaviruses, 325
applied behavior analysis (ABA), 374–376
arrhenoblastomas, 332

arthritis, 245
arthrocentesis, 256
articular gout, 426, 430
ascites, **27–29**
  coelomic distension, 107
  egg yolk coelomitis, 158
  iron storage disease, 239
  ovarian diseases, 330, 332
  renal diseases, 380
aspergillosis, **30–32**
  amyloidosis, 15
  respiratory infections of backyard
    chickens, 389–390
  tracheal and syringeal diseases,
    457–459
aspiration pneumonia, **33–35**, 379
aspiration rhinitis, 379
*Atadenovirus* spp., 1
ataxia
  algal biotoxins, 13
  avian vacuolar myelinopathy, 43
ataxic myoglobinuric syndrome, 74
atherosclerosis, **36–39**
  airborne toxicosis, 434–435
  algal biotoxins, 13
  congestive heart failure, 114–115
  dyslipidemia/hyperlipidemia, 140
  lameness, 245
  obesity, 312
  toe and nail diseases, 426, 430
atoxoplasmosis, 198
automutilation *see* self-injurious behavior
avascular necrosis, 426, 428
avermectins, 9, 445–447
*Aviadenovirus* spp., 1
avian avulaviruses (AAvV), 323–326
avian bornavirus (ABV)
  aquatic birds, **56–57**
  enteritis and gastritis, 165
  psittacines, **58–61**
  regurgitation and vomiting, 378–379
avian circovirus
  bursa of Fabricius diseases, 66–69
  feather disorders, 174–175
  non-psittacine birds, **87–88**
  psittacines, **85–86**
  thymus diseases, 422
avian influenza, **40–42**
avian intestinal spirochetosis (AIS),
    413–414
avian leukosis and reticoendotheliosis virus,
    422
avian leukosis virus (ALV), 330–332
avian polyomavirus (APV), **365–366**
  ascites, 28
  feather disorders, 174–175
  myocardial diseases, 280
  pneumonia, 355
avian reovirus (AVR), **384–385**
  bursa of Fabricius diseases, 66–69
avian vacuolar myelinopathy (AVM), **43–44**
avioserpensosis, 188–189
azoles, 73

**B**

*Baylisascaris* spp., 300–301
B cell lymphoma, 288
beak injuries, **45–47**, 462
beak malocclusion
  lateral beak deformity, **48–50**
  mandibular prognathism, **51–52**
behavioral changes
  aggression, biting, and screaming,
    **374–377**
  air sac mites, 8
  anemia, 17
  aspergillosis, 30
  avian vacuolar myelinopathy, 43
  beak injuries, 45
  body cavity and cardiovascular
    helminthiasis, 188–189
  bornaviral disease, 58
  columbid herpesvirus 1, 208
  enteritis and gastritis, 165
  feather cyst, 168
  gastrointestinal helminthiasis, 190
  heavy metal toxicosis, 443–444
  hemoparasites, 196
  ingested toxicosis, 449
  myocardial diseases, 279
  neural larva migrans, 300
  neurologic disorders, 302, 305
  oil exposure, 316
  oral plaques, 320
  pain, 337
  polydipsia, 362
  regurgitation and vomiting, 378
  renal diseases, 380
  respiratory helminthiasis, 193
  rodenticide toxicosis, 436
  sick-bird syndrome, 411–412
  trauma, 461
  usutu virus, 476
  *see also* self-injurious behavior
benzimidazoles, 445–447
benzodiazepines, 25
beta blockers, 281
biliary adenocarcinoma, 250
biosecurity
  air sac mites, 9
  bursa of Fabricius diseases, 68
  chlamydiosis, 80
  colibacillosis, 113
  diarrhea, 135
  duck enteritis virus, 211
  oral plaques, 321
  orthoavulaviruses, 325
  passerid herpesvirus-1, 214
  polyomavirus, 365
  respiratory infections of backyard
    chickens, 391
  retroviruses in Galliformes, 394
  salmonellosis, 400–401
  thymus diseases, 423
  toe and nail diseases, 429
  tongue diseases, 433

tracheal and syringeal diseases, 459
trichomoniasis, 465–466
West Nile virus, 480
bird flu *see* avian influenza
biting, **374–377**
black spot disease, 87–88
bleeding *see* hemorrhage
blood transfusion
  hemorrhage, 201
  hypotension and hypovolemia, 229
  ingested toxicosis, 450
body cavity helminthiasis, **188–189**
body wall herniation, 107
bone deformity, 263–264
bordetellosis, **53–55**
bornaviral disease
  aquatic birds, **56–57**
  enteritis and gastritis, 165
  psittacines, **58–61**
  regurgitation and vomiting, 378–379
*Borrelia anserina*, 413–414
botulism, **62–63**
brachial plexus injury, **64–65**
*Brachyspira* spp., 413–414
brevetoxins, 13–14
bronchodilators
  aspiration pneumonia, 34
  ingested toxicosis, 450
  lung diseases, 254
  respiratory distress, 387
brown hypertrophy of the cere, 77–78
bulking agents, 34
bumblefoot *see* pododermatitis
bursa of Fabricius diseases, **66–69**
bursectomy, 68
bursitis, 462

**C**

calcium deficiency *see* hypocalcemia
campylobacteriosis, **70–71**
canary circovirus (CaCV), 87–88
candidiasis, **72–73**
  enteritis and gastritis, 165
  oral plaques, 320–322
  tongue diseases, 432
  undigested food in droppings, 469
candling, 154–155
cannabinoids, 445–447
cannibalism, 461, 463
capnometry, 458
capture myopathy (CM), **74–76**
capture shock syndrome, 74
carbamate toxicosis, 439–441
carcinomatosis
  ascites, 28
  ovarian diseases, 332
cardiac neoplasms, 280
cardiomegaly
  ascites, 28
  coelomic distension, 108
cardiovascular disease
  duck enteritis virus, 210

myocardial diseases, **279–281**
cardiovascular helminthiasis,
    **188–189**
cataracts, 313–314
cathartics, 450
celioscopy, 355
central diabetes insipidus, 130–131
central nervous system (CNS), 58–60
cerebral edema, 303
cerebrospinal fluid analysis, 406
cere color changes, **77–78**
cervicocephalic diverticula, 10
cervicocephalic–clavicular air sac
    shunt, 11
chelation therapy
  aspiration pneumonia, 34
  heavy metal toxicosis, 444
  renal diseases, 382
  undigested food in droppings, 470
chemotherapy
  gastrointestinal and hepatic neoplasia, 283
  integumental neoplasia, 285
  lymphoproliferative neoplasia, 287–288
  ovarian diseases, 333
  renal neoplasia, 293
  respiratory neoplasia, 298–299
  tongue diseases, 433
  uropygial gland disease, 474–475
chlamydiosis, **79–81**
  enteritis and gastritis, 165
  neurologic disorders, 303
  spleen diseases, 415–416
  tracheal and syringeal diseases, 457–459
choanal swab, 396
choroid plexus tumors, 290–291
chronic egg laying, **82–84**
chronic hepatitis, 15
chronic lymphocytic leukemia, 288
chronic obstructive pulmonary disease
    (COPD), 253–255
  airborne toxicosis, 434–435
chronic pulmonary interstitial fibrosis
    (CPIF), 253–255
circovirus
  bursa of Fabricius diseases, 66–69
  feather disorders, 174–175
  non-psittacine birds, **87–88**
  psittacines, **85–86**
  thymus diseases, 422
citrinin, 274–275
cloacal atony, 89–91
cloacal bursa *see* bursa of Fabricius diseases
cloacal diseases, **89–91**
  clostridiosis, 95
cloacal neoplasia, 89–91
cloacal obstruction, 89–91
cloacal prolapse, **92–94**
  clinical algorithm, 540
cloacitis, 89–91
cloacopexy, 93
cloacoscopy, 472
clomipramine, 172
clostridiosis, **95–97**

*Clostridium botulinum*, 62–63
coagulation factor deficiency, 98
coagulation therapy, 436–437
coagulopathies and coagulation, **98–100**
coccidiosis
  enteritis and gastritis, 165
  intestinal, **101–103**
  systemic, **104–106**
cochlosomiasis, 177–178
coelomic distension, **107–110**
  ascites, 27
  clinical algorithm, 527
  dystocia and egg binding, 142
  pancreatic diseases, 340
  polyostotic hyperostosis, 367
coelomic hernias, 206–207
colchicine, 16, 29
colibacillosis, **111–113**
colisepticemia, 112
colonic prolapse, 92
colopexy, 93
columbid herpesvirus 1, **208–209**
computed tomography (CT)
  air sac rupture, 10
  anorexia, 24
  aspergillosis, 31
  atherosclerosis, 37
  beak injuries, 45
  brachial plexus injury, 64
  cloacal diseases, 90
  discospondylitis, 137
  egg yolk coelomitis, 158
  enteritis and gastritis, 166
  feather-damaging, 171
  fractures, 183
  functional gastrointestinal ileus, 234
  gastrointestinal and hepatic neoplasia, 282
  gastrointestinal foreign bodies, 180
  hepatic lipidosis, 203
  hernia/pseudohernia, 206
  hypocalcemia and hypomagnesemia, 226
  integumental neoplasia, 284
  iron storage disease, 239
  joint diseases, 241
  liver disease, 251
  lung diseases, 253
  lymphoproliferative neoplasia, 287
  neural larva migrans, 300
  neurologic disorders, 303, 305
  neurologic neoplasia, 291
  ocular lesions, 314
  oral plaques, 321
  ovarian diseases, 331
  oviductal diseases, 334–336
  pancreatic diseases, 341
  perosis/slipped tendon, 349
  pneumonia, 355
  pododermatitis, 359
  regurgitation and vomiting, 378
  renal diseases, 382
  renal neoplasia, 293
  reproductive neoplasia, 296
  respiratory distress, 386

computed tomography (*Continued*)
  rhinusitis and sinusitis, 396
  seizures, 406
  toe and nail diseases, 427
  toxoplasmosis, 454
  tracheal and syringeal diseases, 458
  trauma, 461
  undigested food in droppings, 469
  xanthoma/xanthogranulomatosis, 484
congestive heart failure (CHF), **114–115**
  ascites, 28–29
  myocardial diseases, 279–280
conjunctivitis, 313–314
  passerid herpesvirus-1, 213
  toxoplasmosis, 454
constricted toe syndrome, 426, 428
conure bleeding syndrome, 98
corticosteroids
  neurologic disorders, 306
  ocular lesions, 315
  tracheal and syringeal diseases, 459
  trauma, 463
  West Nile virus, 479
  xanthoma/xanthogranulomatosis, 485
coryza, 54
coxiellosis, **116–117**
cranial nerve (CN) examination, 302, 305,
  327
creatinine, 381
crop burn, **118–119**
  cere and skin color changes, 77–78
crop lavage, 449–450
crop stasis, **233–235**
crossmatching, 201
cryptococcosis, **120–121**
cryptosporidiosis, **122–124**
  undigested food in droppings, 468–470
Cushing syndrome, 4–7
cutaneous papillomatosis, **343–344**
cutaneous pox, 371–373
cutaneous xanthoma, 484–485
cyanotoxins, 13–14
cyclosporines, 59–60
cystic ovarian disease, 330–333
cystic pancreas, 340

D

dantrolene sodium, 75–76
degenerative disease
  egg abnormalities, 154, 157
  functional gastrointestinal ileus, 233
  liver disease, 250
  myocardial diseases, 280
  pododermatitis, 360
  renal diseases, 380
dehydration, **125–126**
  duck enteritis virus, 210–211
  egg yolk coelomitis, 159
  enteritis and gastritis, 165, 167
  flagellate enteritis, 177
  hyperuricemia, 222
  polyuria, 369–370
  regurgitation and vomiting, 379

renal diseases, 380
  retroviruses in Galliformes, 393
  salmonellosis, 400
delayed peracute syndrome, 74
dermal stents, 10–11
dermatitis, **127–129**
  hemorrhage, 199
  mites, 148–149
  ticks, lice, dipterans, 151–152
diabetes insipidus (DI), **130–131**
  polyuria, 370
diabetes mellitus (DM), **132–133**
  dyslipidemia/hyperlipidemia, 139
  iron storage disease, 239
  pancreatic diseases, 341
diarrhea, **134–135**
  campylobacteriosis, 70
  clinical algorithm, 524
  coccidiosis, 104
  cryptococcosis, 120
  duck enteritis virus, 210–211
  enteritis and gastritis, 165
  flagellate enteritis, 177
  gastrointestinal helminthiasis, 190
  histomoniasis, 218
  phallus prolapse, 351
  polyuria, 369
  rotavirus, 398
  salmonellosis, 400
  undigested food in droppings, 468
dietary management
  adrenal gland diseases, 6
  aggression, biting, and screaming, 375
  air sac mites, 8
  angel wing, 20
  angular limb deformity, 22
  anorexia, 24–26
  aspiration pneumonia, 34
  atherosclerosis, 37–38
  beak injuries, 45–46
  bornaviral disease, 59–60
  bursa of Fabricius diseases, 68
  capture myopathy, 74–75
  chlamydiosis, 80
  clostridiosis, 95
  coagulopathies and coagulation, 99–100
  coccidiosis, 102
  coelomic distension, 108
  columbid herpesvirus 1, 208
  congestive heart failure, 115
  coxiellosis, 117
  crop burn, 119
  cryptosporidiosis, 123
  dehydration, 126
  dermatitis, 128
  diabetes insipidus, 131
  diabetes mellitus and hyperglycemia, 133
  diarrhea, 134–135
  duck enteritis virus, 211
  dyslipidemia/hyperlipidemia, 140
  dystocia and egg binding, 142–143
  Eastern and Western equine encephalitis
    virus, 146
  egg yolk coelomitis, 159

emaciation, 162–164
  enteritis and gastritis, 166
  feather-damaging, 172
  feather disorders, 175
  functional gastrointestinal ileus,
    233–234
  gastrointestinal foreign bodies, 181
  heat stroke, 186
  heavy metal toxicosis, 443–444
  hemorrhage, 199–200
  hepatic lipidosis, 203–204
  hernia/pseudohernia, 206–207
  hypocalcemia and hypomagnesemia,
    225–226
  hypotension and hypovolemia, 229
  hypothermia, 231–232
  iatrogenic toxicosis, 447
  infertility, 237
  ingested toxicosis, 450
  integumental neoplasia, 285
  iron storage disease, 239–240
  joint diseases, 241
  lameness, 244
  lateral beak deformity, 48
  liver disease, 251
  lung diseases, 254
  lymphoproliferative neoplasia, 287
  mandibular prognathism, 52
  metabolic bone disease, 264
  mycobacteriosis, 269
  mycotoxicosis, 274–276
  myiasis, 277
  myocardial diseases, 281
  neurologic disorders, 303, 306
  nutritional imbalances, **308–310**
  obesity, 311–312
  ocular lesions, 314
  oil exposure, 318
  ovarian diseases, 332
  oviductal diseases, 335–336
  pain, 337
  pancreatic diseases, 341
  patagium diseases, 347
  perosis/slipped tendon, 349–350
  pneumonia, 354–355
  pododermatitis, 359
  polydipsia, 363
  polyostotic hyperostosis, 367
  polyuria, 370
  regurgitation and vomiting, 379
  renal diseases, 382–383
  respiratory distress, 387
  rhinusitis and sinusitis, 396
  salmonellosis, 400
  sarcocystosis, 403
  sepsis, 409
  sick-bird syndrome, 412
  spirochete infection, 413
  spleen diseases, 415
  thymus diseases, 423
  thyroid diseases, 424–425
  toe and nail diseases, 428
  tongue diseases, 431–433
  toxoplasmosis, 455

trichomoniasis, 466
vitamin D toxicosis, 452–453
West Nile virus, 479
wound management, 482
xanthoma/xanthogranulomatosis, 484
digital egg monitors, 155
digital image capture, 155
dilated cardiomyopathy (DCM), 279–280
dimethyl sulfoxide (DMSO), 16
diphtheroid pox, 371–373
respiratory infections of backyard chickens, 389–391
dipterans, **151–153**
discospondylitis, **136–138**
disinfection
cryptosporidiosis, 123
mites, 149
oil exposure, 317–318
disseminated intravascular coagulation (DIC), 98–100
disseminated xanthogranulomatosis, 484–485
distributive shock, 228
diuretics
congestive heart failure, 115
diabetes insipidus, 131
lung diseases, 254
polyuria, 370
renal diseases, 382
vitamin D toxicosis, 452–453
dobutamine, 229
domoic acid (DA), 13–14
doxycycline, 80
duck circovirus (DuCV), 87–88
duck enteritis virus (DEV), **210–212**
bursa of Fabricius diseases, 66–69
thymus diseases, 422
ductus deferens, 295
dynamic viscoelastic coagulometry, 99
dyslipidemia/hyperlipidemia, **139–141**
atherosclerosis, 37–39
coelomic distension, 108
hepatic lipidosis, 203–204
neurologic disorders, 303
obesity, 311–312
pancreatic diseases, 340–341
dysphagia
duck enteritis virus, 211
oral plaques, 320
dyspnea
air sac mites, 8
ascites, 27
dystocia and egg binding, 142–143
egg yolk coelomitis, 158
hepatic lipidosis, 203
oral plaques, 320
ovarian diseases, 330
passerid herpesvirus-1, 213
psittacid herpesviruses, 215
reproductive neoplasia, 295–296
respiratory helminthiasis, 193–194
sarcocystosis, 402–403
toxoplasmosis, 454–455

tracheal and syringeal diseases, 457
trauma, 461–462
dystocia, **142–144**

## E

early embryonic death (EED), 155–156, 236–237
Eastern equine encephalitis virus (EEEV), **145–147**
echocardiography
congestive heart failure, 114
ingested toxicosis, 449
lung diseases, 253
toe and nail diseases, 427
ectoparasites
air sac mites, **8–9**
feather-damaging, 170–171
mites, **148–150**
ticks, lice, dipterans, **151–153**
toe and nail diseases, 426–427
tracheal and syringeal diseases, 457, 459
ectopic eggs, 144
edema
dermatitis, 127–128
reovirus, 384
egg abnormalities, **154–157**
infertility, 236
egg binding, **142–144**
clinical algorithm, 528
egg necropsy, 155
egg yolk coelomitis, **158–159**
*Eimeria* spp., 101–103
electrocardiography (ECG/EKG)
atherosclerosis, 38
congestive heart failure, 114–115
hypotension and hypovolemia, 228
myocardial diseases, 281
electrocautery, 200
electrocution, **160–161**
electroencephalography (EEG), 406
electromyography, 305
emaciation, **162–164**
flagellate enteritis, 177
histomoniasis, 218–219
*Macrorhabdus ornithogaster*, 259
pancreatic diseases, 340
passerid herpesvirus-1, 213
psittacid herpesviruses, 215
regurgitation and vomiting, 379
renal diseases, 380
retroviruses in Galliformes, 393
embryonal tumors, 290–291
embryonic death, 155–156, 236–237
encephalitis, 454
*Encephalitozoon* spp., **266–267**
endocarditis, 280
endocrine disorders
egg yolk coelomitis, 158
feather-damaging, 170
ovarian diseases, 330
endoparasites
egg abnormalities, 154

enteritis and gastritis, 165
feather-damaging, 170–171
functional gastrointestinal ileus, 233
pneumonia, 355
sarcocystosis, **402–404**
endoscope-assisted gastric lavage, 166, 378–379
endoscopy
airborne toxicosis, 434
air sac rupture, 10
aspergillosis, 31
aspiration pneumonia, 33
atherosclerosis, 38
bursa of Fabricius diseases, 68
cryptosporidiosis, 123
diarrhea, 134
dystocia and egg binding, 143
egg abnormalities, 155
feather-damaging, 172
functional gastrointestinal ileus, 234
gastrointestinal foreign bodies, 180
hepatic lipidosis, 203
infertility, 237
lung diseases, 253–254
otitis, 328
reproductive neoplasia, 296
respiratory distress, 386–387
respiratory helminthiasis, 194
rhinusitis and sinusitis, 396
sepsis, 409
spleen diseases, 415
thyroid diseases, 424
tracheal and syringeal diseases, 458
undigested food in droppings, 469
enteral nutrition, 25
enteritis and gastritis, **165–167**
duck enteritis virus, **210–212**
flagellate enteritis, **177–179**
rotavirus, 398
undigested food in droppings, 469
*Enterococcus* spp., discospondylitis, 137
environmental toxicosis, **439–442**
renal diseases, 381
enzyme-linked immunosorbent assay (ELISA)
bornaviral disease, 59
retroviruses in Galliformes, 393
tendinitis and tenosynovitis, 419
eosinophilia
leukocytosis, 247–248
seizures, 406
eosinophilic intranuclear inclusions, 211
epdidymis, 295
ependymoma, 291
epicarditis, 280
ergotism, 274–275
erosions, 127–128
erythema, 127
erythrocytes
anemia, 17–18
coagulopathies and coagulation, 99
*Escherichia coli*, 111–113
*Eustrongylides* spp., 188–189

euthanasia
  feather disorders, 175
  mycobacteriosis, 269
  neurologic neoplasia, 291
  pododermatitis, 360
  respiratory neoplasia, 298
exertional rhabdomyolysis, **74–76**
exocrine pancreatic insufficiency (EPI),
  340–341
external skeletal fixator intermedullary
  (ESF-IM), 184
extrahepatic biliary obstruction, 341
eyelids, 77

F

fatty liver syndrome *see* hepatic lipidosis
feather cyst, **168–169**
feather disorders, **174–176**
  circovirus, 85
  retroviruses in Galliformes, 393
feather duster disease, 174–175
feather loss/damage
  clinical algorithm, 534
  self-injurious behavior, **170–173**
  trauma, 461–462
  uropygial gland disease, 474
fecal contamination, 111
fecal discoloration, **471–473**
fecal matting, 165
fibrates
  atherosclerosis, 38–39
  dyslipidemia/hyperlipidemia, 140
fibrinogen, 99
filarioidiasis, 188–189
finch circovirus (FiCV), 87–88
fine needle aspiration (FNA)
  discospondylitis, 137
  hepatic lipidosis, 203–204
  renal neoplasia, 293
  respiratory neoplasia, 298
  sepsis, 409
flagellate enteritis, **177–179**
  undigested food in droppings, 469
fluid therapy
  aspiration pneumonia, 34
  beak injuries, 45
  capture myopathy, 75
  coccidiosis, 105
  colibacillosis, 112
  columbid herpesvirus 1, 208
  crop burn, 118–119
  dehydration, 125–126
  diabetes mellitus and hyperglycemia,
    132–133
  diarrhea, 134–135
  duck enteritis virus, 211
  dystocia and egg binding, 143
  egg yolk coelomitis, 159
  emaciation, 162–164
  enteritis and gastritis, 166
  feather cyst, 168–169
  fractures, 183
  functional gastrointestinal ileus, 234

gastrointestinal foreign bodies, 181
gastrointestinal helminthiasis, 191
heat stroke, 186
heavy metal toxicosis, 443–444
hemorrhage, 200–201
hepatic lipidosis, 204
hyperuricemia, 223
hypotension and hypovolemia, 229
hypothermia, 231
iatrogenic toxicosis, 447
ingested toxicosis, 450
lameness, 244
liver disease, 251
luxations, 256
lymphoproliferative neoplasia, 287
*Macrorhabdus ornithogaster*, 259–260
mycoplasmosis, 272
mycotoxicosis, 275
neurologic disorders, 303, 306
nutritional imbalances, 309
ocular lesions, 314
oil exposure, 317–318
oral plaques, 321
oviductal diseases, 335
pancreatic diseases, 341
pasteurellosis, 346
pesticide toxicosis, 440
polydipsia, 363
polyuria, 370
poxvirus, 372
regurgitation and vomiting, 379
renal diseases, 382
reovirus, 384
respiratory distress, 387
respiratory helminthiasis, 194
rodenticide toxicosis, 437
rotavirus, 398
salmonellosis, 400
sarcocystosis, 403–404
spirochete infection, 413
thyroid diseases, 424
toe and nail diseases, 428
tongue diseases, 432
toxoplasmosis, 455
trauma, 462–463
trichomoniasis, 466
West Nile virus, 479
wound management, 482
fluoroscopy
  anorexia, 24
  bornaviral disease, 59
  cloacal diseases, 90
foreign bodies
  gastrointestinal, **180–182**
  ocular lesions, 314
  pneumonia, 355
  respiratory distress, 387
  sick-bird syndrome, 412
  tracheal and syringeal diseases, 458
  undigested food in droppings,
    468, 470
fowl cholera, 389–391
fractures, **183–185**
  electrocution, 160

hypocalcemia and hypomagnesemia,
  225–227
lameness, 245
metabolic bone disease, 264
myiasis, 277
neurologic disorders, 305
toe and nail diseases, 428–429
trauma, 461–463
free thoracic vertebrae (FTV), 136–137
frostbite
  hypothermia, 232
  toe and nail diseases, 428
fructosamines, 132
functional gastrointestinal ileus, **233–235**
fusarotoxins, 274–275

G

gabapentin, 445–447
gape worm, 389–391
gastrointestinal bleeding, 167
gastrointestinal disease
  cryptosporidiosis, 122–123
  myocardial diseases, 279
  oil exposure, 316
  regurgitation and vomiting, 378–379
  undigested food in droppings, 468–470
  *see also* enteritis and gastritis
gastrointestinal foreign bodies, **180–182**
gastrointestinal helminthiasis, **190–192**
gastrointestinal neoplasia, **282–283**
gastrointestinal toxicosis, **448–451**
germ cell tumors, 290–291
giardiasis
  enteritis and gastritis, 165
  flagellate enteritis, 177–178
glaucoma, 315
glioma, 290–291
glomerulonephritis, 381
glucagon, 163–164
glucocorticoids
  adrenal gland diseases, 6–7
  iatrogenic toxicosis, 445–447
glucosuria, 362
gonadotropin-releasing hormone (GnRH)
  agonists
  aggression, biting, and screaming, 376
  atherosclerosis, 39
  chronic egg laying, 83
  cloacal diseases, 91
  cloacal prolapse, 94
  coelomic distension, 108–109
  dystocia and egg binding, 144
  egg yolk coelomitis, 159
  feather-damaging, 172
  hernia/pseudohernia, 207
  ovarian diseases, 332–333
  oviductal diseases, 335
  polyostotic hyperostosis, 367
  reproductive neoplasia, 296
goose circovirus (GoCV), 87–88
gradual water deprivation test, 363
granulomatous disease
  coccidiosis, 105

colibacillosis, 112
cryptococcosis, 120
granulosa cell tumors, 332

## H

*Haemoproteus* spp., 196–198
halitosis, 320
harmful algal blooms (HAB), 13–14
head trauma, 462
heat stroke, **186–187**
heavy metal toxicosis, **443–444**
    anemia, 17–18
    anorexia, 24
    aspiration pneumonia, 34
    diabetes insipidus, 130
    emaciation, 162
    enteritis and gastritis, 165
    feather-damaging, 171
    feather disorders, 174
    gastrointestinal foreign bodies, 180–181
    hemorrhage, 200–201
    hypocalcemia and hypomagnesemia,
        225–226
    lameness, 245
    myocardial diseases, 280
    neurologic disorders, 302
    pancreatic diseases, 341
    pneumonia, 355
    renal diseases, 381
    seizures, 407
    undigested food in droppings, 469
    urate and fecal discoloration, 471–473
helminthiasis
    body cavity and cardiovascular, **188–189**
    gastrointestinal, **190–192**
    respiratory, **193–195**
hematochezia, 165
hematuria
    coagulopathies and coagulation, 99
    urate and fecal discoloration, 471–473
hemochromatosis, 250
hemoglobinuria, 197
hemoglobulinemia, 180
hemoglobinuric nephrosis, 381
hemoparasites, **196–198**
    anemia, 17
*Hemoproteus* spp., 17
hemorrhage, **199–202**
    anemia, 17
    coagulopathies and coagulation, 98–99
    duck enteritis virus, 211
    enteritis and gastritis, 167
    feather cyst, 168–169
    feather-damaging, 170, 173
    gastrointestinal helminthiasis, 191
    hypotension and hypovolemia, 228–230
    neurologic disorders, 303
    pasteurellosis, 345
    pneumonia, 355
    polyomavirus, 365
    rodenticide toxicosis, 436–437
    tongue diseases, 432

toxoplasmosis, 455
trauma, 461–463
wound management, 482
hemorrhagic enteritis
    adenoviruses, 2
    campylobacteriosis, 70
hemorrhagic hypovolemic shock, 229
hemorrhagic septicemia, 112
hepatic cirrhosis/fibrosis, 28–29
hepatic lipidosis, **203–205**
    anorexia, 25
hepatic necrosis, 2
hepatic neoplasia, **282–283**
hepatobiliary disease
    clinical algorithm, 537
    dyslipidemia/hyperlipidemia, 139
    oil exposure, 316
hepatomegaly
    adenoviruses, 2
    chlamydiosis, 79
    hemoparasites, 197
    hepatic lipidosis, 203
    iron storage disease, 239
    liver disease, 251
    myocardial diseases, 279
    passerid herpesvirus-1, 213
    reovirus, 384
    sarcocystosis, 402–403
    sepsis, 409
    toxoplasmosis, 454
    urate and fecal discoloration, 472
    yersiniosis, 486
hernia/pseudohernia, **206–207**
herniorrhaphy, 207
herpesvirus
    columbid herpesvirus 1, **208–209**
    duck enteritis virus, **210–212**
    passerine birds, **213–214**
    pneumonia, 355
    psittacid herpesviruses, **215–217**
heterophilia
    leukocytosis, 247–248
    seizures, 406
heterophilic splenitis, 117
heterotrophic cardiomyopathy (HCM),
    280–281
hinged linear external skeletal fixation
    (HLESF), 257
histomoniasis, **218–219**
hormone stimulation, 333
Horner syndrome, **220–221**
human chorionic gonadotropin (hCG),
    332–333
husbandry *see* socioenvironmental factors
hydrotherapy
    angular limb deformity, 22
    toe and nail diseases, 428
    wound management, 482
hyperadrenocorticism, 4–7
hyperaldosteronism, 4–7
hyperbaric oxygen, 75
hypercalcemia
    chronic egg laying, 82
    dystocia and egg binding, 143

egg yolk coelomitis, 158
lymphoproliferative neoplasia, 286
polydipsia, 362
polyostotic hyperostosis, 367
renal neoplasia, 293
vitamin D toxicosis, 452–453
hypercholesterolemia
    chronic egg laying, 82
    dyslipidemia/hyperlipidemia, 139
    dystocia and egg binding, 143
    obesity, 312
    polyostotic hyperostosis, 367
hyperglobulinemia
    chronic egg laying, 82
    dystocia and egg binding, 143
    egg yolk coelomitis, 158
    lymphoproliferative neoplasia, 286
hyperglycemia, **132–133**
    hypotension and hypovolemia, 228
hyperkalemia, 362
hyperkeratosis
    dermatitis, 127
    mites, 148–149
hyperlipidemia *see* dyslipidemia/
    hyperlipidemia
hypernatremia
    hypotension and hypovolemia, 228
    polydipsia, 362
hyperostosis, 330
hyperproteinemia, 228
hypersensitivity syndrome, 434–435
hypertension, 39
hyperthermia, 186
hyperthyroidism, 424–425
hypertonic sugar solution, 352
hypertriglyceridemia
    chronic egg laying, 82
    dyslipidemia/hyperlipidemia, 140
hyperuricemia, **222–224**
    clinical algorithm, 536
    hypotension and hypovolemia, 228
    polydipsia, 362
    polyostotic hyperostosis, 367
    toe and nail diseases, 426
    vitamin D toxicosis, 452–453
hyperviscosity syndrome, 426–427,
    429–430
hypervitaminosis A, 320
hypervitaminosis D, 452–453
hypervitaminosis E-associated
    coagulopathy, 98
hypoadrenocorticism, 4–7
hypocalcemia, **225–227**
    angular limb deformity, 22
    dystocia and egg binding, 143
    lameness, 245
    metabolic bone disease, 263–264
    neurologic disorders, 303
    nutritional imbalances, 308–309
    seizures, 406
hypochloremia, 228
hypoglycemia, 203
hypomagnesemia, **225–227**
hyponatremia, 362

hypoproteinemia
  ascites, 27
  coagulopathies and coagulation, 99
hypotension and hypovolemia, **228–230**
hypothermia, **231–232**
  anorexia, 25
  sepsis, 408–409
hypothyroidism, 139, 424–425
hypovolemic shock, 228–229, 463

**I**

iatrogenic toxicosis, **445–447**
ileus, **233–235**
immunohistochemistry, 56
immunosuppression
  chlamydiosis, 79, 81
  mycotoxicosis, 274
  neurologic disorders, 306
  renal diseases, 382
  thymus diseases, 422–423
infectious bronchitis, 389
infectious bursal disease virus (IBDV),
    66–69, 422
infectious laryngotracheitis (ILT),
    389–391
infectious myocarditis, 280
infertility, **236–238**
ingested toxicosis, **447–451**
insulin, 132–133
integument
  ascites, 27
  cutaneous papillomatosis, **343–344**
  electrocution, 160
  feather cyst, **168–169**
  feather-damaging, **170–173**
  feather disorders, **174–176**
  myiasis, 277
  nutritional imbalances, 308
  oil exposure, 316
  poxvirus, 371–373
integumental neoplasia, **284–285**
intensive care
  coccidiosis, 105
  hypotension and hypovolemia, 229
  ingested toxicosis, 449
  rodenticide toxicosis, 437
  sepsis, 409
internal papillomatosis, 215–216
intestinal coccidiosis, **101–103**
intracoelomic mass effect, 107
iodine deficiency, 424
iron deficiency anemia, 17–18
iron storage disease (ISD), **239–240**
  ascites, 29
  coelomic distension, 109
*Isospora* spp., 101–103
itraconazole, 445–447
ivermectin
  iatrogenic toxicosis, 445–447
  ticks, lice, dipterans, 152

**J**

joint diseases, **241–242**
  luxations, **256–258**
  perosis/slipped tendon, **349–350**

**K**

ketonuria, 362
*Knemidokoptes* spp., 148–150

**L**

lameness, **243–246**
  clinical algorithm, 535
  dystocia and egg binding, 143
  mites, 148
  renal neoplasia, 293
  reovirus, 384
  tendinitis and tenosynovitis, 418
  toe and nail diseases, 426
laparoscopy
  oviductal diseases, 335
  urate and fecal discoloration, 472
lateral beak deformity, **48–50**
laughing dove circovirus (LDCV), 87–88
leukemia, 426
leukocytosis, **247–249**
  anorexia, 24
  bursa of Fabricius diseases, 67
  chlamydiosis, 79
  coelomic distension, 107–108
  diarrhea, 134
  duck enteritis virus, 211
  dystocia and egg binding, 143
  egg yolk coelomitis, 158
  histomoniasis, 218
  joint diseases, 241
  pneumonia, 354
  seizures, 406
  tracheal and syringeal diseases, 457
*Leukocytozoon* spp., 17, 196–198
leukopenia, 286
lice, **151–153**
limb deformities, 349
lipid pneumonia, 355
lipoma, 284
liver disease, **250–252**
  urate and fecal discoloration, 471–473
local anesthesia, 338
lockjaw *see* bordetellosis
lung diseases, **253–255**
luxations, **256–258**
  toe and nail diseases, 428
lymphatic disease
  duck enteritis virus, 210
  oil exposure, 316
lymphocytosis, 247–248
lymphohistiocytic meningoencephalitis, 455
lymphohistiocytic splenitis, 117
lymphoid disorders, 66
lymphoid leukosis virus (LLV), 393

lymphoma
  integumental neoplasia, 284–285
  liver disease, 250
  lymphoproliferative neoplasia, 286–288
lymphoproliferative neoplasia, **286–289**

**M**

*Macrorhabdus ornithogaster*, **259–260**
  undigested food in droppings, 469–470
  urate and fecal discoloration, 472
magnesium sulfate, 181
magnetic resonance imaging (MRI)
  aspiration pneumonia, 33
  atherosclerosis, 37–38
  capture myopathy, 75
  discospondylitis, 137
  functional gastrointestinal ileus, 234
  iron storage disease, 239
  joint diseases, 241
  lymphoproliferative neoplasia, 287
  neural larva migrans, 300
  neurologic disorders, 303, 305
  neurologic neoplasia, 291
  pancreatic diseases, 341
  renal diseases, 382
  reproductive neoplasia, 296
  respiratory distress, 386
  rhinusitis and sinusitis, 396
  seizures, 406
  toe and nail diseases, 427
  trauma, 461
magnetic resonance spectroscopy, 140
mandibular prognathism, **51–52**
mandibular ramp orthosis, 49
manganese deficiency, 22
Marek's disease virus (MDV), 248,
    **261–262**
  ovarian diseases, 330–332
  retroviruses in Galliformes, 393
  thymus diseases, 422
medulloblastoma, 291
melena, 165
meningioma, 290–291
meningoencephalitis, 443
metabolic bone disease (MBD), **263–265**
  beak injuries, 45
  lateral beak deformity, 48
  polyostotic hyperostosis, 367
metabolic disease
  egg abnormalities, 154
  egg yolk coelomitis, 158
  feather-damaging, 170
  feather disorders, 174
  functional gastrointestinal ileus, 233
  hemorrhage, 199
  liver disease, 250
  myocardial diseases, 280
  polydipsia, 362
metastatic pancreatic neoplasia, 340
microsporidiosis, **266–267**

mites, **148–150**
mononuclear phagocytes, 116
moxidectin, 152
muscle necrosis, 197
muscle relaxants, 75–76
musculoskeletal disorders
    mycoplasmosis, 271–273
    oil exposure, 316
    perosis/slipped tendon, **349–350**
mycobacteriosis, **268–270**
    amyloidosis, 15
    ascites, 28
    joint diseases, 241–242
    lameness, 245
    liver disease, 250
    oral plaques, 320–322
    pneumonia, 355
    spleen diseases, 415–416
    thymus diseases, 422
    undigested food in droppings, 468–469
mycoplasmosis, **271–273**
    amyloidosis, 15
    joint diseases, 241–242
    pneumonia, 355
    respiratory infections of backyard
        chickens, 389–391
    thymus diseases, 422
mycotoxicosis, **274–276**
myiasis, **277–278**
myocardial diseases, **279–281**

### N

nasal discharge
    airborne toxicosis, 434
    pasteurellosis, 345
nasal flush, 387
nasal swab, 396
nebulization therapy
    aspiration pneumonia, 34
    pneumonia, 356
    respiratory distress, 387
    rhinusitis and sinusitis, 396–397
    tracheal and syringeal diseases, 458
neonicotinoid toxicosis, 439–441
neoplastic reproductive disease, 154, 157
nephrogenic diabetes insipidus, 130–131
neural larva migrans (NLM), **300–301**
neuroblastoma, 291
neurologic disorders
    clinical algorithm, 531
    feather-damaging, 171
    hypotension and hypovolemia, 228
    non-traumatic diseases, **302–304**
    oil exposure, 316
    orthoavulaviruses, 323–324
    seizures, 405–407
    trauma, **305–307**
neurologic neoplasia, **290–292**
neuromuscular disorders
    Marek's disease virus, 261–262

metabolic bone disease, 263
myocardial diseases, 279
nutritional imbalances, 308
neuronal ceroid lipofuscinosis, 303
neurotoxins
    algal biotoxins, 13
    avian vacuolar myelinopathy, 43
    botulism, 62
Newcastle disease
    neurologic disorders, 303–304
    orthoavulaviruses, 323–325
nitroimidazoles, 466
nocardiosis, 355
nonsteroidal anti-inflammatory drugs
        (NSAID)
    anorexia, 25
    beak injuries, 46
    cloacal prolapse, 93
    dermatitis, 128–129
    enteritis and gastritis, 167
    feather cyst, 169
    feather-damaging, 172
    fractures, 184
    functional gastrointestinal ileus, 234–235
    hyperuricemia, 222–223
    infertility, 237
    lung diseases, 254
    luxations, 257
    ocular lesions, 314
    otitis, 328
    oviductal diseases, 335
    pain, 338
    pancreatic diseases, 341–342
    perosis/slipped tendon, 349
    phallus prolapse, 352
    pododermatitis, 360
    renal diseases, 381
    toe and nail diseases, 429
    wound management, 483
nutritional imbalances, **308–310**
nystatin, 73

### O

obesity, **311–312**
    coelomic distension, 107, 109
    hepatic lipidosis, 203–204
    lameness, 243
    nutritional imbalances, 308
    pancreatic diseases, 340
    pododermatitis, 358
    toe and nail diseases, 427
ochratoxin
    mycotoxicosis, 274–275
    thymus diseases, 422
ocular injury, 160
ocular larva migrans (OLM), 300–301
ocular lesions, **313–315**
oesophagostomy, 166
oil exposure, **316–319**
oligoastrocytoma, 291

oligodendroglioma, 291
oophoritis, 237, 330–333
oosporein, 274–275
ophthalmic disease
    duck enteritis virus, 210
    Horner syndrome, **220–221**
    Marek's disease virus, 261
    microsporidiosis, 266–267
    mycoplasmosis, 271–273
    neural larva migrans, 300–301
    ocular lesions, **313–315**
    oil exposure, 316
opioids
    functional gastrointestinal ileus,
        234–235
    hypotension and hypovolemia, 229
    luxations, 257
    pain, 338
    phallus prolapse, 352
    renal diseases, 382
oral injury, 160
oral plaques, **320–322**
orchidectomy, 296
organomegaly
    coelomic distension, 108
    egg yolk coelomitis, 158
    lymphoproliferative neoplasia, 287
organophosphate toxicosis, 439–441
    functional gastrointestinal ileus, 233
    neurologic disorders, 302
oropharyngeal lesions, 530
orthoavulaviruses (OAvV), **323–326**
orthopedic surgery, 184
orthotic maxillary beak extension, 51–52
osteomalacia, 263
osteomyelosclerosis
    chronic egg laying, 82
    polyostotic hyperostosis, 367
osteopenia, 244–245
osteotomy, 21
ostrich circovirus (OCV), 87–88
otitis, **327–329**
ovarian diseases, **330–333**
ovarian neoplasia, 295–297, 330–333
    lameness, 245
ovariectomy
    hernia/pseudohernia, 207
    oviductal diseases, 335
oviductal diseases, **334–336**
oviductal prolapse, 92
oxygen therapy
    hernia/pseudohernia, 206
    lung diseases, 254
    neurologic disorders, 306
    nutritional imbalances, 309
    poxvirus, 372
    respiratory distress, 387
    sick-bird syndrome, 412
    spirochete infection, 413
    thyroid diseases, 424
    toe and nail diseases, 428
    tongue diseases, 432

oxygen therapy (*Continued*)
　trauma, 462
　wound management, 482
oxytocin, 144

## P

Pacheco's disease, 215–216
pain management, **337–339**
　beak injuries, 46
　bursa of Fabricius diseases, 68
　capture myopathy, 75–76
　cloacal prolapse, 93
　crop burn, 119
　duck enteritis virus, 211
　dystocia and egg binding, 144
　feather cyst, 169
　fractures, 184
　functional gastrointestinal ileus,
　　234–235
　hernia/pseudohernia, 207
　hyperuricemia, 223
　hypotension and hypovolemia, 229
　lameness, 245
　lateral beak deformity, 49
　lung diseases, 254
　luxations, 257
　metabolic bone disease, 263–264
　oral plaques, 321
　otitis, 328
　pancreatic diseases, 341–342
　perosis/slipped tendon, 349
　phallus prolapse, 352
　pododermatitis, 359–360
　renal diseases, 382
　renal neoplasia, 293
　reproductive neoplasia, 295–296
　respiratory distress, 387
　tendinitis and tenosynovitis, 420
　toe and nail diseases, 429
　tongue diseases, 433
　trauma, 463
pancreatic atrophy, 341
pancreatic diseases, **340–342**
pancreatic necrosis, 340–341
pancreatic neoplasia, 340–341
pancreatitis, 340
　dyslipidemia/hyperlipidemia, 139
papillomatosis
　cutaneous, **343–344**
　toe and nail diseases, 427–428
　tongue diseases, 432
paralysis, 261–262
parathyroid hormone (PTH), 263
paratyphoid *see* salmonellosis
paresis
　dystocia and egg binding, 143
　gastrointestinal foreign bodies, 180
passerid herpesvirus-1 (PHV-1), 213–214
pasteurellosis, **345–346**
patagium diseases, **347–348**
penetration injury, 64–65
perforations, 181

periocular swelling, 313–314
peripheral vasodilators, 39
permethrin, 152
perosis/slipped tendon, **349–350**
persistent halogenated pollutants (PHP),
　439–441
pesticide toxicosis, **439–442**
phalangeal amputation *see* pinioning
phallus prolapse, 92, **351–353**
phenobarbital
　neurologic disorders, 303–304, 306
　seizures, 406
phenylephrine, 220
photosensitization, 127–128
physical therapy, 75
pigeon circovirus (PiCV), 66–69, 87–88
pigeon paramyxovirus serotype-1 (PPMV-1),
　324–325
pigmented dermal mass, 77
pineal tumors, 290–291
pinioning, 21
pituitary tumors, 290–291
*Plasmodium* spp., 17, 196–198
pneumoconiosis, 243–244
pneumonia, **354–357**
　toxoplasmosis, 454–455
pododermatitis, **358–361**
　lameness, 243
　toe and nail diseases, 429
polychlorinated biphenyl (PCB) toxicosis,
　439–441
polycythemia, 253
polydipsia, **362–364**
　clinical algorithm, 532
　diabetes insipidus, 130–131
　diabetes mellitus and hyperglycemia,
　　132
　polyuria, 362–363, 369–370
　vitamin D toxicosis, 452
polymerase chain reaction (PCR)
　bordetellosis, 53
　bornaviral disease, 56, 59
　botulism, 63
　bursa of Fabricius diseases, 68
　candidiasis, 72
　chlamydiosis, 79
　circovirus, 85
　columbid herpesvirus 1, 208
　coxiellosis, 116
　cutaneous papillomatosis, 343
　egg abnormalities, 154
　lymphoproliferative neoplasia, 286
　mycobacteriosis, 268
　neurologic disorders, 303, 305
　orthoavulaviruses, 324
　regurgitation and vomiting, 378
　respiratory infections of backyard
　　chickens, 390
　tendinitis and tenosynovitis, 419
　tracheal and syringeal diseases, 458
　West Nile virus, 478–479
polyomavirus, **365–366**
　ascites, 28
　feather disorders, 174–175

myocardial diseases, 280
　pneumonia, 355
polyostotic hyperostosis, 295, **367–368**
　chronic egg laying, 82
　egg yolk coelomitis, 158
polyserositis, 112
polysulfated glycosaminoglycans
　(PSGAG), 98
polyuria, **369–370**
　clinical algorithm, 533
　diabetes insipidus, 130–131
　diabetes mellitus and hyperglycemia,
　　132
　hepatic lipidosis, 203
　phallus prolapse, 351
　polydipsia, 362–363, 369–370
　vitamin D toxicosis, 452
porphyrinuria, 223
positron emission tomography (PET), 38
poxvirus, **371–373**
　respiratory infections of backyard
　　chickens, 389–391
　toe and nail diseases, 427
probiotics
　emaciation, 163
　renal diseases, 382–383
problem behaviors, **374–377**
protein electrophoresis
　aspergillosis, 30
　mycobacteriosis, 268
　pneumonia, 355
　renal diseases, 381
proteinuria
　hyperuricemia, 223
　polydipsia, 362
　renal diseases, 381
prothrombin time, 99
proventricular dilatation disease (PDD)
　enteritis and gastritis, 165
　gastrointestinal foreign bodies, 180
　neurologic disorders, 303
proventricular lavage, 449–450
pruritus
　dermatitis, 128
　mites, 148
pseudoanorexia, 24
pseudohernia, **206–207**
pseudolymphoma, 288
psittacid herpesviruses, **215–217**
psittacine beak and feather disease (PBFD)
　bursa of Fabricius diseases, 66–69
　circovirus, 85–86
　enteritis and gastritis, 165
　feather-damaging, 170–171
　thymus diseases, 422
psittacosis, 237
psychoactive/mood-altering drugs, 172–173
PTFE toxicosis, 434–435
pulse oximetry, 458

## Q

quarantine *see* biosecurity

**R**

radiography/contrast radiography
  airborne toxicosis, 434
  anorexia, 24
  ascites, 28
  aspergillosis, 31
  aspiration pneumonia, 33
  atherosclerosis, 37
  beak injuries, 45
  brachial plexus injury, 64
  campylobacteriosis, 70
  candidiasis, 72
  chronic egg laying, 82
  cloacal diseases, 90
  cloacal prolapse, 92
  coagulopathies and coagulation, 99
  coccidiosis, 104–105
  coelomic distension, 108, 109
  congestive heart failure, 114
  discospondylitis, 137
  duck enteritis virus, 211
  dystocia and egg binding, 143
  egg abnormalities, 155
  egg yolk coelomitis, 158
  electrocution, 160
  enteritis and gastritis, 166
  fractures, 183–184
  functional gastrointestinal ileus, 234
  gastrointestinal and hepatic neoplasia, 282
  gastrointestinal foreign bodies, 180
  heavy metal toxicosis, 443
  hemorrhage, 200
  hernia/pseudohernia, 206
  hypocalcemia and hypomagnesemia, 226
  infertility, 237
  ingested toxicosis, 449
  integumental neoplasia, 284
  iron storage disease, 239
  joint diseases, 241
  lameness, 244
  leukocytosis, 248
  liver disease, 251
  lung diseases, 253
  luxations, 256
  *Macrorhabdus ornithogaster*, 259
  microsporidiosis, 266
  mycobacteriosis, 268
  mycoplasmosis, 272
  myocardial diseases, 281
  neurologic disorders, 303, 305
  nutritional imbalances, 309
  obesity, 311
  ocular lesions, 314
  oil exposure, 317
  oral plaques, 321
  ovarian diseases, 331
  oviductal diseases, 334–335
  perosis/slipped tendon, 349
  pneumonia, 355
  pododermatitis, 359
  polyostotic hyperostosis, 367–368
  polyuria, 369
  regurgitation and vomiting, 378

renal diseases, 382
renal neoplasia, 293
reproductive neoplasia, 295
respiratory distress, 386
rhinusitis and sinusitis, 395–396
rodenticide toxicosis, 437
seizures, 406
sepsis, 409
sick-bird syndrome, 411–412
spleen diseases, 415
tendinitis and tenosynovitis, 419
thyroid diseases, 424
toe and nail diseases, 427
toxoplasmosis, 454
tracheal and syringeal diseases, 458
trauma, 461
trichomoniasis, 465–466
undigested food in droppings, 469
vitamin D toxicosis, 452
xanthoma/xanthogranulomatosis, 484
yolk sac retention/infection, 488
radiotherapy
  gastrointestinal and hepatic neoplasia, 283
  lymphoproliferative neoplasia, 287
  respiratory neoplasia, 298–299
  uropygial gland disease, 474–475
ramp orthotics, 49
refeeding syndrome, 163
regenerative microcytic hypochromic anemia, 443
regurgitation and vomiting, **378–379**
  aspiration pneumonia, 33–34
  clinical algorithm, 525
  undigested food in droppings, 468
release evaluation, 318
renal diseases, **380–383**
  polydipsia, 362
  polyuria, 369
renal neoplasia, **293–294**, 380
renomegaly, 452
reovirus, **384–385**
  bursa of Fabricius diseases, 66–69
reproductive disorders
  anorexia, 26
  ascites, 27–28
  bornaviral disease, 57, 60
  chlamydiosis, 81
  chronic egg laying, 82–84
  coelomic distension, 108–109
  duck enteritis virus, 210, 212
  dyslipidemia/hyperlipidemia, 141
  dystocia and egg binding, 142–144
  egg abnormalities, **154–157**
  egg yolk coelomitis, **158–159**
  infertility, **236–238**
  mycoplasmosis, 273
  nutritional imbalances, 308, 310
  oil exposure, 316
  ovarian diseases, **330–333**
  pesticide toxicosis, 441
  phallus prolapse, **351–353**
  sepsis, 410
reproductive neoplasia, **295–297**
respiratory colisepticemia, 112

respiratory disease
  cryptosporidiosis, 122–123
  duck enteritis virus, 210
  egg yolk coelomitis, 158
  lung diseases, **253–255**
  mycobacteriosis, 268
  mycoplasmosis, 271–273
  myocardial diseases, 279
  oil exposure, 316
  pneumonia, **354–357**
respiratory distress, **386–388**
  air sac mites, 8
  air sac rupture, 10
  algal biotoxins, 13
  ascites, 27
  aspergillosis, 30–32
  aspiration pneumonia, 33–35
  clinical algorithm, 526, 539
respiratory helminthiasis, **193–195**
respiratory infections of backyard chickens, **389–392**
respiratory neoplasia, **298–299**
retention sutures, 93
reticuloendotheliosis virus (REV), 393
retinal disease, 313–314
retroviruses in Galliformes, **393–394**
rhinusitis, **395–397**
rodenticide toxicosis, **436–438**
  coagulopathies and coagulation, 98, 100
  hemorrhage, 200
rotavirus, **398–399**
ruptured muscle syndrome, 74
Russell viper venom time, 99

**S**

salivary gland impaction/abscess, 432–433
salmonellosis, **400–401**
  joint diseases, 241–242
  thymus diseases, 422
salpingohysterectomy
  chronic egg laying, 83
  cloacal prolapse, 93
  dystocia and egg binding, 143
  oviductal diseases, 335
  reproductive neoplasia, 296
salvage wing amputation, 64–65
sarcocystosis, **402–404**
  pneumonia, 355
schistosomiasis
  body cavity and cardiovascular helminthiasis, 188–189
  respiratory helminthiasis, 193
scintigraphy, 461
screaming, **374–377**
seizures, **405–407**
  gastrointestinal foreign bodies, 180
  hypocalcemia and hypomagnesemia, 225, 227
  mycotoxicosis, 275
  myocardial diseases, 279–280
  neurologic disorders, 303–304, 305–306
selamectin, 152

selective serotonin reuptake inhibitors
      (SSRI), 376, 407
self-injurious behavior
   feather cyst, 169
   feather-damaging, **170–173**
   hemorrhage, 199
   patagium diseases, 347
   renal diseases, 380
   trauma, 461–462
   uropygial gland disease, 474
   West Nile virus, 479
   xanthoma/xanthogranulomatosis, 484
sepsis, **408–410**
   lymphoproliferative neoplasia, 286
septicemia, 483
septicemic pox, 371–373
septicemic shock, 410
serology
   avian influenza, 41
   bornaviral disease, 56
   chlamydiosis, 79
sexual behavior, 92–93
shaping, 375
shell gland prolapse, 92
*Siadenovirus* spp., 1
sick-bird syndrome, **411–412**
   clinical algorithm, 523
   liver disease, 250
sinus aspiration and lavage, 396
sinusitis, **395–397**
skin color changes, **77–78**
slipped tendon, **349–350**
small intestinal prolapse, 92
smoke inhalation, 434–435
socioenvironmental factors
   aggression, biting, and screaming,
      374–377
   airborne toxicosis, 434–435
   feather-damaging, 171, 173
   flagellate enteritis, 178
   gastrointestinal helminthiasis, 190
   hepatic lipidosis, 203
   histomoniasis, 218
   infertility, 236–237
   lung diseases, 253
   mycotoxicosis, 274–276
   obesity, 311–312
   oil exposure, 318–319
   pain, 337
   pasteurellosis, 345–346
   pneumonia, 354
   pododermatitis, 358–360
   regurgitation and vomiting, 378
   renal diseases, 381
   respiratory infections of backyard
      chickens, **389–392**
   retroviruses in Galliformes, 393–394
   rhinusitis and sinusitis, 395–397
   rotavirus, 398
   sepsis, 408
   thymus diseases, 423
   toe and nail diseases, 429
   toxoplasmosis, 454–455

   trichomoniasis, 465–466
   undigested food in droppings, 469–470
   wound management, 481–483
sodium benzoate, 260
sodium bicarbonate, 75–76
spinal trauma, 462
   discospondylitis, 137
spirochete infection, **413–414**
spironucleosis
   enteritis and gastritis, 165
   flagellate enteritis, 177–178
splay leg *see* angular limb deformity
spleen diseases, **415–417**
splenomegaly
   adenoviruses, 2
   chlamydiosis, 79
   hemoparasites, 197
   myocardial diseases, 279
   passerid herpesvirus-1, 213
   reovirus, 384
   sepsis, 409
   toxoplasmosis, 454
   yersiniosis, 486
squamous cell carcinoma (SCC)
   gastrointestinal and hepatic neoplasia,
      282–283
   integumental neoplasia, 284
   respiratory neoplasia, 298
*Staphylococcus* spp., 136–137
statins
   atherosclerosis, 38
   dyslipidemia/hyperlipidemia, 140
   neurologic disorders, 303
*Sternostoma tracheacolum*, 8
straw feather disease, 174
*Streptococcus* spp., 137
stress-associated immune depression, 422
subcutaneous emphysema, air sac rupture,
      10–11
sudden/unexpected death
   adenoviruses, 1
   duck enteritis virus, 210
   myocardial diseases, 279
   passerid herpesvirus-1, 213
   pasteurellosis, 345
   psittacid herpesviruses, 215
   reproductive neoplasia, 296–297
   usutu virus, 476
sulfonamides, 105–106
superficial chronic ulcerative dermatitis
      (SCUD), 347
syncope, 405–406
syringeal diseases, **457–460**
syringe-feeding, 25
systemic coccidiosis, **104–106**


**T**

T-2 toxin, 422
T-cell lymphocytic leukemia, 288
temporary tarsorrhaphy, 314
tendinitis and tenosynovitis, **418–421**

tendonorhaphy, 349
tension band technique, 49, 52
teratoma, 291
testicular neoplasia, 295–297
   lameness, 245
thermal trauma, 77–78
thermography
   discospondylitis, 137
   electrocution, 160–161
   lameness, 244
thiamine supplementation, 164
thrombocytes, 99
thrombocytopenia, 98
thymus diseases, **422–423**
thyroid diseases, **424–425**
thyroid hyperplasia, 424–425
thyroid neoplasia, 424–425
ticks, **151–153**
toe and nail diseases, **426–430**
   cere and skin color changes, 77
tongue diseases, **431–433**
toxoplasmosis, **454–456**
tracheal diseases, **457–460**
tracheal neoplasia, 457
tracheoscopy, 458–459
tracheotomy, 458–459
traditional water deprivation test, 363
transfrontal pin and tension band, 49
trauma, **461–464**
   air sac rupture, 10
   anemia, 17
   angular limb deformity, 22
   beak injuries, 45–46
   brachial plexus injury, 64–65
   cere and skin color changes, 77–78
   cutaneous papillomatosis, 343
   discospondylitis, 137
   egg abnormalities, 154, 156
   electrocution, **160–161**
   emaciation, 162
   feather-damaging, 171–172
   feather disorders, 174
   fractures, **183–185**
   gastrointestinal foreign bodies, 181
   hemorrhage, 199
   hernia/pseudohernia, 206
   Horner syndrome, 220–221
   hypotension and hypovolemia, 228
   joint diseases, 241
   lameness, 243–244
   luxations, 256
   myiasis, 277
   neurologic disorders, **305–307**
   patagium diseases, 347
   phallus prolapse, 351
   pododermatitis, 358–360
   renal diseases, 381
   seizures, 405
   tendinitis and tenosynovitis, 418
   toe and nail diseases, 426–428
   tracheal and syringeal diseases, 457
   uropygial gland disease, 474–475
   wound management, 481–483

trichomoniasis, **465–467**
  oral plaques, 320–322
  tongue diseases, 432
trilostane, 6
tuberculosis (TB) *see* mycobacteriosis
typhlitis, 165
typhoid *see* salmonellosis

## U

ulceration, 127–128
ultracentrifugation, 139–140
ultrasonography
  anorexia, 24
  ascites, 28
  aspiration pneumonia, 33
  chlamydiosis, 79
  cloacal diseases, 90
  cloacal prolapse, 92
  coccidiosis, 105
  coelomic distension, 108
  congestive heart failure, 114
  duck enteritis virus, 211
  dystocia and egg binding, 143
  egg abnormalities, 155
  egg yolk coelomitis, 158
  enteritis and gastritis, 166
  functional gastrointestinal ileus, 234
  gastrointestinal and hepatic
    neoplasia, 282
  gastrointestinal foreign bodies, 180
  gastrointestinal helminthiasis, 191
  hepatic lipidosis, 203
  hernia/pseudohernia, 206
  integumental neoplasia, 284
  iron storage disease, 239
  lameness, 244
  liver disease, 251
  lung diseases, 253
  ocular lesions, 314
  ovarian diseases, 331
  oviductal diseases, 335–336
  pancreatic diseases, 341
  pododermatitis, 359
  polyuria, 369
  regurgitation and vomiting, 378
  renal diseases, 382
  renal neoplasia, 293
  reproductive neoplasia, 295
  respiratory distress, 386
  rhinusitis and sinusitis, 396
  rodenticide toxicosis, 437
  xanthoma/xanthogranulomatosis,
    484
ultraviolet light
  hypocalcemia and hypomagnesemia,
    225–227
  metabolic bone disease, 263–264
undigested food in droppings, **468–470**
unexpected death *see* sudden/unexpected
    death
unilateral paresis, 261
urate discoloration, **471–473**

urea:uric acid ratio, 381
uric acid (UA), 222–224
uropygial gland disease, **474–475**
usutu virus (USUV), 476–477
uveitis, 313–314

## V

vaccination
  avian influenza, 41
  botulism, 63
  coccidiosis, 102–103, 106
  columbid herpesvirus 1, 208
  duck enteritis virus, 211
  Eastern and Western equine encephalitis
    virus, 146
  egg abnormalities, 156
  hemoparasites, 198
  Marek's disease virus, 262
  mycoplasmosis, 272–273
  ocular lesions, 315
  orthoavulaviruses, 325
  pasteurellosis, 346
  polyomavirus, 366
  poxvirus, 373
  reovirus, 384
  rotavirus, 398
  tendinitis and tenosynovitis, 419–420
  West Nile virus, 479
vaccine-induced amyloidosis, 15–16
VAC therapy, 359
vascular aneurysm, 38
vascular disease, 154
vasopressin/desmopressin response test, 363
vasopressors, 229
ventplasty, 93
virions, 372–373
virus isolation, 41
virus neutralization, 393
visceral injury, 160
vitamin A deficiency
  dermatitis, 127
  feather cyst, 168
  functional gastrointestinal ileus, 233
  nutritional imbalances, 308–310
  pododermatitis, 358
  rhinusitis and sinusitis, 396–397
  toe and nail diseases, 426
  tongue diseases, 431–433
vitamin A toxicosis, 445–447
vitamin D deficiency
  angular limb deformity, 22
  hypocalcemia and hypomagnesemia,
    225–227
  metabolic bone disease, 263
  nutritional imbalances, 308–310
vitamin D toxicosis, **452–453**
vitamin E deficiency, 308
vitamin K deficiency, 99–100
vitamin supplementation
  emaciation, 164
  hepatic lipidosis, 204
  lung diseases, 254

metabolic bone disease, 264
mycotoxicosis, 275
nutritional imbalances, 309
psittacid herpesviruses, 227
thymus diseases, 423
vitellogenesis, 139, 141
vomiting *see* regurgitation and vomiting

## W

water deprivation tests, 130, 363,
    369–370
Western blot analysis, 59
Western equine encephalitis virus (WEEV),
    **145–147**
West Nile virus (WNV), **478–480**
  seizures, 405–407
wing droop, 538
wound management, **481–483**
  feather cyst, 168–169
  fractures, 183
  hypothermia, 232
  myiasis, 277
  patagium diseases, 347
  pododermatitis, 359–360
  ticks, lice, dipterans, 152
  toe and nail diseases, 428
  trauma, 462
  uropygial gland disease, 474

## X

xanthoma/xanthogranulomatosis, **484–485**
  integumental neoplasia, 284

## Y

yersiniosis, **486–487**
yolk sac retention/infection, **488–489**

## Z

zoonotic disease
  anorexia, 26
  aspergillosis, 32
  avian influenza, 42
  body cavity and cardiovascular
    helminthiasis, 189
  bordetellosis, 54
  bornaviral disease, 57, 60
  bursa of Fabricius diseases, 69
  campylobacteriosis, 71
  candidiasis, 73
  chlamydiosis, 80–81
  clostridiosis, 96
  colibacillosis, 113
  cryptococcosis, 120–121
  cryptosporidiosis, 122–124
  diarrhea, 135
  duck enteritis virus, 212
  Eastern and Western equine encephalitis
    virus, 147

zoonotic disease (*Continued*)
  egg abnormalities, 157
  mites, 150
  mycobacteriosis, 269
  mycoplasmosis, 273
  mycotoxicosis, 276, 278
  neurologic disorders, 304
  ocular lesions, 315

oil exposure, 318–319
oral plaques, 322
orthoavulaviruses, 325
pneumonia, 356
renal diseases, 383
respiratory infections of backyard
    chickens, 391
rhinusitis and sinusitis, 397
salmonellosis, 400–401

sepsis, 410
sick-bird syndrome, 411–412
spleen diseases, 415
ticks, lice, dipterans, 152
toxoplasmosis, 455
undigested food in droppings, 470
usutu virus, 476
West Nile virus, 480